Critical Care Echocardiography

Roshni Sreedharan • Sandeep Khanna
Ajit Moghekar • Siddharth Dugar
Patrick Collier
Editors

Critical Care Echocardiography

A Self- Assessment Book

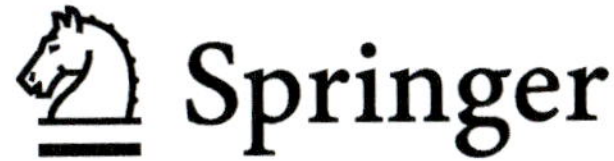

Editors
Roshni Sreedharan
Intensive Care and Resuscitation/Multispecialty Anesthesiology
Cleveland Clinic
Cleveland, OH, USA

Ajit Moghekar
Department of Critical Care Medicine
Respiratory Institute, Cleveland Clinic
Cleveland, OH, USA

Patrick Collier
Robert and Suzanne Tomsich Department of Cardiovascular Medicine
Sydell and Arnold Miller Family Heart and Vascular Institute
The Cleveland Clinic Foundation
Cleveland, OH, USA

Sandeep Khanna
Cardiothoracic Anesthesiology, Multispecialty Anesthesiology & Outcomes Research
Cleveland Clinic
Cleveland, OH, USA

Siddharth Dugar
Department of Critical Care Medicine
Respiratory Institute, Cleveland Clinic
Cleveland, OH, USA

ISBN 978-3-031-45730-2 ISBN 978-3-031-45731-9 (eBook)
https://doi.org/10.1007/978-3-031-45731-9

This Springer imprint is published by the registered company Springer Nature Switzerland AG
The registered company address is: Gewerbestrasse 11, 6330 Cham, Switzerland

Foreword 1

The explosion of Ultrasound use in the Point of Care Setting in the past decade and more importantly the tremendous uptake and interest in Cardiac Ultrasound in the Critical Care setting has been nothing short of revolutionary to the field of Cardiac diagnostics and Critical Care Medicine.

Cardiologists and Echocardiologists have long recognized the truly unique value of this rapid, portable, noninvasive diagnostic tool with virtually no adverse effects/consequences in the care of cardiac patients when applied appropriately. Echocardiography can identify life-threatening diagnoses enabling life-saving treatments and/or interventions to be implemented literally, within minutes of image acquisition. This capability is truly unique in the world of cardiac diagnostics. The unfortunate reality is that unlike other CV diagnostic modalities echo image acquisition is less structured and standardized specifically because it is uniquely user dependent, "shades of grey" are aplenty in the world of Echocardiography, and therefore interpretation on occasion can be simply, wrong, with potentially devastating consequences. As a result every echocardiographer has learned that humility is an acquired trait in this field. The responsibility of the user to learn to acquire diagnostic images, including identifying potentially confounding artifacts and correctly interpreting challenging images, particularly in the often difficult environment of the intensive care unit, is one of the most challenging aspects of performing/practicing POCUS.

This textbook sets out to teach, train, and emphasize the basics as well as the nuances of ultrasound diagnostics specifically as they relate to and are impacted by the critical care environment. Fundamentals of image acquisition and optimization which incorporate the physics of US as well as knobology are covered in this textbook as well as important topics such as valvular heart disease, interpretation of cardiac function, and using US for procedural guidance including mechanical circulatory support. This book is a "must read" for a wide range of medical practitioners from the seasoned Cardiac Sonographer to the Critical Care Intensivist and Cardiologist.

Richard A. Grimm

Heart, Vascular and Thoracic Institute
Cleveland Clinic
Cleveland, OH, USA

Foreword 2

I have the great honor and privilege of serving Cleveland Clinic along with over 1000 caregivers within the Anesthesiology Institute. Our vision is to be a recognized leader in perioperative care through education, research, and innovation within an environment that creates a safe, effective, efficient, and best possible experience for our patients and caregivers. We accomplish this vision by collaborating with each other, other institutes, and outside entities. This comprehensive textbook is a shining example of this vision whereby anesthesiologists within our institute have collaborated with an outstanding team of contributors from other disciplines to review all aspects of critical care ultrasound. Their format utilizes questions and cases to prepare the reader to demonstrate mastery of knowledge expected in the practice of critical care ultrasound.

Drs. Roshni Sreedharan, Sandeep Khanna, Ajit Moghekar, Siddharth Dugar, and Patrick Collier, all staff physicians with the Cleveland Clinic, serve as co-editors and authors for *Critical Care Echocardiography: A Self-Assessment Book*. The book is comprised of over 20 chapters that cover the full spectrum of ultrasonography in critical care, beginning with ultrasound physics and knobology, cardiac disorders of all valves and chambers, and extending to hemodynamics, pulmonary and abdominal disorders, vascular, and other procedural guidance. The authors represent a multidisciplinary team of highly experienced clinicians facile with performing and interpreting ultrasound evaluation among critically ill patients with cardiopulmonary disease, shock, cardiac arrest, and requiring procedural guidance. They utilize a very clinically oriented approach with cases and questions that probe understanding of key concepts and important principles.

Critical care ultrasound is such an important aspect of caring for the critically ill patients, because of its wide availability, ease of use, and providing data that direct the most appropriate clinical care. This tool can answer simple questions such as whether the hypotensive patient needs volume or an inotrope, but also less obvious diagnoses that require surgical intervention, such as cardiac tamponade, pneumothorax, pneumoperitoneum, or intracardiac embolism. The potential for surgical intervention emphasizes the importance for the clinician performing and interpreting the ultrasound in having the requisite knowledge to make an accurate diagnosis of the ultrasound data. This book confirms fundamental knowledge, which when mastered and combined with clinical experience provides the framework for confirming the acquisition of this knowledge, ultimately demonstrated by passing a high-stakes examination.

It gives me great pleasure to highlight the importance of this work and to recommend *Critical Care Echocardiograph : A Self-Assessment Book* to those planning to demonstrate their knowledge in this important aspect of critical care management.

Cleveland Clinic
Cleveland, OH, USA

Christopher A. Troianos

Preface

This book is the culmination of a collaborative effort of editors whose collective experiences span across various medical specialties but are united by a common goal: to provide a comprehensive and accessible resource for those seeking to navigate the complex world of critical care echocardiography and take the certifying board examination. As the field of critical care medicine continues to evolve, the role of echocardiography and ultrasonography in providing rapid and accurate clinical assessments has become pivotal. The imaging modalities are not just tools in the critical care physician's arsenal; they are essential instruments for guiding clinical decisions and management.

In developing this book, our aim was to create a resource that caters to a wide range of readers—from trainees preparing for board examinations to experienced physicians looking to refresh their knowledge and sharpen their skills. The questions within these pages encompass a spectrum of complexity, mirroring the diverse scenarios encountered in critical care practice. The detailed explanations for every question not only elucidate the correct answers but offer insights into underlying concepts and its clinical relevance.

As editors, we would like to extend our sincere appreciation to all the authors. This book wouldn't be a reality without their hard work and expertise. We are immensely grateful for the opportunity to contribute to the education and development of physicians practicing critical care and invite you to embark on this journey with us, to explore the world of critical care echocardiography. We hope that this book will serve as a valuable companion.

Cleveland, OH, USA — Roshni Sreedharan
Cleveland, OH, USA — Sandeep Khanna
Cleveland, OH, USA — Ajit Moghekar
Cleveland, OH, USA — Siddharth Dugar
Cleveland, OH, USA — Patrick Collier

Contents

Contributors

Greg Adams, DO Division of Emergency Ultrasound, Department of Emergency Medicine, MetroHealth Medical Center, Cleveland, OH, USA

Department of Emergency Medicine, University of Colorado Health, Aurora, CO, USA

Oriade K. Adeoye, MD, MPH Departments of Pulmonary, Critical Care, and Sleep Medicine, MetroHealth Medical Center, Cleveland, OH, USA

Sahar Ahmad, MD Division of Pulmonary, Critical Care and Sleep Medicine, Department of Medicine, Stony Brook University Center, Stony Brook, NY, USA

Thamer Alaifan, MBBS, FRCPC Department of Intensive Care Medicine, King Abdulaziz Medical City-National Guard, King Saud bin Abdulaziz University for Health Sciences (KSAU-HS), Jeddah, Saudi Arabia

Division of Critical Care Medicine, Department of Medicine, London Health Sciences Centre, Western University, London, ON, Canada

Saqer Alkharabsheh, MD, MPH Robert and Suzanne Tomsich Department of Cardiovascular Medicine, Sydell and Arnold Miller Family Heart and Vascular Institute, The Cleveland Clinic Foundation, Cleveland, OH, USA

Balaram Anandamurthy, MD Department of Intensive Care and Resuscitation, Cleveland Clinic, Cleveland, OH, USA

Enrico Boero, MD Department of Anesthesiology and Intensive Care, San Giovanni Bosco Hospital, Turin, Italy

Somnath Bose, MD Department of Anesthesia, Critical Care and Pain Medicine, Harvard Medical School, Beth Israel Deaconess Medical Center, Boston, Massachusetts, United States

Jason T. Bouhenguel, MD, MS, MSc Cardiothoracic Anesthesiology, Kaiser Permanente Santa Clara Medical Center, Palo Alto, CA, USA

Neal F. Chaisson, MD Respiratory Institute, Cleveland Clinic, Cleveland, OH, USA

Patrick Collier, MD, PhD, FASE, FACC, FESC Robert and Suzanne Tomsich Department of Cardiovascular Medicine, Sydell and Arnold Miller Family Heart and Vascular Institute, The Cleveland Clinic Foundation, Cleveland, OH, USA

Alexander Daves, DO Division of Emergency Ultrasound, Department of Emergency Medicine, MetroHealth Medical Center, Cleveland, OH, USA

Department of Emergency Medicine, Mountain View Hospital, Las Vegas, NV, USA

Matthew R. Dettmer, MD Emergency Services Institute, Respiratory Institute, Cleveland Clinic Health System, Cleveland, OH, USA

Siddharth Dugar, MD, FASE, FCCP, FCCM Department of Critical Care Medicine, Respiratory Institute, Cleveland Clinic, Cleveland, OH, USA

Ibrahim El husseini, MD Department of Medicine, Division of Pulmonary and Critical Care Medicine, Rutgers University, Robert Wood Johnson Medical School, New Brunswick, NJ, USA

Andrea Elliott, MD University of Minnesota, Minneapolis, USA

Steven Fox, MD Respiratory Institute, Cleveland Clinic, Cleveland, OH, USA

Orlando Garner, MD Division of Pulmonary and Critical Care Medicine, Baylor College of Medicine, Houston, TX, USA

Katarzyna Gil, MD Ohio State University Wexner Medical Center, Columbus, OH, USA

Tarik Hanane, MD Department of Critical Care Medicine, Respiratory Institute, Cleveland Clinic, Cleveland, OH, USA

Kristen Holler, DO Department of Cardiothoracic Anesthesiology, Cleveland Clinic, Cleveland, OH, USA

Shawana Hussain, MD Department of Critical Care Medicine, Cooper University Hospital, Camden, NJ, USA

Division of Critical Care, Cooper University Hospital, Camden, PA, USA

David R. Jury, MD, MS Department of Intensive Care & Resuscitation, Cleveland Clinic Foundation, Cleveland, OH, USA

Matthew C. Kostura, MD Emergency Services Institute, Cleveland Clinic Health System, Cleveland, OH, USA

Michael Kouch, MD Department of Critical Care Medicine, Cooper University Hospital, Cooper Medical School at Rowan University, Camden, NJ, USA

Division of Critical Care, Cooper University Hospital, Camden, PA, USA

Nakul Kumar, MD Department of Intensive Care & Resuscitation, Cleveland Clinic Foundation, Cleveland, OH, USA

Ran Lee, MD Cleveland Clinic, Cleveland, OH, USA

Akiva Leibowitz, MD Department of Anesthesia, Critical Care and Pain Medicine, Harvard Medical School, Beth Israel Deaconess Medical Center, Boston, Massachusetts, United States

Javier Lorenzo, MD Department of Anesthesiology, Stanford School of Medicine, Stanford, CA, USA

Milad Matta, MD Department of Internal Medicine, Cleveland Clinic, Cleveland, OH, USA

Charles McCombs, MD Division of Emergency Ultrasound, Department of Emergency Medicine, MetroHealth Medical Center, Cleveland, OH, USA

Department of Pediatric Emergency Medicine, Nationwide Children's Hosptial, Columbus, OH, USA

James E. Mitchell, MD Department of Critical Care, Stanford University Hospital, Stanford, CA, USA

Rob Montgomery, MD Robert and Suzanne Tomsich Department of Cardiovascular Medicine, Sydell and Arnold Miller Family Heart and Vascular Institute, The Cleveland Clinic Foundation, Cleveland, OH, USA

Simon R. Mucha, MD Department of Critical Care Medicine, Respiratory Institute, Cleveland Clinic, Cleveland, OH, USA

Oncology Intensive Care Unit, Respiratory Institute, Cleveland Clinic, Cleveland, OH, USA

Ronny Munoz-Acuna, MD Department of Anesthesia, Critical Care and Pain Medicine, Harvard Medical School, Beth Israel Deaconess Medical Center, Boston, Massachusetts, United States

Department of Anesthesia, Critical Care and Pain, Yale New Haven Hospital, Yale School of Medicine, New Haven, United States

Tarig Omer, MD Department of Critical Care and Resuscitation, Anesthesia Institute, Cleveland Clinic, Cleveland, OH, USA

Department of Intensive Care and Resuscitation, Cleveland Clinic, Cleveland, OH, USA

Ali Omranian, MD Division of Pulmonary and Critical Care Medicine, Baylor College of Medicine, Houston, TX, USA

Purvesh R. Patel, MD Division of Pulmonary and Critical Care Medicine, Baylor College of Medicine, Houston, TX, USA

Sharad Patel, MD Department of Critical Care, Cooper University Hospital, Camden, NJ, USA

Division of Critical Care, Cooper University Hospital, Camden, PA, USA

Jason Phillips, MD Division of Cardiology, Department of Medicine, University of Texas Health San Antonio, San Antonio, TX, USA

Nitin Puri, MD Department of Medicine/Critical Care, Cooper University Hospital, Camden, NJ, USA

Division of Critical Care, Cooper University Hospital, Camden, PA, USA

Vidya K. Rao, MD, MBA Divisions of Cardiothoracic Anesthesiology and Critical Care Medicine, Department of Anesthesiology, Perioperative and Pain Medicine, School of Medicine, Stanford University, Stanford, CA, USA

Haris Riaz, MD Citizens Memorial Hospital, Heart Institute Clinic, Bolivar, MO, USA

Serena Rovida, MD Department of Emergency and Trauma Center, Linköping University, Linköping, Sweden

Shiva Sale, MD Department of Cardiothoracic Anesthesiology, Cleveland Clinic, Cleveland, OH, USA

Pralay K. Sarkar, MD, FRCP (Edin, UK), FCCP Division of Pulmonary, Critical Care and Sleep Medicine, Department of Medicine, Baylor College of Medicine, Ben Taub General Hospital, Houston, TX, USA

Division of Pulmonary and Critical Care Medicine, Baylor College of Medicine, Houston, TX, USA

Mark Schmidhofer, MD University of Pittsburgh Medical Center, Pittsburgh, PA, USA

Mourad H. Senussi, MD, MS Baylor College of Medicine, Houston, TX, USA

Texas Heart Institute, Houston, TX, USA

Ziad S. Shaman, MD, RDMS Departments of Pulmonary, Critical Care, and Sleep Medicine, MetroHealth Medical Center, Cleveland, OH, USA

Matthew T. Siuba, DO Critical Care Medicine, Respiratory Institute, Cleveland Clinic Foundation, Cleveland, OH, USA

Courtney M. Smalley, MD Emergency Services Institute, Cleveland Clinic Health System, Cleveland, OH, USA

Nilam J. Soni, MD, MS Division of Pulmonary Diseases & Critical Care Medicine/Division of Hospital Medicine, Department of Medicine, University of Texas Health San Antonio, San Antonio, TX, USA

Madiha Syed, MD Department of Intensive Care & Resuscitation, Cleveland Clinic Foundation, Cleveland, OH, USA

Matthew Tabbut, MD, FACEP Division of Emergency Ultrasound, Department of Emergency Medicine, MetroHealth Medical Center, Cleveland, OH, USA

Case Western Reserve University School of Medicine, Cleveland, OH, USA

Samuel J. Tate, MD Department of Emergency Medicine, University of California Davis Health, Davis, CA, USA

Carlos E. Trombetta, MD, MEd Department of Cardiothoracic Anesthesiology, Cleveland Clinic, Cleveland, OH, USA

Chiedozie Udeh, MBBS, MHEcon Department of Intensive Care and Resuscitation, Cleveland Clinic, Cleveland, OH, USA

Rishik Vashisht, MD Cardiac Surgery Intensive Care Unit, Sentara Norfolk General Hospital, Norfolk, VA, USA

Ana Luisa Silveira Vieira, MD, PhD Department of Point of Care Ultrasound, Faculty of Medicine of Barbacena, Barbacena, Minas Gerais, Brazil

Ariel Vinas, MD Division of Cardiology, Department of Medicine, University of Texas Health San Antonio, San Antonio, TX, USA

Giovanni Volpicelli, MD Emergency Medicine, Department of Medical and Surgical Science, Magna Graecia University, Catanzaro, Italy

Brett J. Wakefield, MD Department of Cardiothoracic Anesthesiology, Cleveland Clinic, Cleveland, OH, USA

Tom Kai Ming Wang, MBChB, MD Robert and Suzanne Tomsich Department of Cardiovascular Medicine, Sydell and Arnold Miller Family Heart and Vascular Institute, The Cleveland Clinic Foundation, Cleveland, OH, USA

Mark H. Zahniser, MD Department of Intensive Care and Resuscitation, Cleveland Clinic, Cleveland, OH, USA

Ultrasound Physics

1

Ziad S. Shaman and Oriade K. Adeoye

Question 1
Propagation speed of ultrasound would MOST likely be maximum in which of the following materials?

A. A
B. B
C. C
D. D

Material/medium	Density	Stiffness
A	Low	High
B	High	Low
C	Low	Low
D	High	Low

Answer: A. Low density, high stiffness

Key point: Speed of sound is directly proportional to stiffness and inversely proportional to density of the medium in which it travels. Paradoxically, sound usually travels faster in higher-density materials because they also tend to be stiffer. For example, the velocity of ultrasound in soft tissue is 1540 m/s and in bone the propagation speed is approximates 4100 m/s. Bone, is both denser and stiffer than soft tissue. However, stiffness differences among materials are usually larger than density differences. In general, the propagation speed of sound is low in gases, higher in liquids, and highest in solids.

Question 2
Increasing the depth of interrogation from 10 to 20 cm during transthoracic echocardiography, will MOST likely lead to a decrease in:

A. Pulse Repetition Period
B. Pulse Duration
C. Pulse repetition frequency
D. Amplitude

Answer: C. Pulse repetition frequency is decreased

Key point: Increasing the depth increases the pulse repetition period (PRP) which decreases the pulse repetition frequency (PRF). Pulse duration (PD), amplitude and spatial pulse length, are inherent characteristics of the transducer and cannot be altered.

Question 3
Axial resolution is MOST likely determined by which of the following characteristics of the ultrasound beam:

A. Beam width
B. Pulse repetition period
C. Pulse duration
D. Spatial pulse length

Answer: D. Spatial pulse length

Key point: Axial resolution is determined as one half the Spatial Pulse Length or SPL/2. Spatial pulse length is the product of wavelength and number of cycles in the pulse. The shorter the spatial pulse length, the better the axial resolution.

Question 4
Lateral resolution is MOST likely determined by which of the following characteristics of the ultrasound beam:

A. Beam width
B. Pulse repetition period
C. Pulse duration
D. Amplitude

Supplementary Information The online version contains supplementary material available at https://doi.org/10.1007/978-3-031-45731-9_1.

Z. S. Shaman (✉) · O. K. Adeoye
Departments of Pulmonary, Critical Care, and Sleep Medicine, MetroHealth Medical Center, Cleveland, OH, USA
e-mail: zss@case.edu

R. Sreedharan et al. (eds.), *Critical Care Echocardiography*, https://doi.org/10.1007/978-3-031-45731-9_1

Answer: A. Beam width

Key point: Lateral resolution is determined by beam width. Narrower beams have superior lateral resolution. Axial resolution is determined by spatial pulse length (SPL). Axial resolution = SPL/2. A smaller number has better resolution, therefore shorter pulses provide superior axial resolution.

Question 5

A 55-year-old female with alcoholic cirrhosis is admitted to the ICU with a distended abdomen. Examination reveals an indwelling peritoneal catheter. Bedside ultrasound is performed to assess the ascites (See Video 1.1). Interaction between the ultrasound beam and the peritoneal dialysis catheter is leading to which of the following imaging artifacts?

A. Electrical interference artifact
B. Drop out artifact
C. Stitching artifact
D. Reverberation artifact

Answer: D. Reverberation artifact.

Key point: The presence of a strongly echogenic surface (in this case the peritoneal dialysis catheter), causes ultrasound beams striking this device to bounce back and forth multiple times before returning to the receiver. The delay in time is erroneously interpreted by the transducer as a straight line distance between the object and the transducer. Consequently, despite the presence of only one peritoneal dialysis catheter, due to the reverberation artifact, it appears multiple catheters are present.

Question 6

2D ultrasound imaging and Color flow Doppler interrogation of the axillary vessels is shown in the video (see Videos 1.2 and 1.3). Measurement of the axillary artery diameter is BEST done at which line?

A. A
B. B
C. C
D. D

Answer: A. A

Key point: The patient has an echogenic structure in the axillary vein (Structure X) consistent with a venous thrombus. Structure Y represents the axillary artery. As axial resolution is superior to lateral resolution, measurement of the axillary artery diameter is best done at line A.

Question 7

Angular resolution refers to:

A. Axial resolution
B. Temporal resolution
C. Contrast resolution
D. Lateral resolution

Answer: D. Lateral resolution

Key point: Lateral resolution (also called angular, transverse or azimuthal resolution) is defined as the minimum distance between two structures that are separated side-to-side or perpendicular to the sound beam producing two distinct echoes. Lateral resolution is best at the preset focal length of transducer, and is better with a narrower beam.

Question 8

The accompanying video (Video 1.4) demonstrates a parasternal long axis view during transthoracic echocardiography. Temporal resolution can be BEST improved by:

A. Decreasing depth of imaging
B. Increasing wavelength
C. Decreasing frequency of transmission
D. Increasing sector width

Answer: A. Decreasing depth of imaging

Key point: Temporal resolution depends upon time needed to generate a frame or image. Greater the depth of imaging, longer the time needed to generate a frame. Consequently, temporal resolution can be improved by decreasing the depth of imaging and decreasing sector width. Additionally, temporal resolution in maximal in M mode. Decreasing the depth will also eliminate mirror image artifact at the bottom of the screen (arrow).

Question 9

A sonographer would like to optimize imaging of the aortic valve in the apical 5 chamber view. Which of the following interventions will help her improve the image quality?

A. Increasing depth of imaging
B. Decreasing wavelength of transmitted ultrasound waves
C. Increasing frequency of transmitted ultrasound waves
D. Decreasing frequency of transmitted ultrasound waves

Answer: D. Decreasing frequency of transmitted sound waves

Key point: Use of a lower frequency transducer will help optimize image resolution. While resolution is mostly improved using higher frequency ultrasound, when imaging deep structures using high frequency, much of the ultrasound energy will dissipate to heat before reaching the targeted area. Therefore, lower frequency ultrasound is preferred in this situation.

Question 10

Ultrasound signal deteriorates to heat in the tissue parenchyma by:

A. Absorption
B. Reflection
C. Refraction
D. Scatter

Answer: A. Absorption

Key point: All of the above cause attenuation of the ultrasound beam energy; however, only absorption causes the energy to turn into heat, and that depends on the Acoustic Absorption Coefficient of the medium.

Question 11 (Fig. 1.1)

What interventions would help optimize the image of the internal jugular vein shown below?

A. Increase gain and increase depth
B. Decrease gain and increase depth
C. Increase gain and decrease depth
D. Decrease gain and decrease depth

Answer: D. Decrease gain and decrease depth

Key point: Decreasing depth is important to keep the area of interest in the middle of the screen where the beam is focused. The gain needs to be decreased to allow for better detail definition and less beam diffraction leading to better lateral resolution.

Question 12 (Fig. 1.2)

Below is an apical 2 chamber (A2C) view of the heart showing the left ventricle (LV) and left atrial (LA) chambers in addition to the inferior wall. The red arrow is pointing to the inferior wall, which appears bright. Which of the following interactions of the ultrasound signal with tissue interfaces is MOST likely leading to bright appearance of the inferior wall?

A. Higher speed of ultrasound through inferior wall than blood
B. Higher acoustic impedance of inferior wall than blood
C. Lower attenuation of the ultrasound beam by the inferior wall than blood
D. Greater Rayleigh scattering of the ultrasound beam by the inferior wall than blood

Answer: B. Higher acoustic impedance of inferior wall than blood

Key point: Higher acoustic impedance of inferior wall than blood in LV/LA chambers. The inferior wall of the left ventricle appears bright due to "acoustic enhancement" or "posterior enhancement". This occurs because the acoustic impedance of the inferior wall is greater than that of blood in the cardiac chambers. The time gain compensation (TGC) overcompensates deeper to the fluid-filled structure causing deeper tissues to be assigned a brighter signal on the screen.

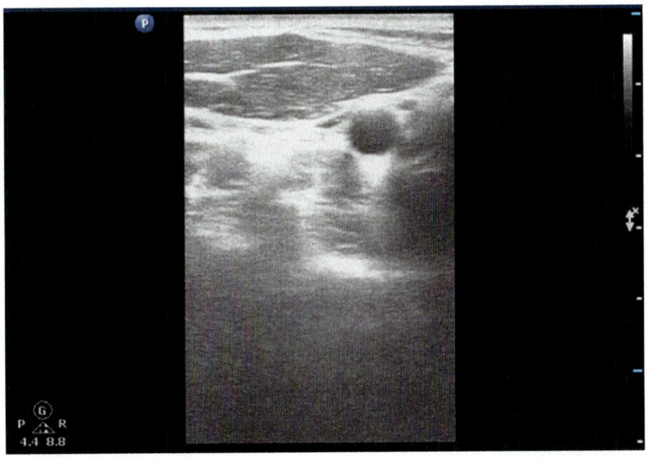

Fig. 1.1 A short axis image of the carotid artery and the internal jugular vein (compressed)

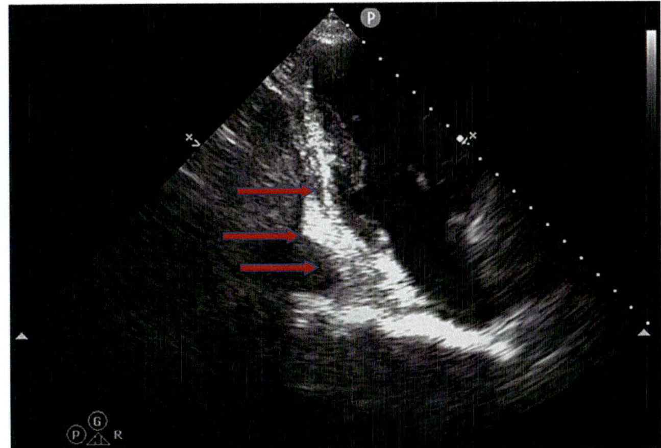

Fig. 1.2 Apical 2 chamber view of the left ventricle and left atrium. The red arrows point to the inferior wall

Table 1.1 Acoustic impedances of various tissues

Tissue	Acoustic impedance
Lung	0.0004
Fat	1.34
Liver	1.65
Muscle	1.71
Bone	7.8

Question 13

The acoustic impedance is the product of:

A. Speed of sound and reflection coefficient
B. Speed of sound and beam amplitude
C. Tissue density and beam wavelength
D. Tissue density and speed of sound

Answer: D. Tissue density and speed of sound

Key point: Acoustic impedance, density × speed, i.e., $Z = \rho \times c$. The lung has low density and slow propagation velocity, whereas bone has a high density and fast propagation velocity. Ultrasound is reflected from boundaries between tissues with differences in acoustic impedance. The acoustic impedances of different tissues is outlined below in Table 1.1.

Question 14

A 10 MHz ultrasound transducer is being used to interrogate the heart. The wavelength generated is:

A. 0.015 mm
B. 0.15 mm
C. 1.5 mm
D. 15 mm

Answer: B. 0.15 mm

Key point: Wavelength = Speed/Frequency

The speed of sound in soft tissue = 1540 m/s (memorize this!)

= 1540 m/s = 154,000 cm/s = 1.54 mm/μs

Wavelength = (1.54 mm/μs)/(10 cycles/μs) = 0.154 mm

Question 15

Which of the following interventions leads to generation of ultrasonic frequencies by a modern piezoelectric transducer?

A. Application of a pressure pulse
B. Application of an electrical pulse
C. Addition of damping material
D. Addition of a matching plate

Answer: B. Application of an electrical pulse

Key point: An ultrasound beam is generated by transforming electrical activity to pressure waves using certain crystals with piezoelectric properties. The effect is known to occur naturally in quartz, and also in other materials like lead-zirconate-titanate crystals that are currently used in commercial ultrasound transducers.

Question 16

Which of the following factors can increase temporal resolution?

A. Decreased depth
B. Increased scan width
C. Increased line density
D. Apodization

Answer: A. Decreased depth

Key point: Temporal resolution is the time from the beginning of one frame to the next; it is the ability of the ultrasound system to distinguish between near instantaneous events of rapidly moving structures such as during echocardiography. Temporal resolution, AKA frame rate = 15,400/(2 × penetration in cm × number of foci × number of scan lines). Frame rate can be increased by:

1. reduced depth of penetration, since pulses have to travel a short distance;
2. reduced number of focal points, since scan lines do not have to be duplicated; and
3. reduced scan lines per frame, that is using narrow frames rather than wide frames.

Apodization refers to the process of minimizing grating lobes by driving the elements at variable voltages. This improves lateral resolution, not temporal resolution.

Question 17

In a sound wave, peak pressure is BEST represented by:

A. Amplitude
B. Wavelength
C. Frequency
D. Power

Answer: A: Amplitude

Key point: Sound is a mechanical, longitudinal wave comprised of compressions (increases in pressure or density) and rarefactions (decreases in pressure or density). Amplitude represents peak pressure and loudness of the sound wave. Power represents rate of energy transfer.

Question 18
How long does it take for a sound pulse to travel to and from a reflector that is 1 cm deep in tissue?

A. 0.13 μs
B. 1.3 μs
C. 13 μs
D. 130 μs

Answer: C: 13 μs
Key point: Since the sound pulse must travel round-trip, the total distance travelled is 2 cm (to the reflector at a depth of 1 cm and back to the transducer).
Time = distance/speed
Distance = 2 cm, speed = 1540 m/s
Time (in μs) = distance (in mm)/speed (mm/μs) = 20/1.54 = 13 μs
This is called "The 13 μs rule" which is the time needed for sound to travel 1 cm round-trip (memorize this!)
This is also known as time-of-flight or go-return time.

Question 19
Time gain compensation (TGC) compensates for sound:

A. Propagation speed
B. Attenuation
C. Reflection
D. Refraction

Answer: B. Attenuation
Key point: Time gain compensation (TGC) is an instrument setting that amplifies echo signals coming from distant reflectors are more than echo signals originating from reflectors close to the transducer. As near field structures are usually brighter (reflected signals are stronger), TGC in the near field can be set low and is increased for far-field structures, so imaging of distant structures can be optimized.

Question 20
Lowest thermal index can be achieved by choosing:

A. Highest frequency and lowest intensity
B. Lowest frequency and lowest intensity
C. Highest frequency and highest intensity
D. Lowest frequency and highest intensity

Answer 20: B. Lowest frequency and lowest intensity
Key point: Low intensity results in low energy transmission into the body. Low frequency results in low absorption.

Question 21
According to the United States Food and Drug Administration (FDA) recommendations, bioeffects of ultrasound are BEST avoided when the Mechanical Index is less than:

A. 4.1
B. 3.2
C. 2.8
D. 1.9

Answer: D. 1.9
Key point: The Mechanical Index (MI) is a measure of the power of an ultrasound beam and determines possibility of non-thermal bioeffects of the acoustic field, such as cavitation. Cavitation is the expansion and contraction or collapse of bubbles because of the acoustic pressure of the ultrasound beam. MI is defined as peak negative pressure divided by the square root of the frequency of the ultrasound wave.

Question 22
Low frequency transducers have:

A. Shorter wavelengths and less penetration
B. Longer wavelengths and greater penetration
C. Shorter wavelengths and greater penetration
D. Longer wavelengths and less penetration

Answer: B. Longer wavelengths and greater penetration
Key point: Frequency is inversely related to wavelength. Therefore, lower frequency means longer waves. Penetration depends on attenuation which is inversely related to the frequency where (attenuation = coefficient × distance travelled × beam frequency). Therefore, lower frequency ultrasound waves suffer lower attenuation and can penetrate deeper into tissue before the energy turns into heat.

Question 23 (Fig. 1.3)
Measurement of Left Ventricular wall thickness in the image shown below, is BEST optimized by implementing changes in which of the following parameters:

A. Gain
B. Orientation
C. Harmonics
D. Depth

Answer: D. Depth
Key point: The gain and the orientation are set correctly. Harmonics imaging is post processing and does not affect resolution. Decreasing the depth will bring the area of interest (the heart in this case) to the center of the image and to the area of most beam focus, therefore improving spatial resolution. Decreasing the depth will increase the frame rate and therefore improve temporal resolution, which is important when imaging fast moving structures such as the heart.

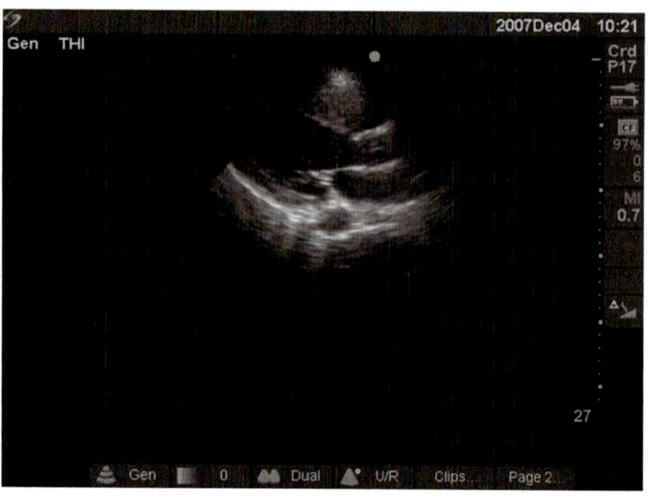

Fig. 1.3 Parasternal long axis view of the heart. Here, the image is very deep relative the area of interest. Decreasing depth will improve resolution

Question 24
Tissue harmonic imaging (THI) uses echoes of:

A. Lower frequencies than the fundamental wave to generate images
B. Higher frequencies than the fundamental wave to generate images
C. Side lobes and grating lobes to generate central field images
D. Reverberations from the incident wave to generate central field images

Answer: B. Higher frequencies than the fundamental wave to generate images

Key point: Tissue harmonics imaging utilize second harmonic echoes of the fundamental frequency of the transmitted beam to generate better resolution images than is possible from the low frequency fundamental wave echoes. Post processing is used to eliminate the fundamental frequency echoes. With THI there are lower side lobe, grating lobe, and reverberation artifacts. These artifacts are known to degrade image quality.

Question 25
With regards to tissue harmonic imaging, which of the following is MOST likely correct?

A. Harmonic waves are generated by ultrasound induced vibration of tissues
B. Harmonic waves are responsible for generating side lobe artifacts
C. Harmonic imaging decreases axial and lateral resolution
D. Harmonic waves suffer greater attenuation compared to the transducer-generated ultrasound waves

Answer: A. Harmonic waves are generated by ultrasound induced vibration of tissue

Key point: The transducer emitted ultrasound beam travels through tissues, causing the tissues to vibrate. Tissue vibration leads to formation of harmonic waves that travel back to the transducer. These waves typically have frequencies that are multiples of the originally transmitted or fundamental frequency. For example, a 6 MHz transducer, will create tissue generated harmonic waves of 12 and 18 MHz frequencies. As these waves travel only once to get back to the transducer, they are attenuated less and have greater acoustic energy. Consequently, tissue harmonic imaging improves axial and lateral resolution while decreasing formation of side lobe artifacts.

Further Reading

Edelman S. Ultrasound physics (Ch. 1-5). ESP Inc.; 2016.
Rengasamy S, Subramaniam B. Basic physics of transesophageal echocardiography. Int Anesthesiol Clin. 2008;46(2):11–29.
Shriki J. Ultrasound physics. Crit Care Clin. 2014;30(1):1–24.

Doppler

2

Chiedozie Udeh, Tarig Omer, and Mark H. Zahniser

Question 1
Which of the following is LEAST likely associated with Pulsed Wave Doppler interrogation:

A. Aliasing
B. Measurement of highest velocity along a beam path
C. Doppler frequency shift is in the audible range
D. Leads to generation of an empty spectral envelope

Answer: B. Measurement of highest velocity along a beam path

Key point: Pulsed wave Doppler is used for estimating velocity of flow at a defined location.

Rationale: Pulsed wave Doppler transmits pulses along a single line of interest using the same crystal for sending and receiving signals. However, signal reception is gated so that only signals from the preset sample volume position are processed, permitting velocity estimation at that position. This is why the spectral envelope is empty as velocities from all other locations are ignored. Aliasing can occur with PWD if the Doppler frequency exceeds the Nyquist limit. Doppler frequency shift is typically in kilohertz and are audible [1].

The following images in panels A and B apply to questions 2 and 3 (Fig. 2.1a, b).

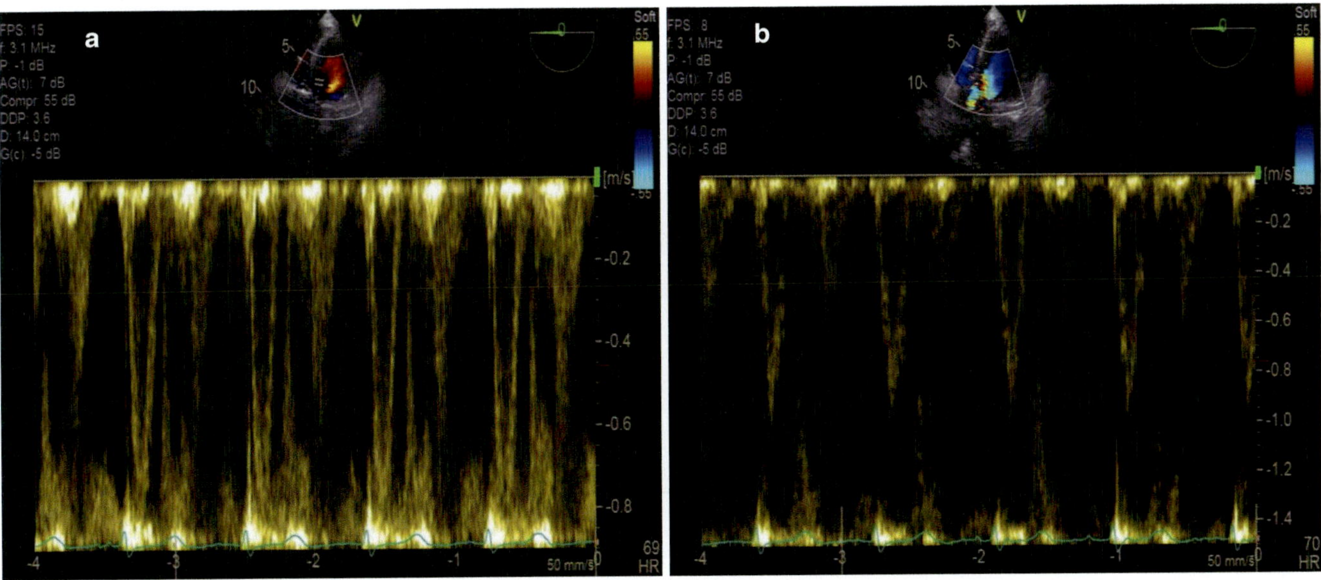

Fig. 2.1 (**a**, **b**) Pulsed wave doppler interrogation in the deep transgastric long axis view

C. Udeh (✉) · T. Omer · M. H. Zahniser
Department of Intensive Care and Resuscitation, Cleveland Clinic, Cleveland, OH, USA
e-mail: udehc@ccf.org; omert@ccf.org; zahnism@ccf.org

R. Sreedharan et al. (eds.), *Critical Care Echocardiography*, https://doi.org/10.1007/978-3-031-45731-9_2

Question 2

The figure in panel A above, is a trans-esophageal image depicting

A. CWD interrogation of the LVOT with aliasing
B. PWD interrogation of the LVOT with aliasing
C. CWD interrogation of the mitral valve with aliasing
D. PWD interrogation of the mitral valve with aliasing

Answer: B. PWD interrogation of the LVOT with aliasing

Key Point: The image depicts spectral analysis from PWD interrogation of the LVOT with signal aliasing. Note the sample gate along the cursor line, positioned in the LVOT and the Doppler spectral envelope pointing away from the baseline consistent with flow away from the transducer.

Rationale: Signal aliasing occurs when the direction of flow cannot be determined because the Doppler frequency exceed the Nyquist limit. In that event, the signal is truncated at the edge of the display and the excised portion appears on the opposite edge. This 'wraparound" continues until the difference in the Doppler frequency and the Nyquist limit is exhausted. Aliasing is not seen with continuous wave Doppler [1].

Question 3

In the panel B above, what is the effect of adjusting the velocity scale to mitigate aliasing?

A. Raises the baseline for flow towards the transducer
B. Increases the pulse repetition frequency
C. Decreases the Nyquist limit
D. Decreases the pulse repetition frequency

Answer B. Increases the pulse repetition frequency

Key Point: Adjusting the velocity scale to its maximum for that depth is effectively maximizing the pulse repetition frequency.

Rationale: Aliasing occurs when the sampled velocities exceed the Nyquist limit, which is the maximum detectable velocity. In clinical imaging, the Nyquist limit can be adjusted as a function of the pulse repetition frequency. Nyquist limit will be exceeded when the Doppler frequency is greater than half the pulse repetition frequency. Maximizing the velocity scale will reduce sensitivity to lower velocities. Also note that the deeper the site of interest, the lower the pulse repetition frequency. As such, Nyquist limit will decrease as depth of interest increases [1].

Question 4

Optimal angles for incident wave for flow velocity assessment are

A. 0° and 20°
B. 0° and 30°
C. 0° and 90°
D. 0° and 180°

Answer: D. 0° and 180°

Key Point: Optimal angles for maximal and accurate assessment of velocity are 0° and 180°.

Rationale: Optimal angle for imaging in B-Mode ultrasonography is 90° in order to achieve maximal reflection of ultrasound. This is unlike Doppler ultrasonography imaging in which maximum Doppler frequency detection occurs when the transducer is interrogating flow at an angle parallel to the direction of flow. Consequently, optimal angle is either 180° or 0° because the cosine of both angles, is 1. At 90°, no velocity is detected because cosine 90 = 0. Interrogation at 20° or less is considered acceptable as the underestimation error in the calculated velocity is less than 6% and can be ignored. For arterial ultrasound imaging, use of angle correction is acceptable up to 60°; however, the use of angle correction is discouraged in cardiac imaging because significant errors can be introduced [1].

The following image applies to question 5 (Fig. 2.2)

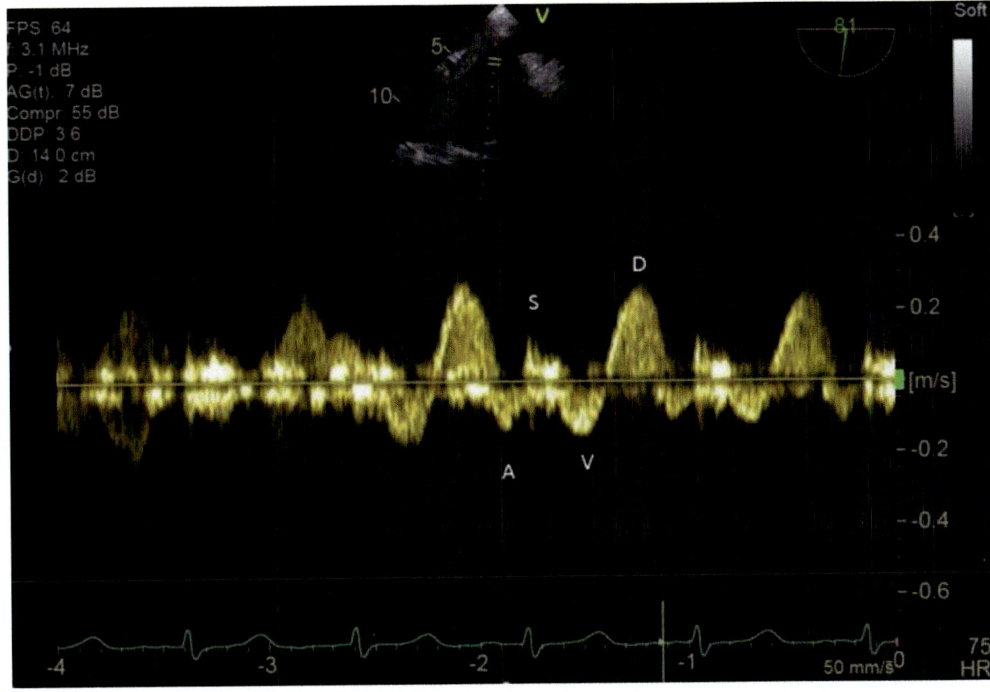

Fig. 2.2 Pulsed wave Doppler spectral analysis of hepatic vein flow

Question 5
This pulsed wave Doppler spectral analysis of hepatic vein flow is LEAST likely to represent:

A. Right heart failure with tricuspid regurgitation
B. Infective endocarditis with tricuspid regurgitation
C. Normal hepatic flow pattern
D. Mild Right Ventricular dysfunction

Answer: C. Normal hepatic flow pattern

Key Point: With normal hepatic vein flow, the 'S' wave is larger than the 'D' wave

Rationale: Spectral Doppler analysis of hepatic vein flow is useful in assessing the severity of tricuspid regurgitation. The normal flow profile has retrograde 'AR' waves and antegrade 'S' and 'D' waves. These respectively reflect hepatic flow waves associated with atrial contraction at end of diastole, descent of the tricuspid annulus in early systole, and ventricular filling during diastole. Normally the systolic flow velocity is higher than diastolic flow velocity or S > D. Blunting or S < D, occurs in mild to moderate tricuspid regurgitation and right ventricular dysfunction. The 'V" wave tends to become more prominent in moderate to severe tricuspid regurgitation, when the ventricles begin to relax and the tricuspid annulus returns to its usual position. With severe tricuspid regurgitation and right ventricular dysfunction, the 'S' wave is often reversed [2].

Question 6
Doppler analysis of blood flow is LEAST dependent upon

A. Blood flow velocity
B. Specular reflection
C. Angle of insonation between the beam and blood flow
D. Speed of sound in tissue

Answer: B. Specular reflection

Key point: Scattering reflection from red blood cells forms the basis of their Doppler Analysis.

Rationale: The Doppler frequency is the change in frequency of a reflected wave when it encounters a moving object. Specular reflection occurs when the beam encounters a large object with a relatively smooth surface and is important for generating images of cardiac structures. Scattering reflection occurs when the beam encounters small and irregular objects such as red blood cells. The reflected wave has a higher frequency if the red blood cell is moving towards the transducer, and vice versa [1].

The following scenario and image apply to questions 7–9 (Fig. 2.3).

Patient is a 28-year-old female with past history of intravenous drug abuse. She had been drug-free for 8 months prior to presentation and is actively enrolled in a methadone program. She presents with shortness of breath on mild exertion. She has also noted a pulsatile feeling in her neck all the time and she also feels that her abdomen and legs are swollen.

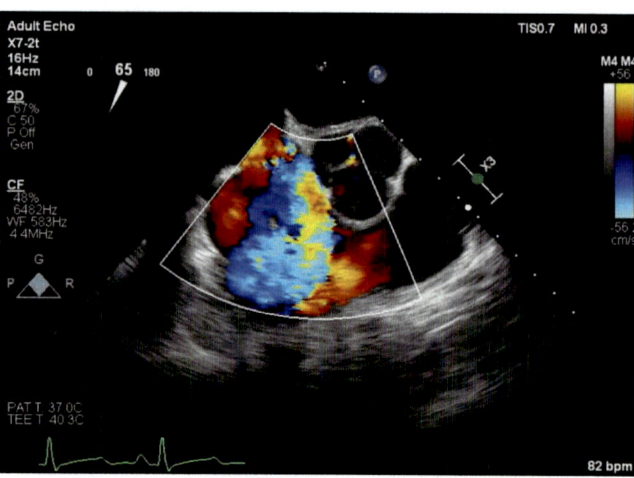

Fig. 2.3 Color flow doppler evaluation of the tricuspid valve

Question 7
The images above depict:

A. Mid-esophageal, bicaval view with severe tricuspid regurgitation
B. Mid-esophageal 4-chamber, RV focus, color flow Doppler of mild tricuspid regurgitation
C. Transthoracic parasternal short axis view with moderate mitral stenosis
D. Mid-esophageal RV inflow–outflow with color flow Doppler of severe tricuspid regurgitation

Answer: D. Mid-esophageal RV inflow–outflow with color flow Doppler of severe tricuspid regurgitation

Key point: The view is obtained with the TEE probe at a depth of 30–40 cm, with 60°–75° image rotation

Rationale: The image depicts severe regurgitant flow through an incompetent tricuspid valve into the right atrium during systole. Tricuspid regurgitation is qualitatively described as severe if the ratio of the regurgitant jet area relative to the right atrium exceeds 0.67 [1, 3].

Question 8
If the patient's tricuspid regurgitant (TR) jet peak velocity is measured at 4.2 m/s by continuous wave Doppler, which of the following is the best estimate of pulmonary artery systolic pressure? (Assume a right atrial pressure = 15 mmHg)

A. 85 mmHg
B. 70 mmHg
C. 34 mmHg
D. 55 mmHg

Answer: A. 85 mmHg

Key Point: The best estimate for this patient's pulmonary artery pressure is 85 mmHg

Rationale: Assuming there is no gradient across the pulmonary valve or RV outflow tract, then the right ventricular systolic pressure (RVSP) is a good surrogate for the pulmonary artery systolic pressure. RVSP can be calculated using the modified Bernoulli equation and then adding the right atrial pressure [3].

$$\text{RSVP} = 4^{*}\text{V}^{2} + \text{RAP}$$

V TR peak velocity, *RAP* right atrial pressure.

Question 9
Which of the following is least likely correct about tricuspid valve endocarditis?

A. The most common causative organism is staphylococcus aureus
B. Surgical treatment in patients with large vegetations is reasonable.
C. Medical therapy with antibiotics is the primary mode of treatment
D. Temporal pattern of fever helps in diagnosis

Answer: D. Temporal pattern of fever helps in diagnosis

Key Point: Tricuspid valve endocarditis is most commonly caused by S. aureus and is amenable to medical therapy as the primary mode of treatment.

Rationale: Right-sided infective endocarditis accounts for only 5–10% of infective endocarditis, and 90% of these cases involve the tricuspid valve. Tricuspid valve endocarditis is commonly associated with intravenous drug abuse, and also with indwelling vascular access catheters. S. Aureus is the most common causative organism and most cases can be successfully treated with intravenous antibiotics. Surgery is reserved for cases with severe tricuspid regurgitation, large vegetations (>2 cm), persistent bacteremia, or recurrent pulmonary septic emboli. Surgery related mortality is on par with medical therapy at less than 15%. While fever greater than 38 °C is a minor Duke criteria, temporal patterns vary widely in infective endocarditis and are of no diagnostic utility [4].

Question 10
Color flow Doppler

A. Has good temporal resolution
B. Is not subject to the Nyquist effect
C. Calculates peak velocities using autocorrelation
D. Is a multi-gated form of pulse wave Doppler

Answer: D. Is a multi-gated form of pulse wave Doppler

Key point: Color flow Doppler is based on the principles of pulsed wave Doppler and it analyses multiple sample volumes along each scan line.

Rationale: Color flow Doppler (CFD) is a multi-gated form of pulse wave Doppler and is subject to all the limitations and features of pulse wave Doppler (PWD). Ultrasound pulses are sent along multiple adjacent scan lines with gates set at different depths within the specified sector, to generate a color-coded map of velocities, superimposed on a B-mode image. Because of the large amount of Doppler data generated, CFD uses autocorrelation to resolve and calculate mean velocity [1].

Question 11
Tissue Doppler imaging uses filters to extract

A. High velocity, low amplitude signals
B. High amplitude, low velocity signals
C. Low velocity, low amplitude signals
D. High velocity, high amplitude signals

Answer: B. High amplitude, low velocity signals

Key point: Tissue Doppler imaging is used to assess diastolic function by isolating and analyzing the high amplitude, low velocity signals emanating from the myocardium.

Rationale: Tissue Doppler imaging (TDI) is an adaptation of Doppler imaging used to assess cardiac systolic or diastolic function by measuring cardiac wall motion velocity, which is normally about 10 cm/s. Cardiac muscle movement results in ultrasound reflections that are high amplitude, and low velocity relative to red cell flow-induced reflections. Accordingly, TDI uses filters to extract velocities less than 20 cm/s [3].

Question 12
Pulsed Wave Doppler interrogation

A. Has multiple scan lines
B. Can over-estimate red blood cell velocity
C. Requires multiple piezo-electric crystals
D. Is affected by the depth of the sample volume

Answer: D. Is affected by the depth of the sample volume

Key Point: Pulse wave Doppler (PWD) interrogation is limited by inability to resolve high velocity particularly in deeper locations.

Rationale: PWD uses one crystal to send pulses down along one scan line, then pauses to listen for reflected waves, using a time gate to focus on signals returning from the imaging depth of interest. Red cell velocity can never be over-estimated. However, under-estimation is expected if the angle of insonation is not parallel to the direction of flow [1].

The following scenario applies to questions 13 and 14

A 54-year-old patient presents in heart failure. A pan-diastolic murmur is detected on examination. Clinicians are unable to place a pulmonary artery catheter. An echocardiogram with spectral Doppler analysis is performed with attention to the mitral valve. The following parameters are obtained.

1. Velocity Time Integral (VTI) is 54 cm
2. HR is 90/min
3. Mean diastolic gradient 20 mmHg
4. Pressure half time (PHT) of the MV is 270 ms

Question 13
Assuming that the aortic valve is normal, what is the best estimate of cardiac output in liters/minute?

A. 5
B. 4
C. 2.5
D. 3

Answer: B. 4

Key Point: Cardiac output is determined by heart rate (HR) and stroke volume (SV). CO = HR × SV (where SV = Cross-sectional area (CSA) * velocity time integral (VTI))

Rationale: Stroke volume is estimated using spectral Doppler interrogation of any point in the heart where the blood flow can be measured accurately. Then multiplying the VTI by the cross-sectional area of that point in the heart. The underlying assumption is that the VTI approximates the volume of blood within the presumed approximate cylinder/column (with a circular base) of blood ejected with each contraction. Given this assumption that the point of measurement is a circle, whose area can be calculated, it is crucial to ensure accurate measurement of the diameter for calculation of the cross-sectional area. If not, large errors will be introduced when the radius is squared. Typically, the left ventricular outflow tract (LVOT) offers the best option for aligning ultrasound and Doppler signals to ensure accurate measurements of the diameter and VTI. These LVOT measurements are also used in calculating the aortic valve area. Flow through the mitral valve will equal flow through the LVOT in the absence of aortic valvular disease.

MV area is calculated as MVA = 220/270 by the Pressure Half Time method. This area is then multiplied with MV VTI given as 54 cm to calculate the volume of blood passing through the MV. This is multiplied by Heart Rate (90/min) to yield Cardiac Output [1].

Question 14
What is the mitral valve area in cm^2?

A. 1.2
B. 2.2
C. 0.8
D. 1.76

Answer: C. 0.8

Key Point: In mitral stenosis, valve area can be calculated from the pressure half time (PHT). The applicable formula for mitral valve area is 220/ PHT. 220 is a constant.

Rationale: In mitral stenosis, left atrial to left ventricular flow is impaired. This leads to the development of high left atrial pressure that in turn drives an elevated peak velocity due to the stenotic valve. Left atrial emptying is slowed, as is the rate of equalization of the pressure difference between both chambers. The pressure half time (PHT) is the time it takes for this pressure differential to drop in half from its peak. The constant (220) was derived from a cohort of patients with mitral stenosis whose valve area was close to 1 cm^2. This formula is not validated for normal native mitral valves, or prosthetic valves. Estimation of aortic valve area (AVA) is typically done using the Continuity equation, based on the assumption that flow through the LVOT equals flow through the AV. The applicable formula is $AVA = (CSA_{LVOT} * VTI_{LVOT})/VTI_{AV}$. The data inputs will require continuous wave spectral Doppler analysis of the LVOT and aortic root [1].

Question 15

Which of the following is LEAST likely correct about duty factor:

A. It is determined by pulse repetition period
B. It is determined by pulse duration
C. It is measured in units of Hertz
D. Increasing depth of imaging, decreases value of duty factor

Answer: C. It is measured in units of Hertz

Key point: Duty factor is a unit less measure.

Rationale: Duty Factor or DF is defined as a percent of time that the ultrasound system is on while transmitting a pulse.

DF = {pulse duration (s)/pulse repetition period (s)} × 100. It has units of % and ranges from 0 (the system is off) to 100 (the system is on continuously).

Typical valued of DF in clinical imaging are 0.1–1% Depending on the imaging depth, the system may spend more time waiting to receive reflected waves. As such deeper imaging depth will reduce the duty factor [1].

Question 16

Nyquist limit is a factor of

A. Pulse repetition period
B. Pulse duration
C. Pulse repetition frequency
D. Transmitted frequency

Answer: C. Pulse repetition frequency

Key point: Nyquist limit is equal to half the pulse repetition frequency

Rationale: The Nyquist limit is the maximum detectable velocity. It is dependent on the frequency of sampling, not the frequency of the transmitted wave. Nyquist limit is reached when the Doppler shift exceeds half the pulse repetition frequency. Aliasing occurs when the velocity exceeds the Nyquist limit [1].

Question 17

Decreasing the angle of insonation toward zero will have the following effect

A. Increase the pulse repetition frequency
B. Increase the Nyquist limit
C. Increase the maximum measurable frequency
D. Increase the accuracy of the measured velocity

Answer: D. Increase the accuracy of the measured velocity

Key Point: Maximal Doppler shift detection occurs when the angle of insonation is parallel to the direction of flow at 180° or 0°.

Rationale: Decreasing the angle of insonation toward zero will decrease the error in estimation of the velocity. Under-estimation error is 6% when the insonation angle is less than 20° and in clinical practice, this can be ignored. Under-estimation error rises to 13% when angle is at 30°. Whereas above 60°, excessive error is introduced [1].

Question 18

Peripheral pulses can be identified using an ultrasound machine because

E. The transmitted ultrasound is reflected off the moving myocardium
F. The transmitted ultrasound is reflected off the moving red blood cells
G. The doppler shift is within the audible range
H. Only for flow towards the probe

Answer: G. The doppler shift is within the audible range

Key Point: The Doppler shift lies within the audible range.

Rationale: The change in frequency when ultrasound encounters a moving object is a small fraction of the transmitted frequency (typically about 0.1%). Accordingly, the Doppler frequency will fall well within the range which humans can hear (2–20 kHz). This is the underlying principle for simple bedside Doppler machines for monitoring peripheral pulses [1].

Question 19
The minimum sampling frequency required to avoid aliasing is

A. At least half the doppler frequency
B. At least 2 times the transmitted frequency
C. At least 2 times the doppler frequency
D. At least half the transmitted frequency

Answer: C. At least 2 times the doppler frequency

Key point: Sampling frequency for the returning signals must be at least twice per cycle in order to accurately determine the wavelength.

Rationale: In order for the frequency of the ultrasound waveform to be accurately measured, it has to be sampled no less than twice per wavelength. The pulse repetition frequency is the sampling frequency. If the sampling rate is slower than twice the Doppler shift, it will result in aliasing [1].

Question 20
Which of the following parameters CANNOT be adjusted by the sonographer

A. Pulse repetition frequency
B. Pulse repetition period
C. Spatial pulse length
D. Duty factor

Answer: C. Spatial pulse length

Key Point: The spatial pulse length cannot be adjusted by the sonographer.

Rationale: The spatial pulse length is the distance in space occupied by an ultrasound pulse. Each pulse comprises several cycles, the wavelength for each is determined by the source of the ultrasound and the medium in which it is being propagated. Consequently, spatial pulse length cannot be adjusted by the sonographer [3].

Question 21
Which of the following parameters is LEAST likely to change when depth of imaging is adjusted:

A. Pulse duration
B. Pulse repetition period
C. Duty factor
D. Pulse repetition frequency

Answer: A. Pulse duration

Key Point: Pulse duration is solely determined by the source of the ultrasound and like spatial pulse length is independent of depth of imaging.

Rationale: Pulse duration is determined by the number of cycles in an ultrasound pulse, multiplied by the period for each cycle. The number of cycles per pulse is set by the manufacturer, depending on the intended use of the transducer. All the other options listed in the question can be adjusted by the sonographer by changing the depth [1].

The following scenario and images in panels A and B apply to questions 22 and 23.

Patient is a 67-year-old female, who presented with months-long history of progressive shortness of breath and palpitations. She has a remote history of cigarette smoking, equivalent to 10-pack years. Physical examination revealed an ejection systolic murmur in the right upper sternal border, radiating up the neck. Trans-esophageal echocardiogram was performed as part of her evaluation (Fig. 2.4a, b).

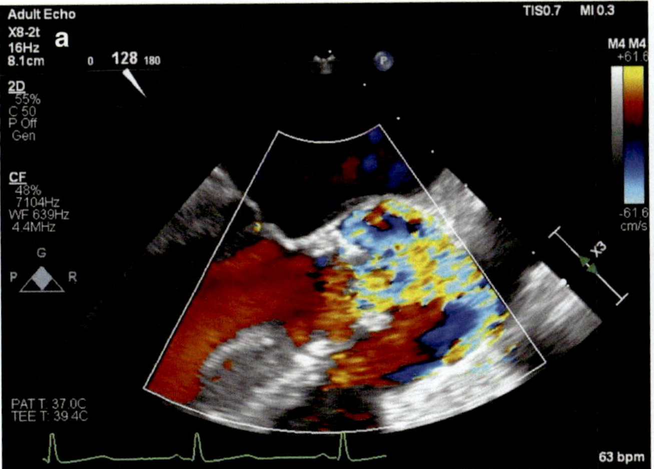

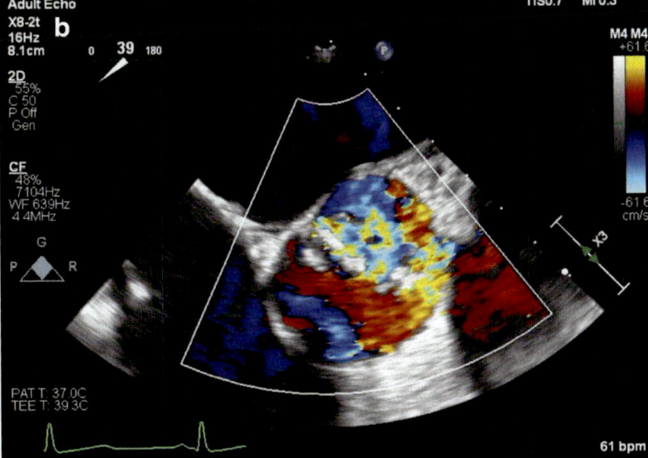

Fig. 2.4 (**a**, **b**) Color flow doppler interrogation of the aortic valve in long and short axes views

Question 22

Which description of the still image in panel A is most accurate?

A. Continuous wave doppler, left ventricular outflow tract depicting aortic regurgitation
B. Continuous wave doppler, left ventricular outflow tract depicting severe aortic stenosis
C. Color flow Doppler, depicting aortic regurgitation in Left ventricular outflow tract
D. Color flow Doppler, depicting turbulent flow due to aortic stenosis

Answer: D. Color flow Doppler, depicting turbulent flow due to aortic stenosis

Key Point: Panel A depicts color flow Doppler (CFD) interrogation of the aortic valve (AV) in the mid-esophageal AV long axis view. Panel B depicts the same valve in a short axis view.

Rationale: These views allow evaluation of the aortic valve leaflets. The color mosaic just distal to the plane of the aortic valve indicates turbulent flow due to rapidly changing velocities and/or directions of flow. Proximal to AV, flow appears reasonably laminar without turbulence in the LV outflow tract. The degree of aortic stenosis cannot accurately be judged qualitatively by CFD. Quantification of severity can be done by calculation of the aortic valve area using the continuity equation, or by measuring the peak velocity (>4 m/s is severe), or the mean pressure gradients across the valve (<20 mmHg is mild; 21–49 mmHg is moderate; >50 mmHg is severe) [1].

Question 23

Which of the following hemodynamic goals would be optimal for the medical management of this patient?

	Preload	Afterload	Heart rate
A.	Normal	Low	90–120
B.	Low	Normal	90–120
C.	Normal	Low	40–60
D.	Normal	Normal	60–90

Answer: D. Normal; Normal; 60–90

Key point.

Rationale: Patients with severe aortic stenosis develop left ventricular (LV) hypertrophy with consequent increased myocardial oxygen demand, decreased LV compliance and increased LV end-diastolic pressure. Thus, such patients are intolerant of hypotension which impairs coronary perfusion. Also, they do best with sinus rhythm, euvolemia, and normal heart rate to allow for adequate filling of the non-compliant LV [5].

Question 24

The duty factor is determined by

A. Propagation speed
B. Insonation angle
C. Ultrasound power
D. Imaging depth

Answer: D. Imaging depth

Key Point: Imaging depth is the main determinant of the duty factor.

Rationale: Duty factor is the proportion of time during which ultrasound pulses are being transmitted into the medium. Accordingly, the deeper the site of image of interest, the longer the time required to be spent in listening mode, awaiting the reflected signals. Duty factor is typically about 5% for pulsed wave Doppler compared to 100% for continuous wave Doppler because the latter dedicates one crystal each for continuous transmission and reception [1].

Question 25

Doppler frequency is inversely related to

A. Transmitted frequency
B. Red blood cell velocity
C. Cosine of the angle of insonation
D. Speed of sound in tissue

Answer: B. Speed of sound in tissue

Key point: The Doppler shift (frequency) is inversely proportional to the speed of sound in the propagation medium.

Rationale: In clinical imaging, Doppler frequency is inversely proportional to the speed of sound in tissues. It is directly proportional to the velocity of the red cells, the transmitted frequency, and the cosine of the angle of insonation. The Doppler equation depicting these relations is as follow.

$$F_D = (F_R - F_T) = (V^* \cos\theta^* 2F_T)/C$$

where F_D = Doppler frequency; F_R = Received frequency; F_T = Transmitted frequency; V = velocity of red cells in blood; Cos θ = angle of insonation; C = speed of sound in blood [1].

Question 26

Range ambiguity is a feature of continuous wave Doppler because

A. It uses only one crystal for transmission and receiving ultrasound

B. It uses separate crystals for transmitting and receiving ultrasound
C. It is simultaneously transmitting and receiving ultrasound
D. It accurately measures high velocities

Answer: C. It is simultaneously transmitting and receiving ultrasound

Key point: Continuous wave Doppler imaging is characterized by range ambiguity

Rationale: Continuous wave Doppler (CWD) uses at least 2 crystal for estimating velocities. Because one crystal is continuously in listening mode, it is impossible to determine the depth (range) from which the returning signals emanate. CWD allows accurate measurement of high velocity flow without aliasing of the signal. Clinically, CW Doppler is used whenever a high velocity signal is present, with aortic stenosis, tricuspid regurgitation, mitral regurgitation, or VSD [3].

Question 27
Axial resolution is

A. Variable throughout an image
B. A factor of the pulse repetition frequency
C. Is equal to twice the spatial pulse length
D. Equal to half the spatial pulse length

Answer: D. Equal to half the spatial pulse length

Key point: Axial resolution in clinical imaging is typically about half the spatial pulse length

Rationale: Axial resolution is the ability to distinguish between two adjacent objects along the beam's main axis. Given the characteristics of the ultrasound beam, axial resolution determines how close two adjacent objects can be and yet appear as two distinct objects in the image. It is dependent on transducer frequency, transducer bandwidth and pulse length. These features are preset by the manufacturer. Axial resolution is better with higher frequencies and shorter pulses. It is independent of the imaging depth, and so is fixed throughout the image [1].

Question 28
Which of the following combinations is associated with better axial resolution?

A. More cycles per pulse, higher frequency
B. Fewer cycles per pulse, lower frequency
C. Fewer cycles per pulse, higher frequency
D. More cycles per pulse, lower frequency

Answer: C. Fewer cycles per pulse, higher frequency

Key point: Higher frequencies with smaller wavelengths improve the ability to resolve the distance between adjacent reflectors. Higher frequencies allow the use of shorter pulses.

Rationale: Axial resolution is better with shorter pulses. Accordingly, fewer cycles and higher frequencies (and so shorter wavelengths) will improve axial resolution. This feature is set by the manufacturer and cannot be adjusted by the sonographer. Consequently, different ultrasound probes are required for imaging tissues at different depths [1].

Question 29
M-mode imaging has the greatest favorable effect on

A. Temporal resolution
B. Lateral resolution
C. Axial resolution
D. Elevation resolution

Answer: A. Temporal resolution

Key Point: M-mode imaging is particularly effective in resolving movement of tissues over time.

Rationale: In M-mode imaging the transmit time / receiver cycle is very rapid because the transducer only sends and receives an ultrasound signal along a single scan line. This optimizes the temporal resolution of the image and allow evaluation of rapidly moving structures [1].

Question 30
Early closure of the aortic valve in hypertrophic cardiomyopathy is best demonstrated by which of the following imaging modalities

A. Color Doppler
B. M-Mode
C. Pulsed Doppler
D. B-mode ECHO

Answer: B. M-Mode

Key Point: M-mode imaging is evaluating moving structures.

Rationale: In M mode imaging the transmit time/receiver cycle is very rapid because the transducer sends and receive an ultrasound signal along a single scan line which improve the temporal resolution of the image and allow evaluation of rapidly moving structures. The frame rate in M mode is much higher than in 2D or 3D because M mode does not sweep through the imaging sector [1].

Question 31
Which imaging modality offers the best diagnostic data for assessment of the severity of mitral regurgitation?

A. Color Flow Doppler imaging
B. M mode imaging
C. Continuous Wave Doppler imaging
D. 2 D imaging

Answer: A. Color Flow Doppler imaging

Key Point: Color flow Doppler imaging is used in quantifying the severity of mitral regurgitation (MR)

Rationale: Color Doppler imaging is useful for evaluating the spatial distribution of flow. This is especially helpful in determining the severity and mechanism of regurgitant flow. Useful metrics include the regurgitant jet area within the left atrium and vena contracta width (VCW), both of which are validated for mild and severe MR. Note severity of MR is affected by left ventricular afterload, so this should be considered during imaging [3].

Question 32
Which of the following statements regarding tissue harmonic imaging is true?

A. Increases reverberation artifact
B. Reduces lateral resolution
C. Reduces slide lobe artifacts
D. Increases axial resolution

Answer: C. Reduces slide lobe artifacts

Key Point: Side lobe artifacts can be reduced using harmonic imaging

Rationale: Tissue harmonic imaging is a technique for isolating the higher harmonic frequencies generated by body tissues being insonated by ultrasound. These harmonic frequencies occur because the ultrasound wave propagates faster through compressed regions of tissues impacted by the compressive phase of the ultrasound, and vice versa. Because these harmonic frequencies only have to travel one-way back to the transducer, the resulting images are clearer. Harmonic frequencies are proportional to the strength of the fundamental frequency and increase with depth of propagation. Harmonic imaging improves endocardial definition and decreases near field and side lobe artifacts. However, axial resolution is reduced in harmonic imaging [1, 6].

The following image applies to question 33 (Fig. 2.5)

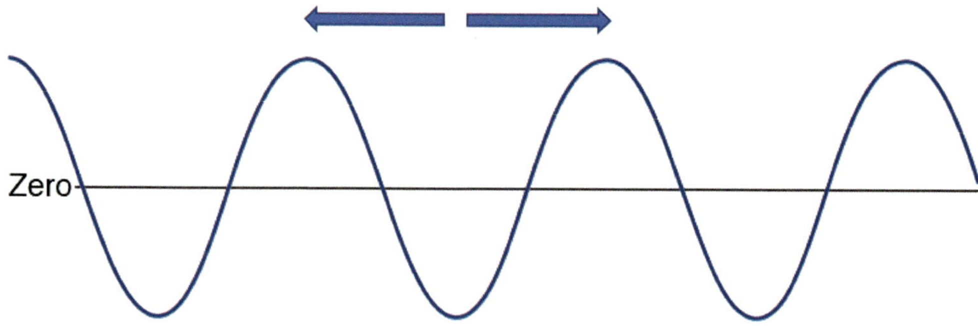

Fig. 2.5 Characteristics of ultrasound waveforms

Question 33
Name the distance shown above

A. Amplitude
B. Frequency (f)
C. Wavelength (λ)
D. Spatial pulse length

Answer: C Wavelength (λ)

Key point: Wavelength (λ) is the distance between any two successive peak to peak (or trough to trough) of an ultrasound wave.

Rationale: Ultrasound waves are characterized by certain properties—frequency, wavelength, amplitude, and the propagation velocity through physical media. The wavelength of an ultrasound influences axial resolution, and depth of propagation. Propagation velocity, frequency and wavelength are inter-related as follows: $\lambda = c/f$. Propagation velocity will depend on the physical properties of the medium, being faster in denser tissues [1].

Question 34
Axial resolution is improved by which of the following

A. Decreasing bandwidth
B. Increasing frequency
C. Using time gain compensation
D. Increasing the gain

Answer: B. Increasing frequency

Key point: Axial resolution can be improved by increasing transducer frequency.

Rationale: Axial resolution refers to the smallest resolvable distance between two objects along the longitudinal axis of the ultrasound beam. Conceptually, the shortest resolvable axial distance between two objects will equal one wavelength. Therefore, axial resolution will be depend on the ultrasound wavelength. In practice, axial resolution approximates twice the transmitted frequency, so higher frequencies and shorter wavelengths will improve axial resolution. Further, wider transducer bandwidth allows incorporation of higher frequencies within a shorter pulse length [1].

Question 35
Good temporal resolution is important for distinguishing:

A. Structures perpendicular to ultrasound
B. Moving structures
C. Two structures that are close to each other
D. Superficial from deeper structures

Answer: B. Moving structures

Key point: M-mode imaging offers the best temporal resolution in assessing moving structures.

Rationale: In M mode imaging the transmit time /receiver cycle is very rapid because the transducer only sends and receives an ultrasound pulse along a single scan line. This improves the temporal resolution of the image and allows evaluation of rapidly moving structures [3].

Question 36
The average velocity of ultrasound in soft tissue is about:

A. 1200 m/s
B. 1840 m/s
C. 1540 m/s
D. 1400 m/s

Answer: C. 1540 m/s

Key point: Average velocity of sound in body soft tissue is about 1540 m/s

Rationale: The speed of sound is a factor of the physical characteristics of the medium in which it is traveling. In general, velocity is faster in denser tissues. For example, in air sound travels at 345 m/s whereas it is much faster in water (1430 m/s), and up to 4080 m/s through bone. Accordingly, on average propagation speed through body soft tissues (made up mostly of water) is about 1540 m/s [3].

Question 37
Calculate wavelength in the heart using 4 MHz transducer

A. 0.385 mm
B. 3.080 mm
C. .770 mm
D. 0.002 mm

Answer: A. 0.385 mm

Key point: Ultrasound velocity, frequency and wavelength are inter-related as follows: $\lambda = c/f$. Using a 4 MHz transducer, wavelength would be 1.54/4 = 0.385 mm.

Rationale: In general, the propagation speed of sound is faster in denser tissues. Propagation speed in slowest speeds in gases, faster, in liquids, and fastest in solids. In clinical imaging of soft tissues, the average propagation speed is 1540 m/s because body soft tissue is mostly made of water [3].

The following image applies to question 38 (Fig. 2.6).

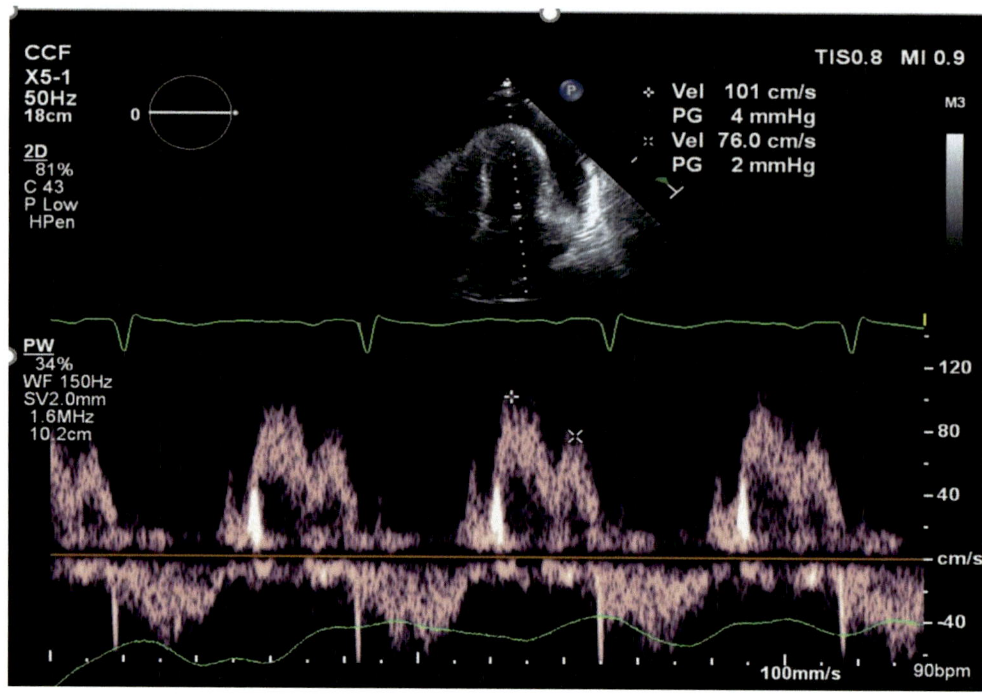

Fig. 2.6 Pericardial effusion in Apical 4-chamber mitral inflow interrogation view

Question 38
Which feature of this image best supports the absence of pericardial tamponade?

A. E wave > A wave
B. E/A ratio 1.25
C. Absence of RV free wall collapse in systole
D. Absence of RV free wall collapse in diastole

Answer: D. Absence of RV free wall collapse in diastole

Key Point: Despite the large effusion surrounding the heart in this apical 4 chamber mitral inflow view, the right ventricular free wall does not appear collapsed during diastole with the tricuspid valve open.

Rationale: Pericardial tamponade is a clinical diagnosis. However, echocardiography can provide strong supportive evidence. In tamponade, pericardial pressures exceed the filling pressures of the cardiac chambers. Supportive echocardiographic findings include right atrial collapse during systole; right ventricular diastolic collapse; plethoric inferior vena cava without respiratory variation; >25% variation with respiration in mitral inflow E wave velocity or >40% tricuspid inflow E wave velocity. Applicable views include the apical 4-chamber mitral inflow view or parasternal long axis with M-mode view at the mitral leaflet tips [1].

Question 39
Which of the following can decrease the mitral inflow E wave velocity?

A. Decreased afterload
B. Hypovolemia
C. Young age
D. Mitral regurgitation

Answer: B. Hypovolemia

Key Points: Hypovolemia can manifest as decreased mitral inflow E wave velocity.

Rationale: Loading conditions and intrinsic left ventricular properties interact to affect the mitral inflow profile in a manner that could mimic abnormal states such as left ventricular diastolic dysfunction. These should be kept in mind in analyzing the mitral inflow spectral display. The E wave reflects the left atrial to left ventricular (LV) gradient in early diastole and thus is preload dependent. As such, hypovolemia will lead to decrease in the peak E wave velocity. Similar effect is seen with increased afterload and with age-related changes in LV compliance [3, 7].

Question 40
Which combination of Doppler derived variables best supports a diagnosis of severe diastolic dysfunction?

	E/A	E/e′	Lat TDI e′	Pulm vein S/D
A.	1.5	12	8	S < D
B.	3	16	6	S < D
C.	1.5	6	12	S > D
D.	0.75	11	9	S > D

Answer: B. 3; 16; 6; S < D

Key point: Severe diastolic dysfunction is characterized by restrictive LV filling pattern**.** Applicable Doppler indices will include a lateral TDI e′ velocity < 10 cm/s, blunted pulmonary venous S wave, mitral inflow E/A ratio >2 and E/e′ ratio >14.

Rationale: Diastolic dysfunction is marked by progressive abnormalities in several Doppler derived indices of left ventricular filling and relaxation as well as pulmonary venous flow. These Doppler indices have facilitated the diagnosis of diastolic dysfunction and in the assessment of LV filling pressures. Whereas the profile of mitral inflow spectral analysis can be load dependent, the tissue Doppler analysis of mitral annulus motion is less so. Accordingly, the inotropic state of the LV should also be considered [3, 7, 8].

Question 41
Which of the following options is the most appropriate in the management of hypotensive patients with acute decompensated diastolic heart failure?

A. Low dose vasoconstriction with phenylephrine
B. High dose inotropic support with dobutamine
C. Aggressive diuresis with furosemide
D. Induce bradycardia with a beta blocker

Answer: A. Low dose vasoconstriction with phenylephrine
Key Point: Low dose vasoconstriction with phenylephrine is the most appropriate of the listed choices in the setting of hypotension due to acute decompensated diastolic heart failure.

Rationale: The hemodynamic considerations in the management of acute decompensated diastolic heart failure are complex. Management priorities differ depending on the exact scenario and which symptoms are predominant. Diastolic heart failure is characterized by elevated LV end-diastolic pressures (LVEDP) associated with impaired LV relaxation, and necessitating higher filling pressures. Consequently any therapeutic approaches which exacerbate these should be avoided. Avoidance of extremes of physiologic states or therapeutic interventions is crucial. In general inotropic support is relatively contra-indicated unless there is co-existing systolic failure. Extremes of heart rate should be avoided to ensure adequate diastolic filling time without raising LVEDP. Euvolemia is probably the most difficult to achieve given the fine line between meeting the required higher filling pressures without precipitating or worsening pulmonary edema [8, 9].

Question 42
Which of the following is LEAST likely correct regarding Pulsed Wave Doppler:

A. Sample volume is adjustable
B. Good for measuring low velocities
C. Measures velocity at a specific point delimited by the sample gate
D. Best measured with high transmitted frequency

Answer: D. Best measured with high transmitted frequency
Key Point: Pulsed wave Doppler (PWD) imaging is unable to resolve higher velocities.

Rationale: PWD allows spatial localization of a velocity signal. It is best used for lower velocity signals and with maximum velocity that is below the Nyquist Level. Examples include LV inflow, and outflow velocity proximal to aortic valve. Typically pulse wave Doppler cannot resolve velocities greater than 1.5 m/s unless high pulse repetition frequency mode is in use, which raises resolvable velocities to 4 m/s. In contrast continuous wave Doppler can measure velocities up to 12 m/s. Use of low transmitted frequency provides a stronger signal secondary to decreased tissue attenuation [1].

Question 43
Ultrasound beams that encounter moving red blood cells are MOST likely to exhibit:

A. Refraction
B. Specular reflection
C. Attenuation
D. Backscattering

Answer: D. Backscattering
Key point: Incident ultrasound waves are backscattered by red blood cells.

Rationale: Red blood cells are poor reflectors of ultrasound because of their shape and size: They have irregular surfaces and their diameters are less than the wavelengths of transmitted ultrasound. Accordingly, any incident ultrasound waves are scattered in all directions rather than being directly reflected back in relation to the angle of insonation. Consequently, only a small proportion of transmitted ultrasound returns to the transducer during Doppler interrogation. This has implications for the power requirements and gain adjustment for Doppler ultrasonography, compared to B-mode imaging [1].

Question 44
Flow through the left ventricular outflow tract is interrogated with Pulse Wave Doppler. Which of the following is LEAST likely to represented by the Doppler spectral display

A. Signal amplitude
B. Red blood cell velocity
C. Red blood cell direction
D. Velocity distance plot

Answer: D. Velocity distance plot
Key Point: The Doppler spectral display is a time velocity plot that helps discern red blood cell velocity and direc-

tion as well as the amplitude of the backscattered signals from the red blood cells.

Rationale: The Doppler spectral analysis is used to convert the frequencies of backscattered signals into flow velocities that are then plotted on a vertical axis against time on the horizontal axis. The loudness (amplitude) of each of these signals is depicted using a gray scale. The deeper the shade of gray, the greater the amplitude and/or the number of red cells creating those frequencies. By convention, flow toward the transducer is displayed above the zero baseline, and vice versa [1].

Question 45

In other to accurately calculate frequency shifts, Doppler ultrasonography requires

A. Broad transducer bandwidth
B. Reflection of most of the transmitted signals
C. Wide range of transmitted frequencies
D. Longer ultrasound pulses

Answer: D. Longer ultrasound pulses

Key Point: Accurate calculation of Doppler frequency shifts requires longer ultrasound pulses

Rationale: Doppler ultrasonography is used to determine intra-cardiac and intra-vascular blood flow velocities. This depends on the change in frequency when transmitted ultrasound waves encounter a moving object, in this case, red blood cells. However, red blood cells are small and only scatter the transmitted sound waves in all directions. Therefore, only small amounts of the transmitted signal return to the transducer, with a change in frequency. In order to accurately determine the change, the transducer has to compare the transmitted and received waveforms. Because multiple changed frequencies will be present, accurate determination of frequency shift is facilitated by transmitting a narrow bandwidth of sound frequencies, which requires longer pulses. Indeed, continuous wave Doppler transmission is at only one frequency with zero bandwidth [1].

Question 46

Color flow mapping of a mitral regurgitation jet is undertaken as shown in the accompanying picture. Which of the following is MOST likely correct with respect to the color scale in the image? (Fig. 2.7).

A. Color variation depends on the direction of flow
B. Zone of red color denotes blood going away from the transducer
C. Zone of blue color denotes blood coming towards the transducer
D. Zone of black color represents maximum velocity

Answer: A. Color variation depends on the direction of flow

Key Point: With respect to Color Flow Mapping by convention, flow toward the transducer is depicted red and flow away from the transducer is depicted blue.

Rationale: The blue and red colors used in color flow Doppler imaging have been set by convention. In addition, lighter shades of the colors are used to encode higher velocities. Further some machines allow the addition of green or yellow to the velocity scale to indicate the variation in estimated mean velocities detected by the pulses along each scan line. Black color denotes no Doppler shift [1].

The following scenario and image apply to question 47

Patient is a 67-year-old female with a remote history of rheumatic fever. She complains of undue fatigue, occasional dizziness over several months. Physical examination revealed a blood pressure of 105/38 mmHg. Trans-esophageal echocardiogram was performed as part of her evaluation (Fig. 2.8).

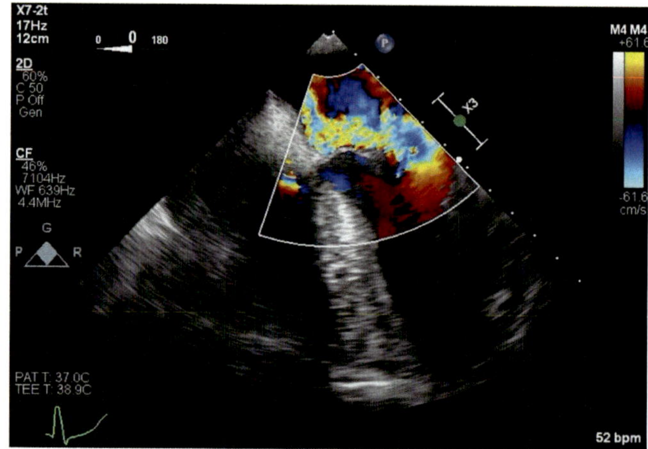

Fig. 2.7 Color flow Doppler interrogation of the mitral valve

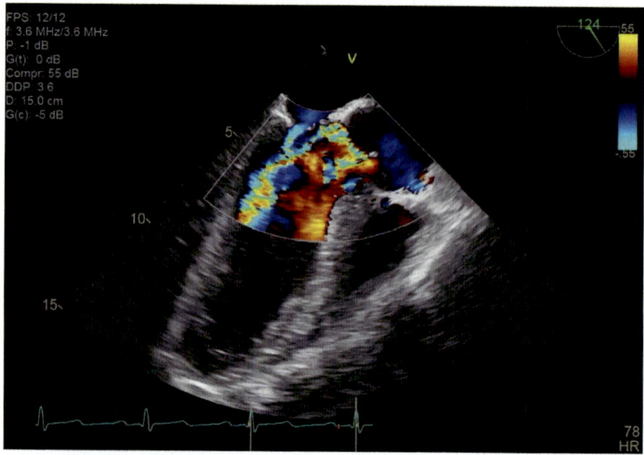

Fig. 2.8 Color flow Doppler interrogation of in mid-esophageal long axis view

Question 47

What is the severity of the valvular lesion depicted in the image?

A. Moderate to severe Mitral Stenosis
B. Moderate to severe Mitral Regurgitation
C. Moderate to severe Aortic Regurgitation
D. Moderate to Severe Aortic stenosis

Answer: C. Moderate to severe Aortic Regurgitation

Key Point: The image depicts the mid-esophageal long axis view of the aortic valve. The eccentric nature of the jet represents moderate to severe aortic regurgitation.

Rationale: The image represents a large eccentric jet occurring across the aortic valve in diastole. The red marker on the ECG tracing in the image depicts timing of when the image was acquired. The severity of aortic regurgitation (AR) can be graded by measuring the regurgitant jet size (relative to the left ventricular outflow tract—LVOT), the regurgitant fraction, or the pressure half time of the pressure gradient in diastole. Using the regurgitant jet size for grading, mild AR has a jet area ratio of 0.25–0.30, moderate AR has a jet area ratio of 0.3–0.60, while severe AR would have a jet area ratio >0.6. However, these criteria apply only to central jets. Eccentric jets may not fulfill these criteria as they travel obliquely in the LVOT. Eccentric dense jets that exhibit flow convergence represent moderate to severe aortic regurgitation. In AR, spectral Doppler interrogation of the descending aorta will show some early diastolic flow reversal in mild AR, up to holodiastolic flow reversal in severe AR. Also note that afterload at the time of the echocardiogram, will affect the degree of AR observed [3].

Question 48

Which of the following is contraindicated in the management of patients with acute aortic regurgitation?

A. Afterload reduction with nitroprusside
B. Inotropic support with dobutamine
C. Preload control with nitroglycerin infusion
D. Afterload reduction with intra-aortic balloon pulsation

Answer: D. Afterload reduction with intra-aortic balloon pulsation

Key Point: Intra-aortic balloon counter pulsation is contra-indicated in patients with decompensated heart failure due to aortic regurgitation.

Rationale: The hemodynamic considerations in the management of acute aortic regurgitation include preload control, afterload reduction, and inotropic support as indicated. Diuretics and vasodilators such as nitroglycerin, nitroprusside, and ACE inhibitors all have role. However, unlike in acute mitral regurgitation, intra-aortic counter-pulsation is contra-indicated because it can worsen the aortic regurgitation, exacerbating ventricular volume overload and further impairing left ventricular function [10].

Question 49

Continuous Wave Doppler is MOST likely to be useful for evaluating

A. Tricuspid regurgitation velocity
B. Vena contracta of mitral regurgitation jet
C. Vena contracta of aortic regurgitation jet
D. Mitral annular Doppler velocities

Answer: A. Tricuspid regurgitation velocity

Key Point: Continuous Wave Doppler (CWD) imaging allows accurate measurement of high velocity flow without aliasing of the signal.

Rationale: Clinically, CW Doppler is used whenever a high velocity signal is present, such as with aortic stenosis, tricuspid regurgitation, mitral regurgitation, or ventricular septal defects. CWD can resolve velocities as high as 12 m/s. However, with CW Doppler, sampling occurs along the line of interrogation without localization of the point of maximum velocity along the line. The clinical context is generally sufficient for interpreting and pinpointing the likely source of the peak velocities identified. Vena contracta is the narrowest part of the neck of a regurgitation jet identified with color flow mapping. Color flow mapping utilizes Pulse Wave Doppler. Mitral annular velocities on tissue Doppler imaging also utilize PWD [1].

The following scenario and image apply to question 50

A 47-year-old male presented with sudden onset of severe chest pain, shortness of breath and a feeling of doom. He is a current smoker with a 30-pack year history. His EKG showed ST elevation in the inferior leads. During emergent cardiac surgery, intraoperative trans-esophageal echocardiogram was performed (Fig. 2.9).

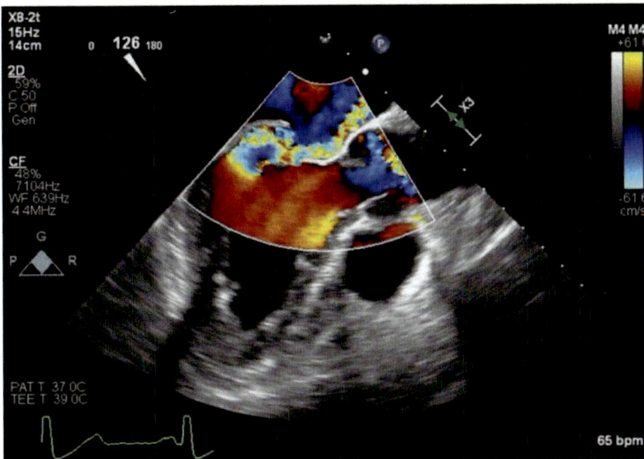

Fig. 2.9 Color flow Doppler interrogation of the LVOT and mitral valve in mid-esophageal long axis view

Question 50
Which of the following is MOST likely correct?

A. The eccentric jet indicates mild mitral regurgitation
B. High velocity flow away from the transducer is displayed as cyan
C. The eccentric jet represents a posteriorly directed mitral regurgitation jet
D. There is significant left ventricular outflow tract obstruction

Answer: B. High velocity flow away from the transducer is displayed as cyan

Key point: The image depicts mid-esophageal long axis view with the color box centered on the mitral valve and left ventricular outflow tract. It shows systolic flow through the left ventricular outflow tract and an eccentric regurgitant jet through the mitral valve.

Rationale: Eccentric regurgitant jets through the mitral valve can appear misleadingly smaller than actual size due to the coanda effect. Accordingly, they are always upgraded to at least the next higher severity grade. Such eccentric jets are typically due to a flail mitral valve leaflet, with the jet directed away from the affected valve. The mosaic color of the eccentric jet reflects the turbulence in the regurgitant stream. In the image in the question, there is posterior mitral leaflet prolapse/flail leading to an anteriorly directed jet. The right side of the image represents anterior structures and the left side represents inferior or posterior structures. The color scale to the right of the image shows that high velocity flows away from the transducer are represented by various shades of cyan/blue [1].

References

1. Otto CM. Textbook of clinical echocardiography. 5th ed. Philadelphia: Saunders; 2013.
2. Luxford J, Bassin L, D'Ambra M. Echocardiography of the tricuspid valve. Ann Cardiothorac Surg. 2017;6(3):223–39. https://doi.org/10.21037/acs.2017.05.15.
3. Brown SM, Blaivas M, Hirshberg EL, et al. Comprehensive critical care ultrasound. Mount Prospect: Society of Critical Care Medicine; 2015.
4. Hussain S, Witten J, Shrestha N, et al. Tricuspid valve endocarditis. Ann Cardiothorac Surg. 2017;6(3):255–61.
5. Brown J, Morgan-Hughes NJ. Aortic stenosis and non-cardiac surgery. Contin Educ Anaesth Crit Care Pain. 2005;5(1):1–4.
6. Uppal T. Tissue harmonic imaging. Austral J Ultrasound Med. 2010;13(2):29–31.
7. Porter TR, Shillcutt SK, Adams MS, et al. Guidelines for the use of echocardiography as a monitor for therapeutic intervention in adults: a report from the American Society of Echocardiography. J Am Soc Echocardiogr. 2015;28:40–56.
8. Shillcutt SK, Chacon MM, Brakke TR, et al. Heart failure with preserved ejection fraction: a perioperative review. J Cardiothorac Vasc Anesth. 2017;31(5):1820–30.
9. Alsaddique AA, Royse AG, Royse CF, et al. Management of diastolic heart failure following cardiac surgery. Eur J Cardiothorac Surg. 2009;35(2):241–9.
10. Krishna M, Zacharowski K. Principles of intra-aortic counterpulsation. Contin Educ Anaesth Crit Care Pain. 2009;9(1):24–8.

Knobology, Image Acquisition, Optimization and Artifacts

3

Jason T. Bouhenguel, James E. Mitchell, Vidya K. Rao, and Javier Lorenzo

Abbreviations

A2C	Apical two chamber
A3C	Apical three chamber
A4C	Apical four chamber
A5C	Apical five chamber
ED	Emergency department
EROA	Effective regurgitant orifice area
FAST	Focused assessment with sonography for trauma
Hz	Hertz
IVC	Inferior vena cava
MHz	Megahertz
MI	Mechanical index
MR	Mitral regurgitation
PRF	Pulse repetition frequency
PSLX	Parasternal long axis
PSSX	Parasternal short axis
ROI	Region of interest
RUQ	Right upper quadrant
S4C	Subcostal four chamber
TAPSE	Tricuspid annular plan systolic excursion
TEE	Transesophageal echo
TGC	Time gain compensation
TI	Thermal index
TTE	Transthoracic echo
VCW	Vena contracta width

Supplementary Information The online version contains supplementary material available at https://doi.org/10.1007/978-3-031-45731-9_3.

J. T. Bouhenguel
Cardiothoracic Anesthesiology, Kaiser Permanente Santa Clara Medical Center, Palo Alto, CA, USA

J. E. Mitchell
Department of Critical Care, Stanford University Hospital, Stanford, CA, USA
e-mail: jmitchell34@mgh.harvard.edu

V. K. Rao
Divisions of Cardiothoracic Anesthesiology and Critical Care Medicine, Department of Anesthesiology, Perioperative and Pain Medicine, School of Medicine, Stanford University, Stanford, CA, USA
e-mail: vknayak@stanford.edu

J. Lorenzo (✉)
Department of Anesthesiology, Stanford School of Medicine, Stanford, CA, USA
e-mail: javierl@stanford.edu

Question 1
To obtain an apical two chamber view, what is the approximate probe position?

A. Along the left sternal border, between the 3rd to 5th intercostal spaces, with the probe indicator pointing to patient's right shoulder.
B. Inferolateral to nipple/breast fold, between the 4th to 5th intercostal spaces, with the probe indicator pointing to the patient's left shoulder (approximately 12 to 1 o'clock) and a slight tilt of the probe tail towards the patient's right flank.
C. 1–2 cm below the xiphoid process, tilted nearly horizontal, with the probe indicator pointing to the patient's left flank (3 o'clock).
D. Inferolateral to nipple/breast fold, between the 4th to 5th intercostal spaces, with the probe indicator pointing to the patient's left flank (approximately 3–5 o'clock).

Answer B. Inferolateral to nipple/breast fold, between the 4th-5th intercostal spaces, with the probe indicator pointing to the patient's left shoulder (approximately twelve-one o'clock) and a slight tilt of the probe tail towards the patient's right flank.

Explanation: See Table 3.1.

Question 2
What probe manipulation is being demonstrated in Video 3.1?

A. Rocking
B. Tilting
C. Sliding
D. Rotating

R. Sreedharan et al. (eds.), *Critical Care Echocardiography*, https://doi.org/10.1007/978-3-031-45731-9_3

Table 3.1 Standard views and associated probe position

View	Probe position	Indicator orientation	Probe finessing
Parasternal long axis (PSLX)	Position the probe along the left sternal border in the 3rd to 5th intercostal spaces	Towards patient's right shoulder (approximately 10–11 o'clock)	
Parasternal short axis (PSSX)	Same as PSLX view	Towards patient's left shoulder (approximately 1–2 o'clock)	From PSLX view, rotate the probe 90° CW
Apical four (or five) chamber (A4C or A5C)	Position the probe at the patient's PMI (if palpable), inferolateral to nipple/breast fold, or along the mid-clavicular line in the 4th to 5th intercostal space	Towards patient's left flank (approximately 3–5 o'clock)	To obtain A5C view: from A4C tilt the probe tail down slightly bringing the LVOT and AV into view
Apical two chamber (A2C)	Same as A4C view	Towards patient's left-shoulder (approximately 12 o'clock)	From the A4C view rotate the probe 60–90° CCW tilting the probe tail slightly towards the patient's right flank until the right-heart structures are no longer visible
Apical three chamber (A3C)	Same as A4C view	Towards patient's right-shoulder (approximately 12 o'clock)	From the A2C view, rotate the probe an additional 45–60° CCW, with a slight tail tilt to the patient's feet bringing the LA, LV, and LVOT into view
Subcostal four chamber (S4C)	Place the probe 1–2 cm below the patient's xiphoid process, slightly patient-right of midline	Toward the patient's left flank (approximately three o'clock)	Tilt probe tail as flat as possible (nearly horizontal)
Subcostal IVC view (IVC)	Same as S4C view	Towards patient's head (approximately 12 o'clock)	From S4C view rotate the probe 90° CCW

Based on data from [1]

Answer B. Tilting

Explanation: To obtain an apical 5 axis view, which allows for visualization of the left ventricular outflow tract, from an apical 4 axis, the probe the tail is tilted downward. **Tilting** is the movement of the face of the transducer while maintaining a fixed position. **Rocking** refers to moving toward or away from the probe orientation marker, while maintaining the same plain or view. Sliding is moving the probe across the patient to a new position. Lastly **rotating** occurs when the probe is kept in the same position but moving the indicator marker to a new position [2].

Question 3

To achieve adequate depth while performing a lung ultrasound examination, which of the following probe properties is most important?

A. Large Footprint
B. Low frequency
C. Ability to perform M-Mode
D. Less radiation

Answer B. Low frequency

Explanation: (B) Lower frequency probes, such as the phased-array and curvilinear allow for greater depth of penetration at the expense of resolution. Exams of deeper structures (e.g. kidney, liver, pancreas, spleen, aorta) benefit from lower-frequency transducers (e.g. 2–5 MHz curvilinear probe), while more superficial structures (e.g. appendix, liver surface, lung pleura, vascular structures) are better visualized with higher-frequency transducers (e.g. 6–13 MHz linear probe). Ultrasound transducers are generally capable of emitting several frequencies which can be selected from; presets often toggle between these frequencies based on the anticipated structures of interest, but one should be able to adjust the probe frequency based on the structure of interest being imaged and the patient's specific body habitus in order to optimize image acquisition. For example, in a thin patient or child using the higher end of an abdominal probe's frequency spectrum (e.g. 5 MHz) would provide better spatial resolution as compared to 2 or 3 MHz which would be more ideal for an obese adult in assessing a deeper ROI. (A) Footprint refers to the size of the area that sends and receives the ultrasound waves. (C) The three commonly used probes in critical care ultrasound (phased-array, curvilinear, and linear) have the ability to perform m-mode imaging. (D) Ultrasound is an imaging modality that lacks radiation [3]).

Question 4

In performing the FAST exam, probes with a curvilinear footprint are preferred over linear probes because:

A. The perpendicularly oriented soundwaves produced by curvilinear probes are ideal for visualizing large deep organs such as the kidneys.
B. Curvilinear probes yield the greatest spatial resolution of the two probe types.

C. The diverging/fanning soundwaves produce an image with a wider field of view than the footprint of the probe itself, facilitating visualization of deeper broader structures.
D. Curvilinear probes are always smaller than linear probes and thus allow for easier maneuverability between rib spaces.

Answer C. The diverging/fanning soundwaves produce an image with a wider field of view than the footprint of the probe itself, facilitating visualization of deeper broader structures.

Explanation: Ultrasound transducer probes characteristically differ from one another based on the size and shape of their footprint and their operational frequency range. The most commonly used probes include curvilinear array, straight linear array, and phased array probes.

Curvilinear array probes have a curved surface with sound wave emitting piezoelectric crystals arranged accordingly in a curved fashion resulting in a diverging sound wave propagation. This diverging feature results in a field of view which is wider than the footprint of the probe itself. Combining this property with a lower frequency range (typically 1–8 MHz) makes these probes ideal for imaging deeper structures, albeit sacrificing image quality (ideal for visualizing deeper abdominal/pelvic structures e.g. kidney, liver, pancreas, spleen, aorta).

Straight linear array probes emit higher frequency soundwaves (5–15 MHz) oriented perpendicular to the probe's surface. Although only capable of producing a field of view as wide as its footprint, the higher-resolution images make it ideal for imaging superficial structures (e.g. appendix, liver surface, lung pleura, vascular structures) and ultrasound-guided procedures [4].

Question 5
Which of the following regarding phased-array probes is NOT true? Phased-array probes:

A. Use constructive interference approaches to "steer" soundwaves to focus on regions of interest in the acquired image.
B. Typically have a linear footprint making them ideal for positioning in tight spaces (e.g. between ribs).
C. Produce a field of view wider than the footprint itself.
D. Span a wide range of operational frequencies making them useful for imaging both high-resolution structures and deeper anatomical structures.

Answer B. Typically have a linear footprint making them ideal for positioning in tight spaces (e.g. between ribs).

Explanation: Phased array probes use the concept of constructive interference to "steer" soundwaves to focus on specified regions of interest within an acquired image; unique to these probes are particular image optimization features and tunable spectral doppler options (such as pulsed and continuous wave). Phased array probes feature a smaller curved surface which emits diverging soundwaves (similar to the curvilinear probe) producing a field of view wider than the footprint of the probe itself, ideal for maneuvering between ribs. Probe frequencies span higher and lower frequencies (2–8 MHz) allowing these probes to be used for both higher-resolution cardiac imaging and deeper abdominal or pelvic structures depending on the selected preset or manually specified transducer frequency [4].

Question 6
Which of the following changes would increase the frame rate and improve the temporal resolution of the image?

A. Increasing imaging depth
B. Increasing doppler box window size
C. Narrowing sector width
D. Increasing the number of focal zones

Answer C. Narrowing sector width

Explanation: Maximizing the framerate of an image is desirable as it increases the temporal resolution (number of acquired frames/images per second). Only narrowing the sector width would increase the frame rate. Other maneuvers that would increase the frame rate include decreasing the image depth and decreasing the number of focal zones [5].

Question 7
In the following Fig. 3.1, what can be said about the sample volume size (10 mm) in the following image?

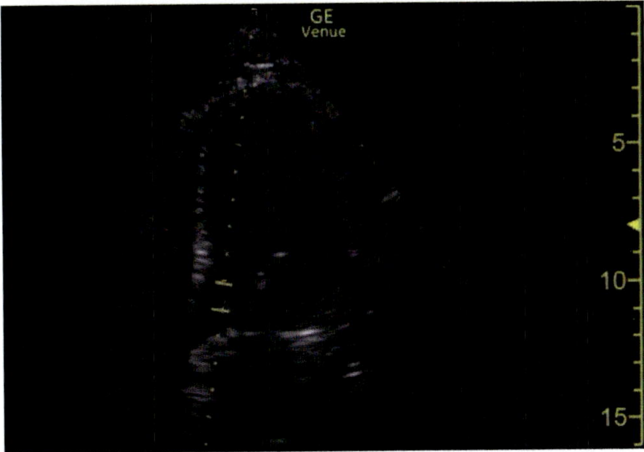

Fig. 3.1 Volume/gate size

A. It is too small
B. It is too large
C. It makes no difference in the doppler tracing

Answer B. It is too large

Explanation: In this Apical 5 chamber view, the sample gate is set at 10 mm. This is too large, as it typically should be set between 3–5 mm. When the sample gate is set too large it allows for increasing "noise" within the doppler signal. This can make it difficult to distinguish laminar flow from turbulent flow [6].

Question 8

When optimizing the display of a spectral doppler tracing one should:

A. Use as little gain as possible to avoid the introduction of noise.
B. Minimize the size of the tracing to avoid aliasing at all costs.
C. Always represent velocity flows toward the probe with upward deflections.
D. Use a sweep setting of at least 100 mm/s when performing velocity and/or time measurements.

Answer D. Use a sweep setting of at least 100 mm/s when performing velocity and/or time measurements.

Explanation: When optimizing a spectral doppler tracing one can adjust the tracing's baseline, velocity scale, sweep speed, and gain. The **doppler velocity scale** (vertical axis: maximum/minimum velocity display limits) should be decreased sufficiently to accommodate the largest tracing possible while avoiding aliasing (wrap around artifact). **Doppler sweep speed** (horizontal axis: time scale), typically set to 100 mm/s, can be adjusted to accommodate for faster or slower heart rates–ideally two to three spectral beats should span the entire horizontal axis to allow for beat-to-beat comparison and more accurate time measurements. While all velocity and time measurements should be performed at a sweep speed of ≥100 mm/s, slower sweep speeds (e.g. 25 mm/s) can be used to assess for respiratory variation in the doppler tracing. **Doppler gain**, similar to gain in B-Mode, should be adjusted to display the clearest doppler signal possible: sufficient gain to avoid missing important low-amplitude information, without obscuring the true spectral envelope with excessive noise [1].

Question 9

True or False: Increasing the ultrasound probe's output power always results in better image quality.

A. True
B. False

Answer B. False

Explanation: By increasing the ultrasound output power one may gain both increased depth of penetration and higher soundwave frequency, but these increases do not always yield detectable improvements in image quality. With increased power, however, one always increases the risk of deleterious biologic effects due to the increased energy transmission. Sometimes increasing the gain (the sensitivity of the receiver) which does not increase the output power, results in as a similar improvement in image quality without the added risk [7].

Question 10

Select the most appropriate parameter to adjust for each of the situations described below.

1. While trying to assess cardiac function, you note the heart motion appears choppy, and there is a noticeable lag each time you move the probe 2. While in the apical four chamber view, you have great resolution of the RV and LV apexes, but suboptimal mid-field resolution; you're hoping to get a better view of the tricuspid, mitral, and LVOT 3. Performing the RUQ portion of a FAST exam you're clearly able to make out the hepatorenal recess laterally, but the image quality darkens considerably more medially, making the diaphragm less visible 4. Upon rotating away from a subcostal four chamber view of the heart, you easily identify the IVC in the image's near field but are having difficulty assessing for respiratory variation in the vessel 5. While trying to optimize your subcostal four chamber view you accidentally toggle an option resulting in an intensely hyperechoic appearing liver and myocardium and hypoechoic cardiac chambers	A. Gain/time gain compensation (TGC) B. Image framing/depth control C. Focal zone D. Frame rate E. Dynamic range

Answer: 1-D; 2-C; 3-A; 4-B; 5-E

Explanation:

Frame rate: Frame rate determines the temporal resolution of the ultrasound. The frame rate can be increased by decreasing the depth of the image or narrowing the sector width, decreasing the number of focal zones, or using preprocessing zoom [1]. (Exemplified in Videos 3.2, 3.3, and

3.4: narrowing the sector width increases the temporal resolution aka frame rate—from 28 Hz to 40 Hz)

Focal zone: Soundwaves emitted from the ultrasound probe converge and diverge forming an hourglass shape, with the narrowest part of beam representing the focal point and the region spanning just proximal and distal to the focal point comprising the focal zone [8]. While some ultrasound systems use automated dynamic focusing based on the selected preset and image depth, others allow the user to manually set the depth of the focal zone, enhancing the resolution of a desired region of interest [1]. (Exemplified in Videos 3.5 and 3.6: Observe how the moving the focal zone from the apex to the level of the tricuspid/mitral valves effects the local resolution of the acquired clips).

Gain: Gain refers to the amount of amplification applied to the returned echo signal; visually, changes to gain affect the overall image brightness. Optimizing overall gain may improve contrast resolution and thus the overall image quality and visual experience. Excessive gain may distort the image by amplifying not only the echogenic portions of the image (the signal) but also the non-echogenic portions (the noise) yielding an over-exposed appearing image. Increasing gain does not increase the overall output power of the transducer. In contrast to overall gain, **time gain compensation (TGC)** allows one to set different gain values at different depths of the image. TGC helps to make up for energy loss due to attenuation that occurs at greater image depths [1].

Image framing/depth control: Image framing/depth control indicate how wide and how deep into the body the ultrasound images, respectively. The depth should be adjusted to include only slightly beyond the region of interest (33%, beyond is a good rule of thumb); the deeper the depth and wider the frame the longer it takes to produce each image, the slower the frame rate, and the lower the temporal resolution. When imaging a rapidly moving structure like the heart, lower temporal resolution may result in unsatisfactory clips [1] (Exemplified once again in Videos 3.2 and 3.5, as described above).

Dynamic range (aka Compression): Dynamic range is a visualization setting which specifies the grayscale color content the ultrasound image. A low dynamic range yields an image that is very black and white appearing, eliminating subtle details in the image--this is sometimes necessary for images of marginal quality. A high dynamic range, on the other hand, produces an image with more shades of grey and less black and white which if too high may cause the image to appear washed out [1].

Question 11

When performing ultrasound, zooming on a region of interest (ROI) prior or subsequent to image capture results in the same magnified image.

A. True
B. False

Answer B. False

Explanation: On most ultrasound machines the zoom options exists in two flavors: pre- and post-processing. Zooming prior to image capture (preprocessed zoom) results in a higher resolution image and a higher frame rate clip of the selected ROI than the post-processed zoom does. Pre-processing zoom (See Video 3.7) is a powerful albeit underutilized feature, which allows the user to magnify a specific ROI prior to image capture; because the ultrasound probe focuses its energy on a smaller ROI, the acquired image is ultimately higher resolution with an increased frame rate compared to its post-processed zoom counterpart. Post-processing zoom (see Video 3.8) is an option which allows for magnification of an image or clip post-capture; these magnifications are simply enlargements of original images with the same number of pixels, resulting in larger dimensioned images of poorer resolution [1].

Question 12

While initially performing a focused cardiac exam, you notice the digital indicator dot is on the opposite side of the screen and the image quality is markedly worse than expected (poorer resolution and inappropriate gain settings). Which of the following is the best initial choice to remedy this?

A. Center image over aortic valve and adjust the TGC sliders until the optimal gain is achieved.
B. Rotate the probe 180° in your hand.
C. Change the selected ultrasound preset from Abdominal to Cardiac.
D. Perform a hard reboot of the ultrasound machine.

Answer C. Change the selected ultrasound preset from Abdominal to Cardiac.

Explanation: Presets are used to initialize ultrasound settings depending on the specified exam type; predefined settings include transducer frequency, acoustic output power, gain, dynamic range, and depth based on the presumed ROI, tissue-type, and size of organs/structures. Compared to an abdominal imaging preset, cardiac presets classically switch the probe's operating frequency to a higher band (optimizing resolution over penetration), a faster frame-rate (to capture the moving organ by decreasing the preset depth and sector width), and adjusts the gain/dynamic range setting one more optimal for viewing relevant cardiac features (e.g. valves, endocardium, etc.) [1].

Question 13
Which of the following regarding Tissue Harmonic Imaging is TRUE?

A. Tissue harmonic imaging is not recommended for use by ultrasound societies.
B. Tissue harmonic imaging allows for improved visualization of deeper structures than conventional ultrasound technologies.
C. The generated tissue harmonics are higher frequency, unidirectional waves.
D. Tissue harmonic imaging has numerous disadvantages including a high burden of artifacts particularly reverberation artifacts.

Answer C. The generated tissue harmonics are higher frequency, unidirectional waves.

Explanation: **Tissue harmonic imaging** is an ultrasound imaging technique intended to enhance image quality, particularly the visualization of tissue borders. This feature is available on select modern imaging systems and is recommended for use by the ASE when performing cardiac ultrasound. In brief, harmonics are soundwaves whose frequencies are multiples of the parent soundwave's frequency. When the parent soundwave strikes tissues, multiple harmonic soundwaves are created. Because these generated harmonics are higher frequency and unidirectional (originating from the tissue and not the probe), the image quality obtained is higher resolution and free of certain artifacts (including reverberation, beam width, and side-lobe artifacts) [9]. **D**isadvantages of tissue harmonic imaging include lower-penetration and increased acoustic shadowing artifacts [1].

Question 14
Which of the following regarding Mechanical Index (MI) is INCORRECT?

A. MI represents the likelihood of mechanical bioeffects occurring given the current ultrasound settings.
B. MI is a function of the probe's operating frequency.
C. MI values >1–1.5 are considered safe.
D. The FDA mandates MI values be displayed during B-mode imaging.

Answer C. MI values >1–1.5 are considered safe.

Explanation: Bioeffects refer to the biological impact ultrasound pressure waves have on living tissues. Classically, these effects are categorized as either thermal or mechanical (non-thermal) in nature. **Mechanical (MI) and Thermal (TI) indices** are frequency-dependent calculated values which indicate the likelihood of clinically relevant bioeffects (given the current ultrasound probe settings). MI or TI values <0.5 are unlikely to exert significant bioeffects, while values >1–1.5 indicate likely bioeffects and require careful attention. As part of the FDA's effort to limit the harmful effects of diagnostic imaging, the Output Display Standard (1992) was created, mandating that all ultrasound machines display the Mechanical Index (MI) when operating in B-mode and the Thermal (TI) when performing adult orbital/cephalic or obstetrical ultrasound examinations [10, 11].

Question 15
What is the optimal patient position to perform both parasternal and apical cardiac examination?

A. Supine
B. Left lateral decubitus
C. 30° of Trendelenburg
D. Sitting up at a 45-degree angle

Answer B. Left lateral decubitus

Explanation: Left lateral decubitus position is the optimal position for both the parasternal and apical views. This allows the heart to move more directly adjacent to the thorax and therefore closer to the transducer. Many times, this position is difficult to achieve due to the limited mobility of critically ill patients. Supine is idea for subcostal examination. Reverse Trendelenburg and sitting up is not a standard recommendation for optimizing windows [5, 12, 13].

Question 16
Which of the following is not a fundamental assumption made when interpreting an ultrasound image?

A. Soundwaves emitted from the ultrasound probe travel in a straight path.
B. Ultrasound waves originate from the main beam.
C. Soundwaves return to the transducer after a at least two reflections
D. Travel at a uniform speed, 1540 m/s, and are uniformly attenuated by all tissues

Answer C. Soundwaves return to the transducer after a at least two reflections

Explanation: Emitted ultrasound waves pass into tissue and are either transmitted, reflected, or refracted depending on the densities of the tissue medium. Transmitted waves pass through the tissue medium in a straight line, while reflected waves are accelerated straight back to the ultrasound transducer and refracted waves are deflected at an angle as the waves pass through one tissue into another of differing density. Waves that ultimately make it back to the ultrasound probe are processed based on the travel time and signal intensity to generate the observed 2D image.

Artifacts in ultrasound imaging are important to recognize and understand in order to avoid misinterpretation and misdiagnosis of the clinical scenario being evaluated. Artifacts are classically divided into two categories: those that arise as a consequence of (1) violations of assumptions built into the ultrasound equipment [namely: soundwaves travel in a straight path, originate from the main beam, **return to the transducer after a single reflection**, travel at a uniform speed 1540 m/s, and are uniformly attenuated by all tissues 0.5 dB/cm/MHz] or (2) external interference generated by other devices [14].

Question 17

An 18-years old male with history of severe asthma presents to the ED with acute onset shortness of breath. Upon further evaluation the patient is noted to have unilateral breath sounds and absence of B-lines (aka "comet tail artifacts") on an ultrasound of his left chest. B-lines which are hyperechoic lines extending from the pleural surface to the bottom of ultrasound image, are an example of what of the following ultrasound artifacts:

A. Side-lobe artifact
B. Mirror image artifact
C. Reverberation artifact
D. Acoustic enhancement artifact

Answer C. Reverberation artifact

Explanation: Reverberations artifacts are a consequence of violation of the assumption that "soundwaves return to the transducer after a single reflection". **Simple reverberation artifacts** are produced when a reflected ultrasound wave is reflected a second time by a second surface back to the primary reflector surface and then back to the transducer probe–commonly this second surface is the plastic housing of the ultrasound probe itself (as diagramed in Fig. 3.2). A circuitous path which results in doubling of the soundwave's travel time would result in the appearance of a "ghost object" (in addition to the "real object") at twice the distance below the original structure. **Complex reverberation artifacts** are produced through multiple rounds of reflection between two closely apposed reflector surfaces; an example of this is comet tail artifacts–e.g. B-lines observed in interstitial pulmonary diseases [14, 15].

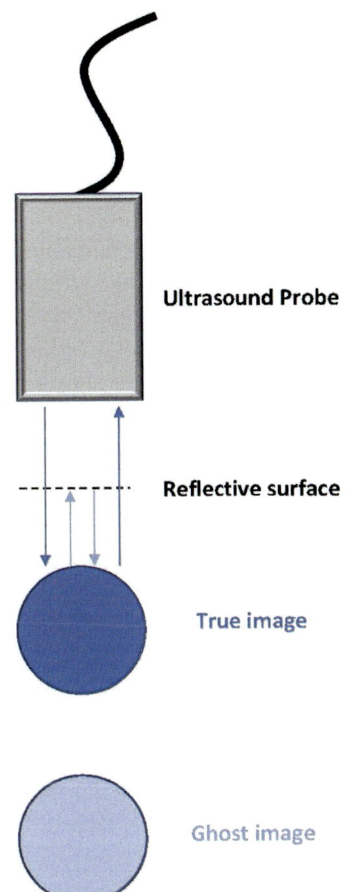

Fig. 3.2 Reverberation diagram

Question 18

A 55-year-old male with a history of hypertension and tobacco smoking presented to the ED with new onset chest pain and a syncopal episode. In the ED, his heart rate was 125 bpm and his blood pressure 182/90 mmHg. Bedside TTE demonstrated what looked like an aortic root dissection flap, but on subsequent CT-angiogram no dissection flap could be visualized. Which type of artifact likely caused this misdiagnosis of a Type A Dissection on TTE?

A. Side-lobe artifact
B. Mirror image artifact
C. Refraction artifact
D. Acoustic enhancement artifact

Answer A. Side-lobe artifact

Explanation: The **side lobe artifact** is produced when higher-energy reflections from offshoot soundwaves return to the probe violating the assumption that all returned soundwaves originate from the main ultrasound beam. Side lobes are collections of unintended offshoot soundwaves produced by the ultrasound probe due to constructive interference patterns; these side lobes are low energy and off axis, traveling at an angle relative to the main central ultrasound beam. When a side lobe reflects off a strong reflector (e.g. a calcified plaque/stone or bowel tissue: gas interface) the returned soundwaves are comparable in energy to reflected soundwaves originating from the higher energy main ultrasound beam (albeit often still less energetic). Because of the higher-than-expected energies of these strong reflections, the ultrasound probe misinterprets these waves as originating from the main beam and shifts the location of the strong reflective surface from its actual lateral position to an artifactual position coincident with the main central beam. On parasternal long axis view, side lobe artifacts due to reflection of the sinotubular junction can result in curvilinear artifact within the lumen of the aorta which may be misinterpreted as an aortic dissection flap [14].

Question 19
Vessel duplication is a phenomenon sometimes observed when imaging vasculature, particularly the abdominal aorta or carotid arteries. If unrecognized, this artifact can lead to the mistaken diagnosis of a vessel dissections in an otherwise normal vasculature. Vessel duplication of this sort is an example of which of the following categories of artifacts?

A. Mirror image artifact
B. Side-lobe artifact
C. Refraction artifact
D. Beam width artifact

Answer A. Mirror image artifact

Explanation: The **mirror image artifact** is produced when ultrasound waves return to the probe via an indirect path, violating two core assumptions: (1) "soundwaves travel in a straight line" and (2) "return to the transducer after a single reflection". This artifact is produced when emitted ultrasound waves encounter a reflective surface and instead of being reflected back are deflected at an angle; these deflected soundwaves next encounter a second highly reflective surface laying between the first surface and the probe; the soundwaves are reflected back towards the first surface and ultimately deflected along the original incident path back to the transducer (as diagramed in Fig. 3.3). Because of the assumptions made the ultrasound probe misinterprets the actual path and constructs a "mirror image" of the second reflector downfield from the first surface at a distance equal to the distance between the two reflected surfaces [14].

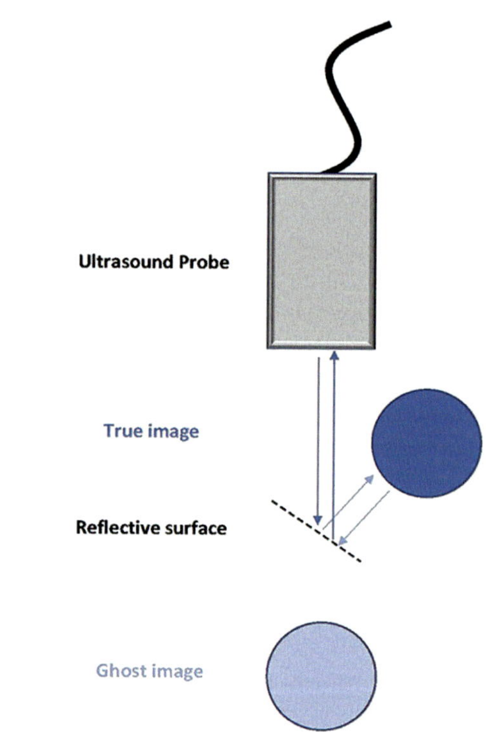

Fig. 3.3 Mirror-image diagram

Question 20
Which of the following basic ultrasound assumptions are violated to produce refraction artifacts? (Select all that apply)

A. Soundwaves travel in a straight path
B. Originate from the main beam
C. Return to the transducer after a single reflection
D. Travel at a uniform speed through all tissues (1540 m/s)
E. Are uniformly attenuated by all tissues 0.5 dB/cm/MHz

Answer A. Soundwaves travel in a straight path; **D.** Travel at a uniform speed through all tissues (1540 m/s)

Explanation: The **refraction artifact** occurs due to violation of two core assumptions: (1) "soundwaves travel in a straight path" and (2) "soundwaves travel at a uniform speed through all tissues". Like the mirror image artifact, refraction artifacts occur when initially deflected soundwaves are ultimately, albeit indirectly, returned to the probe via the original incident path. Unlike the mirror image artifact, this deflection occurs due to refraction of the soundwaves as they travel through a tissue medium with different physical properties. Similar to how light refracts through a prism, some of the emitted soundwaves are deflected along a different path; these soundwaves are then reflected off a surface of interest and ultimately deflected back to the probe through re-refraction of the soundwaves. Rather than a mirror image (which produces a downfield artifact), a refraction artifact produces a carbon-copy of a structure of interest adjacent to said structure of interest [14] (as depicted in Fig. 3.4).

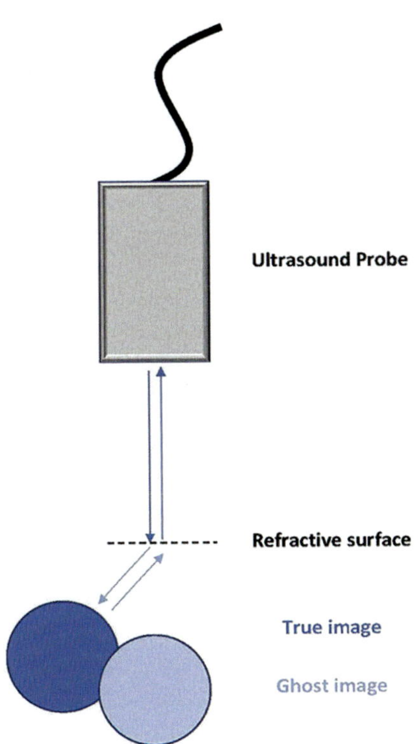

Fig. 3.4 Refraction diagram

Question 21
The acoustic shadowing artifact is classically present in which of the following ultrasound scenarios?

A. RUQ abdominal ultrasound in patient without gallstones
B. Subprapubic longitudinal view of FAST exam in a patient with a full bladder
C. Vascular ultrasound of aorta in patient with significant atherosclerotic disease
D. Lung ultrasound on patient with a significant amount of pulmonary edema

Answer C. Vascular ultrasound of aorta in patient with significant atherosclerotic disease

Explanation: The **acoustic shadowing artifact** occurs due to violation of the assumption that "soundwaves are uniformly attenuated by all tissues". The artifact is produced when soundwaves encounter a highly reflective surface (e.g. a calcified plaque or stone); a "shadow" (hypoechoic band) is produced deep to this surface which can be misinterpreted by the ultrasonographer as a hypoechoic structure if the artifact goes unrecognized. Inversely, **acoustic enhancement** occurs when soundwaves pass through a less attenuating structure (e.g. a simple fluid-filled cyst), producing hyperechoic enhancement deep to the hypo-attenuating surface [14].

Question 22
Aliasing occurs when:

A. The reflected sound wave is greater than the Nyquist limit
B. Reversal of blood flow is present
C. The reflected sound wave is less than the Nyquist limit
D. The probe is aligned perpendicular to blood flow

Answer A. The reflected sound wave is greater than the Nyquist limit

Explanation: Doppler shift is a phenomenon that occurs when a wave's frequency is changed (or shifted) following reflection by a moving surface. The magnitude of this frequency shift is a function of the velocity of the moving surface: this is how we can calculate blood flow velocity through a valve, for example, using ultrasound. An ultrasound probe's upper limit of detection of sound wave frequencies is referred to as the Nyquist limit of the probe; the Nyquist limit is equal to one-half of the probe's sampling frequency, a value determined by the probe's operating frequency and the depth of the sample volume. **Aliasing** is an artifact that occurs (while using pulsed-wave spectral doppler or color doppler) when the doppler-shifted soundwave is greater than the probe's calculated Nyquist limit; this reality results in a "wrap around" phenomenon where the ultrasound machine displays an artifactually speckled color map (with color doppler) or a noisy over-saturated velocity-time graph (with spectral doppler). Recognition of aliasing is important to avoid misdiagnosing this artifact for reversal of flow or turbulence. Of note, doppler-shift is greatest (and most accurate) when the emitted and returned soundwaves are parallel to the measured blood flow and least, when perpendicular to blood flow [14].

Question 23
Which of the following are true with regards to electrical interference? (Select all that apply)

A. It results from nearby shielded electronics.
B. It manifests as scattered random patterning in color or spectral doppler modes.
C. When present, it appears across all acoustic windows.
D. It can be seen with bovie use, pacemaker discharge, and TOF/twitch monitor firing.

Answer C. When present, it appears across all acoustic windows; **D.** It can be seen with bovie use, pacemaker discharge, and TOF/twitch monitor firing.

Explanation: **Electrical interference** artifacts occur as a result of nearby unshielded electronics. Typically, these artifacts appear in both spectral and color doppler modes and manifest as band-like jets or streams, in geometrical patterns across all acoustic windows [14].

Question 24
Which of the following is true regarding modern ultrasound probes?

A. Modern ultrasound probes use quartz crystals
B. Piezoelectric crystals are arranged linearly throughout the length of the probe
C. Plumbium zirconium titanate crystals provide better image quality
D. Misalignment of crystals is a complication of moisture accumulation.

Answer C. Plumbium zirconium titanate crystals provide better image quality

Explanation: Piezoelectric crystals are located at the footprint of the probe and are arranged according to the shape of the probe tip. The footprint is a transmitter and receiver of the US beam during scanning. Most modern probes use synthetic plumbium zirconium titanate, compared with quartz crystals that were used in earlier units. These plumbium zirconium titanate crystals are integral in the image quality obtained during the scan and can be damaged or misaligned when probes are dropped, crushed, or thrown against other objects [16].

Table 3.2 Transducer type and clinical use

Probe type	Frequency (MHz)	Applications
Curvilinear	2–5	FAST, renal, IVC, pelvic, bladder, blower, appendicitis
Linear	6–15	Ocular, trachea, DVT, soft tissue, thyroid, thoracic, vascular access
Intracavitary	8–13	Pelvic, intra vaginal, pelvic
Phased array	1–5	Cardiac, abdominal, renal, IVC, pediatric abdomen

Question 25
When considering the principle of tissue penetration of the ultrasonic beam, which of the following statements is most accurate?

A. Lower frequency probes provide less penetration of the ultrasound waved but generate higher-resolution images.
B. A linear transducer has a higher frequency range and provides detailed anatomic resolution for evaluating superficial structures.
C. The phased array transducer has a uniform crystal arrangement providing a rectangular image in the ultrasound machine screen.
D. Higher frequency ultrasound waves penetrate tissues easier and provide better resolution of deeper structures.

Answer B. A linear transducer has a higher frequency range and provides detailed anatomic resolution for evaluating superficial structures.

Explanation: The principle of tissue penetration of the ultrasonic beam, expressed in megahertz (MHz), determines the type of transducer that should be used. Higher-frequency probes provide less penetration of the US waves through the tissue planes but generate higher-resolution images.

High-frequency probes include the linear probe and the intracavitary probe. These probes should be used to visualize superficial structures, such as vascular structures for line placement, pulmonary pleura, muscle, or structures in the pelvis. Conversely, probes with a lower spectrum frequency, such as the curvilinear probe, should be used to visualize deeper structures. The ability to visualize deeper structures comes at the expense of resolution. Lower-frequency probes are useful in evaluating the abdominal aorta, the gallbladder, the inferior vena cava (IVC), pelvic organs, and so forth [16].

The phased or sector array transducer has a frequency range of 1–5 MHz. The crystal arrangement in the footprint is bundled in the center and fans out creating a pielike image on the US machine screen. Because of the smaller footprint, this probe is commonly used for echocardiography and is particularly useful in the evaluation of pediatric patients. The phased array probe can also be used for the FAST examination in patients with tight intercostal spaces. The most commonly used US probes and beside US applications are summarized in the Table 3.2 below [16, 17].

Question 26
Which of the following statements is true regarding the piezoelectric effect?

A. It is the property that allows ultrasound technology to convert electrical energy into mechanical energy.
B. It is the physical principle that describes the changes of position of an electron in the atom
C. Allows the creation of an image from all the beams rarefracted and reflected by the medium
D. Sound waves traveling through a vacuum are reflected orthogonally to the direction of movement.

Answer A. It is the property that allows ultrasound technology to convert electrical energy into mechanical energy.

Explanation: The piezoelectric effect is the cornerstone of traditional ultrasound. In the ultrasound system, the sound source is a piezoelectric crystal, such as quartz. The piezoelectric effect allows for crystals to vibrate when an electrical voltage is applied across it and subsequently creates sound waves. Conversely, piezoelectric crystals also can convert sound waves back into electrical energy so that the sound waves can be converted into data that can be processed into anatomic images.

The piezoelectric effect allows ultrasound probes to convert electrical energy into mechanical energy (sound waves). Sound should be thought of as the interaction of energy and matter. In contrast to electromagnetic energy which comes from alternating electron position in an atom, sound is mechanical energy transmitted by pressure waves in a medium. Which means that sound exists in the form of particles moving in a medium. In diagnostic ultrasound, the media can be air, blood, or soft tissue. In the absence of media (i.e., a vacuum), sound cannot propagate [18].

Every time the sound waves pass through a different medium, the beam is **rarefracted** and some of the waves can change direction/velocity. The ultrasound can only create an image with sound waves that are **reflected** back to the probe's transducer. A computer analyzes the time delay between when the pulse was sent, when the echo was received, as well as properties of the sound itself (amplitude, pitch, etc.) to calculate velocities and create images [18].

Question 27
Which of the following statements is true regarding the use of the "auto gain" function in most advanced ultrasound machines?

A. "Auto gain" adjusts the gain preset based on the frequency of the waves reflected back to the probe.
B. It might increase the gain leading to a brighter image with increase image noise and artifact.
C. Increasing gain at a specific depth is not a functionality of most modern ultrasound machines.
D. Increasing gain compensate for attenuation by amplifying the receive and the send signal.

Answer B. It might increase the gain leading to a brighter image with increase image noise and artifact.

Explanation: The gray scale of the image can be manipulated by adjusting the gain. By increasing the gain, the ultrasound machine allows processing of more incoming echoes, thereby creating a brighter image. Increasing the gain leads to a brighter image on the screen, but it also increases image noise and artifact, with loss of contrast and finer details.

As the ultrasound beam travels deeper into a medium, the returning echoes are attenuated, resulting in less resolution. The gain function compensates for attenuation by amplifying the receive signal (not the send signal). A feature known as time gain compensation allows for the adjusting of brightness at specific depths. The top row of buttons controls nearfield gain, whereas the bottom row of buttons controls farfield gain. Advanced ultrasound machines have an "***auto gain***" button, which resets the machine back to standard gain presets for the type of scan being performed (i.e. abdominal) [18].

Question 28
An ultrasound probe has a frequency of 5 MHz. Which of the following is true

A. It produces 50 amplitudes/s
B. It produces 5000 cycles/s
C. It produces 5,000,000 cycles/min
D. It produces 5,000,000 cycles/s

Answer D. It produces 5,000,000 cycles/s

Explanation: A Herz (Hz) is a measure of frequency per unit of time, or the number of cycles per second. One megahertz is abbreviated MHz, and it is equal to one million Hz. The most well-known acoustic variables are period and frequency. Period is the time to complete a single cycle. It can also be stated as the time from the start of 1 cycle to the start of the next cycle. In ultrasound, period is the time from the start of 1 peak, including 1 valley, to the next peak. Typical values in diagnostic ultrasound for period are expressed in microseconds. Frequency is the number of events that occur in a particular time frame. In ultrasound, the frequency of a wave is the number of cycles that occur in 1 s. Typical frequencies in diagnostic ultrasound are expressed in megahertz. Ultrasound transducer frequencies vary from 1 MHz to 15 MHz. Given this inverse relationship, period and frequency are the reciprocal of each other [19].

Questions 29 and 30 please use Fig. 3.5 below:

Question 29

What is the frequency of the sound wave depicted in Fig. 3.5?

A. 1 Hz
B. 3 Hz
C. "A" divided by "B"
D. "A" multiplied by "B"

Question 30

Which of the following statements is true of the depicted sound wave in Fig. 3.5?

A. "A" represents a wavelength and not a cycle
B. "A" represents a wavelength and a cycle
C. "A" represents the amplitude
D. "A" × "B" is the speed of sound

Question 29: Answer B. 3 Hz

Question 30: Answer B. "A" represents a wavelength and a cycle

Explanation: The distance between one peak and the next represents 1 cycle ("A" in Fig. 3.5); it is the distance between 2 similar points on corresponding waves and represents 1 wavelength. Period is the time to complete a single cycle. In ultrasound, period is the time from the start of 1 peak, including 1 valley, to the next peak. Typical values in diagnostic ultrasound for period are expressed in microseconds. Frequency is the number of events that occur in a particular time frame. Figure 3.5 shows a sound wave that has completed 3 cycles in 1 s. The frequency is 3 cycles/s which is 3 Hz.

Typical frequencies in diagnostic ultrasound are expressed in megahertz. Ultrasound transducer frequencies vary from 1 MHz to 15 MHz. Given this inverse relationship, period and frequency are the reciprocal of each other. "A" in Fig. 3.5 represents both a cycle and a wavelength. "B" is the amplitude of the wave.

Typical diagnostic ultrasound wavelengths are in the millimeter range. Wavelength (λ) and frequency (f) are also inversely related to one another. The higher the frequency the shorter the wavelength. The speed of sound is the product of frequency and wavelength ($v = f \times \lambda$).

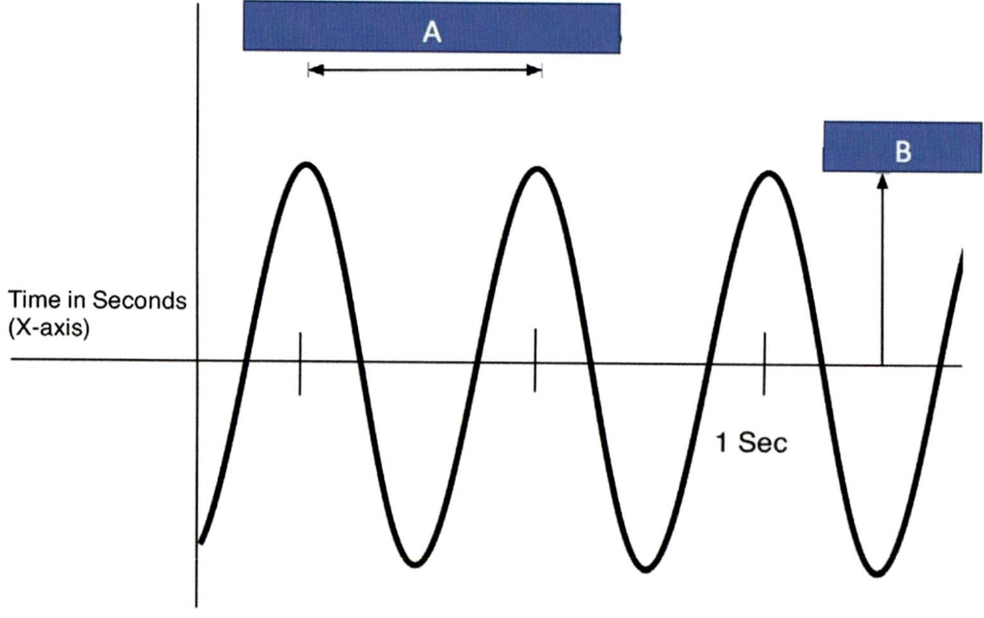

Fig. 3.5 Sound wave

Question 31
Which of the following statements best explains the rationale for using color power Doppler in the evaluation of testicular or ovarian torsion?

A. It allows for the audible representation of blood flow.
B. It provides more sensitive information about the direction of flow.
C. It does not allow color signal to be superimposed on the B-mode image.
D. It is more sensitive to detect flow in organs with typically low flow states

Answer D. It is more sensitive to detect flow in organs with typically low flow states

The use of the Doppler principle in ultrasonography includes color Doppler, pulse wave Doppler, and color power Doppler. Color Doppler detects the overall blood flow and its direction of flow under a region of interrogation. The energy of the returning waves is displayed as an assigned color on the ultrasound screen. By convention, echoes demonstrating flow toward the transducer are seen in shades of red and those representing flow away from the transducer are seen as shades of blue. The color display is usually superimposed on the B-mode image.

In pulse wave Doppler, the direction and velocity of the blood flow can be displayed graphically and audibly. If blood is moving away from the transducer, a lower frequency (negative shift) is detected. If blood is moving toward the transducer, a higher frequency (positive shift) is detected.

Color power Doppler identifies the amplitude or power of the Doppler signals rather than the frequency shifts. It is more sensitive than pulse wave Doppler to detect blood flow in organs with typically low-flow states, such as the ovaries or testicles. Power Doppler is more sensitive than color Doppler for the detection and demonstration of blood flow but provides no information about the direction of flow [18].

Question 32
The creation of an ultrasound image relies on several physical assumptions of the wave produced by the ultrasound wave and the returning echoes. When assumptions are not maintained it can lead to imaging artifacts. Which of the following statements accurately describes one of these assumptions?

A. The speed of sound in human tissue is different for blood rich organs (i.e. kidney and heart) than for blood poor organ (i.e. bone and cartilage).
B. The depth of an object is independent to the time of flight for an ultrasound pulse to return to the transducer as an echo.
C. The acoustic energy in an ultrasound field is uniformly attenuated.
D. The echo returns to the transducer after several reflections depending on the density of the medium.

Answer C. The acoustic energy in an ultrasound field is uniformly attenuated.

Explanation: The creation of an ultrasound image is based on the physical properties of ultrasound pulse formation, propagation of sound in matter, interaction of sound with reflective interfaces, and echo detection and processing by the probe. Ultrasound display relies on physical assumptions to assign the location and the intensity of each received echo. These assumptions are as follows [20]:

1. The echoes detected originated from within the main ultrasound beam.
2. An echo returns to the transducer after a single reflection.
3. The depth of an object is directly related to the time of flight for an ultrasound pulse to return to the transducer as an echo.
4. The speed of sound in human tissue is constant.
5. The sound beam and its echo travel in a straight path.
6. The acoustic energy in an ultrasound field is uniformly attenuated.

Question 33
An 18-year-old trauma patient undergoes a FAST exam in the trauma bay. The provider conducting the exam is worried of a potential diaphragmatic injury as liver is visualized deep to the diaphragm. No free fluid is seen and no pneumothorax appreciated. Findings are NOT confirmed by computer tomography scan of the chest. Which of the following artifacts could have explained this finding?

A. Mirror image artifact
B. Reverberation
C. Shadowing
D. Comet Tail

Answer A. Mirror image artifact

Explanation: The error in diagnosis in the FAST exam was most likely due to a mirror-image artifact. This artifact is seen between an object adjacent to a strong reflector (such as the diaphragm), which prolongs the time of flight for the ultrasound beam. Reverberations develop between the object and the strong reflector, which prolongs the time of flight for the ultrasound beam. This phenomenon can register the echoes created by the object as equidistant to, but on the opposite side of, the reflector, creating a mirror image. In this case the liver was reflected on the opposite side of the diaphragm.

Reverberation artifact is caused by significant differences in the acoustic impedance of 2 adjacent tissues at their interface. They are usually seen as bright parallel lines at uniform intervals occurring between different tissue interfaces, that is, fluid-gas, solid-gas, and solid-fluid. For a perpendicular sound beam, the amount reflected at an interface is related to the acoustic impedance difference between the adjacent media the portion reflected is maximized. The reflected beam strikes the transducer and returns back to the subject tissue [21, 22].

For Questions 34–39, select the artifact most likely depicted by the diagram and match it the choices listed A–F.

Question 34	(Fig. 3.6)	A. Speed error artifact
Question 35	(Fig. 3.7)	B. Mirror image artifact
Question 36	(Fig. 3.8)	C. Reverberation artifact
Question 37	(Fig. 3.9)	D. Shadowing artifact
Question 38	(Fig. 3.10)	E. Directional ambiguity artifact
Question 39	(Fig. 3.11)	F. Acoustic enhancement artifact

Question 34: Answer C. Reverberation artifact
Question 35: Answer B. Mirror image artifact
Question 36: Answer D. Shadowing artifact
Question 37: Answer F. Acoustic enhancement artifact
Question 38: Answer A. Speed error artifact
Question 39: Answer E. Directional ambiguity artifact

Reverberation Artifact: Reverberation artifact is caused by significant differences in the acoustic impedance of 2 adjacent tissues at their interface. Reverberation artifacts are usually seen as bright parallel lines at uniform intervals occurring between different tissue interfaces, that is, fluid-gas, solid-gas, and solid-fluid. For a perpendicular sound beam, the amount reflected at an interface is related to the acoustic impedance difference between the adjacent media the portion reflected is maximized. The reflected beam strikes the transducer and returns back to the subject tissue.

Mirror Image Artifact: This artifact is seen between an object adjacent to a strong reflector, which prolongs the time of flight for the ultrasound beam. Strong reflectors in the body that tend to create mirror-image artifacts include the diaphragm, the bladder, the pleura and the bowel. Earlier a similar question tested this artifact when liver was visualized deep to the diaphragm in a trauma FAST exam.

Shadowing Artifact: The shadowing artifact is caused by partial or complete attenuation of the ultrasound beam along its path due to absorption or reflection by an object. Deep into the object, the amplitude of the sound beam is considerably diminished, resulting in loss of signal, creating a shadow on the screen display. Ribs have high attenuation and cause shadowing artifacts.

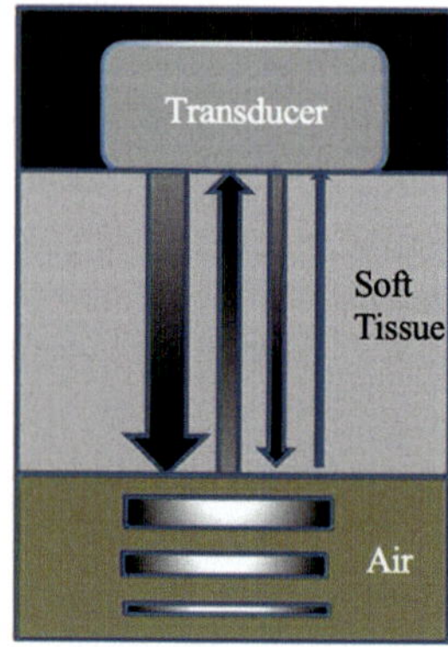

Fig. 3.6 Artifacts

Acoustic Enhancement Artifact: The acoustic enhancement artifact can be seen when a fluid-filled structure such as cystic lesion causes increased through-transmission of the ultrasound beam and enhanced visualization of deeper structures. This artifact can be thought of as a opposite to the shadowing artifact. When the ultrasound beam encounters an object in its path that is more weakly attenuating than the surrounding tissue, the amplitude of the beam deep into this object is increased compared with the amplitude of the beam at similar depth in the remainder of the tissue in the field. Therefore, echoes returning from tissue deep into the object will display increased signal, resulting in the enhancement artifact [23].

Speed Error Artifact: The speed error artifact occurs because of the assumption of the ultrasound hardware that the velocity of sound in tissue is uniformly 1540 m/s. The image processor calculates the depth of an object from the roundtrip time of flight for the sound beam and returning echo. In fatty tissue, where the velocity of sound is less than 1540 m/s, shallow objects will be misrepresented as deeper; in tissue with little fat, that is, skeletal muscle, where the velocity of sound is greater than 1540 m/s, deeper objects will be misrepresented as being shallower.

Directional Ambiguity Artifact: The directional ambiguity artifact is primarily caused by operator error. When the ultrasound beam intercepts a vessel at a 90-degree angle, with the beam side lobes interrogating flow both upstream and downstream, the resulting signal is manifested as a spectral tracing both above and below the baseline. Altering the transducer position to change the beam angle away from perpendicular will correct for the direction ambiguity [23].

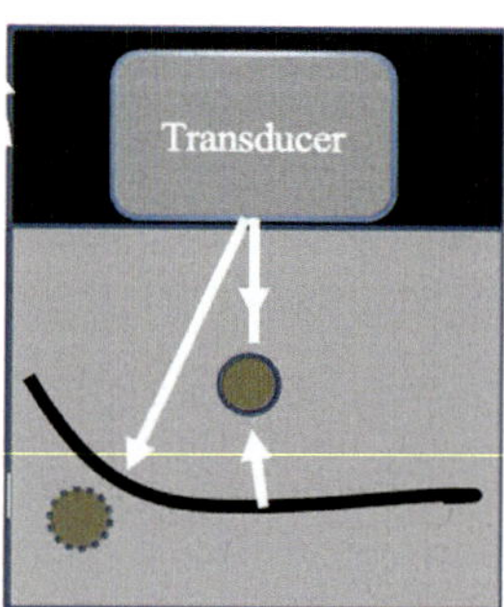

Fig. 3.7 Artifacts

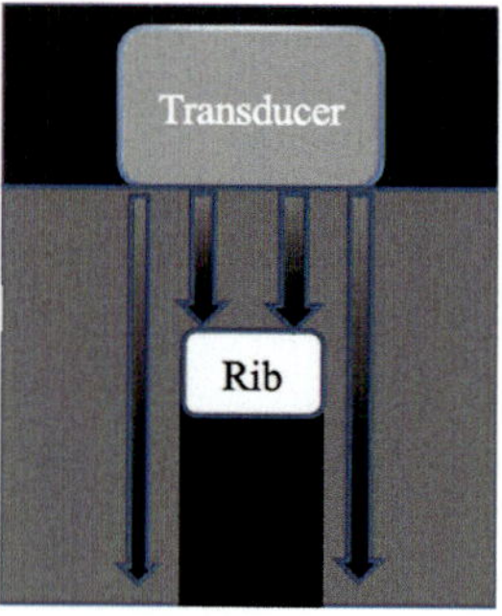

Fig. 3.8 Artifacts

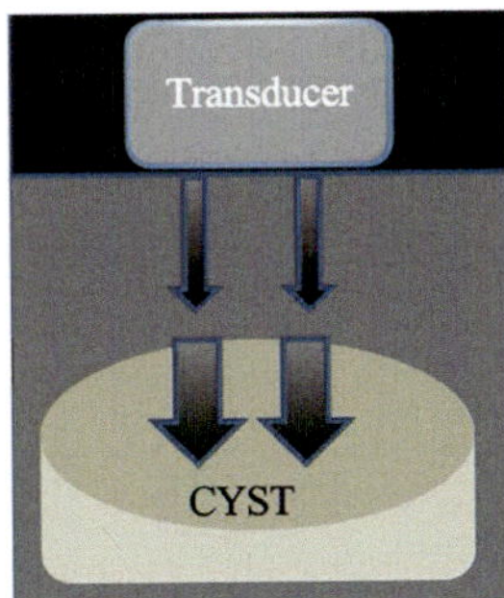

Fig. 3.9 Artifacts

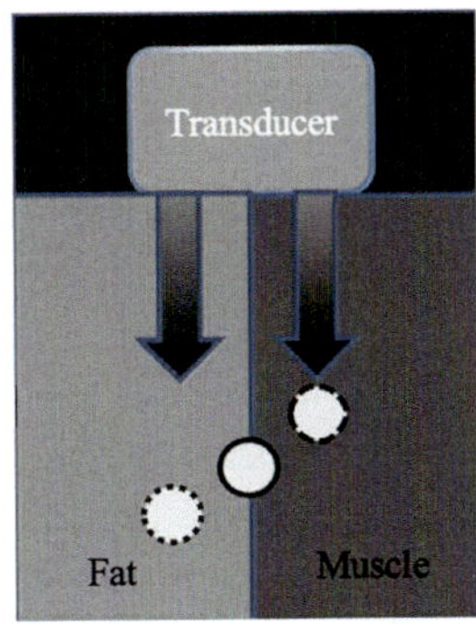

Fig. 3.10 Artifacts

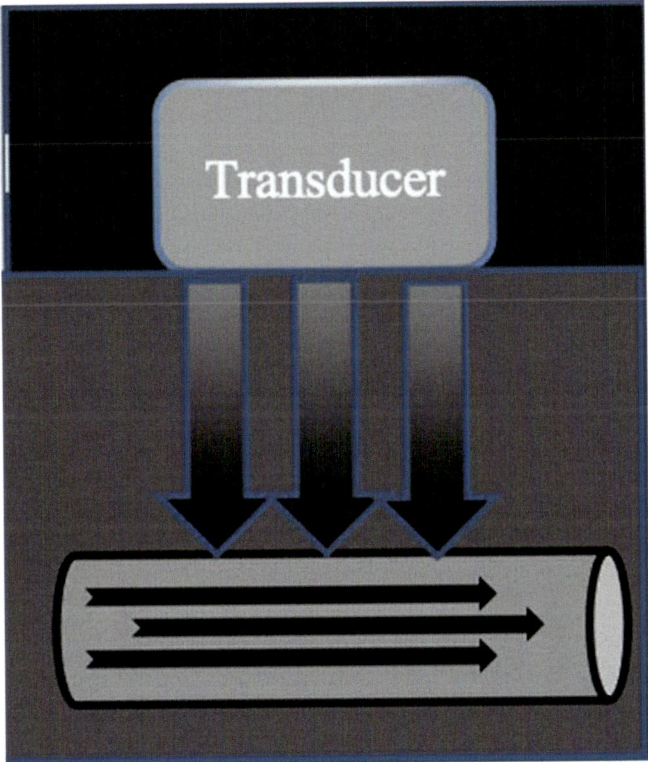

Fig. 3.11 Artifacts

Question 40
Which of the following is true regarding A-lines seen in lung ultrasound?

A. They are always indicate lung pathology such as lung edema or consolidation
B. They are a reverberation artifact resulting in a bright white, hyperechoic, semicircular repeating horizontal lines which are found deep to the pleural line.
C. They slide back and forth with respiration
D. They are best visualized with a higher frequency probe (10–13 MHz)

Answer B. They are a reverberation artifact resulting in a bright white, hyperechoic, semicircular repeating horizontal lines which are found deep to the pleural line.

Explanation: A-lines are a normal ultrasound finding of the lung and do not indicate pathology. They are caused by a reverberation artifact that causes a bright white, hyperechoic semicircular repeating horizontal lines, which are found deep to the pleural line. In contrast to the comet-tail artifact, A-lines do not slide back and forth with respirations. These lines are best visualized with a lower-frequency probe (3–5 MHz) [24].

Question 41
You are conducting a lung ultrasound in an intubated trauma patient with several rib fractures. Which of the following is true regarding the interpretation of this exam?

A. Subcutaneous emphysema may make it difficult to visualize pleural sliding
B. The presence of rib fractures is a contraindication to lung ultrasound
C. A right mainstem intubation will not affect the interpretation of the exam.
D. Lung contusions cannot be visualized by ultrasound.

Answer A. Subcutaneous emphysema may make it difficult to visualize pleural sliding

Explanation: Because the lung ultrasound examination relies on evaluation of the pleural line and lung sliding, there are several conditions that may make the examination unreliable. The presence of extensive subcutaneous emphysema will make it difficult for ultrasound beams to travel through this subcutaneous air to find the pleural line. If a pleural effusion or hemothorax has developed together with a pneumothorax, fluid may be widely present between the visceral and parietal pleura, effectively prohibiting lung sliding. In most cases of small to moderate-sized pleural effusions, the fluid preferentially layers posteriorly and if the probe is positioned on the anterior chest, lung sliding should still be present. Pleural thickening or scarring can make it difficult to discern pleural sliding.

The presence of a loculated pneumothorax or large pulmonary bleb can also make the examination unreliable, because the pleural line can be split in defined areas of the lung. A large pneumonia or lung contusion may further result in a lack of lung sliding because of pulmonary consolidation, but the consolidated parenchyma can still be visualized. In intubated patients, a right mainstem intubation results in atelectasis of the left lung, resulting in a lack of lung sliding on that side. Lung ultrasound can be safely performed on patients with rib fracture by minimizing the pressure placed on the chest with the probe [25, 26].

Question 42

Which of the following is true regarding B-lines seen in lung ultrasound?

A. They result from intralobular septa thickening.
B. B-lines remain static through the respiratory cycle.
C. They represent a good estimate of pulmonary wedge pressure.
D. They may be best appreciated in the anterior chest segments.

Answer C. They represent a good estimate of pulmonary wedge pressure.

Explanation: In patients with alveolar fluid an artifact known as *B-lines* develops. B-lines appear as well-defined bright hyperechoic lines arising from the pleural line and extending vertically into the lung. B-lines move with sliding of the lung and through the respiratory cycle. The development of B-lines results from the thickening of the interlobular septa, because extravascular fluid accumulates within the pulmonary interstitial area and alveoli [27]. The B-line pattern has been shown to correlate with pulmonary artery occlusion pressure [24] and resolves after adequate diuresis has been instituted. B-lines may best be appreciated by positioning the probe in a more posterior position. This increased sensitivity of a posterior approach is a result of the movement of fluid to the dependent areas due to gravity.

Question 43

What is the best position to place the pulse wave Doppler sample volume for mitral inflow?

A. At the tips of the mitral valve in diastole
B. At the tips of the mitral valve in systole
C. In the middle of the mitral leaflets
D. At the mitral valve annulus

Answer A. At the tips of the mitral valve in diastole

Explanation: The best view to record the mitral inflow signal is the apical four-chamber view (or an apical long-axis view). The Doppler sample volume should be placed between the anterior and the posterior leaflet, making sure that the sample volume is at the tip of the leaflets and parallel to mitral inflow.

Question 44

What of the following is the primary determinant of mitral inflow E-wave and A-wave velocities?

A. Transmitral pressure gradient
B. Mitral valve area
C. Left ventricular compliance
D. Left atrial compliance

Answer A. Transmitral pressure gradient

Explanation: Out of the variables listed, the pressure gradient between the left atrium and the left ventricle during diastolic filling, is the primary single determinant of the mitral inflow velocities. Other variables such as preload, LV compliance, LV lusitropy (relaxation), LA contractile state, and mitral inflow obstruction (stenosis) will also affect mitral E-wave and A-wave velocities but to a lesser extent [28].

Question 45

What is an advantage of continuous wave Doppler over pulsed wave Doppler?

A. Aliasing
B. Range resolution
C. Assessing the severity of regurgitant flow
D. Detection of high velocities

Answer D. Detection of high velocities

Explanation: With continuous-wave Doppler ultrasound, the emitting and receiving crystals function continuously and display information representative of all moving targets along the ultrasound beam. The continuous mode has no limitation of recordable velocities and therefore allows accurate measurement of high velocities. The signal, however, is not gated (it receives all underlying velocities); thus, spatial localization of the abnormal velocities is poor.

Pulsed-wave Doppler echocardiography uses short bursts of ultrasound with a process called range gating to facilitate signal analysis from a small area at a specified depth from the transducer. This sample volume can be moved or repositioned along the path of the ultrasound beam for examination of the spatial extent of the Doppler signals in relationship to the two-dimensional image (Doppler mapping). Because the pulsed-wave Doppler technique sends and receives ultrasound intermittently, accurate recording of high-velocity signals is more difficult than with continuous-wave studies (because of aliasing). Thus, pulsed-wave Doppler has signal aliasing at high frequencies but has depth acuity, whereas continuous-wave Doppler has no signal aliasing but does have depth ambiguity [29].

Question 46
Which of the following is not a quantitative measurement of mitral regurgitation severity?

A. Vena contracta width
B. Regurgitant volume and fraction
C. Effective regurgitant orifice area
D. Continuity equation valve area

Answer D. Continuity equation valve area
Explanation: Quantitative parameters of mitral regurgitation include vena contracta width, regurgitant volume and fraction, and effective regurgitant orifice area. All have prognostic significance and are recommended to be obtained on patients with more than mild moderate regurgitation. Although these quantitative techniques are described in the literature there can be significant interobserver variability when measuring them [30]. The continuity equation valve area, along with mean gradient and jet velocity, are quantitative assessments of aortic stenosis.

Question 47
Which of the following is true regarding the measurement of the vena contracta?

A. The vena contracta is the widest portion of the mitral regurgitant jet.
B. The transducer should be adjusted as necessary to obtain the smallest mitral regurgitant jet size.
C. A modified parasternal short axis view is the best to image the vena contracta.
D. Vena contracta width measurements are less influenced by instrument settings than other quantitative techniques.

Answer D. Vena contracta width measurements are less influenced by instrument settings than other quantitative techniques.
Explanation: The vena contracta is the narrowest portion of the MR jet, at or just downstream of the mitral regurgitant orifice. The vena contracta width (VCW) is a measure of the effective regurgitant orifice area (EROA). VCW measurements are less influenced by instrument settings than other quantitative techniques [30] and are accurate indicators of MR severity, regardless of the MR etiology and jet direction. A modified parasternal long-axis view is best to image the VC with the transducer laterally translated or angulated, if necessary, to allow complete visualization of the MR jet and to capture the largest MR jet [31].

Question 48
Which of the following is true when considering the Doppler shift?

A. If the blood is approaching the ultrasound source the reflected frequency is shifted upward.
B. If the blood is moving away from the ultrasound source, then the returning frequency is higher.
C. A negative Doppler shift is represented as red on the color screen.
D. As the angle of incidence approaches 90°, the Doppler shift increases maximally

Answer A. If the blood is approaching the ultrasound source the reflected frequency is shifted upward.
Explanation: The Austrian physicist Christian Doppler is credited with reporting the phenomenon that the apparent pitch of sound was affected by motion either toward or away from the listener. You may have experienced this with the sound of an ambulance sounding differently when approaching you versus when the ambulance is driving away from you. Similarly, the frequency of the wave reflected by a moving object increases if the moving object (i.e., blood) is moving towards the transducer. By convection, a positive Doppler shift (increased in frequency) is represented as red on the color screen, and a negative Doppler shift, such as the wave reflected back from blood moving away from the transducer, is represented as blue on the color screen.

The angle of incidence affects Doppler shift, as the angle approaches 90°, no Doppler shift is detected and color may not be present where flow exists, causing an artifactual loss of color information [32].

Question 49 (Refers to Fig. 3.12 Depicted Below)
Which of the following accurately depicts the angle of incidence?

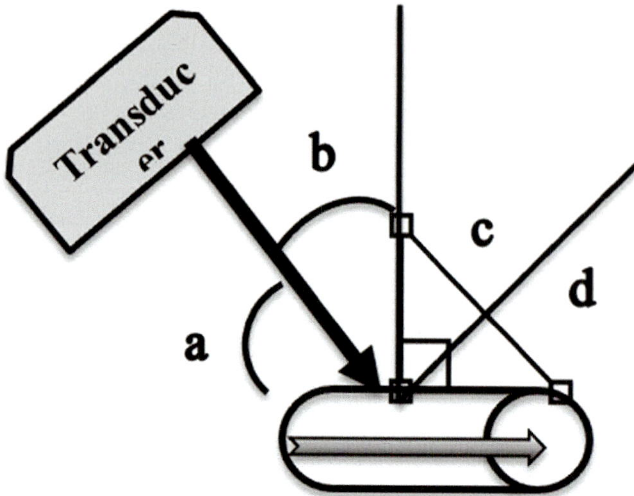

Fig. 3.12 Angle of incidence

A. a
B. b
C. a + b
D. a + d

Answer A. a

Explanation: The angle of incidence is the angle between the ultrasound beam and the vector of red blood cell flow. In the above diagram that angle is depicted by angle a. The impact of the angle on the Doppler shift will be greatest when the angle of incidence is 0°, since the cos 0° is 1, and least when the angle of incidence is 90° (the probe is exactly perpendicular to the source), since the cosine of a 90° angle is 0 [32].

Question 50

Which of the following accurately depicts the equation to calculate the velocity of blood when using Doppler?

A. $v = f \times c/2\ f_0 \times \cos\theta$
B. $v = 2\ f_0 \times \cos\theta$
C. TRvel2 = PAP/4
D. $v = Q/\pi R^2$

Answer A. v = f × c/2 f0 × cos θ

Explanation: The ultrasound beam hits moving red blood cells and reflects the beam back at a different frequency and angle, based on how the beam (probe) is positioned. The change in frequency of the reflected wave allows for the measurement of the velocity of blood. That equation is:

$$v = f \times c / 2 f_0 \times \cos\theta$$

v = velocity of red blood cell targets, f = Doppler shift frequency, f_0 = transmitted ultrasound beam frequency, θ = angle between the ultrasound beam and the vector of red blood cell flow, c = velocity of ultrasound in blood (approximately 1570 m/s)

Choice C depicts a variation of the modified Bernoulli's equation used to estimate pulmonary pressure from the peak velocity in the tricuspid regurgitation jet. Choice D is the basic volumetric Doppler equation where Q is flow (ml/s) and the πR^2 represents the cross-sectional area (cm^2) and v is the velocity of blood in cm/s [33].

Question 51

Aliasing occurs with pulsed-wave Doppler due to which of the following?

A. High Nyquist limit
B. High pulse repetition frequency
C. Angle of incidence approaches 90°
D. Sample signal used over continuous recording.

Answer D. Sample signal used over continuous recording.

Explanation: During pulsed-wave Doppler ultrasound beams are emitted in "pulses". The same transducer element receives the reflected signal from each pulse. As every emitted pulse is paired with a corresponding return signal, it is possible to determine where the reflection has occurred and calculate the distance of the "reflector". The frequency of these pulses is the pulse repetition frequency (PRF), which is the number of pulses within one second. The PRF limit within which aliasing occurs is known as the aliasing or Nyquist limit. Specifically, aliasing occurs when the velocity is more than one half of the pulse repetition frequency. In this case velocities above this limit will be displayed on the tracing opposite to the true direction of blood flow.

Question 52

Which of the following is the recommended Nyquist limit for color-flow Doppler?

A. 30–40 cm/s
B. 40–50 cm/s
C. 50–60 cm/s
D. 60–70 cm/s

Answer C. 50–60 cm/s

Explanation: The Nyquist limit for cardiac imaging as recommended by the American Society of Echocardiography (ASE) guidelines should be set between 50 cm/s and 60 cm/s. This limit may be adjusted higher for faster heart rate or increased hemodynamic flows or lower to visualize lower flow velocities. Nyquist limits below 40 cm/s may be too low for cardiac imaging and will overestimate quantification of regurgitant flow. Similarly, a color Nyquist limit above 60 cm/s is too high and may underestimate quantification of regurgitant flow [34].

Question 53

A 56-year-old man is intubated for increased work of breathing and hypoxia. The lung ultrasound (see Video 3.9) shows a large pleural effusion (blue arrow) surrounding consolidated lung tissue, and the thoracic spine located posteriorly (orange arrows). The "spine sign" represents which of the following artifacts?

A. Acoustic shadowing
B. Posterior acoustic enhancement
C. Reverberation
D. Mirror image

Answer B. Posterior acoustic enhancement

Explanation: The "spine sign", in which the thoracic spine is seen cephalad to the diaphragm, occurs as a result of posterior acoustic enhancement. In normally aerated lung, ultrasound waves are almost completely reflected due to high acoustic mismatch between tissue and air, precluding visualization of deeper structures. By contrast, fluid is poorly attenuating and allows increased through transmission of ultrasound waves, which results in a brighter, more hyperechoic appearance of structures immediately posterior to the fluid-containing space. Thus, in the presence of a pleural effusion, ultrasound waves are able to pass through the thoracic cavity with resultant acoustic enhancement and visualization of the thoracic spine [35].

Question 54

Decreasing power and increasing overall gain will do which of the following?

A. Increase energy transmitted to the tissue and decrease the returning signal amplitude
B. Increase energy transmitted to the tissue and increase the returning signal amplitude
C. Decrease energy transmitted to the tissue and decrease the returning signal amplitude
D. Decrease energy transmitted to the tissue and increase the returning signal amplitude

Answer D. Decrease energy transmitted to the tissue and increase the returning signal amplitude

Explanation: Increasing the power increases the energy and the heat transmitted to the patient's tissue. Adjusting gain manipulates the brightness of the field by adjusting the amplitude of the received signal; increasing overall gain will amplify the signal returning to the machine [36].

Question 55

Tissue Doppler imaging quantifies the velocities of myocardial structures by assessing which of the following types of signals?

A. Low velocity, low amplitude
B. Low velocity, high amplitude
C. High velocity, low amplitude
D. High velocity, high amplitude

Answer B. Low velocity, high amplitude

Explanation: Blood cells move at a faster speed and have lower amplitude signals than cardiac structures. Thus, conventional Doppler imaging quantifies the velocity of blood cells by filtering out lower velocity, higher amplitude signals. Tissue doppler imaging reverses these filters to allow for quantification of the slower velocity, higher amplitude signals from myocardial tissue [7].

Question 56

Which of the following statements most accurately describes the differences between continuous-wave (CWD) and pulsed-wave doppler (PWD)?

A. CWD measures slower velocities than PWD but allows for depth specification
B. CWD measures slower velocities than PWD but does not allow for depth specification
C. CWD measures higher velocities than PWD but allows for depth specification
D. CWD measures higher velocities than PWD but does not allow for depth specification

Answer D. CWD measures higher velocities than PWD but does not allow for depth specification

Explanation: Continuous-wave Doppler utilizes two separate crystals to continuously transmit and receive ultrasound signals, which allows for the measurement of high velocities. This modality measures all velocities along a specified line and does not allow for quantification at a specific depth. In pulsed-wave Doppler, a single crystal sends and receives signals, which limits the velocity that can be quantified. Signals are analyzed from a specific depth along the Doppler line, which allows for localization of velocities and better depth perception [37].

Question 57

In this lung ultrasound video (see Video 3.10), which of the following combinations of arrows indicate reverberation artifact?

A. Red and green arrows
B. Red and blue arrows
C. Green and yellow arrows
D. Yellow and blue arrows

Answer D. Yellow and blue arrows

Explanation: Reverberation artifacts occur when an ultrasound beam is reflected back and forth between two highly reflective surfaces multiple times. A-lines (yellow and blue arrows) are an example of a reverberation artifact, where the ultrasound beam is reflected back and forth between the pleural interface and the transducer. The initial ultrasound beam is reflected from an intact pleural line back to the transducer, which provides an image of the pleural line with lung sliding (green arrow). However, the returning beam is reflected off of the transducer and back into the tissue, where it is once again reflected from the pleural line. This second signal returns to the transducer after a time delay, and the machine interprets this delay as the presence of a deeper structure. This cycle may repeat multiple times. A-lines appear as parallel hyperechoic lines that are spaced at intervals equivalent to the distance between the transducer and the pleural line: the distance between the lines indicated by the yellow and blue arrows is equivalent to the distance between the transducer and the pleural line. The red arrow indicates the surface of the rib [21].

Question 58

Doppler assessment of flow across the aortic valve is performed (See Fig. 3.13). The maximum velocity is associated with which of the following locations?

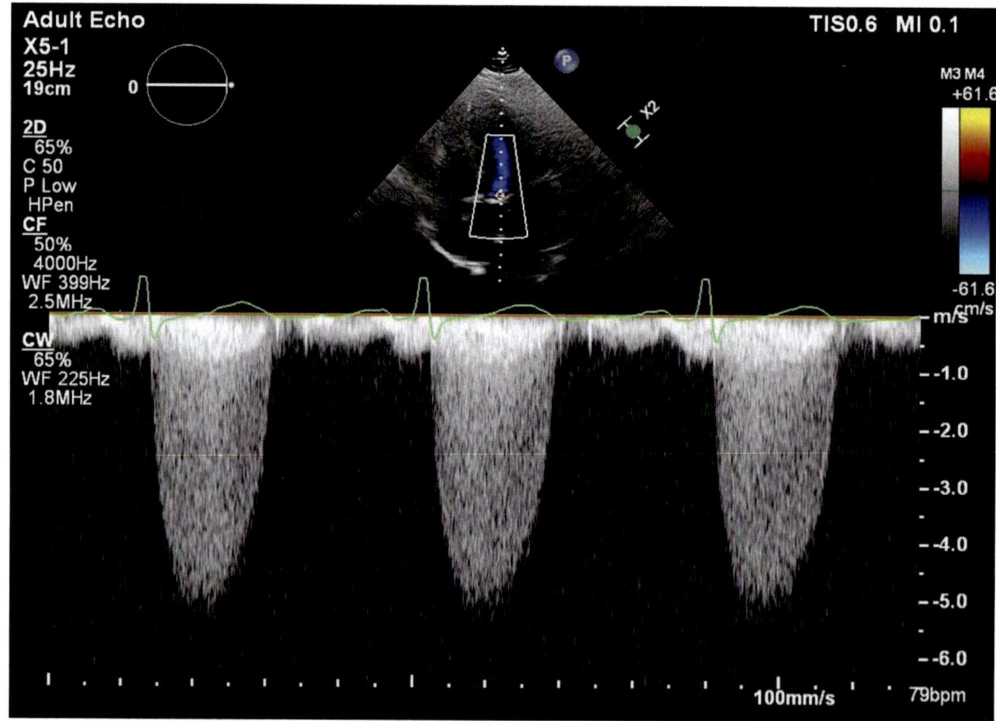

Fig. 3.13 Doppler assessment of flow across the aortic valve

A. The level of the aortic valve
B. At a set sampling location along the interrogation line
C. The ventricular outflow tract
D. At some location along the interrogation line

Answer D. At some location along the interrogation line

Explanation: Continuous-wave Doppler measures all velocities along the dotted interrogation line. This modality can quantify high velocities but cannot specify the location of the peak velocity. In pulsed-wave Doppler, a sampling location is specified, allowing for the localization of peak velocity [37].

Question 59
In the spectral Doppler profile below (Fig. 3.14), which of the following statements is most accurate?

A. The Doppler profile shows the velocity of blood at a specified location along the interrogation line
B. The Doppler profile shows the velocity of a cardiac structure at a specified location along the interrogation line
C. The Doppler profile shows the velocity of blood at some unknown location along the interrogation line
D. The Doppler profile shows the velocity of a cardiac structure at some unknown location along the interrogation line

Answer A. The Doppler profile shows the velocity of blood at a specified location along the interrogation line

Explanation: This spectral Doppler profile (Fig. 3.14) shows pulsed-wave Doppler interrogation of blood flow across the mitral valve. The velocities shown are for a **specific** sampling location on the dotted interrogation line. Continuous-wave Doppler shows **all** blood flow

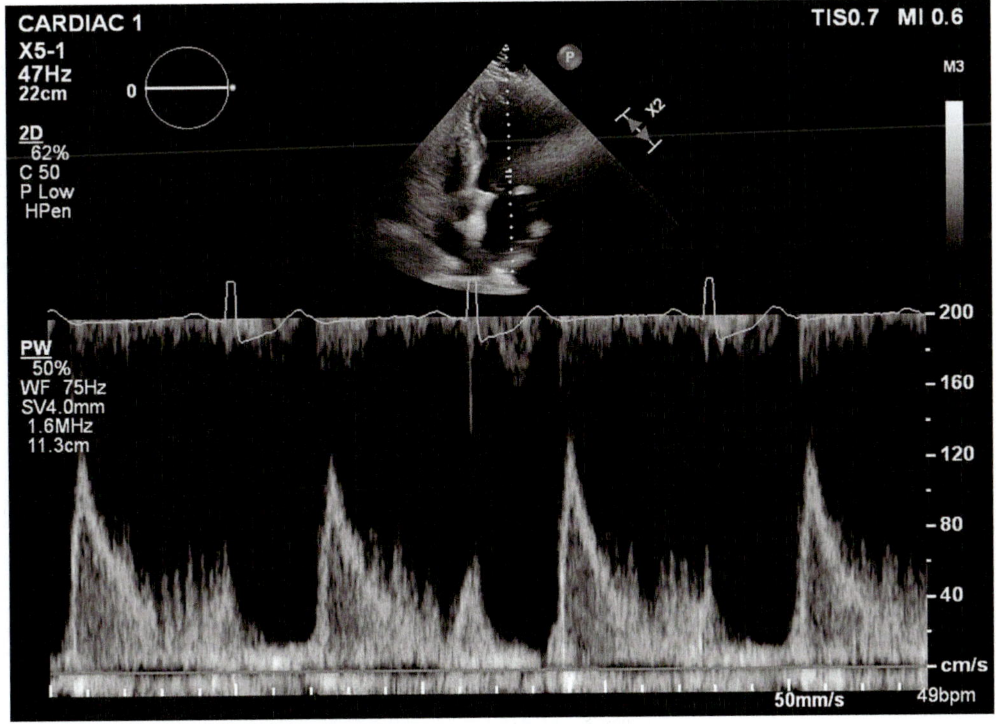

Fig. 3.14 PW Doppler interrogation of blood flow across the mitral valve

velocities along the interrogation line and will therefore have a solid, 'filled-in' appearance. Tissue Doppler imaging can be used to quantify myocardial velocity at a specific location.

Question 60

The modality used in the image below (Fig. 3.15) displays which of the following?

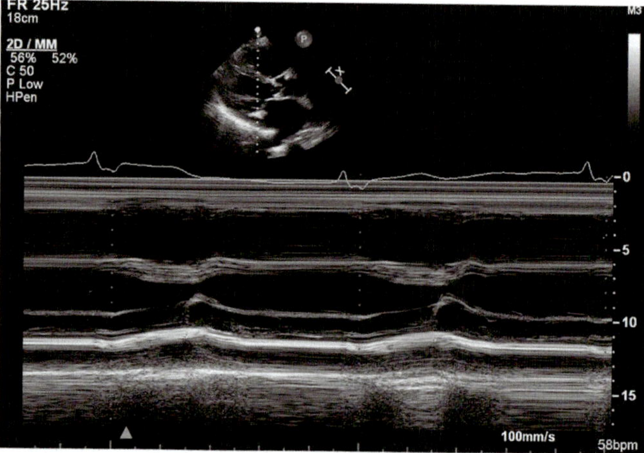

Fig. 3.15 M-mode though the parasternal long axis view

A. Movement of all cardiac structures located along a single line over time.
B. Movement of all cardiac structures located in the sector over time
C. Movement of blood flow along a single line over time
D. Movement of blood flow throughout the sector over time

Answer A. Movement of all cardiac structures located along a single line over time.

Explanation: M-mode imaging displays the movement of tissues **along a single line** over time. Given its high frame rate in excess of 1000 frames/s, it is an ideal modality to evaluate the timing and motion of cardiac structures.

Question 61

Which of the following is true regarding the measurements shown in Fig. 3.16?

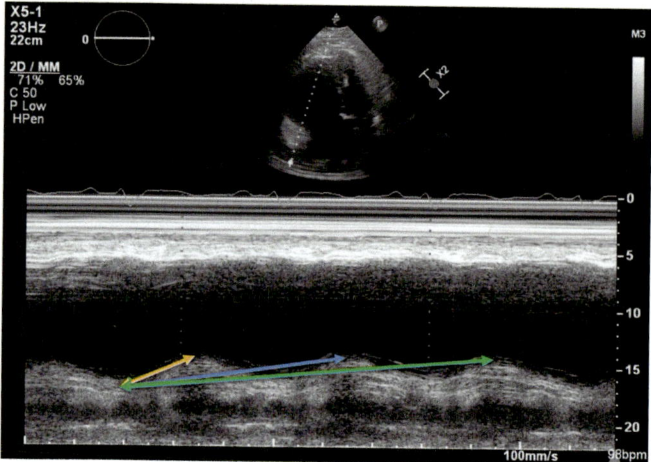

Fig. 3.16 TAPSE measurement

A. Yellow arrow shows a measurement smaller than green arrow
B. Yellow arrow shows a measurement smaller than blue arrow
C. **Yellow arrow shows a measurement approximately the same size as all arrows**
D. Yellow arrow shows a measurement of no diagnostic value

Answer C. Yellow arrow shows a measurement approximately the same size as all arrows

Explanation: Figure 3.16 shows an apical four chamber view with an M-mode cursor parallel with the RV free wall as it meets the tricuspid annulus. The displacement of this measurement is the tricuspid annular plane systolic excursion, also known as TAPSE. Values <17 mm are abnormal and has strong association with outcomes in pulmonary hypertension. In the M-mode window, the x-axis is time, and the y-axis is the position along the M-mode (translational distance over time). Since all arrows are measuring approximately the same position of the tricuspid annular plane, all measurements are likely to be the similar [38].

Question 62

Which of the following is true regarding the measurement in Fig. 3.17?

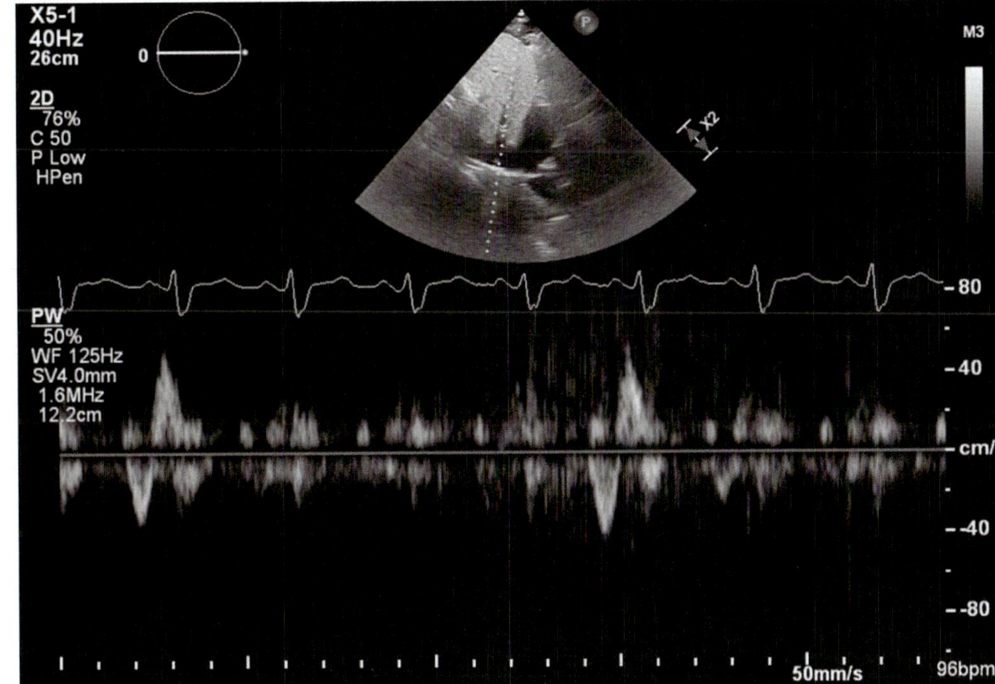

Fig. 3.17 Hepatic vein flow with pulse wave Doppler

A. It is influenced by aliasing
B. It can measure velocities of high speed
C. Changes of left atrial pressure will be transmitted into this structure
D. Cardiac tamponade will reverse the flow

Answer D. Cardiac tamponade will reverse the flow

Explanation: Figure 3.17 shows a pulse wave Doppler sample taken at the hepatic vein in a subcostal inferior vena cava window. Pulse wave Doppler unlike continuous-wave Doppler is limited in the velocities it can measure. Aliasing will occur with pulse wave Doppler when the velocity exceeds the Nyquist limit, or one half of the pulse repetition frequency (PRF). An exaggerated expiratory decrease in diastolic forward ***flow*** and increase in ***reverse flow*** in the ***hepatic vein*** is a characteristic of patients with ***cardiac tamponade*** [39].

Question 63

Which of the following is true regarding the echo loop in Video 3.11?

A. Measurement of tricuspid regurgitation is not possible in this view
B. Measurement of pulmonary insufficiency is not possible in this view
C. The aortic valve is not well visualized in this view
D. Tilting the probe caudally will attain the short axis view of the mitral valve

Answer D. Tilting the probe caudally will attain the short axis view of the mitral valve

Explanation: The echo loop shows a parasternal short axis view at the aortic level. There is right ventricular hypertrophy and a moderately enlarged right ventricle. The aortic valve is well visualized at its short axis and there is good aortic opening. This short axis view at the aortic level allows the continuous Doppler bean to align well with the tricuspid valve and the pulmonic valve. It is one of the views that allows for tricuspid and pulmonic valve interrogation. The **Parasternal Short Axis view** at the **mitral** valve **level** shows the **short axis** of the **mitral** valve. This **view** is obtained by tilting the tip of the transducer caudally, to scan inferiorly beneath the **aortic** valve in **short axis.**

Question 64

Which of the following is true regarding the echo loop depicted in Video 3.12?

A. The right ventricular function is normal, and the left ventricular function is reduced
B. The right ventricular function is normal, and the left ventricular function is normal
C. There are prominent trabeculations in the right ventricle
D. There is a prominent pericardial effusion

Answer C. There are prominent trabeculations in the right ventricle

Explanation: Video 3.12 shows a parasternal short axis mid papillary view of a patient with moderately enlarged right ventricle with markedly reduced ejection fraction. The left ventricle has a normal ejection fraction. The loop also shows prominent trabeculations in the right ventricle. A prominent trabeculation in the right ventricle is the moderator band. Trabeculations are cardiac muscle bundles that extends into the ventricular chamber and it is a normal remnant of heart development. There is no pericardial effusion seen on this view.

Question 65

Which of the following is true regarding the echo loop depicted in Video 3.13?

A. Tilting the probe cephalad will attain the mitral valve at its short axis.
B. Tilting the probe caudal will attain the mid papillary view
C. The structure between the right atrium and right ventricle is not an artifact
D. The structure between the left atrium and left ventricle is an artifact

Answer C. The structure between the right atrium and right ventricle is not an artifact

Explanation: Video 3.13 shows the parasternal short axis view at the level of the aortic valve. There is a serpiginous thrombus extending from the right atrium to the right ventricle. There is also a severely dilated right ventricle with severely reduced function. You can rest assured this structure is not an artifact since it moves appropriately with the cardiac cycle. It's shape is also irregular and does not violate myocardial borders. In this view, the left ventricle is not well visualized. From this parasternal short axis level, tilting the probe caudal (towards feet) will attain the mitral valve at its short axis. Tilting the probe cephalad (towards the head) will attain the pulmonary artery view.

References

1. Mitchell C, Rahko PS, Blauwet LA, Canaday B, Finstuen JA, Foster MC, et al. Guidelines for performing a comprehensive transthoracic echocardiographic examination in adults: recommendations from the American Society of Echocardiography. J Am Soc Echocardiogr. 2019;32(1):1–64.
2. American Institute of Ultrasound in Medicine. Transducer manipulation for echocardiography. J Ultrasound Med. 2005;24(5):733–6.
3. Enriquez JL, Wu TS. An introduction to ultrasound equipment and knobology. Crit Care Clin. 2014;30(1):25–45.
4. Markowitz J. Probe selection, machine controls, and equipment. In: Carmody KA, Moore CL, Feller-Kopman D, editors. Handbook of critical care and emergency ultrasound. New York: McGraw-Hill Medical; 2011. p. 25–38.
5. Otto CM. Principles of echocardiographic image acquisition and doppler analysis. In: Textbook of clinical echocardiography. 5th ed. Philadelphia: Saunders; 2013. p. 1–30.
6. Quiñones MA, Otto CM, Stoddard M, Waggoner A, Zoghbi WA. Recommendations for quantification of Doppler echocardiography: a report from the Doppler quantification task force of the nomenclature and standards committee of the American Society of Echocardiography. J Am Soc Echocardiogr. 2002;15(2):167–84.
7. Wiafe YA, Badu-Peprah A. The influence of ultrasound equipment knobology in abdominal sonography. In: Gamie SAA, Foda EM, editors. Essentials of abdominal ultrasound. London: IntechOpen; 2019. https://doi.org/10.5772/intechopen.83713. https://www.intechopen.com/chapters/65515.
8. Lieu D. Ultrasound physics and instrumentation for pathologists. Arch Pathol Lab Med. 2010;134(10):1541–56.
9. Uppal T. Tissue harmonic imaging. Australas J Ultrasound Med. 2010;13(2):29–31.
10. American Institute of Ultrasound in Medicine. Section 7–discussion of the mechanical index and other exposure parameters. J Ultrasound Med. 2000;19(2):143–8.
11. O'Brien WD. Standard means for the reporting of the acoustic output of medical diagnostic ultrasonic equipment. Proceeding of the Society of Diagnostic Medical Sonographers Conference; 1994, p. 317–26.
12. Otto CM. Normal anatomy and flow patterns on transthoracic echocardiography. In: Textbook of clinical echocardiography. 5th ed. Philadelphia: Saunders; 2013. p. 31–64.
13. Henry WL, Demaria A, Gramiak R, King DL, Kisslo JA, Popp RL, et al. Report of the American Society of Echocardiography Committee on nomenclature and standards in two-dimensional echocardiography. Circulation. 1980;62(2):212–7.
14. Quien MM, Saric M. Ultrasound imaging artifacts: how to recognize them and how to avoid them. Echocardiography. 2018;35(9):1388–401.
15. Picano E, Scali MC, Ciampi Q, Lichtenstein D. Lung ultrasound for the cardiologist. J Am Coll Cardiol Img. 2018;11(11):1692–705.
16. Enriquez JL, Wu T. An introduction to ultrasound equipment and knobology. Crit Care Clin. 2014;30:25–45.
17. American Institute of Ultrasound in Medicine. AIUM practice guidelines for the performance of the focused assessment with sonography for trauma (FAST) examination. J Ultrasound Med. 2008;27(2):313–8.
18. Shriki J. Ultrasound physics. Crit Care Clin. 2014;30:1–24.
19. Zagzebski JA. Essentials of ultrasound physics. St. Louis: Mosby; 1996.
20. Mahesh M. The essential physics of medical imaging, third edition. Med Phys. 2013;40:7.
21. Prabhu SJ, Kanal K, Bhargava P, Vaidya S, Dighe MK. Ultrasound artifacts: classification, applied physics with illustrations, and imaging appearances. Ultrasound Q. 2014;30(2):145–57.
22. Scanlan KA. Sonographic artifacts and their origins. AJR Am J Roentgenol. 1991;156(6):1267–72.
23. Pozniak MA, Zagzebski JA, Scanlan KA. Spectral and color Doppler artifacts. Radiographics. 1992;12(1):35–44.
24. Lichtenstein DA, Mezière GA, Lagoueyte JF, Biderman P, Goldstein I, Gepner A. A-lines and B-lines: lung ultrasound as a bedside tool for predicting pulmonary artery occlusion pressure in the critically ill. Chest. 2009;136(4):1014–20.
25. Slater A, Goodwin M, Anderson KE, Gleeson FV. COPD can mimic the appearance of pneumothorax on thoracic ultrasound. Chest. 2006;129(3):545–50.
26. Blaivas M, Tsung JW. Point-of-care sonographic detection of left endobronchial main stem intubation and obstruction versus endotracheal intubation. J Ultrasound Med. 2008;27(5):785–9.
27. Soldati G, Copetti R, Sher S. Sonographic interstitial syndrome: the sound of lung water. J Ultrasound Med. 2009;28(2):163–74.
28. Appleton CP, Hatle LK, Popp RL. Relation of transmitral flow velocity patterns to left ventricular diastolic function: new insights from a combined hemodynamic and Doppler echocardiographic study. J Am Coll Cardiol. 1988;12(2):426–40.
29. Reeder GS, Currie PJ, Hagler DJ, Tajik AJ, Seward JB. Use of Doppler techniques (continuous-wave, pulsed-wave, and color flow imaging) in the noninvasive hemodynamic assessment of congenital heart disease. Mayo Clin Proc. 1986;61(9):725–44.
30. Thavendiranathan P, Phelan D, Collier P, Thomas JD, Flamm SD, Marwick TH. Quantitative assessment of mitral regurgitation: how best to do it. JACC Cardiovasc Imaging. 2012;5(11):1161–75.
31. Zoghbi WA, Enriquez-Sarano M, Foster E, Grayburn PA, Kraft CD, Levine RA, et al. Recommendations for evaluation of the severity of native valvular regurgitation with two-dimensional and Doppler echocardiography. J Am Soc Echocardiogr. 2003;16(7):777–802.
32. Rubens DJ, Bhatt S, Nedelka S, Cullinan J. Doppler artifacts and pitfalls. Radiol Clin N Am. 2006;44(6):805–35.
33. Hoskins PR. A review of the measurement of blood velocity and related quantities using Doppler ultrasound. Proc Inst Mech Eng. 1999;213:391–400.
34. Zoghbi WA, Enriquez-Sarano M, Foster E, Grayburn PA, Kraft CD, Levine RA, Nihoyannopoulos P, Otto CM, Quinones MA, Rakowski H, Stewart WJ, Waggoner A, Weissman NJ, American Society of Echocardiography. Recommendations for evaluation of the severity of native valvular regurgitation with two-dimensional and Doppler echocardiography. J Am Soc Echocardiogr. 2003;16(7):777–802.
35. Goffi A, Kruisselbrink R, Volpicelli G. The sound of air: point-of-care lung ultrasound in perioperative medicine. Can J Anesth. 2018;65:399–416.
36. Ho C, Solomon S. A clinician's guide to tissue doppler imaging. Circulation. 2006;113:e396–8.
37. Harris P, Kuppurao L. Quantitative Doppler echocardiography. BJA Educ. 2016;16(2):46–52.
38. Alerhand S, Hickey SM. Tricuspid annular plane systolic excursion (TAPSE) for risk stratification and prognostication of patients with pulmonary embolism. J Emerg Med. 2020;58(3):449–56.
39. Burstow DJ, Oh JK, Bailey KR, Seward JB, Tajik AJ. Cardiac tamponade: characteristic Doppler observations. Mayo Clin Proc. 1989;64(3):312–24.

4 LV Segments and Chamber Quantification

Saqer Alkharabsheh and Patrick Collier

Question 1
Which segmental model of the left ventricle is highlighted in Fig. 4.1?

A. 16 segment model
B. 17 segment model
C. 18 segment model
D. All of these
E. None of these

Answer: B. 17 segment model. Figure 4.1 provides a classical graphical representation of the relevant segments within a 17 segmental model of the left ventricle. The outer circle divisions represent 6 basal wall segments. Moving inwards, the next circle divisions represent 6 mid-wall segments, inside which are a further 5 apical segments. It is a frequently used segmentation model as it includes a central true apical segment (unlike the 16-segment model which has 4 apical segments), without relative over-representation of the apex (unlike the 18-segment model which has 6 apical segments).

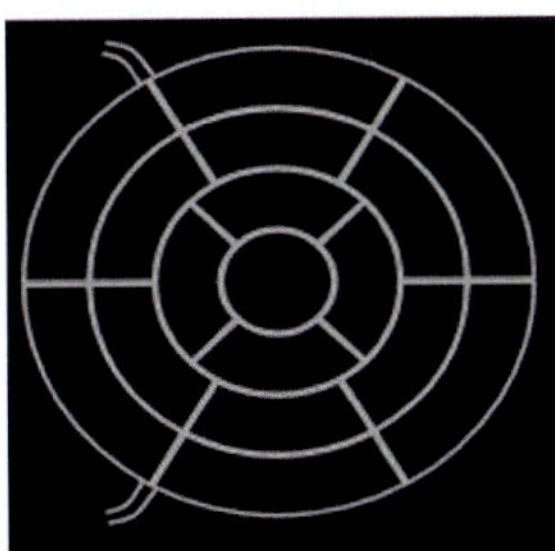

Fig. 4.1 Graphical representation of segments of the left ventricle

Question 2
Which left ventricular segments are highlighted in Fig. 4.2?

A. Anterior
B. Antero-septal
C. Infero-septal
D. Antero-lateral
E. Infero-lateral (posterior)

Answer: D. Antero-lateral. Figure 4.2 highlights the antero-lateral left ventricular segments. Starting from the bottom left, the highlighted green segments are the apical lateral wall, the mid antero-lateral wall and the basal antero-lateral wall respectively. This territory is typically supplied by the left circumflex coronary artery. It forms the anterior part of the "free wall of the left ventricle" as it opposes (is opposite to) the infero-septum. The apical 4-chamber view delineates segments of the antero-lateral cardiac wall (and the opposing infero-septum).

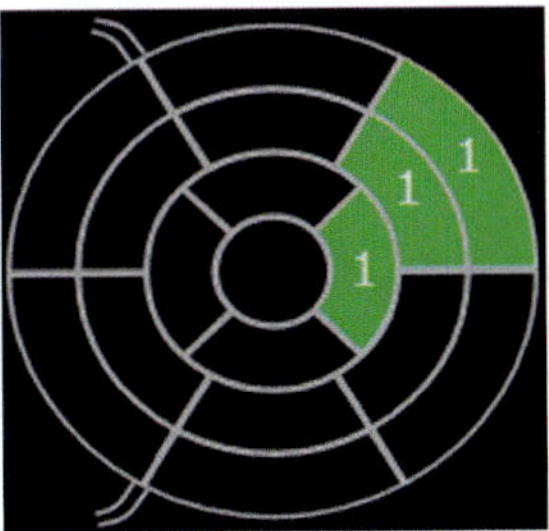

Fig. 4.2 Graphical representation of specific segments of the left ventricle

Supplementary Information The online version contains supplementary material available at https://doi.org/10.1007/978-3-031-45731-9_4.

S. Alkharabsheh · P. Collier (✉)
Robert and Suzanne Tomsich Department of Cardiovascular Medicine, Sydell and Arnold Miller Family Heart and Vascular Institute, The Cleveland Clinic Foundation, Cleveland, OH, USA
e-mail: ALKHARS@ccf.org; colliep@ccf.org

R. Sreedharan et al. (eds.), *Critical Care Echocardiography*, https://doi.org/10.1007/978-3-031-45731-9_4

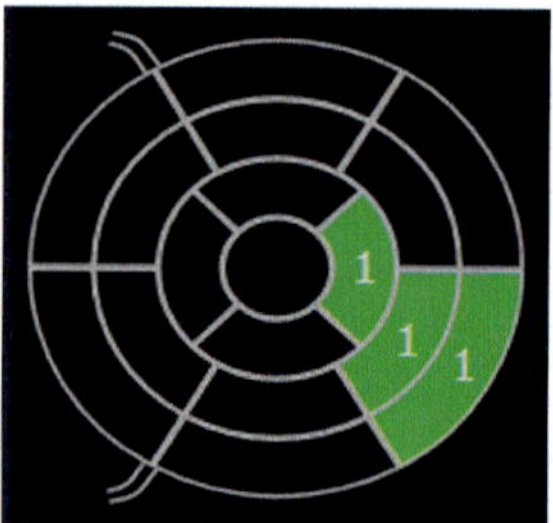

Fig. 4.3 Graphical representation of specific segments of the left ventricle

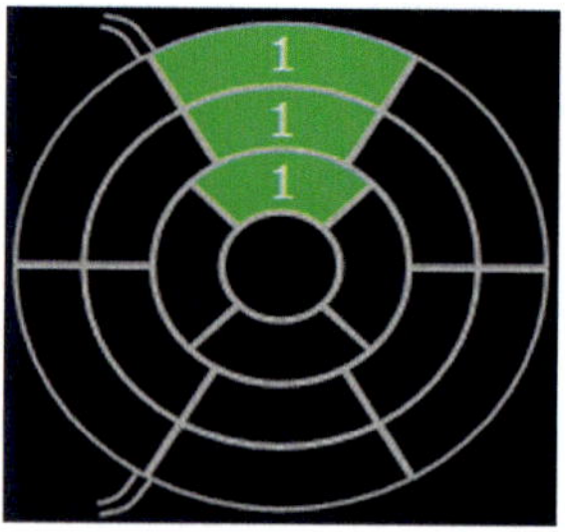

Fig. 4.4 Graphical representation of specific segments of the left ventricle

Question 3
Which left ventricular segments are highlighted in Fig. 4.3?

A. Inferior
B. Antero-septal
C. Infero-septal
D. Antero-lateral
E. Infero-lateral (posterior)

Answer: E. Infero-lateral (posterior). Figure 4.3 highlights the infero-lateral (posterior) left ventricular segments. Starting from the top left, the highlighted green segments are the apical lateral wall, the mid infero-lateral (posterior) wall and the basal infero-lateral (posterior) wall respectively. This territory is typically supplied by the left circumflex coronary artery. It forms the posterior part of the "free wall of the left ventricle" as it opposes (is opposite to) the antero-septum. The apical 3-chamber view delineates segments of the infero-lateral (posterior) cardiac wall (and the opposing antero-septum).

Question 4
Which left ventricular segments are highlighted in Fig. 4.4?

A. Anterior
B. Antero-septal
C. Infero-septal
D. Antero-lateral
E. Infero-lateral (posterior)

Answer: A. Anterior. Figure 4.4 highlights the anterior left ventricular segments. Starting from the top, the highlighted green segments are the basal anterior wall, the mid anterior wall and the apical anterior wall respectively. This territory is typically supplied by the left anterior descending coronary artery. The apical 2-chamber view delineates segments of the anterior cardiac wall (and the opposing inferior wall).

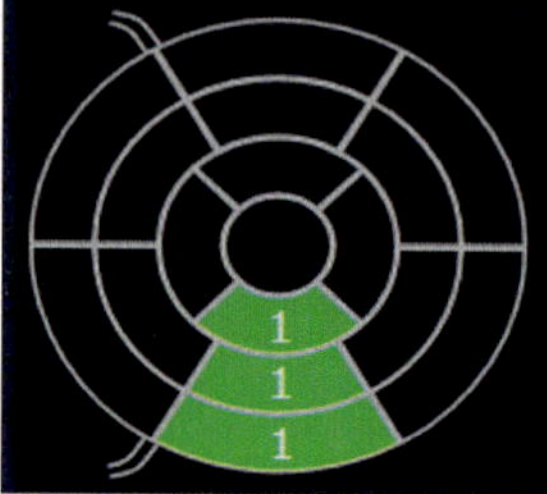

Fig. 4.5 Graphical representation of specific segments of the left ventricle

Question 5
Which left ventricular segments are highlighted in Fig. 4.5?

A. Inferior
B. Antero-septal
C. Infero-septal
D. Antero-lateral
E. Infero-lateral (posterior)

Answer: A. Inferior. Figure 4.5 highlights the inferior left ventricular segments. Starting from the bottom, the highlighted green segments are the basal inferior wall, the mid inferior wall and the apical inferior wall respectively. This territory is typically supplied by the right coronary artery. The apical 2-chamber view delineates segments of the inferior cardiac wall (and the opposing anterior wall).

Question 6
Which left ventricular segments are highlighted in Fig. 4.6?

A. Anterior
B. Antero-septal
C. Infero-septal
D. Antero-lateral
E. Infero-lateral (posterior)

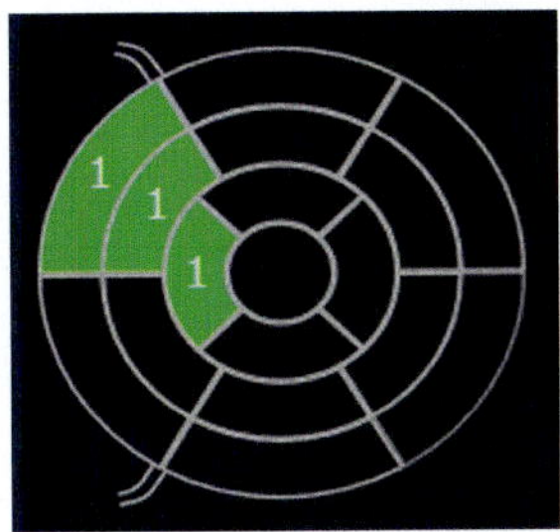

Fig. 4.6 Graphical representation of specific segments of the left ventricle

Answer: B. Antero-septal. Figure 4.6 highlights the antero-septal left ventricular segments. The double lines extending from the outer circle demarcate septal segments with the antero-septum on top and the infero-septum on the bottom. Starting from the top left, the highlighted green segments are the basal antero-septal wall, the mid antero-septal wall and the apical septal wall respectively. This territory is typically supplied by the left anterior descending coronary artery. The apical 3-chamber view delineates segments of the antero-septal cardiac wall (and the opposing infero-lateral or posterior wall).

Question 7
Which left ventricular segments are highlighted in Fig. 4.7?

A. Inferior
B. Antero-septal
C. Infero-septal
D. Antero-lateral
E. Infero-lateral (posterior)

Answer: C. Infero-septal. Figure 4.7 highlights the infero-septal left ventricular segments. The double lines extending from the outer circle demarcate septal segments with the antero-septum on top and the infero-septum on the bottom. Starting from the bottom left, the highlighted green segments are the basal infero-septal wall, the mid infero-septal wall and the apical septal wall respectively. This territory is typically supplied by the right coronary artery. The apical 4-chamber view delineates segments of the infero-septal cardiac wall segments (and the opposing antero-lateral wall).

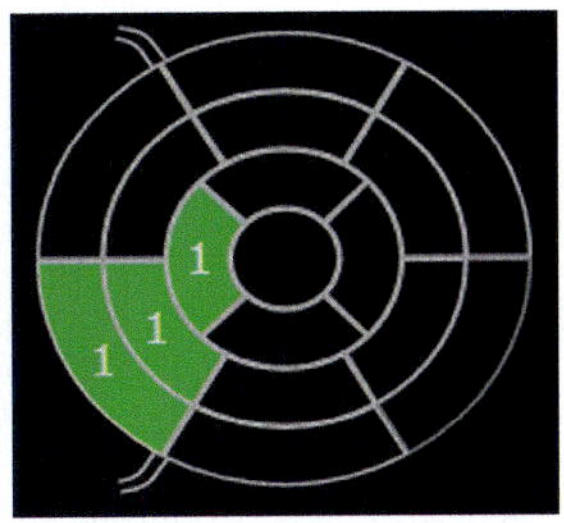

Fig. 4.7 Graphical representation of specific segments of the left ventricle

Question 8
The apical 4 chamber view demonstrates which walls highlighted in Fig. 4.8?

A. A&B
B. C&D
C. E&F
D. A&F
E. B&E

Answer: D. A&F. The apical 4-chamber view delineates segments of the antero-lateral (A) and the infero-septal (F) cardiac walls.

Question 9
The apical 3 chamber view demonstrates which walls highlighted in Fig. 4.8?

A. A&B
B. C&D
C. E&F
D. A&F
E. B&E

Answer: B. C&D. The apical 3-chamber view delineates segments of the antero-septum (C) and the infero-lateral or posterior (D) cardiac walls.

Question 10
The apical 2 chamber view demonstrates which walls highlighted in Fig. 4.8?

A. A&B
B. C&D
C. E&F
D. A&F
E. B&E

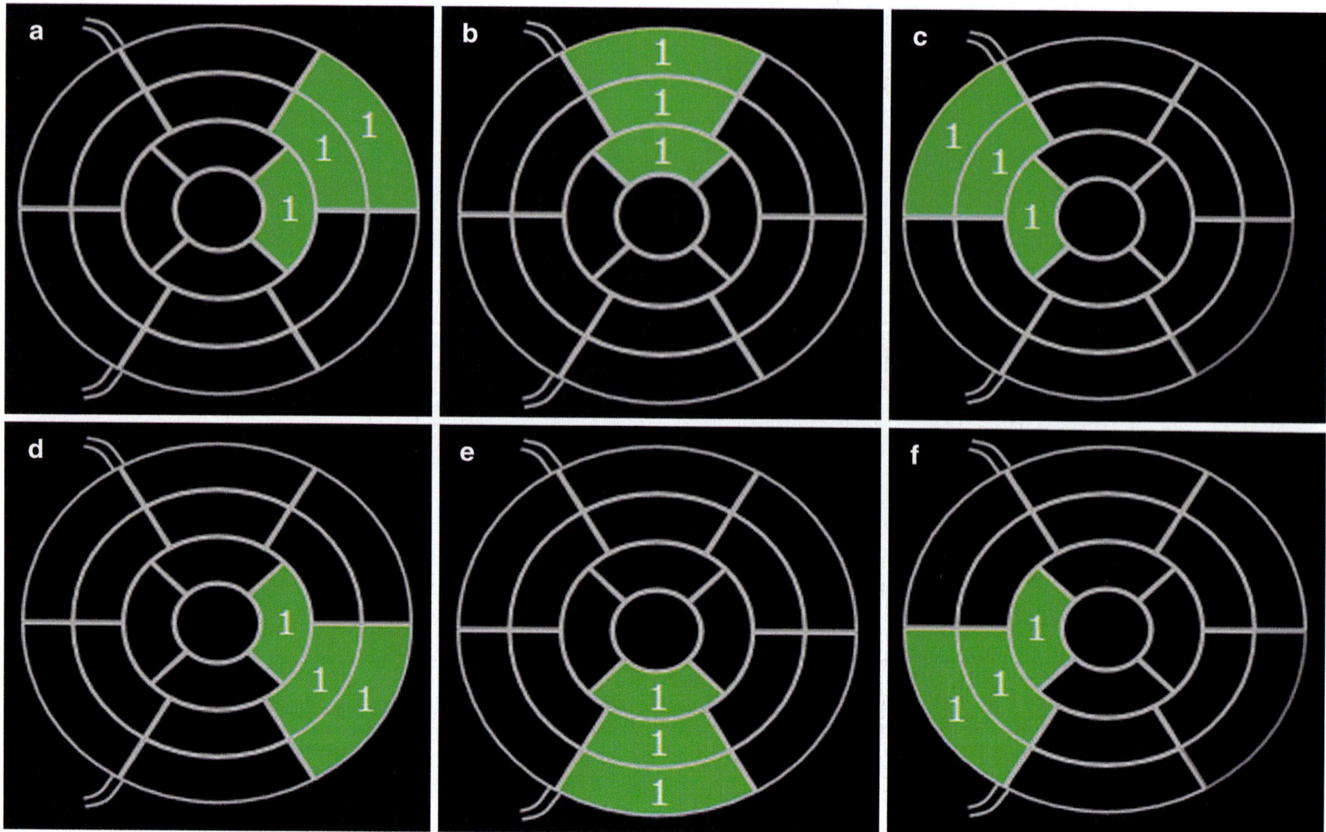

Fig. 4.8 Graphical representation of specific segments of the left ventricle

Answer: E. B&E. The apical 2-chamber view delineates segments of the anterior (B) and the inferior (E) cardiac walls.

Question 11

Which echocardiographic view is highlighted in Fig. 4.9 (and Video 4.1)?

A. Parasternal long axis
B. Parasternal short axis
C. Apical 4-chamber view
D. Apical 2-chamber view
E. Apical 3-chamber view

Answer: C. Apical 4-chamber view. Figure 4.9 highlights the apical 4-chamber view (center panel) which is a horizontal long axis view of the heart (the plane created by slicing the heart along the white line in the right panel), sometimes called the 0^0 view. In the left panel, the highlighted green segments in the apical 4-chamber view (starting from the bottom left) are the basal infero-septum, the mid infero-septum, the apical septum, the true apex, the apical lateral wall, the mid antero-lateral wall and the basal antero-lateral wall respectively. The apical 4-chamber view is best obtained by placing the echo transducer in the fourth or fifth intercostal space with the orientation marker facing the patient's left shoulder.

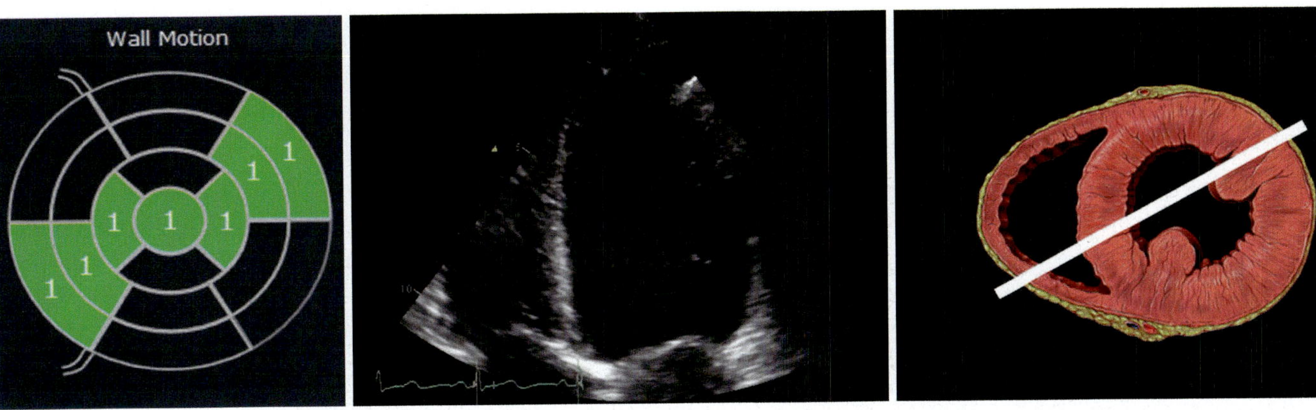

Fig. 4.9 Graphical representation of specific segments of the left ventricle (left panel), with the corresponding echo image (middle panel), and the equivalent slice of the left ventricle in a 3d short axis model (right panel)

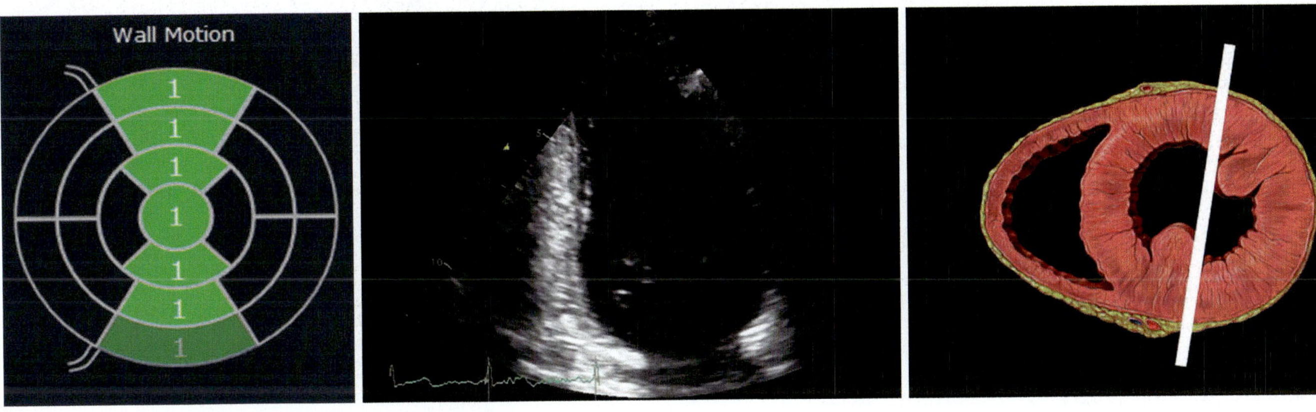

Fig. 4.10 Graphical representation of specific segments of the left ventricle (left panel), with the corresponding echo image (middle panel), and the equivalent slice of the left ventricle in a 3d short axis model (right panel)

Question 12
Which echocardiographic view is highlighted in Fig. 4.10 (and Video 4.2)?

A. Parasternal long axis
B. Parasternal short axis
C. Apical 4-chamber view
D. Apical 2-chamber view
E. Apical 3-chamber view

Answer: D. Apical 2-chamber view. Figure 4.10 highlights the apical 2-chamber view (center panel) which is a vertical long axis view of the heart (the plane created by slicing the heart along the white line in the right panel), sometimes called the 90^0 view. In the left panel, the highlighted green segments in the apical 4-chamber view (starting from the top) are the basal anterior wall, the mid anterior wall, the apical anterior wall, the true apex, the apical inferior wall, the mid inferior wall and the basal inferior wall respectively. The apical 2-chamber view is best obtained by rotating the echo transducer approximately 60 degrees or more in a counterclockwise direction from the apical 4-chamber view.

Question 13
Which echocardiographic view is highlighted in Fig. 4.11 (and Video 4.3)?

A. Parasternal long axis
B. Parasternal short axis
C. Apical 4-chamber view
D. Apical 2-chamber view
E. Apical 3-chamber view

Answer: E. Apical 3-chamber view. Figure 4.11 highlights the apical 3-chamber view (center panel) which is a long axis outflow view of the heart (the plane created by slicing the heart along the white line in the right panel), sometimes called the 120° view. In the left panel, the highlighted green segments in the apical 3-chamber view (starting from the top left) are the basal antero-septum, the mid antero-septum, the apical septum, the true apex, the apical lateral wall, the mid infero-lateral (posterior) wall and the basal infero-lateral (posterior) wall respectively. The apical 3-chamber view is best obtained by rotating the transducer counterclockwise from the two-chamber view.

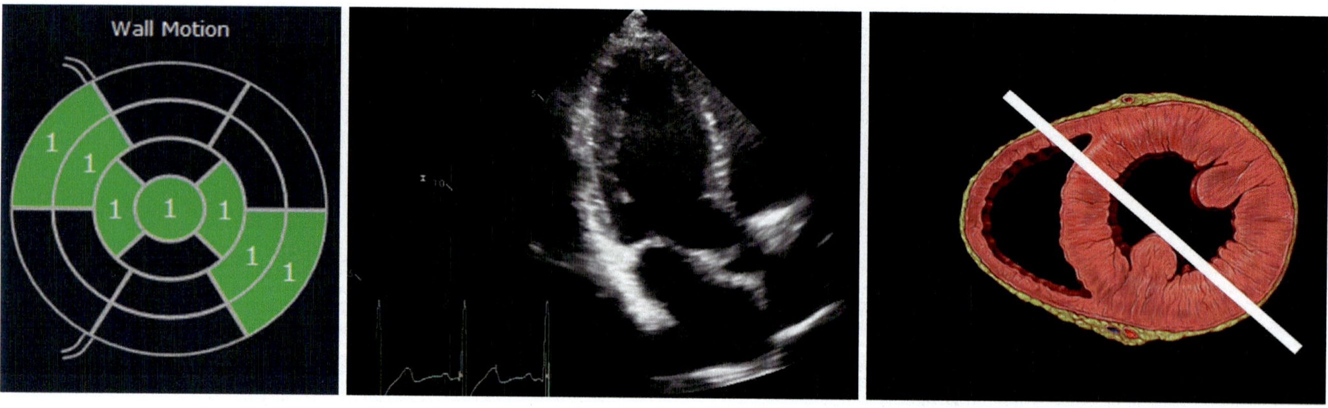

Fig. 4.11 Graphical representation of specific segments of the left ventricle (left panel), with the corresponding echo image (middle panel), and the equivalent slice of the left ventricle in a 3d short axis model (right panel)

Question 14

A 65-year-old woman undergoes an echocardiogram to evaluate chest pain. The resting images in Fig. 4.12 (and Video 4.4) show wall motion abnormalities in:

A. Left anterior descending artery territory
B. Left circumflex artery territory
C. Right coronary artery territory
D. Multi-vessel territory
E. A non-coronary artery distribution

Answer: A. Left anterior descending artery territory. Video 4.4 demonstrates an apical 4-chamber view showing septal and apical wall akinesis consistent with a left anterior descending artery territory regional wall motion abnormality. Figure 4.12 demonstrates this regional wall motion abnormality with relevant visualized segments color- and numerically- coded as shown, whereby segment with normal function are coded in green and numbered 1, and akinetic segments are coded in orange and numbered 3.

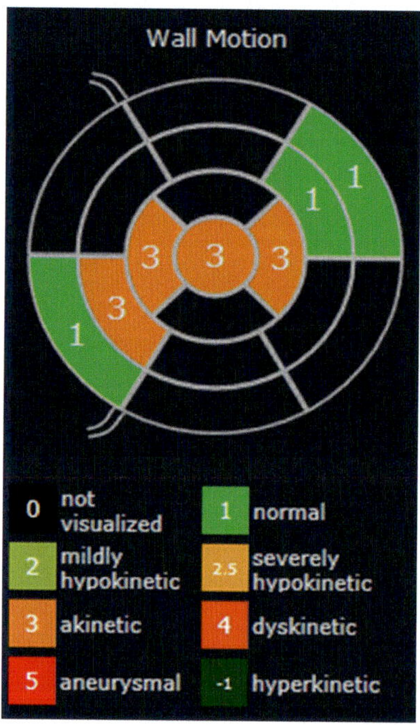

Fig. 4.12 Graphical representation of specific segments of the left ventricle

Question 15

A 75-year-old man undergoes an echocardiogram to evaluate chest pain. The resting images in Fig. 4.13 (and Video 4.5) show wall motion abnormalities in:

A. Left anterior descending artery territory
B. Left circumflex artery territory
C. Right coronary artery territory
D. Multi-vessel territory
E. A non-coronary artery distribution

Answer: C. Right coronary artery territory. Video 4.5 demonstrates an apical 2-chamber view showing inferior wall akinesis/severe hypokinesis consistent with a right coronary artery territory regional wall motion abnormality. Figure 4.13 demonstrates this regional wall motion abnormality with relevant visualized segments color- and numerically- coded as shown, whereby segments with normal function are coded in green and numbered 1, a severely hypokinetic segment is coded in light orange and numbered 2.5, and an akinetic segment is coded in orange and numbered 3.

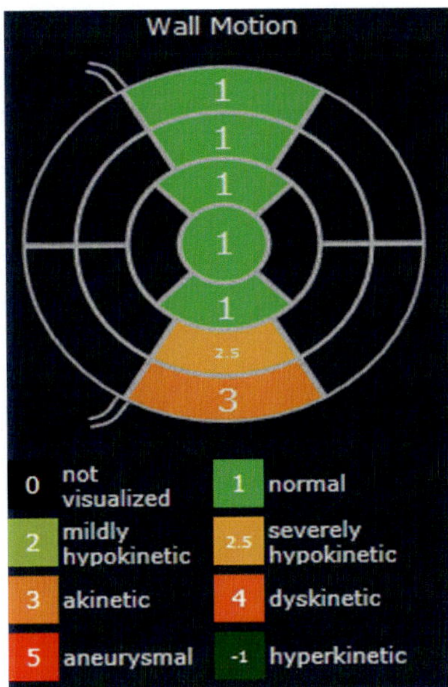

Fig. 4.13 Graphical representation of specific segments of the left ventricle

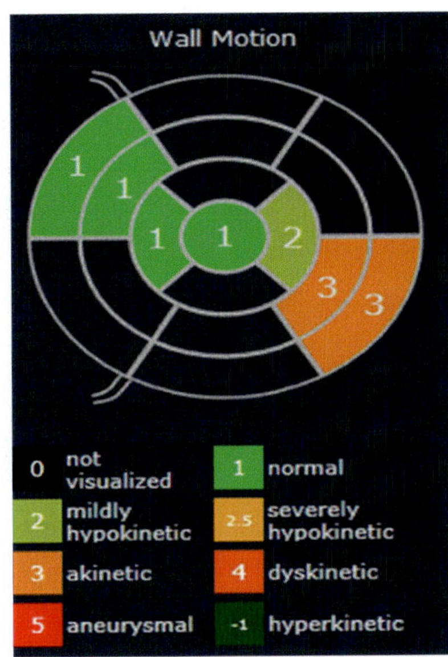

Fig. 4.14 Graphical representation of specific segments of the left ventricle

Question 16

A 55-year-old man undergoes an echocardiogram to evaluate chest pain. The resting images in Fig. 4.14 (and Video 4.6) show wall motion abnormalities in:

A. Left anterior descending artery territory
B. Left circumflex artery territory
C. Right coronary artery territory
D. Multi-vessel territory
E. A non-coronary artery distribution

Answer: B. Left circumflex artery territory. Video 4.6 demonstrates an apical 3-chamber view showing infero-lateral (posterior) wall akinesis/hypokinesis consistent with a left circumflex artery territory regional wall motion abnormality. Figure 4.14 demonstrates this regional wall motion abnormality with relevant visualized segments color- and numerically- coded as shown, whereby segments with normal function are coded in green and numbered 1, a mildly hypokinetic segment is coded in light green and numbered 2, and akinetic segments are coded in orange and numbered 3.

Question 17

Which of the following is true in the setting of normal left ventricular contraction?

A. The anterior wall contributes twice more than the inferior wall
B. Normal left ventricular contraction is symmetrical with relatively equal contribution by all walls
C. The inferior wall contributes twice more than the anterior wall
D. The septal wall contributes twice more than the free wall
E. The free wall contributes twice more than septal wall

Answer: B. Normal left ventricular contraction is symmetrical with relatively equal contribution by all walls. If one assumes that normal ejection fraction is roughly 60%, then each wall contributes about 10% which can be a helpful simple way of working out visual ejection fraction (Fig. 4.15). In disease states, sometimes the wall opposing a regional wall motion abnormality hyper-compensates (mechanism via pre-systolic stretch). For example, with circumflex territory infarction, septal wall hyperkinesis may

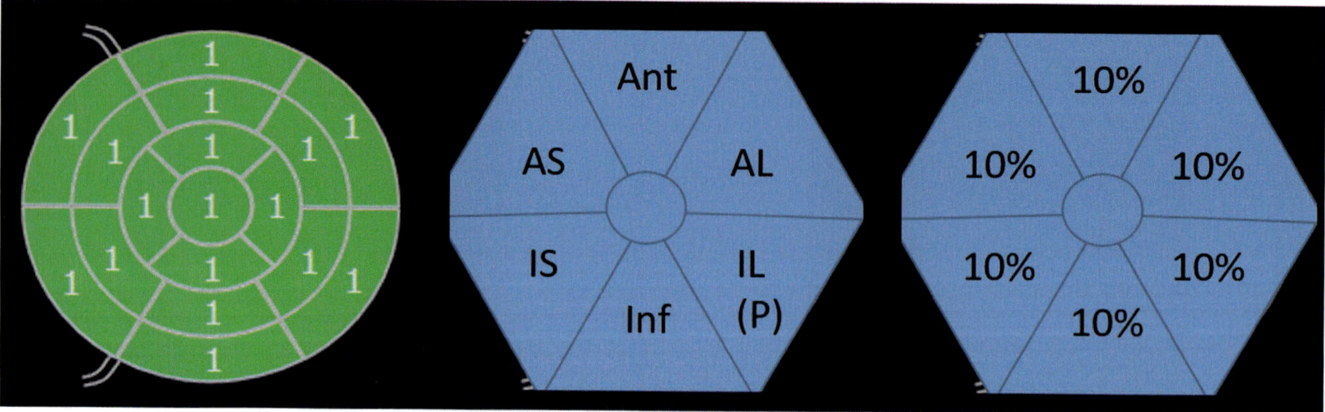

Fig. 4.15 Graphical representation of specific segments of the left ventricle (left panel), names of 6 walls of the heart and their relative contribution to ejection fraction assuming equivalency

compensate for free wall akinesis. Of note, such compensatory hyperkinetic function may be easier to identify than the original regional wall motion abnormality. Thus, a helpful rule of thumb is to have a high degree of suspicion for a regional wall motion abnormality in the wall opposing hyperkinetic segments.

Question 18
A 30-year-old male patient in the intensive care unit with mixed septic and cardiogenic shock. Echocardiogram is performed and the report states severe left ventricular dysfunction, severe global left ventricular hypokinesis, and an ejection fraction of 20%. Which of the following regional wall motion plots in Fig. 4.16 best represents this clinical report?

A. Plot A
B. Plot B
C. Plot C
D. Plot D
E. None of these

Answer: D. Plot D. The regional wall motion plot D in Fig. 4.16 shows all segments coded in orange and numbered 2.5 representing severe global hypokinesis, and in keeping with the reported ejection fraction of 20%.

Question 19
A 20-year-old female patient in the intensive care unit with pulmonary embolism. Echocardiogram is performed and the report states hyperdynamic left ventricular dysfunction, global left ventricular hyperkinesis, and an ejection fraction of 75%. Which of the following regional wall motion plots in Fig. 4.16 best represents this clinical report?

A. Plot A
B. Plot B
C. Plot C
D. Plot D
E. None of these

Answer: A. Plot A. The regional wall motion plot A in Fig. 4.16 shows all segments coded in dark green and numbered −1 representing global left ventricular hyperkinesis, and in keeping with the reported ejection fraction of 75%.

Question 20
A 40-year-old male patient in the intensive care unit with COVID related respiratory failure. Echocardiogram is performed and the report states normal left ventricular dysfunction, no regional wall motion abnormality, and an ejection fraction of 60%. Which of the following regional wall motion plots in Fig. 4.16 best represents this clinical report?

A. Plot A
B. Plot B
C. Plot C
D. Plot D
E. None of these

Answer: B. Plot B. The regional wall motion plot B in Fig. 4.16 shows all segments coded in green and numbered 1 representing normal left ventricular dysfunction, and in keeping with the reported ejection fraction of 60%.

Question 21
An 80-year-old male patient in the intensive care unit with urosepsis. Echocardiogram is performed and the report states mild left ventricular dysfunction, mild global left ventricular hypokinesis, and an ejection fraction of 45%. Which of the following regional wall motion plots in Fig. 4.16 best represents this clinical report?

A. Plot A
B. Plot B
C. Plot C
D. Plot D
E. None of these

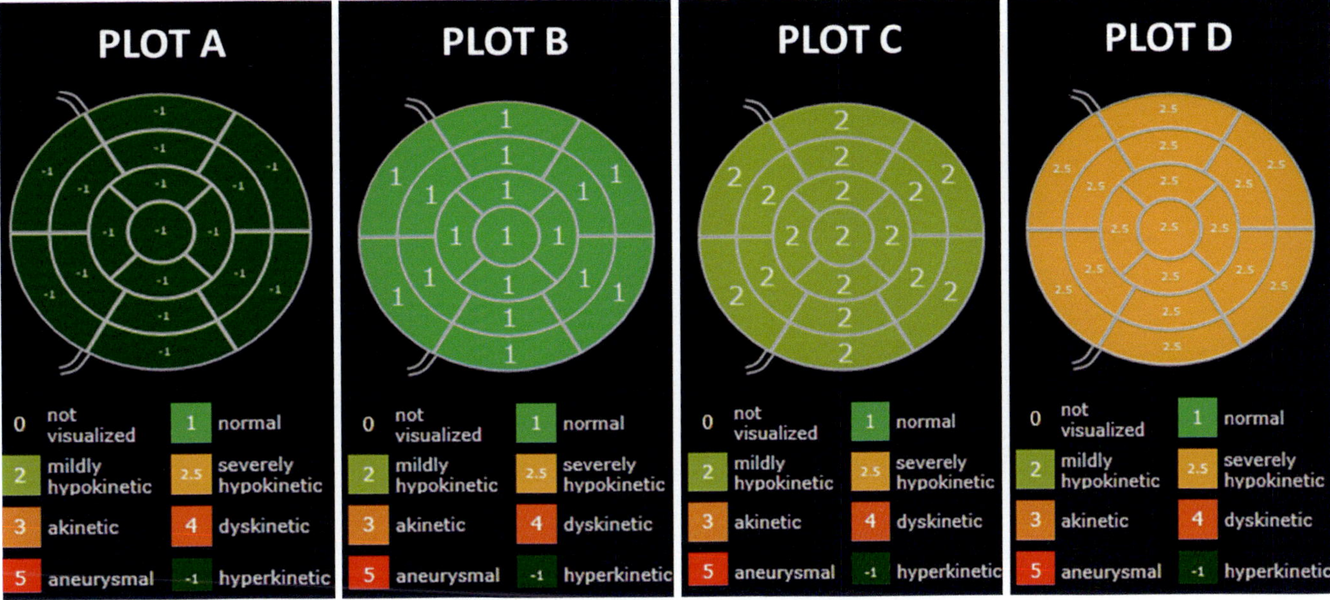

Fig. 4.16 Graphical representation of different regional wall motion plots of the left ventricle

Answer: C. Plot C. The regional wall motion plot C in Fig. 4.16 shows all segments coded in light green and numbered 2 representing mild global hypokinesis, and in keeping with the reported ejection fraction of 45%.

Question 22
An 85-year-old female patient in the intensive care unit with suspected apical ballooning syndrome, (otherwise known as broken heart syndrome, classical stress cardiomyopathy or Takotsubo cardiomyopathy). Echocardiogram is performed and the report states severe apical left ventricular dysfunction, severe apical akinesis, and an ejection fraction of 35%. Which of the following regional wall motion plots in Fig. 4.16 best represents this clinical report?

A. Plot A
B. Plot B
C. Plot C
D. Plot D
E. None of these

Answer: E. Plot E. The regional wall motion plots in Fig. 4.16 show symmetrical global heart function/dysfunction, without regional wall motion abnormality, unlike this patient who was noted to have apical akinesis.

Question 23
A 70-year-old woman in the intensive care unit is diagnosed with apical ballooning syndrome, (otherwise known as broken heart syndrome, classical stress cardiomyopathy or Takotsubo cardiomyopathy). Which regional wall motion segmental plot in Fig. 4.17 would be most consistent with that diagnosis?

A. Segmental plot A
B. Segmental plot B
C. Segmental plot C
D. Segmental plot D
E. None of these

Answer: A. Segmental plot A. Figure 4.17 demonstrates four discrete regional wall motion segmental plots with relevant visualized segments color- and numerically- coded as shown in the right panel. Panel A shows a regional wall motion segmental plot consistent with apical akinesis (segments are coded in orange and numbered 3), with normal function of all other visualized segments (coded in green and numbered 1).

Question 24
A 55-year-old man in the intensive care unit is diagnosed with left circumflex ischemia/infarction. Which regional wall motion segmental plot in Fig. 4.17 would be most consistent with that diagnosis?

A. Segmental plot A
B. Segmental plot B
C. Segmental plot C
D. Segmental plot D
E. None of these

Answer: D. Segmental plot D. Figure 4.17 demonstrates four discrete regional wall motion segmental plots with relevant visualized segments color- and numerically- coded as shown in the right panel. Panel D shows a regional wall motion segmental plot consistent with left circumflex ischemia/infarction, with akinetic free wall segments coded in orange and numbered 3, with normal function of all other visualized seg-

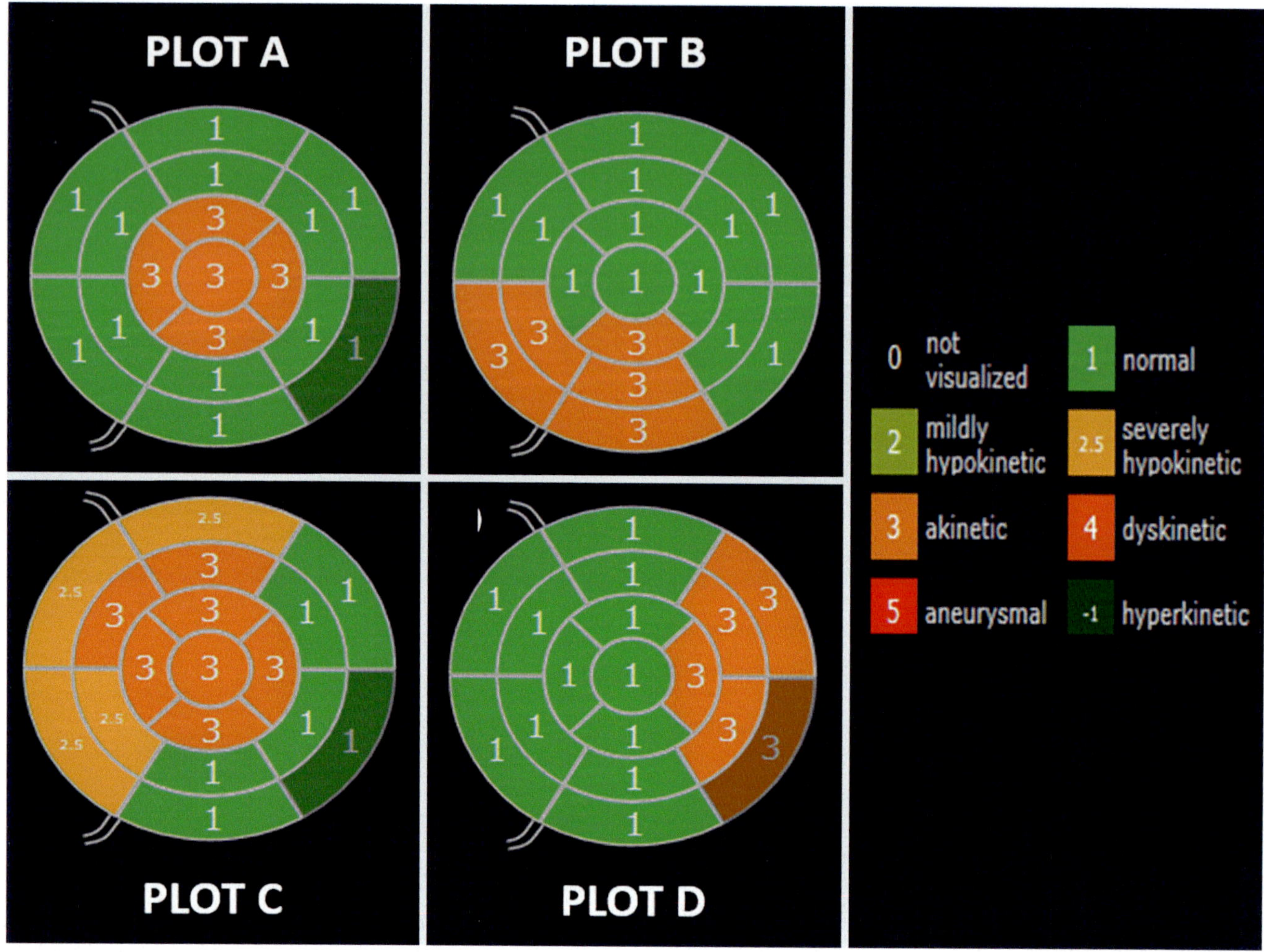

Fig. 4.17 Graphical representation of different regional wall motion plots of the left ventricle

ments (coded in green and numbered 1). Left circumflex related acute coronary syndrome can be the most challenging to diagnose as ST changes are not always apparent in standard lead electrocardiography and posterior leads (V7–V9) may be required to better identify. There are additional diagnostic challenges in this setting with echocardiography also, as the free wall is generally more difficult to visualize than the septum, while ejection fraction may not be significantly impaired in the acute setting. In that regard, compensatory hyperkinesis of opposing septal segments may be present and provide an important cue to make this diagnosis.

Question 25

A 65-year-old woman in the intensive care unit is diagnosed with left anterior descending artery ischemia/infarction. Which regional wall motion segmental plot in Fig. 4.17 would be most consistent with that diagnosis?

A. Segmental plot A
B. Segmental plot B
C. Segmental plot C
D. Segmental plot D
E. None of these

Answer: C. Segmental plot C. Figure 4.17 demonstrates four discrete regional wall motion segmental plots with relevant visualized segments color- and numerically- coded as shown in the right panel. Panel C shows a regional wall motion segmental plot consistent with left anterior descending artery ischemia/infarction with akinetic segments coded in orange and numbered 3, severely hypokinetic segments coded in light orange and numbered 2.5, and segments with normal function coded in green and numbered 1. Restriction motion of both leaflets of the mitral valve due to apical tethering with associated centrally-directed mitral regurgitation is most likely to be seen with anterior descending artery ischemia/infarction.

Question 26

A 55-year-old man in the intensive care unit is diagnosed with right coronary artery ischemia/infarction. Which regional wall motion segmental plot in Fig. 4.17 would be most consistent with that diagnosis?

A. Segmental plot A
B. Segmental plot B
C. Segmental plot C
D. Segmental plot D
E. None of these

Answer: B. Segmental plot B. Figure 4.17 demonstrates four discrete regional wall motion segmental plots with relevant visualized segments color- and numerically- coded as shown in the right panel. Panel A shows a regional wall motion segmental plot consistent with infero-septal and inferior akinesis (segments are coded in orange and numbered 3), with normal function of all other visualized segments (coded in green and numbered 1). Because the right coronary artery lies in an anterior position, it is considered relatively more susceptible to embolic events. Restriction of the posterior leaflet of the mitral valve with associated posteriorly-directed mitral regurgitation is most likely to be seen with non-left anterior descending artery ischemia/infarction.

Question 27
Which echocardiographic view is highlighted in Fig. 4.18 (and Video 4.7)?

A. Parasternal long axis
B. Parasternal short axis—basal
C. Parasternal short axis—mid
D. Parasternal short axis—apical
E. None of these

Answer: B. Parasternal short axis—basal. Figure 4.18 highlights the parasternal short axis—basal view. The highlighted green segments in the parasternal short axis—basal view (starting at the bottom and going clockwise) are basal inferior, infero-septal, antero-septal, anterior, antero-lateral and infero-lateral (posterior) respectively. The parasternal short axis—basal view is best obtained by placing the echo transducer left of the left sternal border at the fourth intercostal space with the transducer indicator pointed towards patient's left shoulder.

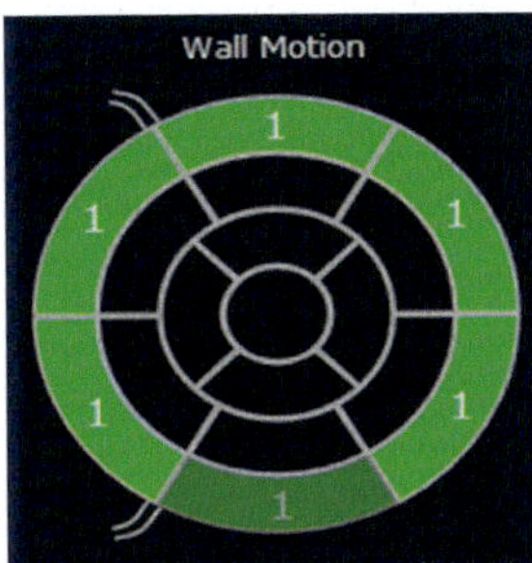

Fig. 4.18 Graphical representation of specific segments of the left ventricle

Question 28
Which echocardiographic view is highlighted in Fig. 4.19 (and Video 4.8)?

A. Parasternal long axis
B. Parasternal short axis—basal
C. Parasternal short axis—mid
D. Parasternal short axis—apical
E. None of these

Answer: C. Parasternal short axis—mid. Figure 4.19 highlights the parasternal short axis—mid view. The highlighted green segments in the parasternal short axis—mid view (starting at the bottom and going clockwise) are mid inferior, infero-septal, antero-septal, anterior, antero-lateral and infero-lateral (posterior) respectively. The parasternal short axis—mid view is best obtained by placing the echo transducer left of the left sternal border at the fourth intercostal space with the transducer indicator pointed towards patient's left shoulder, gradually tilting down the heart axis.

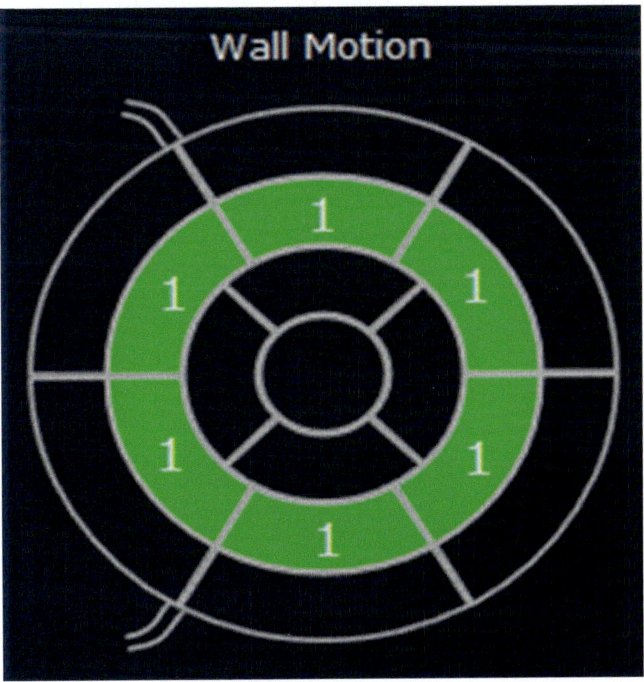

Fig. 4.19 Graphical representation of specific segments of the left ventricle

Question 29

Which echocardiographic view is highlighted in Fig. 4.20 (and Video 4.9)?

A. Parasternal long axis
B. Parasternal short axis—basal
C. Parasternal short axis—mid
D. Parasternal short axis—apical
E. None of these

Answer: D. Parasternal short axis—apical. Figure 4.20 highlights the parasternal short axis—apical view. The highlighted green segments in the parasternal short axis—apical view (starting at the bottom and going clockwise) are apical inferior, septal, anterior and lateral respectively. The parasternal short axis—apical view is best obtained by placing the echo transducer left of the left sternal border at the fifth intercostal space with the transducer indicator pointed towards patient's left shoulder, gradually tilting down the heart axis.

Question 30

A 55-year-old man is admitted to the intensive care unit with right heart failure. Which is the cause of the regional wall motion abnormality highlighted in Video 4.10?

A. Left anterior descending artery ischemia/infarction
B. Left circumflex artery ischemia/infarction
C. Right coronary artery ischemia/infarction
D. Multi-vessel ischemia/infarction
E. A non-coronary cause

Answer: E. A non-coronary cause. Video 4.10 highlights the parasternal short axis—mid view in a patient with pericardial constriction. The classical finding here is a septal bounce caused by abrupt cessation of mitral and tricuspid inflow as the filling heart comes up against the abrupt constricting force of the diseased pericardium in diastole repeatedly with each beat (cardio-phasic). There is also present an abnormal septal shift, leftward in inspiration when intra-thoracic pressures fall and the right heart fills preferentially at the expense of the left heart, and reversed rightward in expiration when the opposite happens (respiro-phasic ventricular interdependence).

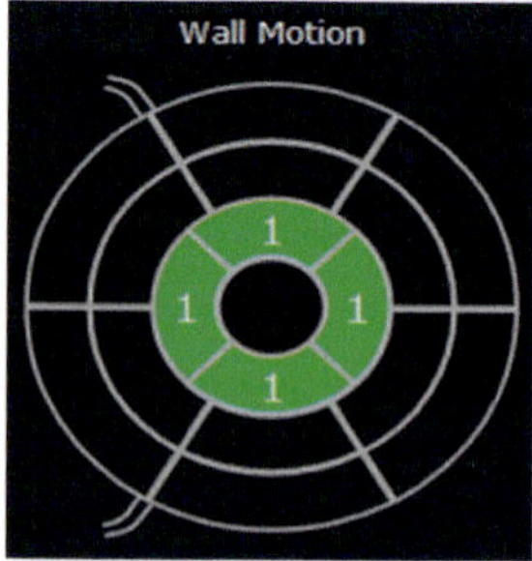

Fig. 4.20 Graphical representation of specific segments of the left ventricle

Question 31

The motion of the basal posterior segment in Video 4.11 is consistent with

A. Left anterior descending artery ischemia/infarction
B. Left circumflex artery ischemia/infarction
C. Right coronary artery ischemia/infarction
D. Multi-vessel ischemia/infarction
E. A non-coronary cause

Answer: E. A non-coronary cause. Video 4.11 highlights the parasternal short axis—mid view in a patient with pseudo-dyskinesis. The classical finding here is the inferior wall moving inwards in diastole (dyskinesis), not because of an intrinsic heart issue (the affected segments still thicken appropriately with systole), but rather secondary to a mechanical force exerted outside the heart such as tense ascites, raised hemi-diaphragm, morbid obesity etc.

Question 32

Which echocardiographic view is highlighted in Fig. 4.21?

A. Parasternal long axis
B. Parasternal short axis—basal
C. Parasternal short axis—mid
D. Parasternal short axis—apical
E. None of these

Answer: A. Parasternal long axis view. Figure 4.21 highlights the parasternal long axis view. The highlighted green segments in the parasternal long axis view (starting at the top left) are basal antero-septum, the mid antero-septum, the apical septum, the true apex (not seen—hence the coding as black 0), the apical lateral wall, the mid infero-lateral (posterior) wall and the basal infero-lateral (posterior) wall respectively. The parasternal long axis view is best obtained by placing the echo transducer left of the left sternal border at the fourth intercostal space with the transducer indicator pointed towards patient's right shoulder.

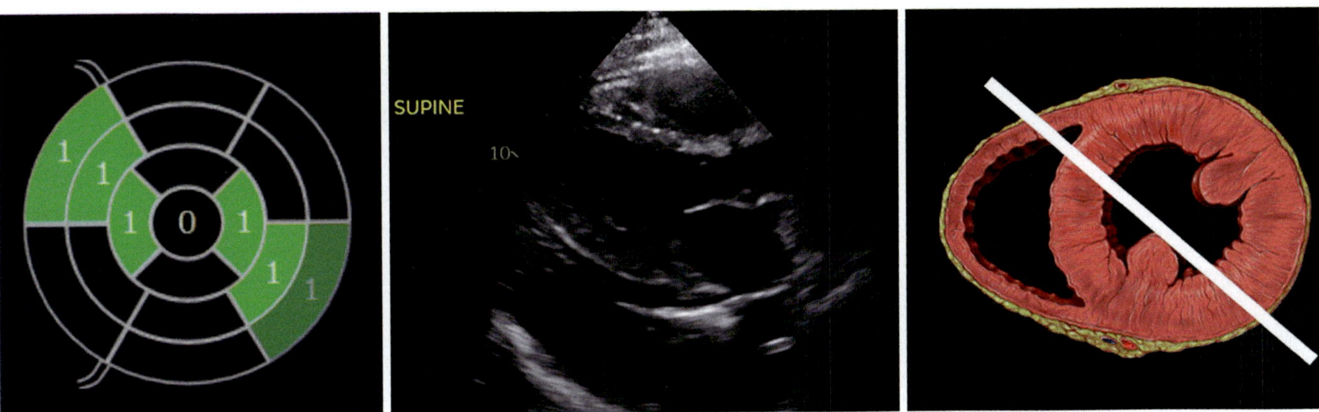

Fig. 4.21 Graphical representation of specific segments of the left ventricle

Question 33

A 60-year-old man is admitted to the intensive care unit with shortness of breath. How would you best describe the motion of the basal infero-lateral (posterior) wall in the parasternal long axis view in Video 4.12?

A. Normal/Hyperkinetic
B. Mildly hypokinetic
C. Severely hypokinetic
D. Akinetic
E. Dyskinetic

Answer: A. Normal/Hyperkinetic. The basal infero-lateral (posterior) wall in the parasternal long axis view in Video 4.12 demonstrates normal/hyperkinetic motion.

Question 34

A 60-year-old man is admitted to the intensive care unit with shortness of breath. How would you best describe the motion of the basal infero-lateral (posterior) wall in the parasternal long axis view in Video 4.13?

A. Normal/Hyperkinetic
B. Mildly hypokinetic
C. Severely hypokinetic
D. Akinetic
E. Dyskinetic

Answer: D. Akinetic. The basal infero-lateral (posterior) wall in the parasternal long axis view in Video 4.13 demonstrates akinesis. While this segment moves, the movement represents displacement (secondary motion due to its attachment to adjacent kinetic segments), without deformation/thickening (as every muscle should do if it contracting normally). This akinetic segment also appears thin and so most likely represent chronic scar.

Question 35

A 60-year-old non-diabetic woman is admitted to the intensive care unit with shortness of breath. On exam, blood pressure is normal and there are no audible rest or inducible murmurs. You review previously acquired echo images as in Fig. 4.22 where there is discrepant measurement of septal wall thickness between views, namely 1.3 cm in a parasternal long axis view (left panel), and 0.9 cm in a parasternal basal axis view (right panel). You suspect findings are most consistent with which of the following?

A. Under-measured parasternal short axis view measurement
B. Over-measured parasternal long axis view measurement
C. Hypertrophic cardiomyopathy
D. Aortic stenosis
E. Mild concentric left ventricular hypertrophy

Answer: B. Over-measured parasternal long axis view measurement. Normal left ventricular septal wall thickness is less than 1.1 cm. While the parasternal long axis view is considered the standard view for measurement of posterior and septal wall thickness, it is not without limitations. Inaccurate measurements may be as a result of oblique measurement (the septum is a curved structure) or inadvertent inclusion of right ventricular structures (such as trabeculations, a tricuspid valve papillary muscle, or even the moderator band). True left ventricular septal wall thickness is typically replicable in other views. Thus, in this case, it is most likely that the parasternal long axis view measurement was over-measured.

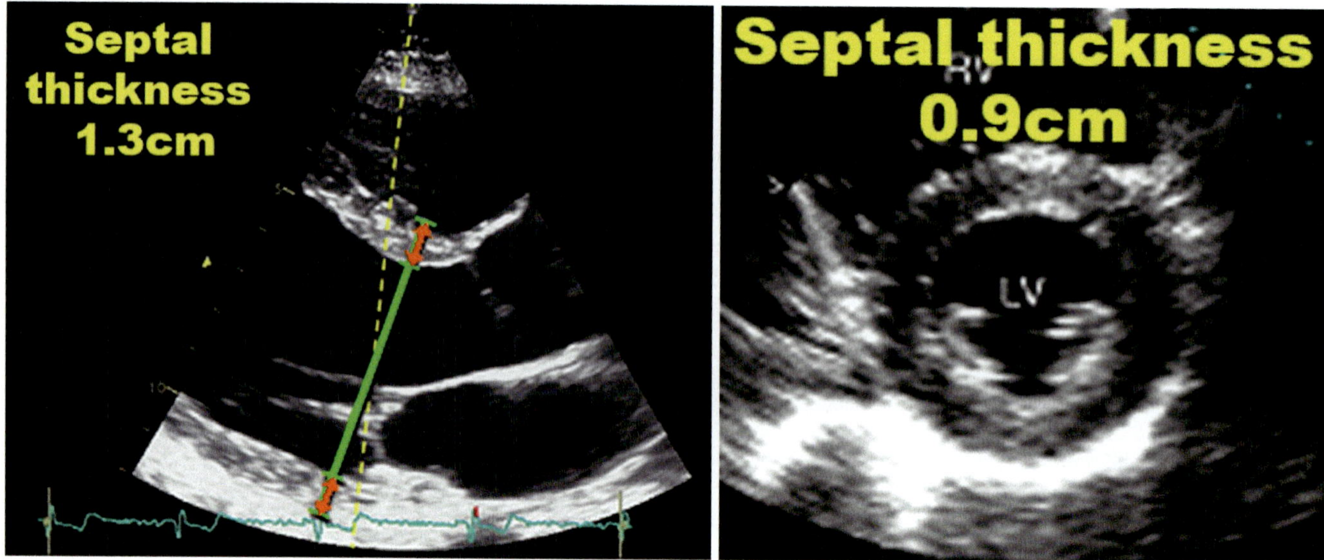

Fig. 4.22 Parasternal long axis view (left panel), and parasternal basal axis view (right panel) of the left ventricle

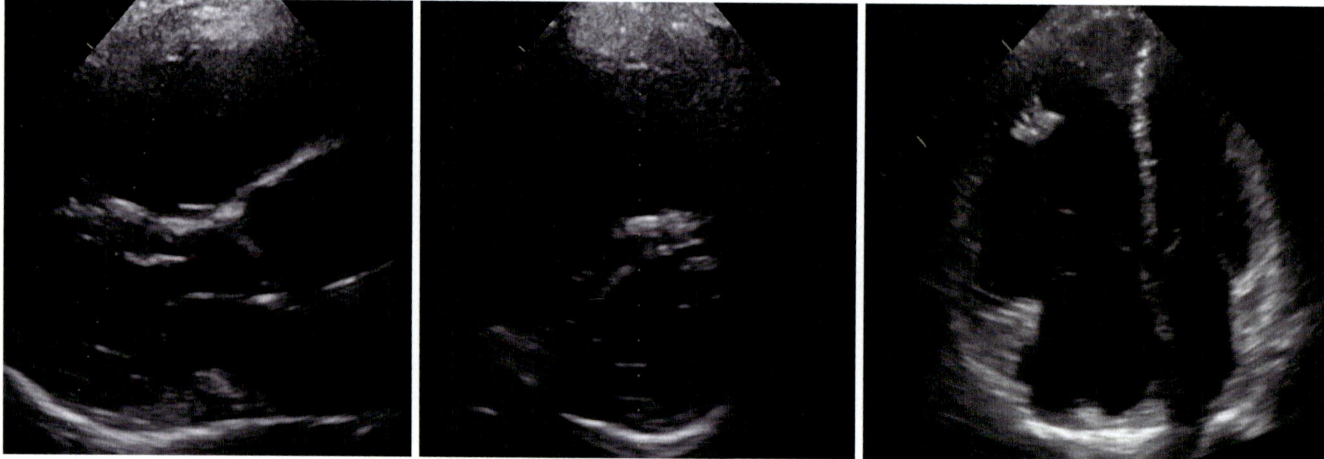

Fig. 4.23 Parasternal long axis view (left panel), a parasternal short axis view (middle panel) and an apical 4 chamber view (right panel)

Question 36
A 60-year-old man is admitted to the intensive care unit with shortness of breath and acute pulmonary embolism. Right ventricular strain is suspected on the pulmonary embolism protocolled computer tomography scan. A bedside echo is performed and right ventricular dilation is suspected based upon visual assessment of the relative ratios of the right ventricular size to the left ventricular size in Fig. 4.23, namely a parasternal long axis view (left panel), a parasternal short axis view (middle panel) and an apical 4 chamber view (right panel). Which of the following scenarios is suspicious for right ventricular dilation?

A. RV:LV < 1:1 in both apical 4 chamber and parasternal long axis views
B. RV:LV > 1:1 in both apical 4 chamber and parasternal long axis views
C. RV:LV < 2/3:1 in an apical 4 chamber view
D. RV:LV = 1/3:2/3 in a parasternal long axis view
E. RV:LV = 1/3:2/3 in a parasternal short axis view

Answer: B. RV:LV > 1:1 in both apical 4 chamber and parasternal long axis views. If the right ventricle is visually bigger than the left ventricle in parasternal and apical 4 chamber views, then it is highly likely that right ventricular dilation is present. Indeed, right ventricle width is usually less than half that of the left ventricular on qualitative (visual) assessment in a parasternal long axis view and less than two thirds in an apical 4 chamber view.

Question 37
An echocardiogram is performed on a 55-year-old man with hypotension in the intensive care unit. The resting images in Fig. 4.24 (and Video 4.14) show a regional wall motion abnormality that can be seen with:

A. Left bundle branch block
B. Left anterior descending artery territory infarction
C. Non-ischemic cardiomyopathy
D. Right ventricular pacing
E. All of these

Answer: E. All of these. Figure 4.24 (and Video 4.14) demonstrate an apical 4-chamber view with a classical left bundle branch block regional wall motion abnormality including septal hypokinesis (segments shown in light green and numbered 2) and basal free wall hyperkinesis (segment shown in dark green and numbered −1). Left bundle branch block can be present in multiple settings including acute left anterior descending artery territory infarction, non-ischemic cardiomyopathy, right ventricular pacing and even in a rate-dependent manner in tachycardia. Comparing a current electrocardiogram with a prior electrocardiogram (to see whether the left bundle branch block is a new finding, versus a long-standing or chronic finding) can be helpful clinically to better understand the etiology of the left bundle branch block.

Question 38
Figure 4.25 demonstrates which of the following?

A. Apical 4-chamber view with apical hypokinesis
B. Apical 2-chamber view with apical hypokinesis
C. Apical 3-chamber view with apical hypokinesis
D. Apical 4-chamber view with apical akinesis
E. Apical 2-chamber view with apical akinesis

Answer: D. Apical 4-chamber view with apical akinesis. Figure 4.25 demonstrates an apical 4-chamber view with apical akinesis (akinetic segments are shown in orange and numbered 3).

Question 39
Figure 4.25 could represent which clinical scenario(s)?

A. Left anterior descending artery ischemia/infarction
B. Left circumflex artery ischemia/infarction
C. Right coronary artery ischemia/infarction
D. A non-coronary artery process
E. A or D

Answer: E. A or D. Figure 4.25 demonstrates apical akinesis consistent with either a left anterior descending artery ischemia/infarction or a non-coronary artery process specifically affecting the apex (such as apical ballooning syndrome, otherwise known as broken heart syndrome, classical stress cardiomyopathy or Takotsubo cardiomyopathy).

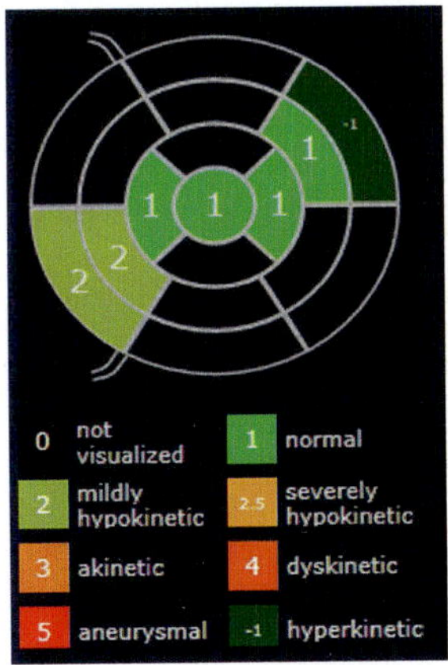

Fig. 4.24 Graphical representation of a regional wall motion plot of the left ventricle

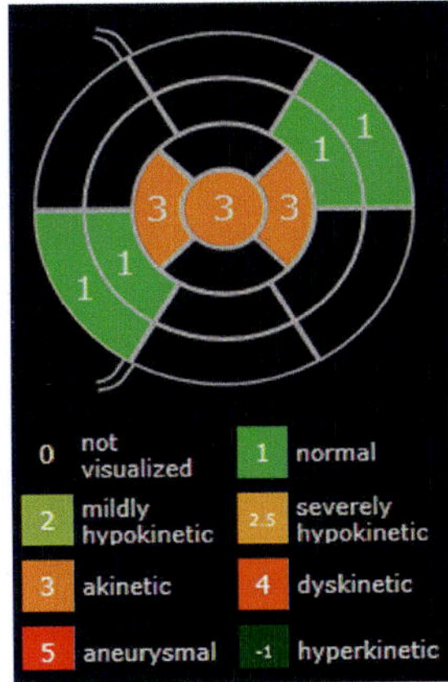

Fig. 4.25 Graphical representation of a regional wall motion plot of the left ventricle

Question 40
What complication of acute coronary syndrome is suspected in Video 4.15?

A. Ruptured papillary muscle
B. Free wall rupture
C. Ventricular septal rupture
D. Mural thrombus
E. Right ventricular infarction

Answer: D. Mural thrombus. Apical left ventricular thrombus is not uncommon in any patient with severe apical wall motion abnormalities. Following a large anterior myocardial infarction, apical left ventricular thrombus has a reported incidence of up to 15%. Apical left ventricular thrombus can also arise as a complication of apical ballooning syndrome, (otherwise known as broken heart syndrome, classical stress cardiomyopathy or Takotsubo cardiomyopathy). Given the high risk of an embolic complication in this setting, it is important to have a high suspicion for this complication in any patient with severe apical wall motion abnormalities.

Question 41
After reviewing Video 4.15, what would be the most appropriate next step in the management of this patient?

A. Use of an ultrasound enhancer agent
B. Continuous wave Doppler through the mitral valve
C. Trans-esophageal echocardiography
D. Cardiac magnetic resonance imaging
E. Non-contrast computed tomography

Answer: A. Use of an ultrasound enhancer agent. Given suspected mural apical LV thrombus in Video 4.8, the best next step would be to obtain similar views using an ultrasound enhancer agent to better demonstrate the thrombus (see Video 4.16). Trans-esophageal echocardiography would not be an ideal modality for imaging the left ventricular apex, as it is in the far field for this modality. Non-contrast computed tomography would typically fail to detect mural apical LV thrombus. Gated contrast computed tomography and cardiac magnetic resonance imaging would be high yield alternative modalities that could demonstrate mural thrombus, but are less commonly performed in the acute setting than echocardiography.

Question 42
A 72-year-old male with no significant past medical history who presented with a 1 week history of epigastric tightness and nausea. On physical examination, blood pressure 94/60, heart rate 93. Lungs are clear. Cardiac auscultation revealed a 3/6 harsh pan-systolic murmur in the lower left sternal border with an associated thrill. An electrocardiogram showed inferior ST depressions and a transthoracic echocardiogram was done. What complication of acute coronary syndrome is suspected in Fig. 4.26 (Video 4.17)?

A. Ruptured papillary muscle
B. Free wall rupture
C. Ventricular septal rupture
D. Mural thrombus
E. Right ventricular infarction

Answer: C. Ventricular septal rupture. The transthoracic echocardiogram shows an inferior ventricular septal rupture. This is a rare complication in the current era of revascularization (less than 1% of patients presenting with acute myocardial infarction), but carries a high mortality rate. Patients with ventricular septal rupture can appear stable early in the course however they can decompensate quickly and suddenly, hence the importance of early identification of this complication. Auscultation is helpful tool, however in cases of low cardiac output the murmur may be harder to appreciate.

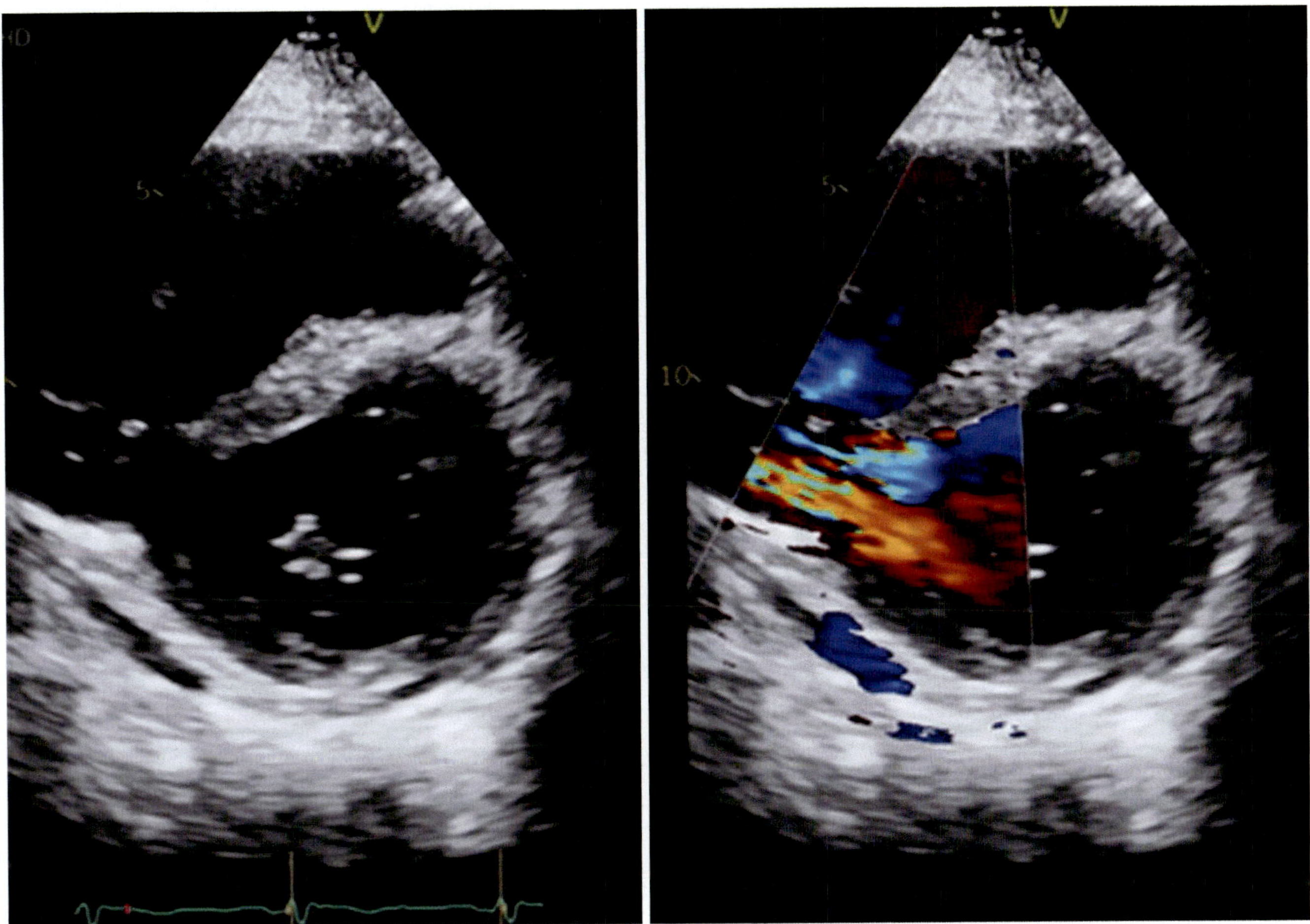

Fig. 4.26 Parasternal short axis view of the left ventricle without color Doppler (left panel) and with color Doppler (right panel)

Question 43

A 60-year-old male with no significant past medical history, presents with substernal chest tightness of 2 h duration. Physical exam showed blood pressure 85/55 mmHg, heart rate 110, bilateral lung crackles and no cardiac murmur. Electrocardiogram showed inferior ST depression and a transthoracic echocardiogram was done. What complication of acute coronary syndrome is suspected in Fig. 4.27 (Video 4.18)?

A. Ruptured papillary muscle
B. Free wall rupture
C. Ventricular septal rupture
D. Mural thrombus
E. Right ventricular infarction

Answer: A. Ruptured papillary muscle. The echocardiogram shows hyperdynamic basal and mid septal segments and an akinetic basal inferolateral (posterior) segment consistent with acute left circumflex artery occlusion. There is posteriorly directed mitral regurgitation and a highly mobile echodensity associated with the posteromedial papillary muscle within the left ventricle consistent with a partially ruptured papillary muscle head. This mechanical complication of acute coronary syndrome is more common with an inferior myocardial infarction, because the posteromedial papillary muscle receives blood supply from the posterior descending artery which usually arises from the right coronary artery, whereas the anterolateral papillary muscle has dual blood supply from the left anterior descending artery and circumflex artery. The typical pan-systolic murmur of mitral regurgitation may be absent in such an acute setting due to elevated left atrial pressure and rapid equalization of pressures between the left atrium and the left ventricle. Acute severe mitral regurgitation is associated with hemodynamic compromise and pulmonary edema and represents a surgical emergency.

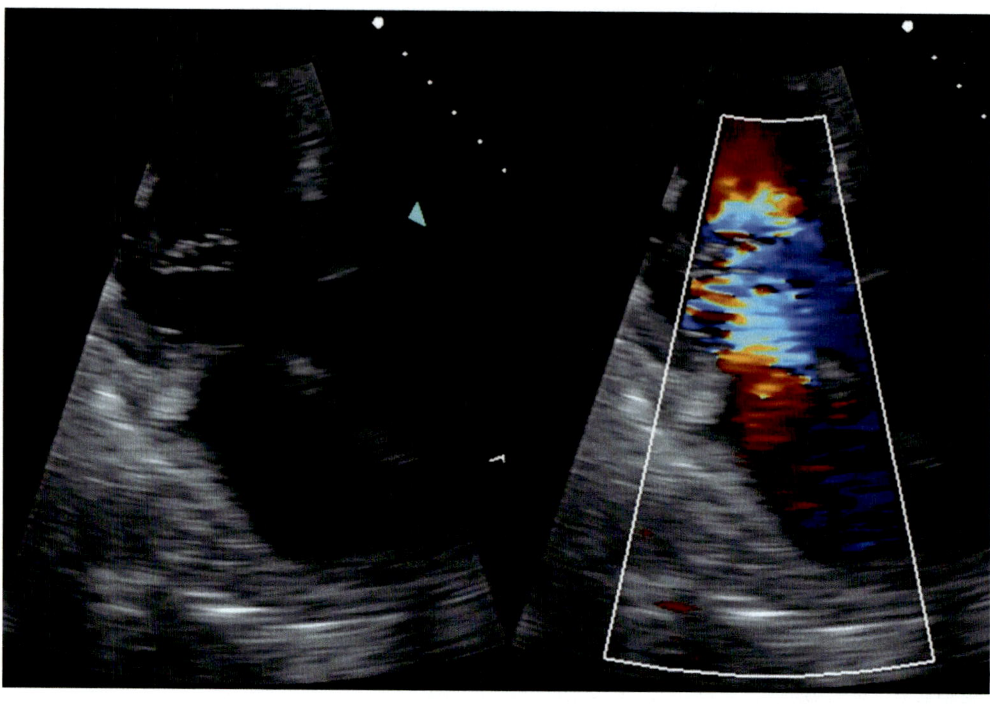

Fig. 4.27 Modified apical 3 chamber view of the left ventricle without color Doppler (left panel) and with color Doppler (right panel)

Question 44
A 90-year-old female with past medical history of hypertension and diabetes presents to the emergency department with chest pain. Electrocardiogram showed inferior ST elevation and she underwent primary percutaneous coronary intervention to the right coronary artery. A few hours after the procedure, the patient became hypotensive. Physical exam showed jugular venous distension, clear lung fields, and no cardiac murmur. A repeat electrocardiogram showed no new changes and a bedside transthoracic echocardiogram was performed. What complication of acute coronary syndrome is suspected in Video 4.19?

A. Ruptured papillary muscle
B. Free wall rupture
C. Ventricular septal rupture
D. Mural thrombus
E. Right ventricular infarction

Answer: E. Right ventricular infarction. The patient has the classic triad of hypotension, jugular venous distension, and clear lung fields which are most suggestive of right ventricular infarction complicating inferior myocardial infarction in this setting. The echocardiogram shows right ventricular systolic dysfunction with sparing of the apex. Look to the body of the right ventricle (mid & basal segments) to properly appreciate the regional wall motion abnormality. The left ventricular apex of the heart is hyperdynamic as it compensates for the opposing regional wall motion. Sometimes the right ventricular apex is more influenced by the left ventricular apical motion than what is going on in the rest of the right ventricle. Hypercontractile apical right ventricular function despite akinesia of the basal and mid right ventricular free wall is also seen in pulmonary embolism (McConnell's sign).

Question 45
What is the next most appropriate next step in the management of the patient in Video 4.19?

A. Urgent heart catheterization
B. Start pressors
C. Place an intra-aortic balloon pump
D. Intravenous fluid resuscitation
E. Urgent cardio-thoracic consultation

Answer: D. Intravenous fluid resuscitation. The immediate goal of treatment for patients with right ventricular infarction complicating inferior myocardial infarction is to maintain preload to the right ventricle to ensure adequate cardiac output, blood pressure, coronary artery filling pressures and to prevent shock. In this setting, intravenous fluids (normal saline) should be started. Vasodilators such as nitroglycerin and morphine, beta-blockers and ACE inhibitors all may worsen the hemodynamics. Pressors may be started if cardiac output cannot be maintained with fluids alone. Atropine and pacing may be indicated to support acute bradycardia or heart block. Mechanical support may be necessary in more refractory cases.

Question 46
An 80-year-old female with past medical history of hypertension presents to the emergency department reporting of grumbling chest pain for a week. Electrocardiogram showed antero-lateral ST elevation. Physical exam showed blood

pressure 80/50 mmHg, heart rate 110, bilateral lung crackles and a systolic murmur. Transthoracic echocardiogram was performed. What complication of acute coronary syndrome is suspected in Fig. 4.28?

A. Ruptured papillary muscle
B. Free wall rupture
C. Ventricular septal rupture
D. Mural thrombus
E. Right ventricular infarction

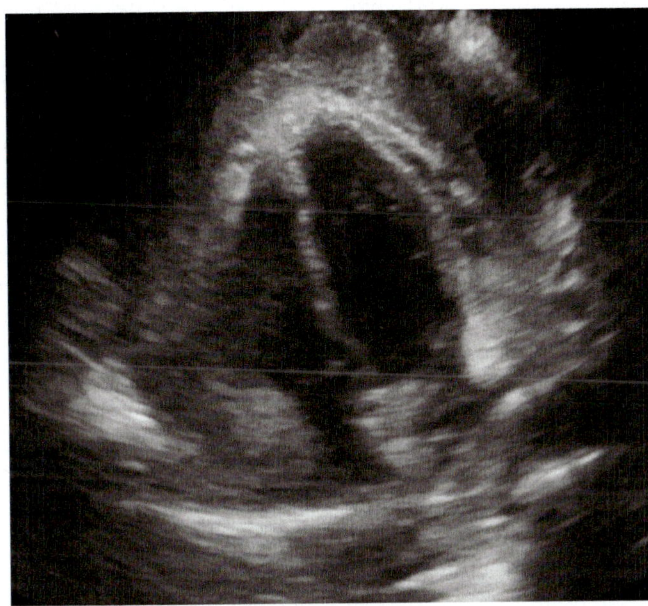

Fig. 4.28 Modified apical 4 chamber view of the left ventricle

Answer: A. Free wall rupture. The echocardiogram shows a very large organizing pericardial effusion (suspected hemopericardium) in the setting of acute coronary syndrome and cardiogenic shock due to pericardial tamponade, and is suspicious for free wall rupture (Fig. 4.28). Free wall rupture is more common in female, elderly patients with a history of hypertension, presenting with a first antero-lateral myocardial infarction, and in particular those with a lack of collateral circulation/ischemic preconditioning. The definitive treatment for free wall rupture is emergency surgical repair. Among patients with ST elevation myocardial presentation, free wall rupture is the least common of the mechanical ruptures that can complicate myocardial infarction.

Question 47

A 65-year-old male with no significant past medical history, presents with substernal chest tightness of 2 h duration. Physical exam showed blood pressure 85/55 mmHg, heart rate 110, bilateral lung crackles and a prominent holosystolic murmur. Electrocardiogram showed ST elevation in inferior leads and a transthoracic echocardiogram was done. What complication of acute coronary syndrome is suspected in Fig. 4.29 and Video 4.20?

A. Ruptured papillary muscle
B. Free wall rupture
C. Ventricular septal rupture
D. Mural thrombus
E. Right ventricular infarction

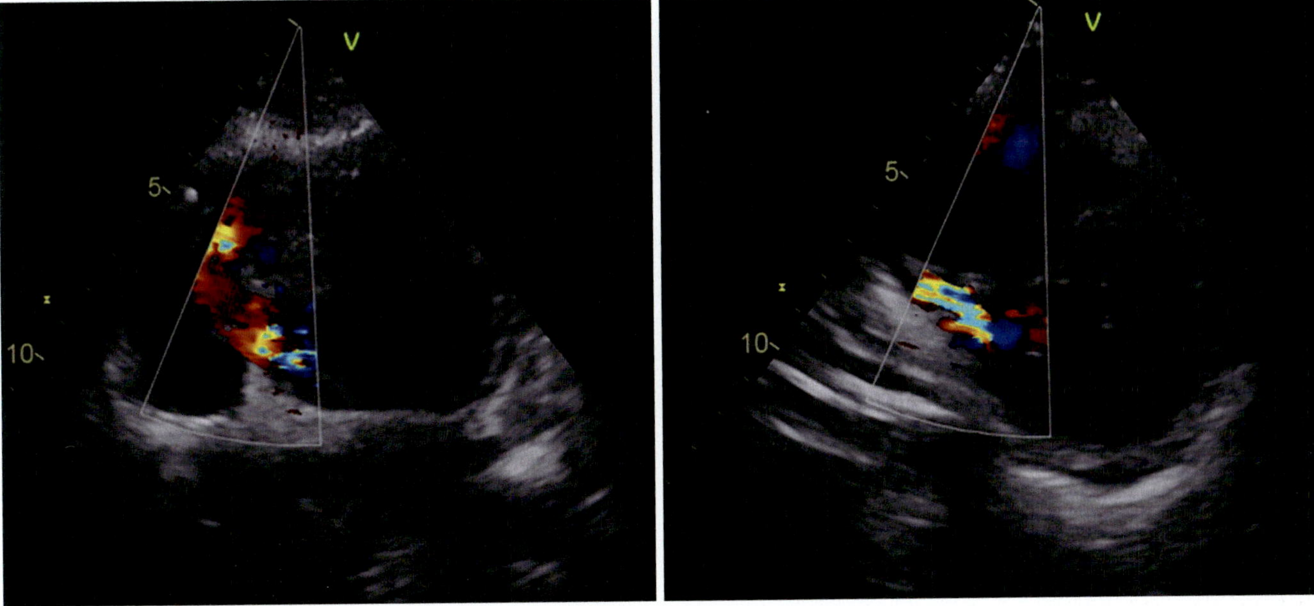

Fig. 4.29 Modified apical 4 chamber view of the left ventricle with color Doppler (left panel) and modified parasternal short axis view of the left ventricle with color Doppler (right panel)

Answer: C. Ventricular septal rupture. Figure 4.29 and Video 4.20 demonstrate echocardiographic views with (holosystolic) flow across the basal interventricular septum, in the setting of an inferior regional wall motion abnormality. Echocardiography also demonstrated severe right ventricular dilation and dysfunction. Among patients with ST elevation myocardial presentation, ventricular septal rupture is the most common of the mechanical ruptures that can complicate myocardial infarction, and occurs with a frequency of about 1 in 500 and is associated with high mortality.

Question 48

A 60-year-old male with prior anterior ST elevation myocardial infarction is admitted with shortness of breath felt to be related to congestive heart failure. Echocardiography reveals findings in Fig. 4.30. This is most consistent with which of the following?

A. Severe prosthetic valvular mitral regurgitation
B. Severe prosthetic paravalvular mitral regurgitation
C. Left ventricular pseudoaneurysm
D. Left ventricular aneurysm
E. Ventricular septal rupture

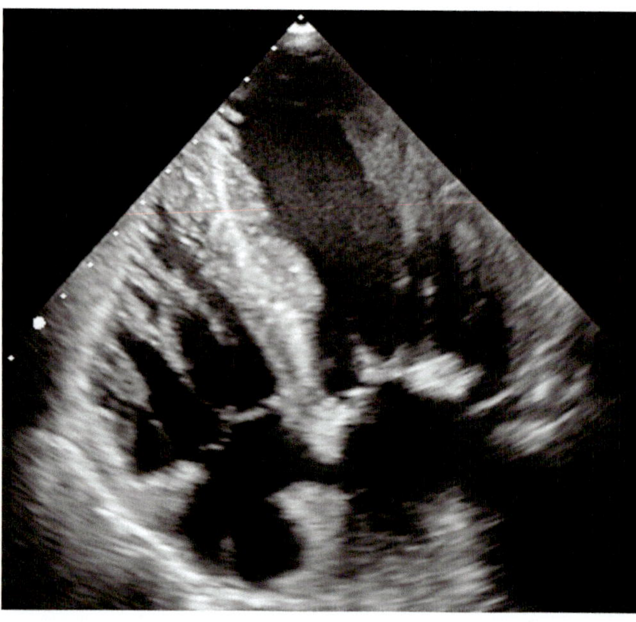

Fig. 4.30 Modified apical 4 chamber view of the left ventricle

Answer: D. Left ventricular aneurysm. A left ventricular aneurysm forms as a result of a healed transmural myocardial infarction and has a well delineated, thin, scarred wall, and most commonly affects the apex and anterior walls (Fig. 4.30). With improvements in the early management of patients with acute myocardial infarction, this complication is less often seen. Left ventricular aneurysms are associated with a high incidence of mural thrombus. Calcification may occur chronically as the area remodels overtime. Left ventricular aneurysm are also associated with increased risks of developing heart failure, ventricular arrhythmias, and thromboembolism. Left ventricular aneurysms are usually treated by medical therapy of the complications that can occur, and consideration of aneurysmectomy in refractory cases.

Question 49

A 60-year-old male with remote mitral valve replacement complicated by left circumflex artery occlusion and postoperative myocardial infarction is admitted with shortness of breath and noted to have a new systolic murmur. Echocardiography reveals parasternal long axis imaging findings in Fig. 4.31. This is most consistent with which of the following?

A. Severe prosthetic valvular mitral regurgitation
B. Severe prosthetic paravalvular mitral regurgitation
C. Left ventricular pseudoaneurysm
D. Left ventricular aneurysm
E. Ventricular septal rupture

Answer: C. Left ventricular pseudoaneurysm. Figure 4.31 shows echocardiographic findings in a parasternal long axis image of flow through the basal infero-lateral (posterior) wall into a pseudoaneurysm cavity behind the heart.

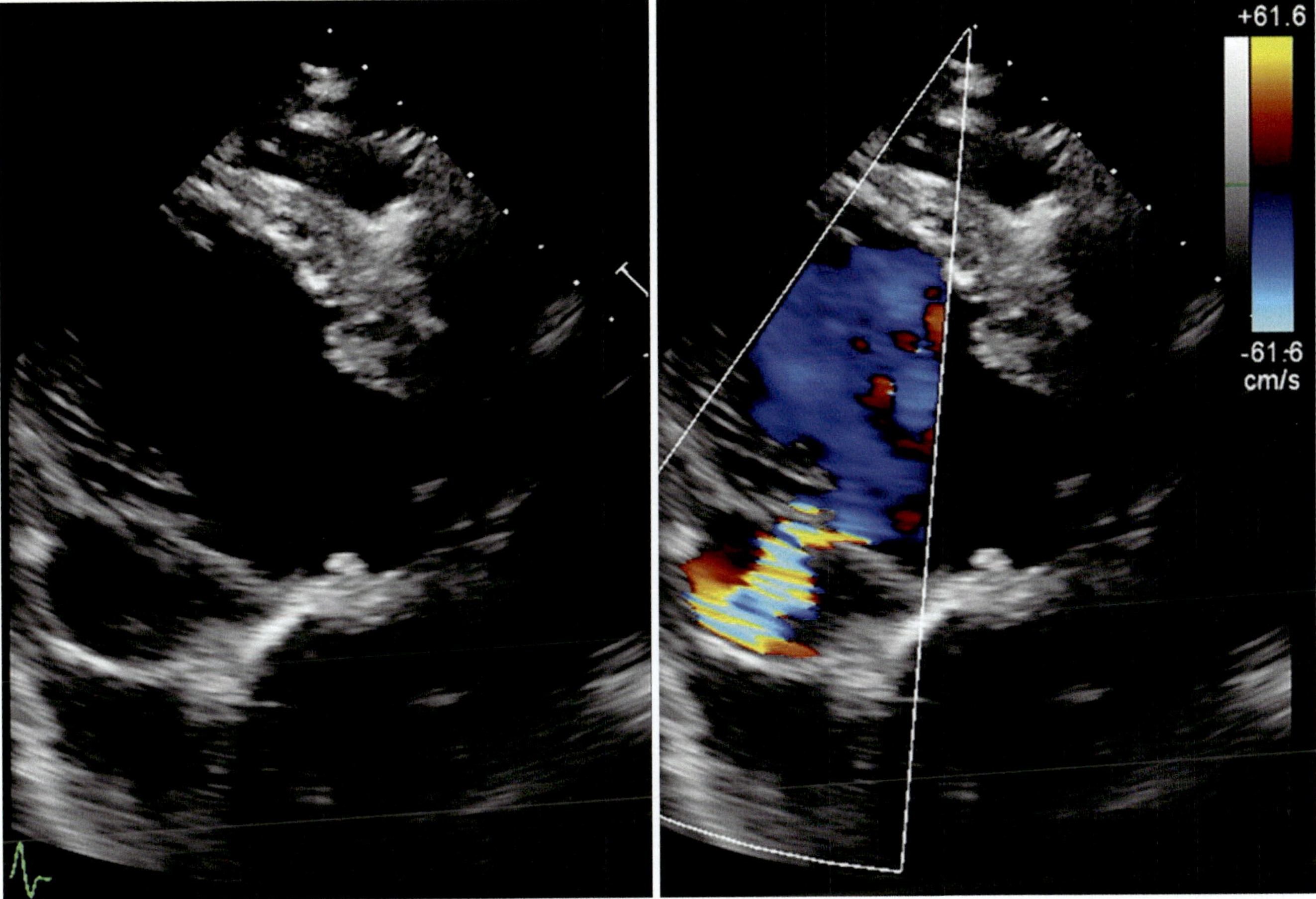

Fig. 4.31 Modified parasternal long axis view of the left ventricle without color Doppler (left panel) and with color Doppler (right panel)

Question 50

A 60-year-old male with a history of prior myocardial infarction is admitted to the intensive care unit with shortness of breath. What findings on an echocardiogram may help distinguish a left ventricular (false) pseudoaneurysm from a left ventricular (true) aneurysm?

A. The neck of the aneurysm
B. Shortness of breath
C. Age of the patient
D. Sex of the patient
E. History of prior myocardial infarction

Answer: A. The neck of the aneurysm. Compared to a (true) left ventricular aneurysm, a left ventricular (false) pseudoaneurysm has a narrow neck. This makes sense when you think that a left ventricular pseudoaneurysm is a consequence of free wall cardiac rupture that is contained by adherent pericardium or scar tissue, and therefore must have a narrow neck, given that only small free wall ruptures of the ventricular wall are compatible with survival. Unlike a true aneurysm, a (false) pseudoaneurysm contains no endo- or myocardium, is more prone to (and high risk for) rupture, so that surgery is the preferred therapeutic option.

Further Reading

Lang RM, Badano LP, Mor-Avi V, et al. Recommendations for cardiac chamber quantification by echocardiography in adults: an update from the American Society of Echocardiography and the European Association of Cardiovascular Imaging. J Am Soc Echocardiogr. 2015;28(1):1–39.e14.

Mor-Avi V, Lang RM, Badano LP, et al. Current and evolving echocardiographic techniques for the quantitative evaluation of cardiac mechanics: ASE/EAE consensus statement on methodology and indications endorsed by the Japanese Society of Echocardiography. J Am Soc Echocardiogr. 2011;24(3):277–313.

Rudski LG, Lai WW, Afilalo J, Hua L, et al. Guidelines for the echocardiographic assessment of the right heart in adults: a report from the American Society of Echocardiography endorsed by the European Association of Echocardiography, a registered branch of the European Society of Cardiology, and the Canadian Society of Echocardiography. J Am Soc Echocardiogr. 2010;23(7):685–713.

Left Ventricle Systolic Function

5

Steven Fox, Milad Matta, and Siddharth Dugar

1. In the parasternal short axis view, which level is most recommended for assessment of LV systolic function?

   A. Aortic valve
   B. Mitral valve
   C. Papillary muscle
   D. Apex

   Answer: C. Papillary Muscle Level.

   Explanation: The papillary muscle level is the recommended level for assessment of LV systolic function in parasternal short axis. The mitral valve level may appear to have less cavity closure due to the presence of the mitral valve annulus; this may lead to underestimation of LV systolic function. The utilization of PSAX view at LV apex level for assessment may lead to overestimation of LV systolic function. The aortic valve level typically does not allow visualization of left ventricular cavity. Notably, in presence of wall motion abnormalities, individual planes may not accurately estimate global LV systolic function [1, 2].

2. Under which of the following conditions is mitral regurgitant jet dp/dt most likely to provide an inaccurate estimate of LV systolic function?

   A. Presence of mitral regurgitation
   B. **Presence of markedly elevated left atrial pressure**
   C. Presence of wall motion abnormalities
   D. Presence of aortic regurgitation

   Answer: B. Presence of markedly elevated left atrial pressure.

   Explanation: The dp/dt estimate of LV systolic function is based on the understanding that higher left ventricular contractility would be associated with a steeper increase in the pressure gradient of the mitral regurgitant jet. However, in case of elevated left atrial pressure, the dp/dt of mitral regurgitant pressure gradient would not solely be influenced by LV contraction but also on the left atrial pressure, thus leading to a reduced slope (change in pressure over change in time) for the mitral regurgitant jet. This would result in reduced dp/dt and thus an underestimation of LV systolic function [3–5].

3. Mitral regurgitant jet dp/dt is used to estimate LV systolic function in setting of normal left atrial pressure. 320 milliseconds elapses between a velocity of 1 m/s and a velocity of 3 m/s. This would correspond to which of the following interpretations for LV systolic function?

   A. **Normal**
   B. Mildly reduced
   C. Moderately reduced
   D. Severely reduced

   Answer A. Normal. dp/dt represents the slope of change in pressure over change in time for the mitral regurgitant jet. The interval to be evaluated is defined by convention as the interval between a regurgitant velocity of 1 m/s and 3 m/s. The change in pressure across this interval is 32 mmHg (4 × 3^2–4 × 1^2), thus in this case the change in pressure divided by change in time is 32 mmHg divided by 0.320 s which equals 1000 and is within the

Supplementary Information The online version contains supplementary material available at https://doi.org/10.1007/978-3-031-45731-9_5.

S. Fox
Cleveland Clinic, Respiratory Institute, Cleveland, OH, USA

M. Matta
Department of Internal Medicine, Internal Medicine, Cleveland Clinic, Cleveland, OH, USA
e-mail: MATTAM@ccf.org

S. Dugar (✉)
Department of Critical Care Medicine, Respiratory Institute, Cleveland Clinic, Cleveland, OH, USA
e-mail: dugars@ccf.org

R. Sreedharan et al. (eds.), *Critical Care Echocardiography*, https://doi.org/10.1007/978-3-031-45731-9_5

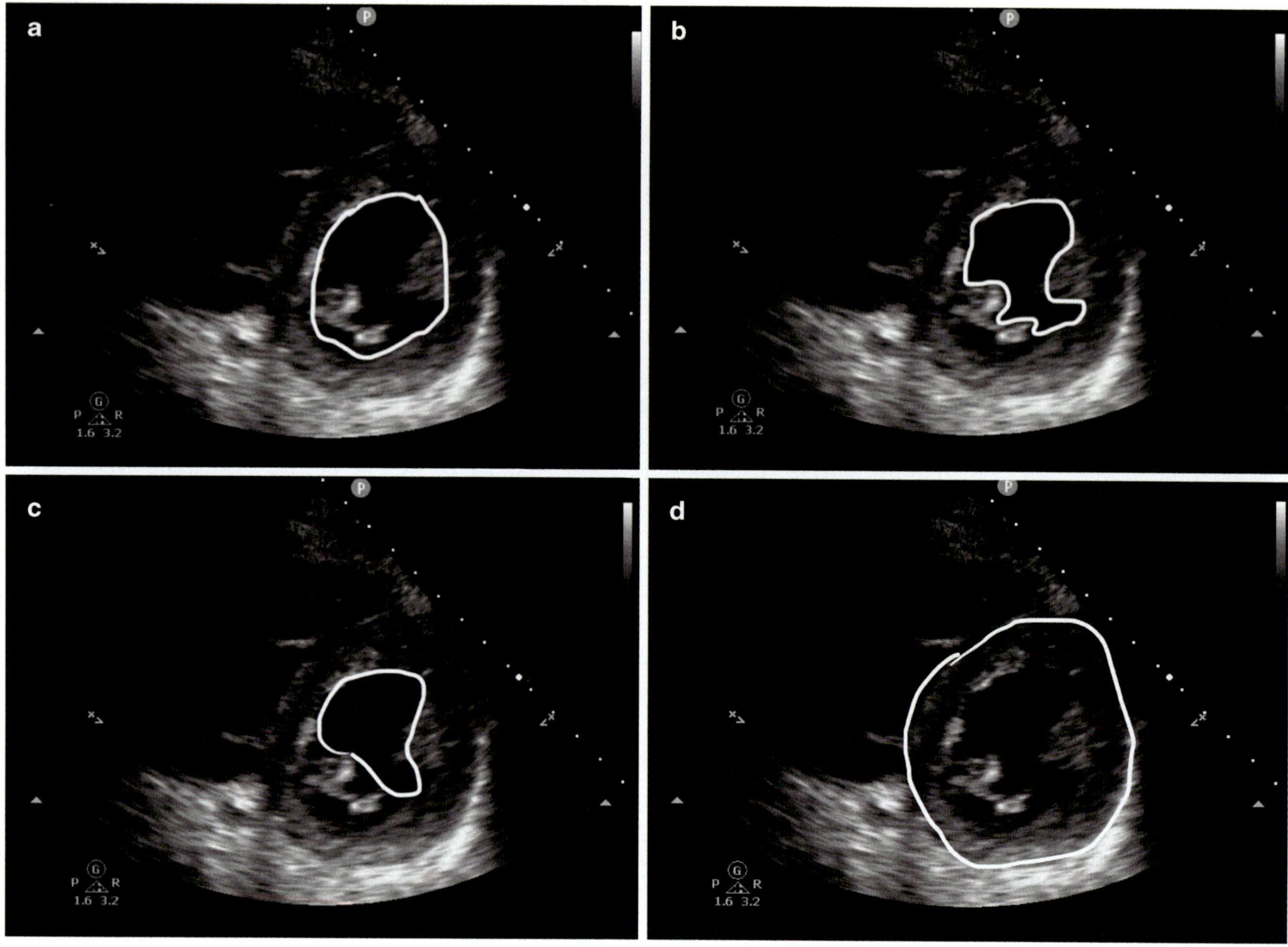

normal range (800–1200). A higher dp/dt represents greater systolic function and a lower dp/dt represents lower systolic function [3, 5].

4. Which of the following is the most correct tracing for evaluation LV fractional area change?

   Answer A. The papillary muscles should not be considered part of the LV endocardium when performing the tracing, as rightly shown in Figure A. In Figure B and C, the papillary muscle was considered part of endocardium, hence are incorrect. The tracing should include the cavity but not the LV wall, as shown in tracing D [5, 6].

5. Which of the following represents a normal range for fractional shortening and fractional area change?

   A. Fractional shortening: 12–24%. Fractional area change 38–60%
   B. **Fractional shortening: 24–36%. Fractional area change 38–60%**
   C. Fractional shortening: 36–48%. Fractional area change 24–36%
   D. Fractional shortening: 12–24%. Fractional area change 24–36%
   E. Fractional shortening: 36–48%. Fractional area change 38–60%

   Answer B. The normal range for **Fractional shortening is 24–36% and the normal range for fractional area change is 38–60%** [7].

6. A 30-year-old female patient with type 1 diabetes mellitus presents with nausea, vomiting is admitted to the ICU with severe anion gap metabolic acidosis, hypotension, elevated lactate, minimal urine output, and lethargy. She is administered 2 L of crystalloid with no improvement in blood pressure and is started on norepinephrine. Critical care echocardiography reveals a hyperdynamic left ventricle. Which of the following statements is most true with the information provided?

   A. The cardiac output is normal or high
   B. The cardiac output is low

C. The patient is volume responsive
D. **No conclusion can be drawn regarding the cardiac output with this information alone**

Answer D. Left ventricular systolic function assessed by qualitative or quantitative change in LV cavity size is a separate variable from cardiac output. A hyperdynamic LV can exist with high, normal, or low cardiac output, depending on preload and afterload conditions. A hyperdynamic left ventricle is observed in distributive, hypovolemic, obstructive, or cardiogenic shock (from right heart failure or valvular disease). Of these, distributive shock states typically have a normal to high cardiac output, while the others have a low cardiac output. Volume responsiveness cannot be concluded solely from observing a hyperdynamic left ventricle alone [8–10].

7. A 50-year-old male is admitted to the intensive care unit with shortness of breath. Lung Ultrasound showed diffuse B lines pattern. Critical care echocardiography reveals severely reduced LV systolic function with anterior-septal wall hypokinesia. Which of the following methods of quantifying LV systolic function is expected to be most accurate in this case?

A. **Biplane Simpson method**
B. Teicholz method
C. LV fractional area change
D. E point septal separation
E. Area-length method

Answer A. Quantification of LV systolic function is challenging in cases of regional wall motion abnormalities. The biplane Simpson method assumes the left ventricular cavity is made up of multiple stacked discs. This method has some ability to account for irregularities in shape and contraction of different regions of the ventricle. The remaining methods are very inaccurate, particularly in the setting of regional wall motion abnormalities. The Teicholz method (Answer B) is based on a single measurement of the LV cavity at the tip of mitral valve and assumes a simple ellipsoid shape of the left ventricle. LV fractional area change (Answer C) similarly assesses LV systolic function in a single plane (parasternal short axis, papillary muscle level). E point septal separation (Answer D) only evaluates mitral valve approximation to the septum. Area-length method (Answer E) assumes a bullet-shaped left ventricle. Given the other methods than Biplane Simpson assesses LV systolic function at one site and then assumes it represent the global function, they have higher rate of inaccuracies which is exaggerated in cases of regional wall motion abnormality [5, 6].

8. A 45 year female is admitted to the ICU with acute cardiogenic pulmonary edema and cardiogenic shock due to infective endocarditis of the mitral valve with acute severe regurgitation. Critical care echocardiography reveals normal LV systolic function and severe mitral regurgitation, with a left ventricular outflow tract velocity time integral of 6 (averaged over 5 beats). She undergoes successful mitral valve replacement. Postoperatively compared to preoperatively, which of the following changes would be expected for LV systolic function and for LVOT VTI.

A. LV systolic function: Increased. LVOT VTI: Increased
B. LV systolic function: Increased. LVOT VTI: Unchanged
C. LV systolic function: Unchanged. LVOT VTI: Unchanged.
D. **LV systolic function: Decreased. LVOT VTI: Increased.**
E. LV systolic function: Decreased. LVOT VTI: Decreased

Answer: D. The left ventricle systolic function and output is load dependent. LV afterload is low in the setting of severe MR due to a significant fraction of Regurgitant flow. This is expected to elevate the LV systolic function while reducing the systemic cardiac output. Correction of the problem will typically lead to a reduction in LV systolic function and an increase in cardiac output [11].

9. Which of the following views are used for the Biplane Simpson method of estimating LV ejection fraction?

A. **Apical 4 chamber and Apical 2 chamber**
B. Apical 4 chamber and Apical 3 chamber
C. Parasternal long axis and parasternal short axis
D. Apical 3 chamber and parasternal short axis
E. Apical 2 chamber and parasternal short axis

Answer A. The Simpson method relies on the principle that the left ventricular volume can be approximated by the summation of multiple stacked cylindrical discs of varying diameters with the same height. A tracing of the left ventricle is obtained at end-diastole and end-systole, which is used to calculate the end-diastolic and end-systolic volume, which are then used to calculate LV EF. Preferably both apical 4 chamber and apical 2 chamber views are used for measurement, often described as the Biplane Simpson method. This is the recommended method for evaluation of LV EF using 2D echocardiography. Assessment can be limited in cases with beat-to-beat variability in stroke volume, arrhythmia, dyssynchronous contraction, or regional wall motion abnormalities [6].

10. A 70-year-old male develops acute chest pain while sitting in traffic and is brought into the ED. On arrival, BP is 90/60, HR 130, SpO_2 94% on room air, T 37.0, RR 22/min. He undergoes left heart catheterization which reveals no coronary artery obstruction. He is admitted to the ICU. Critical care echocardiography reveals the following parasternal long and apical 5 chamber view. E point septal separation is subsequently measured in the parasternal long axis view to be 4 mm. Which of the following statements is most accurate?

    A. Based on the EPSS of 4 mm, the LV systolic function is most likely normal.
    B. Based on the EPSS of 4 mm, the LV systolic function is most likely reduced.
    C. **The EPSS does not accurately represent the LV systolic function in this case.**
    D. 4 mm is a borderline value for EPSS so the interpretation is unclear (Videos 5.1 and 5.2).

    Answer C. This image demonstrates apical hypokinesia. Apical hypokinesia in this clinical setting may be due to ischemia (typically a lesion in the left anterior descending artery) or stress-induced cardiomyopathy. Left heart catheterization is necessary in such a case to exclude ischemia. In this case, with the clinical picture described, the echocardiographic findings shown, and the normal coronary angiography, the diagnosis of stress-induced cardiomyopathy can be made. In such cases with focal or segmental asymmetric hypokinesia or akinesis, assessment of LV systolic function can be difficult with regional measurement. Some methods of evaluation are particularly prone to error in such situations, including E-point septal separation (EPSS). EPSS is a measurement of how closely the anterior leaflet of the mitral valve approaches the septum. This value is more affected by more vigorous contraction at the LV base compared to the LV apex. Thus, in a case like this, the EPSS may be normal (<0.6 cm) despite a significantly reduced LV systolic function [12, 13].

11. Which of the following values of MAPSE would be considered normal?

    A. 8 mm
    B. **13 mm**
    C. 18 mm
    D. 23 mm
    E. 28 mm

    Answer B. Mitral annular plane systolic excursion (MAPSE) is used in the evaluation of LV systolic function, with higher values indicating more vigorous LV systolic function. MAPSE is obtained by placing the M-mode cursor through the lateral annulus of the mitral valve in apical 4 chamber view. The normal range for MAPSE is 12–15 mm. A MAPSE value below 8 mm is associated with LVEF <50%, with sensitivity of 98% and specificity of 80% [14, 15].

12. You are caring for a 65-year-old female admitted with severe COVID-19 pneumonia, respiratory failure on mechanical ventilation. She develops worsening shock on day 3 of hospital stay. Critical care echocardiography is used to evaluate for LV systolic dysfunction. Views are obtained in parasternal long axis, parasternal short axis, and apical 4 chamber. The chambers are seen but endocardial definition is extremely limited. Which of the following methods of categorizing LV systolic function would be most applicable?

    A. Biplane Simpson
    B. LV fractional area change
    C. LV fractional shortening
    D. Area length method
    E. **Eyeball semi quantitative classification**

    Answer E. In a 2006 study of critically ill patients found eyeball semi quantitative classification classified patients more accurately compared with actual measurements of left ventricular ejection fraction by fractional area change (Answer B) or area-length method (Answer D). The same applies for LV fractional shortening (Answer C). Biplane Simpson method is difficult and less likely to be accurate when endocardial definition is poor, as in this case. This is a common limitation of the biplane Simpson method in critically ill patients [16].

13. Which of the following M-mode cursor positions is recommended for assessment of MAPSE (lateral annulus)

    Answer C. The MAPSE cursor should pass through the LV apex and the lateral annulus of the mitral valve (the M-mode cursor in Answer A and B do not pass through the apex). If the M-mode cursor is directed too lateral and into the LV lateral wall (Answer D), excursion may be over- or under-estimated. Care should also be taken not to place the m-mode cursor through the mitral valve leaflet itself (Answer E). If the window does not allow optimum positioning of the M-mode cursor, Anatomic M-mode can be applied to optimize M-mode cursor position [14, 17].

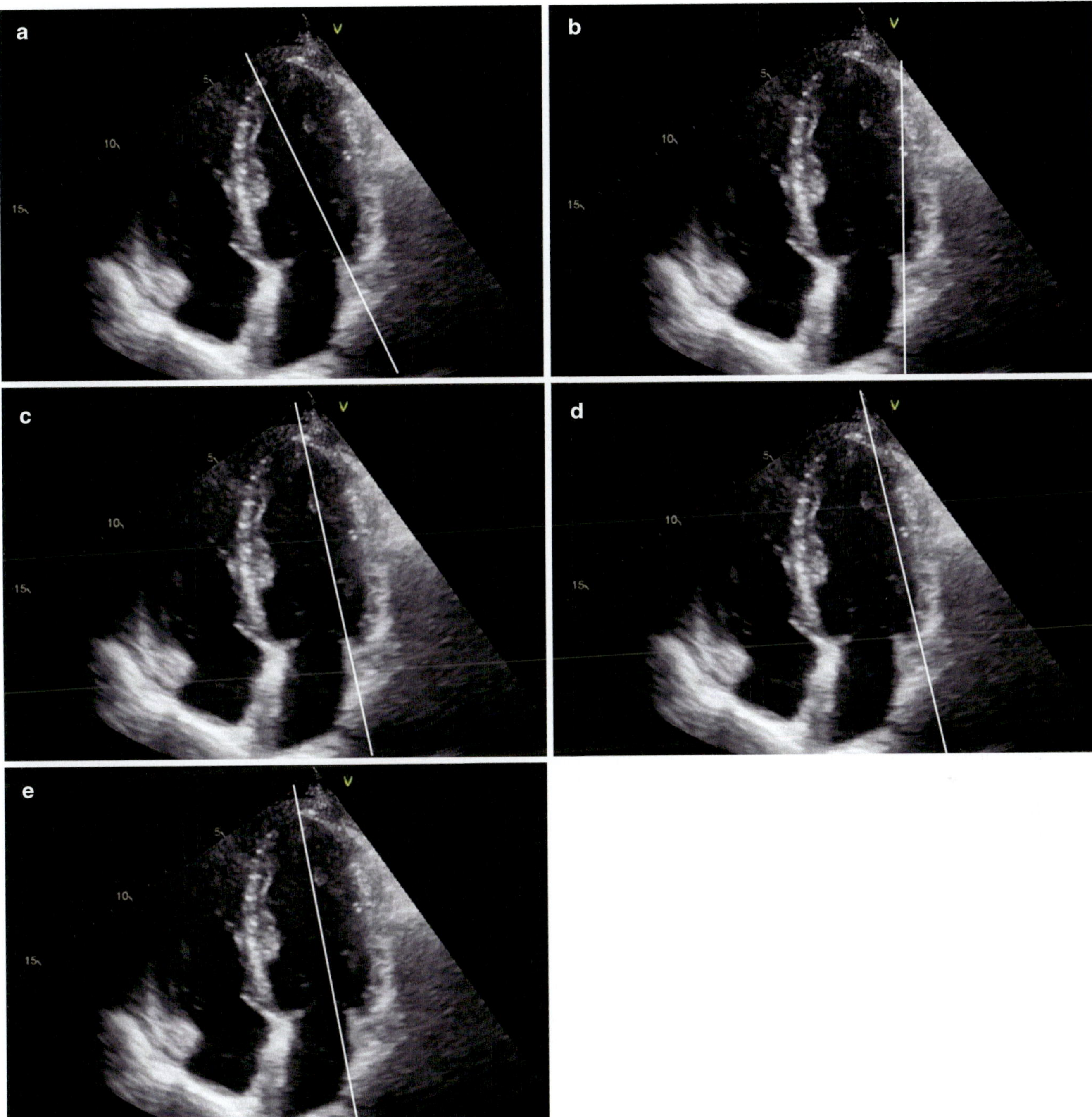

14. Of all the following potential methods for evaluating LV contractility, which one is most afterload dependent?

   A. Speckle Tracking
   B. Maximal Elastance
   C. Acceleration of Aortic Blood Flow
   D. **Measurement of the slope of the mitral Regurgitant jet**
   E. Rate corrected velocity of circumferential fiber shortening

Answer D. LV systolic function is dependent on contractility as well as afterload. Higher afterload will lead to lower ejection fraction if contractility remains constant. Several methods are being used to evaluate contractility, including speckle tracking, maximal elastance, acceleration of aortic blood flow, and rate corrected velocity of circumferential fiber shortening (Answers A, B, C, and E) which is less affected by afterload. dP/dT (measurement of the slope of the mitral Regurgitant jet) can be used to evaluate LV systolic function but does not evaluate contractility independent of afterload (Answer D) [3].

Questions 15 and 16.

A 40-year-old female is admitted with high fevers and several days of nausea and vomiting and is noted to be hypotensive and hypoxic with bilateral lower extremity edema and is admitted to the medical ICU and initiated on broad spectrum antibiotics for sepsis. She receives 30 cc/kg of crystalloid and is subsequently initiated on norepinephrine for ongoing shock. Critical care echocardiography reveals the following in parasternal long axis view (Video 5.3).

15. How would you describe the LV systolic function?

 A. Hyperdynamic
 B. Normal
 C. Moderately Reduced
 D. Severely Reduced

Answer A. The LV systolic function is hyperdynamic by eyeball semi-quantitative estimation in this clip. There is significant reduction in LV cavity size during systole. In addition, the anterior mitral valve leaflet contacts the septum in early diastole (EPSS). The mitral annular excursion appears normal. All walls appear to thicken by a factor of >1.5. When quantitative measurement is used, hyperdynamic refers to a LV EF greater than or equal to 70%. The distinction between normal and hyperdynamic LV systolic function on eyeball semi quantitative estimation is sometimes not very clear. Features to suggest a hyperdynamic LV include complete or near-complete cavity obliteration as well as contact of the mitral valve anterior leaflet with the septum. Sometimes a fast heart rate may give an observer the impression of a hyperdynamic LV when in fact systolic function is normal. Caution should be taken not to mistake tachycardia with a normal LV systolic function for a hyperdynamic left ventricle [1].

16. Which of the following can be concluded from the information given?

 A. The patient is volume down and will benefit from additional fluid administration.
 B. The patient is volume up and will benefit from fluid removal
 C. The shock is most likely cardiogenic
 D. The shock may be distributive, obstructive, or hypovolemic
 E. Distributive, cardiogenic, obstructive, and hypovolemic shock all remain on the differential.

Answer E. A hyperdynamic left ventricle indicates a high ratio of stroke volume to end diastolic volume. This can occur in settings of low LV filling, increased contractility, septal hypertrophy, reduced LV afterload, or valvular disease. This profile is routinely observed in septic shock, cardiogenic shock from acute aortic or mitral valve regurgitation, obstructive shock from a pulmonary embolus with acute Cor-pulmonale, and hypovolemic shock. A hyperdynamic left ventricle does not by itself indicate volume responsiveness (for example in the case of pulmonary embolus with severe right ventricular dilation). In order to distinguish the different causes of shock and to determine volume responsiveness, additional evaluation is required.

The following images apply to questions 17, 18 (Videos 5.4 and 5.5).

17. Which of the following is correct regarding LV systolic function for the clips shown?

 A. Hyperdynamic
 B. Normal
 C. Mildly reduced
 D. Moderately to severely reduced

Answer D. This clip demonstrates reduced wall thickening, reduced cavity reduction, reduced excursion of the anterior leaflet of the mitral valve, and reduced excursion of the lateral annulus of the mitral valve, indicating reduced LV systolic function. Guidelines define severe LV systolic dysfunction as LV EF < 30%, and moderate systolic dysfunction as LV EF 30–39%, mild LV systolic dysfunction as 40–49%, normal as 50–69%, and hyperdynamic as 70% or more [18].

18. Which of the following is present for the image shown?

 A. Global akinesis
 B. A heterogeneous pattern of LV wall thickening
 C. Normal LV systolic function
 D. Hyperdynamic LV

Answer **B.** Wall thickening is reduced throughout (hypokinesia) but is most notably reduced (akinesis) in the antero-septal, septal, and infero-septal regions. Thus a heterogeneous pattern of LV wall thickening is present, often referred to as regional wall motion abnormality. The left ventricle is thus not globally akinetic (answer A). The LV systolic function is moderately to severely reduced (Answers C and D are incorrect).

19. Which of the following is correct regarding LV systolic function for the image shown?

    A. Hyperdynamic
    B. Normal
    C. Moderately reduced
    D. Severely reduced (Video 5.6)

    Answer D. Guidelines define severe LV systolic dysfunction as LV EF < 30%, moderate systolic dysfunction as LV EF 30–39%, mild LV systolic dysfunction as 40–49%, normal as 50–69%, and hyperdynamic as 70% or more. The distinction between moderately and severely reduced LV systolic function on eyeball qualitative assessment can be difficult to define. In a case such as this, the LV wall thickening, cavity closure, and mitral valve excursion are reduced significantly, with all walls being nearly akinetic and minimal motion of the mitral valve. This would be consistent with severe LV systolic dysfunction, which would correlate with LVEF <30%.

20. How would you grade the LV systolic function for the following study?

    A. Hyperdynamic
    B. Normal
    C. Mildly reduced
    D. Severely Reduced (Videos 5.7, 5.8, 5.9)

    Answer C. Guidelines define severe LV systolic dysfunction as LV EF < 30%, moderate systolic dysfunction as LV EF 30–39%, mild LV systolic dysfunction as 40–49%, normal as 50–69%, and hyperdynamic as 70% or more. In a case such as this, the LV wall thickening, cavity closure, and mitral valve excursion are mildly reduced, with mildly reduced motion of the mitral valve. This would be consistent with mild LV systolic dysfunction, which would correlate with LVEF <40–39%.

21. Contractility on a TTE can be assessed by the dp/dt formula by evaluating the time required for the left ventricle to generate what pressure difference?

    A. 12 mmHg
    B. 32 mmHg
    C. 35 mmHg
    D. 40 mmHg

    Answer B. Using the Bernoulli Equation (P = 4 × V^2) we can determine the gradient pressures using the velocities: Pressure at 1 m/s = 4 × 1^2 = 4 mmHg. Pressure at 3 m/s = 4 × 3^2 = 36 mmHg. dp = 36–4 = 32 mmHg. Making the equation dp/dt = 32/1 (in seconds). Based on this calculation we can deduce that the dp/dt formula is actually the time it is takes for the ventricle to generate a pressure difference of 32 mmHg.

22. What type of Doppler needs to be used to evaluate contractility using mitral Regurgitant dp/dt?

    A. Tissue doppler
    B. Continuous wave doppler
    C. Color doppler
    D. Pulse wave doppler

    Answer B. For dp/dt continuous wave Doppler should be used. Pulse wave Doppler applies intermittent pulses of sound waves in order to evaluate the velocities at a set distance (within the sample volume gate). The frequency at which pulses are emitted is the pulse repetition frequency (PRF). Doppler shifts greater than half of the PRF will exceed the Nyquist limit and aliasing will occur, limiting the ability to quantify high velocities. Continuous wave Doppler applies continuous sound waves, so it does not evaluate the velocity at a set distance, but rather along the entire axis. Because pulses are continuously emitted and received, the Nyquist limit does not apply to continuous wave Doppler, making it better than pulse wave Doppler for higher velocity movement, such as the mitral Regurgitant jet. Color Doppler (Answer C) would not enable quantification of the dp/dt because a waveform is not produce. Tissue doppler (Answer A) amplifies and displays low velocity signals from tissue, while filtering out high velocity signals from fluid, so this is not used for dp/dt.

23. 69-year-old male is admitted to the Intensive Care Unit in the setting of undifferentiated shock. His past medical history is significant for ischemic cardiomyopathy with echocardiogram 2 months ago showing normal EF at 50%, complete heart block s/p pacemaker placement, hypertension, and hyperlipidemia. EKG shows atrial fibrillation with paced rhythm. To further elucidate the cause of his shock, you perform critical care echocardiography and observe EPSS of 11 mm and MAPSE of 7 mm. You conclude the following:

    A. This patient has an abnormal EPSS and abnormal MAPSE meaning his EF is likely lower than his prior echocardiogram.
    B. Neither EPSS nor MAPSE can be used to evaluate EF in this patient
    C. EPSS can be used to estimate EF in this patient but the use of MAPSE is not valid here
    D. MAPSE can be used to estimate EF in this patient but the use of EPSS is not valid here

Answer B. EPSS cannot be reliably used in the setting of atrial fibrillation due to absence of synchronized atrial activity and will have beat to beat variability. In addition, EPSS cannot also be used in the setting of significant mitral stenosis, significant aortic regurgitation where movement of mitral valve is impacted by factors other than pressure gradient between left atrium and left ventricle during early diastolic filling phase. MAPSE cannot be used in patients with dyssynchrony, including left bundle branch block, Wolf-Parkinson-White syndrome, and paced rhythm [12, 13].

24. Fractional shortening assessed in the parasternal long axis view estimates contraction in which region of the heart?

    A. Apical part of the septum and lateral wall
    B. Apical part of the antero-septal and inferior walls
    C. Basal part of the septum and lateral wall
    D. Basal part of the antero-septal and inferior walls

    Answer A. Parasternal long axis view is recommended for measurement of fractional shortening. Parasternal short axis view can also be used for measurement of fractional shortening. The M-mode cursor should be placed at the level of the papillary muscles. Care should be taken to keep the M-mode cursor perpendicular to the LV chamber axis. This axis evaluates the basal antero-septal and the basal inferio-lateral wall [6].

25. Mitral annular plane systolic excursion of <6 mm reflects an ejection fraction of?

    A. >55%
    B. <50%
    C. <30%
    D. 20%

    Answer C. Mitral annular plane systolic excursion (MAPSE) is routinely referred to as atrioventricular displacement. MAPSE has been suggested as a surrogate measurement for left ventricular function given the ease of its measurement. It is a simple regional measurement assessing longitudinal function of left ventricle that can even be performed by novice practitioners. In addition, its measurement is less dependent on endocardial resolution and can be performed even in technically challenging studies. Routinely, an average value of MAPSE from septal and lateral mitral for decision making. However, studies have also used measurement either from the septal or lateral annulus to predict outcome in critically ill patients. MAPSE>10 mm is highly reflective of an EF >55%. MAPSE <6 mm predicts LV EF of <30% with positive predictive value of 100% in men and 88% in women [14].

26. 65-year-old male with past medical history significant for coronary artery disease with ischemic cardiomyopathy and heart failure with reduced ejection fraction, along with chronic kidney disease presented to the intensive care unit with shock of unclear etiology. The patient has been feeling unwell with fever and new onset cough and sputum production for the last few days. The following conclusions can be made based on the Video? (Video 5.10)

    A. Patient is in cardiogenic shock based on his images showing decreased LV systolic function
    B. A cardiac component could be playing a role in his shock, but further assessment is required
    C. Patient is known to have low ejection fraction thus this is not a new finding, his current cardiac status is not playing a role in his shock
    D. Echocardiography could not be used to help determine cause of shock

    Answer B. Images of this patient show a severely reduced LV systolic function based on the eyeball method. However, it will be erroneous to deem his shock to be related to his low ejection fraction. This patient is known to have heart failure with reduced Ejection fraction. It cannot be assumed that his shock is related to his markedly reduced LV systolic function in setting of pre-existing heart disease. The current differential diagnosis in this patient based on history and echocardiography findings suggest either cardiogenic shock or septic shock in a patient with known chronic heart failure. A thorough assessment of cardiac function including measurement of LVOT VTI/stroke volume along with an assessment of the patient's hemodynamic extending beyond critical care echocardiography is needed to clearly identify the cause of shock [3, 19, 20].

27. 75-year-old patient with known ischemic cardiomyopathy (an echocardiogram from two days ago showed an ejection fraction of 25%) on standard goal directed medical treatment with Carvedilol, Lisinopril and Spironolactone comes into the ICU with fever, chills and low blood pressure and is suspected to be in septic shock. The patient was adequately fluid resuscitated, started on broad spectrum antibiotics. Critical care echocardiography was performed after resuscitation goal was achieved with good endocardial definition and uses the Biplane Simpson method to calculate an ejection fraction of 40%. The discordance between recent formal echocardiography and critical care echocardiography in this case is most likely due to

A. Improved cardiac function in the setting of GDMT use
B. Ejection fraction can be affected by afterload and his ejection fraction is likely a reflection of decreased afterload from vasoplegia
C. Ejection fraction can be affected by afterload and his ejection fraction is likely a reflection of decreased afterload from vasoplegia.
D. The critical care echocardiography findings are erroneous

Answer is B. It is highly unlikely for GDMT to improve ejection fraction in such a short duration given that the patient had a prior echocardiography recently (Answer A). Ejection fraction is dependent on contractility, but it is also directly related to preload and inversely related to afterload. A decrease in the afterload which is likely to be seen in distributive shock (i.e. septic shock), will increase LV ejection measurement and even lead to pseudonormalization of LV function as assessed by LVEF. In study, assessing influence of loading conditions in septic shock, the author found contractility indices to be not associated with preload indices once adequate fluid resuscitation was achieved, but inversely correlated with afterload indices as in this case (Answer C). In case of significantly reduced preload, echocardiogram performed prior to resuscitation in patient with normal systolic function, the LV ejection fraction will appear higher as ejection fraction assess stroke volume standardized to end diastolic volume, which is reduced in setting of severe hypovolemia. The ejection fraction should always be interpreted in the settings of patient's hemodynamics. Though there is potential for error on any echocardiography study, the discrepancy in ejection fraction can be explained by difference in clinical condition, so we cannot conclude that either study was erroneous based on the information provided (Answer D).

28. Bedside echocardiography performed on a male patient shows a left ventricular end diastolic diameter (LVEDD) of 50 mm along with a left ventricular end systolic diameter (LVESD) 40 mm obtained in the parasternal long axis view. In the absence of asymmetric wall motion, based on those numbers you would qualify the LV systolic function as:

A. Hyperdynamic
B. Normal
C. Mildly reduced
D. Severely reduced

Answer C. LV systolic function can be estimated using M-mode by measuring end diastolic and end systolic diameters to get to the fractional shortening.

Fractional shortening = (LVEDD-LVESD)/LVEDD × 100.

Fractional shortening in this patient = (50–40)/50 × 100 = 20%.

Based on the table below, a fractional shortening of 20% in a man corresponds to a mildly abnormal (approaching moderately abnormal) LV systolic function [5, 21].

29. Which of the following statements is true regarding fractional shortening (FS):

A. Fractional shortening can be used to assess LV function in patients with septal wall motion abnormality
B. Fractional shortening can overestimate LV function in patient with posterior wall motion abnormality.
C. The endpoints of the measurement should be the innermost endocardium of the papillary muscles.
D. Fractional shortening of 40% typically corresponds to an ejection fraction of greater than 55%.
E. If the M mode cursor cannot be aligned perpendicular to the endocardium; then there fractional shortening cannot be measured.

Answer C. Fractional shortening provides a rough estimate of left ventricular ejection fraction (LVEF), with a reference range of 27–45% for women and 25–43% for men. Thus, a fractional shortening of 40% corresponds with normal LV systolic function (Answer D). This method has several limitations. FS assesses septal wall and posterior wall motions, making it inaccurate in the setting of posterior/septal wall motion abnormalities (Answers A and B). FS also relies heavily on the ability to delineate septal and posterior wall endocardial border so having poor image quality will affect FS measurement. The measurement are obtained from endocardial blood interface of the ventricular wall of the heart (not the inner border of the papillary muscle) (Answer C). If M-mode is used, the M-mode cursor must be perpendicular to the endocardium. If the M-mode cursor cannot be aligned perpendicular to the endocardium, there are other ways to perform the measurement (Answer E): (1) The image can be paused at end-diastole (and end-systole) with the calipers applied to perform the measurement, or (2) anatomic M-mode (a method of image processing that adjusts the angle of the M-mode cursor) may be used to make the M-mode cursor in the correct axis.

30. Bedside echocardiography performed on a female patient shows a left ventricular end diastolic area (LVEDA) of 75 cm^2 along with a left ventricular end systolic area (LVESA) 45 cm^2. Based on measurements, how will one grade LV systolic function?

    A. Hyperdynamic
    B. Normal
    C. Mildly reduced
    D. Severely reduced

    Answer B. Fractional area change (FAC) can be estimated by measuring end diastolic and end systolic areas.

    FAC = (LVEDA-LVESA)/LVEDA × 100.

    Fractional area changes in this patient = (75–40)/75 × 100 = 40%.

    FAC >35% is correlated with normal function, and FAC <15% is correlated with severe LV systolic dysfunction. Thus, for this patient, FAC of 40% would qualify the LV systolic function as normal, within the limitations of the method.

31. What is true regarding speckle tracking:

    A. This method of estimation of the systolic function is less prone to error compared to other quantitative methods of the left ventricular function in the setting of regional wall motion abnormality and desynchrony.
    B. The best parameter of this method is the global longitudinal strain with a normal value close to −10%
    C. This method functions in the same way across different vendor software.
    D. A change in LV systolic function will be noted earlier on the ejection fraction measurement compared to speckle tracking method.

    Answer A. Speckle tracking offer the advantage of being less prone to error compared to other quantitative methods of the left ventricular systolic function assessment in the setting RWMA and dyssynchrony (Answer A). It is true that the global longitudinal strain (GLS) is currently considered the best parameter to assess cardiac function given its limited dependence on loading condition. However, normal values are close to −18%, so −10% would represent an abnormal GLS (Answer B). Speckle tracking is affected by the vendor software on which it is performed (Answer C). A change in LV systolic function will be picked up on speckle tracking earlier compared to ejection fraction, which is especially relevant in certain conditions including chemotherapy-related subclinical dysfunction, sepsis induced cardiomyopathy and infiltrative diseases [22–24].

Fractional Shortening (%)	Men	Women
Reference Normal	25–43%	27–45%
Mildly Abnormal	20–24%	22–26%
Moderately Abnormal	15–19%	17–21%
Severely Abnormal	≤ 14%	≤ 16%

References

1. Soni NJ, Arntfield R, Kory P. Point-of care-ultrasound. 2nd ed. Philadelphia, PA: Elsevier; 2019.
2. Zerbib Y, Maizel J, Slama M. Echocardiographic assessment of left ventricular function. J Emerg Crit Care Med. 2019;3:33.
3. de Backer D, Cholley BP, Slama M, Vieillard-Baron A, Vignon P. In: de Backer D, Cholley BP, Slama M, Vieillard-Baron A, Vignon P, editors. Hemodynamic monitoring using echocardiography in the critically ill [electronic resource]. 1st ed. Berlin, Heidelberg: Springer Berlin Heidelberg; 2011.
4. Bargiggia GS, Bertucci C, Recusani F, Raisaro A, de Servi S, Valdes-Cruz LM, et al. A new method for estimating left ventricular dP/dt by continuous wave Doppler-echocardiography. Validation studies at cardiac catheterization. Circulation. 1989;80(5):1287–92.
5. Chengode S. Left ventricular global systolic function assessment by echocardiography. Ann Card Anaesth. 2016;19(Supplement):S26–34.
6. Lang RM, Badano LP, Mor-Avi V, Afilalo J, Armstrong A, Ernande L, et al. Recommendations for cardiac chamber quantification by echocardiography in adults: an update from the American Society of Echocardiography and the European Association of Cardiovascular Imaging. J Am Soc Echocardiogr. 2015;28(1):1–39.e14.
7. Quinones MA, Waggoner AD, Reduto LA, Nelson JG, Young JB, Winters WL Jr, et al. A new, simplified and accurate method for determining ejection fraction with two-dimensional echocardiography. Circulation. 1981;64(4):744–53.
8. Bednarczyk JM, Fridfinnson JA, Kumar A, Blanchard L, Rabbani R, Bell D, et al. Incorporating dynamic assessment of fluid responsiveness into goal-directed therapy: a systematic review and meta-analysis. Crit Care Med. 2017;45(9):1538–45.
9. Cherpanath TG, Geerts BF, Lagrand WK, Schultz MJ, Groeneveld AB. Basic concepts of fluid responsiveness. Neth Heart J. 2013;21(12):530–6.
10. Boissier F, Razazi K, Seemann A, Bedet A, Thille AW, de Prost N, et al. Left ventricular systolic dysfunction during septic shock: the role of loading conditions. Intensive Care Med. 2017;43(5):633–42.
11. Huikuri HV. Effect of mitral valve replacement on left ventricular function in mitral regurgitation. Br Heart J. 1983;49(4):328–33.
12. Ginzton LE, Kulick D. Mitral valve E-point septal separation as an indicator of ejection fraction in patients with reversed septal motion. Chest. 1985;88(3):429–31.
13. Silverstein JR, Laffely NH, Rifkin RD. Quantitative estimation of left ventricular ejection fraction from mitral valve E-point to septal separation and comparison to magnetic resonance imaging. Am J Cardiol. 2006;97(1):137–40.
14. Matos J, Kronzon I, Panagopoulos G, Perk G. Mitral annular plane systolic excursion as a surrogate for left ventricular ejection fraction. J Am Soc Echocardiogr. 2012;25(9):969–74.
15. Hu K, Liu D, Herrmann S, Niemann M, Gaudron PD, Voelker W, et al. Clinical implication of mitral annular plane systolic excursion for patients with cardiovascular disease. Eur Heart J Cardiovasc Imaging. 2013;14(3):205–12.
16. Vieillard-Baron A, Charron C, Chergui K, Peyrouset O, Jardin F. Bedside echocardiographic evaluation of hemodynamics in sepsis: is a qualitative evaluation sufficient? Intensive Care Med. 2006;32(10):1547–52.

17. Prada G, Vieillard-Baron A, Martin AK, Hernandez A, Mookadam F, Ramakrishna H, et al. Echocardiographic applications of M-mode ultrasonography in anesthesiology and critical care. J Cardiothorac Vasc Anesth. 2019;33(6):1559–83.
18. Dugar S, Sato R, Chawla S, Young J, Wang X, Grimm R, et al. Is left ventricular systolic dysfunction associated with increased mortality among patients with sepsis and septic shock? Chest. 2023;163:1437.
19. Cecconi M, De Backer D, Antonelli M, Beale R, Bakker J, Hofer C, et al. Consensus on circulatory shock and hemodynamic monitoring. Task force of the European Society of Intensive Care Medicine. Intensive Care Med. 2014;40(12):1795–815.
20. Davies SJ, Yates DR, Wilson RJT, Murphy Z, Gibson A, Allgar V, et al. A randomised trial of non-invasive cardiac output monitoring to guide haemodynamic optimisation in high risk patients undergoing urgent surgical repair of proximal femoral fractures (ClearNOF trial NCT02382185). Perioper Med (Lond). 2019;8(1):8.
21. Johansson Blixt P, Chew MS, Ahman R, de Geer L, Blomqwist L, Astrom Aneq M, et al. Left ventricular longitudinal wall fractional shortening accurately predicts longitudinal strain in critically ill patients with septic shock. Ann Intensive Care. 2021;11(1):52.
22. Mondillo S, Galderisi M, Mele D, Cameli M, Lomoriello VS, Zaca V, et al. Speckle-tracking echocardiography: a new technique for assessing myocardial function. J Ultrasound Med. 2011;30(1):71–83.
23. Orde S, Huang SJ, McLean AS. Speckle tracking echocardiography in the critically ill: enticing research with minimal clinical practicality or the answer to non-invasive cardiac assessment? Anaesth Intensive Care. 2016;44(5):542–51.
24. Sanfilippo F, Corredor C, Fletcher N, Tritapepe L, Lorini FL, Arcadipane A, et al. Left ventricular systolic function evaluated by strain echocardiography and relationship with mortality in patients with severe sepsis or septic shock: a systematic review and meta-analysis. Crit Care. 2018;22(1):183.

Left Ventricular Diastolic Function in the Critically Ill

6

Mourad H. Senussi, Ran Lee, Andrea Elliott, and Mark Schmidhofer

Abbreviations

Ao	Aorta
ASE	American Society of Echocardiography
BMI	Body Mass Index
BP	Blood pressure
BSA	Body surface area
DT	Deceleration time
ECG	Electrocardiogram
HR	Heart rate
ICU	Intensive care unit
IVCT	Isovolumic contraction time
IVRT	Isovolumic relaxation time
JVP	Jugular venous pressure
LA	Left atrium
LAD	Left anterior descending
LV	Left ventricular
LVEF	Left ventricular ejection fraction
LVOT	Left ventricular outflow tract
NSAIDs	Non-steroidal anti-inflammatory agents
NSTEMI	Non ST-elevation myocardial infarction
PASP	Pulmonary artery systolic pressure
PCI	Percutaneous coronary intervention
RAP	Right atrial pressure
RCA	Right coronary artery
RR	Respiratory rate
RVOT	Right ventricular outflow tract
RVSP	Right ventricular systolic pressure
T	Temperature
TDI	Tissue doppler imaging
TR	Tricuspid regurgitation
VSD	Ventricular septal defect

Supplementary Information The online version contains supplementary material available at https://doi.org/10.1007/978-3-031-45731-9_6.

M. H. Senussi (✉)
Baylor College of Medicine, Houston, TX, USA

Texas Heart Institute, Houston, TX, USA
e-mail: Mourad.Senussi@bcm.edu

R. Lee
Cleveland Clinic, Cleveland, OH, USA
e-mail: leer2@ccf.org

A. Elliott
University of Minnesota, Minneapolis, USA
e-mail: elliotta@umn.edu

M. Schmidhofer
University of Pittsburgh Medical Center, Pittsburgh, PA, USA
e-mail: schmidhoferm@upmc.edu

Question 1. A 65-year-old man with known coronary artery disease s/p Percutaneous coronary intervention (PCI) to the LAD and RCA previously is admitted to the medical ICU with hypoxemic respiratory failure from likely community-acquired pneumonia. His other medical history is notable for hypertension, diabetes, and ongoing tobacco use. His ECG shows sinus tachycardia and an old anterior infarction but is otherwise unremarkable for acute ischemic changes. His echocardiogram demonstrates a severely reduced LVEF (Video 6.1). The following doppler waveforms were interrogated (Figs. 6.1 and 6.2).

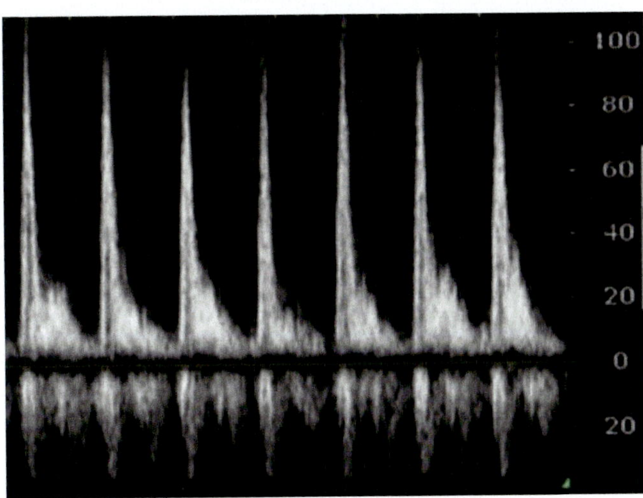

Fig. 6.1 Mitral inflow Doppler with fused E-A wave

R. Sreedharan et al. (eds.), *Critical Care Echocardiography*, https://doi.org/10.1007/978-3-031-45731-9_6

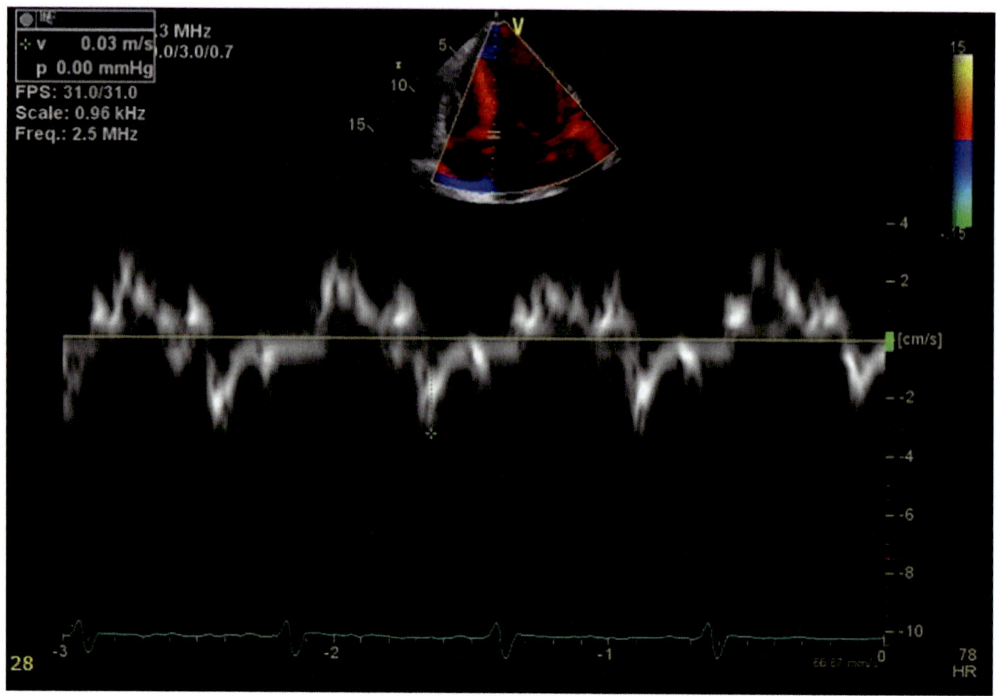

Fig. 6.2 Septal mitral tissue Doppler waveform

On examination, vital signs are T 37.7 C, BP 105/60, HR 105, and RR 28. He is using accessory muscles. JVP is estimated at 10 cm H_2O. He has bibasilar rales. Heart rate is tachycardic, rhythm is regular, and he has normal heart sounds without murmurs. His abdomen is benign and there is no lower extremity edema.

Based on the above information, which of the following is an accurate assessment of the patient's diastolic function on echocardiogram?

A. Normal diastolic function
B. Indeterminate diastolic function
C. Grade I diastolic dysfunction
D. Grade II diastolic dysfunction
E. Grade III diastolic dysfunction

Answer to Question 1: The answer is E.

Rationale: Based on the 2016 ASE Guidelines, the following algorithm should be used for assessment of diastolic function (Fig. 6.3). In patients with depressed EF, algorithm B should be followed. In this patient, the E/A ratio is well above 2:1, indicating grade III diastolic dysfunction. Other signs of diastolic dysfunction include an elevated E/e' when factoring in the septal e' measurement [1, 2].

Question 2. What is the pathophysiological explanation for the flow pattern in Fig. 6.4 in this patient?

A. Increased atrial afterload, decreased atrial compliance, increased blood flow in the pulmonary vein during diastole, and increased flow reversal into the pulmonary veins during atrial systole
B. Decreased atrial afterload, decreased atrial compliance, severe mitral regurgitation leading to pulmonary vein flow reversal
C. Decreased atrial afterload, increased atrial compliance, LVOT outflow obstruction leading to systolic anterior motion of the mitral valve
D. Increased atrial afterload, increased atrial compliance, rheumatic mitral disease leading to mixed mitral stenosis and regurgitation

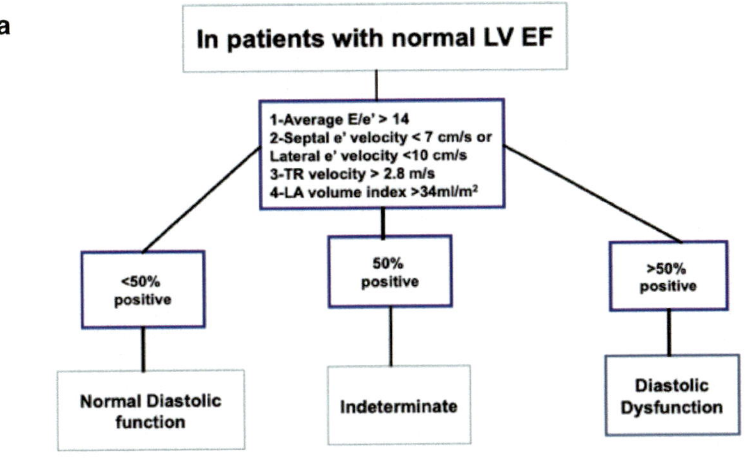

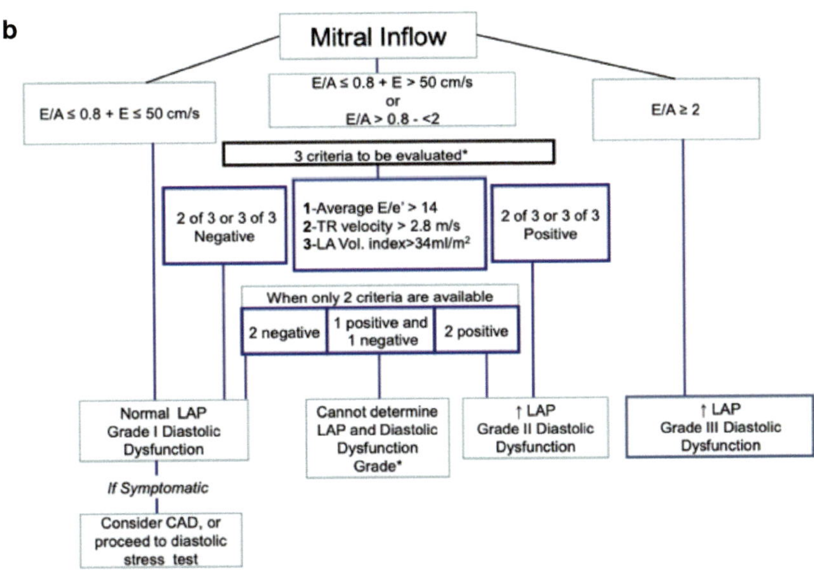

Fig. 6.3 (**a**) Algorithm for diagnosis of LV diastolic dysfunction in subjects with normal LVEF. (**b**) Algorithm for estimation of LV filling pressures and grading LV diastolic function in patients with depressed LVEFs and patients with myocardial disease and normal LVEF after consideration of clinical and other 2D data

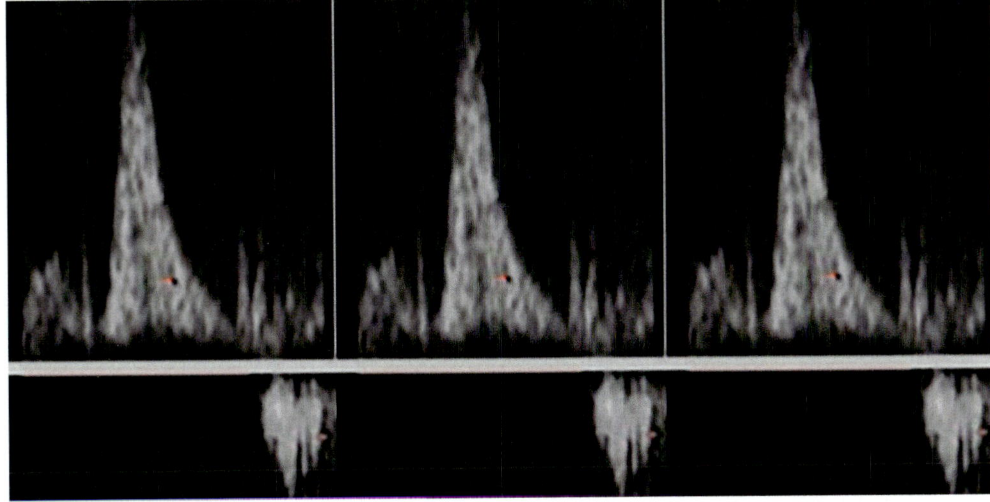

Fig. 6.4 Pulmonary vein flow pattern

Answer to Question 2: A.

Rationale: Pulmonary vein waveforms are a useful adjunct in assessment of diastolic dysfunction, though its utility in guidelines and daily practice has been de-emphasized. The feasibility of optimal imaging may be limited, especially in patients who are critically ill. On interrogation of the pulmonary vein, the s-wave velocity corresponds to atrial relaxation and ventricular systole. The d-wave corresponds to early diastole. The Ar-wave corresponds to atrial contraction. In pseudonormal and restrictive filling patterns, increased atrial pressures, lower atrial compliance, and impaired atrial relaxation leads to blunted velocity in the pulmonary veins during atrial relaxation (s-wave), and a shift of pulmonary vein flow predominantly to early diastole (elevated d-wave, moving in parallel with the mitral E velocity) (Fig. 6.5). The Ar-wave deflection becomes more prominent due to increased ventricular stiffness, as atrial contraction against a noncompliant ventricle forces blood back into the pulmonary veins [3–5].

Question 3. Which of the following echocardiographic views and pulse wave Doppler positions are most appropriate for obtaining mitral inflow velocities?

A. Apical 4 chamber view; mid-cavity of left ventricle
B. Apical 2 chamber view; above mitral leaflets within the left atrium
C. Apical 4 chamber view; at the level of the mitral leaflets
D. Apical 5 chamber view; left ventricular outflow tract

Answer to Question 3: B.

Rationale: The apical 4 chamber view represents the most optimal view for obtaining mitral inflow velocities. The pulse wave doppler is placed at the level of the tip of the mitral leaflets. Improper placement of PW doppler may lead to suboptimal and inaccurate inflow velocities [6].

Question 4. A 70-year-old-man with hypertension, sleep apnea, and obesity presents with increasing exertional dyspnea over the past several months. An echocardiogram is ordered demonstrating the following mitral inflow pattern (Fig. 6.6). The LVEF is 65%. A Valsalva maneuver is performed (Fig. 6.7).

Based on the above information, how would you characterize the baseline mitral inflow filling pattern?

A. Normal
B. Impaired relaxation
C. Pseudonormal
D. Restrictive

Answer to Question 4: C.

Rationale: The Valsalva maneuver can differentiate a normal LV filling pattern from a pseudonormal LV filling pattern, in which LV filling pressures would be elevated. In patients with a pseudonormal LV filling pattern, the

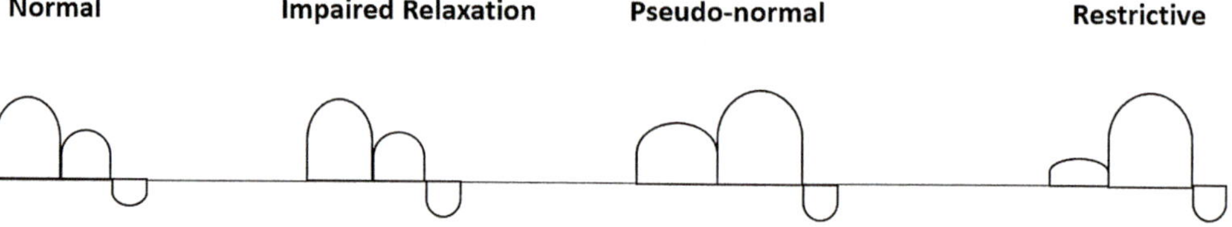

Fig. 6.5 Change in pulmonary vein flow pattern with increased ventricular stiffness

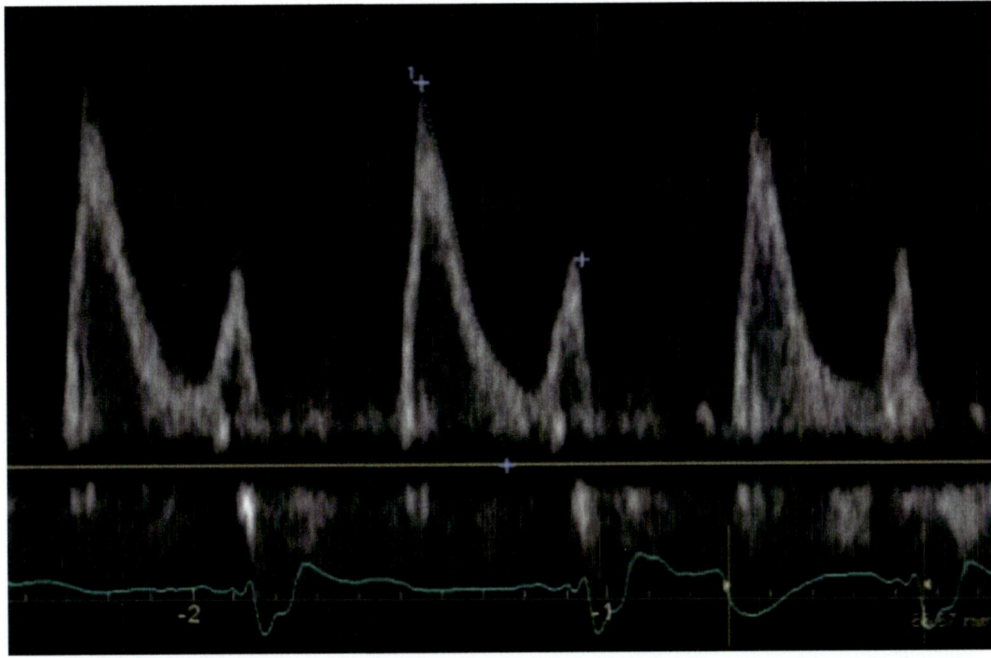

Fig. 6.6 Mitral inflow Doppler with E > A

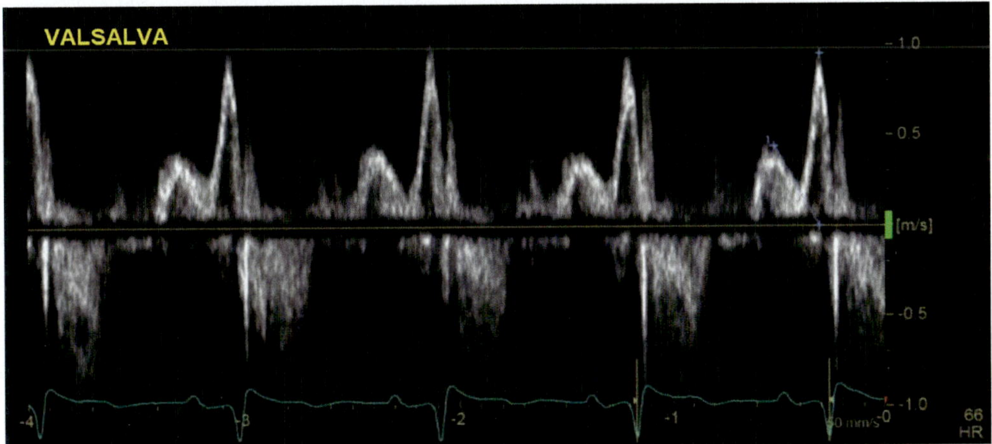

Fig. 6.7 Mitral inflow Doppler after performing Valsalva maneuver

Valsalva maneuver leads to an increase in intrathoracic pressure, reducing venous return, lowering the E:A ratio, and thus unmasking underlying impaired ventricular relaxation [1].

Question 5. A 58-year-old woman with hypertension and diabetes undergoes an echocardiogram (Videos 6.2 and 6.3). Further echocardiographic measurements reveal the following:

Septal e′: 8 cm/s.

Lateral e′: 8 cm/s.

E velocity: 80 cm/s.

TR velocity: 2.5 m/s.

LA volume index: 30 ml/m^2.

Based on the above information, how would you characterize her diastolic function?

A. Normal diastolic function
B. Indeterminate diastolic function
C. Grade I diastolic dysfunction
D. Grade II diastolic dysfunction
E. Grade III diastolic dysfunction

Answer to Question 5: A.

Rationale: Based on the 2016 ASE guidelines for diastolic function assessment, this patient has a normal LVEF and thus algorithm A should be followed. She fulfills only one of the four criteria (lateral e′ velocity < 10 cm/s) but otherwise has an E/e′ < 14, a TR jet velocity < 2.8 m/s, and a LA volume index <34 ml/m^2 [1] (Fig. 6.3).

Question 6. Which of the following are causes of diastolic dysfunction?

A. Hypertension
B. Diabetes Mellitus
C. Aging
D. Cardiac Amyloidosis
E. All of the above

Answer to Question 6: E.

Rationale: There are a multitude of causes of diastolic dysfunction which include ischemic heart disease, systemic hypertension, hypertrophic cardiomyopathy, aortic valve stenosis, diabetes mellitus, obesity, aging, infiltrative, and pericardial diseases [7, 8].

Question 7. A 75-year-old woman with diabetes on insulin, rheumatoid arthritis on low-dose corticosteroids, essential hypertension, previous tobacco abuse, and obesity presents with several days of stuttering substernal chest pressure and associated dyspnea on exertion. On examination, she is afebrile, her BP is 100/60, and HR is 90. She is breathing 22 breaths per minute on 2 liters per minute of oxygen on nasal canula. Heart rate is normal, rhythm is regular, S1 and S2 are normal, and she has a holosystolic murmur at the apex. ECG shows ST elevations in the anterior precordial leads. Echocardiogram was performed (Video 6.4). She undergoes emergent coronary angiography which demonstrates a significant proximal LAD lesion which is intervened upon with angioplasty and placement of a drug-eluting stent. Follow-up echocardiography reveals an LVEF of 35% and shows the following doppler waveforms and data (Figs. 6.8 and 6.9).

E velocity: 80 cm/s.

A velocity: 95 cm/s.

Septal e′: 5 cm/s.

Lateral e′: 6 cm/s.

TR Jet: 3.4 m/s.

LA volume index: 38 ml/m^2.

Which of the following is a true statement regarding diastolic dysfunction?

A. Normal diastolic function
B. Indeterminate diastolic function
C. Grade I diastolic dysfunction
D. Grade II diastolic dysfunction
E. Grade III diastolic dysfunction

Answer to Question 7: D.

Rationale: Based on the 2016 ASE guidelines for diastolic function assessment, this patient has a depressed EF after MI and algorithm B should be followed. There is elevated LV filling pressure due to an E/e′ ratio of 16. The E/A ratio is 0.84, the TR velocity is greater than 2.8 m/s, and the LA volume index is greater than 34 ml/m^2. Thus, the patient

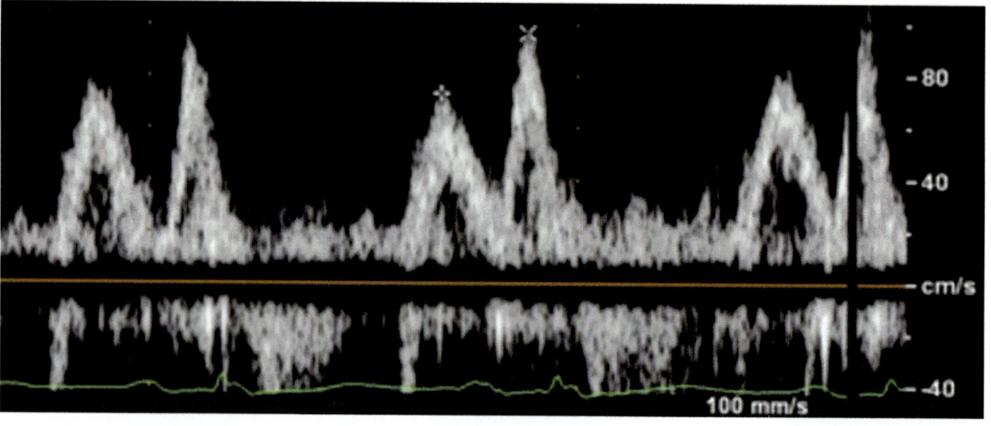

Fig. 6.8 Mitral inflow Doppler with E < A

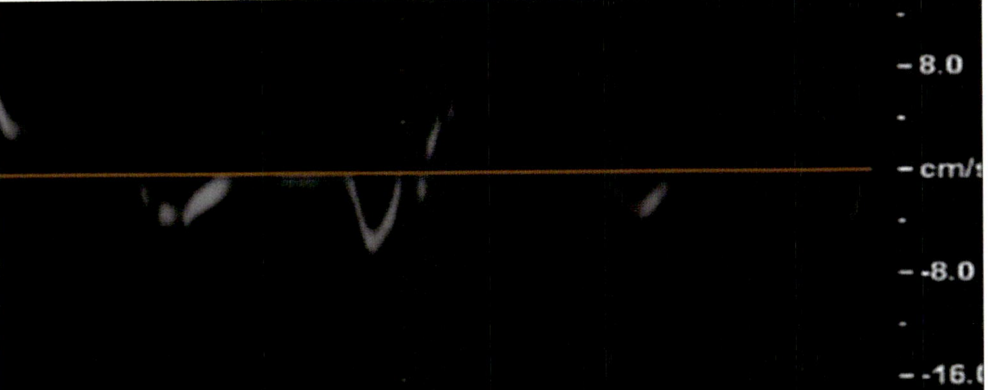

Fig. 6.9 Mitral tissue Doppler waveform through lateral wall

meets 3/3 criteria and can be categorized as having elevated filling pressure and grade II diastolic dysfunction. In patients with myocardial ischemia, relaxation abnormalities and diastolic dysfunction precede changes in systolic function. These changes in diastolic function may persist after revascularization. E/e′ is a powerful predictor of survival after acute MI and is useful in prognostication [8, 9] (Fig. 6.3).

Question 8. A 72-year-old woman with hypertension, sleep apnea, and obesity is referred for echocardiography due to worsening exertional dyspnea with simple household activities over the past 4 months. On exam, she is afebrile, blood pressure is 157/80, HR is 90, and she is breathing 20 times a minute. Her body habitus precludes an accurate JVP assessment. Her heart sounds are normal and do not feature additional murmurs, rubs, or gallops. Her lower extremities are without edema. A transthoracic echocardiogram is performed (Video 6.5). The doppler waveforms are shown in Figs. 6.10, 6.11 and 6.12.

E: 120 cm/s.

A: 70 cm/s.

Septal E′: 6 m/s.

Lateral E′: 11 m/s.

Due to diagnostic uncertainty regarding her symptoms, she undergoes a left heart catheterization.

What would her estimated PCWP be based on the above data?

A. 10 mmHg
B. 15 mmHg
C. 20 mmHg
D. 25 mmHg
E. 30 mmHg

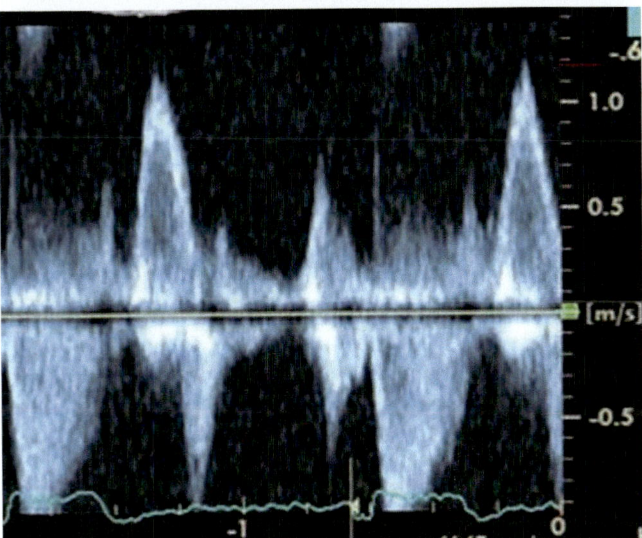

Fig. 6.10 Mitral inflow Doppler with mitral regurgitation

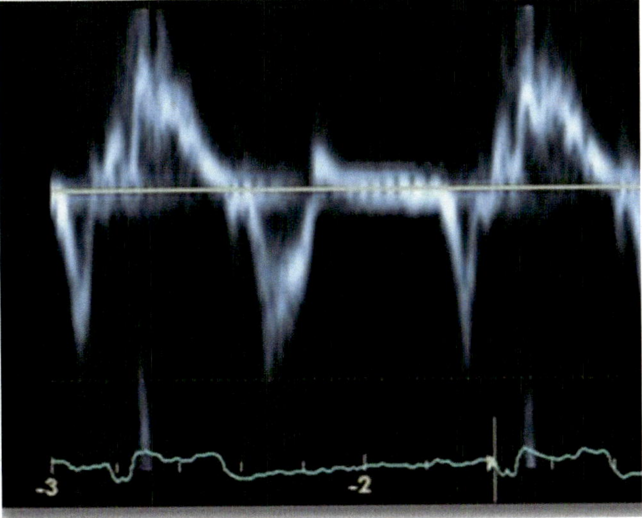

Fig. 6.11 Mitral tissue Doppler septal wall

Answer to Question 8: C.

Rationale: The transthoracic echocardiogram shows evidence of left ventricular hypertrophy. Elevated E/e′ ratios >14 have a high specificity for increased LV filling pressures and has been validated against mean PCWP using the following formula: PCWP = 1.24 × (E/e′) + 1.9. Utilizing the data from the previous case, PCWP = 1.24 × (120/8.5) + 1.9, which approximately is equal to 20 mmHg. The limitations

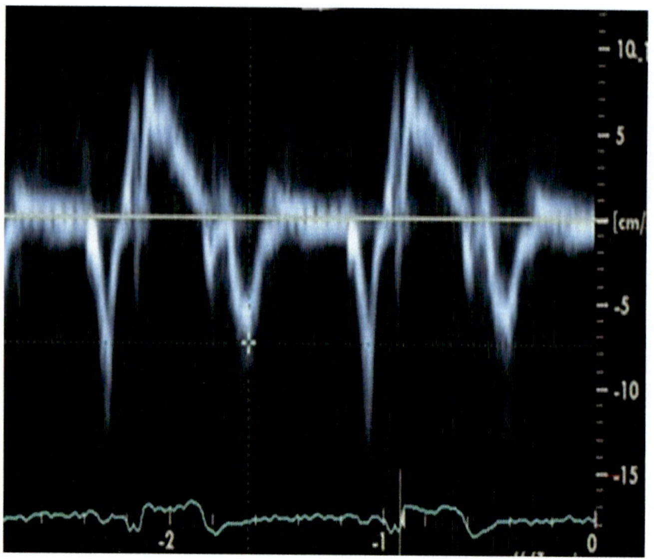

Fig. 6.12 Mitral tissue Doppler lateral wall

to this technique occur in patients with mitral valve disease, mitral annular calcification, and pericardial disease, where E/e′ can be inaccurate. Elevated E/A ratios >1.1 have also been validated to correlate with PCWP >12 mmHg [10, 11].

Question 9. Which the following diastology characteristics is more consistent with normal diastolic function:

A. IVRT 50 ms, DT 100 ms
B. IVRT 80 ms, DT 200 ms
C. IVRT 140 ms, DT 270 ms
D. IVRT 100 ms, DT 200 ms

Answer to Question 9: B.

Rationale: The isovolumic relaxation time is the interval between aortic valve closure and mitral valve opening, or the time it takes from the end of systole for the pressure in the LV to drop below the LA to proceed with LV filling. Normal is between 70 ms–100 ms (Fig. 6.13). The deceleration time is

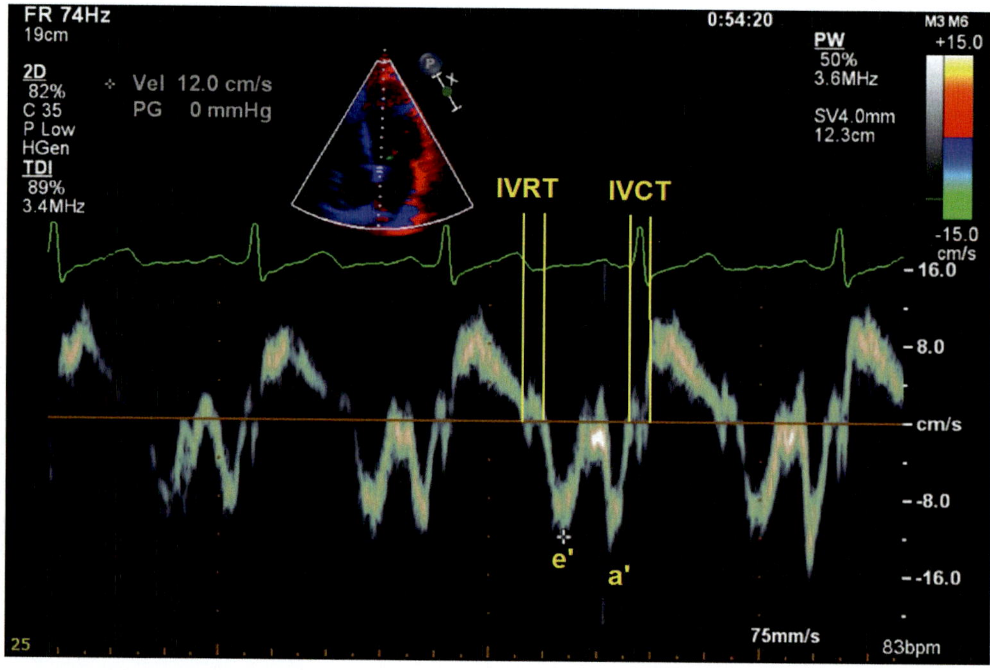

Fig. 6.13 Mitral tissue Doppler. *IVRT* isovolumic relaxation time, *IVCT* isovolumic contraction time

how rapidly the flow velocity declines in the early phase of diastole. Normal is between 140–240 ms. Normal IVRT is between 70–100 and normal DT between 140–240. In impaired relaxation there is prolonged IVRT and DT (Option C). Pseudonormal pattern shows Upper-normal IVRT and normal DT (Option D). Restrictive pattern shows a short IVRT and short DT (Option A). In patients with impaired relaxation, a stiffened ventricle will prolong the time it takes for atrial pressure to exceed LV pressure and thus proceed the filling process. The deceleration time is also prolonged. In patients with pseudonormal relaxation, progressive diastolic dysfunction leads to higher left sided filling pressures and an elevation in the early diastolic pressure gradient. While IVRT can be normal or slightly prolonged, deceleration time should normalize. In patients with restrictive filling pattern, significantly elevated left sided filling pressures lead to both early filling and early termination of early diastole.

Question 10. A 57-year-old woman with systemic sclerosis is referred for an echocardiogram due to worsening exertional dyspnea. The following doppler waveform is obtained (Fig. 6.14). The estimated RAP is 15 mmHg based on IVC assessment.

What is the approximate right ventricular systolic pressure (RVSP)?

A. 55 mmHg
B. 70 mmHg
C. 85 mmHg
D. 100 mmHg
E. 115 mmHg

Answer to Question 10: E.

Rationale: The RVSP can be calculated using the following equation:

$$\text{RVSP} = 4(\text{TR Vmax})^2 + \text{RAP}$$

The Vmax of the TR jet in the figure is 5 m/s. In situations where there is no significant stenosis at the RVOT or pulmonic valve, the RVSP is equivalent to the pulmonary artery systolic pressure (PASP).

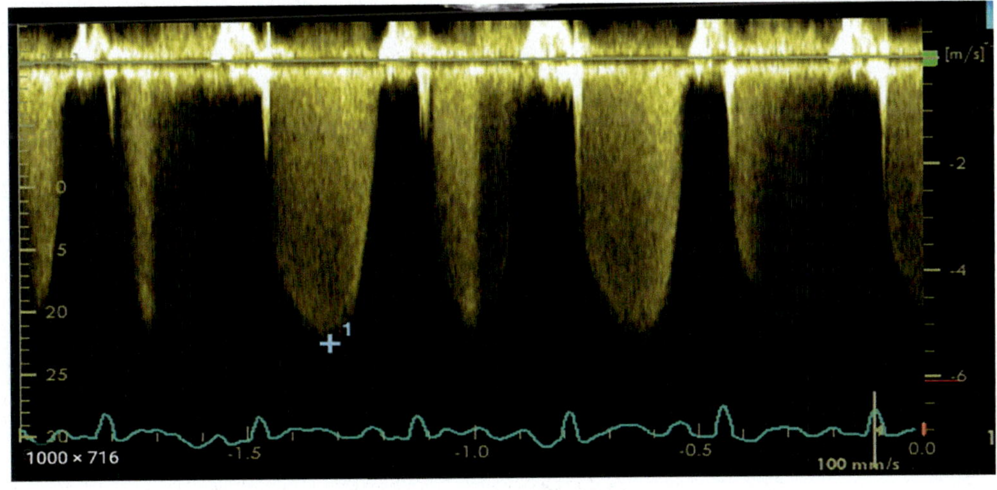

Fig. 6.14 Continuous wave Doppler of Tricuspid regurgitant jet

Question 11. A 68-year-old man is referred for an echocardiogram due to increasing exertional dyspnea. He has a medical history including obesity, diabetes, essential hypertension, and obstructive sleep apnea. His BMI is 39 and BSA is 2.42. The following echocardiographic images and measurements are obtained (Figs. 6.15 and 6.16).

What is this patient's left atrial volume index?

A. 25 ml/m^2
B. 30 ml/m^2
C. 35 ml/m^2
D. 40 ml/m^2
E. 45 ml/m^2

Answer to Question 11: C.

Rationale: Left atrial volume index by Biplane Area-Length Method can be calculated with the following equation:

$$\text{LA Volume} = 0.85 \times (A_1 \times A_2 / L)$$

A1 = area from 4-chamber view. A2 = area from 2-chamber view. L = length, the shortest length in either view.

Dividing the LA volume by the body surface area yields the LA volume index. When obtaining this measurement, planimetry measurements should be made keeping in mind to exclude the pulmonary veins and LA appendage from view.

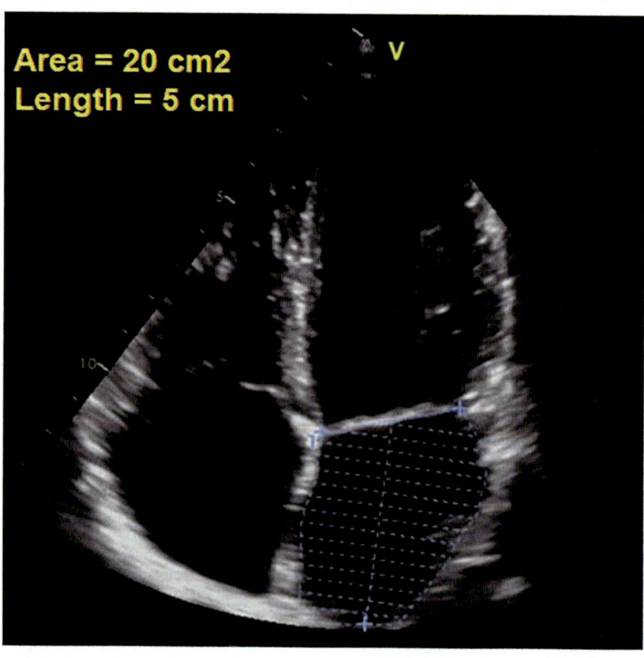

Fig. 6.15 Apical view estimating left atrial size

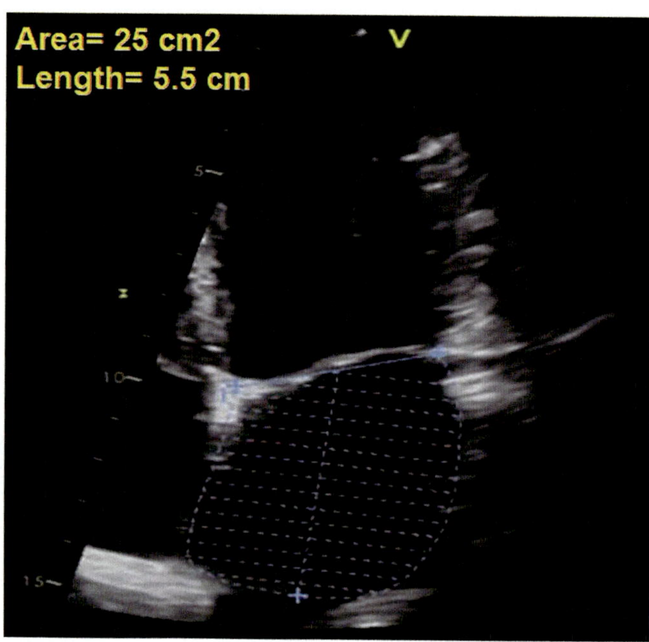

Fig. 6.16 Zoomed in Apical view estimating left atrial size

Question 12. A 72-year-old man with longstanding essential hypertension, previous tobacco use, paroxysmal atrial fibrillation, previous coronary artery disease s/p PCI to the RCA for exertional angina, and obstructive sleep apnea is admitted to the hospital for hypoxemic respiratory failure. On examination, he is afebrile, BP of 160/80, HR of 90, and RR of 24. He has bibasilar rales and new lower extremity edema. Cardiac exam is significant for a normal rate, regular rhythm, normal S1 and S2 and an S3. A transthoracic echocardiogram is performed (Video 6.12, Fig. 6.17). The following measurements were obtained:

E velocity: 80 cm/s.
A velocity: 45 cm/s.
Septal E′ velocity: 8 cm/s.
Lateral E′ velocity: 10 cm/s.
TR velocity: incomplete envelope, not obtained.
LA volume index: 32 ml/m^2.

Based on the above information, which of the following is an accurate assessment of the patient's diastolic function on echocardiogram?

A. Normal diastolic function
B. Indeterminate diastolic function
C. Grade I diastolic dysfunction
D. Grade II diastolic dysfunction
E. Grade III diastolic dysfunction

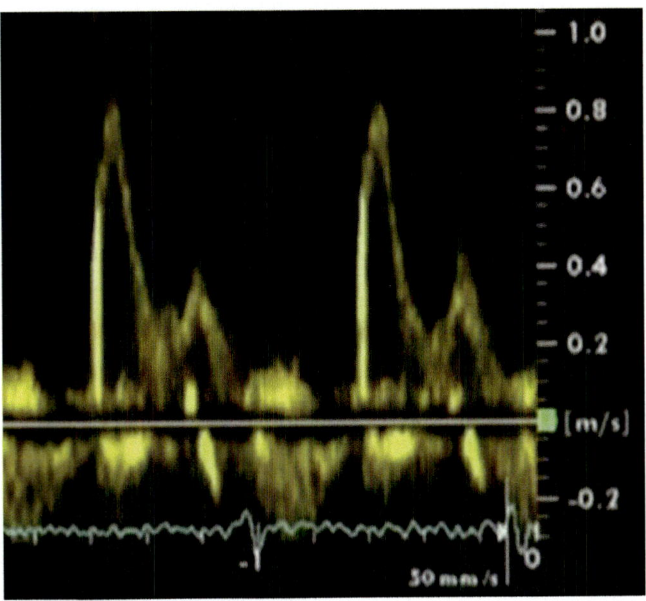

Fig. 6.17 Mitral inflow Doppler with E > A

Answer to Question 12: C.

Based on the 2016 ASE Guidelines, the following algorithm should be used for assessment of diastolic function. Algorithm B should be followed due to the depressed LVEF. In this patient, the E/A ratio is 1.7. Out of three criteria to be evaluated, the average E/e′ is <14, and the LA volume index is <34 ml/m^2. The TR jet velocity is not available. Despite the pseudonormal filling pattern, there are no surrogate measures of elevated LV filling pressures present, and the two existing criteria are negative. Thus, the patient has grade 1 diastolic dysfunction [11]. Note the inferior wall hypokinesis consistent with right coronary artery ischemia (Video 6.6 and Fig. 6.3).

Question 13. A 62-year-old man with a history of coronary artery disease, type 2 diabetes mellitus, and hypertension presents to the intensive care unit with respiratory distress and hypoxemia. Blood pressure is 198/78 mmHg, pulse 105/min, respiratory rate 32/min, saturating 92% on 6 liters of oxygen via nasal cannula. Lung ultrasonography is performed with representative images of the anterior lung fields shown in (Video 6.7). A limited transthoracic echocardiogram is performed (Video 6.8, Figs. 6.18, 6.19, 6.20 and 6.21).

Mitral E-wave velocity: 132 cm/s.

Mitral A-wave velocity: 6 cm/s.

E/A ratio: 2.2.

Septal e′: 3 cm/s.

Lateral e′: 3 cm/s.

Which of the following best describes the point-of-care ultrasound findings?

A. Lung US: B-profile, Systolic function: normal, Diastolic dysfunction: Grade III
B. Lung US: B-profile, Systolic function: mildly decreased, Diastolic dysfunction: Grade I

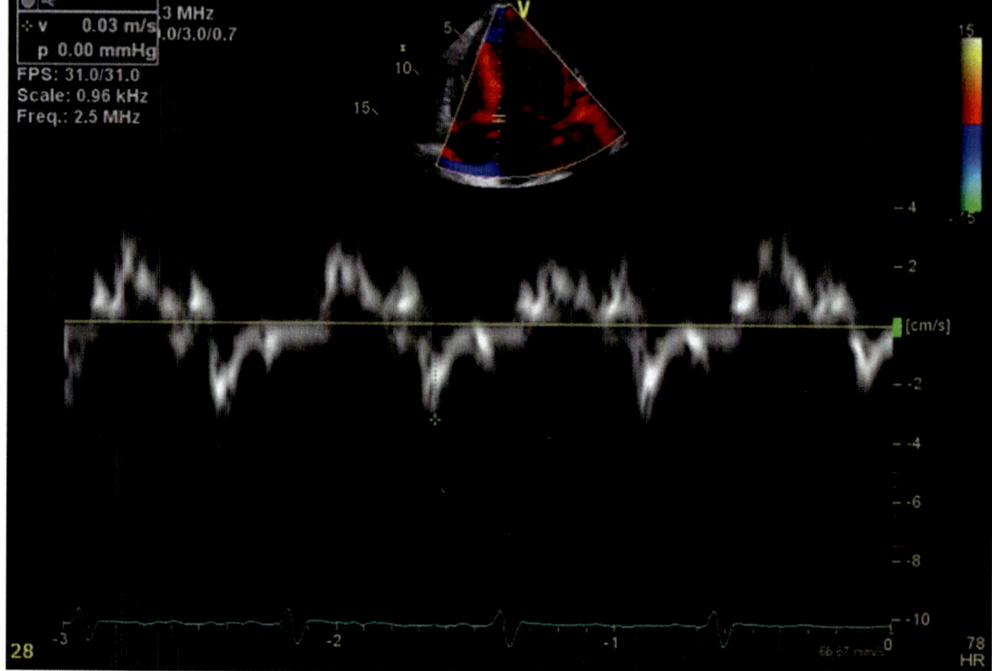

Fig. 6.18 Tissue Doppler, septal wall

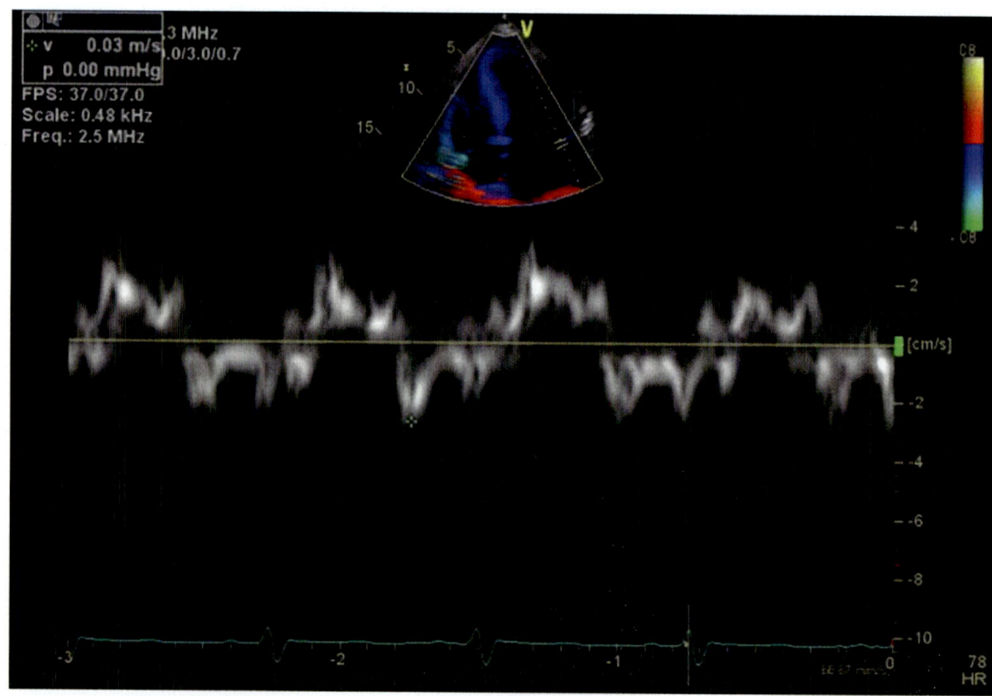

Fig. 6.19 Mitral tissue Doppler, lateral wall

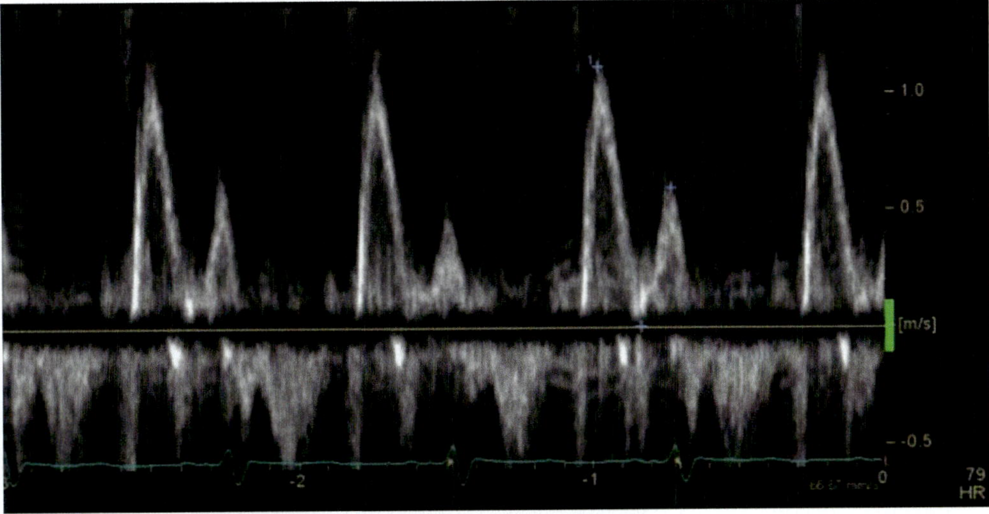

Fig. 6.20 Mitral inflow Doppler with normal E/A pattern

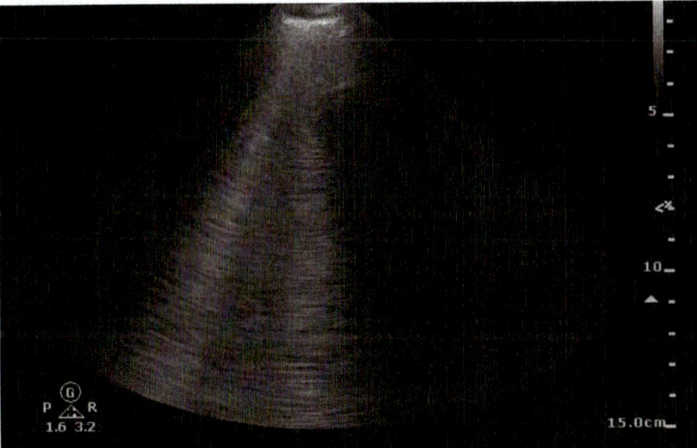

Fig. 6.21 Apical four chamber view

C. Lung US: A/B-profile, Systolic function: decreased, Diastolic dysfunction: Indeterminate
D. Lung US: A-profile, Systolic function: normal, Diastolic dysfunction: Grade II

Answer to Question 13: A.

Key Point: Diastolic dysfunction is common in the intensive care unit and can contribute to elevated filling pressures of the heart. Patients may present acutely with pulmonary edema in the setting of hypertensive crisis.

Rationale: The patient has several risk factors for diastolic dysfunction which includes age, coronary artery disease, hypertension, and diabetes mellitus. The patient is presenting with undifferentiated hypoxemia in the setting of elevated blood pressure with positive lung sliding and normal pleural line structure on point-of-care lung ultrasound. Options C and D are incorrect as the lung ultrasound is showing a predominant bilateral B-line profile of the anterior lung fields. These findings are all consistent with cardiogenic pulmonary edema. However, transthoracic echocardiography reveals preserved systolic function (Option B is incorrect). There is echocardiographic evidence of severe left ventricular hypertrophy and left atrial enlargement. Therefore, one should suspect the possibility of diastolic dysfunction playing a major role in this patient's presentation. Mitral inflow velocities are consistent with Grade III diastolic dysfunction (E/A > 2, short deceleration time). Furthermore, E/e′ > 14 which is consistent with high left atrial pressures. Therefore, Option A is correct. Patients with diastolic dysfunction commonly present to the intensive care unit with acute hypertensive pulmonary edema with no evidence of systolic dysfunction [12–14].

Question 14. The patient is managed in the intensive care unit and improves clinically. He is normotensive. A repeat transthoracic echocardiogram (Fig. 6.22) and lung ultrasound (Video 6.9, Fig. 6.23) is performed at day 4 of hospitalization and he is discharged to the medical floor.

E-wave velocity: 70 cm/s.

A-wave velocity: 12 cm/s.

Septal e′ = 3 cm/s.

Which of the following therapeutic interventions most likely caused the interval changes seen from day 1 to day 4?

A. Intravenous fluid resuscitation and empirical antibiotic coverage
B. Intravenous diuresis
C. Non-invasive positive pressure ventilation
D. Afterload reduction

Answer to Question 14: B.

Key Point: Diastolic dysfunction represents a spectrum with progressive predictable changes in mitral spectral waveform velocities with intravenous diuresis and volume removal.

Rationale: Option A is incorrect. There is no compelling clinical evidence of sepsis. The interval changes shown in the lung ultrasound reveal an improved bilateral B to A-line profile after the therapeutic intervention. This is not consistent with intravenous fluid resuscitation. Lung ultrasound findings in pneumonia may show subpleural changes, an

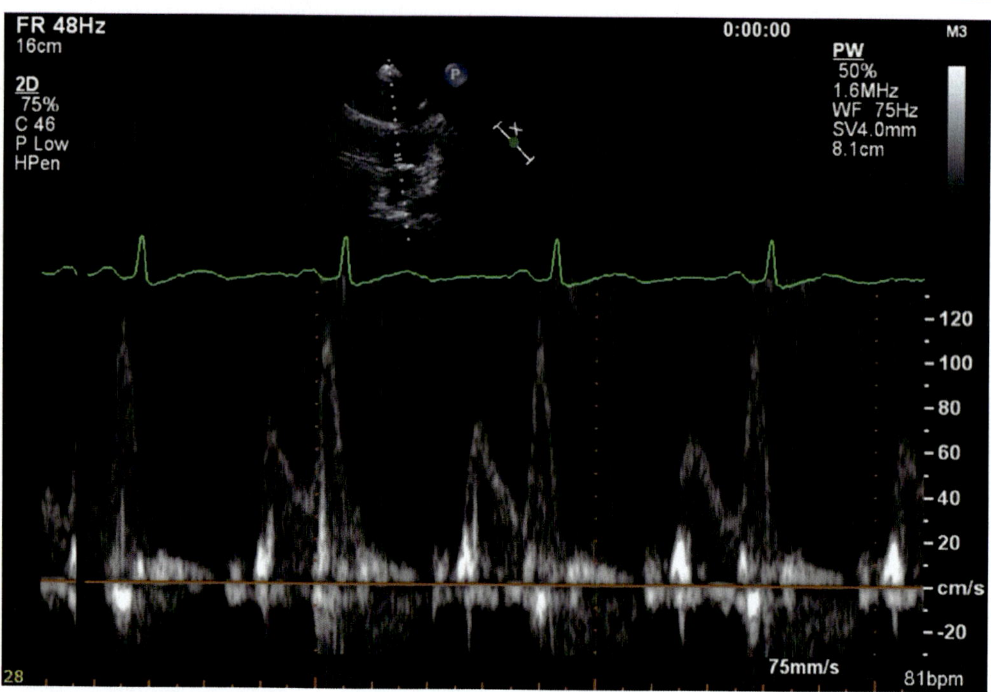

Fig. 6.22 Mitral inflow Doppler with E < A

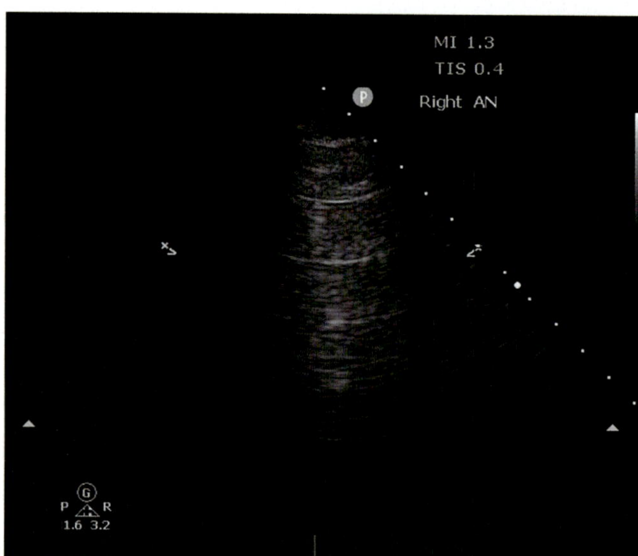

Fig. 6.23 Lung ultrasound of anterior lung field

irregular pleural line, A/B profile in unilateral pneumonia, scattered B-lines across both lung fields in multifocal pneumonia, or consolidation with pathognomonic sonographic air bronchograms. Option C is incorrect. Although the use of non-invasive positive pressure ventilation can lead to alveolar recruitment and diminish the number of B-lines to the point of an A-line pattern, this would not explain the improved changes seen in diastolic function. Option D is incorrect. Afterload reduction plays an important role in optimizing hemodynamics in patients with diastolic dysfunction with hypertension however is not markedly elevated on the subsequent days and would not lead to the changes noted on point-of-care ultrasound. As the patient is diuresed there is progressive improvement in diastolic function as evidenced by progressive decrease of the "preload dependent" E- wave velocities. With aggressive diuresis the patient has improved over the spectrum of diastology from Grade III to Grade I. Also noted is the decrease in E/e′ ratio which is a useful surrogate for left atrial and pulmonary capillary wedge pressures. Mitral annular tissue Doppler velocities remain constant (preload independent) and thus progressive decrease in E-wave velocities with diuresis will lead to a lower E/e′ ratios. Therefore, option B is correct [15, 16].

Question 15. A 27-year-old athletic man presents with a Methicillin resistant Staphylococcus aureus soft tissue infection. Blood pressure is 122/62 mmHg, Pulse 62/min, respiratory rate is 12/min, saturating at 98% on room air. Lactate 0.5 mmol/L. A limited transthoracic echocardiogram is performed (Video 6.10, Figs. 6.24, 6.25 and 6.26).

E-wave velocity: 146 cm/s.
A-wave velocity: 25 cm/s.
E/A ratio: 5.85.
Septal e′: 15 cm/s.
Lateral e′: 6 cm/s.

What do the echocardiographic findings represent in this patient?

A. Grade I diastolic dysfunction
B. Grade II diastolic dysfunction
C. Grade III diastolic dysfunction
D. Normal Variant

Answer to Question 15: D.

Key Point: High E-wave velocities may be seen in young patients with supraphysiological early filling and does not indicate diastolic dysfunction.

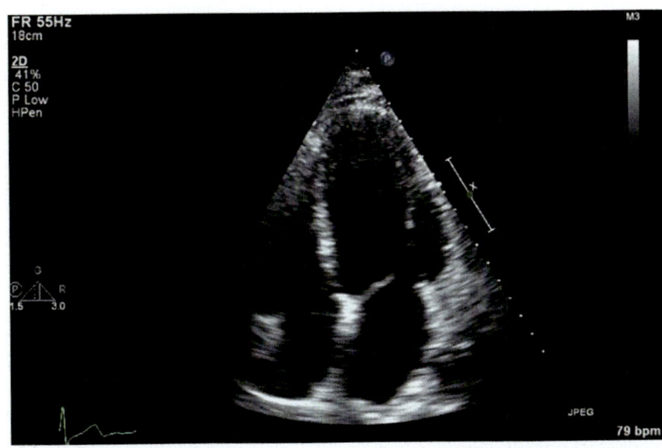

Fig. 6.24 Apical four chamber view

Rationale: The assessment and interpretation of diastology should be considered in its totality. An apical four chamber view reveals a normal appearing heart with preserved systolic function and no clear evidence of left ventricular hypertrophy or left atrial enlargement (Video 6.10, Fig. 6.24). The patient has 'supraphysiological' early diastolic filling which can be seen in younger patients (note a high E = 75 cm/s). The increased E-wave velocity is not due to an increase in left atrial pressure but rather more prominent suction force during the relaxation of the heart. Thus, using E/A velocities alone will lead to a mis-categorization as Grade III diastolic dysfunction (E/A > 2). A helpful clue is the tissue Doppler velocities which are robust (e′ > 15) and indicative of a normal variant of diastolic function [1, 17].

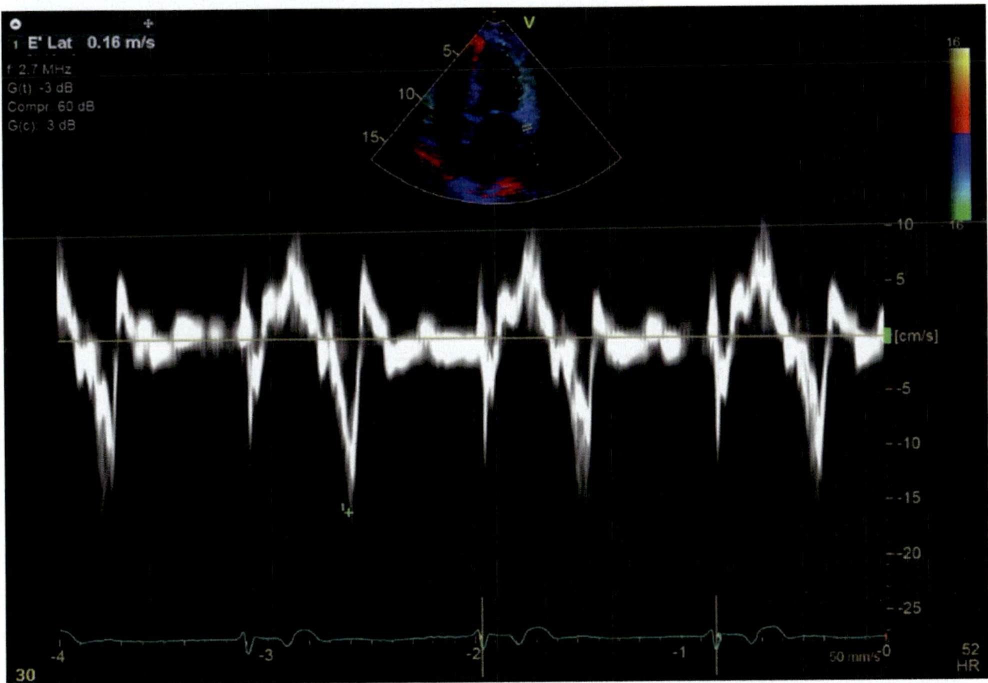

Fig. 6.25 Tissue Doppler, septal wall

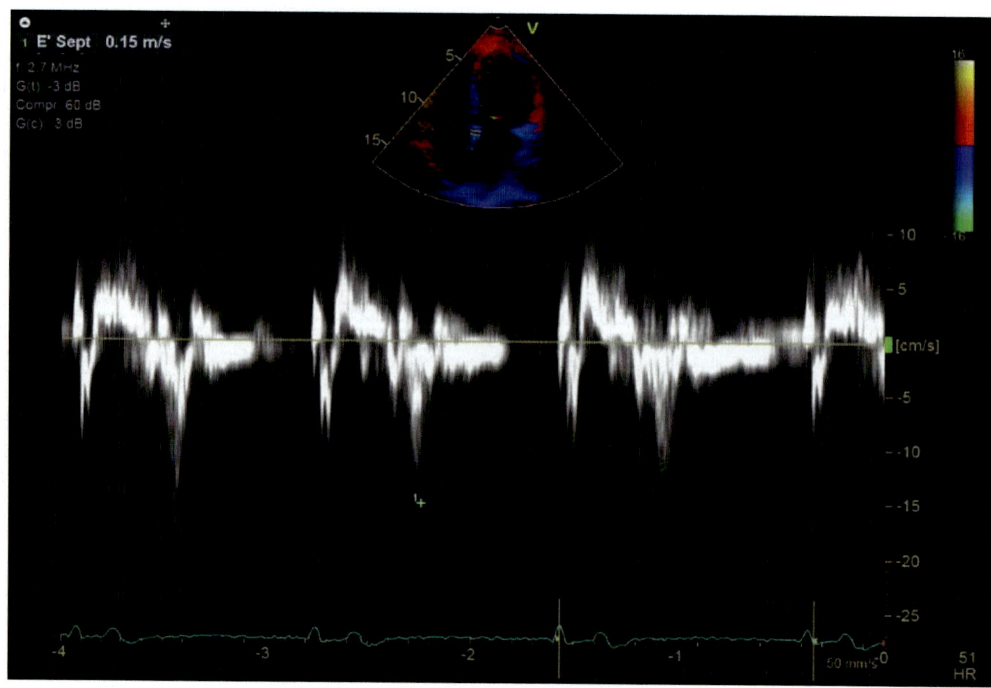

Fig. 6.26 Mitral tissue Doppler, lateral wall

Question 16. A 22-year-old woman with no past medical history undergoes a transthoracic echocardiogram. She has normal systolic function, normal sized atria, and no evidence of tricuspid regurgitation. She is asked to perform a Valsalva maneuver. Baseline and post Valsalva mitral inflow velocities are shown in Figs. 6.27 and 6.28 respectively.

Which of the following best describes the changes that have occurred?

A. Impaired relaxation to pseudonormal pattern
B. Pseudonormal to impaired relaxation pattern
C. No changes; Normal Diastolic function
D. Grade III to Grade II diastolic dysfunction

Answer to Question 16: C.

Key Point: The Valsalva maneuver can be used to distinguish normal diastolic function from pseudonormal pattern which can help in determining the grade of diastolic dysfunction.

Rationale: The Valsalva is a simple maneuver that can be used to determine the reversibility along the diastolic spectrum between grades. It becomes especially useful when a pseudonormal pattern (grade 2 diastolic dysfunction) is unmasked and an impaired relaxation pattern (grade 1 diastolic dysfunction) is seen. This is denoted by a significant decrease in E-wave velocities noted during the straining phase of the Valsalva maneuver which coincides with decreased venous return, cardiac filling and preload. In higher grades of diastolic dysfunction, the Valsalva maneuver is unlikely to revert to an impaired relaxation stage with characteristic E/A ratio [18, 19].

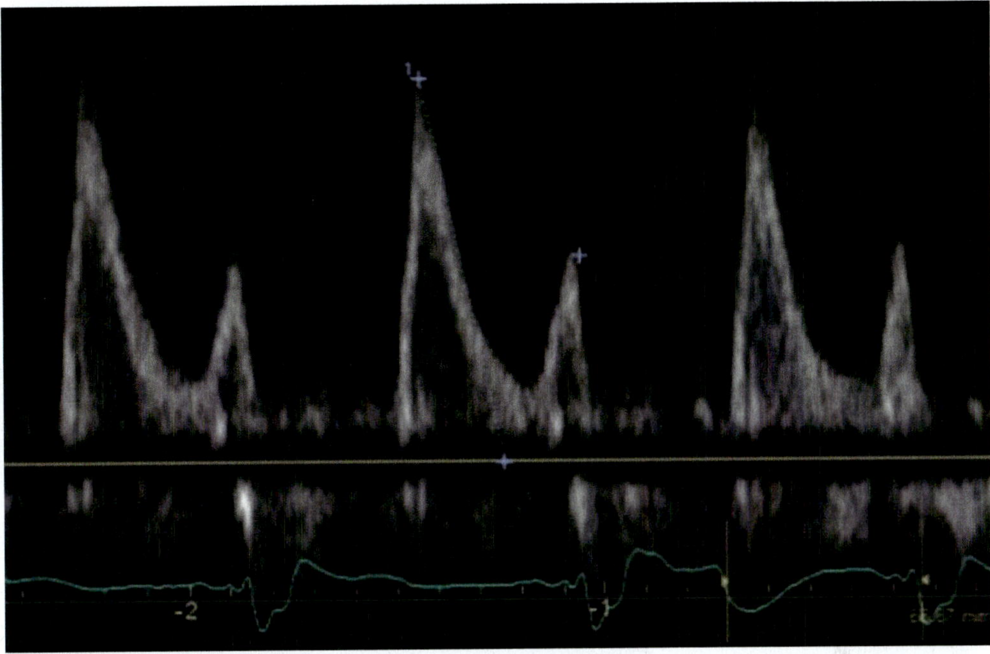

Fig. 6.27 Mitral inflow Doppler with normal E/A pattern

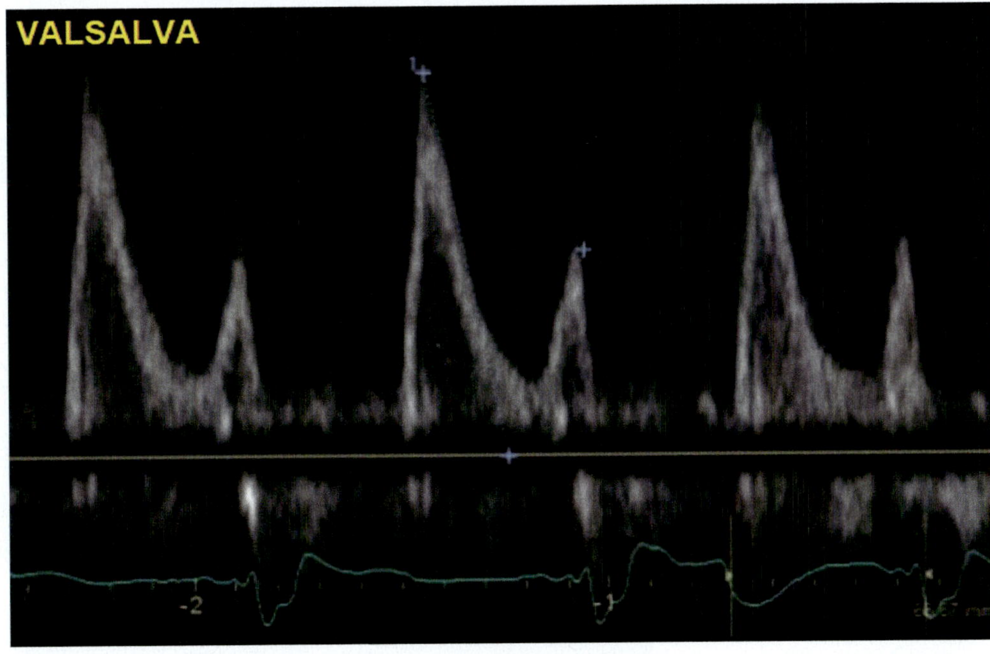

Fig. 6.28 Mitral inflow Doppler with Valsalva maneuver

Question 17. Which of the following mitral deceleration times are likely associated with severe diastolic dysfunction?

A. 150 ms
B. 240 ms
C. 120 ms
D. All of the above

Answer to Question 17: C.

Key Point: Deceleration time is a helpful adjunct to determining the severity of diastolic dysfunction.

Rationale: In patients with normal diastolic dysfunction deceleration times are usually >140 ms. With impaired relaxation, deceleration times may be more prolonged >230 ms (Fig. 6.29). With severe restrictive filling, deceleration time shortens significantly and is associated with high E/A ratios >2 (Fig. 6.30). Using deceleration times in conjunction with other echocardiographic parameters is helpful in determining the stage of diastolic dysfunction and estimation of left atrial pressures [1].

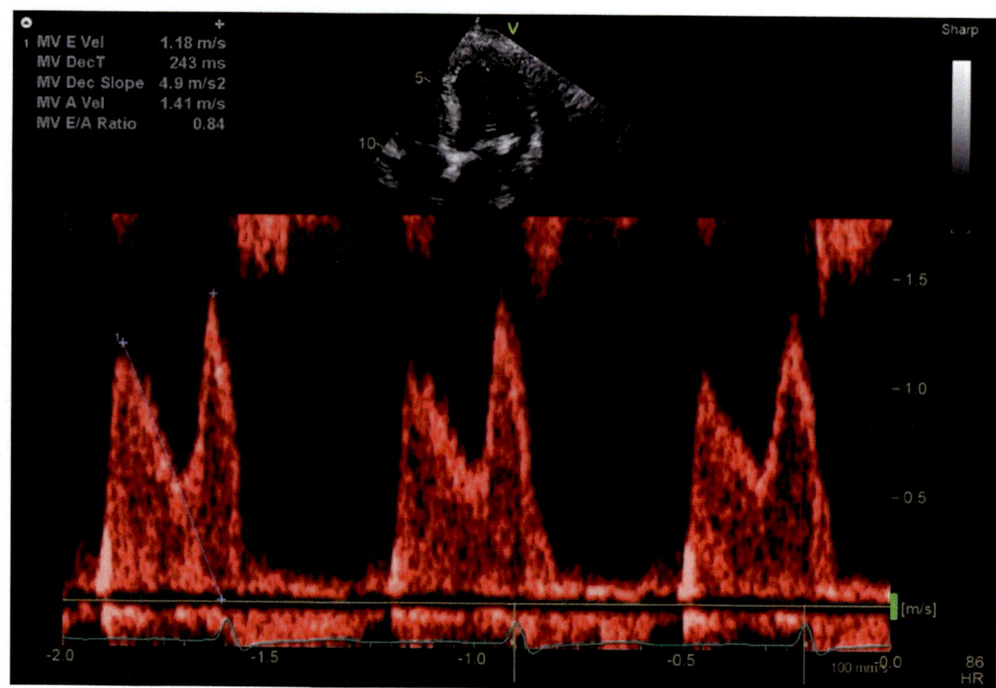

Fig. 6.29 Mitral inflow Doppler, fused E/A wave

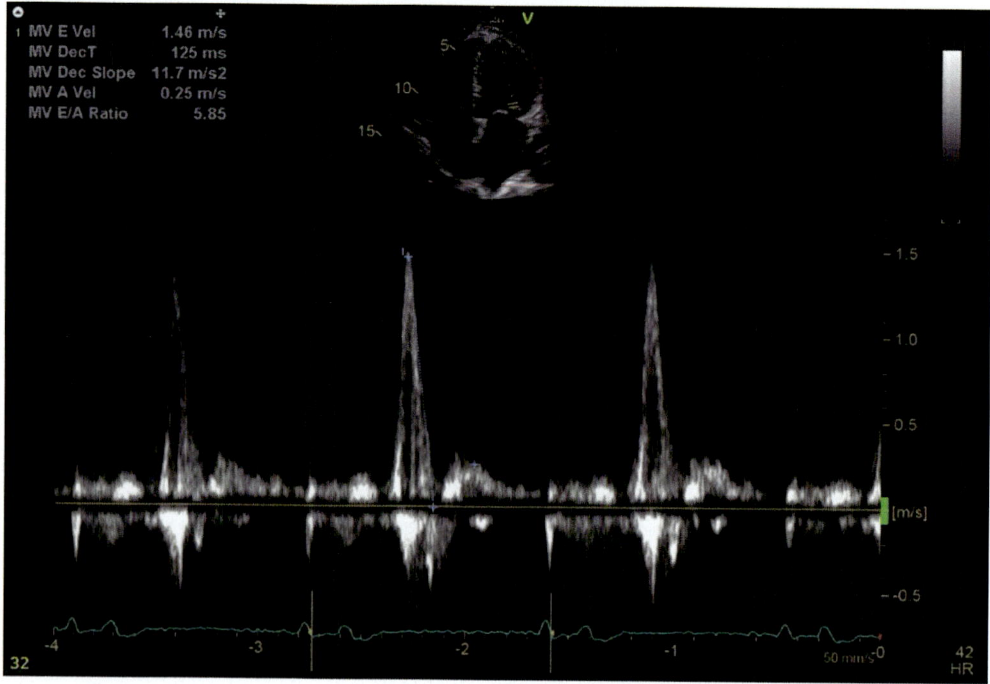

Fig. 6.30 Mitral inflow Doppler, with high E A Ratio

Question 18. A 62-year-old woman with a past medical history of paroxysmal atrial fibrillation, hypertension, and stable chronic kidney disease is being evaluated for hypotension. Review of her medical records reveals an outpatient transthoracic echocardiogram two months prior (Fig. 6.31). Interval changes in mitral inflow velocities are shown in Fig. 6.32.

What is the most likely explanation for the changes seen?

A. Progressive worsening of systolic function
B. Interval worsening of diastolic dysfunction
C. Development of atrial fibrillation
D. Left ventricular outflow tract obstruction

Answer to Question 18: C.

Key Point: Loss of the A-wave and variability and irregularity of the E-wave is indicative of the development of atrial fibrillation. Patients with impaired relaxation pattern

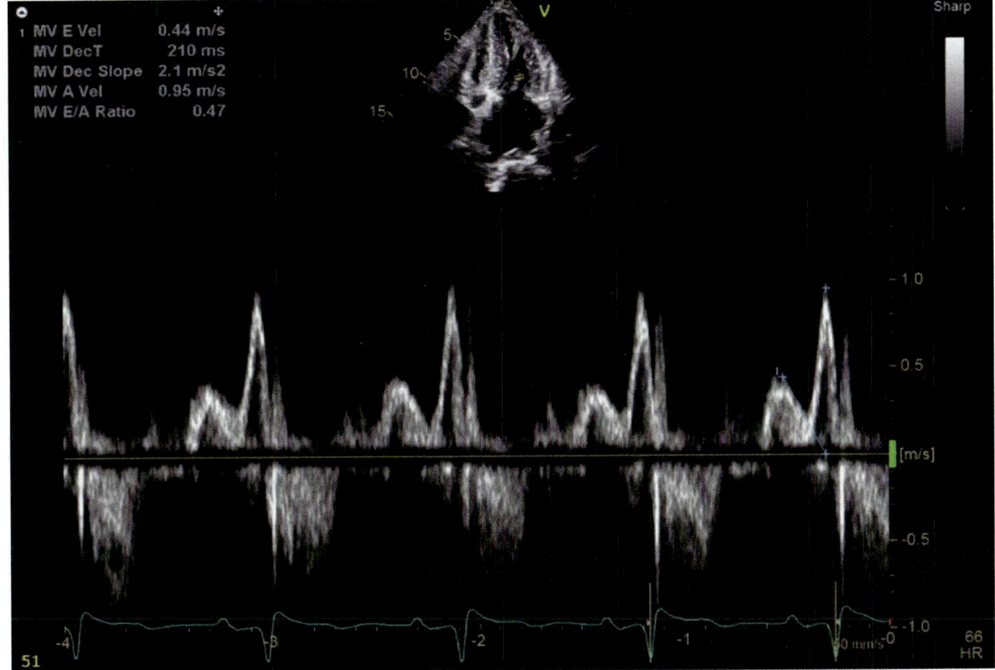

Fig. 6.31 Mitral inflow Doppler, with reveresed E A Ratio

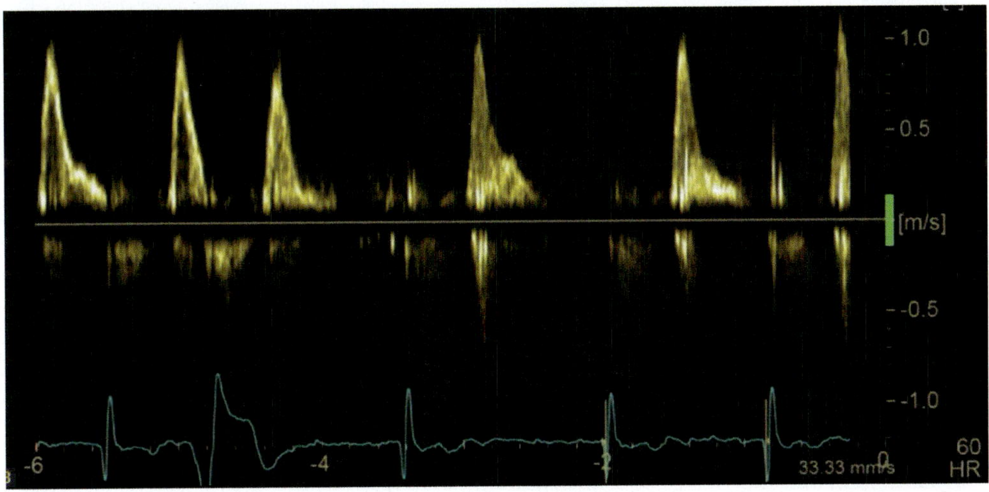

Fig. 6.32 Mitral inflow Doppler in atrial fibrillation

are dependent on their atrial kick for diastolic filling and may develop hemodynamic compromise with atrial dysrhythmias.

Rationale: The outpatient transthoracic echocardiogram shows a smaller E than A-wave with an E/A ratio < 0.5. Given the clinical context, this patient likely has Grade I diastolic dysfunction (impaired relaxation pattern). The interval changes seen on the repeat study shows loss of the A-wave. There is variability in the R-R interval and the magnitude of the E-wave. There are no p-waves seen on the simultaneous EKG tracing on the echocardiogram. This is consistent with the development of atrial fibrillation in this patient with a known history of paroxysmal atrial fibrillation (Option C is correct). This leads to complete loss of the atrial kick responsible for late filling in diastole. Given the limited early filling that occurs during diastole, patients with impaired relaxation are often dependent on late filling via atrial contraction and do not tolerate atrial fibrillation well from a hemodynamic standpoint. Therapeutic measures to restore sinus rhythm in these patients are important in managing hypotension. Diastolic assessment in atrial fibrillation is challenging, however, high E velocities, presence of a mitral L-wave, low e′, short deceleration time, high E/e′ ratio, and lack of variability of E wave despite irregular R-R intervals are all signs consistent with increased left atrial pressures [1, 20, 21].

Question 19. A 56-year-old man with no known medical history is being evaluated for hypotension in the setting of atrial fibrillation with a rapid ventricular rate. Blood pressure is 89/62 mmHg, Pulse 156 beats per minute and irregular, respiratory rate is 18 breaths per minute, saturating 98% on room air. He undergoes cardioversion. The following mitral inflow velocities were obtained before and after cardioversion (Fig. 6.33).

What is the best explanation for the changes noted?

A. Unsuccessful cardioversion; patient remains in atrial fibrillation
B. E/A > 2, Grade 3 diastolic dysfunction
C. Mitral regurgitation
D. Atrial stunning after cardioversion

Answer to Question 19: D.

Key Point: A-waves are absent in patients with atrial fibrillation.

Rationale: A-waves during late diastole are present after cardioversion albeit low amplitude. This is consistent with restoration of sinus rhythm and successful cardioversion (Option A is incorrect) and the presence of atrial contraction. The low amplitude A-wave is reflective of stunning of the myocardium that may occur with electrical cardioversion and usually recovers over the course of several days. This may be miscategorized as Grade 3 diastolic dysfunction given low A-wave velocities and subsequent high E/A ratios (Fig. 6.33). Figure 6.34 shows the representative mitral spectral waveform changes that occur in atrial fibrillation, post cardioversion stunning and recovery thereafter [22, 23].

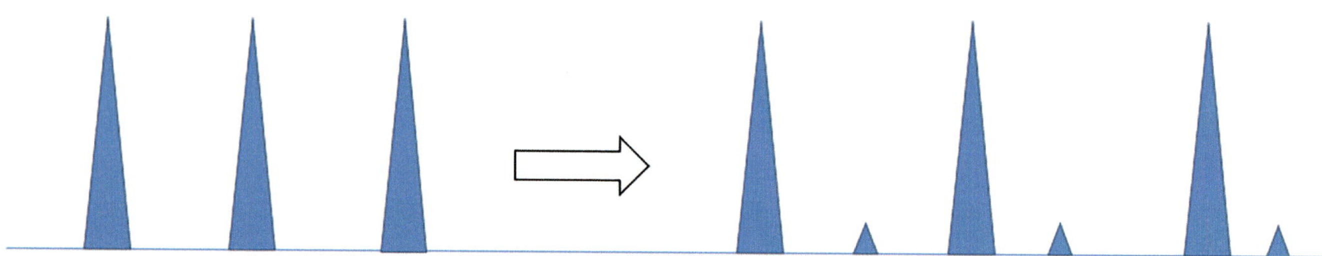

Fig. 6.33 Changes in mitral inflow Doppler patterns from atrial fibrillation to sinus rhythm

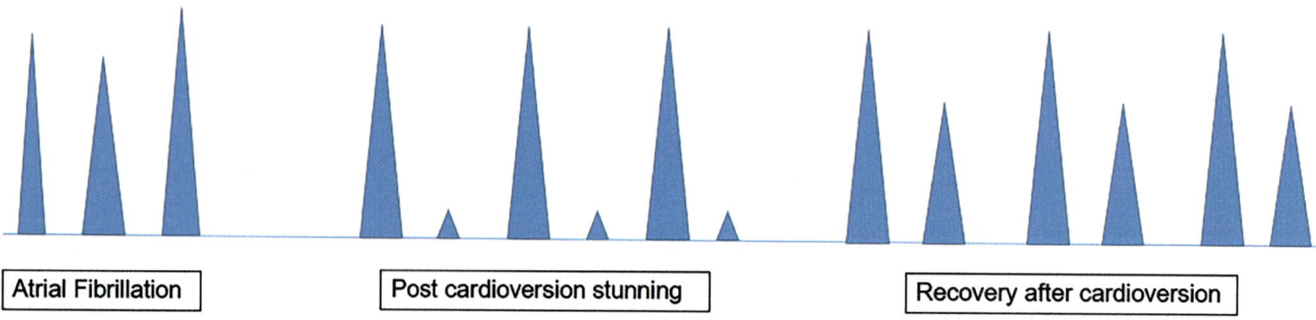

Fig. 6.34 Changes in mitral inflow doppler patterns with cardioversion

Question 20. A 66-year-old man with a history of long-standing hypertension, coronary artery disease, and heart failure with preserved ejection fraction presents to the ICU with septic shock secondary to a urinary tract infection. Blood pressure is 80/60 mmHg and pulse 121/min. He has received 3 liters of intravenous fluid resuscitation. A limited transthoracic echocardiogram is performed to assess volume responsiveness, and mitral spectral velocities obtained after a passive leg raise is performed (Table 6.1).

Before passive leg raise:

E-wave: 66 cm/s.

A-wave: 42 cm/s.

E/A: 1.57.

E/e′: 10.

After passive leg raise:

E-wave: 119 cm/s.

A-wave: 42 cm/s.

E/A: 2.83.

E/e′: 18.

What is the next best step in management?

A. Administer IV fluid bolus
B. Start inotropes
C. Start norepinephrine
D. IV diuresis

Table 6.1 Change in echocardiographic parameters with passive leg raise test

	Before passive leg raise	After passive leg raise
E-wave	66 cm/s	119 cm/s
A-wave	42 cm/s	42 cm/s
E/A	1.57	2.83
E/e′	10	18

Answer to Question 20: C.

Key Point: Increase in E/e′ with a fluid bolus or passive leg raising can help identify patients who may be non-responders to volume loading.

Rationale: This is a patient with known history of diastolic dysfunction who remains hypotensive despite receiving intravenous fluid resuscitation. Although the presence of diastolic dysfunction does not preclude the use of intravenous fluids, clinicians should be cognizant of the dangers of volume loading in this patient population. With passive leg raising, diastolic dysfunction has worsened and the E/e′ has increased accordingly. These findings are helpful in identifying non-responders who are no longer volume responsive. Therefore, further fluid loading may be detrimental in this patient (Option A is incorrect). There is no indication for inotropes (Option B is incorrect). Norepinephrine would be the first line vasopressor of choice in this patient with septic shock who is no longer volume responsive (Option C is correct). Although intravenous diuresis will play an important role during the medical optimization of this patient, it would not be the initial strategy in this hypotensive patient [24].

Question 21. A 58-year-old man was admitted to the intensive care unit with hypoxemic respiratory failure in the setting of acute exacerbation of COPD requiring intubation and mechanical ventilation. The patient responded well to antibiotics and steroids. On day 3, the patient becomes acutely hypoxic and agitated shortly after starting a spontaneous breathing trial. BP 196/100 mmHg. Representative examples of lung ultrasound are shown in Video 6.11. Mitral inflow velocities are obtained before and during the weaning trial (Figs. 6.35 and 6.36).

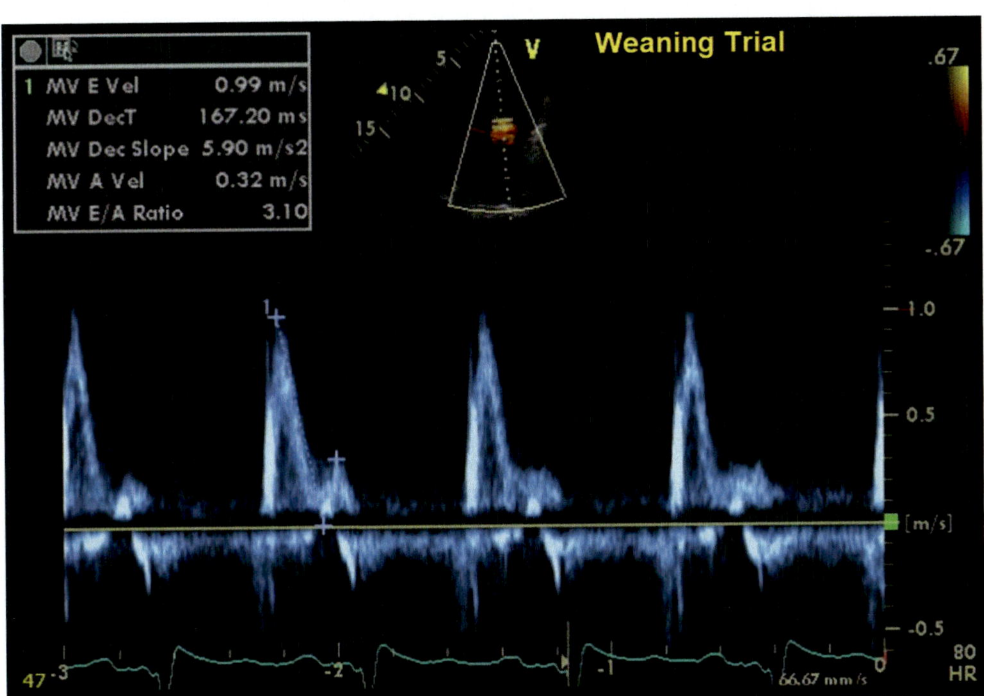

Fig. 6.35 Mitral inflow Doppler pre ventilator weaning trial

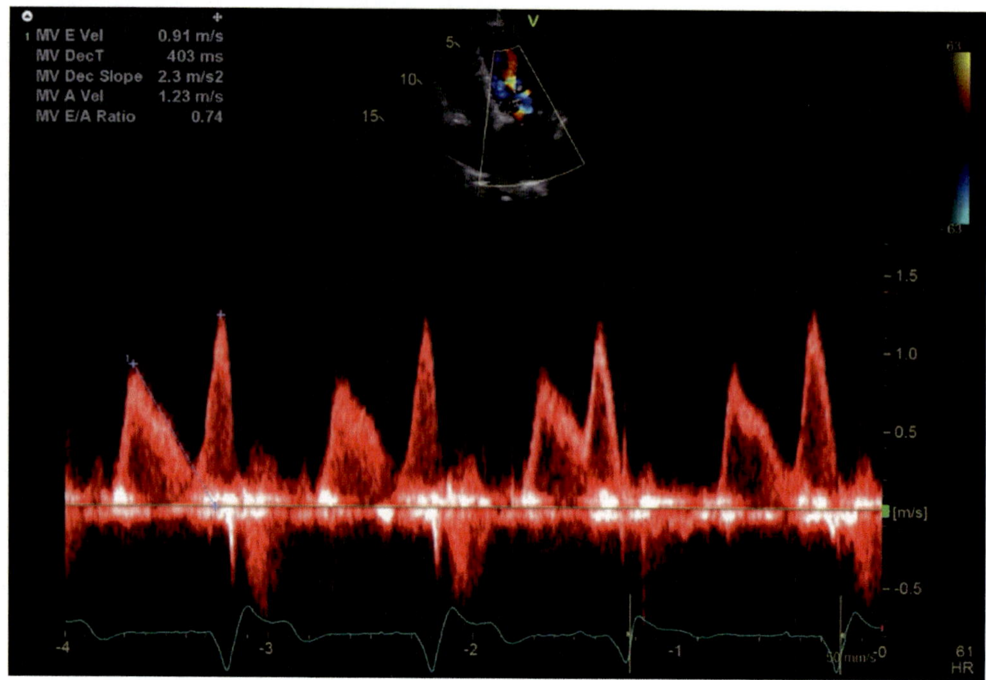

Fig. 6.36 Mitral inflow Doppler post ventilator weaning trial

What is the most likely cause of this patient's respiratory distress?

A. Diastolic Dysfunction
B. Pulmonary Embolism
C. Pneumonia
D. Pneumothorax

Answer to Question 21: A.

Key Point: Diastolic dysfunction is common in the intensive care unit with incidence that varies between 40–80% and can contribute to failure of weaning from mechanical ventilation.

Rationale: The clinical vignette presents a patient with chronic obstructive pulmonary disease with risk factors for diastolic dysfunction who develops heart failure symptoms shortly after initiation of spontaneous breathing trial. Patients with diastolic dysfunction have exaggerated shifts in left ventricular end diastolic pressure with small changes in afterload and preload due to deviations in the left ventricular pressure-volume curve. Patients with diastolic dysfunction are thus susceptible to hypertensive crisis and acute cardiogenic pulmonary edema with small increases in afterload or preload. Conversely, these patients may develop hypotension or renal dysfunction with small decreases in afterload and preload. Prior to the spontaneous breathing trial, lung ultrasound images show a predominant A-line pattern. There is an increase in venous return, increased sympathetic activity, decreased left ventricular compliance, and increased left ventricular afterload when transitioning from positive pressure ventilation to a spontaneous breathing trial. This will manifest clinically as worsening respiratory distress. Left sided filling pressures will increase as evidenced by the predominant B-line pattern in lung ultrasonography. Despite limited echocardiographic views, clinicians should be alerted to the potential for diastolic dysfunction. Higher E/e′ and E/A ratios after a spontaneous breathing trial were associated with weaning induced pulmonary edema [25, 26].

Question 22. A 52-year-old woman with a history of morbid obesity, diabetes mellitus, and hypertension was admitted to the intensive care unit with pneumonia. Her hospital course was prolonged and complicated by acute respiratory distress syndrome and acute kidney injury. She required paralysis and remains anuric. She is unresponsive to high doses of intravenous diuretics. She is ultimately extubated. Blood pressure 90/70 mmHg. A point-of-care ultrasound is performed. Mitral Doppler inflow E velocity to annular tissue Doppler e′ wave velocity (E/e′) = 21. Lung ultrasound shows a predominant bilateral B-line profile. Inferior vena cava and hepatic veins are shown in Video 6.12. Hepatic waveforms are also obtained (Fig. 6.37).

What is the next best step in management?

A. Nebulized β2-agonist
B. Dobutamine infusion
C. Aggressive IV diuresis
D. Continuous renal replacement therapy

Answer to Question 22: D.

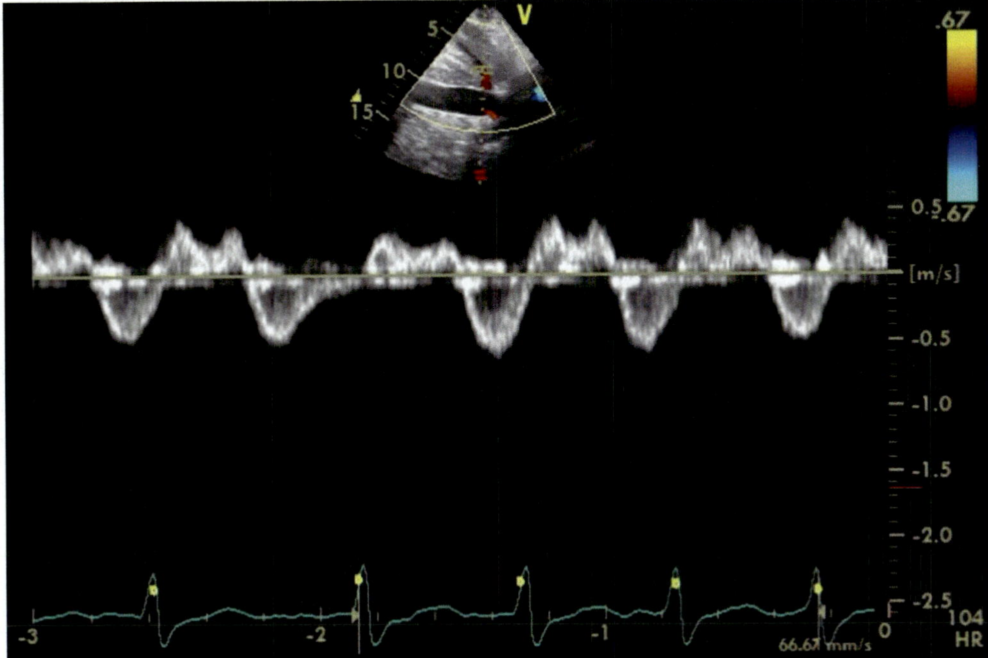

Fig. 6.37 Hepatic Vein Doppler waveforms

Key Point: Diastolic parameters in conjunction with other congestive indices are useful in assessing volume status and response to volume removal.

Rationale: There is clear evidence of elevated left sided filling pressures (high E/e′). These pressures are transmitted along the congestion cascade. Evidence that may support a volume overloaded state can include (a) systolic flow reversal of the pulmonary veins, (b) bilateral B-line profile on lung ultrasound, (c) plethoric inferior cava with minimal respiratory variation, (d) systolic flow reversal of hepatic vein waveforms (e) pulsatile portal vein flow, and (f) more pulsatile or biphasic/monophasic intrarenal venous doppler flow. Understanding the changes that occur with higher filling pressures in various organs along the congestion cascade can be helpful in optimizing volume status. In this patient, there is systolic flow reversal in the hepatic veins. These findings are all consistent with increased venous congestion. The patient is unlikely to benefit from intravenous diuresis given anuria and will require continuous renal replacement therapy for volume removal. (Option D is correct). After adequate volume removal, the hepatic veins show a normal biphasic pattern (Fig. 6.38) [27–29].

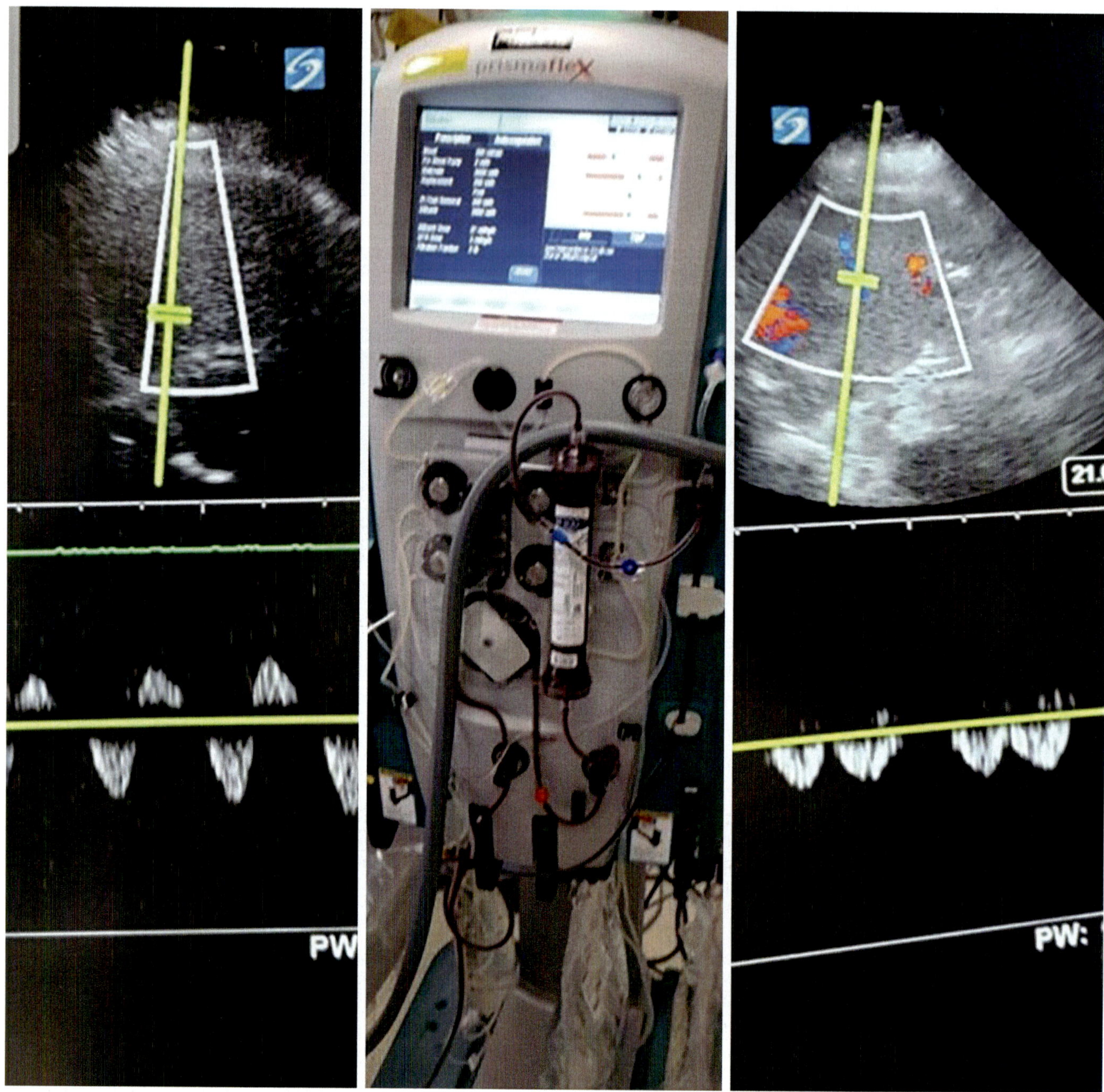

Fig. 6.38 Hepatic vein Doppler waveforms changes with volume removal

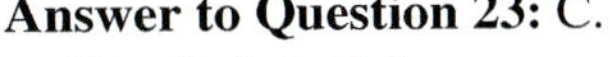

Question 23. A limited transthoracic echocardiogram is performed and the following pulmonary vein waveforms (Fig. 6.39) and mitral tissue Doppler velocities (Figs. 6.40 and 6.41) are obtained.

These findings are most consistent with?

A. Pulmonary embolism
B. Elevated left atrial pressures
C. Normal pulmonary waveforms
D. Severe mitral regurgitation

Answer to Question 23: C.

Key Point: Pulmonary vein waveforms can be useful in assessing left atrial pressures.

Rationale: Pulmonary vein waveforms can be interrogated with transthoracic echocardiography usually in the apical four chamber view. Sample volumes for pulse wave Doppler are placed within 10 mm proximal to the vein's junction with the left atrium. Normal pulmonary waveforms are usually triphasic with an S wave (during ventricular systole), D wave (during early diastole), and A reversal wave

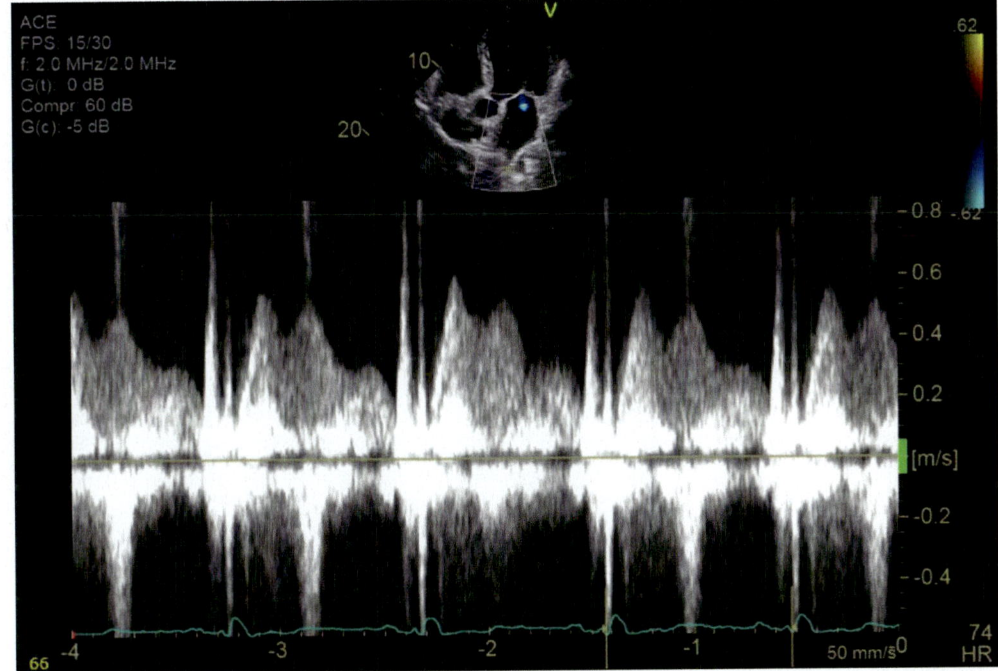

Fig. 6.39 Pulmonary vein Doppler waveform

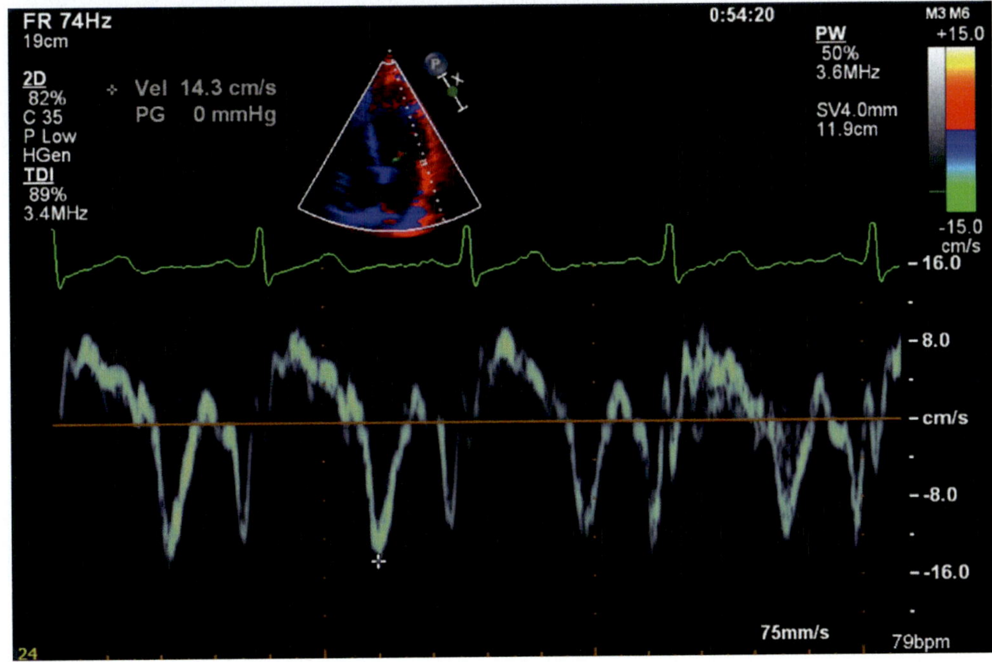

Fig. 6.40 Lateral mitral tissue Doppler

(during atrial contraction). A pulmonary vein first (S1) and second (S2) systolic wave may be seen and is a normal variant (Option C is correct) (Fig. 6.42). Normal left atrial pressures are further evidenced by mitral tissue Doppler velocities that are consistent with normal diastolic function. Pulmonary vein velocities can be affected by age, left ventricular function, atrioventricular conduction, and heart rate. Normal S/D ratio is >1. In patients with normal LV function, S/D ratio correlates well with changes in left atrial pressure. Pulmonary embolism will not affect pulmonary vein wave form morphology. (Option A is incorrect). Elevated left atrial pressures or severe mitral regurgitation may show blunting of the S-wave or flow reversal (Option D is incorrect) [5, 6].

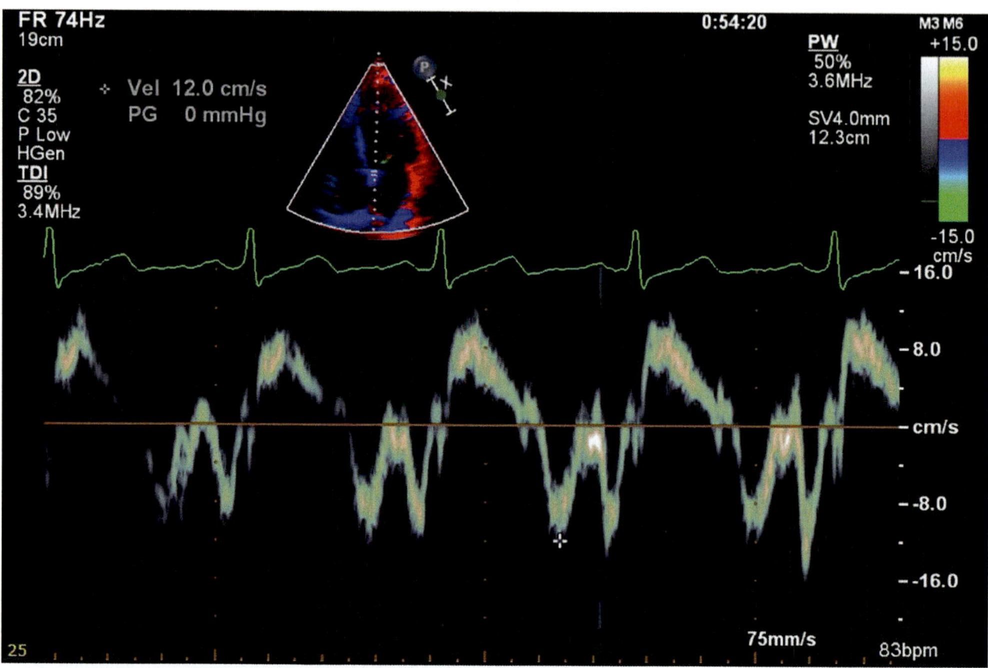

Fig. 6.41 Medial mitral tissue Doppler

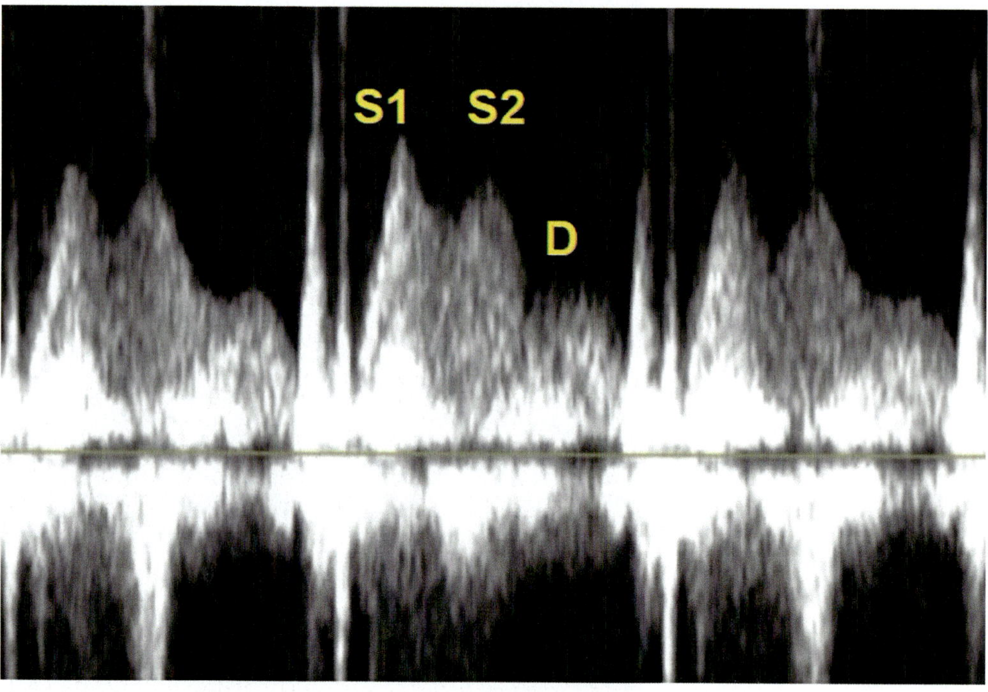

Fig. 6.42 Pulmonary vein Doppler waveform depicting normal S1 and S2 pattern

Question 24. A 67-year-old man with a known history of nonischemic cardiomyopathy (most recent LVEF~25%) presented with respiratory distress and weight gain. The patient is afebrile, BP 117/82 mmHg, HR 98/min RR 26/min. Bilateral widespread crackles are heard on auscultation. CBC is unremarkable, serum creatinine 1.1 mg/dl, BNP 1780. Lung ultrasound revealed a bilateral B-line profile in the anterior lung fields. A limited transthoracic echocardiogram revealed depressed ejection fraction similar to previous scans. Prior to treatment E/e′ = 28. The patient received noninvasive positive pressure ventilation and aggressive intravenous diuresis. A repeat E/e′ = 12 and lung ultrasound demonstrates an A-line pattern.

Which of the following is TRUE?

A. Lung ultrasound and E/e′ ratio is unhelpful in this scenario
B. E/e′ is a useful congestion parameter to assess treatment response
C. BNP levels show rapid initial decline within hours
D. None of the above

Answer to Question 24: B.

Rationale: E/e′ and lung ultrasound are both useful congestion parameters that can be used to monitor early response to treatment and predicts prognostically important resolution of pulmonary congestion. Patients who respond to therapy exhibit significant rapid decline in E/e′ however BNP levels may lag behind clinical resolution. Lung ultrasound response independently predicted both 6-month all-cause mortality and rehospitalization for acute decompensated heart failure. Rapid assessment of patients with focused cardiac and lung ultrasound is useful in the management of acute decompensated heart failure [30].

Question 25. A 59-year-old man with no known medical history presents with an ST-elevation myocardial infarction. He undergoes cardiac catheterization through the right femoral artery with successful stenting of mid LAD culprit lesion. 12 h after PCI, you are called to evaluate for hypotension. BP 88/52 HR 132/min RR 14/min saturating 98% on room air. EKG showing sinus tachycardia. Repeat Hgb 6 g/dl from 14 g/dl on admission. A point of care echocardiogram is performed (Videos 6.13, 6.14, 6.15 and 6.16, Fig. 6.43).

What is the most likely change to mitral inflow velocities in response to tachycardia?

A. Loss of E-wave
B. Decrease in diastasis time
C. Augmentation of A-wave
D. None of the above

Answer to Question 25: B.

Rationale: The diastasis phase decreases with increased heart rates which leads to approximation of the E and A-waves. This represents the time period between E and A waves where little filling occurs. This patient is presenting with hypotension after percutaneous coronary intervention. There is evidence of a hyperdynamic left and right ventricle. The IVC is small and collapsible. Although mechanical complications post myocardial infarction are an important consideration this is not consistent with the findings on point of care echocardiography (no mitral regurgitation, VSD, or pericardial effusion). In the setting of a precipitous drop hemoglobin, this is all consistent with hypovolemic/hemorrhagic shock with compensatory tachycardia. The patient received supportive blood transfusions. A CT Scan was performed and revealed a retroperitoneal hemorrhage likely caused by recent instrumentation for PCI [1].

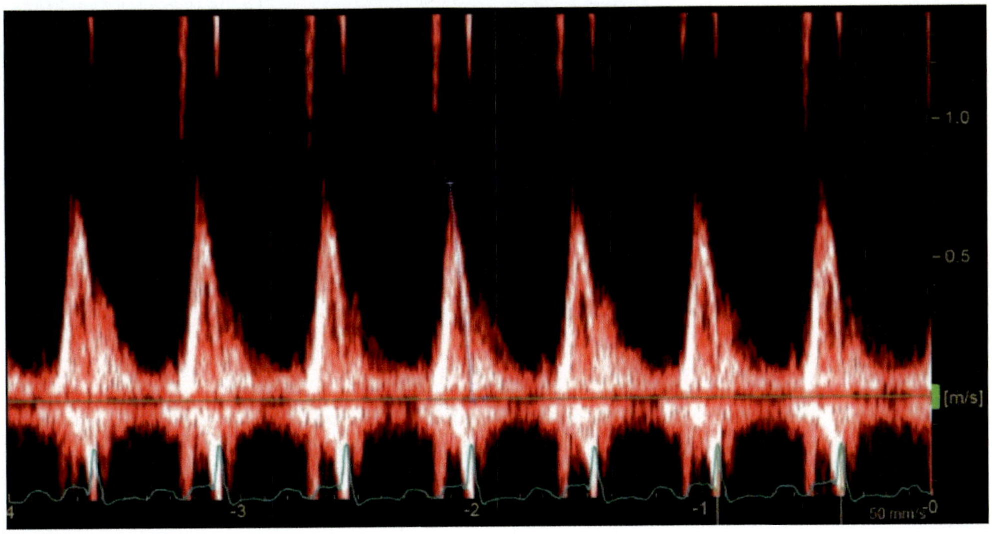

Fig. 6.43 Mitral inflow Doppler with fused E/A Wave

Question 26. A 72-year-old woman with a past medical history of heavy tobacco abuse, uncontrolled hypertension, diabetes, and hyperlipidemia has noted progressive shortness of breath for several months. On evaluation in the emergency room she is found to have a HR 62, BP 188/87, RR 17 and sating 92% on 6 L nasal cannula. As part of her initial work up she has a transthoracic echocardiogram performed which shows, normal ejection fraction without wall motion abnormalities, and mild mitral regurgitation. There is bi-atrial enlargement with severe left ventricular hypertrophy and an atrial septal aneurysm (Video 6.17). The following representative images are also from her exam (Figs. 6.44, 6.45, 6.46 and 6.47).

The following conclusion(s) can be drawn from the above information

A. The patient has high grade diastolic dysfunction and is likely volume overloaded.
B. The patient has an atrial arrythmia and thus her diastolic function cannot be evaluated with the information provided.
C. She has pulmonary hypertension, which, when paired with her atrial septal aneurysm places the women at high risk for a right to left shunt which explains her mild hypoxia.
D. These are normal findings in the elderly, the patient should be worked up for primary pulmonary disease as an etiology for her symptoms.

Answer to Question 26: A.

Rationale: The arrow indicates an "L wave" which can be seen in advanced diastolic dysfunction in the setting of volume overload and low heart rates (Fig. 6.48). The L wave represents persistent mid-diastolic pulmonary vein flow transmitted through the atria and across the mitral valve. The L wave is not related to any atrial electrical or contractile activity, has no relation to elevated pulmonary pressures and is considered pathologic regardless of patient age [20, 31]. Other representative images of L-waves can be seen in Figs. 6.49 and 6.50.

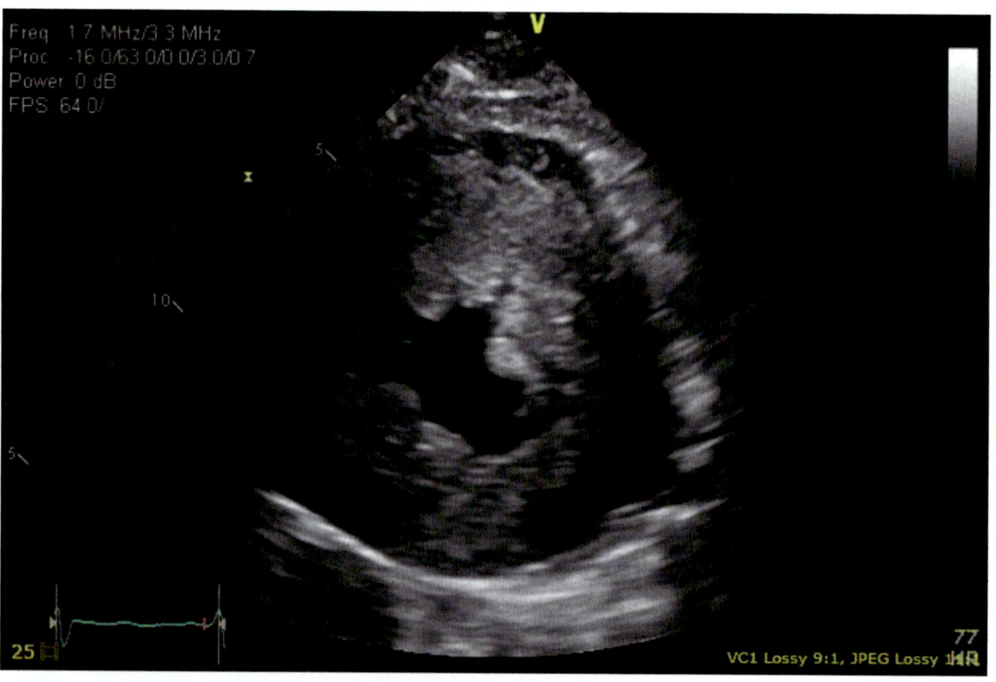

Fig. 6.44 Parasternal short axis view

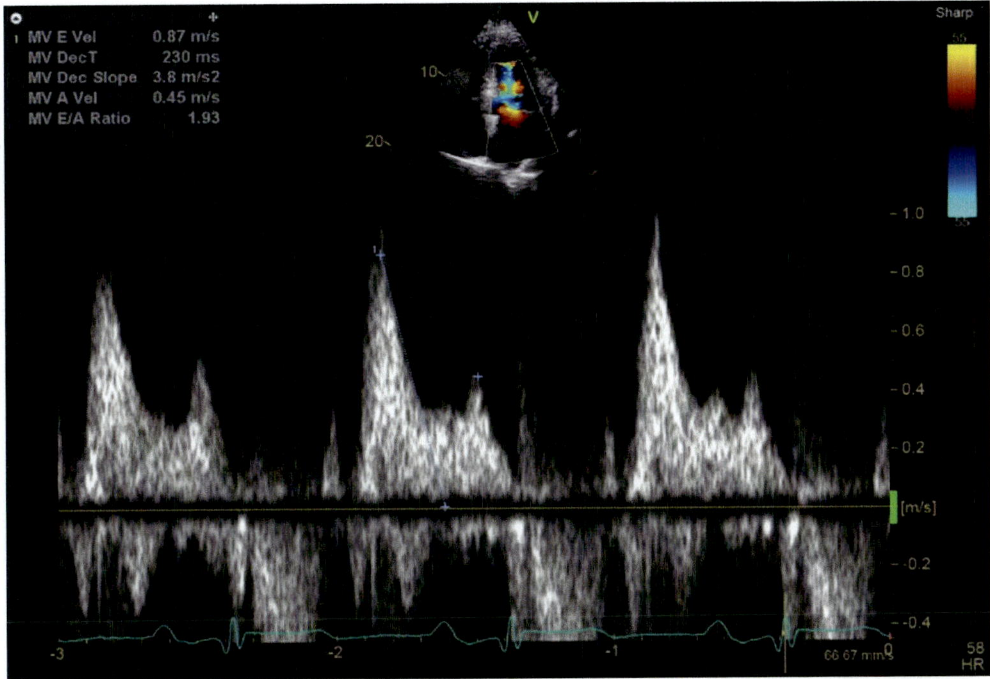

Fig. 6.45 Mitral inflow Doppler with fused E/A wave

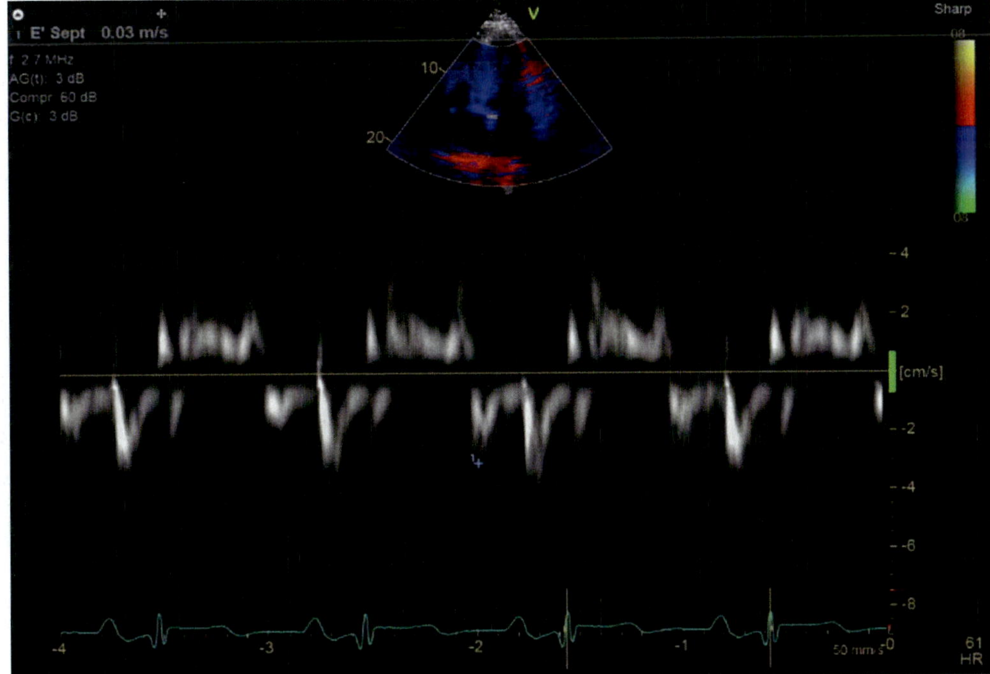

Fig. 6.46 Medial mitral tissue Doppler

Fig. 6.47 Lateral mitral tissue Doppler

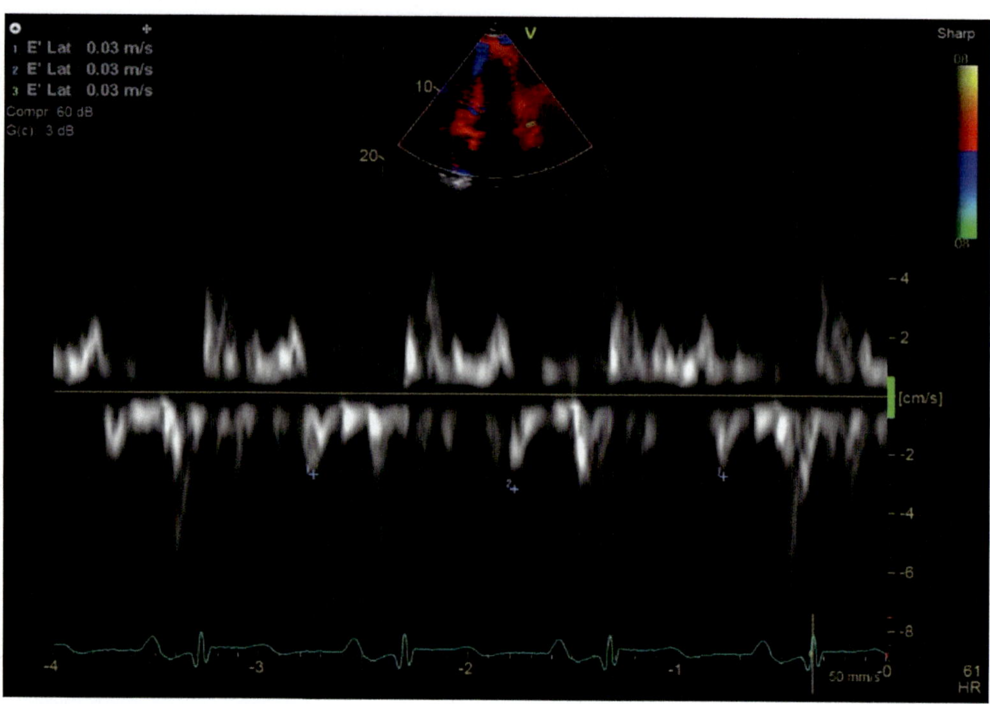

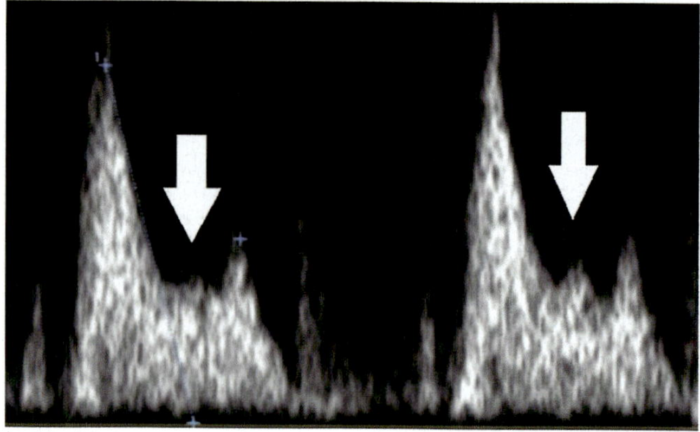

Fig. 6.48 Mitral inflow Doppler with D wave image 1

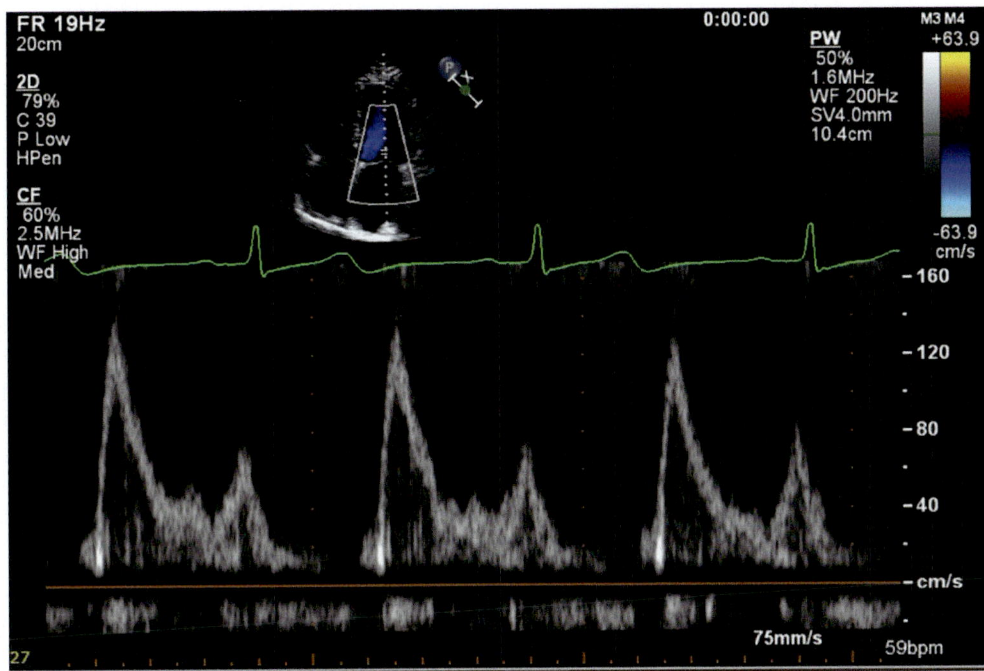

Fig. 6.49 Mitral inflow Doppler with D wave image 2

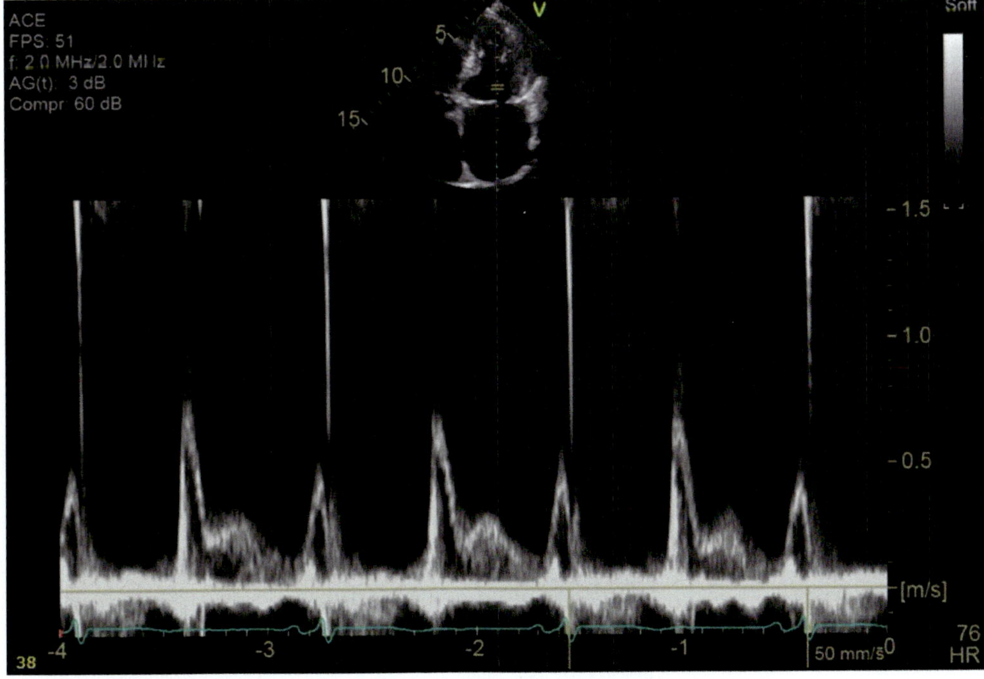

Fig. 6.50 Mitral inflow Doppler with D wave image 3

Question 27. A few days after admission, the patient develops a fever, narrow complex tachycardia with a rate of approximately 120 and a drop in the systolic blood pressure to 90 s. Over the next two hours labs and imaging are collected. Her CXR has evidence of a new right lower lobe infiltrate consistent with a hospital acquired pneumonia. ECG shows sinus tachycardia with S-T depressions in V4–V6. Initial labs show a troponin of 2 ng/ml and creatinine of 1.4 (baseline of 0.9). Her blood pressure is 54/31 mmHg, saturation is 91% on 3 L by nasal cannula. She is initiated on norepinephrine infusion to maintain mean arterial pressure above 65 mmHg. Lactate is 6 mmol/L.

Based on the entirety of her presentation which of the following is most true?

A. This patient should be taken urgently to the cardiac catheterization lab for simultaneous right and left heart evaluation.
B. The patient should urgently receive IV beta blocker therapy, and pulse dose steroids.
C. This patient has a higher mortality than a similar patient with normal diastolic function.
D. An emergent consult should be placed for evaluation by an electrophysiologist.

Answer to Question 27: C.

Rationale: The patient has developed sepsis likely secondary to a hospital acquired pneumonia with a concurrent NSTEMI. While the patient does have some myocardial ischemia the patient likely is experiencing a type II NSTEMI secondary to supply demand mismatch and may not benefit from urgent catheterization especially in the setting of acute renal failure and septic shock. Similarly, the primary issue is not related to any underlying electrical abnormality. The patient clearly has advanced diastolic dysfunction based on the presence of an L wave at the time of her presentation and persistent diastolic dysfunction after diuresis. Diastolic dysfunction is associated with higher mortality in the setting of sepsis [32, 33].

Question 28. An 80-year-old man with a past medical history significant for hypertension, CKD Stage 3, prior myocardial infarction with recent stenting to the circumflex coronary artery, and depressed ejection fraction. Recent transthoracic echocardiogram showed recovery of ejection fraction, no wall motion abnormality, moderate left ventricular hypertrophy, severe mitral annular calcification, moderate aortic stenosis, mild mitral and mild tricuspid regurgitation. Over the past 3-days he has developed intermittent palpitations with persistent shortness of breath prompting his presentation to the ER. His initial troponin was negative. The following are representative echocardiogram images and mitral inflow patterns (Figs. 6.51, 6.52, 6.53, 6.54 and 6.55).

Which of the following conclusions is most accurate?

A. The patient has significant volume overload and should be treated rapidly and aggressively with IV diuretic therapy.
B. Prior myocardial infarction prevents the accurate assessment of diastolic function

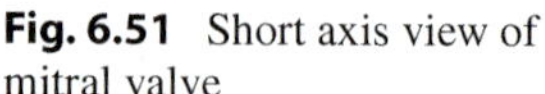

Fig. 6.51 Short axis view of mitral valve

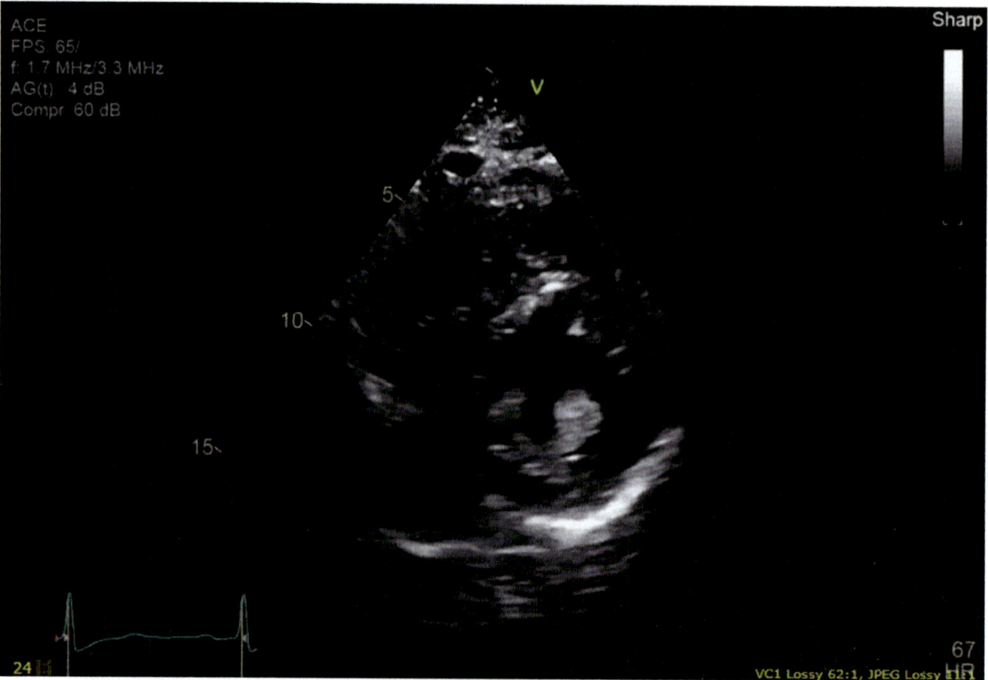

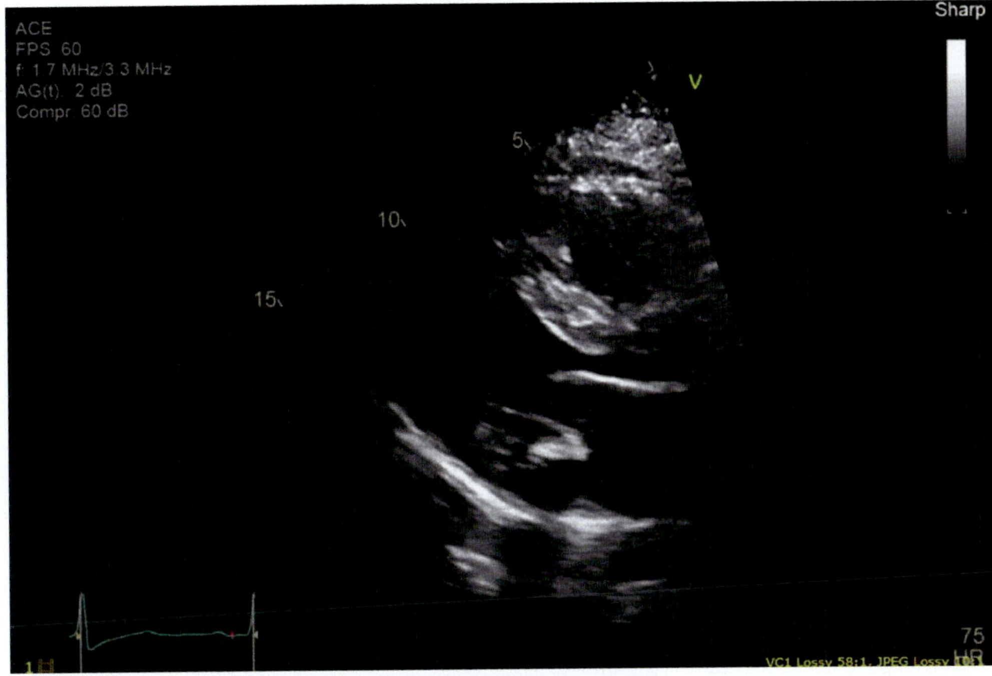

Fig. 6.52 Parasternal long axis view

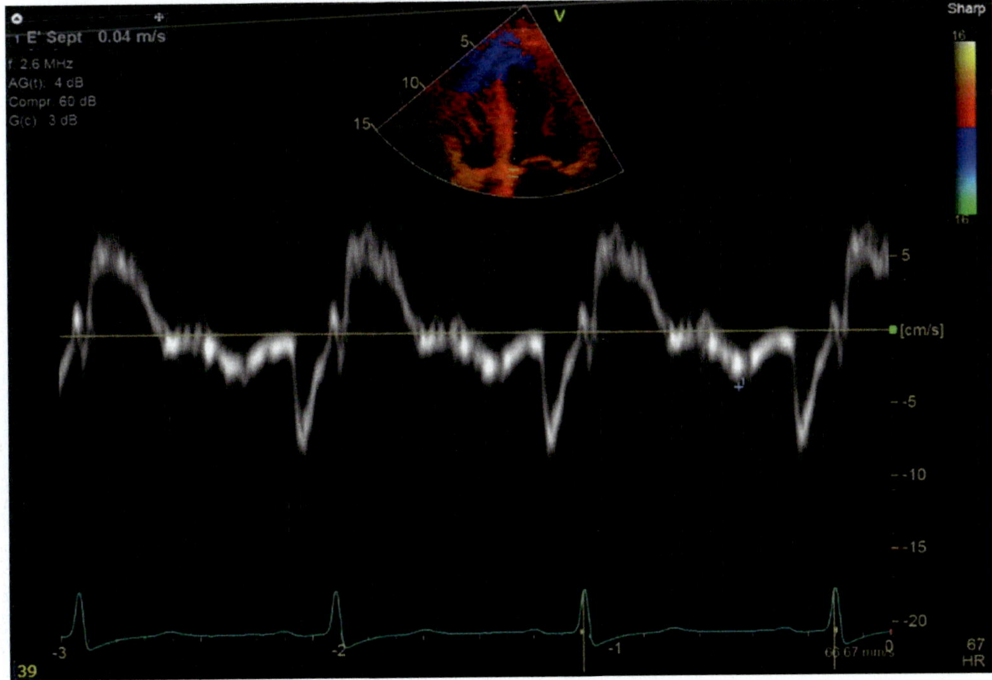

Fig. 6.53 Medial mitral tissue Doppler

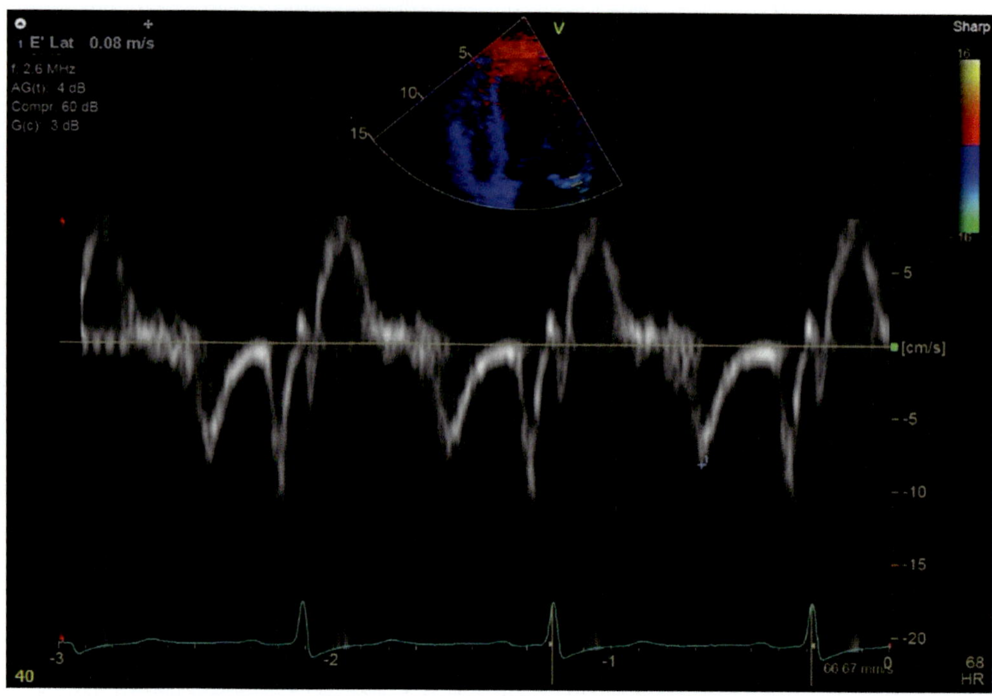

Fig. 6.54 Lateral mitral tissue Doppler

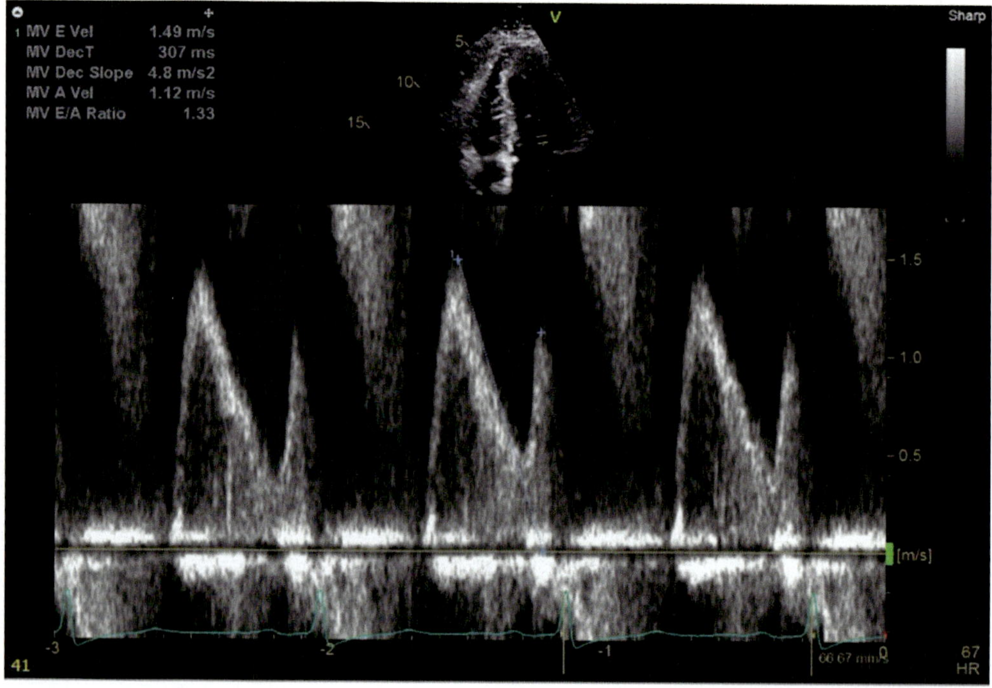

Fig. 6.55 Mitral inflow Doppler with fused E/A wave

C. The patient has findings concerning for cardiac amyloidosis and should undergo cardiac magnetic resonance imaging
D. The patient's volume status and diastolic function cannot be estimated with the provided information.

Answer to Question 28: D.

Rationale: This patient has dense mitral annular calcification (MAC) (Parasternal views Figs. 6.51 and 6.52) which can cause small, non-hemodynamically significant decreases in the mitral orifice area leading to small increases in mitral inflow velocities (increase in E) despite there being no change in the mean gradient. Furthermore, MAC can limit the e′ velocities even in the setting of normal left ventricular relaxation. The two artifactually modified measurements result in an inaccurately increased E/e′ estimate. Thus, diastolic function cannot be estimated given the information provided. While prior myocardial infarction can result in regional wall motion abnormalities and locally abnormal TDI thus limiting the utility of a specific region (ex. lateral e′) as a tool for estimating diastolic function, this patient has had full recovery of ejection fraction post revascularization and presumably has no systolic or diastolic sequalae of the ischemic event [34, 35].

Question 29. A 62-year-old obese female with a past medical history of hypertension presents with a two-week history of palpitations. Her vital signs are significant for a blood pressure of 192/92 and an irregular heart rate of 160–180 s. Her ECG that shows atrial fibrillation with rapid ventricular response. She is given 10 mg IV Diltiazem followed by a second bolus then started on a drip. Her heart rate is still irregular, but rate controlled. The patient was admitted for management and evaluation. Along with appropriate labs the primary team ordered a transthoracic echocardiogram (Fig. 6.56).

Which of the following statements is NOT true regarding her echocardiographic images?

A. Beat to beat variability will cause variable flow across the mitral valve.
B. Pulse Doppler through the mitral valve will have a fused E and A wave.
C. The E/e′ will retain its predictive value regarding left ventricular end-diastolic pressure.
D. Using either septal or lateral e′ TDI is sufficient for the evaluation in this setting.

Answer to Question 29: B.

Rationale: Atrial fibrillation causes beat to beat variability in atrial filling with absence of A-wave, not a fused E-A wave which is usually seen in first degree AV block with PR intervals >280 ms. Despite this, the E/e′ does retain its value in evaluating LVEDP. Atrial fibrillation does not affect TDI [36].

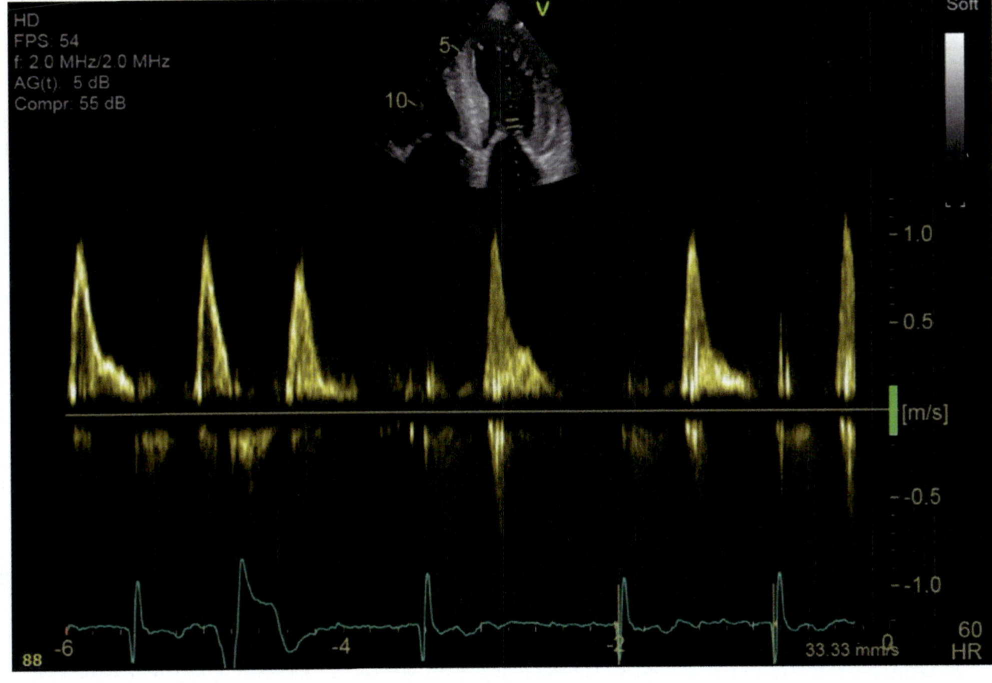

Fig. 6.56 Mitral inflow Doppler in atrial fibrillation

Question 30. A 53-year-old woman with a past medical history of hypertension, rate controlled atrial fibrillation on anticoagulation, and known grade I diastolic dysfunction presents to the ER with shortness of breath and tachycardia one week after running out of her metoprolol. Her vital signs on admission are BP 202/103 HR 119 and Sat 89%. CXR shows bilateral pulmonary edema a small left sided pleural effusion.

Which of the following statements is most correct?

A. Volume status cannot be assessed in the setting of atrial fibrillation.
B. Slowing the HR will improve symptoms by decreasing pulmonary edema.
C. Afterload reduction will improve symptoms by decreasing pulmonary edema.
D. Right pleural drainage to improve oxygenation.
E. Both B and C
F. Both C and D

Answer to Question 30: E.

Rationale: The patient has grade I diastolic dysfunction and is preload sensitive; small increases in volume will increase LVEDP to a greater extent in the setting of impaired LV relaxation. Similarly, tachycardia will lead to shorter filling times and in the setting of significant afterload will exacerbate symptoms associated with diastolic dysfunction by increasing LVEDP, LAP and subsequent pulmonary edema. Thus, decreasing both HR and blood pressure will improve her symptoms. Volume status can be assessed in atrial fibrillation as E/e′ remains accurate. Placing a pigtail catheter will not address the underlying pulmonary edema. Furthermore, a heart failure associated pleural effusion is likely to reaccumulate without addressing the volume overload, tachycardia and afterload [21].

Question 31. 77-year-old man with coronary artery disease, normal EF, and known left bundle branch block presents with respiratory failure. BP 120/60 mmHg HR 78/min RR 14/min. A point of care ultrasound is performed. He is found to have an EF of 55–60% and normal sized atria and no evidence of aortic valve stenosis. Echocardiogram shows a mild central mitral regurgitation with a regurgitant jet with peak velocity of 2.1 m/s.

Which of the following parameters can be utilized to estimate left atrial pressures?

A. Systolic blood pressure
B. Tricuspid regurgitant jet velocity
C. Pulsed wave Doppler thru the mitral valve
D. Left ventricular outflow tract (LVOT) diameter
E. Mitral annular velocities and E/e′

Answer to Question 31: A.

Rationale:

Left atrial pressure can be estimated using the formula:

$$\text{LAP} = \text{LVSP} - 4 \times (\text{MR vel max})^2$$

LVSP approximates SBP in the setting of no significant aortic stenosis or outflow tract obstruction. The tricuspid regurgitant velocity can be used to estimate the right ventricular systolic pressure (RVSP) assuming there is no RVOT stenosis, pulmonary valve stenosis or pulmonary arterial hypertension; however in order to estimate the RVSP it is necessary to also have some estimation of the right atrial filling pressures. Mitral annular velocities and E/e′ may not be accurate in the setting of left bundle branch block. LVOT would be of no utility in this scenario but would be helpful in calculating stroke volume if required [37].

Question 32. A 56-year-old patient with multiple myeloma and known cardiac amyloidosis presents with shortness of breath, weight gain and anasarca. He reports compliance with his medications including his diuretics at home. Creatinine has risen from its baseline of 1.2 up to 2.6 mg/dl. At this time, he is unable to lay flat for any extended periods and refuses a right heart catheterization. He has had a right heart catheterization in the past with a wedge pressure of 16 mmHg, at that time he was feeling well with minimal shortness of breath with exertion. He undergoes a transthoracic echocardiogram that has the following diastolic parameters.

E-wave = 96 cm/s.

Medial e′ = 4 cm/s.

Latera; e′ = 8 cm/s.

Approximately how many mmHg of difference has the left atrial pressure increased from his baseline?

A. >15 mmHg
B. 10 mmHg
C. 6 mmHg
D. 4 mmHg
E. It is less than his baseline, the symptoms are not being driven by volume overload

Answer to Question 32: C.

Rationale: The pulmonary capillary occlusion or wedge pressure during a right heart catheterization is a surrogate measurement for left atrial pressure. In this case we know when he was asymptomatic his LAP was estimated at 16 mmHg. At presentation, the echocardiogram estimates an E of 96 cm/s, medial e′ of 4 cm/s and a lateral e′ of 8 cm/s. The average e′ is 6 cm/s. E/e′ = 96(cm/s)/6 (cm/s) = 16. Applying the formula LAP = 1.9 + 1.24 E/e′ to this case gives a value of 21.74 mmHg. The difference from a baseline wedge of 16 mmHg and 21.74 is 5.74 mmHg (~6 mmHg) [11].

Question 33. A 62-year-old man presents with chest pain which worsens when laying down after a recent viral illness. Physical exam is significant for a rub, troponin is reported as 0.9 ng/ml and the EKG shows diffuse ST segment elevations. Transthoracic echocardiogram at that time confirmed a small pericardial effusion. He was treated with NSAIDs and sent home. He is now returning 3 months later with shortness of breath and increased lower extremity edema. He is found to have a blood pressure of 80/50 and a heart rate of 102 Sat 92%. Troponin is negative. EKG is within normal limits. A limited transthoracic echocardiogram is performed (Videos 6.18, 6.19 and 6.20, Figs. 6.57, 6.58, 6.59, 6.60 and 6.61).

What is the most accurate diagnosis?

A. Volume overload and pleural effusions
B. Pericardial effusion
C. Echocardiographic evidence of tamponade physiology
D. A and B
E. B and C

Answer to Question 33: E.

Rationale: The images show a pericardial effusion NOT a pleural effusion. The descending Aorta (Ao) is outside of the pericardium and is useful in differentiating a pericardial effusion from a pleural effusion. The pericardial fluid is noted with the arrow and the descending Ao is marked with an asterisk (Fig. 6.62). Tamponade physiology is a clinical diagnosis (jugular venous distension, tachycardia, hypotension, pulsus paradoxus) however echocardiographic evidence of tamponade is present in the data presented which shows mitral inflow respiratory variability (decreased with inspiration) >25%, and normal septal and lateral e′ [38].

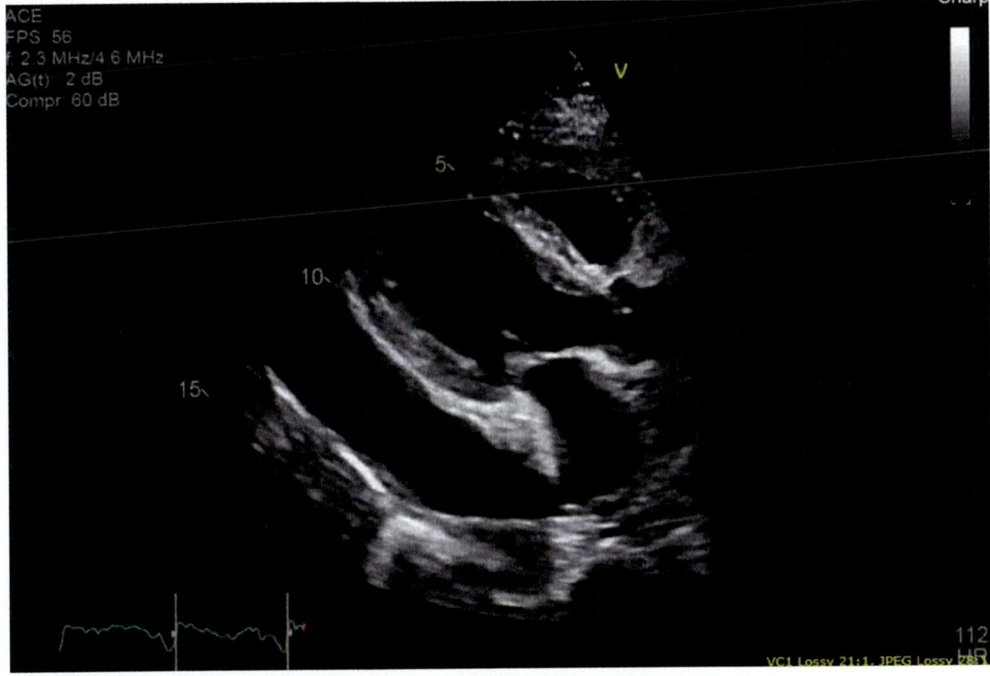

Fig. 6.57 Parasternal long axis view with pericardial effusion

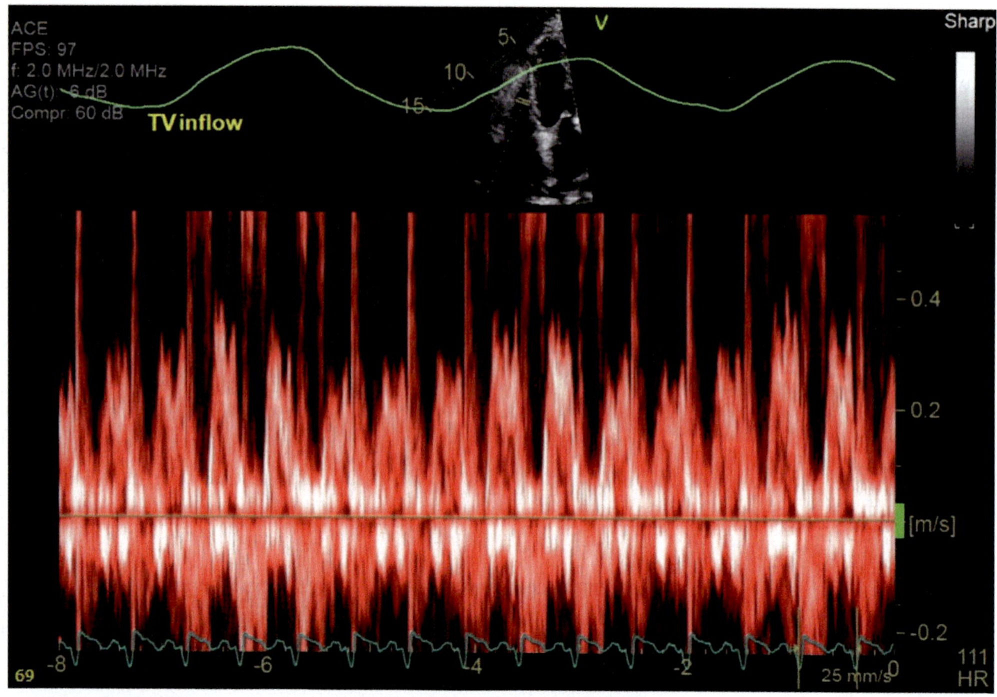

Fig. 6.58 Tricuspid valve inflow Doppler with respirometry

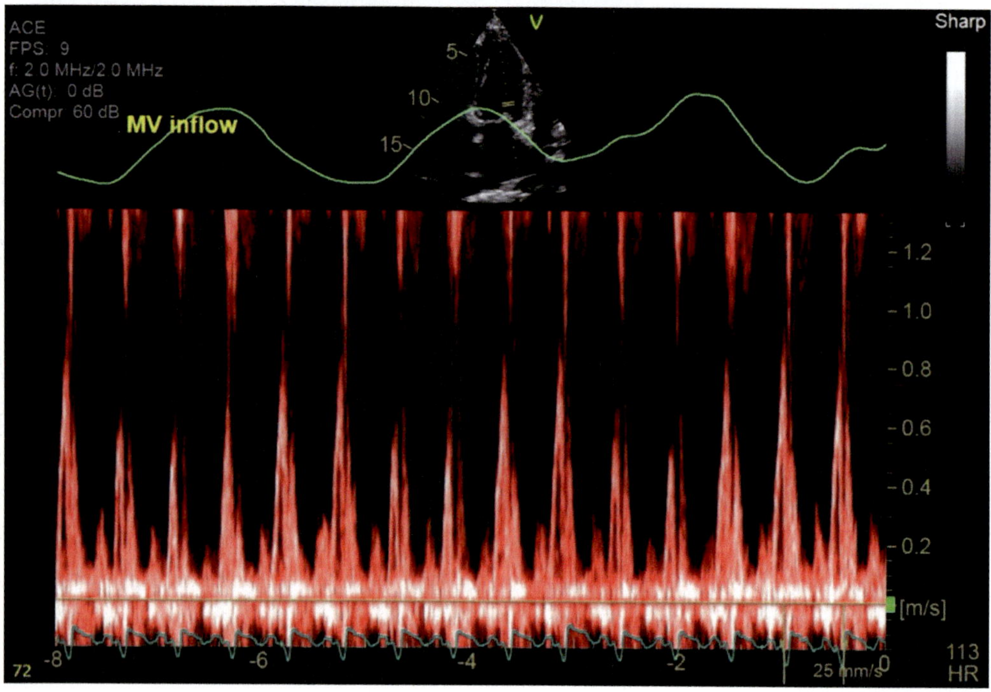

Fig. 6.59 Mitral valve inflow Doppler with respirometry

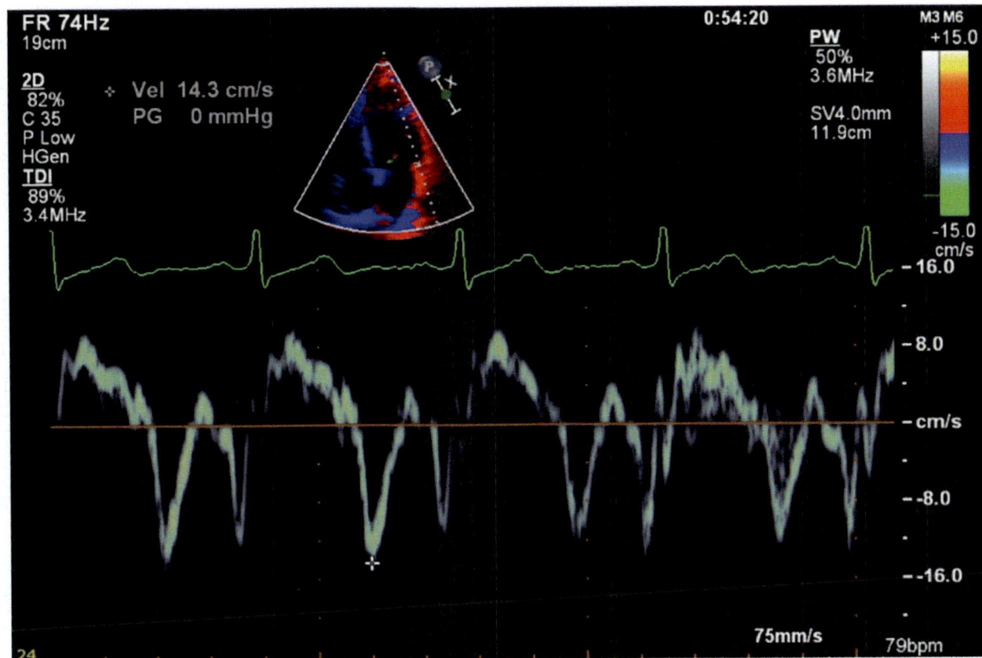

Fig. 6.60 Lateral mitral tissue Doppler with variation

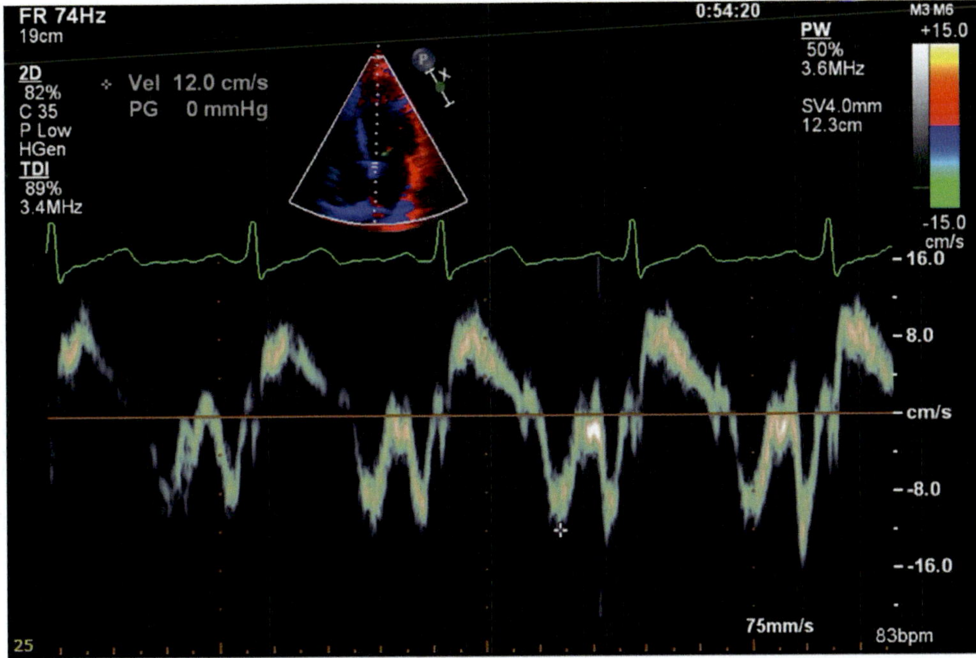

Fig. 6.61 Medial mitral tissue Doppler with variation

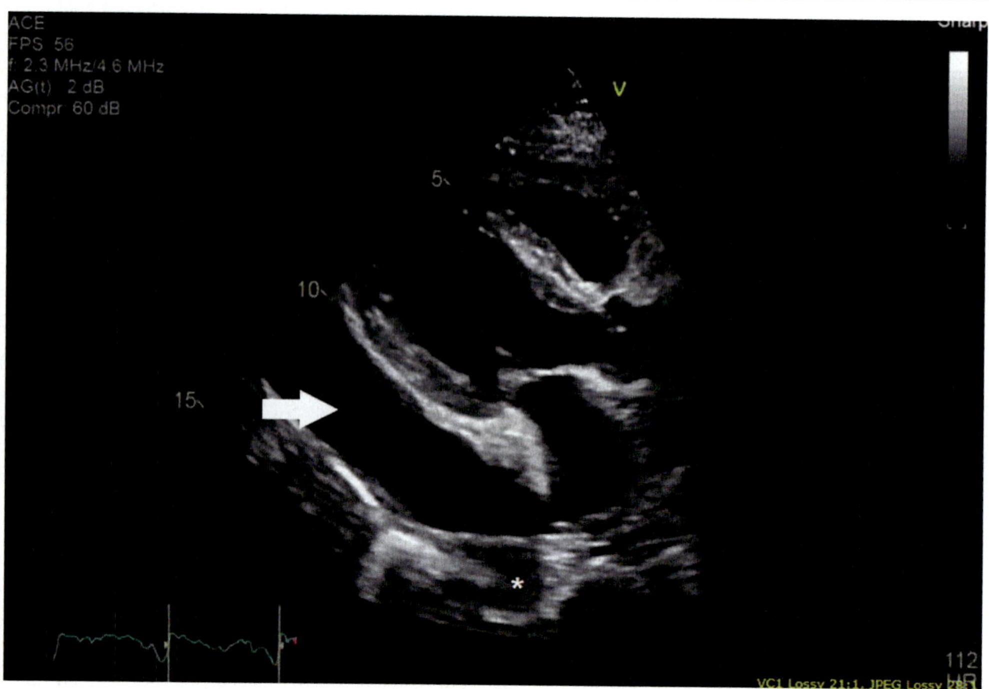

Fig. 6.62 Pericardial effusion (white arrow)

Question 34. The same man is treated and sent home again. After 1 month he returns with symptoms of shortness of breath and volume overload. Again, his troponin is negative and ECG normal. Again, a transthoracic echocardiogram is performed and includes the below images (Figs. 6.63, 6.64, 6.65 and 6.66).

What other data may support the diagnosis of constrictive pericarditis at this time?

A. Hepatic vein flow reversal with inspiration
B. Echocardiographic respiratory related septal bounce or shift
C. Simultaneous left and right heart catheterization with evidence of right ventricular and left ventricular (wedge) concordance
D. Elevated RVSP

Answer to Question 34: B.

Rationale: The patient has now developed constriction as evidenced by the development of annulus reversus. This is characterized by a decrease in the lateral annular e′ velocity while the medial mitral annulus e′ remains the same or elevated (Figs. 6.63 and 6.64). In addition, constrictive pericardial disease is associated with hepatic vein flow reversal which is present during EXPIRATION not inspiration (Fig. 6.65), septal bounce and the mitral inflow variation noted (Fig. 6.66). Representative echocardiograms demonstrating a septal bounce can be seen in Videos 6.21 and 6.22 associated with a complex pericardial effusion. Simultaneous right and left heart catheterization will result in discordance of left ventricular and right ventricular pressures in the setting of constriction [39].

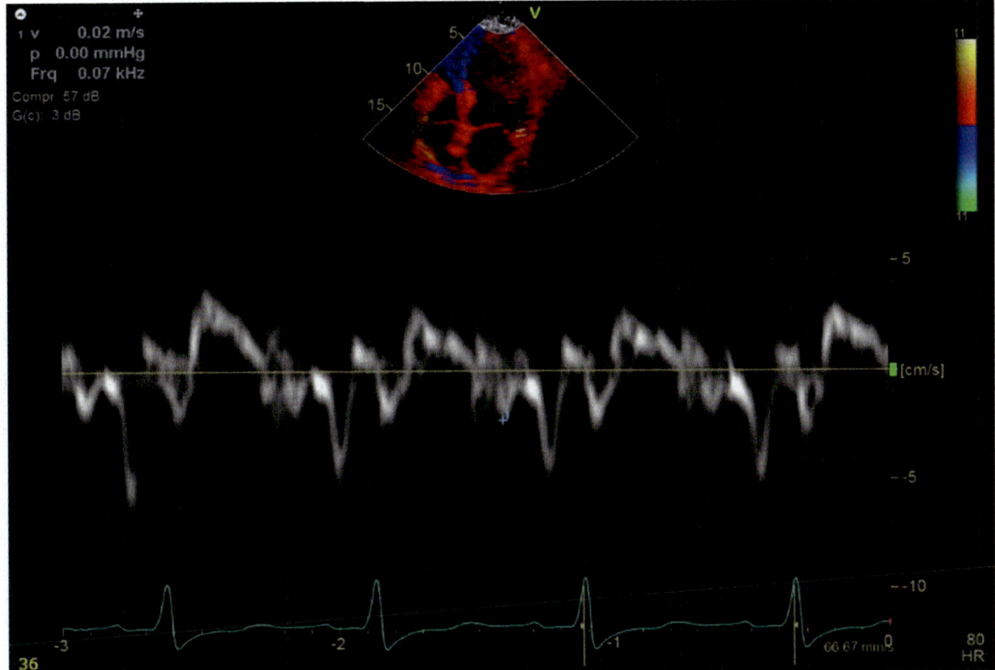

Fig. 6.63 Lateral mitral tissue Doppler

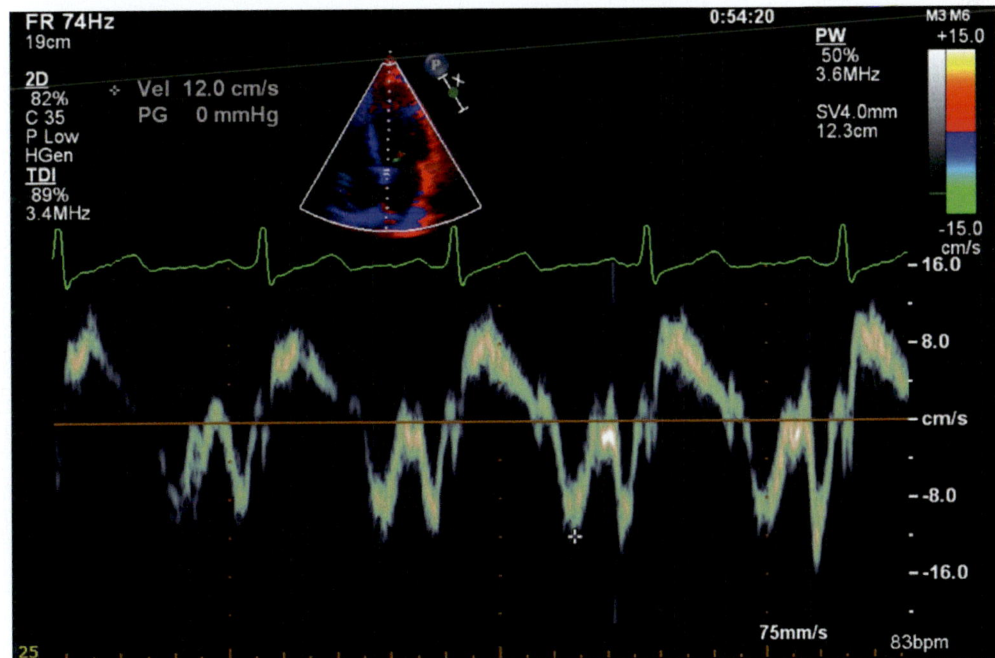

Fig. 6.64 Medial mitral tissue Doppler

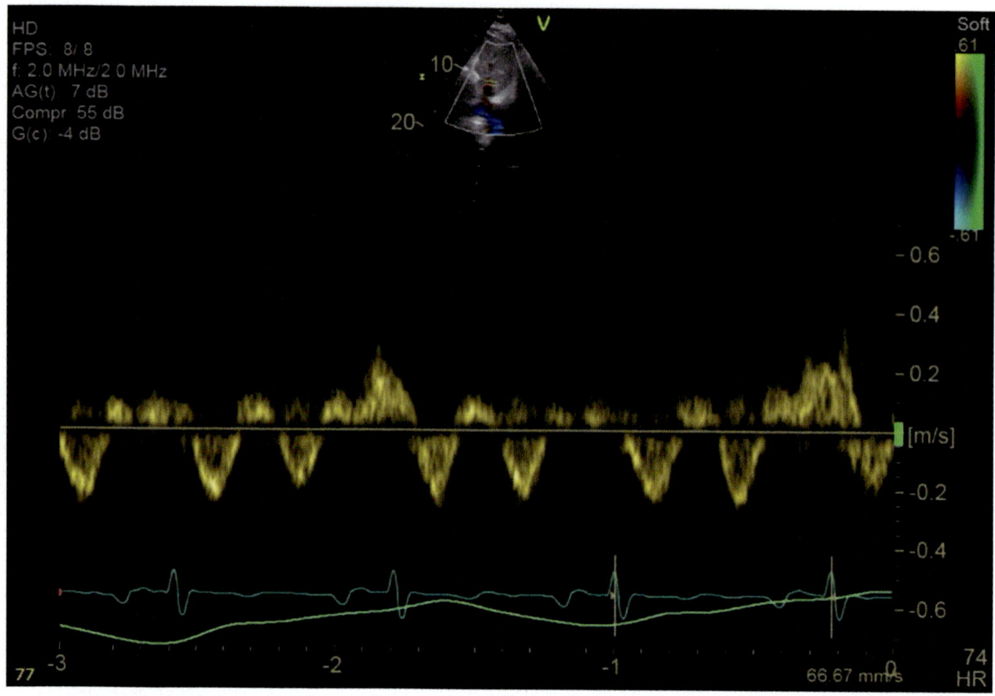

Fig. 6.65 Hepatic Vein Doppler

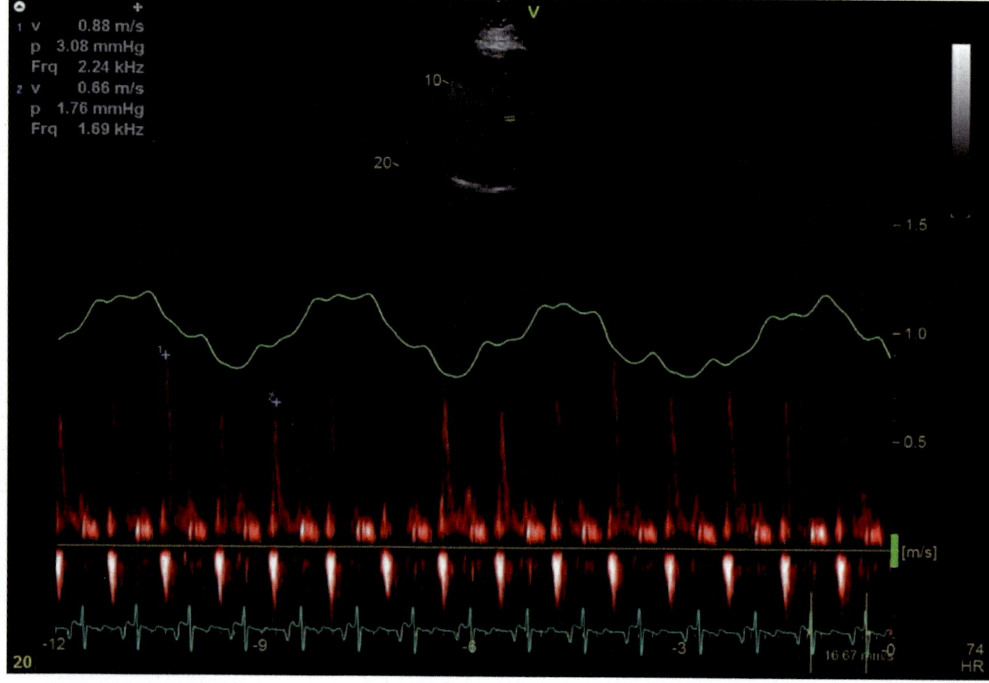

Fig. 6.66 Mitral inflow Doppler

Question 35. A morbidly obese 50-year-old female with a history of intravenous drug abuse is being evaluated for shortness of breath with exertion. Transthoracic echocardiography was completed (Fig. 6.67). She undergoes a transesophageal echocardiogram which reveals no evidence of infective endocarditis. Pulmonary veins are interrogated (Fig. 6.68).

Which of the following statements are true given the above images?

A. The patient has significant mitral regurgitation.
B. The left atrial pressure is increased.
C. The patient has pulmonary hypertension.
D. The patient has constriction.

Answer to Question 35: B.

Rationale: Ar (~70 ms), or the duration of the Atrial wave in the pulmonary vein pulse Doppler images indicates the duration of retrograde flow during atrial systole. 'A' duration (~30 ms, is the length of time the atria contraction results in

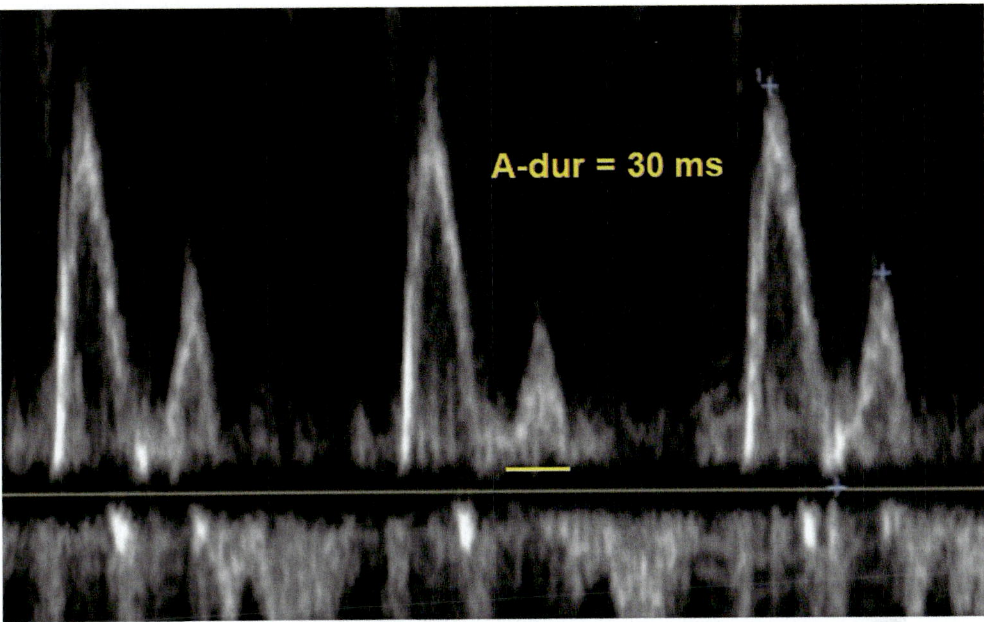

Fig. 6.67 Mitral inflow Doppler. A-dur: atrial wave duration

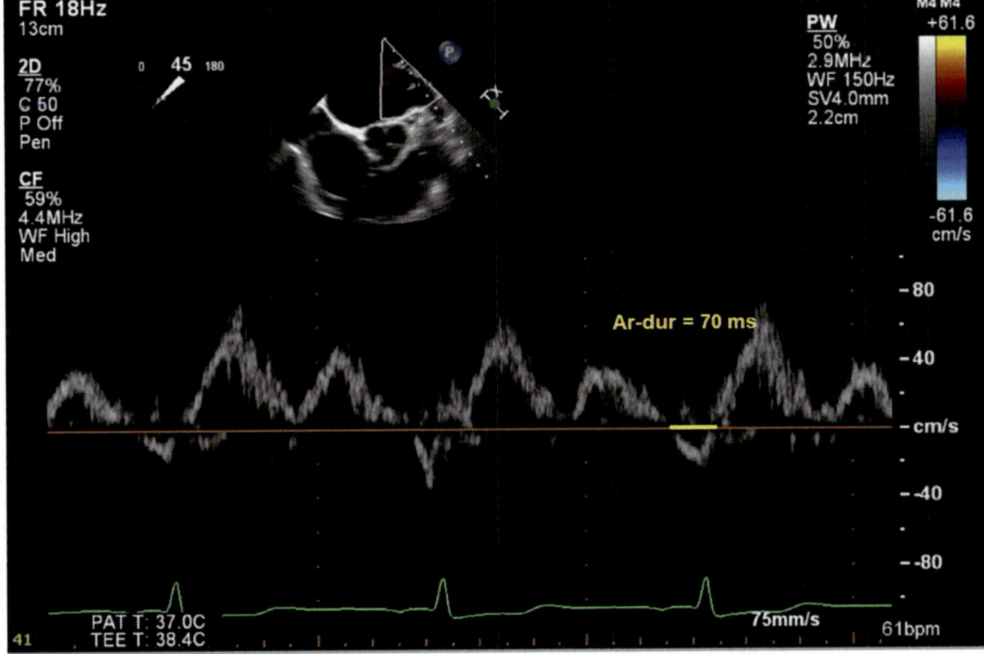

Fig. 6.68 Transesophageal echocardiogram pulmonary vein Doppler showing atrial wave duration

flow thru the mitral valve. LVEDP is significantly increased if Ar-A > 30 ms. There is unlikely to be any significant mitral regurgitation because there is no blunting or systolic flow reversal in the pulmonary vein. There is no data presented to support elevated pulmonary arterial pressures or constriction [4].

Clinical Pearls

1. Diastolic dysfunction is highly prevalent in the intensive care unit, risk factors include age, hypertension, ischemic heart disease, valvular heart disease and diabetes mellitus.
2. Diastolic dysfunction is almost invariably present in those patients with systolic dysfunction. However, in patients with preserved ejection fraction, diastolic dysfunction is often overlooked as a cause of decompensation.
3. Due to the deviation in the left ventricular pressure-volume curve, patients with diastolic dysfunction are sensitive to small changes in afterload/preload leading to exaggerated responses in left ventricular pressure. Acute pulmonary edema can be precipitated by volume overload, tachycardia, dysrhythmias, and hypertensive crisis.
4. Mitral inflow velocities show characteristic early (E) and late diastolic filling waves (A). With increasing severity

of diastolic dysfunction there is a predictable progression through the various stages of diastolic dysfunction from Grade 1 (impaired relaxation) to Grade 2 (pseudonormal pattern) to Grade 3 (restrictive filling pattern).

5. Mitral annular tissue Doppler velocities (e′), mitral inflow velocities (E, A, deceleration time, E/A ratio), left atrial volume index, and tricuspid regurgitant velocity are all important diastolic parameters that help in grading the severity of diastolic dysfunction and estimating left atrial pressures.
6. Elevated E/e′ ratios >14 have a high specificity for increased LV filling pressures and has been validated against mean PCWP
7. Diastolic parameters may change between different grades along the diastolic continuum in response to changes in afterload and preload. This can be demonstrated after therapeutic interventions such as volume loading, volume removal, and afterload reduction.
8. The Valsalva is a simple maneuver that can impede venous return, decrease preload and cardiac filling that helps distinguish normal diastolic function from pseudonormal pattern.
9. Diastolic assessment in atrial fibrillation is challenging and characterized by lack of A-waves, however, high E wave velocities, short deceleration times, presence of a mitral L-wave, Low e′, high E/e′ ratio, and lack of variability of E wave despite irregular R-R intervals are all signs consistent with increased left atrial pressures.
10. Increase in E/e′ ratio in response to a fluid bolus or passive leg raise may identify non-responders. Similarly, high E/e′ in response to a spontaneous breathing trial may identify patients likely to fail a weaning trial or used to diagnose weaning induced cardiogenic pulmonary edema.
11. Diastolic dysfunction plays an important role in prognostication, evidence of severe dysfunction is associated with worse outcomes in the intensive care unit population.

References

1. Nagueh SF, Smiseth OA, Appleton CP, Byrd BF, Dokainish H, Edvardsen T, et al. Recommendations for the evaluation of left ventricular diastolic function by echocardiography: an update from the American Society of Echocardiography and the European Association of Cardiovascular Imaging. J Am Soc Echocardiogr. 2016;29(4):277–314.
2. Maurer MS, Spevack D, Burkhoff D, Kronzon I. Diastolic dysfunction: can it be diagnosed by Doppler echocardiography? J Am Coll Cardiol. 2004;44(8):1543–9.
3. Keren G, Sherez J, Megidish R, Levitt B, Laniado S. Pulmonary venous flow pattern—its relationship to cardiac dynamics. A pulsed Doppler echocardiographic study. Circulation. 1985;71(6):1105–12.
4. Rossvoll O, Hatle LK. Pulmonary venous flow velocities recorded by transthoracic Doppler ultrasound: relation to left ventricular diastolic pressures. J Am Coll Cardiol. 1993;21(7):1687–96.
5. Tabata T, Thomas JD, Klein AL. Pulmonary venous flow by doppler echocardiography: revisited 12 years later. J Am Coll Cardiol. 2003;41(8):1243–50.
6. Mitchell C, Rahko PS, Blauwet LA, Canaday B, Finstuen JA, Foster MC, et al. Guidelines for performing a comprehensive transthoracic echocardiographic examination in adults: recommendations from the American Society of Echocardiography. J Am Soc Echocardiogr. 2019;32(1):1–64.
7. Mandinov L, Eberli FR, Seiler C, Hess OM. Diastolic heart failure. Cardiovasc Res. 2000;45(4):813–25.
8. Hillis GS, Møller JE, Pellikka PA, Gersh BJ, Wright RS, Ommen SR, et al. Noninvasive estimation of left ventricular filling pressure by E/e′ is a powerful predictor of survival after acute myocardial infarction. J Am Coll Cardiol. 2004;43(3):360–7.
9. Farhad H, Murthy VL. Pharmacologic manipulation of coronary vascular physiology for the evaluation of coronary artery disease. Pharmacol Ther. 2013;140(2):121–32.
10. Appleton CP, Galloway JM, Gonzalez MS, Gaballa M, Basnight MA. Estimation of left ventricular filling pressures using two-dimensional and Doppler echocardiography in adult patients with cardiac disease. Additional value of analyzing left atrial size, left atrial ejection fraction and the difference in duration of pulmonary venous and mitral flow velocity at atrial contraction. J Am Coll Cardiol. 1993;22(7):1972–82.
11. Nagueh SF, Middleton KJ, Kopelen HA, Zoghbi WA, Quiñones MA. Doppler tissue imaging: a noninvasive technique for evaluation of left ventricular relaxation and estimation of filling pressures. J Am Coll Cardiol. 1997;30(6):1527–33.
12. Kumar R, Gandhi SK, Little WC. Acute heart failure with preserved systolic function. Crit Care Med. 2008;36(1 Suppl):S52–6.
13. Gandhi SK, Powers JC, Nomeir AM, Fowle K, Kitzman DW, Rankin KM, et al. The pathogenesis of acute pulmonary edema associated with hypertension. N Engl J Med. 2001;344(1):17–22.
14. Zile MR, Baicu CF, Gaasch WH. Diastolic heart failure—abnormalities in active relaxation and passive stiffness of the left ventricle. N Engl J Med. 2004;350(19):1953–9.
15. Ettles DF, Williams GJ. Changes in transmitral flow velocity pattern with diuretic therapy. Eur Heart J. 1988;9(5):561–2.
16. Mitter SS, Shah SJ, Thomas JD. A test in context: E/A and E/e′ to assess diastolic dysfunction and LV filling pressure. J Am Coll Cardiol. 2017;69(11):1451–64.
17. Caballero L, Kou S, Dulgheru R, Gonjilashvili N, Athanassopoulos GD, Barone D, et al. Echocardiographic reference ranges for normal cardiac Doppler data: results from the NORRE study. Eur Heart J Cardiovasc Imaging. 2015;16(9):1031. https://doi.org/10.1093/ehjci/jev083; [cited 2020 Jan 28].
18. Dumesnil JG, Gaudreault G, Honos GN, Kingma JG. Use of Valsalva maneuver to unmask left ventricular diastolic function abnormalities by Doppler echocardiography in patients with coronary artery disease or systemic hypertension. Am J Cardiol. 1991;68(5):515–9.
19. Ghazal SN. Valsalva maneuver in echocardiography. J Echocardiogr. 2017;15(1):1–5.
20. Nakai H, Takeuchi M, Nishikage T, Nagakura T, Otani S. The mitral L wave: a marker of advanced diastolic dysfunction in patients with atrial fibrillation. Circ J. 2007;71(8):1244–9.
21. Suárez JC, López P, Mancebo J, Zapata L. Diastolic dysfunction in the critically ill patient. Med Intensiva. 2016;40(8):499–510.
22. Iuchi A, Oki T, Fukuda N, Tabata T, Manabe K, Kageji Y, et al. Changes in transmitral and pulmonary venous flow velocity patterns after cardioversion of atrial fibrillation. Am Heart J. 1996;131(2):270–5.

23. Xiong C, Sonnhag C, Nylander E, Wranne B. Atrial and ventricular function after cardioversion of atrial fibrillation. Br Heart J. 1995;74(3):254–60.
24. Vignon P, AitHssain A, François B, Preux P-M, Pichon N, Clavel M, et al. Echocardiographic assessment of pulmonary artery occlusion pressure in ventilated patients: a transoesophageal study. Crit Care. 2008;12(1):R18.
25. Moschietto S, Doyen D, Grech L, Dellamonica J, Hyvernat H, Bernardin G. Transthoracic echocardiography with Doppler tissue imaging predicts weaning failure from mechanical ventilation: evolution of the left ventricle relaxation rate during a spontaneous breathing trial is the key factor in weaning outcome. Crit Care. 2012;16(3):R81.
26. de Meirelles Almeida CA, Nedel WL, Morais VD, Boniatti MM, de Almeida-Filho OC. Diastolic dysfunction as a predictor of weaning failure: a systematic review and meta-analysis. J Crit Care. 2016;34:135–41.
27. Iida N, Seo Y, Sai S, Machino-Ohtsuka T, Yamamoto M, Ishizu T, et al. Clinical implications of intrarenal hemodynamic evaluation by Doppler ultrasonography in heart failure. JACC Heart Fail. 2016;4(8):674–82.
28. Beigel R, Cercek B, Luo H, Siegel RJ. Noninvasive evaluation of right atrial pressure. J Am Soc Echocardiogr. 2013;26(9):1033–42.
29. Tang WHW, Kitai T. Intrarenal venous flow: a window into the congestive kidney failure phenotype of heart failure? JACC Heart Fail. 2016;4(8):683–6.
30. Öhman J, Harjola V-P, Karjalainen P, Lassus J. Assessment of early treatment response by rapid cardiothoracic ultrasound in acute heart failure: cardiac filling pressures, pulmonary congestion and mortality. Eur Heart J Acute Cardiovasc Care. 2017;7(4):311. https://doi.org/10.1177/2048872617708974.
31. Ha J-W, Oh JK, Redfield MM, Ujino K, Seward JB, Tajik AJ. Triphasic mitral inflow velocity with middiastolic filling: clinical implications and associated echocardiographic findings. J Am Soc Echocardiogr. 2004;17(5):428–31.
32. Landesberg G, Gilon D, Meroz Y, Georgieva M, Levin PD, Goodman S, et al. Diastolic dysfunction and mortality in severe sepsis and septic shock. Eur Heart J. 2012;33(7):895–903.
33. Sanfilippo F, Scolletta S, Morelli A, Vieillard-Baron A. Practical approach to diastolic dysfunction in light of the new guidelines and clinical applications in the operating room and in the intensive care. Ann Intensive Care. 2018;8(1):100. [cited 2019 Oct 11]. https://annalsofintensivecare.springeropen.com/articles/10.1186/s13613-018-0447-x.
34. Abudiab MM, Chebrolu LH, Schutt RC, Nagueh SF, Zoghbi WA. Doppler echocardiography for the estimation of LV filling pressure in patients with mitral annular calcification. JACC Cardiovasc Imaging. 2017;10(12):1411–20.
35. Codolosa JN, Koshkelashvili N, Alnabelsi T, Goykhman I, Romero-Corral A, Pressman GS. Effect of mitral annular calcium on left ventricular diastolic parameters. Am J Cardiol. 2016;117(5):847–52.
36. Feigenbaum H, Armstrong WF, Ryan T, Feigenbaum H. Feigenbaum's echocardiography. Philadelphia, PA: Lippincott Williams & Wilkins; 2010.
37. Gorcsan J, Snow FR, Paulsen W, Nixon JV. Noninvasive estimation of left atrial pressure in patients with congestive heart failure and mitral regurgitation by Doppler echocardiography. Am Heart J. 1991;121(3 Pt 1):858–63.
38. Rajagopalan N, Garcia MJ, Rodriguez L, Murray RD, Apperson-Hansen C, Stugaard M, et al. Comparison of new Doppler echocardiographic methods to differentiate constrictive pericardial heart disease and restrictive cardiomyopathy. Am J Cardiol. 2001;87(1):86–94.
39. Reuss CS, Wilansky SM, Lester SJ, Lusk JL, Grill DE, Oh JK, et al. Using mitral "annulus reversus" to diagnose constrictive pericarditis. Eur J Echocardiogr. 2009;10(3):372–5.

Right Ventricular Assessment

7

Haris Riaz and Patrick Collier

Question 1
Assessment of the right ventricular size and function by transthoracic echocardiography is best made in the following window(s)?

A. Parasternal long axis
B. Parasternal short axis
C. Retrosternal location
D. Complex contraction mechanism
E. All of the above

Answer: E. All of the above. Assessment of the right ventricle size and function by transthoracic echocardiography is best made in a composite of all the aforementioned windows (Fig. 7.1). The crescentic shape, irregular surface, retrosternal location and complex contraction mechanism of the right ventricle explains why multi-window right ventricular assessment is recommended [1].

Question 2
A 62-year-old-male presents with severe short of breath and is admitted to the medical intensive care unit for the concern of pulmonary embolism. The on call fellow intends to assess the status of the right ventricle. Which factors pose challenges for the assessment of right ventricle via echocardiography?

A. Crescentic shape
B. Irregular surface
C. Retrosternal location
D. Complex contraction mechanism
E. All of the above

Answer: E. All of the above. Assessment of the right ventricle size and function via echocardiography is challenging because of amongst others, its crescentic shape, irregular surface, retrosternal location and complex contraction mechanism. Furthermore, the lack of defined specific reference anatomic landmarks adds variability to measurements.

Question 3
A 38-year-old female is admitted to the medical intensive care unit for respiratory failure. Which of these measurements is most suggestive of right ventricular dilatation on transthoracic echocardiography?

A. Basal right ventricular diameter of 5.2 cm in a right ventricular focused apical view
B. Mid right ventricular diameter of 2.7 cm in a right ventricular focused apical view
C. Longitudinal right ventricular diameter of 7.1 cm in a right ventricular focused apical view
D. Right ventricular outflow tract proximal diameter of 2.8 cm in a parasternal short axis view
E. Right ventricular outflow tract distal diameter of 2.2 cm in a parasternal short axis view

Answer: A. Basal RV dimensions of 5.2 cm in a right ventricular focused apical view. Reference values for RV dimensions have been published [1]. In general, normal values for basal right ventricular diameter < 4.1 cm, mid right ventricular diameter < 3.5 cm, longitudinal right ventricular diameter < 8.3 cm, right ventricular outflow tract proximal diameter 3.5 cm, and right ventricular outflow tract distal diameter < 2.7 cm. Measurements above these thresholds suggest right ventricular dilatation.

Supplementary Information The online version contains supplementary material available at https://doi.org/10.1007/978-3-031-45731-9_7.

H. Riaz
Citizens Memorial Hospital, Heart Institute Clinic, Bolivar, MO, USA
e-mail: Haris.Riaz@citizensmemorial.com

P. Collier (✉)
Robert and Suzanne Tomsich Department of Cardiovascular Medicine, Sydell and Arnold Miller Family Heart and Vascular Institute, The Cleveland Clinic Foundation, Cleveland, OH, USA
e-mail: colliep@ccf.org

R. Sreedharan et al. (eds.), *Critical Care Echocardiography*, https://doi.org/10.1007/978-3-031-45731-9_7

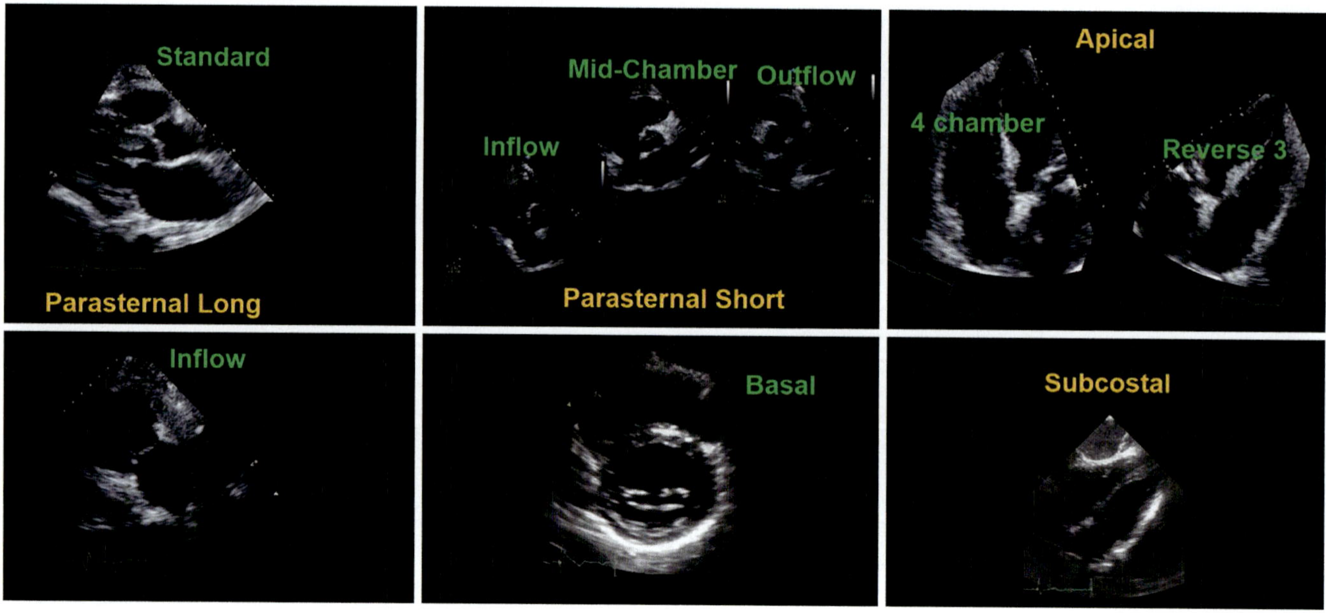

Fig. 7.1 Multiple views of the right ventricle

Question 4

A 66-year-old man is admitted to the medical intensive care unit for the management of hypoxemic respiratory failure. For measurement of the right ventricle, which view will lead to greatest changes in the RV dimensions when the transducer is tilted?

A. Right ventricular inflow view
B. Parasternal long axis view
C. Parasternal short axis view
D. Apical four chamber view
E. Subcostal view

Answer: D. Apical four chamber view. The appearance of the right ventricle is highly dependent on how the apical four chamber view is acquired. A right ventricular focused apical view is obtained by tilting the transducer medially from a standard apical 4-chamber view to show the maximal right ventricular basal dimension.

Question 5

A 42-year-old man with past medical history most significant for idiopathic pulmonary arterial hypertension presents with progressive decline in the functional status as well as shortness of breath. For assessing the right ventricular hypertrophy, which of the following is true?

A. The apical four chamber view is the recommended view for assessment
B. The apical two chamber view is the recommended view for assessment
C. Measurements greater than 5 mm in the subcostal views at end diastole are diagnostic
D. Trabeculae must be included in the measurements for precise estimation
E. Measurements greater than 2 mm in apical views at end diastole are diagnostic

Answer: C. Measurements greater than 5 mm in the subcostal views at end diastole are diagnostic. Right ventricular hypertrophy is more challenging to diagnose compared to left ventricular hypertrophy as appropriate measurements greater than 5 mm (versus 11 mm for the left side) are diagnostic. Furthermore, the right ventricle is highly trabeculated (trabeculae should be excluded from the measurements for precise estimation). Right ventricular hypertrophy is most commonly seen in patients with chronic right ventricular pressure overload.

Question 6

A 42-year-old man with past medical history most significant for idiopathic pulmonary arterial hypertension presents with progressive decline in the functional status as well as shortness of breath. Which of the following is consistent with pressure and volume overload of the right ventricle?

A. Systolic bowing of the interventricular septum towards the right ventricle
B. Diastolic bowing of the interventricular septum towards the right ventricle
C. Diastolic bowing of the interventricular septum away from the right ventricle

D. Systolic and diastolic bowing of the interventricular septum towards the right ventricle
E. Systolic and diastolic bowing of the interventricular septum away from the right ventricle

Answer: E. Systolic and diastolic bowing of the interventricular septum away from the right ventricle. Right ventricular pressure and volume overload causes the interventricular septum to be pushed away from the right ventricle and is an important echocardiographic finding that can be present in both acute and chronic disease states.

Question 7
A 66-year-old man with long standing smoking and chronic obstructive pulmonary disease is admitted for the management of hypoxemic respiratory failure. For the assessment of right ventricular function, which of the following best measurements are required for the estimation of fractional area change?

A. End systolic as well as end diastolic areas
B. Tricuspid valve closure time
C. Ejection time
D. Tricuspid annular plane systolic excursion
E. Right ventricular ejection fraction

Answer: A. End systolic as well as end diastolic areas. Right ventricular fractional area change gives an estimate of global right ventricular systolic function [1]. All of the right ventricle (especially the apex and the free wall) should be contained in the imaging window during both systole and diastole. Right ventricular trabeculae should be included within the right ventricular cavity. Values of right ventricular fractional area change <35% are indicative of right ventricular systolic dysfunction.

Question 8
A 28-year-old female with anti-phospholipid antibody syndrome is admitted for the management of saddle pulmonary embolus. Which of the following measures of right ventricular systolic function is essentially a measure of right ventricular longitudinal displacement and a correlate of global regional right ventricular function?

A. Index of myocardial performance
B. "Eye ball" method for assessment of function
C. Rate of change of pressure (dp/dt)
D. Tricuspid annular plane systolic excursion
E. Fractional area change

Answer: D. Tricuspid annular plane systolic excursion. Tricuspid annular plane systolic excursion is a one-dimensional measurement relative to the transducer position and therefore may over- or under-estimate right ventricular function because of cardiac translation [1]. While this parameter is essentially a measurement of right ventricular longitudinal displacement, it has shown good correlations with parameters estimating right ventricular global systolic function, such as right ventricular ejection fraction and right ventricular fractional area change.

Question 9
A 62-year-old presents with severe short of breath and is admitted to the medical intensive care unit with a suspected diagnosis of pulmonary embolism. An echocardiogram is performed and reveals which distinct finding that has been described in patients with acute, massive pulmonary embolism.

A. Plethoric inferior vena cava
B. McConnell's sign
C. Pulsus alternans
D. Right ventricular apical hypokinesis
E. Right ventricular hypertrophy

Answer: B. McConnell's sign. McConnell's sign is a distinct echocardiographic finding described in patients with acute, massive pulmonary embolism which refers to a distinct regional pattern of right ventricular dysfunction, with akinesia of the mid free wall but normal motion at the apex (which may relate to acute tethering of the right ventricular apex in the setting of hyperdynamic left ventricular function).

Question 10
A 72-year-old female with known non-ischemic cardiomyopathy and septic arthritis of the left knee joint is admitted to the medical ICU. An echocardiogram is obtained as part of pre-operative work up. Which of the following is an incorrect statement about the Doppler tissue imaging derived Tricuspid Lateral Annular Systolic Velocity as a marker of the right ventricular function?

A. It is easy to measure, reliable, and reproducible and assesses right ventricular longitudinal function
B. Values <9.5 cm/s measured are indicative of right ventricular systolic dysfunction.
C. It is measured relative to the transducer and may therefore be influenced by overall heart motion
D. It correlates well with measures of global right ventricular systolic function.
E. All of the above

Answer: E. All of the above. Doppler tissue imaging derived Tricuspid Lateral Annular Systolic Velocity is a useful parameter of right ventricular function. Like tricuspid annular plane systolic excursion, it is essentially a measurement of right ventricular longitudinal function that has also shown good correlations with parameters estimating right ventricular global systolic function, such as right ventricular ejection fraction and right ventricular fractional area change.

Question 11

In the assessment of a patient with acute pulmonary embolus, which of the following is suggestive of poor prognosis?

A. Right ventricular/left ventricular ratio greater than 0.9
B. Tricuspid annular plane systolic excursion greater than 1.6 cm
C. Sinus bradycardia
D. Right ventricular annular velocities greater than 10 cm/s
E. Hypertension

Answer: A. Right ventricular/left ventricular ratio greater than 0.9. A right ventricular/left ventricular ratio greater than 0.9 implies relative right ventricular enlargement (given that the mean right ventricular basal diameter is 33 mm vs. mean diastolic left ventricular internal diameter of 45 mm for females and 50 mm for males). The relatively thin-walled right ventricle is not designed to deal with acute increases in afterload. Thus, right ventricular enlargement in acute pulmonary embolus is generally proportional to the degree of acute pulmonary hypertension and is reflective of poor prognosis.

Question 12

A 26-year-old patient is admitted with septicemia and is found to have infective endocarditis involving the tricuspid valve. The transthoracic echo also reveals torrential tricuspid regurgitation caused by a perforated leaflet. The pulmonary valve is normal. Which of the following is a measure of pulmonary artery systolic pressure in this patient?

A. 4 times the square of the early diastolic pulmonary regurgitation jet velocity plus the right atrial pressure
B. 4 times the square of the end diastolic pulmonary regurgitation jet velocity plus the right atrial pressure
C. 4 times the square of the tricuspid regurgitation jet velocity plus the right atrial pressure
D. Right ventricular systolic pressure cannot be calculated in torrential tricuspid regurgitation
E. A plethoric inferior vena cava

Answer: D. Right ventricular systolic pressure cannot be calculated in torrential tricuspid regurgitation. The Bernoulli equation does not hold up in torrential tricuspid regurgitation as there is not a restrictive orifice and assumptions do not apply. Ordinarily, pulmonary artery systolic pressure can be estimated by 4 times the square of the tricuspid regurgitation jet velocity plus the right atrial pressure; mean pulmonary artery pressure can be estimated by 4 times the square of the early diastolic pulmonary regurgitation jet velocity plus the right atrial pressure; while pulmonary artery end-diastolic pressure can be estimated by 4 times the square of the end diastolic pulmonary regurgitation jet velocity plus the right atrial pressure. A plethoric inferior vena cava is indicative an elevated right atrial pressure (15 mmHg or higher) and typically refers to when the inferior vena cava measures >2.5 cm in diameter and decrements <50% in inspiration.

Question 13

A 76-year-old male with prior history of ischemic cardiomyopathy is admitted for the management of decompensated heart failure. The echocardiogram reveals severely reduced left ventricular function and a dilated right ventricle. Which of the following parameters can be used for the assessment of pulmonary arterial diastolic pressures?

A. Tricuspid regurgitation jet
B. Pulmonary regurgitation jet
C. Aortic regurgitation jet
D. Right ventricular outflow tract velocity time integral
E. A plethoric inferior vena cava

Answer: B. Pulmonary regurgitation jet. Ordinarily, pulmonary artery systolic pressure can be estimated by 4 times the square of the tricuspid regurgitation jet velocity plus the right atrial pressure; mean pulmonary artery pressure can be estimated by 4 times the square of the early diastolic pulmonary regurgitation jet velocity plus the right atrial pressure; while pulmonary artery end-diastolic pressure can be estimated by 4 times the square of the end diastolic pulmonary regurgitation jet velocity plus the right atrial pressure. A plethoric inferior vena cava is indicative an elevated right atrial pressure (15 mmHg or higher) and typically refers to when the inferior vena cava measures >2.5 cm in diameter and decrements <50% in inspiration. The right ventricular outflow tract velocity time integral is a surrogate measure of right ventricular cardiac output. Left ventricular end-diastolic pressure can be estimated subtracting 4 times the square of the end diastolic aortic regurgitation jet velocity from the diastolic blood pressure.

Question 14

A 71-year-old man with past medical history significant for end stage renal disease is admitted for the management of pericardial effusion. An echocardiogram is suggestive of a large, circumferential pericardial effusion. Which of the following echocardiographic features is suggestive of cardiac tamponade?

A. A dilated but collapsible inferior vena cava
B. Diastolic mitral regurgitation
C. Right ventricular diastolic collapse
D. Inspiratory leftward septal shift of the interventricular septum
E. Diastolic bounce of the interventricular septum

Answer: C. Right ventricular diastolic collapse. A highly sensitive sign on transthoracic echocardiography of cardiac tamponade is the presence of right ventricular diastolic collapse. A dilated but collapsible inferior vena cava indicates normal right atrial pressure (~8 mmHg). Diastolic mitral regurgitation is indicative of elevated left ventricular end-diastolic pressure. Inspiratory leftward septal shift of the interventricular septum and a diastolic bounce of the interventricular septum are signs of constrictive pericarditis.

Question 15
A 32-year-old female is admitted for the management of respiratory failure in the context of pulmonary arterial hypertension and is undergoes evaluation for initiation of pulmonary vasodilators. Which view is best suited to assess right ventricular hypertrophy?

A. Subcostal view
B. Parasternal long axis
C. Parasternal short axis
D. Apical four chamber
E. Right ventricular focused apical four chamber

Answer: A. Subcostal view. Right ventricular free wall thickness measurements greater than 5 mm in the subcostal views at end diastole are consistent with right ventricular hypertrophy. Right ventricular hypertrophy is a chronic remodeling change seen in chronic right ventricular pressure overload that can be seen in patients with long-standing pulmonary arterial hypertension.

Question 16
An 82-year-old male is admitted to the medical intensive care unit for the management of septic shock. To gauge the volume status of the patient, the on call fellow measures the inferior vena cava at 1.5 cm and records the following image (Fig. 7.2) of the inferior vena cava at rest (left panel) with inspiration (right panel). Which of the following is the correct interpretation of the images:

A. The estimated right atrial pressure is high, fluids should be withheld
B. The estimated right atrial pressure is 3 mmHg
C. Right atrial pressure cannot be estimated given that the signal is not clear
D. Estimated right atrial pressure is 8 mmHg
E. Estimated right atrial pressure is 15 mmHg

Answer: B. The estimated right atrial pressure is 3 mmHg. The combination of measuring the inferior vena cava diameter at 1.5 cm and demonstrating that the inferior vena cava decrements by >50% with inspiration is indicative of a low right atrial pressure (3 mmHg). Elevated right atrial pressure (15 mmHg) would be suggested by both an inferior vena cava diameter measurement of >2.5 cm and an inferior vena cava decrement of <50% with inspiration. A normal right atrial pressure (8 mmHg) would be suggested by either an inferior vena cava diameter measurement of <2.5 cm or an inferior vena cava decrement of >50% with inspiration.

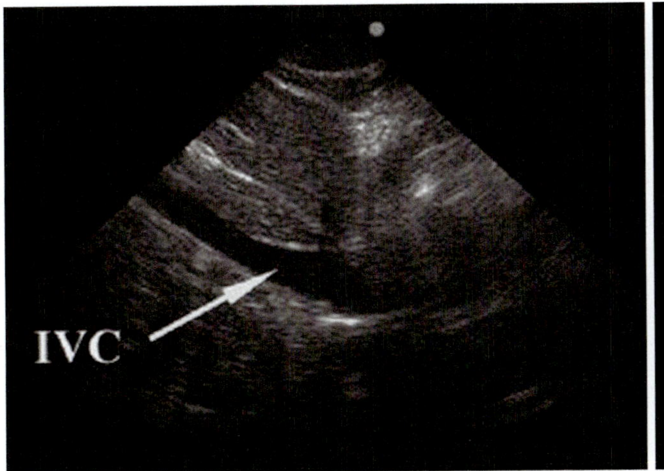

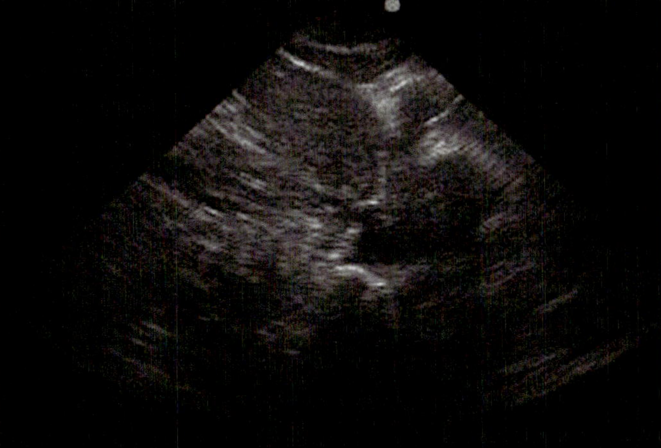

Fig. 7.2 Subcostal views of the inferior vena cava (left panel) with inspiration/sniff (right panel)

Question 17

A 36-year-old female with idiopathic pulmonary hypertension shows good clinical response to pulmonary vasodilators. An echocardiogram is obtained as a follow up (see Fig. 7.3). Which of the following is correct regarding the estimation of right ventricular systolic pressures:

A. 82 mmHg + right atrial pressure
B. 102 mmHg + right atrial pressure
C. 41 mmHg + right atrial pressure
D. RVSP cannot be estimated because of insufficient TR jet
E. 32 mmHg + right atrial pressure

Answer: C. 41 mmHg + right atrial pressure. Estimated right ventricular systolic pressure is 4 times the square of the tricuspid regurgitation jet velocity plus the right atrial pressure which in this example equates to 41 mmHg + right atrial pressure.

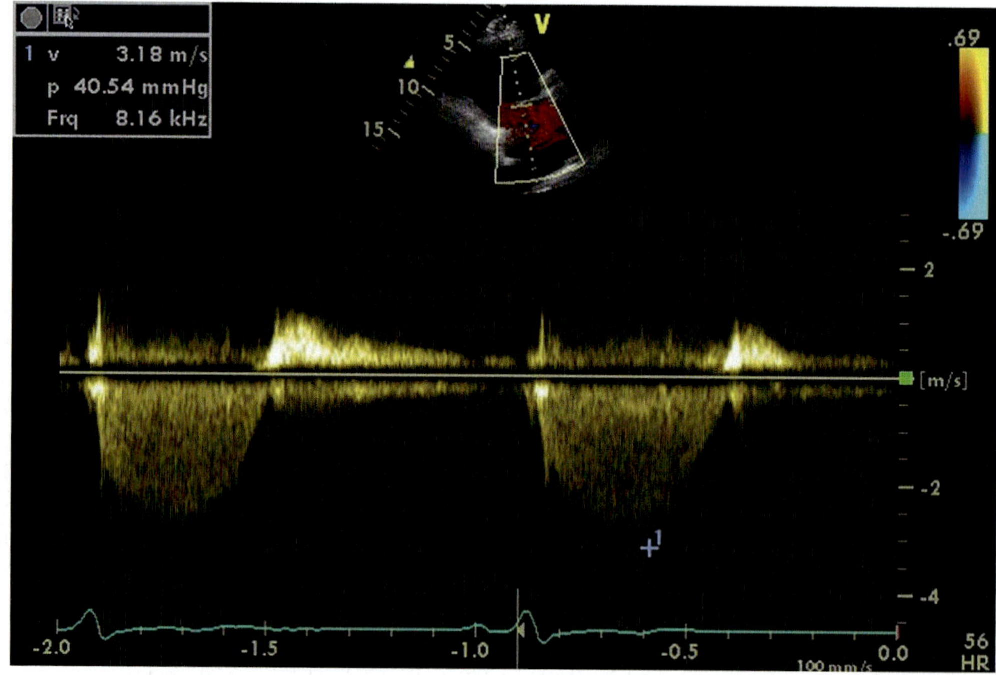

Fig. 7.3 Continuous Wave Doppler of the tricuspid regurgitation jet velocity

Question 18
A 52-year-old male is admitted to the intensive care unit after presenting with shortness of breath. Three days ago he had an episode of chest pain that lasted for hours, however, the patient thought that it was reflux disease and self-medicated himself with antacid medications. Systolic blood pressure was recorded as 106 mmHg. The electrocardiogram reveals Q waves involving the anterior precordial leads. An echocardiogram is obtained and detects a peak systolic velocity of 3 m/s across a ventricular septal defect (Fig. 7.4). The aortic valve opens normally. Which of the following represents an estimated right ventricular systolic pressure:

A. 40 mmHg
B. 50 mmHg
C. 60 mmHg
D. 70 mmHg
E. 80 mmHg

Answer: D. **70 mmHg**. The peak systolic velocity recorded across the ventricular septal defect relates to the difference between left and right ventricular systolic pressures. Assuming no significant gradient across the aortic valve, left ventricular systolic pressure is equal to recorded systolic blood pressure. Thus, estimated right ventricular systolic pressure can be measured by subtracting 4 times the peak systolic velocity recorded across the ventricular septal defect from the systolic blood pressure.

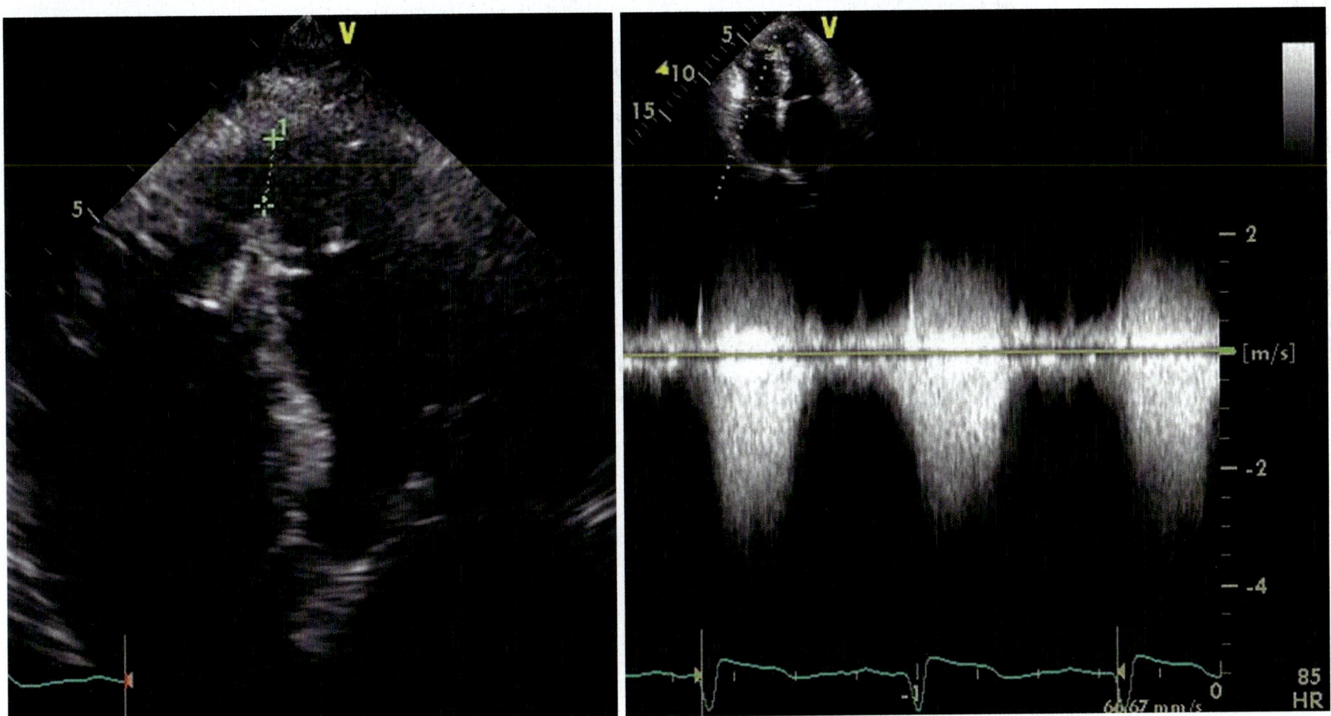

Fig. 7.4 Apical view showing a ventricular septal defect (left panel) and Continuous Wave Doppler of the related flow (right panel)

Question 19

A 45-year-old female with pulmonary hypertension presents with worsening dyspnea on exertion. As part of the follow up, an echocardiogram is obtained. The inferior vena cava is noted to be plethoric. The following signal (Fig. 7.5) is obtained from the right ventricular outflow tract:

Which of the following is the correct diagnosis?

A. Severe pulmonary regurgitation
B. Severe pulmonary stenosis
C. Right sided heart failure
D. Pulmonary hypertension
E. Patent ductus arteriosus

Answer: D. Pulmonary hypertension. The mean pulmonary artery pressure can be estimated by 4 times the square of the early diastolic pulmonary regurgitation jet velocity plus the right atrial pressure. Thus, in this case, mean pulmonary artery pressure can be estimated by 4× $(2.5)^2$ + 15 mmHg or 40 mmHg which is indicative of pulmonary hypertension.

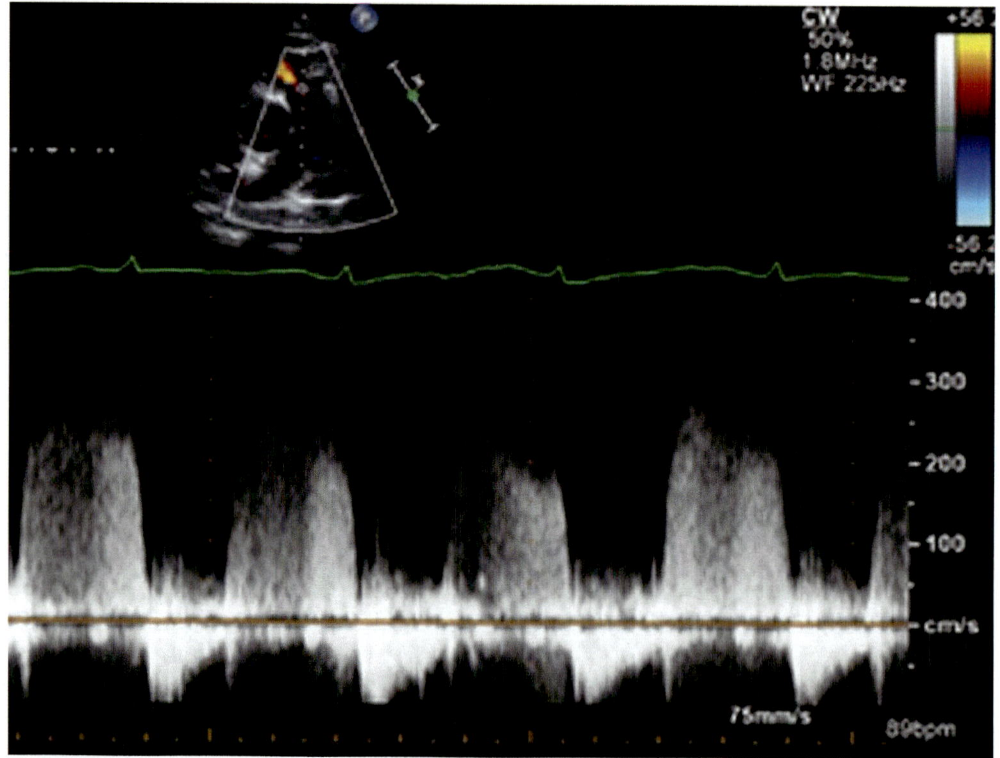

Fig. 7.5 Continuous Wave Doppler across the right ventricular outflow tract

Question 20

A 75-year-old male is admitted to the medical intensive care unit for suspected acute decompensated heart failure. As part of the evaluation, the following echocardiographic signal is obtained (Fig. 7.6) where the inferior vena cava measured 2.6 cm and did not collapse with inspiration. The hepatic veins were noted to be dilated.

The estimated right atrial pressure is:

A. 3 mmHg
B. 8 mmHg
C. 15 mmHg
D. not possible to estimate
E. 20 mmHg

Answer: E. 20 mmHg. Elevated right atrial pressure (15 mmHg) would be suggested by both an inferior vena cava diameter measurement of >2.5 cm and an inferior vena cava decrement of <50% with inspiration. In this situation, if the hepatic veins are noted to be dilated, right atrial pressures are estimated to be even further elevated at 20 mmHg.

Question 21

In right ventricular pressure overload, septal flattening occurs due to:

A. Right ventricular hypertrophy which changes the septal shape
B. Relative equilibration of right and left ventricular diastolic pressures
C. Interventricular conduction delay and septal ischemia

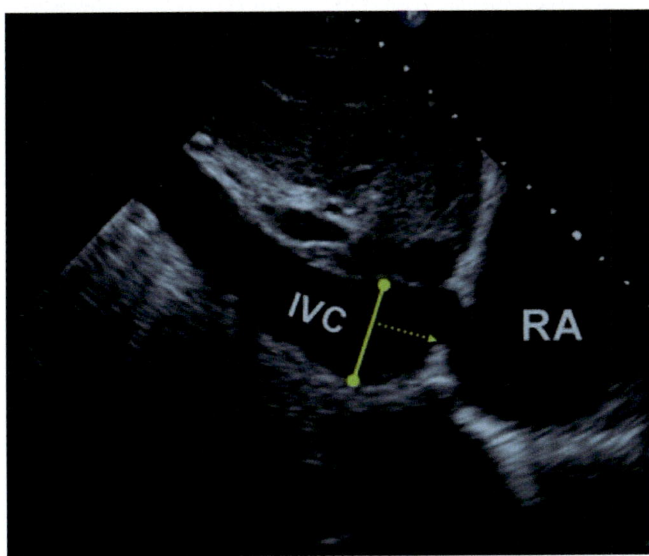

Fig. 7.6 Subcostal views of the inferior vena cava

D. Relative equilibration of right and left ventricular systolic pressures
E. Low left ventricular end-diastolic pressure

Answer: D. Relative equilibration of right and left ventricular systolic pressures. In right ventricular pressure overload, septal flattening occurs due to relative equilibration of RV and LV systolic pressures. Leftward D-shaped flattening of the interventricular septum in systole is an easily recognizable finding in echocardiography indicative of either acute or chronic right ventricular pressure overload states.

Question 22

What would be the most likely clinical scenario in a patient whose echocardiogram reported a dilated right ventricle with leftward D-shape septal flattening in systole, severe tricuspid regurgitation, and a tricuspid regurgitation velocity of 3.5 m/s?

A. Estimated right ventricular systolic pressure is low
B. Pulmonary hypertension
C. Estimated right ventricular systolic pressure of 49 + right atrial pressure
D. Estimated right ventricular systolic pressure of 49 + 15 = 64 mmHg
E. A trans-esophageal echocardiogram is required for more adequate assessment of tricuspid regurgitation velocity

Answer: B. Pulmonary hypertension. Leftward D-shaped flattening of the interventricular septum in systole is an easily recognizable finding in echocardiography indicative of either acute or chronic right ventricular pressure overload states. In this case, the presence of severe tricuspid regurgitation means that the standard calculation for pulmonary artery systolic pressure (estimated by 4 times the square of the tricuspid regurgitation jet velocity plus the right atrial pressure) may turn out to be an underestimate regardless of whether it is measured by trans-thoracic or trans-esophageal echocardiography.

Question 23

A 28-year-old female is admitted to the medical intensive care unit for the management of saddle pulmonary embolus. Which of these measurements is most suggestive of reduced right ventricular function on transthoracic echocardiography?

A. Right ventricular fractional area change of 25%
B. Tricuspid annular plane systolic excursion of 1.8 cm.
C. Doppler tissue imaging derived Tricuspid Lateral Annular Systolic Velocity of 11 cm/s

D. Three-dimensional ejection fraction of 50%
E. Global longitudinal right ventricular free wall stain of −23%

Answer: A. Right ventricular fractional area change of 25%. Values of right ventricular fractional area change <35% are indicative of right ventricular systolic dysfunction. Other values indicative of right ventricular systolic dysfunction include a tricuspid annular plane systolic excursion <1.7 cm, Doppler tissue imaging derived Tricuspid Lateral Annular Systolic Velocity < 9.5 cm/s, three-dimensional ejection fraction <45%, and/or a global longitudinal right ventricular free wall stain of less negative than −20%.

Question 24
A 60-year-old male with a history of severe pulmonary hypertension is admitted to the medical intensive care unit for suspected acute cor pulmonale. As part of the evaluation, a transthoracic echocardiogram is obtained. The right ventricle is severely dilated with systolic flattening of the interventricular septum. Fractional area change is 5%. Right ventricular index of myocardial performance by Doppler Tissue imaging is 0.7. Tricuspid annular plane systolic excursion is measured at 1.8 cm. Doppler tissue imaging derived Tricuspid Lateral Annular Systolic Velocity is measured at 11 cm/s. Which of the following is the most likely correct interpretation of these echocardiographic findings?

A. Severe right ventricular dysfunction
B. It is not possible for such discrepant findings to occur
C. It is not possible to resolve such discrepant findings
D. Only three-dimensional right ventricular ejection fraction can resolve such discrepant findings
E. Only right ventricular global longitudinal strain can resolve such discrepant findings

Answer: A. Severe right ventricular dysfunction. Right ventricular index of myocardial performance by Doppler Tissue imaging refers to the sum of isovolumic contraction and relaxation times divided by the ejection time as measured by Doppler Tissue imaging at the lateral tricuspid valve annulus with values >0.54 indicative of right ventricular dysfunction. This case example shows discrepant findings with very abnormal values for fractional area change and right ventricular index of myocardial performance yet preserved values for tricuspid annular plane systolic excursion and Doppler tissue imaging derived tricuspid lateral annular systolic velocity. Tricuspid annular plane systolic excursion and Doppler tissue imaging derived Tricuspid Lateral Annular Systolic Velocity are focal parameters at the lateral tricuspid valve annulus of right ventricular longitudinal displacement and tissue motion respectively. While both these parameters have shown good correlations with those estimating right ventricular global systolic function (such as right ventricular ejection fraction and right ventricular fractional area change), it is possible for these parameters to have normal or near normal values even in the presence of severe right ventricular dysfunction due to abnormal longitudinal rotation, particularly in severe pulmonary hypertension (see Video 7.1) [2].

Question 25
A 70-year-old female is admitted to the medical intensive care unit for suspected acute pulmonary embolism. As part of the evaluation, a transthoracic echocardiogram is obtained and right heart strain/dysfunction is reported. The need to obtain multiple views of the right ventricle is important because:

A. The right ventricle is a complicated shape
B. Right ventricular dysfunction can be regional
C. The tricuspid annulus, right ventricular free wall and interventricular septum each contribute to right ventricular systolic function and adequate visualization of each requires multiple windows
D. None of the above
E. All of the above

Answer: E. All of the above. It is true that the right ventricle is a complicated shape; right ventricular dysfunction can be regional; and the tricuspid annulus, right ventricular free wall and interventricular septum each contribute to right ventricular systolic function and adequate visualization of each requires multiple windows. Thus, the need to obtain multiple views of the right ventricle is most important.

Question 26
A 50-year-old male is admitted to the medical intensive care unit for acute exacerbation of chronic obstructive airways disease. As part of the evaluation, a transthoracic echocardiogram is obtained but there is limited visualization of the right heart. Next steps to consider include:

A. Reposition the patient and if a brief breath-hold is possible, assess whether a better image may be obtained during a different part of the respiratory cycle
B. Echo contrast can be considered
C. Transesophageal echo can be considered
D. None of the above
E. All of the above

Answer: E. All of the above. Transthoracic echocardiography is a very important tool in the management of acute pulmonary embolism as concomitant right heart strain/dysfunction may modify potential treatment options and prognosis. Limited visualization of the right heart is not an infrequent occurrence given challenges with body habitus, patients positioning and/or potential respiratory distress. In such an event, different strategies can be followed and these include repositioning the patient and if a brief breath-hold is possible, assessment made as to whether a better image might be obtained during a different part of the respiratory cycle; echo contrast can be considered if two contiguous segments of the right ventricle are not visible; in certain situations, transesophageal echocardiography may be helpful to provide adequate views of the right ventricle even when not possible via transthoracic echocardiography.

Question 27

A patient with acute coronary syndrome developed hypotension. Electrocardiography showed inferior ST elevation. Right sided leads also showed ST elevation. Anti-platelet therapy was administered and the cathlab was activated. What treatment is recommended while waiting for transfer?

A. Initiate intravenous fluids
B. Beta-blocker therapy
C. Intravenous nitrates
D. Sublingual nitrates
E. ACE inhibitor therapy

Answer: A. Initiate intravenous fluids. The right ventricle is pre-load sensitive and hypotension in the setting of acute myocardial infarction can be ameliorated with initiation of intravenous fluids. All of the other options would exacerbate hypotension.

Question 28

A patient with metabolic syndrome developed acute chest pain. EKG shows acute ST changes and hypotension. An echocardiogram is obtained. Videos 7.2 and 7.3 are most consistent with which of the following?

A. Ventricular septal defect
B. Right ventricular dysfunction
C. Free wall rupture
D. Echo evidence of cardiac tamponade
E. Acute mitral regurgitation due to papillary muscle rupture

Answer: B. Right ventricular dysfunction. Video 7.2 is a right ventricular inflow view showing gross right ventricular dysfunction and moderate functional tricuspid regurgitation. Video 7.3 is a parasternal basal short axis view showing gross biventricular dysfunction, moderate aortic regurgitation and mild mitral regurgitation.

Question 29

Video 7.4 shows a subcostal view of the inferior vena cava with inspiration. Which of the following statements are true?

A. Right atrial pressure is a surrogate of right ventricular afterload
B. Right atrial pressure is not a surrogate of right ventricular preload
C. Right ventricular preload is low
D. Right ventricular preload is normal
E. Right ventricular preload is high

Answer: E. Right ventricular preload is high. Video 7.4 shows a subcostal view of the inferior vena cava with inspiration which appears dilated >2.5 cm in diameter, and decrements less than 50% with inspiration equating to a right atrial pressure of at least 15 mmHg. Right atrial pressure is a surrogate of right ventricular preload and this example showing elevated right atrial pressure is thus consistent with elevated right ventricular preload.

Question 30

A 54-year-old otherwise healthy man after a transatlantic airflight is admitted acutely to the medical intensive care unit with acute shortness of breath and suspected acute pulmonary embolism. Video 7.5 shows a mobile echodensity in the right ventricular cavity most suspicious for which of the following?

A. Myxoma
B. Cardiac metastasis
C. Thrombus
D. Vegetation
E. Artifact

Answer: C. Thrombus. Video 7.5 is a right ventricular focused apical 4 chamber view showing severe right ventricular dilation and dysfunction with a mobile echodensity in the right ventricular cavity most likely attached to the tricuspid subvalvular chordal apparatus. The clinical scenario and imaging findings are most suspicious for thrombus. Myxomas are most commonly seen in the left atrium, and usually attached to the interatrial septum by a stalk. Cardiac metastasis is a less likely differential here given the clinical scenario and are often found as multiple masses. Vegetations are usually attached to the low pressure side of valves.

Question 31

A 60-year-old male with a history of cardiomyopathy and recent pacemaker implantation is admitted to the medical intensive care unit for suspected urinary tract infection and hypotension. As part of the evaluation, a transthoracic echocardiogram is obtained that demonstrates right ventricular dilation and overall moderate right ventricular dysfunction in a regional pattern. Videos 7.6 and 7.7 respectively demonstrate which pattern of right ventricular dysfunction?

A. Preserved right ventricular outflow tract wall motion and reduced right ventricular free wall motion
B. Reduced right ventricular outflow tract wall motion and preserved right ventricular free wall motion
C. Reduced right ventricular outflow tract wall motion and reduced right ventricular free wall motion
D. Preserved right ventricular outflow tract wall motion and preserved right ventricular free wall motion
E. Echo evidence of cardiac tamponade

Answer: A. Preserved right ventricular outflow tract wall motion and reduced right ventricular free wall motion. The right ventricle has a complicated shape and right ventricular dysfunction can be regional. Thus, the need to obtain multiple views of the right ventricle is most important. In this particular case, right ventricular pacing may (at least in part) account for the regional right ventricular dysfunction.

Question 32

A 40-year-old female is admitted to the medical intensive care unit with hypotension. As part of the evaluation, a transthoracic echocardiogram is obtained. Video 7.8 is a subcostal 4 chamber view which shows what type of right ventricular regional wall motion abnormality?

A. Diastolic flattening consistent with right ventricular volume overload
B. Systolic flattening consistent with right ventricular pressure overload
C. Focal distal right ventricular akinesia
D. Septal bounce and respiro-phasic shift consistent with constrictive physiology
E. Normal septal wall motion

Answer: C. Focal distal right ventricular akinesia. Video 7.8 is a subcostal 4 chamber view showing focal distal right ventricular akinesia. This is the so-called paradoxical or reverse McConnell's sign that can be seen in focal right ventricular stress cardiomyopathy.

Question 33

A 60-year-old male is admitted to the medical intensive care unit with hypotension and hypoxia. Suspected granulomatous lung disease is noted on computed tomography of the chest. As part of the evaluation, a transthoracic echocardiogram is obtained. Video 7.9 demonstrates an apical 4 chamber view with findings most consistent with which of the following?

A. McConnell's sign
B. Apical regional wall motion abnormality
C. Basal and mid interventricular septal wall thinning and akinesis suggestive of cardiac sarcoidosis
D. Right ventricular free wall regional motion abnormality
E. Normal right ventricular wall motion

Answer: C. Basal and mid interventricular septal wall thinning and akinesis suggestive of cardiac sarcoidosis. Cardiac sarcoidosis can present as a wide variety of cardiac phenotypes, but classically is associated with patchy regional wall motion abnormality in a non-coronary distribution with a predilection for the basal septum. Video 7.9 is an apical 4 chamber view showing basal interventricular septal wall thinning and akinesis is suspicious for scar formation and suggestive of cardiac sarcoidosis.

Question 34

A 60-year-old male developed acute hypotension, 3 days post mitral valve surgery and was transfer to the intensive care unit. As part of the evaluation, a transthoracic echocardiogram is obtained. Video 7.10 demonstrates a subcostal view with findings most consistent with which of the following?

A. McConnell's sign
B. Apical regional wall motion abnormality
C. Basal interventricular septal wall thinning and akinesis suggestive of cardiac sarcoidosis
D. Septal wall motion consistent with right ventricular pressure overload
E. Large pericardial effusion with compression of the right heart and cardiac tamponade physiology

Answer: E. Large pericardial effusion with compression of the right heart and cardiac tamponade physiology. Video 7.10 is a subcostal view showing a large pericardial effusion with compression of the right heart and cardiac tamponade physiology. The patient was taken urgently to the operating room to drain the effusion.

Question 35

A 60-year-old male is admitted to the medical intensive care unit with anemia, hypotension and hypoxia after a fall. Prior history of atrial fibrillation on coumadin and beta-blocker therapy. As part of the evaluation, a transthoracic echocardiogram is obtained. Video 7.11 demonstrates an apical 4 chamber view with findings most consistent with which of the following?

A. McConnell's sign
B. Apical regional wall motion abnormality
C. Basal interventricular septal wall thinning and akinesis suggestive of cardiac sarcoidosis
D. Large loculated pericardial effusion with compression of the right ventricular free wall
E. Septal wall motion consistent with right ventricular pressure overload

Answer: D. Large loculated pericardial effusion with compression of the right ventricular free wall. Video 7.11

is an apical 4 chamber view showing a large loculated pericardial effusion with compression of the right ventricular free wall. Coumadin therapy was reversed and the patient was taken to the operating room to drain the effusion and address bleeding.

Question 36
A 70-year-old female is admitted to the medical intensive care unit with hypotension. On auscultation, there is a prominent systolic murmur and V waves in the neck. As part of the evaluation, a transthoracic echocardiogram is obtained. Video 7.12 demonstrates a parasternal basal short axis view. What valve lesion is most likely present and directly responsible for the abnormal septal motion shown?

A. Severe tricuspid regurgitation
B. Severe aortic stenosis
C. Severe mitral regurgitation
D. Severe pulmonary stenosis
E. Severe mitral stenosis

Answer: A. Severe tricuspid regurgitation. Video 7.12 is a parasternal basal short axis view showing septal wall motion consistent with right ventricular volume overload. The leftward septal shift in diastole is cardiophasic (with each beat). Severe tricuspid regurgitation is the valve lesion most likely to be associated with right ventricular volume overload.

Question 37
A 50-year-old female with pulmonary arterial hypertension is admitted to the medical intensive care unit with hypotension. As part of the evaluation, a transthoracic echocardiogram is obtained. Video 7.13 is a parasternal mid-chamber short axis view which shows what type of septal motion?

A. Diastolic flattening consistent with right ventricular volume overload
B. Systolic flattening consistent with right ventricular pressure overload
C. Systolic and diastolic flattening consistent with right ventricular pressure and volume overload
D. Septal bounce and respiro-phasic shift consistent with constrictive physiology
E. Normal septal wall motion

Answer: B. Systolic flattening consistent with right ventricular pressure overload. Video 7.13 is a parasternal mid-chamber short axis view showing systolic flattening consistent with right ventricular pressure overload. The leftward septal shift in systole is cardio-phasic (with each beat). This is a finding consistent with the patient's history of pulmonary arterial hypertension.

Question 38
Additional findings in Video 7.13 obtained in this patient with pulmonary arterial hypertension include which of the following?

A. Atrial fibrillation
B. A large inferior pericardial effusion
C. Right ventricular dysfunction
D. Right ventricular hypertrophy
E. All of the above

Answer: E. All of the above. Video 7.13 is a parasternal mid-chamber short axis view that (in addition to systolic flattening consistent with right ventricular pressure overload) shows atrial fibrillation, a large inferior pericardial effusion, right ventricular dysfunction and right ventricular hypertrophy.

Question 39
A 70-year-old man after a transatlantic airflight is admitted acutely to the medical intensive care unit with acute shortness of breath and suspected acute pulmonary embolism. Video 7.14 shows a mobile echodensity in the right ventricular cavity most suspicious for which of the following?

A. Myxoma
B. Cardiac metastasis
C. Thrombus
D. Vegetation
E. Artifact

Answer: C. Thrombus. Video 7.14 is a subcostal 4 chamber view a mobile echodensity in the right ventricular cavity most likely attached to the tricuspid subvalvular chordal apparatus. The clinical scenario and imaging findings are most suspicious for thrombus.

This echo also shows McConnell's sign is a distinct echocardiographic finding described in patients with acute, massive pulmonary embolism which refers to a distinct regional pattern of right ventricular dysfunction, with akinesia of the mid free wall but normal motion at the apex (which may relate to acute tethering of the right ventricular apex in the setting of hyperdynamic left ventricular function).

Question 40
Additional findings in Video 7.14 obtained in this patient include which of the following?

A. Normal sinus rhythm
B. McConnell's sign
C. Right ventricular dysfunction
D. Right ventricular dilation
E. All of the above

Answer: E. All of the above. Video 7.14 is a subcostal 4 chamber view that to a mobile right ventricular thrombus shows normal sinus rhythm, McConnell's sign, right ventricular dysfunction and right ventricular dilation. McConnell's sign is a distinct echocardiographic finding described in patients with acute, massive pulmonary embolism which refers to a distinct regional pattern of right ventricular dysfunction, with akinesia of the mid free wall but normal motion at the apex (which may relate to acute tethering of the right ventricular apex in the setting of hyperdynamic left ventricular function).

Question 41

Presuming normal right atrial pressure, Fig. 7.7 is most consistent with which of the following hemodynamics?

A. Pulmonary hypertension with normal pulmonary end-diastolic pressure
B. Pulmonary hypertension with high pulmonary end-diastolic pressure
C. Normal pulmonary systolic pressure with high pulmonary end-diastolic pressure
D. Normal pulmonary systolic pressure with normal pulmonary end-diastolic pressure
E. None of the above

Answer: A. Pulmonary hypertension with normal pulmonary end-diastolic pressure. Pulmonary artery pressures can be calculated using the formula $4v^2$ plus right atrial pressure (where v = peak systolic tricuspid regurgitation signal for pulmonary artery systolic pressure; v = peak early diastolic pulmonary regurgitation signal for mean pulmonary artery systolic pressure; v = peak end-diastolic pulmonary regurgitation signal for end-diastolic pulmonary artery systolic pressure). The left panel shows a tricuspid regurgitation signal consistent with pulmonary hypertension (right ventricular systolic pressure of 53 mmHg plus right atrial pressure). The right panel shows a pulmonary regurgitation signal consistent with elevated mean pulmonary artery pressure and normal end-diastolic pulmonary pressure (presuming normal right atrial pressure).

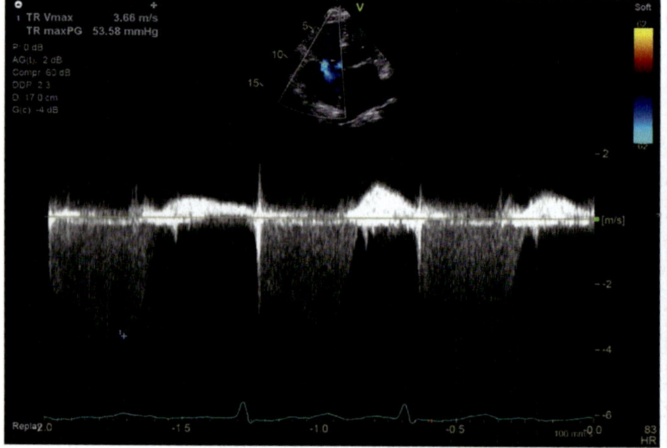

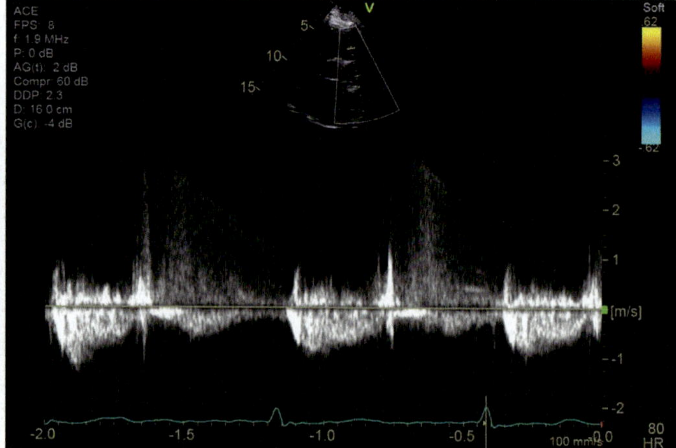

Fig. 7.7 Continuous Wave Doppler of the tricuspid regurgitation jet velocity (left panel) and Continuous Wave Doppler of the pulmonary regurgitation jet velocity (right panel)

Question 42

Presuming a right atrial pressure of 20 mmHg, Fig. 7.8 is most consistent with which of the following hemodynamics?

A. Pulmonary hypertension with normal pulmonary end-diastolic pressure
B. Pulmonary hypertension with high pulmonary end-diastolic pressure
C. Normal pulmonary systolic pressure with high pulmonary end-diastolic pressure
D. Normal pulmonary systolic pressure with normal pulmonary end-diastolic pressure
E. None of the above

Answer: B. Pulmonary hypertension with high pulmonary end-diastolic pressure. Pulmonary artery pressures can be calculated using the formula $4v^2$ plus right atrial pressure (where v = peak systolic tricuspid regurgitation signal for pulmonary artery systolic pressure; v = peak early diastolic pulmonary regurgitation signal for mean pulmonary artery systolic pressure; v = peak end-diastolic pulmonary regurgitation signal for end-diastolic pulmonary artery systolic pressure). The left panel shows a tricuspid regurgitation signal consistent with pulmonary hypertension (albeit somewhat of an incomplete trace). The right panel shows a pulmonary regurgitation signal consistent with elevated mean pulmonary artery pressure and elevated end-diastolic pulmonary pressure (presuming elevated right atrial pressure).

Question 43

A patient with shortness of breath is referred for echocardiography and is noted to have interval tachycardia, hypotension, right ventricular dilation and dysfunction, elevated right ventricular systolic pressures, systolic interventricular septal flattening and functional tricuspid regurgitation. What is the most likely clinical diagnosis?

A. Hypovolemic shock
B. Cardiac Tamponade
C. Septic shock
D. Pulmonary embolism
E. Right ventricular infarction

Answer: D. Pulmonary embolism. Echocardiography is sometimes a test that suggests the diagnosis of pulmonary embolism. Together, the constellation of findings described above have a pre-test probability of pulmonary embolism. Echocardiography is also a helpful test for patients with known pulmonary embolism, the presence of right heart strain can help guide appropriate management decisions.

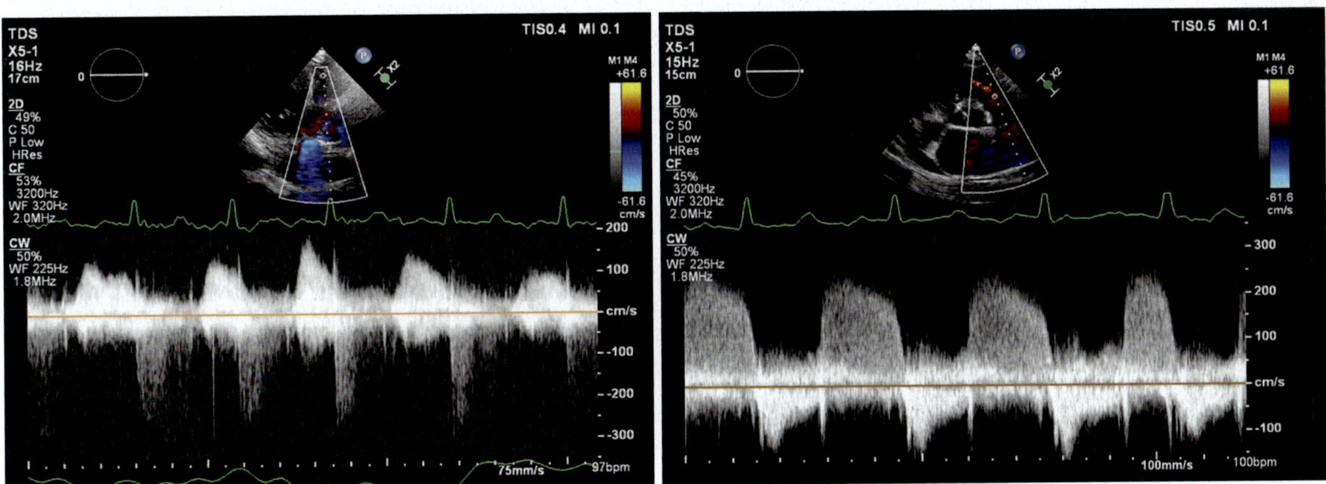

Fig. 7.8 Continuous Wave Doppler of the tricuspid regurgitation jet velocity (left panel) and Continuous Wave Doppler of the pulmonary regurgitation jet velocity (right panel)

Question 44

A patient with chest pain undergoes echocardiography. Figure 7.9 shows longitudinal strain measured in an apical two chamber view and Video 7.15 shows an apical 4 chamber view, both demonstrating a regional wall motion abnormality most likely related to which of the following?

A. Right ventricular pacing
B. Stress cardiomyopathy
C. Acute coronary syndrome involving the left anterior descending artery
D. Acute coronary syndrome involving the left circumflex artery
E. Acute coronary syndrome involving the right coronary artery

Answer: A. Right ventricular pacing. There is a wide QRS complex rhythm and a distal septal to apical regional wall motion abnormality in the setting of right ventricular pacing.

Question 45

A patient with anasarca, hypotension and tachycardia undergoes echocardiography. Video 7.16 shows a parasternal right ventricular inflow view. Video 7.17 shows a right ventricular focused apical 4 chamber view. These videos both demonstrate which of the following?

A. Free (very severe) tricuspid regurgitation
B. Right ventricular volume overload
C. Sinus tachycardia
D. Hyperdynamic right ventricular function
E. All of the above

Answer: E. All of the above. Videos 7.16 and 7.17 both demonstrate free (very severe) tricuspid regurgitation, right ventricular volume overload, sinus tachycardia, hyperdynamic right ventricular function. The color flow jet in free (very severe) tricuspid regurgitation can be brief, as there is rapid equalization of pressures between chambers and hence the associated murmur may potentially be harder to appreciate. Free (very severe) tricuspid regurgitation will augment right ventricular function due to rapid off-loading and hyperdynamic right ventricular function may be present. The corollary of this is that the absence of hyperdynamic right ventricular function in the presence of free (very severe) tricuspid regurgitation typically represents (potentially masked) right ventricular dysfunction.

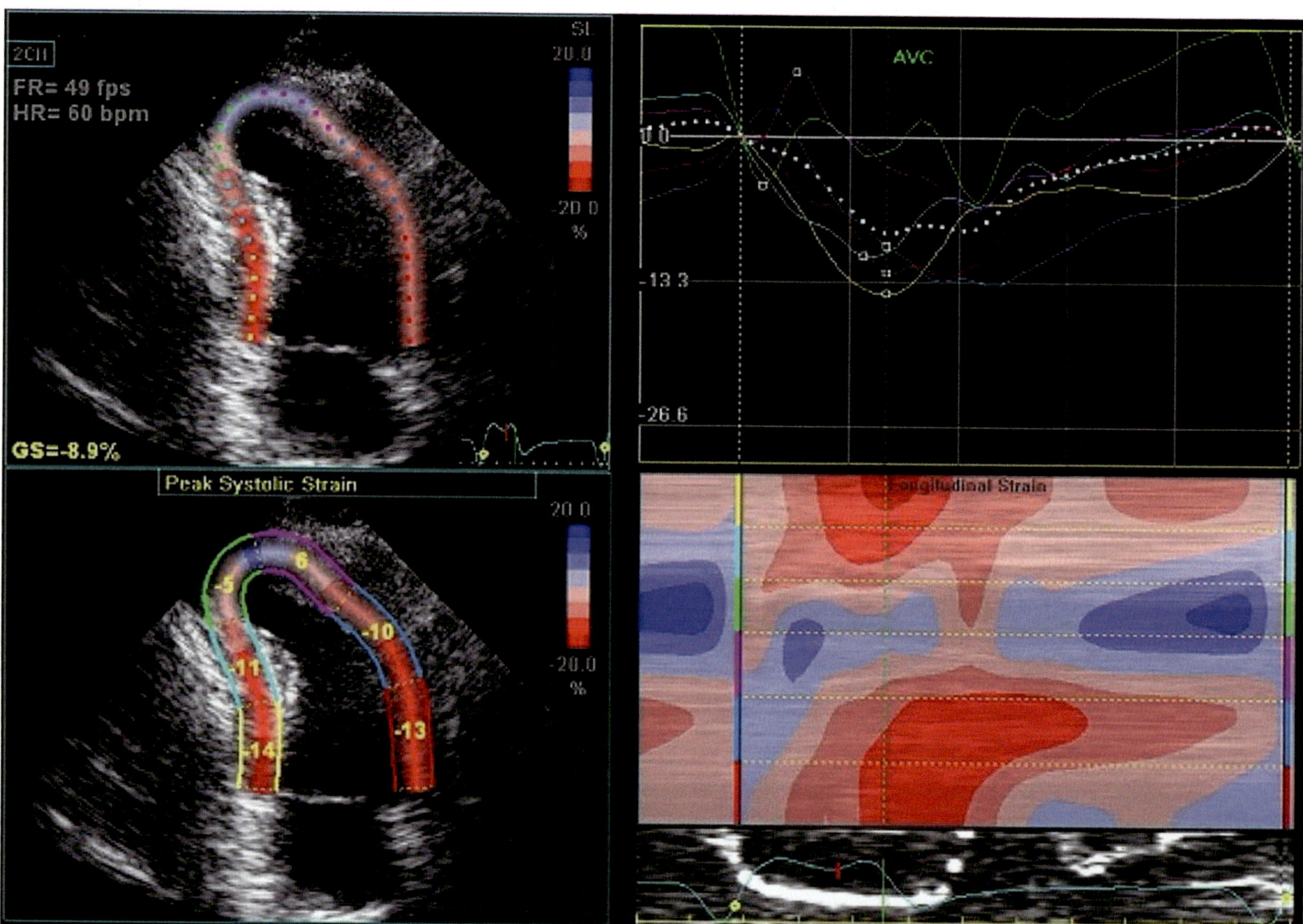

Fig. 7.9 Global Longitudinal Strain measured in an apical two chamber view

Question 46

Figure 7.10 shows a pulse wave Doppler image of the inferior vena cava flow from a subcostal view. Video 7.18 shows a color flow Doppler image of the inferior vena cava flow from a subcostal view. Which of the following conditions are present?

A. Free (very severe) tricuspid regurgitation
B. Severe tricuspid regurgitation
C. Moderate tricuspid regurgitation
D. Mild tricuspid regurgitation
E. Trivial tricuspid regurgitation

Answer: A. Free (very severe) tricuspid regurgitation. Figure 7.10 and Video 7.18 demonstrate "to and fro" flow in a sine wave pattern consistent with free (very severe) tricuspid regurgitation. There is equal intensity of back and forward flow on pulse wave Doppler. The volume of blood that crosses the tricuspid valve is equal to eventual forward flow plus the tricuspid regurgitant volume. Reflecting increased forward flow, the magnitude of the forward flow is increased. The magnitude of the peak systolic tricuspid regurgitation is reduced and cannot be used in the Bernoulli equation to estimate pulmonary artery systolic pressure as there is not a restrictive orifice (a required assumption of the equation).

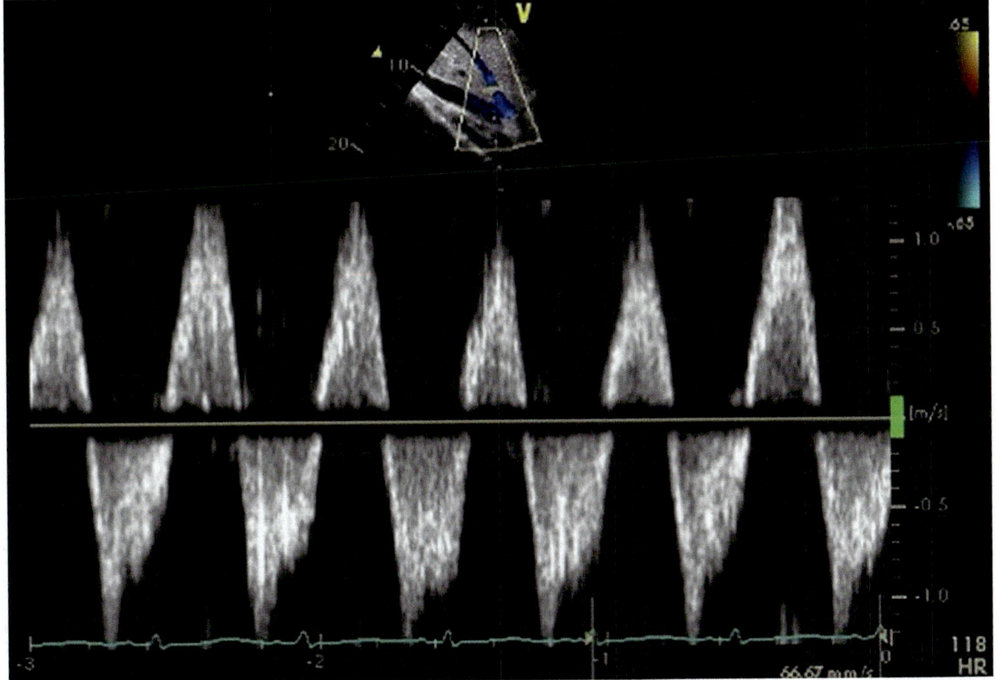

Fig. 7.10 Continuous Wave Doppler of the tricuspid regurgitation jet velocity

Question 47

Which of the following statements are true?

A. Tamponade physiology is more likely to cause compression of right heart chambers rather than left due to their lower pressures
B. The thin-walled right ventricle is less adapted to deal with high afterload compared to the left ventricle
C. The tricuspid valve is more likely susceptible to endocarditis than the pulmonary valve
D. None of the above
E. All of the above

Answer: E. All of the above. Tamponade physiology is more likely to cause compression of right heart chambers (atrium > ventricle) rather than left due to their lower pressures. Elevated pulmonary pressures are typically associated with right ventricular dysfunction as the thin walled right ventricle is poorly adapted to deal with high afterload. Vegetations are more commonly seen on the tricuspid valve than the pulmonary valve.

Question 48

Video 7.19 shows a right ventricular focused apical 4 chamber view. Figure 7.11 shows tricuspid annular plane systolic excursion measurement from the same view. Which of the following statements are true?

A. Tricuspid annular plane systolic excursion is normal/increased. Right ventricular function is normal.
B. Tricuspid annular plane systolic excursion is normal/increased. Right ventricular function is abnormal.
C. Tricuspid annular plane systolic excursion is reduced. Right ventricular function is normal.
D. Tricuspid annular plane systolic excursion is reduced. Right ventricular function is abnormal.
E. None of the above

Answer: B. Tricuspid annular plane systolic excursion is normal/increased. Right ventricular function is abnormal. In this specific (but not uncommon) example, there is abnormal longitudinal rocking motion of the right ventricle in the setting of right ventricular dysfunction and remodeling (dilation and hypertrophy) in the setting of chronic pulmonary hypertension [2]. Thus, tricuspid annular plane systolic excursion is normal/increased yet right ventricular function is abnormal. In such cases, it is important not to underappreciate the right ventricular dysfunction (visually, note that right ventricular fractional area change is markedly reduced). Equally, it is important not to assume normal right ventricular function just because tricuspid annular plane systolic excursion is preserved or even increased. Tricuspid annular plane systolic excursion is essentially a measurement of right ventricular longitudinal displacement only and therefore may over- or under-estimate right ventricular function because of cardiac translation [1].

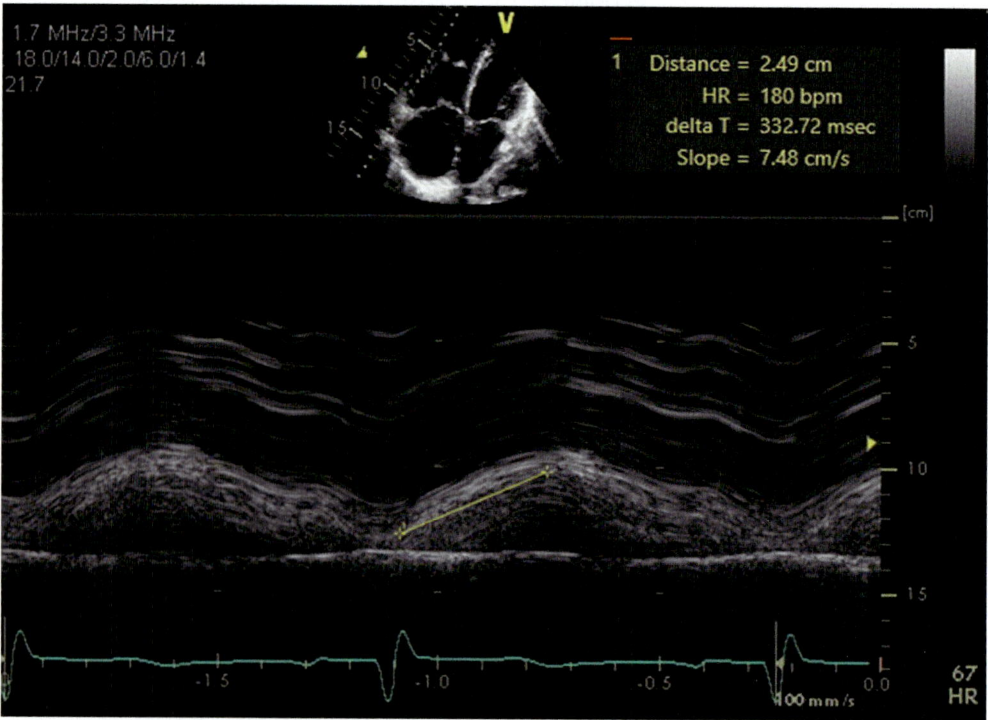

Fig. 7.11 Right ventricular focused apical 4 chamber view showing tricuspid annular plane systolic excursion measurement

Question 49

Figure 7.12 shows a ventricular septal defect with restrictive flow measured at 3.5 m/s. What is the estimated right ventricular systolic pressure in this patient with a systolic blood pressure of 120 mmHg and no aortic stenosis?

A. 49 mmHg.
B. 61 mmHg.
C. 71 mmHg.
D. 81 mmHg.
E. 120 mmHg.

Answer: C. 71 mmHg. Ventricular septal defect systolic gradient equals left ventricular systolic pressure minus right ventricular systolic pressure. Left ventricular systolic pressure equals systolic blood pressure assuming no aortic stenosis. Thus, applying the Bernoulli equation, estimated right ventricular systolic pressure equals 120–4 $(3.5)^2$ or 120–49 = 71 mmHg.

Question 50

Video 7.20 shows three dimensional right ventricular ejection fraction measurement. Which of the following statements are true?

A. Right ventricular systolic function is normal
B. Right ventricular systolic function is mildly abnormal
C. Right ventricular systolic function is moderately abnormal
D. Right ventricular systolic function is severely abnormal
E. Image quality is insufficient for assessment

Answer: A. Right ventricular systolic function is normal. In this example, three dimensional right ventricular ejection fraction measurement is 51% (>45%) and thus in the normal range. In patients with good image quality, three dimensional right ventricular ejection fraction measurements are accurate and reproducible and should be used when available and feasible [1].

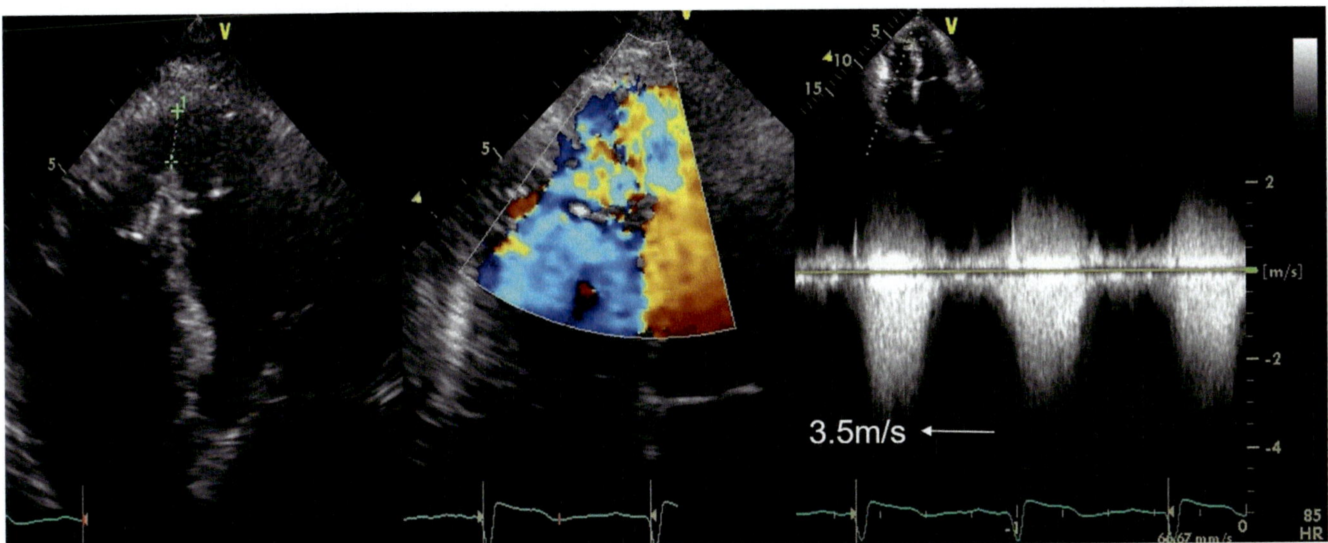

Fig. 7.12 Apical view showing a ventricular septal defect (left panel) and Continuous Wave Doppler of the related flow (right panel)

References

1. Lang RM, Badano LP, Mor-Avi V, Afilalo J, Armstrong A, Ernande L, et al. Recommendations for cardiac chamber quantification by echocardiography in adults: an update from the American Society of Echocardiography and the European Association of Cardiovascular Imaging. J Am Soc Echocardiogr. 2015;28(1):1–39.e14. https://doi.org/10.1016/j.echo.2014.10.003.
2. Collier P, Xu B, Kusunose K, Phelan D, Grant A, Thavendiranathan P, et al. Impact of abnormal longitudinal rotation on the assessment of right ventricular systolic function in patients with severe pulmonary hypertension. J Thorac Dis. 2018;10(8):4694–704. https://doi.org/10.21037/jtd.2018.07.118.

TEE in the Critically Ill

8

Brett J. Wakefield, Balaram Anandamurthy, and Shiva Sale

Question 1
A patient with undifferentiated shock presents to the emergency department. Which of the following is an absolute contraindication to transesophageal echocardiography (TEE):

A. History of gastric bypass
B. Esophageal diverticulum
C. Esophageal varices
D. Symptomatic hiatal hernia

Answer B. Esophageal diverticula are an absolute contraindication to TEE placement due to the significant risk of perforation.

Transesophageal echocardiography (TEE) is an invasive procedure with known complications. The primary indication for TEE in critically ill patients is when TTE does not provide the diagnostic information required, and the course of patient management may be altered by a TEE exam. The majority of contraindications involve the risk of bleeding or damage to the gastrointestinal (GI) tract. Both absolute and relative contraindications are presented in Table 8.1 [1, 2]. Absolute contraindications have an unacceptably high risk of GI tract damage or bleeding. Patients with relative contraindications may undergo a TEE examination; however, the risks and benefits of the procedure must be weighed and discussed due to the increased risk for serious injury.

Esophageal varices are an important complication of chronic liver disease and a leading cause of mortality [3]. The incidence increases with the degree of cirrhosis and the time course of liver disease. Esophageal varices are present in 5–9% of patients with liver cirrhosis at 1 year and up to 44% at 10 years. Hemorrhage is the primary concern, and acute variceal bleeding carries a mortality rate approaching 25% [4]. Despite these concerns, TEE is only a relative contraindication in patients with esophageal varices. Research has demonstrated a very low incidence of bleeding in patients undergoing TEE exam with esophageal varices. Considering varices are typically in the distal esophagus, concerned practitioners may consider avoiding transgastric views in particularly high-risk patients.

A remote history of bariatric surgery is a relative contraindication to TEE. Midesophageal views can be performed safely in these patients; however, transgastric views, if performed, require careful probe manipulation and consideration of the risks and benefits [5].

Question 2
Which of the following is the most common complication from TEE?

Table 8.1 Absolute and relative contraindications to transesophageal echocardiography

Absolute contraindications	Relative contraindications
Patient refusal	Peptic ulcer disease
Active upper GI bleeding	Lower risk esophageal pathology
Esophagectomy	– Varices
Recent esophageal surgery	– Barrett's esophagus
Upper GI perforation	– Esophagitis
High risk esophageal pathology	Dysphagia
– Stricture	Cervical spine restriction
– Tumor	GI surgery
– Diverticulum	Recent upper GI bleeding
– Laceration	Radiation to neck or chest
	Coagulopathy
	Symptomatic hiatal hernia
	Thoracoabdominal aneurysm

Supplementary Information The online version contains supplementary material available at https://doi.org/10.1007/978-3-031-45731-9_8.

B. J. Wakefield (✉) · S. Sale
Department of Cardiothoracic Anesthesiology, Cleveland Clinic, Cleveland, OH, USA
e-mail: wakefib@ccf.org; sales@ccf.org

B. Anandamurthy
Department of Intensive Care and Resuscitation, Cleveland Clinic, Cleveland, OH, USA
e-mail: anandab@ccf.org

R. Sreedharan et al. (eds.), *Critical Care Echocardiography*, https://doi.org/10.1007/978-3-031-45731-9_8

A. Esophageal perforation
B. Dysphagia
C. Pharyngeal trauma
D. Hoarseness

Answer D. Of the listed complications, hoarseness is the most common. Hoarseness may occur in up to 12% of patients.

TEE is not a benign procedure and is associated with complications. Significant complications related to TEE occur in 0.2–0.5% of patients, and mortality is reportedly <0.01% [1]. It is important to note that the incidence of complications may vary depending on the circumstances of the TEE exam. Awake patients undergoing TEE with conscious sedation can assist placement with swallowing and can report pain with TEE-induced distension of the GI tract. On the other hand, in unconscious critically ill patients or patients in the operating room under anesthesia, this is not possible. The top five complications of TEE are presented in Table 8.2 [1, 6]. The most common complications are lip injury (13%) and hoarseness (12%). Esophageal perforation is very rare and occurs <0.01% of patients. The two primary causes of injury are due to probe placement and probe manipulation. During probe placement, the probe may become lodged in one of the piriform sinuses just lateral to the tracheal and esophageal orifices. If advanced from this position, the probe may buckle and cause serious injury to the oropharynx. It is important to avoid forcing the probe during placement. Probe manipulation may result in mucosal injury along the GI tract; however, the gastroesophageal junction is particularly at risk.

Table 8.2 Complications of Transesophageal Echocardiography

Complication	Incidence
Lip injury	13%
Hoarseness	12%
Dysphagia	1.8%
Major bleeding[a]	0.01–0.8%
Arrhythmia	0.06–0.3%

Other complications with <0.2% incidence include: laryngospasm, bronchospasm, esophageal perforation, heart failure, tracheal intubation, pharyngeal injury, odynophagia, and dental injury
[a] Major bleeding is more common with intraoperative TEE

Question 3

A 62-year-old female with no significant past medical history is admitted to the MICU with sepsis. She develops the rhythm presented below, which persists despite pharmacologic maneuvers. Which of the following is true regarding the management of patients with this rhythm? (Fig. 8.1)

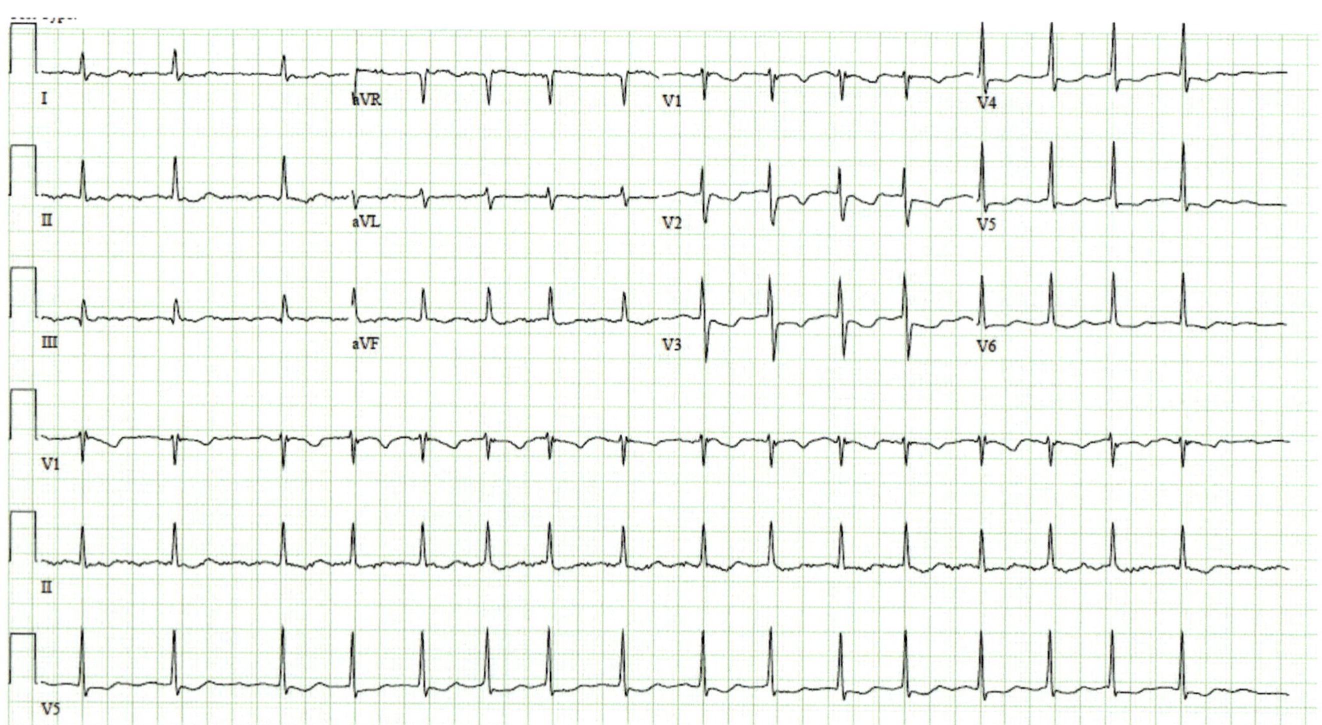

Fig. 8.1 Electrocardiogram demonstrating an arrhythmia

A. TEE is required to rule out left atrial thrombus in all patients prior to direct current cardioversion (DCCV)
B. If this rhythm is new onset and of <48 h duration, TEE is not required prior to DCCV
C. Patients who are converted to sinus rhythm following DCCV do not require further anticoagulation
D. Electrical and pharmacologic cardioversion are more likely to be effective the longer the patient has been in this rhythm

Answer B. Patients with new onset atrial fibrillation for <48 h can be cardioverted without TEE.

Atrial fibrillation is the most common cardiac arrhythmia, and new-onset atrial fibrillation frequently complicates the course of critically ill patients [7]. The American Heart Association has published guidelines regarding the management of patients with atrial fibrillation [8, 9]. Direct current cardioversion (DCCV) is indicated for patients with atrial arrhythmias in order to convert to sinus rhythm. Both pharmacologic and electrical cardioversion are more likely to be successful the shorter the period of atrial fibrillation. The primary concern of DCCV for atrial fibrillation is the embolization of an intracardiac thrombus resulting in stroke, myocardial infarction, or mesenteric or peripheral ischemia.

For hemodynamically stable patients with atrial fibrillation for longer than 48 h (or when the duration is unknown), anticoagulation (warfarin, Xa inhibitor, or direct thombin inhibitor) is recommended for 3 weeks before and 4 weeks after DCCV. A period of atrial stunning can occur after DCCV, which increases the risk of thrombus formation, even in the setting of conversion to normal sinus rhythm. This risk of thrombus formation is highest in the first 72 h after DCCV. TEE guidance can be used as an alternative to 3 weeks of pre-DCCV coagulation, however, therapeutic anticoagulation should be implemented prior to TEE. Once therapeutically anticoagulated, a TEE exam is performed to exclude left atrial appendage clot formation. Once excluded, DCCV can be performed; however, the patient should continue anticoagulation for a minimum of 4 weeks. If atrial fibrillation has been present for less than 48 h, DCCV can be performed without TEE evaluation or anticoagulation. Short term (4 week) anticoagulation should be initiated post-DCCV. The decision to initiate long term anticoagulation after DCCV in patients with atrial fibrillation for less than 48 h should be based on high-risk features and the CHA_2DS_2-VASc score. Therapeutic anticoagulation is recommended in men with a CHA_2DS_2-VASc score of 2 or greater and women with a score of 3 or greater (anticoagulation can be considered in men with a score of 1 and women with a score of 2). Furthermore, it is important to weigh the risks and benefits of initiating therapeutic anticoagulation in critically ill patients. Therefore, not all patients can be anticoagulated after DCCV. Hemodynamically unstable patients with atrial fibrillation and a rapid ventricular response should undergo DCCV without TEE evaluation (Table 8.3).

Table 8.3 CHA_2DS_2VASc score

Risk factor	Score
Congestive heart failure	+1
Hypertension	+1
Age	
– <65	+0
– 65–74	+1
– ≥75	+2
Diabetes mellitus	+1
Stroke/TIA/thromboembolism	+1
Sex	
– Female	+1
– Male	+0
Vascular disease[a]	+1

TIA transient ischemic attack
[a] Prior myocardial infarction, peripheral vascular disease, aortic aneurysm/dissection, carotid stenosis

Question 4

The decision is made for TEE examination prior to cardioversion. The following image of the left atrial appendage is obtained. Which TEE view is shown? (Fig. 8.2)

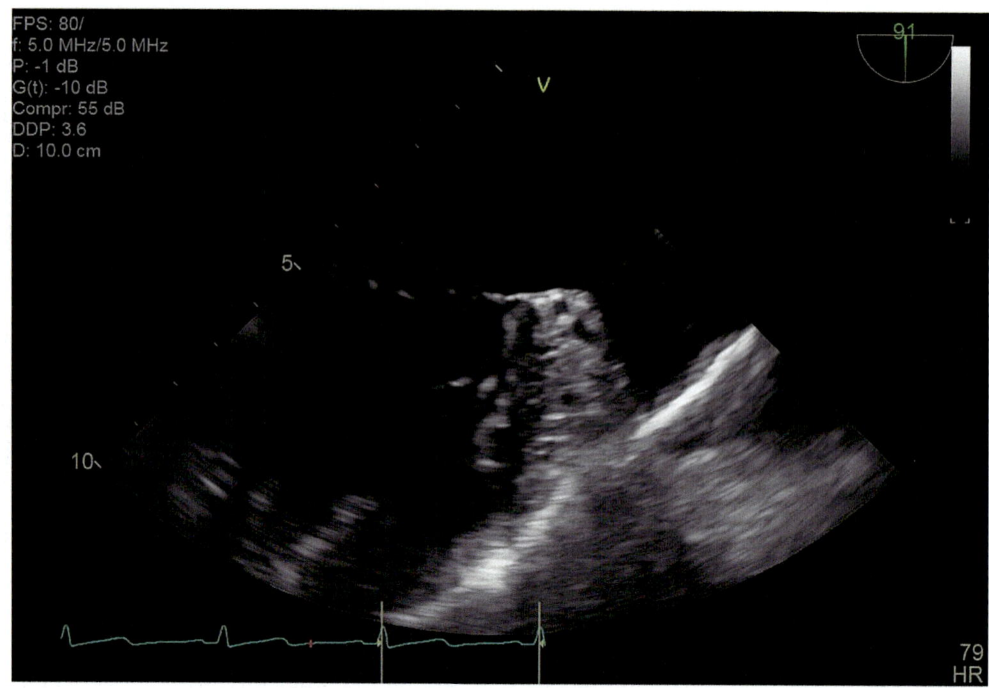

Fig. 8.2 Midesophageal TEE view

A. Midesophageal 4-chamber view
B. Midesophageal mitral commissural view
C. Midesophageal 2-chamber view
D. Midesophageal long axis view

Answer C. Midesophageal 2-chamber view.

In 2013, the American Society of Echocardiography and the Society of Cardiovascular Anesthesiologists published guidelines detailing the comprehensive examination with 28 TEE views [1]. These views can be broken down into upper esophageal, midesophageal, transgastric, and deep transgastric locations [10]. Initially, the probe should be advanced to the midesophageal location (about 30–35 cm - tip of probe to patient incisors). With the omniplane at 0–10°, the mid-esophageal 4-chamber view should be visible (Fig. 8.3). Rotating the omniplane further will reveal the mid-esophageal mitral commissural view at 50–70° (Fig. 8.4), the mid-esophageal 2-chamber view at 80–100° (Fig. 8.2) and the mid-esophageal long axis view at 120–140° (Fig. 8.5).

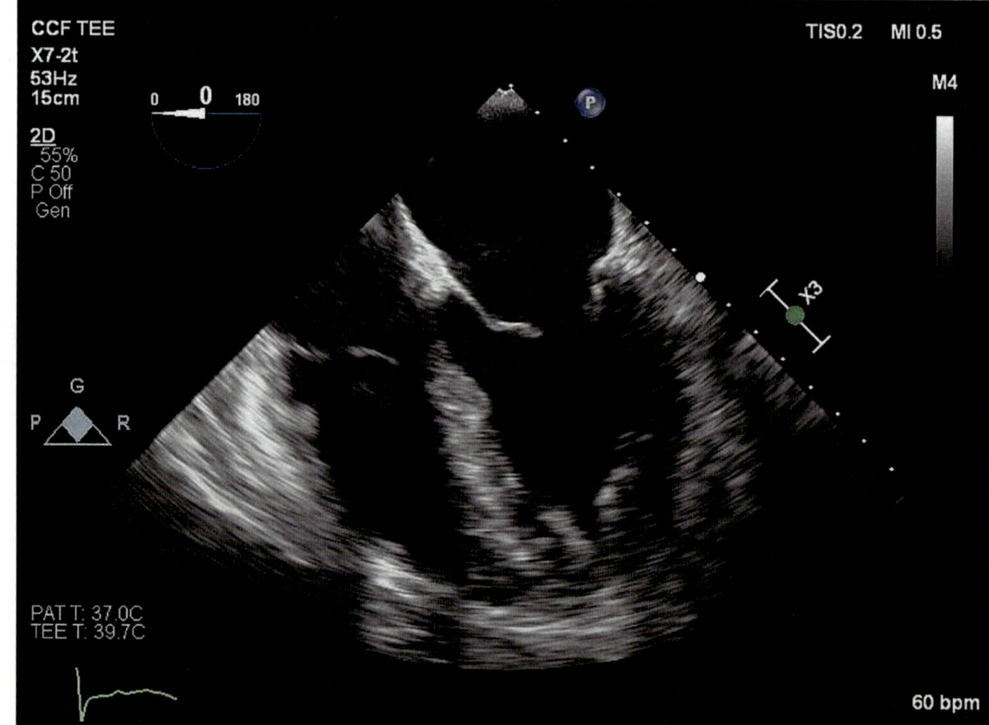

Fig. 8.3 Midesophageal four-chamber view

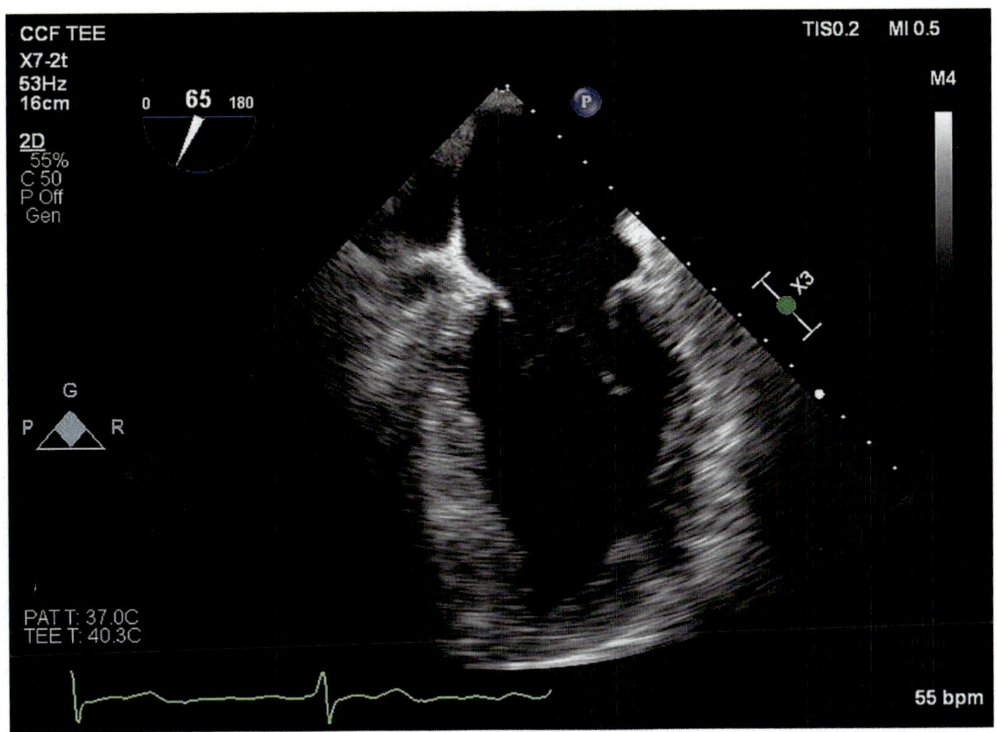

Fig. 8.4 Midesophageal mitral commissural view

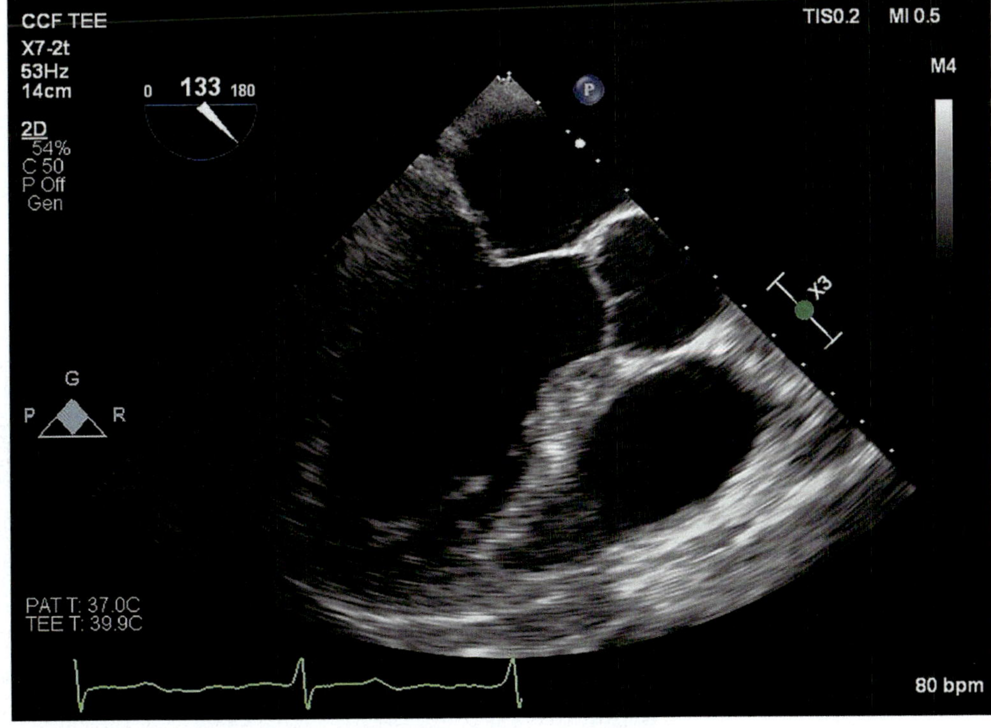

Fig. 8.5 Midesophageal long axis view

Question 5
Which of the following will not be identified on echocardiography in patients with atrial fibrillation?

A. Blunted systolic pulmonary venous flow
B. Mitral inflow pattern demonstrating E- and A-waves
C. Spontaneous echo contrast
D. Abnormal left atrial appendage motility

Answer B. There is no atrial contraction during atrial fibrillation and therefore no A-wave on the mitral inflow spectral Doppler tracing.

Atrial fibrillation results in the loss of coordinated atrial contraction. As a result, any echocardiographic signs of atrial contraction are lost. Pulsed wave Doppler interrogation of the mitral valve (sampling gate at the tip of the mitral valve leaflets during diastole) can reveal blood flow characteristics during diastole [11]. Diastole (and transmitral blood flow) can be divided into four distinct periods: isovolumetric relaxation time, early ventricular filling, diastasis, and atrial contraction. Early ventricular filling is characterized by an E-wave, while atrial contraction is characterized by an A-wave. Considering atrial contraction is lost in atrial fibrillation, the transmitral inflow pattern will only consist of an E-wave.

Spontaneous echo contrast (also called "smoke") is suggestive of blood stasis and is a strong risk factor for thrombus formation. Other findings in patients with atrial fibrillation abnormal motion of the left atrial appendage and blunted systolic pulmonary venous flow [12] (Figs. 8.6 and 8.7).

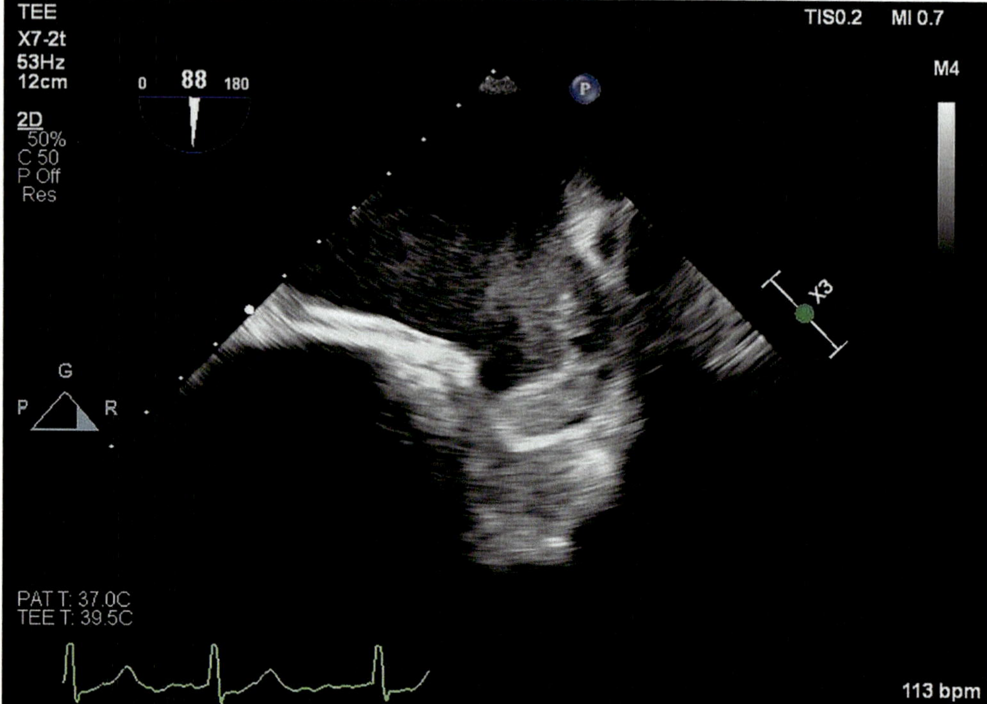

Fig. 8.6 Midesophageal two-chamber view focused on the left atrial appendage. Notice the thrombus in the appendage with spontaneous echo contrast throughout the left atrium

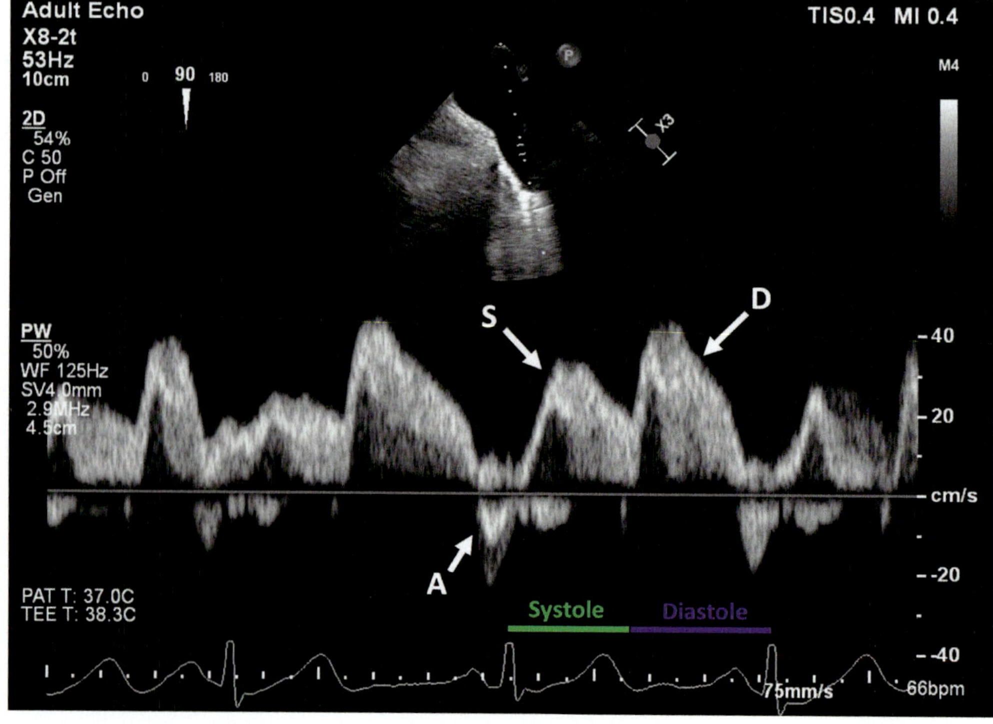

Fig. 8.7 Pulsed wave Doppler interrogation of the left upper pulmonary vein. Note the A, S, and D waves. During normal pulmonary venous flow the S wave is larger than the D wave. In this example, the S wave is shorter than the D wave indicating blunted systolic flow which suggests increased left atrial pressures

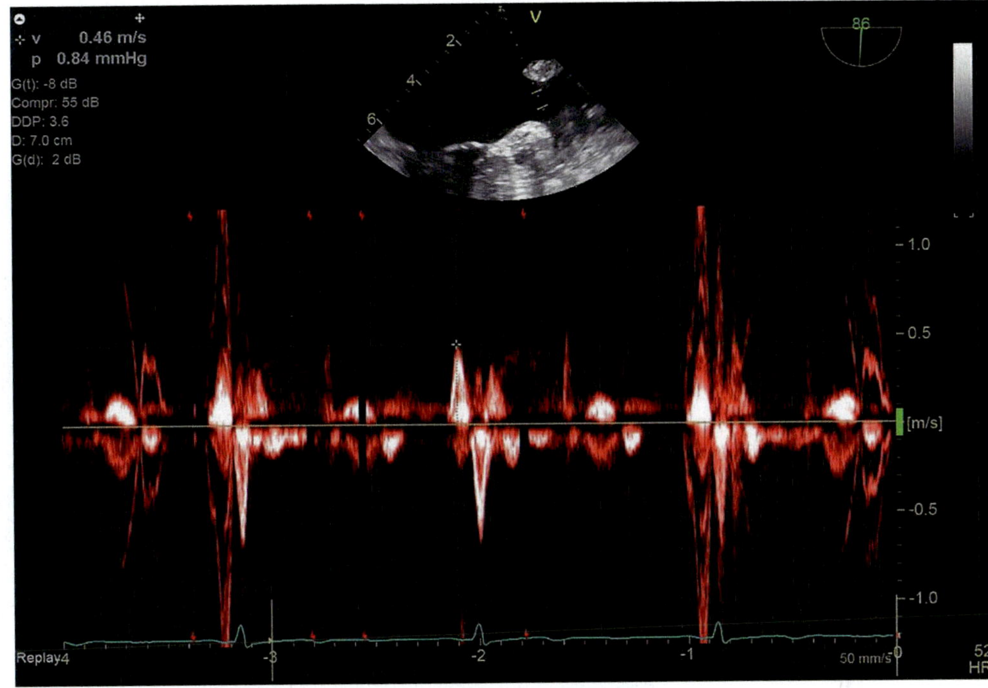

Fig. 8.8 Pulsed-wave Doppler waveform of the left atrial appendage

Question 6
Which of the following echocardiographic findings is a risk factor for left atrial appendage thrombus formation?

A. Left atrial appendage emptying velocity >40 cm/s
B. Mitral regurgitation
C. Severe left ventricular dysfunction
D. Mitral E/e′ < 8

Answer C. Severe left ventricular dysfunction is a risk factor for left atrial appendage thrombus formation.

Due to the proximity of the left atrium to the esophagus, TEE is essential for the evaluation of the left atrial appendage for thrombus formation [13]. The sensitivity and specificity of TEE in the detection of left atrial appendage thrombus is 92–100% and 98–100%, respectively. During atrial fibrillation, left atrial appendage contractility decreases and the appendage dilates, leading to stasis and an increased risk for thrombus formation. Mitral regurgitation results in increased left atrial flow during systole, which decreases blood stagnation and greatly decreases the risk of any thrombus formation [14]. On the other hand, mitral stenosis increases resistance to left atrial emptying and increases the risk of thrombus formation significantly, particularly in the presence of atrial fibrillation. Severe left ventricular systolic function can promote intracardiac stasis and lead to thrombus formation. In addition, left ventricular diastolic dysfunction increases left atrial appendage filling pressures and reduces left atrial appendage emptying, both of which lead to an increased risk of thrombus formation. A mitral E/e′ < 8 is characteristic of normal diastolic function and is therefore not a risk factor for thrombus formation.

The left atrial appendage emptying velocity is evaluated in any midesophageal view with a focus on the left atrial appendage [15]. The pulsed wave Doppler sample gate is placed in the proximal third of the left atrial appendage producing a characteristic spectral Doppler waveform (Fig. 8.8). Emptying velocities >40 cm/s are indicative of a low risk of thrombus formation. Emptying velocities <20 cm/s are associated with thrombus formation and require meticulous evaluation to rule out thrombus.

Question 7
A 75-year-old female with a history of mitral regurgitation presents to CVICU after an uncomplicated mitral valve repair. Her admission CBC is presented. Over the first hour in the ICU her chest tubes drain a total of 400 mL of dark red blood. The bedside nurse has increased the norepinephrine infusion from 2 μg/min to 10 μg/min. Urine output has decreased. A TEE probe is placed emergently due to cardiovascular instability.

CBC		
Component	Value	Range and units
WBC	6.34	3.70–11.00 k/μL
RBC	2.63	4.20–6.00 m/μL
Hemoglobin	7.0	13.0–17.0 g/dL
Hematocrit	23.7	39.0–51.0%
MCV	90.1	80.0–100.0 fL
RDW	13.8	11.5–15.0%
Platelet count	131	150–400 k/μL

WBC white blood cell, *RBC* red blood cell, *MCV* mean corpuscular volume, *RDW* red cell distribution width, *μL* microliters, *dL* deciliters, *fL* femtoliters

The following color-flow Doppler image is obtained. Of the following options, what is the next best step in management? (Fig. 8.9)

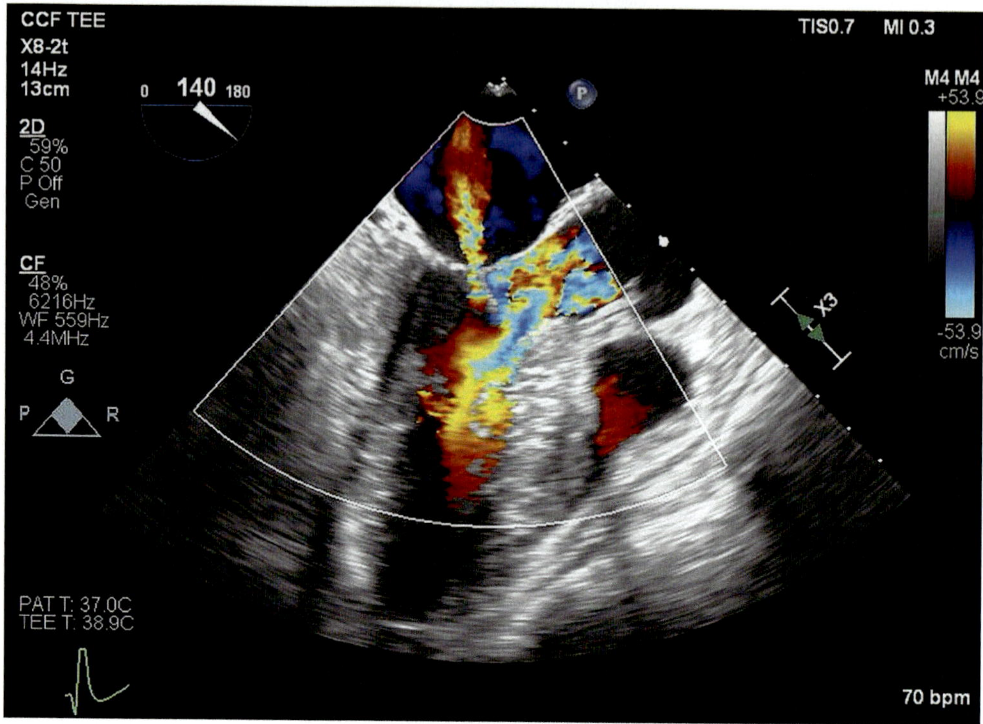

Fig. 8.9 Midesophageal TEE view with color flow Doppler

A. Add epinephrine
B. Continue to titrate up norepinephrine
C. Bolus crystalloid
D. Blood transfusion

Answer D. This patient has evidence of systolic anterior motion (SAM) of the mitral valve. While increasing the afterload with increasing doses of norepinephrine may help reduce the SAM, this patient is bleeding and requires volume. Considering the patient is actively bleeding with a hemoglobin of 7.0 g/dL, a blood transfusion would be preferred over crystalloid.

Systolic anterior motion (SAM) of the mitral valve occurs when one or both mitral valve leaflets are displaced into the left ventricular outflow tract during systole resulting in left ventricular outflow tract obstruction and mitral regurgitation [16]. Classically, SAM occurs in patients with hypertrophic obstructive cardiomyopathy due to the close proximity of the hypertrophied septum and the mitral valve leaflets; however, SAM can also occur in patients without HOCM. Patients with hyperdynamic cardiac function, such as with sepsis or advanced liver disease, can develop SAM, as well as cardiac surgical patients following mitral valve repair. Anatomic factors that increase the risk of SAM include excessive residual anterior or posterior mitral valve leaflets, small left ventricles, and a short distance between the mitral valve coaptation point and the septum. Precipitating factors include hypovolemia, tachycardia, hyperkinesis, and reduced afterload.

The mechanism of SAM is thought to be due to drag forces in the left ventricular outflow tract. Abnormal ventricular blood flow pushes the mitral valve leaflet into the left ventricular outflow tract during early systole. As left ventricular ejection occurs, drag forces continue to push the leaflet into the LVOT, causing obstruction to forward flow.

The management of SAM involves increasing preload and afterload while decreasing the heart rate and contractility [17]. Phenylephrine is an excellent intervention in the hypotensive patient with SAM due to the increase in afterload and reflex bradycardia it causes. Fluid administration can increase the left ventricular cavity size and increase the distance between the mitral valve leaflets and the septum, thus, reducing the incidence or severity of SAM. In the patient presented above, although continuing to increase the afterload with norepinephrine may help temporize the SAM and hypotension, this patient is hypovolemic and bleeding. Therefore, fluid administration is the proper choice. Given the patient's frank blood loss from the chest tubes and the low hemoglobin, a blood transfusion is indicated.

Question 8

Which of the following view(s) can be used to evaluate gradients through the left ventricular outflow tract?

A. Deep transgastric and transgastric long axis views
B. Midesophageal long axis
C. Midesophageal long axis and deep transgastric views
D. Transgastric two-chamber view

Answer A. Deep transgastric and transgastric long axis views.

Proper Doppler evaluation requires the direction of the ultrasound beam to be parallel to the direction of blood flow [18]. As the angle of incidence increases above zero, the Doppler shift becomes underestimated. Therefore, in order to accurately assess the velocity of blood through any cardiac structure, the echocardiographic views must align the blood flow with the ultrasound beam. When the left ventricular outflow tract (LVOT) is the region of interest, only the transgastric long axis and deep transgastric views can allow Doppler interrogation (Fig. 8.10).

From the midesophageal four-chamber view with focus on the left ventricle, the probe is advanced approximately 5 cm (to about 40 cm) [1]. Slight anteflexion will angle the transducer toward the heart. With an omniplane of zero degrees, the transgastric short axis view of the heart should be visible. The transgastric midpapillary short axis view will show the left ventricle cut in cross-section at the level of the papillary muscles. From this view, the omniplane is advanced 80–100° to the transgastric two-chamber view. Further advancement of the omniplane to 120–140° will bring the LVOT and aortic valve into view just anterior to the mitral valve (Fig. 8.10). Once the LVOT is identified, the pulsed wave Doppler sample volume can be placed just proximal to the aortic valve in order to interrogate LVOT velocities and gradients.

After returning the omniplane to zero degrees, the probe is advanced another 10 cm (~50 cm) to image in the deep transgastric window. Additional anteflexion may be required to bring the heart into view. A deep transgastric five-chamber or long axis view (Fig. 8.11) will demonstrate the left atrium, mitral valve, left ventricle, LVOT, and aortic valve allowing Doppler interrogation of the LVOT and aortic valve.

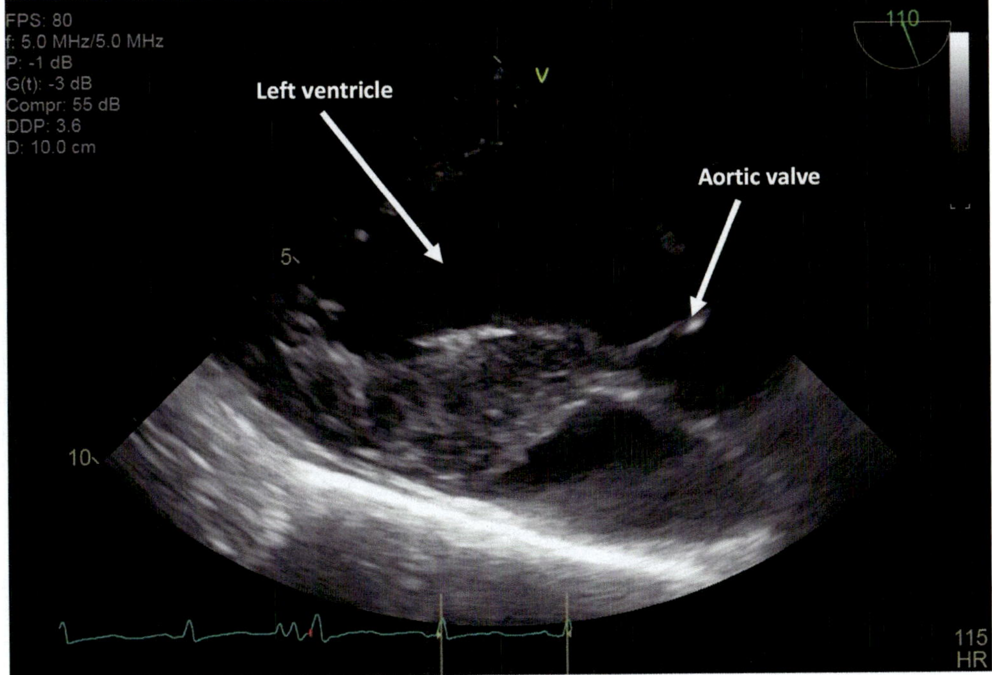

Fig. 8.10 Transgastric long axis view

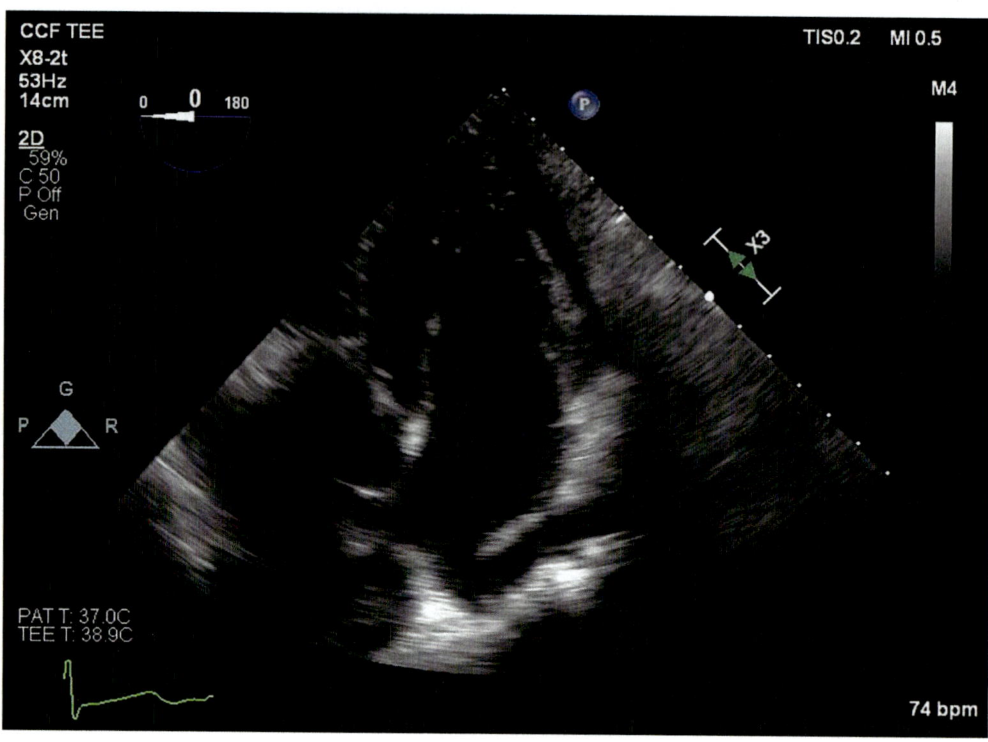

Fig. 8.11 Deep transgastric long axis view

Question 9

Which of the following Doppler waveforms is consistent with LVOT obstruction?

A. Figure 8.12
B. Figure 8.13
C. Figure 8.14
D. Figure 8.15

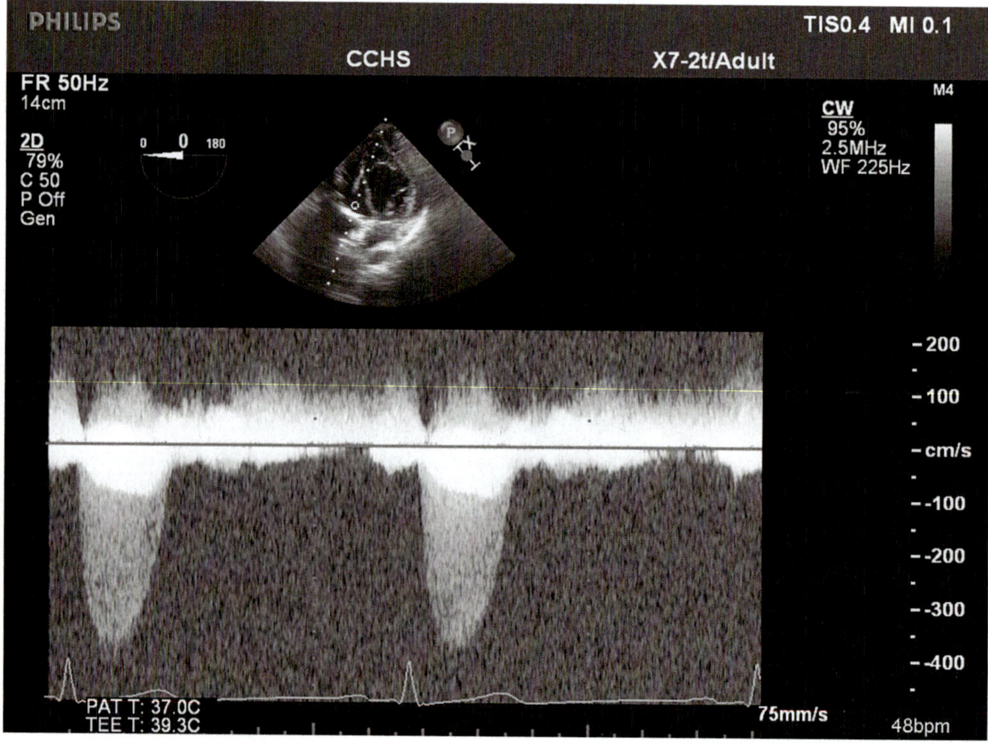

Fig. 8.12 Spectral Doppler envelope

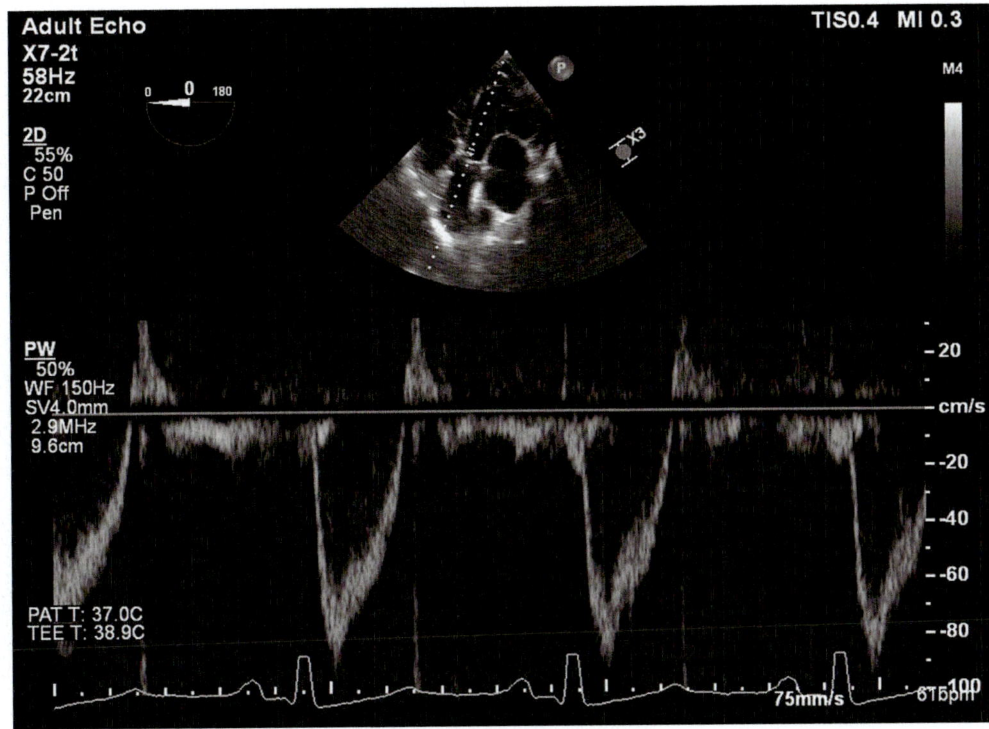

Fig. 8.13 Spectral Doppler envelope

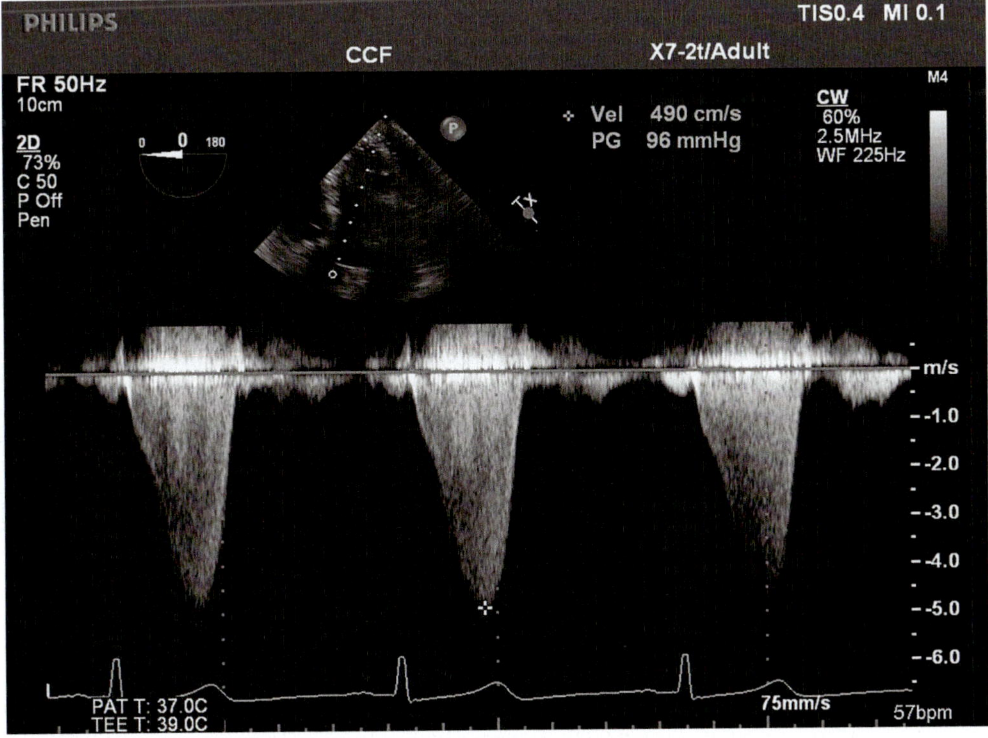

Fig. 8.14 Spectral Doppler envelope

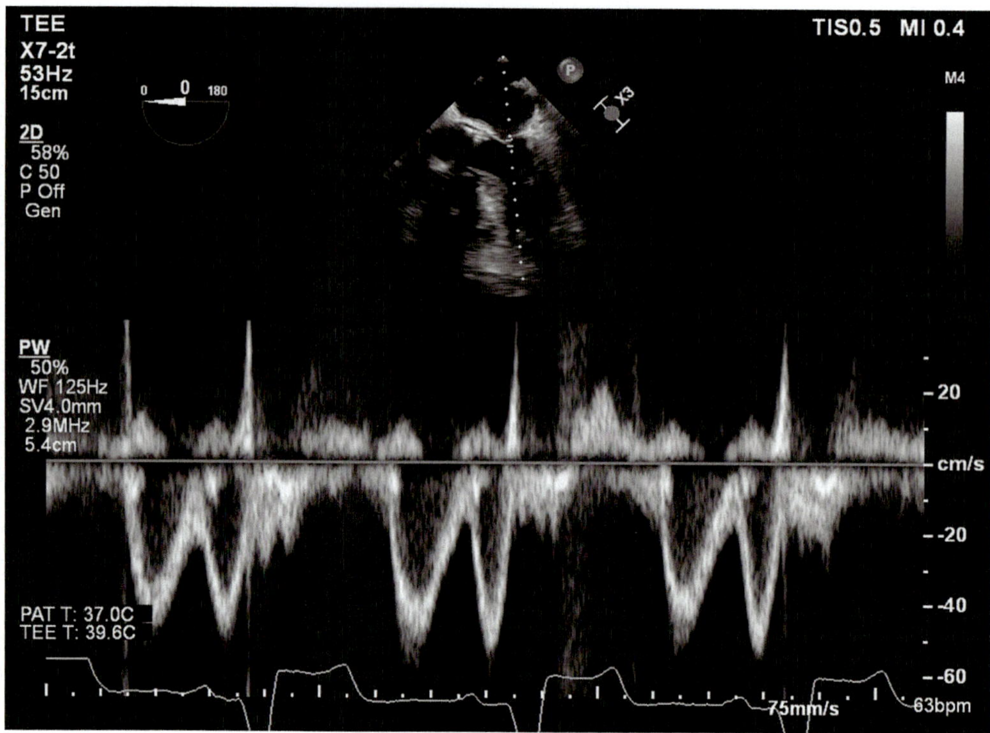

Fig. 8.15 Spectral Doppler envelope

Answer C. This continuous wave Doppler waveform demonstrates LVOT obstruction.

This waveform demonstrates LVOT obstruction. During early systole (prior to the development of obstruction), ejection occurs normally evident as a convex-to-the-left orientation of the waveform. As the mitral valve hits the septum during SAM, obstruction begins. This obstruction is marked by the transition of the waveform from convex-to-the-left to a concave-to-left formation [19]. As systole progresses, the LVOT narrows, and the obstruction worsens, causing flow acceleration. This results in the dagger-shaped pulsed wave Doppler waveform characteristic of LVOT obstruction and SAM.

The waveform in answer A is a continuous wave Doppler waveform in a patient with aortic stenosis. Continuous wave Doppler evaluates all velocities along the entire ultrasound beam as opposed to pulsed wave Doppler, which only evaluates the velocities within the sample volume. A continuous wave Doppler waveform is typically dense and full, while a pulsed wave Doppler waveform typically has a hollowed-out or darkened interior [18]. In patients with a fixed obstruction, such as aortic stenosis, the rise and fall of the spectral waveform will be uniform and symmetrical as opposed to the dagger-shaped waveform of LVOT obstruction.

The waveform in answer B is a pulsed wave Doppler envelope (note the hollowed-out darkened interior) through the LVOT in a normal patient. Answer D is a pulsed-wave Doppler waveform interrogating diastolic inflow through the mitral valve.

Question 10

Which letter on the following TEE image corresponds to the coronary artery territory most at risk during mitral valve surgery (Fig. 8.16)?

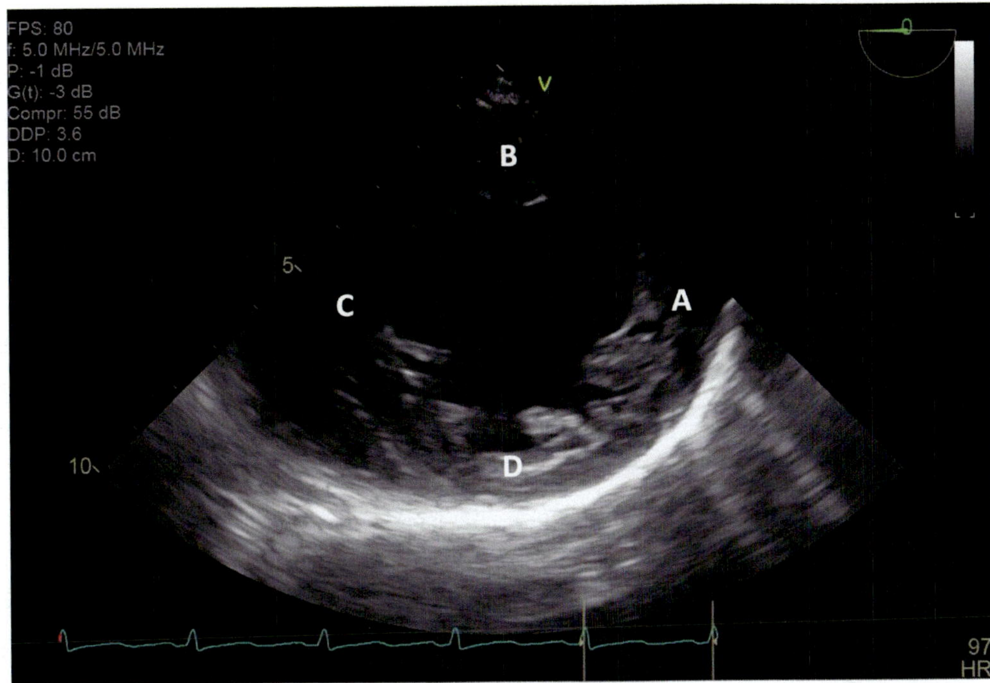

Fig. 8.16 Transgastric TEE view

A. A
B. B
C. C
D. D

Answer A. The left circumflex artery is the most likely coronary artery to be injured during mitral valve surgery. The left circumflex artery territory typically includes the inferolateral and anterolateral walls of the left ventricle (letter A).

The left circumflex artery runs in the left atrioventricular groove in very close proximity to the posterior leaflet of the mitral valve annulus. As a result of this anatomic relationship, injury to the left circumflex artery may occur following mitral valve repair or replacement; particularly, when suturing the posterior mitral valve annulus [20]. Injury may be more common in patients with left-dominant or co-dominant circulation where the left circumflex may be as close as 1 mm to the posterior annulus. Injury may occur due to direct suture line violation of the artery or due to arterial kinking as sutures are tied or tightened. Myocardial compromise is typically detected early either in the operating room or in the first few hours of ICU admission. Management of left circumflex injury following mitral valve surgery can be accomplished with percutaneous coronary intervention and stenting or a return to the operating room.

The left circumflex artery typically supplies the lateral wall of the left ventricle. On the transgastric short axis views, wall motion abnormalities may be apparent in the anterolateral and inferolateral walls [21].

Use the following stem for Questions 11–12. A 60-year-old female with a history of severe COPD presents to the CVICU after a bilateral lung transplantation. Oxygen saturation is 91% on an FiO_2 of 80% with a PEEP of 12 cm H_2O. The initial chest X-ray is presented (Fig. 8.17).

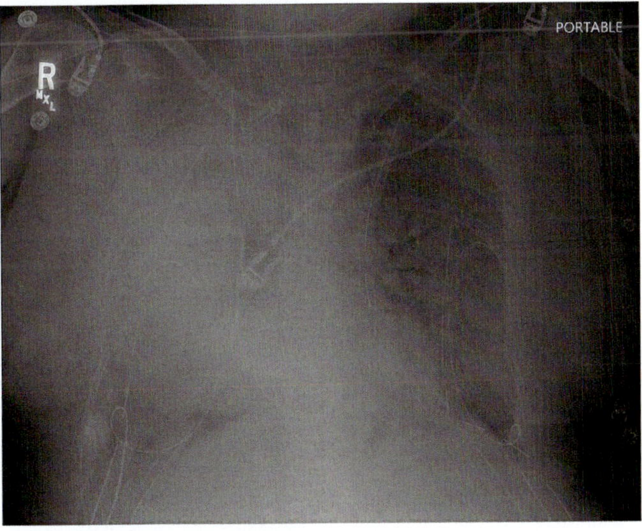

Fig. 8.17 Chest X-ray following bilateral lung transplantation

Question 11

A TEE image is shown below with the corresponding spectral Doppler waveform (Figs. 8.18 and 8.19).

Based on the images, what is the most likely cause of the patient's hypoxemia?

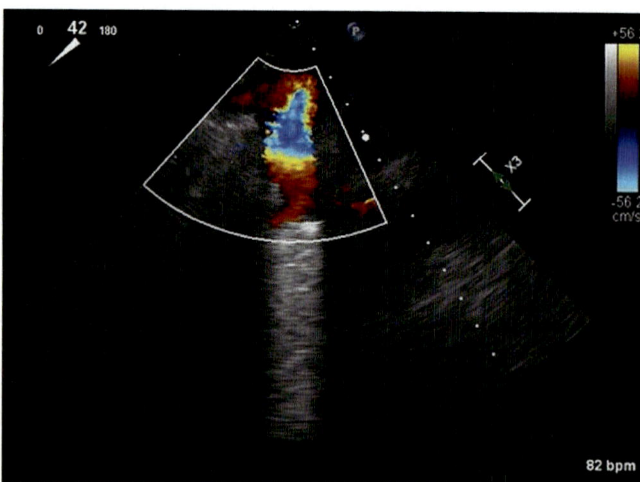

Fig. 8.18 Midesophageal view with color Doppler interrogation

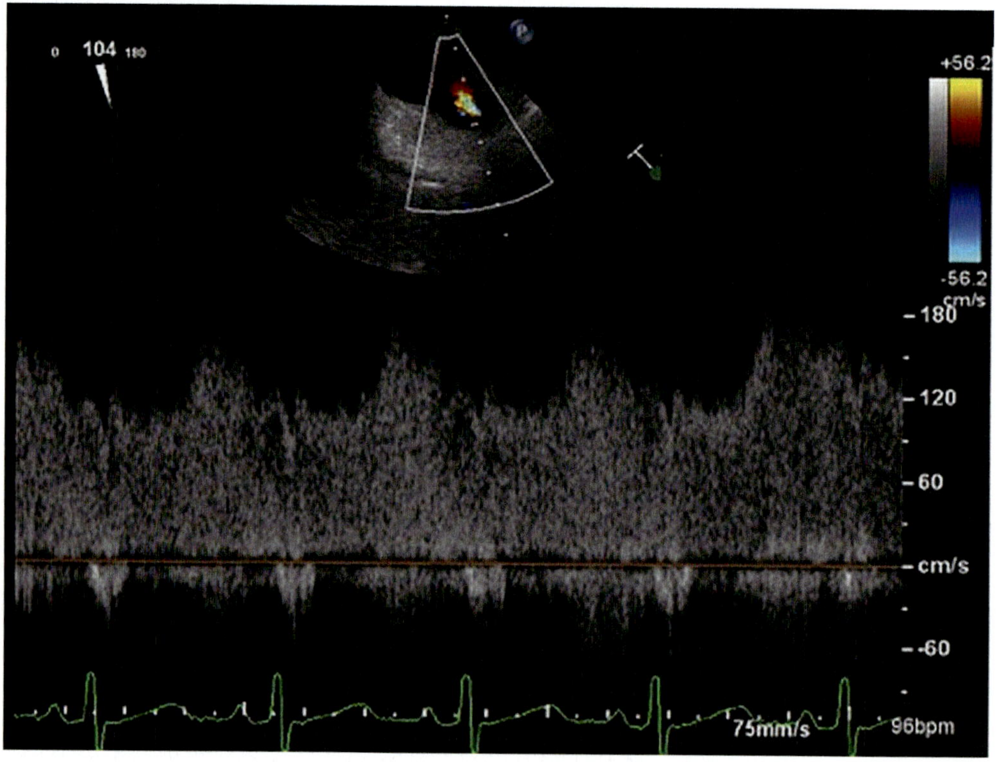

Fig. 8.19 Spectral Doppler envelope

A. Pulmonary edema
B. Pulmonary arterial stenosis
C. Pulmonary venous stenosis
D. Primary graft dysfunction

Answer C. The patient is suffering from right sided pulmonary edema secondary to pulmonary venous obstruction.

Obstruction of the pulmonary veins can occur after lung transplantation due to kinking, thrombus, or stenosis. If this complication is unrecognized, pulmonary edema develops, leading to ischemia, pulmonary hypertension, and eventually, pulmonary infarction. Following implantation of the donor lungs, TEE with pulsed wave and color flow Doppler is used in the operating room to evaluate the pulmonary venous anastomoses and rule out any obstruction [22]. The pulmonary veins are identified with TEE and a pulsed wave Doppler sample volume is placed about 1 cm distal to the left atrial ostia. The normal pulsed wave Doppler spectral waveform can be tri- or quadri-phasic with atrial, systolic, and diastolic waves. In the presence of significant obstruction, turbulence will be noted on color flow Doppler and high velocities will be present on pulsed wave Doppler. While an exact cutoff has not been validated, velocities higher than 170 cm/s may indicate an obstruction. In addition to TEE evaluation, pulmonary perfusion scanning may help narrow the differential diagnosis.

In the ICU, hypoxemia after lung transplantation is primarily due to primary graft dysfunction; however, other causes such as pulmonary edema, pneumonia, atelectasis, and pulmonary venous obstruction can occur [23]. It is important to find the correct diagnosis because the management of these causes of hypoxemia can vary. When noted in the ICU, pulmonary venous complications typically require an expeditious return to the operating room in order to avoid permanent lung damage.

Question 12

Which of the following TEE views can be modified to best evaluate for this complication?

A. Transgastric two-chamber view
B. Deep transgastric long axis view
C. Midesophageal four-chamber view
D. Ascending aortic short axis view

Answer C. The midesophageal views, primarily the four-chamber, two-chamber, and bicaval views, can be modified to evaluate the pulmonary veins.

The left-sided pulmonary veins course between the left atrial appendage and the descending aorta before inserting into the lateral left atrium. From the midesophageal four-chamber view, the left upper pulmonary vein may be seen when turning to the left and withdrawing slightly [22]. Rotation of the omniplane to 20–30° and retroflexion may be required to image the left upper pulmonary vein. The left lower pulmonary vein can prove challenging to view; however, the left lower pulmonary vein may appear if the probe is advanced slightly while turning to the left. The midesophageal two-chamber view is the author's preferred view for imaging the left pulmonary veins. From this view, the probe is withdrawn and turned to the left. The left upper pulmonary vein should be seen coursing posterior to the left atrial appendage (separated by the Coumadin Ridge or ligament of Marshall). Forward rotation of the omniplane to 110° may be required. Advancing the probe until the left atrial appendage disappears may allow for imaging of the left lower pulmonary vein.

The right-sided pulmonary veins course behind the superior vena cava before entering the medial left atrium [24]. The midesophageal four-chamber view is the author's preferred view for imaging the right sided veins. From this view, the probe is turned to the right with slight advancement and retroflexion. Forward rotation of the omniplane to 30–60° may be required. The right-sided veins can also be viewed from the midesophageal bicaval view. From this view, the probe is turned clockwise to the right. The right upper pulmonary vein can be seen entering the left atrium from behind the superior vena cava. Color flow Doppler can be useful in identifying the pulmonary veins if imaging proves difficult (Fig. 8.20).

Use the following stem for Questions 13–15. A 57-year-old male with a history of poorly controlled hypertension presents with acute tearing chest pain which radiates to his shoulder blades. The patient's computed tomography with angiography scan and TEE are shown below (Figs. 8.21, 8.22 and 8.23).

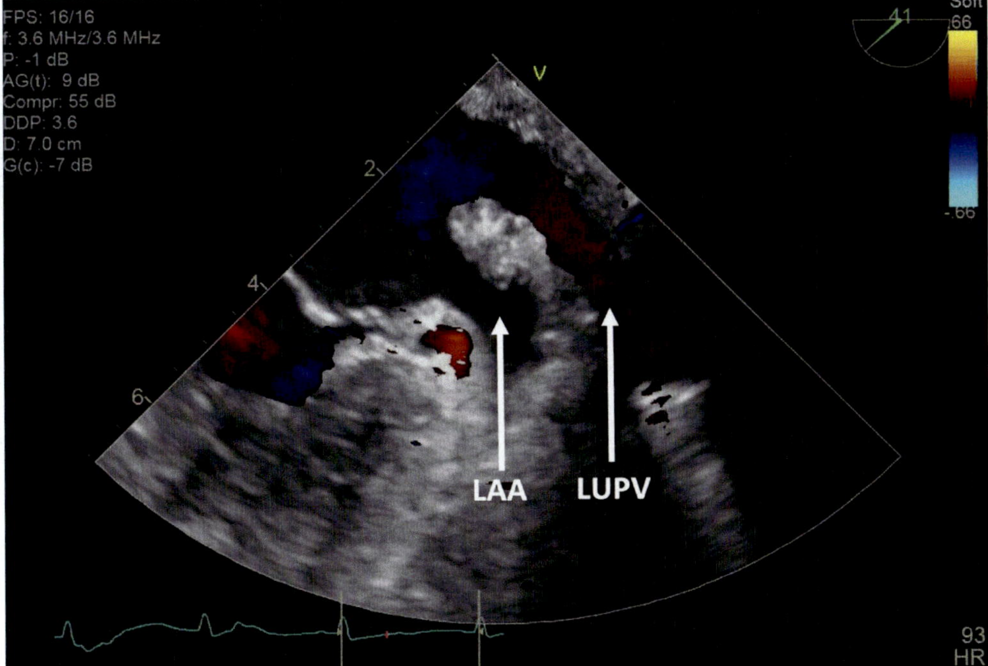

Fig. 8.20 Midesophageal view of the left upper pulmonary vein (LUPV) and the left atrial appendage (LAA)

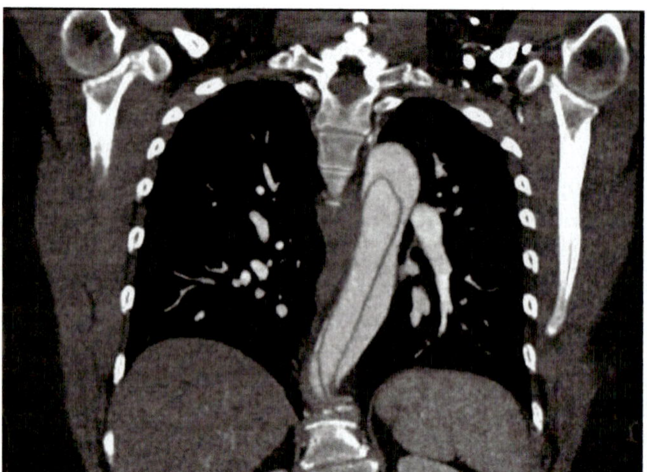

Fig. 8.21 Coronal still image from computed tomography scan with contrast

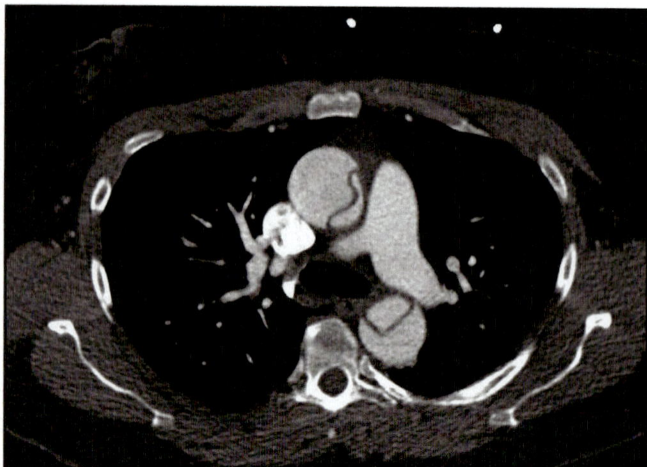

Fig. 8.22 Axial still image from computed tomography scan with contrast

Fig. 8.23 TEE view

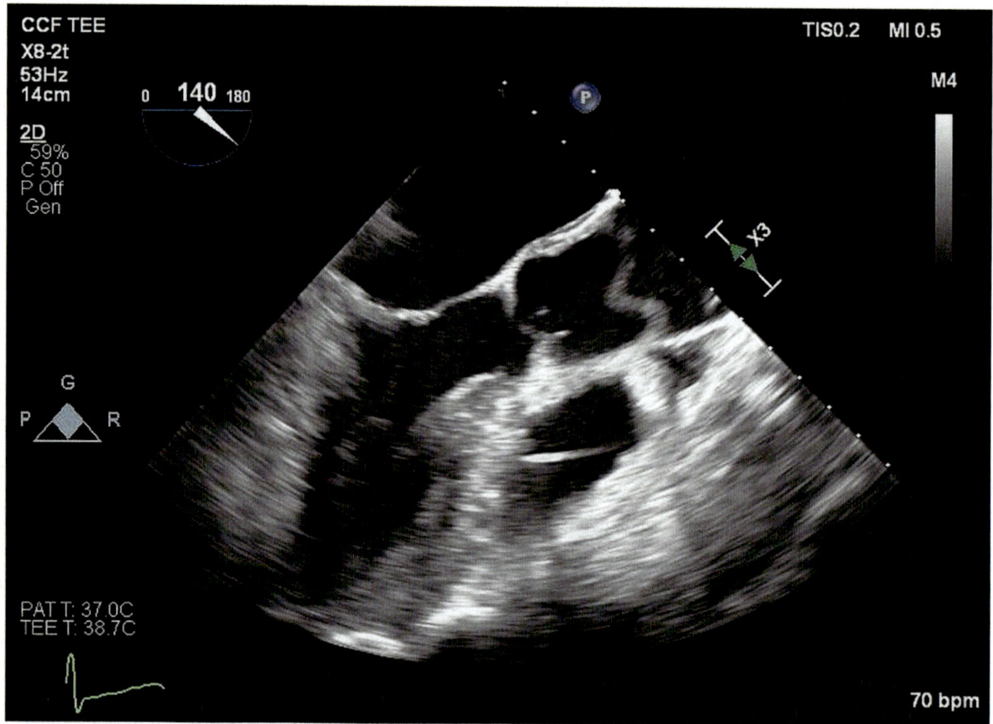

Question 13
Which of the following transesophageal views was obtained?

A. Midesophageal mitral commissural view
B. Midesophageal bicaval view
C. Upper esophageal aortic short axis view
D. Midesophageal long axis view

Answer D. Midesophageal long axis view.

The midesophageal long axis view is found at 30–35 cm at an omniplane of 120–140° [1]. From the midesophageal four-chamber view, the left ventricle is centered in the imaging plane, and the omniplane is advanced until the aortic valve and proximal aorta come into view. This is an important view in the evaluation of a patient with an aortic dissection because it will often identify the dissection flap in type-A dissections while also evaluating for complications such as aortic insufficiency or coronary artery involvement [25].

The midesophageal aortic valve short axis view (Fig. 8.24) is found by centering the aortic valve in the midesophageal long axis view and rotating the omniplane back to 30–50°.

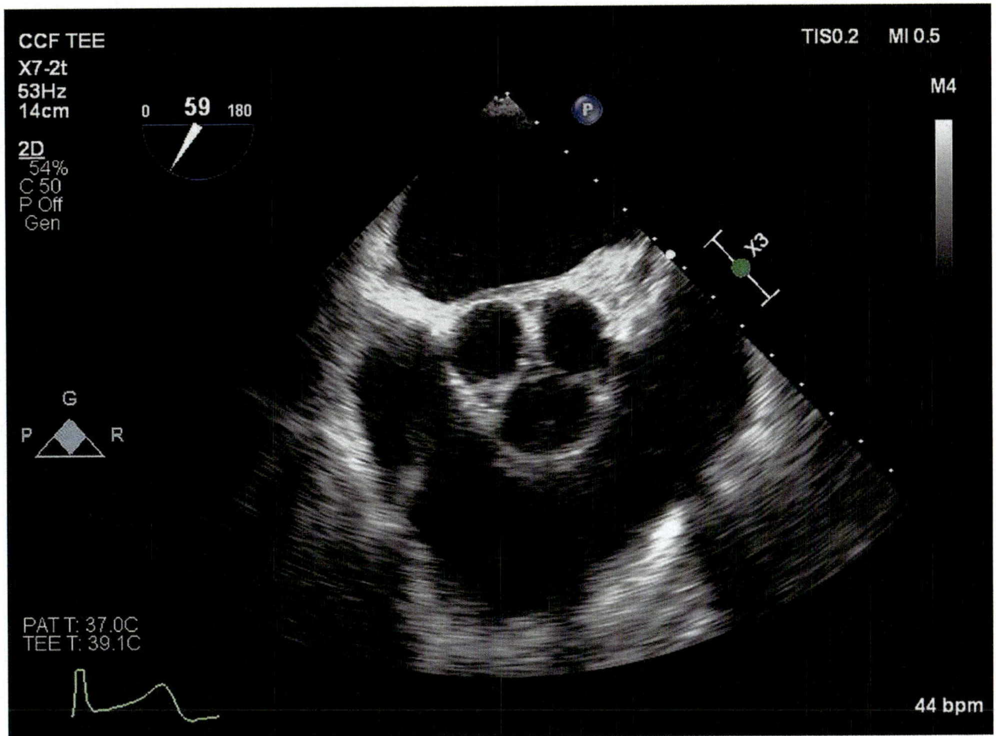

Fig. 8.24 Midesophageal aortic valve short axis view

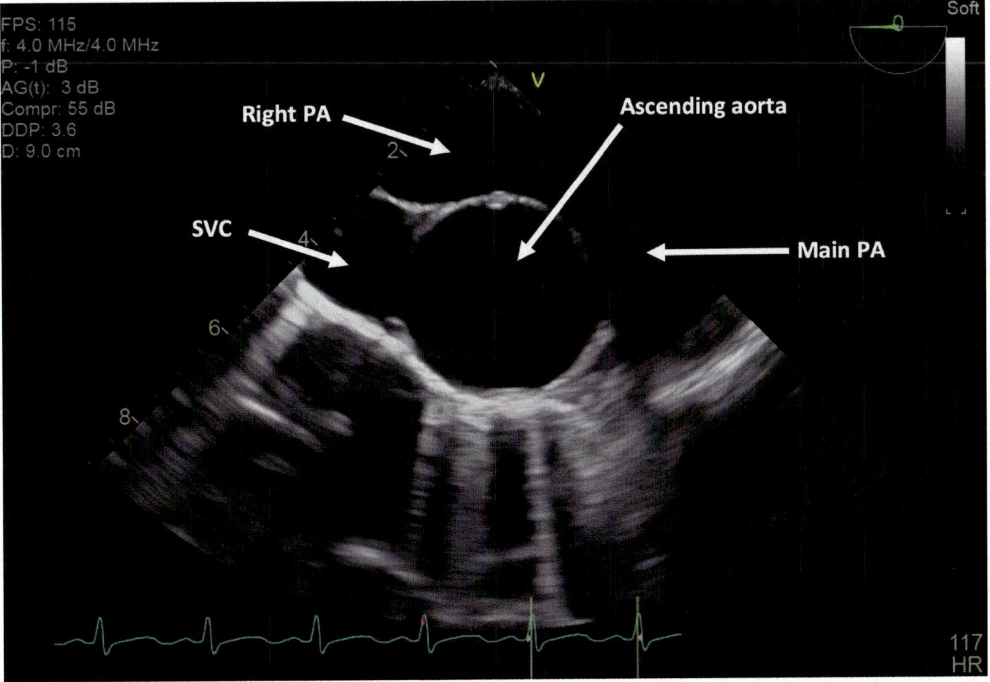

Fig. 8.25 Upper esophageal aortic short axis view. *PA* pulmonary artery, *SVC* superior vena cava

The aortic valve will be seen in short axis view with the three coronary cusps. Slight anteflexion may be required for image optimization. Withdrawal of the probe can identify any involvement of the coronary arteries with the dissection flap.

The midesophageal ascending short axis view (Fig. 8.25) is found by withdrawing the probe slightly from the midesophageal aortic valve short axis or midesophageal five-chamber views. The omniplane is rotated down to zero to 30°, and anteflexion is typically required. The ascending aorta in short axis is seen with the main pulmonary artery and the superior vena cava. Rotating the omniplane forward 90° to 90 to 120° will identify the ascending aorta long axis view. This view allows a detailed assessment of the dissection and may help identify the intimal tear.

The descending aorta short and long axis views are easily found starting from the midesophageal four-chamber view. From this view, the probe is turned counter-clockwise (to the left) until the descending aorta is seen in short axis. A dissection flap is frequently seen in this view. The descending aorta long axis view is found by advancing the omniplane 90°.

Question 14
How would this pathology be classified?

A. DeBakey Type 1
B. DeBakey Type 2
C. DeBakey Type 3
D. DeBakey Type 4

Answer A. DeBakey Type 1 dissection includes both the ascending and descending aorta.

This patient has a dissection flap originating in the ascending aorta and extending down into the descending aorta, which is classified as a DeBakey type I or Stanford type A aortic dissection.

Acute aortic syndromes consist of aortic dissection, penetrating atherosclerotic ulcer, and intramural hematoma [26]. Of these presenting pathologies, acute aortic dissection represents up to 95% of all cases. Hypertension and tobacco use are the primary comorbidities in patients presenting with aortic dissection. Other common comorbidities include male gender, renal insufficiency, chronic obstructive pulmonary disease, and cerebrovascular disease. This condition also affects patients with congenital heart disease and connective tissue diseases such as those with bicuspid aortic valve, Marfan syndrome, Loeys-Dietz syndrome, Ehlers-Danlos syndrome, and Turner syndrome. The most common presenting symptom is sharp chest or back pain. Other presenting signs or symptoms include weak pulses, hypotension, syncope, diastolic heart murmur, heart failure, syncope, and stroke.

Acute aortic dissection can be classified by the Stanford or DeBakey classification systems [27]. The Stanford system separates acute aortic dissection into those affecting the ascending aorta (type-A) or those only affecting the descending aorta (type-B). The DeBakey system is separated into three distinct types. Type I includes the ascending and descending aorta. Type II affects the ascending aorta only. Type III affects the descending aorta only and can be broken up into type IIIa (above the diaphragm) and type IIIb (extends below the diaphragm). DeBakey type I and II aortic dissections are also Stanford type-A. DeBakey type III aortic dissection is akin to a Stanford type B.

Question 15
Which of the following echocardiographic findings is a characteristic of the false lumen?

A. Lumen connected with aortic valve
B. Smallest lumen
C. Systolic expansion
D. Spontaneous echo contrast or thrombus formation

Answer D. Spontaneous echo contrast or thrombus formation can identify the false lumen.

Identification of the true lumen can be of paramount importance, particularly in the operating room prior to aortic cannulation for cardiopulmonary bypass. It is also important to identify the true lumen and any malperfusion prior to endovascular intervention, such as fenestrated graft placement or intimal fenestration [25].

The true lumen will always be the lumen into which blood travels from the left ventricular outflow tract and through the aortic valve; therefore, it is always the lumen connected with the aortic valve [28]. Considering this lumen also experiences antegrade blood flow, the true lumen frequently experiences systolic expansion while the false lumen experiences systolic compression. However, this systolic expansion may not be well evident when there is a wide communication between the two lumens. Furthermore, areas of the dissected aorta may demonstrate systolic expansion of the false lumen, thus, systolic expansion should not be the only measure used to identify the true lumen. If difficulty is encountered differentiating which lumen is expanding during systole, M-mode in conjunction with EKG can be used to identify the expanding and thus true lumen (Fig. 8.26). In addition to systolic expansion, the true lumen should demonstrate forward systolic flow while the false lumen may have slowed flow or even reversal. Due to this low flow in the false lumen, spontaneous echo contrast, or even thrombus, can be seen. If the intimal tear is found, high-velocity flow may be seen from the true lumen into the false lumen. The true lumen is typically smaller than the false lumen; however, this is not entirely consistent. The most valuable method to differentiate the true and false lumen may involve focused echocardiograpic imaging to visualize the layers of the aortic wall. The true lumen will have an intact media throughout its entire circumference, whereas the false lumen will lack this medial continuity. Table 8.4 identifies useful qualities in the differentiation of the true and false lumen.

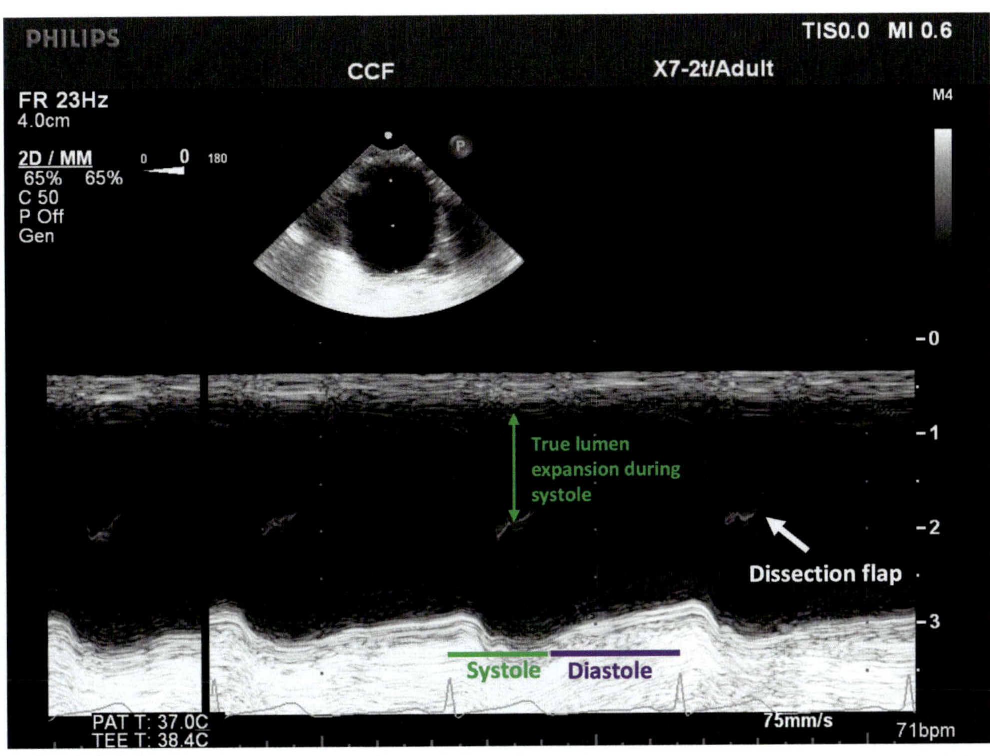

Fig. 8.26 M-mode interrogation of the aorta in the descending aortic short axis view. Note the expansion of the true lumen during systole

Table 8.4 Identification of True Lumen in aortic dissection

	True lumen	False lumen
Size	True lumen typically smaller than false	False lumen typically larger than true
Systolic pulsation	Systolic expansion	Systolic compression
Systolic flow	Forward systolic flow	Slowed or reversed systolic flow
Echogenicity	Hypoechoic—Blood	Spontaneous echo contrast or thrombus formation
Aortic wall	Continuity of medial layer	Discontinuity of medial later

Question 16

The trachea interferes with TEE imaging of the aortic arch with all of the following structures, **EXCEPT**?

A. Left subclavian
B. Left common carotid
C. Right brachiocephalic
D. Distal ascending aorta

Answer A. Imaging of the left subclavian artery is not typically obstructed by the trachea or left mainstem bronchus.

The distal ascending aorta and aortic arch are challenging to image due to the interposition of the trachea or left mainstem bronchus in between the aorta and the esophagus [1]. This will give a characteristic air artifact when withdrawing the probe in order to image the aortic arch. As a result, the distal ascending aorta and the proximal two aortic branches (right brachiocephalic and left common carotid) cannot typically be imaged with TEE. The left subclavian artery, however, can be found by gradually withdrawing the probe from the descending aorta short axis view. With the help of color flow Doppler, the left subclavian artery can be seen as a branch off the lateral aorta [29]. Counterclockwise rotation may be required. This view is important during the placement of an intra-aortic balloon pump because the tip of the balloon should be immediately distal to the origin of the left subclavian artery.

Question 17

An acute ascending aortic dissection is most likely to involve with which coronary artery?

A. Left main coronary artery
B. Left anterior descending coronary artery
C. Left circumflex coronary artery
D. Right coronary artery

Answer D. Right coronary artery.

It is important to evaluate the coronary arteries in patients with proximal type A aortic dissections because the dissection flap could extend into the coronary arteries [30]. The most common coronary artery involved is the right coronary artery resulting in myocardial ischemia of the right coronary artery distribution with subsequent wall motion abnormalities and bradycardia [31].

The coronary arteries can be evaluated in the midesophageal long axis and short axis views with slight probe movements focusing on the distal segments of the sinus of Valsalva. In the midesophageal short axis view, the right coronary artery can be seen arising from the right coronary cusp adjacent to the right ventricle. The coronary cusp directly adjacent to the interatrial septum is the noncoronary cusp. The left main coronary artery can be seen arising from the remaining left coronary cusp (Fig. 8.27).

Use the following stem for Questions 18–20. A 52-year-old male with a history of hypertension, diabetes mellitus, hyperlipidemia, and tobacco abuse arrives in the emergency department in respiratory distress with acute tearing chest pain with radiation to his left shoulder. The EKG demonstrates ST segment elevation in leads V1–V5 with reciprocal ST segment depression in leads III and aVF. His extremities are cool to touch and his blood pressure is 89/51 mmHg. Labs are significant for a lactate of 3.2 mmol/L and troponin I of 2.1 ng/mL. A TEE probe is placed to evaluate his cardiac function (Figs. 8.28 and 8.29).

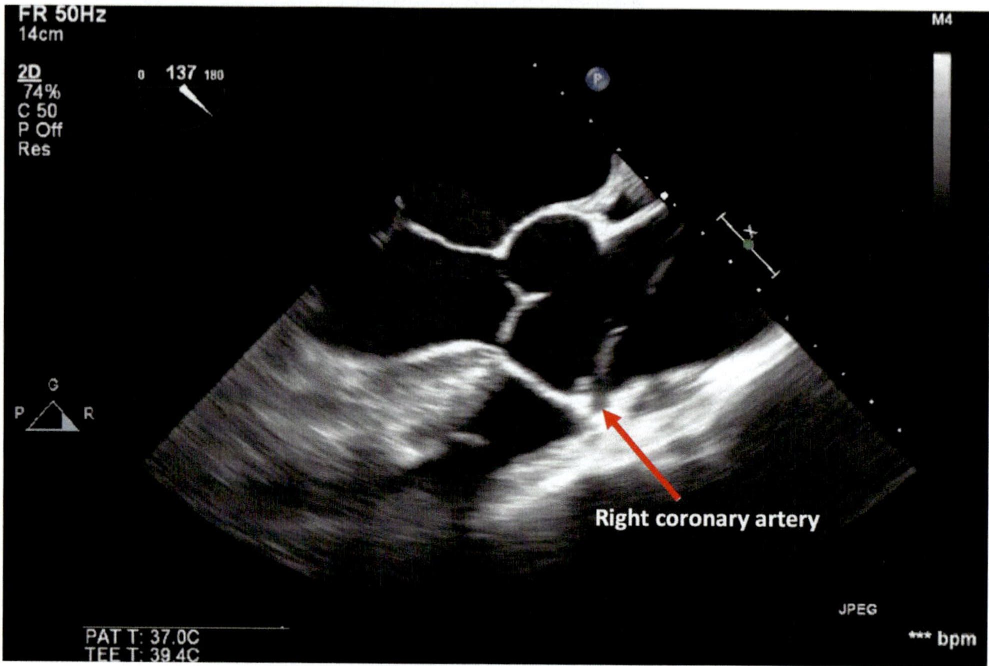

Fig. 8.27 Midesophageal long axis view in a patient with a type A aortic dissection. Note the dissection flap approaching the ostia of the right coronary artery

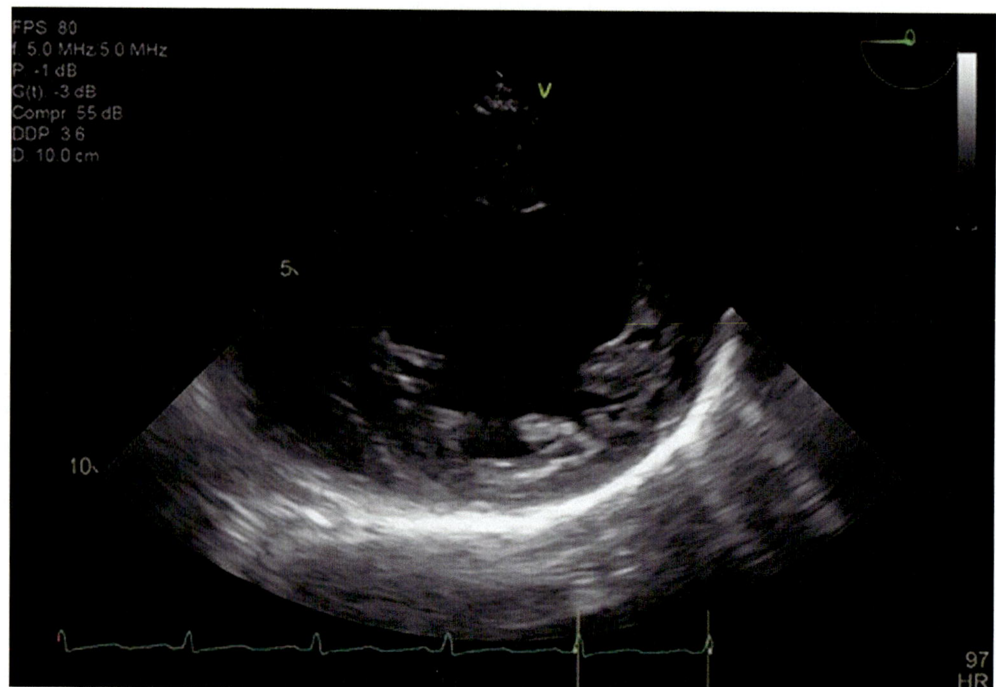

Fig. 8.28 Transgastric TEE view

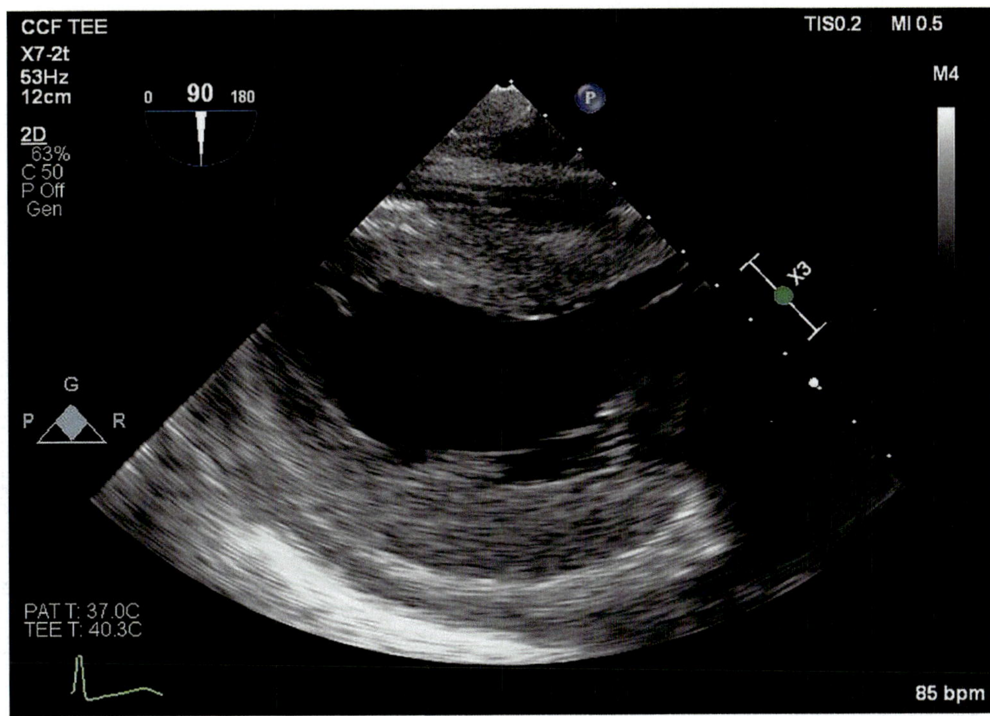

Fig. 8.29 Transgastric TEE view

Question 18
Which of the following TEE views were obtained?

A. Transgastric midpapillary short axis and transgastric basal short axis
B. Transgastric midpapillary short axis and transgastric long axis
C. Transgastric midpapillary long axis and transgastric two-chamber
D. Transgastric midpapillary short axis and transgastric two-chamber

Answer D. Transgastric midpapillary short axis and transgastric two-chamber views.

The transgastric midpapillary short axis view allows the echocardiographer to view all three coronary distributions at once [21]. In addition, left and right ventricular size and function can be evaluated, and volume status may be assessed. This can aid the clinician in diagnosing myocardial infarction, hypovolemia, heart failure, and tamponade efficiently and accurately. The orthogonal view is the transgastric two-chamber view, which shows the anterior and inferior walls of the left ventricle as well as the mitral valve and subvalvular mitral apparatus.

The transgastric views are found by advancing the probe from the midesophageal four-chamber view (zero–20°) into the stomach (about 40 cm from the teeth) [1]. The probe is advanced while maintaining focus on the left ventricle. It is important to avoid probe manipulation as the probe passes through the lower esophageal sphincter in order to avoid esophageal damage. As the left ventricle exits view, the probe is anteflexed to bring the short axis of the left ventricle. Three views can be found with slight insertion and variation of anteflexion: the transgastric basal short axis view, midpapillary view short axis view, and the apical short axis view. Turning the probe to the right from the transgastric midpapillary short axis will typically bring the short axis of the mid-right ventricle into view.

Rotating the omniplane forward 90° from the transgastric midpapillary short axis view will identify the transgastric two-chamber view [10]. The inferior wall is closest to the probe while the anterior wall is furthest. Continuing the omniplane to 120 to 140° will bring the aortic valve and LVOT into view in the transgastric long axis view. This view is useful for Doppler evaluation of the LVOT and aortic valve.

Question 19
Which wall motion abnormalities would be expected given this coronary lesion?

A. Inferior and inferoseptal
B. Inferolateral and anterolateral
C. Anterior and anteroseptal
D. Right ventricular free wall

Answer C. Anterior and anteroseptal wall motion abnormalities will be seen in patients with a left anterior descending artery myocardial infarction.

The left main coronary artery arises from the left coronary cusp and gives rise to the left circumflex artery and the left anterior descending artery (LAD) [32]. The LAD courses around the pulmonary artery and enters the interventricular groove as it courses down and around the apex

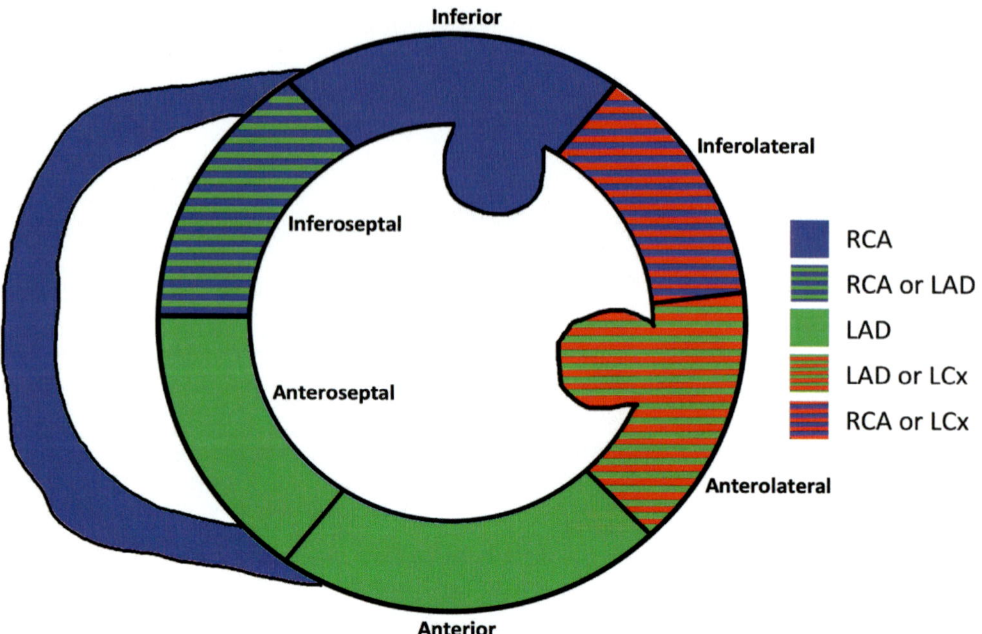

Fig. 8.30 TEE transgastric midpapillary short axis view demonstrating the coronary artery distributions

into the inferior interventricular groove. The LAD gives rise to the diagonal arteries and the deep septal perforator arteries. These arteries supply the anterior and anteroseptal walls of the left ventricle in addition to the apex of the heart. In some patients, the LAD may also supply the anterolateral and inferoseptal walls; however, this is inconsistent [21]. The right coronary artery typically supplies the inferior and inferoseptal walls, while the left circumflex artery typically supplied the inferolateral and anterolateral walls (Fig. 8.30).

Question 20

The patient is emergently transferred to the catheterization laboratory for cardiac catheterization. A complete occlusion of the left anterior descending artery is found and a drug eluting stent is placed. Despite revascularization, the patient decompensates over the next 24 h requiring emergent surgical placement of a temporary microaxial ventricular assist device (Impella 5.5) via the left axillary artery. Based on the following image, how deep should the microaxial ventricular assist device be placed into the left ventricle (Fig. 8.31)?

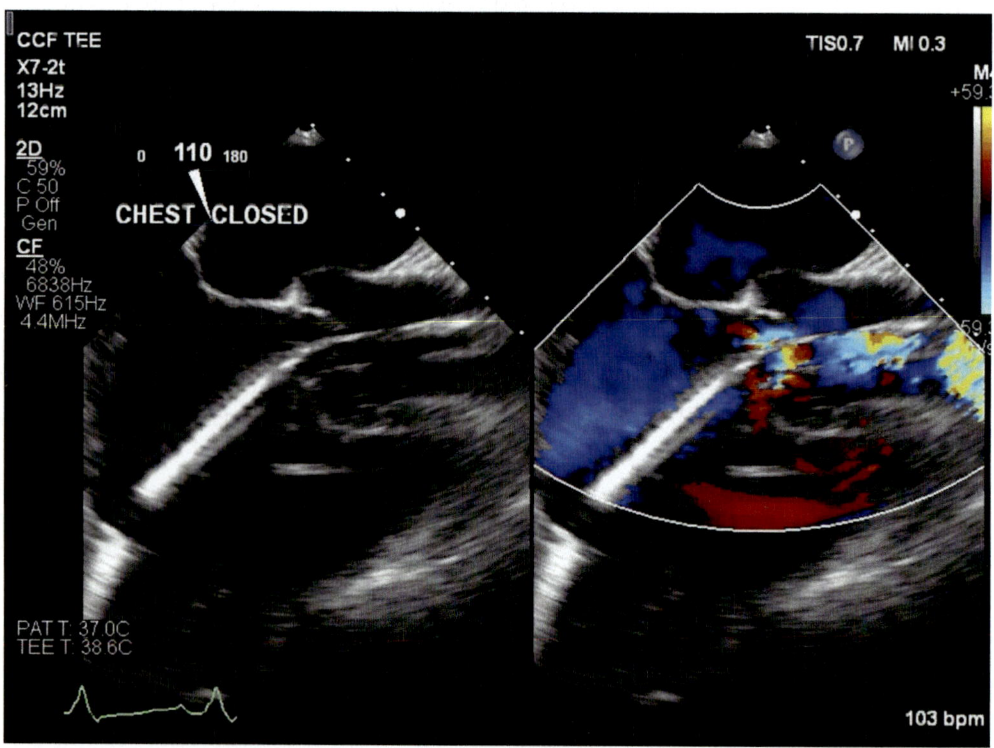

Fig. 8.31 Midesophageal long axis view demonstrating Impella 5.5 microaxial left ventricular assist device

A. 2.0–3.0 cm
B. 3.0–4.0 cm
C. 4.0–5.0 cm
D. 5.0–6.0 cm

Answer C. 4.0–5.0 cm.

Microaxial ventricular assist devices (Impella, Abiomed Inc., Danvers, MA) are temporary pumps placed via the femoral and axillary arteries which traverse the aortic valve and allow decompression of the left ventricle as blood is pumped from the left ventricle into the aorta. The main indications for placement are high risk percutaneous coronary intervention, ventricular tachycardia ablation, reversible myocardial ischemia, and acute severe left ventricular failure [33]. Contraindications include moderate to severe aortic insufficiency, aortic dissection, biventricular failure, mechanical aortic valves, and intracardiac thrombus. The two primary left-heart Impella pumps available are the Impella CP and Impella 5.5. The Impella CP can be placed percutaneously via the femoral artery while the Impella 5.5 requires surgical placement in the operating room via an axillary artery cutdown. The Impella CP pump is composed of three major components: the Archimedes screw pump, a driveline that extends to a console outside the patient, and a pigtail that extends into the left ventricle. The Impella 5.5 is a newer device that allows for higher flows and does not have the pigtail tip at the end (Fig. 8.31).

Correct placement is of paramount importance to ensure that blood is drained from the left ventricle and ejected into the aorta. In the ICU, it is important to verify the position of the pump with TEE or TTE whenever significant changes in hemodynamics or device console alarms occur. In the midesophageal long axis view, the pump can be seen entering the left ventricle via the ascending aorta with the pigtail terminating in the left ventricle. For the Impella 5.5, the distance from the aortic valve to the pump inlet should be 4.0–5.0 cm. For the Impella CP pump, the distance should be 3.5–4.0 cm [34]. Color flow Doppler can be used to assess placement as well. Turbulence should be noted in the ascending aorta, distal to the aortic valve (Video 8.1). Turbulence below the aortic valve may indicate the device is positioned too far into the ventricle (Fig. 8.32).

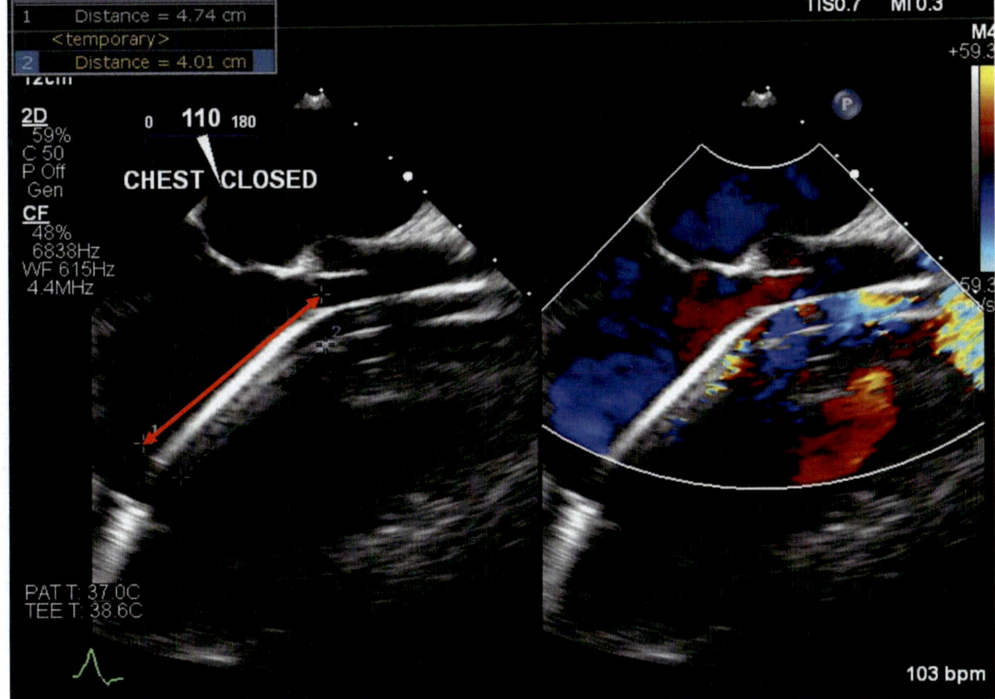

Fig. 8.32 Midesophageal long axis view demonstrating Impella 5.5 microaxial left ventricular assist device in the left ventricle. The Impella 5.5 is placed 4.0–5.0 cm into the left ventricle. Note the distance between the aortic valve and the pump inlet (red line) in this image is 4.74 cm

Question 21

A 52-year-old male with a history of coronary artery disease and ischemic cardiomyopathy undergoes placement of a left ventricular assist device (LVAD, Heartmate III - Abbott Laboratories, Chicago, IL) complicated by coagulopathy and right heart failure requiring multiple transfusions, epinephrine, and milrinone. On the first postoperative day, blood pressure abruptly decreases from 105/60 to 70/35 with an increase in central venous pressure. The LVAD flows decrease significantly and the LVAD alarm sounds. The patient suddenly develops sustained ventricular tachycardia. Due to inadequate TTE images, a TEE probe is placed. What is the best next step in management?

A. Increase RPMs
B. Reduce RPMs
C. Add furosemide drip
D. Add inhaled epoprostenol

Answer B. RPMs should be reduced during a suction event.

Suction events can occur at any time after left ventricular assist device (LVAD) placement. Periods of reduced left ventricular preload, such as hemorrhage, hypovolemia, arrhythmias, and right heart failure, will reduce the size of the left ventricle and allow the pump inlet to suck down and cause a complete collapse of the left ventricle [35]. These suction events may also occur in the perioperative period if LVAD RPMs are set too high. The pump console will demonstrate low flows and typically a low pulsatility index. This may present as complete cardiovascular collapse with hypotension and elevated right-sided filling pressures. Recurrent ventricular tachycardia may occur as well. This event may be diagnosed with bedside ultrasound; however, patients have notoriously difficult TTE images following LVAD implantations, and therefore, TEE may be required [36]. The first step in management is to reduce the RPMs to their lowest safe level. TEE will show a reduced (or obliterated) left ventricular cavity and may be helpful in differentiating the cause of the suction event. Right ventricular failure increases the right ventricular cavity dimensions, which can shift the septum into the left ventricle and closer to the pump inlet, increasing the risk of a suction event. In addition, hypovolemia can contribute to a suction event due to the fall in preload (Figs. 8.33 and 8.34).

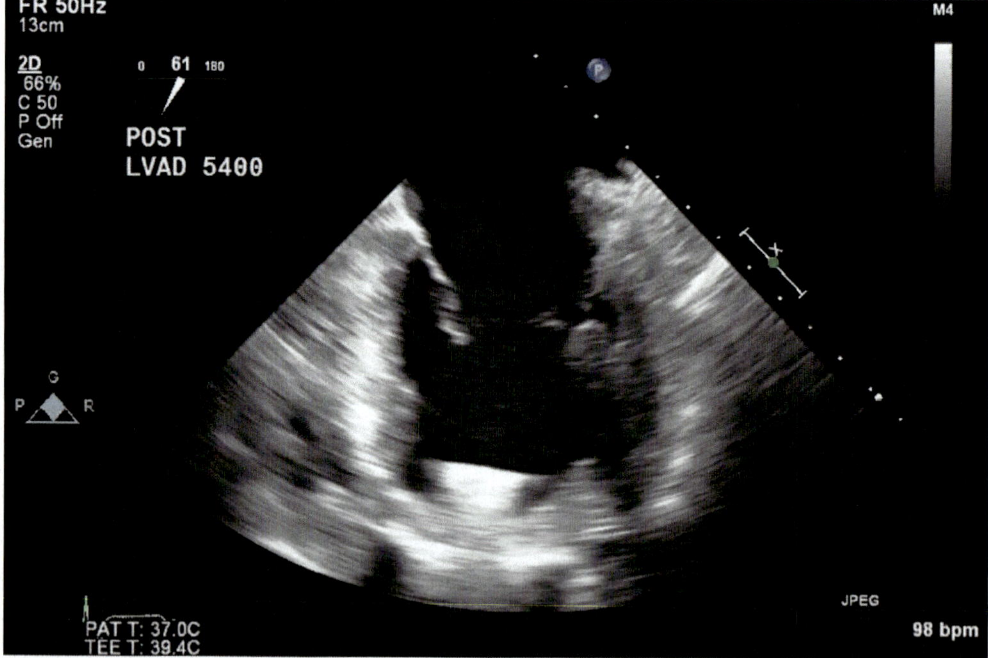

Fig. 8.33 Midesophageal TEE view demonstrating a Heartmate III LVAD inflow canula in the apex of the left ventricle

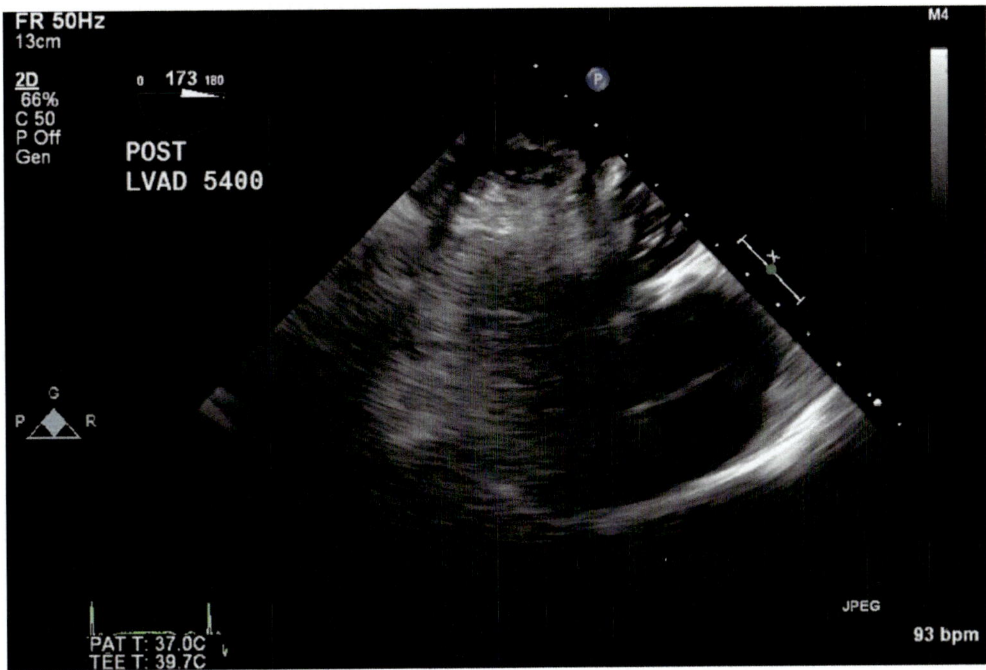

Fig. 8.34 This is a midesophageal view of a suction event occurring in a patient with a Heartmate III LVAD. Note the complete obliteration of the left ventricular cavity

Use the following stem for Questions 22–23. A 45-year-old female with a liver cirrhosis secondary to chronic hepatitis C infection presents to SICU following liver transplantation. On postoperative day 3, she develops acute onset hypotension, tachycardia, and respiratory distress requiring emergent intubation. Epinephrine and norepinephrine are initiated due to hemodynamic collapse. Considering her poor TTE windows, a TEE probe is placed.

Question 22
Which tricuspid valve leaflet is identified by the arrow? (Fig. 8.35)

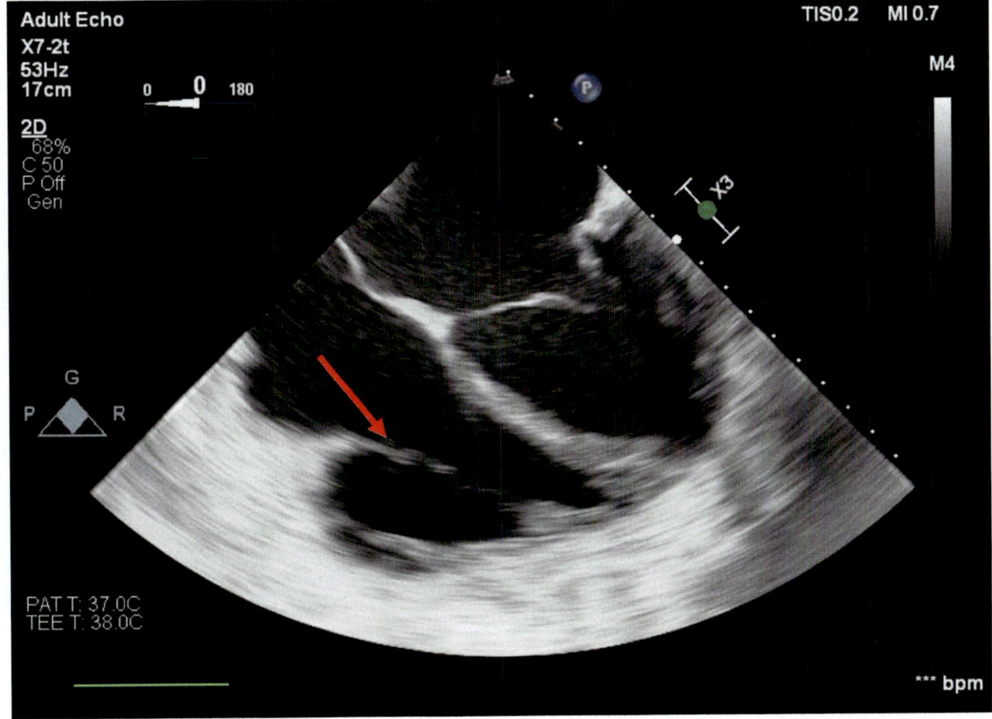

Fig. 8.35 Midesophageal four-chamber view

A. Anterior leaflet
B. Posterior leaflet
C. Septal leaflet
D. Anterior or posterior leaflet

Answer D. The leaflet to the left in the midesophageal four-chamber view is either the anterior or posterior leaflet. The leaflet to the right is the septal leaflet.

The tricuspid valve has the largest orifice of any of the cardiac valves (4–6 cm^2) and contains three leaflets – anterior, posterior, and septal [37]. The septal leaflet inserts into the septum in a more apical location than the mitral valve. The tricuspid valve can be evaluated in three primary midesophageal views: four-chamber, right ventricular inflow-outflow, and modified bicaval view.

In the midesophageal four-chamber view, the leaflet to the left is either the anterior or posterior leaflet, while the leaflet to the right is the septal leaflet. When evaluating for tricuspid pathology in this view, it is essential to image the entire tricuspid valve by advancing and withdrawing the probe until the valve disappears. Advancing the probe will image the posterior leaflet while withdrawing the probe will identify the anterior leaflet. The coronary sinus will come into view when advancing the probe, which suggests the leaflet to the left is the posterior leaflet. The leaflet to the right of the screen will always be the septal leaflet.

From the midesophageal four-chamber view, the tricuspid valve is centered on the screen, and the omniplane is advanced to 50 to 70° [1]. This should bring the right ventricular inflow-outflow view into focus (Fig. 8.36). The aortic valve will also be seen in short axis. This view is extremely similar to the midesophageal aortic valve short axis view; however, the midesophageal aortic valve short axis view is typically optimized at a lower omniplane angle (25–45°). In the midesophageal right ventricular inflow-outflow view, the leaflet attached to the right ventricular free wall (the leaflet to the left) is the posterior leaflet, while the anterior or septal leaflet is seen attaching near the aortic valve.

The midesophageal bicaval view is found by advancing the omniplane to 80 to 100° while turning the probe to the right (clockwise). The superior vena cava will be seen to the right of the screen, and the inferior vena cava will be seen to the left. From this view, the midesophageal modified bicaval view can be found by rotating the omniplane to 110 to 120° to bring the tricuspid valve into view. This view can also be found by centering the tricuspid valve in the midesophageal right ventricular inflow-outflow view and advancing the omniplane to 110 to 120°. In this view, the anterior leaflet is seen on the right side of the screen adjacent to the right atrial appendage. The leaflet on the left side of the screen is either the septal or posterior leaflets.

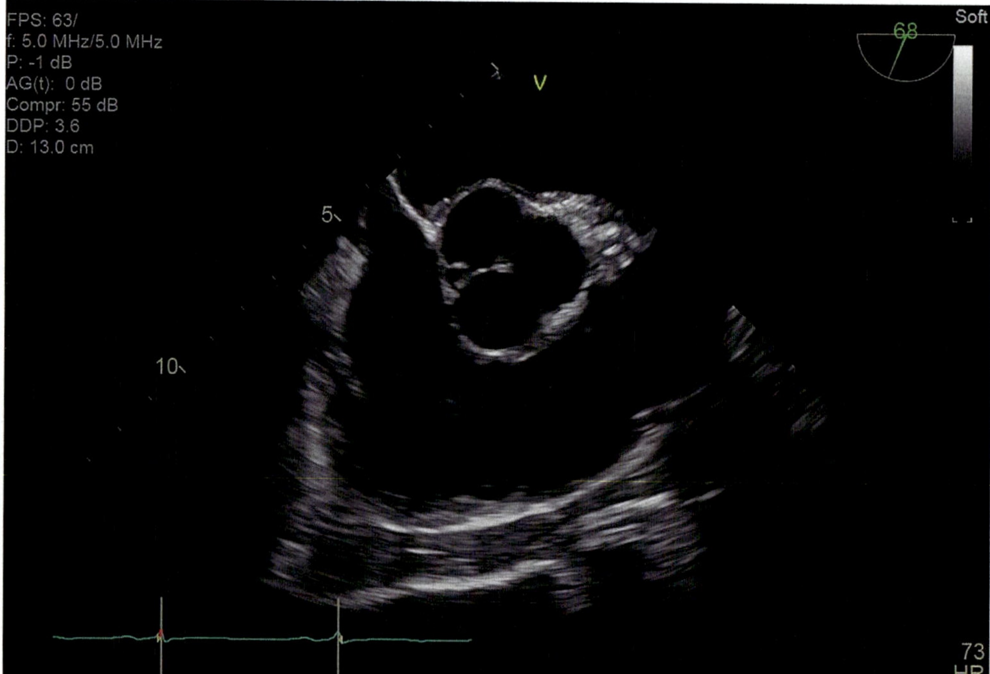

Fig. 8.36 Midesophageal right ventricular inflow-outflow view

Question 23

The following TEE image and spectral Doppler waveform are obtained. What is the patients estimated right ventricular systolic pressure? (Fig. 8.37)

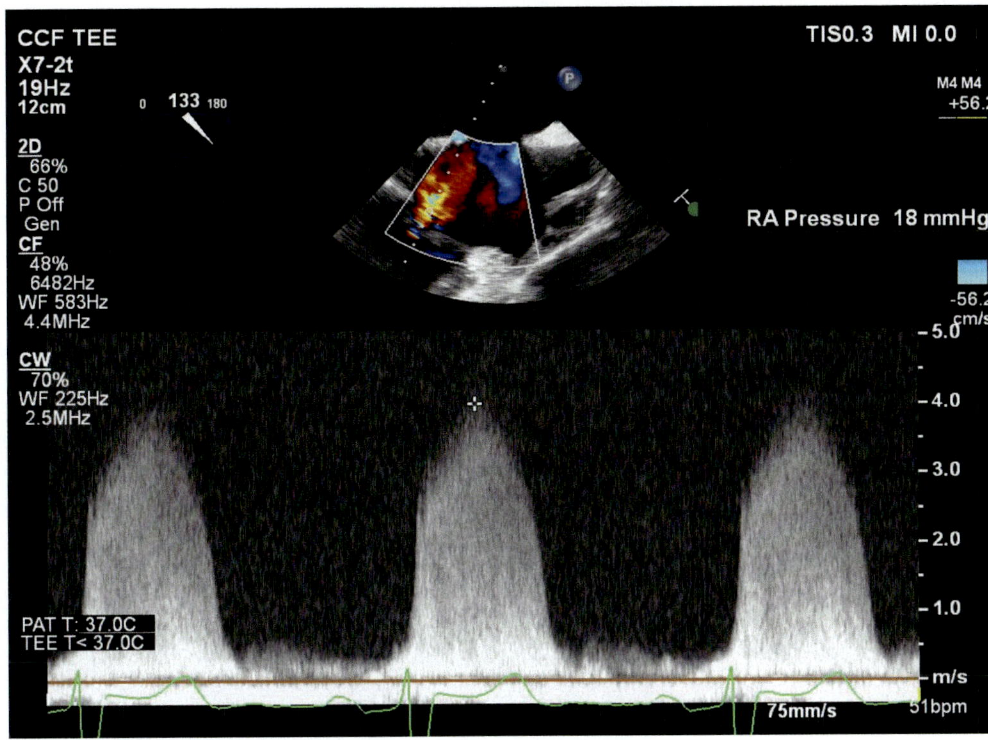

Fig. 8.37 Spectral Doppler envelope. The peak velocity is 4.0 m/s. The right atrial pressure (RA) is 18 mmHg

A. 46 mmHg
B. 64 mmHg
C. 74 mmHg
D. 82 mmHg

Answer D. The estimated right ventricular systolic pressure is equal to the right atrial pressure plus the pressure gradient through the tricuspid valve (Pressure gradient = 4 V^2).

Multiple TEE views can be used to evaluate the tricuspid valve with Doppler echocardiography. The view that provides the best alignment will depend on the direction of the jet, but for central jets, the modified bicaval view typically allows ideal alignment for Doppler analysis [37]. It is important to note that most spectral Doppler waveforms will be flipped 180° from their TTE counterparts. In this view, regurgitant blood flow is directed toward the probe resulting in an upward deflection on the spectral Doppler waveform as opposed to transthoracic views where tricuspid regurgitant flow is directed away from the transducer resulting in a downward deflection.

The simplified Bernoulli equation ($\Delta P = 4 \times V^2$; ΔP = pressure gradient; v = peak velocity) can be used to estimate right ventricular systolic pressure (RVSP) using a continuous wave Doppler spectral waveform [38]. On this waveform we see the velocity corresponding to the peak of the tricuspid regurgitant jet is 4 m/s. When this velocity is entered into the simplified Bernoulli equation, $\Delta P = 4 \times V^2 = 4 \times 4^2$. Therefore, the pressure gradient through that valve is 64 mmHg. However, the right atrial pressure (RAP) must be added to this pressure gradient to generate the estimated RVSP (64 mmHg + 18 mmHg = 82 mmHg)

$$\text{RVSP} = \text{RAP} + \Delta P$$

Question 24

Which view allows for right ventricular quantitative assessment with tricuspid annular plane systolic excursion (TAPSE) and tissue Doppler tricuspid lateral annular systolic velocity (s′)?

(a) Midesophageal four-chamber view
(b) Midesophageal modified bicaval view
(c) Transgastric midpapillary short axis view
(d) Modified deep transgastric five-chamber view

Answer D. The deep transgastric four-chamber view allows optimal alignment for evaluation of the right ventricle with TAPSE and S′.

Several indices can be used to quantify right ventricular function, including tricuspid annular plane systolic excursion (TAPSE), tissue Doppler systolic excursion velocity (S′), fractional area of change, myocardial performance index, 3-D ejection fraction, and strain [39]. Both TAPSE and S′ require optimal alignment with the probe as both measures are angle-dependent. Of the views presented, a modified deep transgastric five-chamber view allows optimal alignment for measurement of angle-dependent calculations for the right ventricle. Slight manipulation of the probe may be required to bring the lateral annulus for the tricuspid valve into an optimal position. A modified transgastric right ventricle inflow view may allow optimal alignment as well.

Considering the majority of right ventricular systolic function is comprised of the longitudinal fibers shortening from the apex to the annulus, measuring the displacement of the lateral annulus of the tricuspid valve (TAPSE) can give strong insights into right ventricular function [40]. TAPSE is measured in the apical four-chamber view in TTE and either the deep transgastric five-chamber or transgastric right ventricular inflow views. Using M-mode, the cursor is placed through the lateral tricuspid valve annulus. The waveform is measured from peak to trough and a TAPSE less than 17 mm indicates right ventricular dysfunction.

While TAPSE measures the movement of the lateral tricuspid annulus, S′ allows for the measurement of the velocity of this tissue. Using tissue Doppler, the sample volume is placed in the myocardium near the lateral tricuspid valve annulus. A value <10 cm/s is indicative of right ventricular dysfunction (Figs. 8.38 and 8.39). It is important to note these measurement cutoffs (TAPSE, S′) were validated using TTE and may not correlate with values derived from TEE imaging.

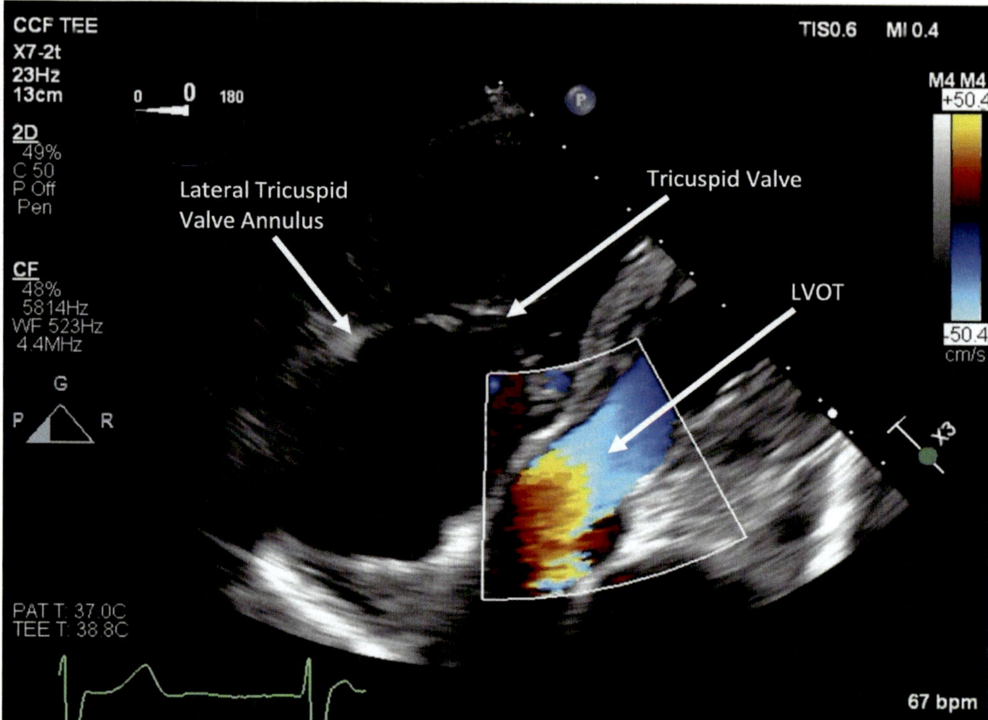

Fig. 8.38 Deep transgastric view. The M-mode cursor is lined up with the lateral tricuspid valve annulus in this view to measure tricuspid annular place systolic excursion (TAPSE)

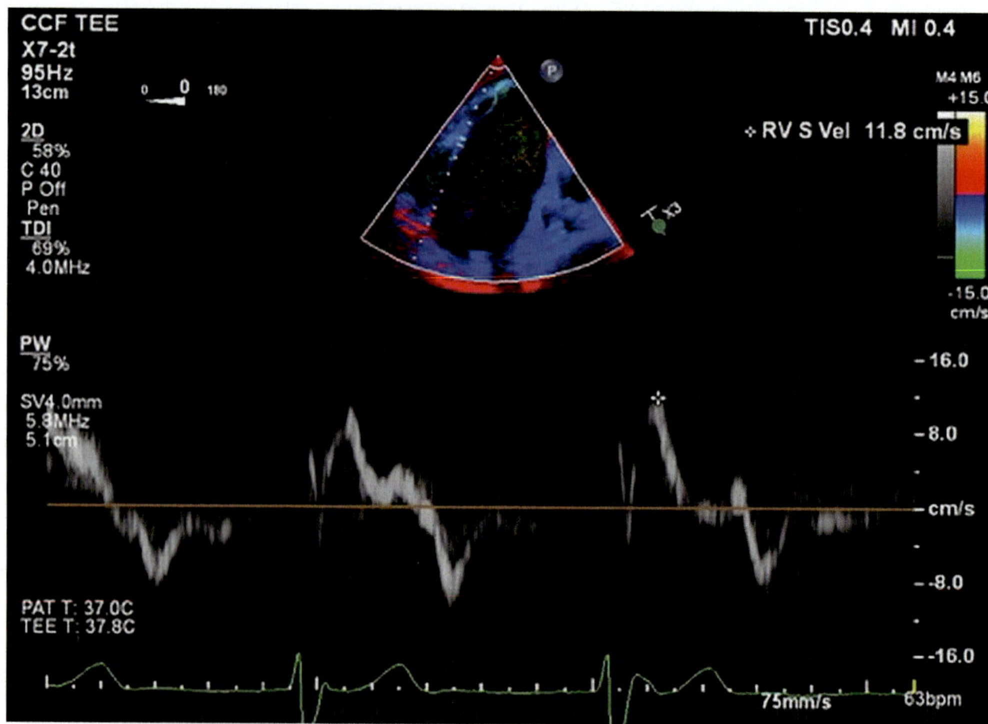

Fig. 8.39 Tissue Doppler spectral envelope demonstrating a right ventricular s prime value of 11.8 cm/s

Question 25
What is demonstrated by the following TEE image? (Fig. 8.40)

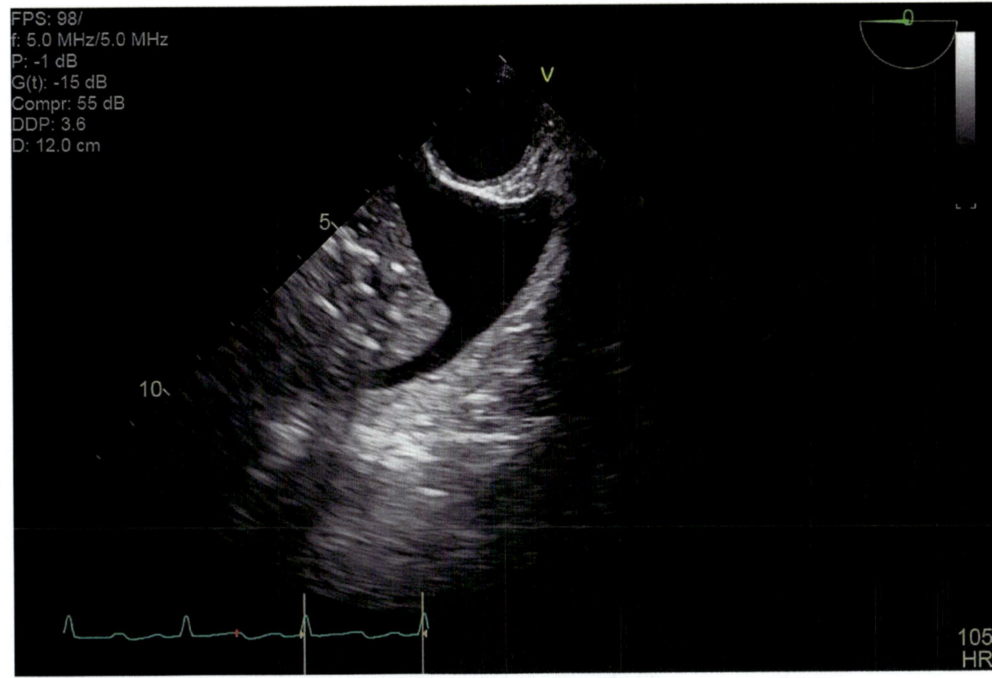

Fig. 8.40 TEE view

A. Left pleural effusion
B. Right pleural effusion
C. Pericardial effusion
D. Ascites

Answer A. Left pleural effusion.

Pleural effusions can be identified on TEE [41]. Left-sided pleural effusions can be found by turning the probe to the left from the midesophageal four-chamber view to find the descending aorta. Left-sides pleural effusions can be seen immediately anterior to the descending aorta as a homogenous hypoechoic fluid pocket [42]. Complicated effusions may have a heterogeneous appearance. The fluid pocket typically has the shape of a "tiger's claw" with the curve directed to the left (Fig. 8.40). Right-sided pleural effusions are slightly more difficult to identify due to the left-sided location of the esophageal in the chest. From the midesophageal four-chamber view with focus on the right atrium, the probe is advanced and rotated clockwise (to the right) following the inferior vena cava to the liver. Right-sided pleural effusions can be seen superior and posterior to the liver. The curve of a right-sided pleural effusion is directed to the right. Ascites may be seen as hypoechoic fluid; however, it will be located below the diaphragm.

Use the following stem for Questions 26–27. A 63-year-old male with a history of two prior cardiac surgeries presents to CVICU after surgical mitral valve replacement. Intraoperative coagulopathy required 4 units of pRBCs, 20 units of cryoprecipitate, and 3 units of platelets. Blood pressure and contractility are maintained with norepinephrine and epinephrine. Immediately upon arrival and after turning the patient, the patient develops bradycardia and severe hypotension requiring escalating doses of norepinephrine. An EKG shows ST elevation in leads II, III, and aVF. Due to cardiovascular collapse, a TEE probe is placed demonstrating hypokinesis in the inferior left ventricular wall and right ventricular free wall.

Question 26
What is the most likely cause of cardiovascular collapse?

A. Acute myocardial infarction
B. Cardiac tamponade
C. Air embolus
D. Hemorrhage

Answer C. Air embolism can occur following cardiac surgery which may embolize to the right coronary artery.

Retained intracardiac air is common when separating from cardiopulmonary bypass. The most common sites of air retainment are the right upper pulmonary vein, left ventricular apex, and the left atrium [43]. Typically the air is removed intraoperatively with de-airing procedures such as Valsalva maneuvers, direct myocardial agitation, or direct needle decompression. However, complete de-airing is not always possible. When this air embolizes past the aortic valve, the air can travel into the coronary arteries causing acute myocardial ischemia [44]. Considering the right coronary artery ostia is anterior when compared to the left coronary ostia; this air preferentially causes ischemia in the right coronary artery distribution resulting in right ventricular failure and inferior wall motion abnormalities.

TEE will demonstrate inferior wall motion abnormalities and a dilated right ventricle with reduced right ventricular function. Rarely, air can be seen in the coronary artery or myocardial wall.

Considering the involvement of the right coronary artery and the timing of cardiovascular collapse (immediately following patient turning), the most likely cause is air embolism due to retained intracardiac air. Treatment primarily involves increasing blood pressure with norepinephrine to increase coronary perfusion and allow time for air resorption. Pulmonary vascular resistance should be optimized with avoidance of hypercarbia, hypoxia, pain, and hypothermia. Temporarily inotropic support with epinephrine may be required as well.

Question 27

Over the next 12-h the patient continued to improve and vasopressor infusions were weaned. However, on postoperative day one, the patient's blood pressure began to fall and vasopressors were reinitiated. The following vitals are recorded.

Time	14:30	15:30	16:30	17:30
Blood pressure (mmHg)	99/55 (76)	90/60 (70)	80/60 (67)	70/55 (60)
Heart rate (bpm)	80	86	98	105
CVP (mmHg)	8	10	14	16
Cardiac index (L/min/m^2)	2.4	2.1	1.7	1.1
SvO_2 (%)	80	70	55	40
NE (μg/min)	0	2	6	12
Lactate (mmol/L)	1.3	2.4	3.2	4.5

Breath sounds are equal bilaterally. There is no evidence of pulsus paradoxus. A TEE probe is placed to evaluate the patient's undifferentiated shock (Video 8.2) (Fig. 8.41).

What is the next step in management?

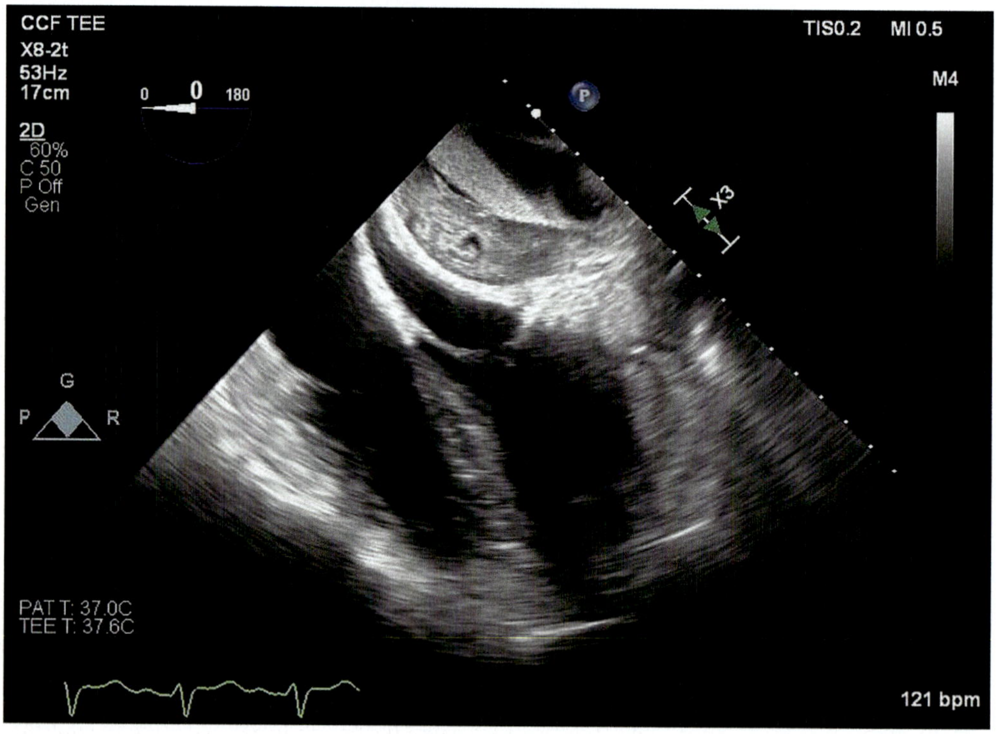

Fig. 8.41 Midesophageal four-chamber view

A. Pericardiocentesis
B. Call cardiac surgery for emergent sternotomy
C. Add vasopressin
D. Add phenylephrine

Answer B. This patient has acute postoperative cardiac tamponade and needs emergent sternotomy.

Postoperative cardiac tamponade occurs in 0.2–8.4% of patients after cardiac surgery [45]. Tamponade is more common after valvular procedures and transplantation than coronary bypass grafting and is typically regional rather than circumferential. Tamponade most commonly involves regional compression of the right atrium with or without compression of the right ventricle. Left-sided regional tamponade occurs less frequently.

Tamponade most commonly presents with signs of decreased cardiac output, hypotension, and tachycardia [46]. Any patient with increasing central venous pressure in the setting of reduced cardiac output and increased lactate concentrations should be evaluated for cardiac tamponade. Transthoracic echocardiography is difficult to use in the perioperative period due to mediastinal air and surgical dressings. As a result, TEE is the confirmatory modality of choice. TEE will demonstrate localized blood or thrombus compressing a cardiac chamber. The classic hemodynamic and echocardiographic signs may be missing in patients with regional tamponade following cardiac surgery.

This patient has evidence of cardiogenic shock with increasing central venous pressure, reduced cardiac output and mixed venous oxygen saturation, as well as increasing vasopressor requirement and lactate concentration. TEE confirmed the presence of regional cardiac tamponade and the patient should undergo emergent re-sternotomy to evaluate blood or thrombus and identify any sources of bleeding [47]. Pericardiocentesis may help temporize an acute cardiac tamponade; however, the blood appears to be thrombosed in this TEE image, and therefore pericardiocentesis would be of no benefit.

Use the following stem for Questions 28–30. A 62-year-old woman with a history of severe COPD is admitted to MICU with pneumonia and septic shock. She was intubated in the emergency department for respiratory distress. A left sided central venous catheter is placed and a norepinephrine infusion (4 μg/min) is started to maintain a mean arterial pressure greater than 65 mmHg. Her hypoxemia worsens (SpO_2 88%) despite a FiO_2 of 100% and 14 mmHg of PEEP. A TEE probe is placed. What view is shown? (Fig. 8.42).

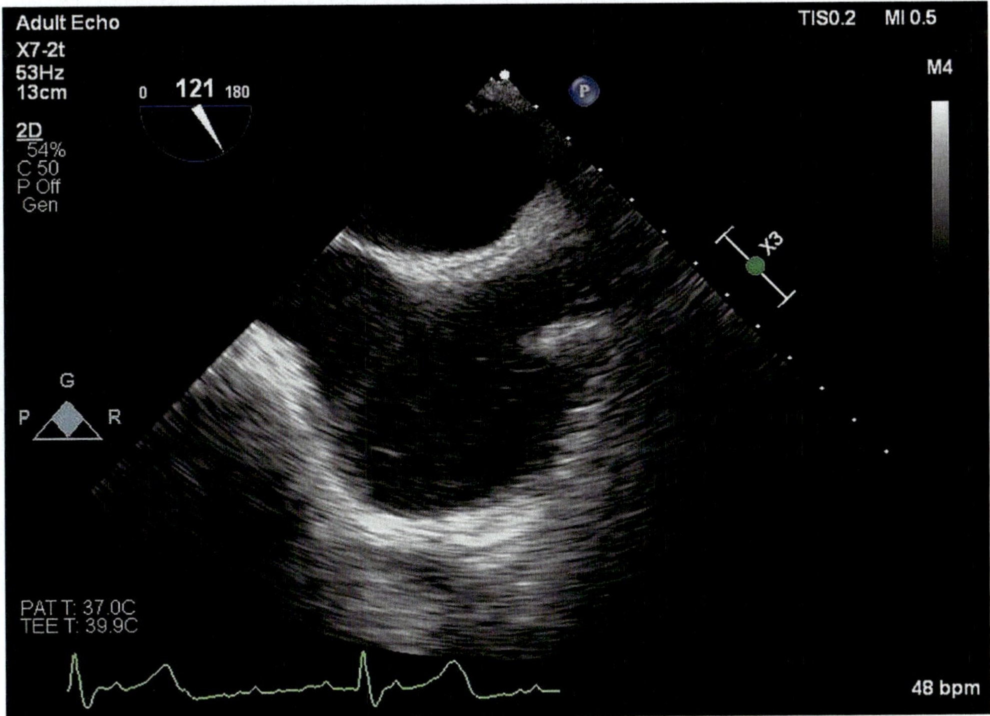

Fig. 8.42 TEE view

Question 28
Which TEE view is shown?

A. Midesophageal ascending aorta short axis view
B. Midesophageal bicaval view
C. Midesophageal right atrial view
D. Transgastric right ventricular inflow view

Answer B. Midesophageal bicaval view.

The midesophageal bicaval view is found by rotating the omniplane to 90–110° from any midesophageal view and turning the probe clockwise (or to the right) [1]. As in any midesophageal view, the left atrium is closest to the TEE probe with the interatrial septum and right atrium in the far-field. The superior vena cava is seen to the right as it enters the right atrium. The inferior vena cava is seen to the left. This view is ideal for the evaluation of the interatrial septum.

Question 29
The following TEE image is obtained. Her oxygen saturation falls to 84%. Given the following settings and values, what is the next best step in management? (Fig. 8.43)

Ventilatory	Arterial blood gas	TEE
FiO_2 100% Tidal volume 8 mL/kg (IBW) Respiratory rate 18 breaths/min PEEP 14 mmHg	PaO_2 50 mmHg $PaCO_2$ 65 mmHg Lactate 3.5 mmol/L	RVSP 65 mmHg

IBW ideal body weight, *PEEP* positive end-expiratory pressure, *RVSP* right ventricular systolic pressure

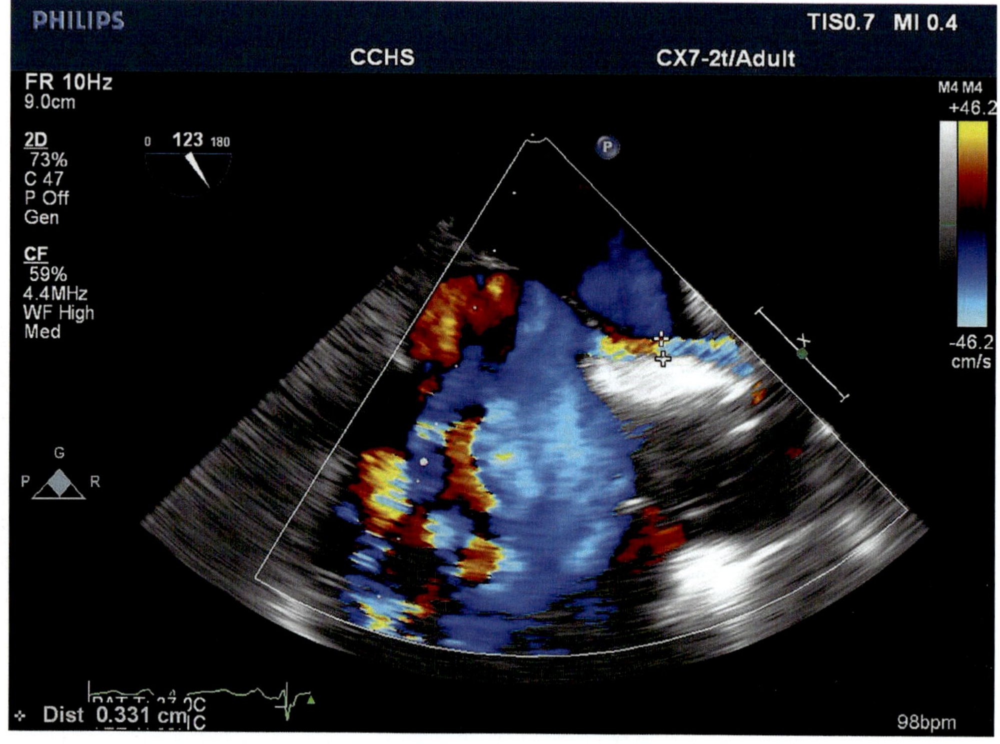

Fig. 8.43 TEE view with color flow Doppler interrogation

A. Venovenous extracorporeal membrane oxygenation support
B. Inhaled epoprostenol
C. Increase PEEP
D. Reduce tidal volume

Answer B. Inhaled epoprostenol.

This patient has a right-to-left shunt resulting in persistent hypoxemia despite an escalation in FiO2. A patent foramen ovale is present in up to 30% of the population and can cause right-to-left shunting in patients with increased right-sided cardiac pressures [48]. This patient likely has increased right-sided cardiac pressures due to hypoxemia and hypercarbia mediated increases in pulmonary vascular resistance and right ventricular afterload. Furthermore, intubation and mechanical ventilation, as well as high levels of PEEP, increase right ventricular afterload by increasing intrathoracic pressures [49]. This can increase right atrial pressure and cause right-to-left shunting in patients with a PFO.

Management of a patient with right-to-left shunting through a PFO involves reducing right atrial pressure [50]. This can be accomplished with reductions in pulmonary vascular resistance. Hypoxemia and hypercarbia should be avoided, and intrathoracic pressures should be minimized. Increasing PEEP will increase intrathoracic pressures further. Reducing the tidal volume will decrease minute ventilation and cause an increase in $PaCO_2$, which will increase her pulmonary vascular resistance. Inhaled epoprostenol will allow for reduced pulmonary arterial pressures and a reduction in right ventricular afterload. This will reduce right atrial pressure and may reduce or eliminate the shunting. Venovenous extracorporeal membrane oxygenation support may be required if hypoxemia worsens despite right ventricular afterload reduction measures. While these interventions may temporarily improve the patient's right-to-left shunting, a cardiology consult may be warranted for potential PFO closure.

Question 30

Following the chest X-ray for central line placement, the radiologist calls and notes the central line may be located in the aorta; however, a venous tracing is seen on the monitor. The following TEE view was obtained on her previous examination (Fig. 8.44).

Where is the central line most likely positioned?

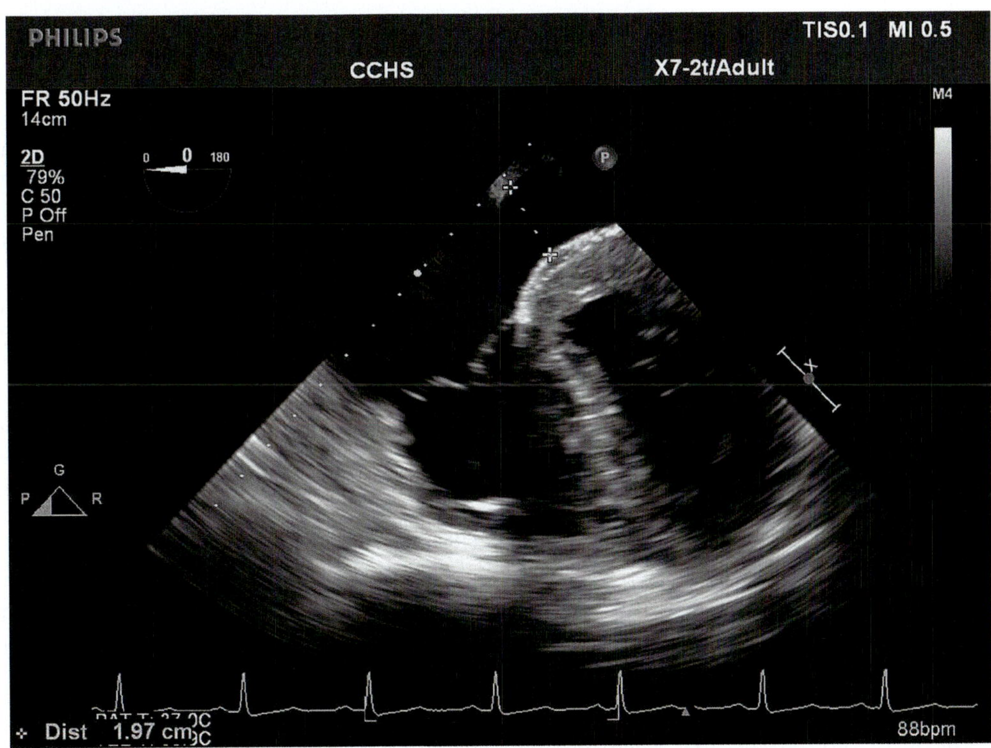

Fig. 8.44 Midesophageal TEE view

A. Brachiocephalic vein
B. Azygous vein
C. Persistent left superior vena cava
D. Aorta

Answer C. A dilated coronary sinus is consistent with a persistent left sided superior vena cava.

Persistent left-sided superior vena cava is the most common venous congenital anomaly and may be present in up to 0.5% of the population [51]. The left-sided SVC drains into the coronary sinus resulting in dilated (>1 cm) coronary sinus [52]. This diagnosis can be confirmed with echocardiography and a left-sided bubble study. During a left-sided bubble study, agitated saline is injected into an intravenous line in the patient's left arm. Identification of agitated saline entering the coronary sinus before the left atrium is diagnostic of a persistent left SVC. Left-sided central venous line placement in patients with persistent left SVC may appear as though the catheter is placed in the aorta.

Question 31

A 34-year-old male with a history of heroin abuse presents with new-onset left-sided facial droop, fever (38.9 °C), and tachycardia. Computed tomography imaging of the brain demonstrates a small acute stroke. Blood cultures are drawn and empiric antibiotics are started. TTE views are inadequate to rule out endocarditis and a TEE exam is performed. A TEE exam is performed and images are presented (Video 8.3 and Fig. 8.45). In this patient, which of the following findings would allow for a diagnosis infective endocarditis according to the modified Duke criteria?

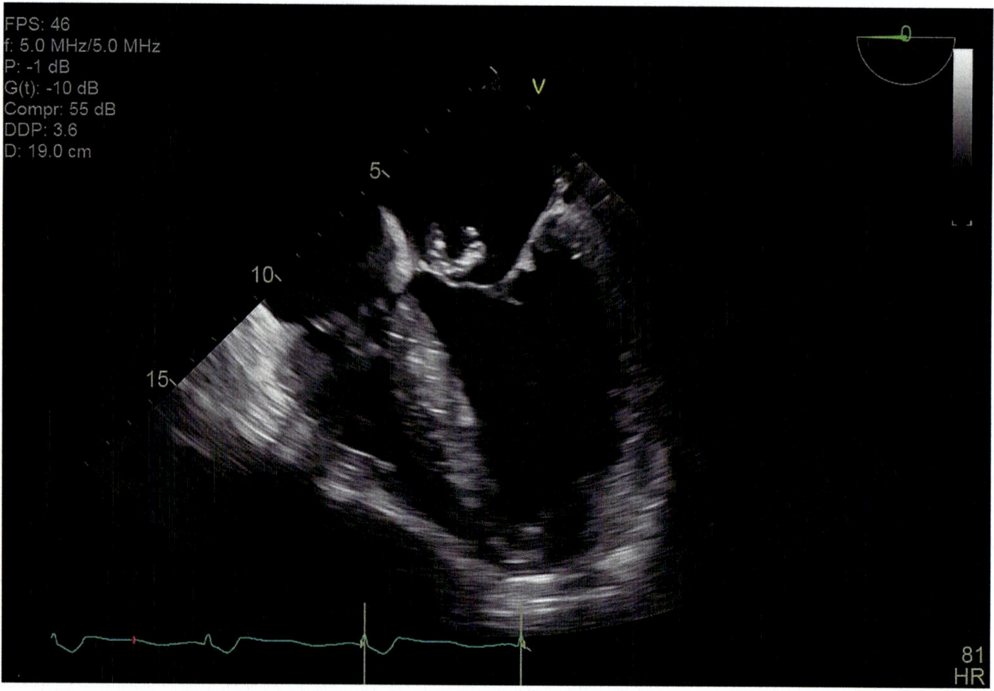

Fig. 8.45 Midesophageal four-chamber view demonstrating a mass on the anterior leaflet of the mitral valve

A. Two positive blood cultures
B. No additional criteria required
C. Glomerulonephritis
D. Conjunctival hemorrhages

Answer B. This patient has one major (TEE evidence of vegetation) and three minor (temperature > 38 °C, arterial emboli, intravenous drug abuse) modified Duke criteria, which fulfills the requirement for a diagnosis of infective endocarditis.

The diagnostic criteria for infective endocarditis are the modified Duke criteria, which is composed of major and minor criteria [53, 54]. In order for a definite diagnosis of infective endocarditis, the patient must have direct pathologic evidence of infective endocarditis, two major criteria, one major and three minor criteria, or five minor criteria. The major criteria include blood culture evidence (two separate positive blood cultures of a typical organism, persistently positive blood cultures, or a single positive blood culture for Coxiella burnetti) and evidence of endocardial involvement (oscillating intracardiac mass, abscess, new valvular regurgitation, or new prosthetic valve dehiscence). There are five minor criteria: a predisposing heart condition or intravenous drug abuse, fever (temperature > 38 °C), microbiologic evidence of infection which does not meet major criteria, vascular phenomena, and immunologic phenomena. Vascular phenomena can include arterial embolism, conjunctival or intracranial hemorrhages, pulmonary infarction, Janeway lesions, and mycotic aneurysms. Immunologic phenomena include Roth spots, Osler nodes, a positive rheumatoid factor, and glomerulonephritis.

Question 32

Which of the following is an indication for medical management of infective endocarditis?

A. Aortic root abscess
B. Fungal endocarditis
C. Bacteremia >3 days after initiation of antibiotics
D. New onset complete heart block

Answer C. Persistent bacteremia >5–7 days after initiation of antibiotics is an indication for surgery.

The decision on whether to operate on patients with infective endocarditis is complex and depends on a multitude of factors [55]. Thus, it is important to involve infectious disease and cardiac surgery in the evaluation of these patients. In 2016, the American Heart Association published a scientific statement endorsed by the Infective Diseases Society of America, which outlined the management of these patients [54]. Class 1 recommendations include early surgery in patients with valve dysfunction resulting in heart failure, infective endocarditis caused by fungi or highly virulent bacteria, mechanical cardiac complications (such as heart block, fistula, penetrating lesions, or abscesses), and persistent infection (>5–7 days after initiation of antibiotics). Additional recommendations (not Class I) support early surgery in patients with recurrent emboli, enlarging vegetations, and large vegetations (>10 mm). It is important to note these recommendations are similar for prosthetic valve endocarditis.

Question 33

A 64-year-old male with a history of a bioprosthetic aortic valve replacement presents with fevers and chills. Blood cultures are positive for Streptococcus salivarius and a TEE is performed. The following TEE image and video (Video 8.4 and Figs. 8.46 and 8.47) demonstrates which of the following complications of infective endocarditis?

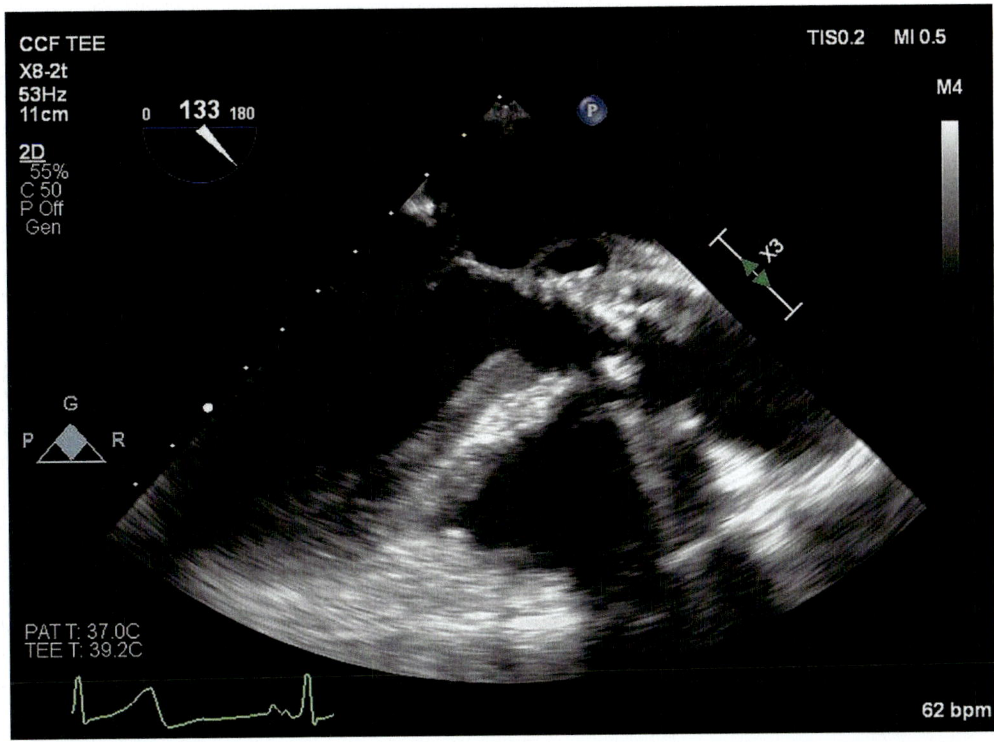

Fig. 8.46 Midesophageal long axis view demonstrating a complication of infective endocarditis

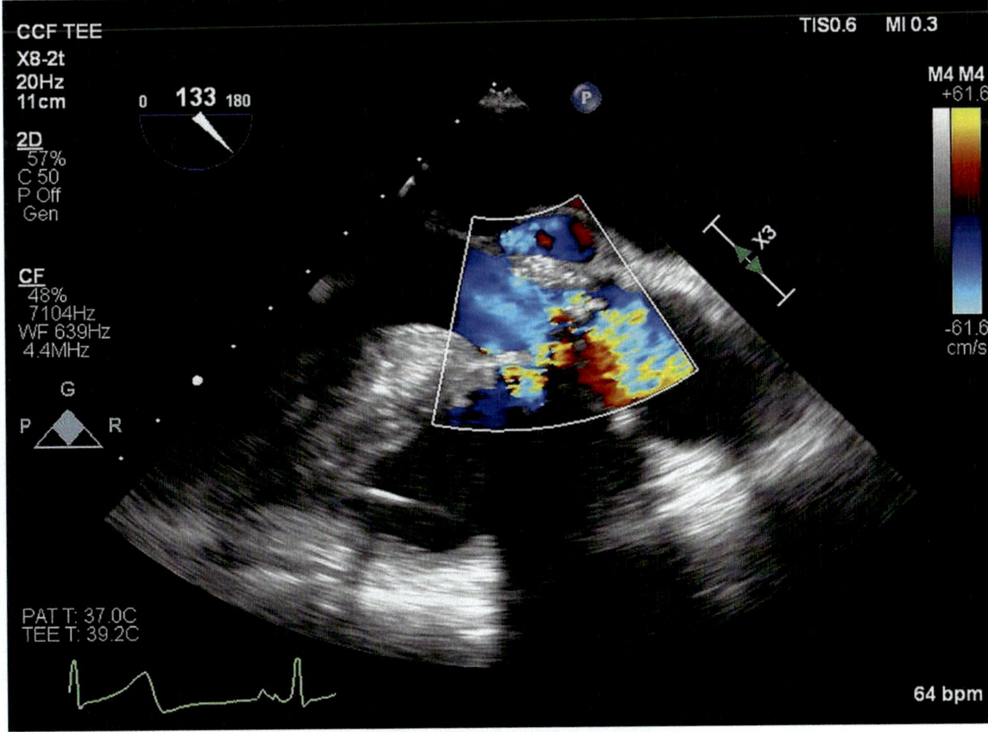

Fig. 8.47 Midesophageal long axis view with color flow Doppler demonstrating a complication of infective endocarditis

A. Mitral regurgitation
B. Aortic regurgitation
C. Aortic root abscess
D. Gerbode defect

Answer C. These midesophageal long axis views demonstrate a hypoechoic fluid filled structure posterior to the aortic valve. This structure experiences turbulent blood flow during systole consistent with an aortic root abscess.

Endocarditis can lead to complications such as valvular regurgitation, paravalvular abscess, valvular perforations, aneurysms, pseudoaneurysms, and fistula formation [56]. Destruction of the valvular apparatus can lead to flail, prolapse, or perforations in the leaflet tissue. This leads to acute severe valvular regurgitation, which typically presents with heart failure symptoms. Abscesses can form near valve structures as well. Staphylococcus aureus is the most common organism associated with intracardiac abscess formation and the aortic valve is the most common valve involved. Abscesses can lead to pseudoaneuerysm formation or fistulous communications. Fistula may occur between any two cardiac chambers involved in infective endocarditis. The Gerbode defect is described as a fistulous communication between the left ventricle and the right atrium [57]. Fistulae between the sinus of Valsalva and the right atrium have been reported as well.

Use the following stem for Questions 34–35. A 46-year-old male with a history of a mechanical mitral valve replacement for rheumatic heart disease presents to the emergency department with respiratory distress, atrial fibrillation, and jugular venous distention. His oxygen saturation is 82% on room air and his chest X-ray demonstrates bilateral pulmonary edema. He recently starting taking over the counter St. John's Worts for depression.

Question 34

What is the most likely diagnosis?

A. Prosthetic valve dehiscence
B. Prosthetic valve thrombosis
C. Prosthetic valve regurgitation
D. Prosthetic valve endocarditis

Answer B. Prosthetic valve thrombosis. He is presenting with heart failure symptoms due to left sided valvular disease. Concomitant St Johns Wort and warfarin use will lower INR thus substantially increasing the risk of thrombosis.

Current guidelines recommendations suggest anticoagulation with vitamin K antagonist for all patients with mechanical aortic and mitral valves [58, 59]. Patients with mechanical mitral valves should target an INR goal of 2.5–3.5. Patients with a mechanical aortic valve and no other risk factors for thromboembolism should target an INR between 2.0–3.0 and those with additional risk factors (atrial fibrillation, left ventricular dysfunction, hypercoagulable states) should target an INR between 2.5–3.5. In addition, aspirin (75–100 mg) is recommended in addition to a vitamin K antagonist. In addition, due to an increased risk of early thromboembolism in patients with bioprosthetic valves, anticoagulation with a vitamin K antagonist is described as reasonable for the first 3–6 months. It is important to note that patients with a particular type of mechanical aortic valve, the On-X valve, can target an INR of 1.5–2.0 if no other thromboembolic risk factors are present. An example of a mechanical mitral valve thrombus is presented in Fig. 8.48 and Video 8.5.

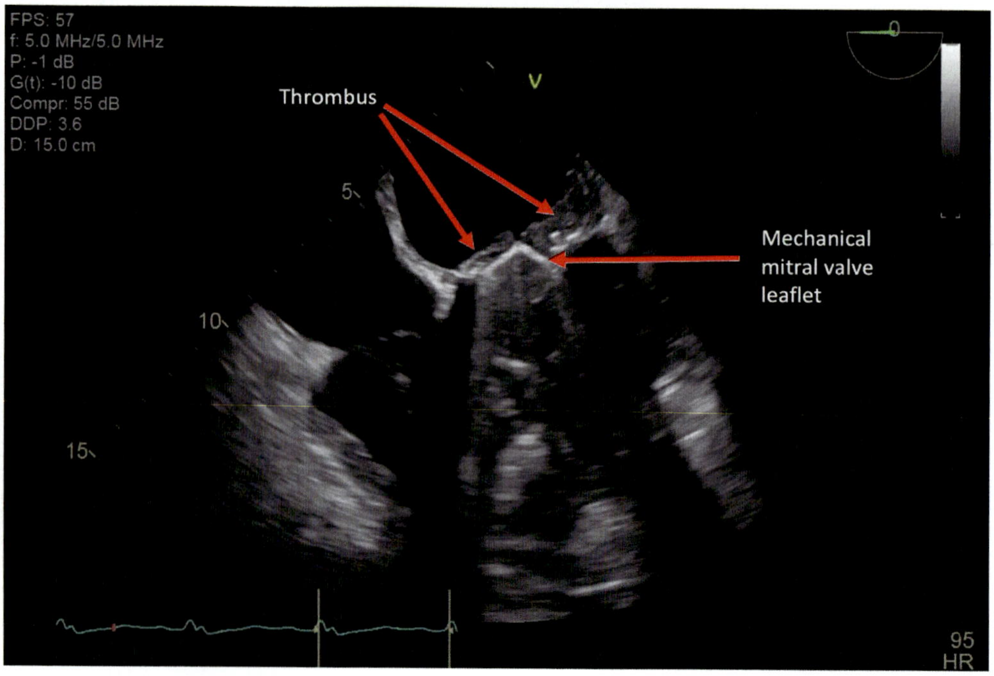

Fig. 8.48 Midesophageal four-chamber view of a patient with a mechanical mitral valve thrombus

There exists a multitude of medications that interfere with the metabolism and action of warfarin. Carbamazepine, Ribavirin, Trazodone, Barbiturates, Cholestyramine, mesalamine, rifampin, and St John's wort all inhibit warfarin activity and result in a lower than expected INR [60]. Considering this patient recently started self-medication with an over the counter medication, St John's wort, his INR is likely subtherapeutic and the cause of her symptoms is most likely mechanical mitral valve thrombosis causing mitral stenosis.

Question 35
Which of the following would be suggestive of significant mechanical mitral valve stenosis?

A. Peak velocity 1.9 m/s
B. Mean gradient 7 mmHg
C. VTI_{PrMV}/VTI_{LVOT} 2.8
D. Pressure half time (PHT) 180 ms

VTI, velocity time integral. PrMV, prosthetic mitral valve. LVOT, left ventricular outflow tract.

Answer C. A VTI (prosthetic mitral valve)/VTI (LVOT) ratio of greater than 2.5 suggests significant mechanical mitral valve stenosis.

Values for stenosis and regurgitation cutoffs for native valves are not always translatable to prosthetic valves. These values are validated only in patients with native valves. As a result, the American Society of Echocardiography, in collaboration with numerous other societies, published recommendations for the evaluation of patients with prosthetic valves [61]. There are five parameters for evaluation of prosthetic

Table 8.5 Recommendations for grading prosthetic mitral valve stenosis

	Normal	Potential stenosis	Significant stenosis
Mean gradient (mmHg)	≤5	6–10	>10
PHT (ms)	<130	130–200	>200
Peak E wave velocity (m/s)	<1.9	1.9–2.4	≥2.5
EOA (cm^2)	≥2.0	1–2	<1.0
VTI_{PrMV}/VTI_{LVOT}	<2.2	2.2–2.5	>2.5

PHT pressure half time, *EOA* effective orifice area, *VTI* velocity time integral, *PrMV* prosthetic mitral valve, *LVOT* left ventricular outflow tract

mitral valve stenosis: mean gradient, pressure half time, peak E wave velocity, effective orifice area, and VTI ratio (Table 8.5).

It is important to note that the mitral valve area equation, which utilizes the pressure half time (220/PHT), was validated for patients with rheumatic mitral stenosis and may not hold for patients with other conditions [62]. When using this equation, associated moderate to severe mitral regurgitation tends to over-estimate the mitral valve area and moderate to severe aortic regurgitation tends to under-estimate the mitral valve area. The number 200 should be used for calculating prosthetic valve area with PHT.

Question 36
In the following midesophageal image, what is identified by the arrows (Fig. 8.49)?

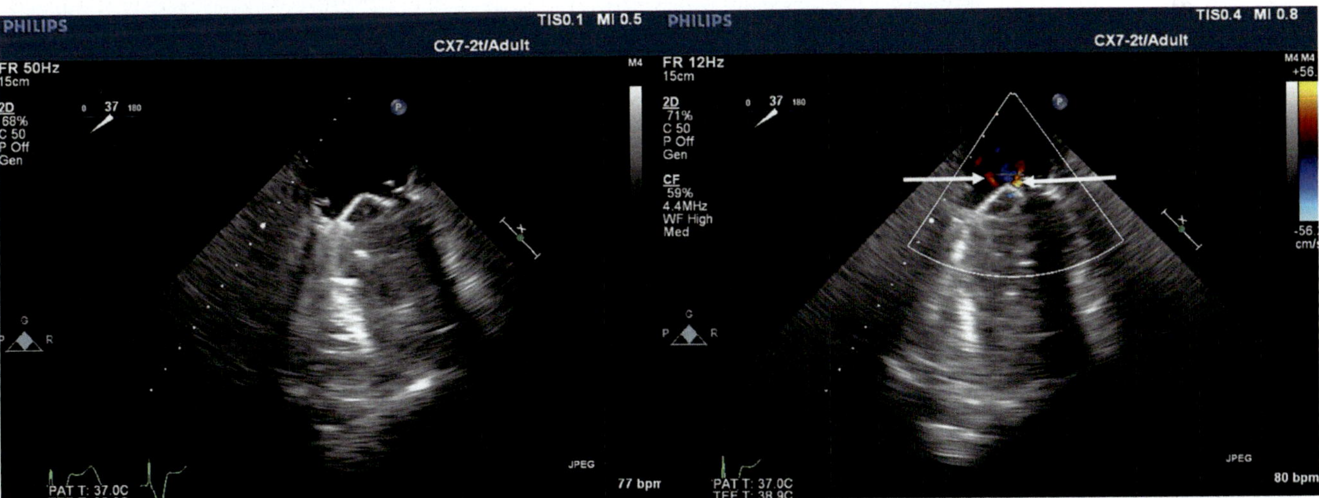

Fig. 8.49 Midesophageal view of a patient with a mechanical mitral valve. Two-dimensional imaging on the left and color flow Doppler on the right

A. Paravalvular leak
B. Intravalvular mitral regurgitation
C. Normal washing jets
D. Mitral stenosis

Answer C. Washing jets are a normal phenomenon noted on echocardiography in patients with mechanical valves.

This is an example of normal physiologic jets that occur with mechanical valves, termed "washing jets." They are typically directed away from the center [61]. In this modified midesophageal view, two red jets are seen directed away from the center of this bileaflet mechanical mitral valve [63]. These jets are considered normal and do not need to be interrogated further.

Question 37

A 53-year-old male with a history of interstitial lung disease was placed on venovenous (VV) extracorporeal membrane oxygenation (ECMO) with a right internal jugular double lumen cannula at an outside hospital due to hypoxia and acute clinical deterioration. He was transferred to CVICU to be listed for lung transplantation. Overnight, the patient was stable with ECMO flows at 4 L/min, sweep at 4 L/min, oxygen saturation >92%, and acceptable arterial blood gas values (pH = 7.35, $PaCO_2$ = 44 mmHg, PaO_2 = 65 mmHg). Upon lightening sedation in the morning, the patient became tachycardic and tachypneic. His oxygen saturation dropped to 70%. The ECMO specialist increased the flow to 6 L/min, however, patient remained hypoxemic. Due to concern regarding the cannula position, a TEE was performed (Fig. 8.50). Which of the following is true?

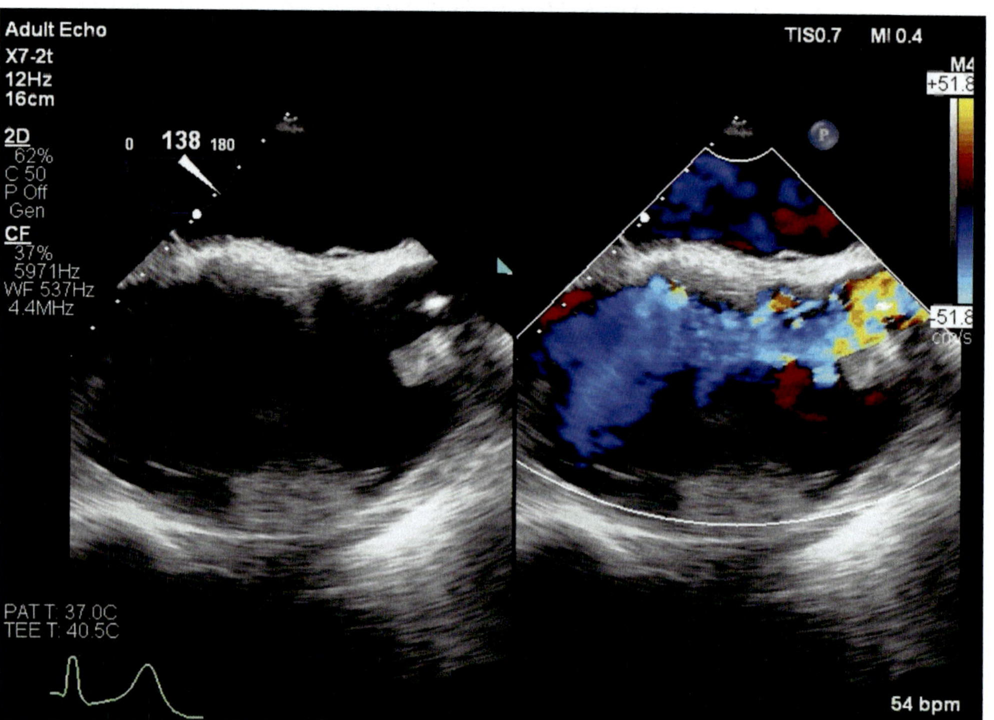

Fig. 8.50 Midesophageal bicaval view with a two-dimensional image on the left and a color flow Doppler image on the right

A. The cannula needs to be advanced and the outflow port should be positioned in the right atrium facing towards tricuspid valve
B. The cannula needs to be pulled back until the lower inflow port is in right atrium to allow for better drainage
C. This is not the ideal view to visualize the cannula position as a midesophageal aortic valve long axis view allows better interrogation of the cannula
D. The patient needs an additional imaging modality (i.e. CXR) to make the decision.

Answer A. The outflow port of the double lumen VV ECMO cannula should be in the right atrium directing blood flow toward the tricuspid valve.

The cannula needs to be advanced with TEE and fluoroscopic guidance to ensure that the return/outflow port is in right atrium is facing the tricuspid valve. In the figure, note the turbulence in the superior vena cava suggesting the return/outflow port is too high and needs to be advanced and repositioned. Malposition of the double lumen ECMO cannula can result in increased recirculation and decreased efficiency of the ECMO circuit. The optimal positioning requires TEE and fluoroscopic guidance during placement. TEE can help to confirm the proper cannula position after insertion if there is any question of abnormal positioning or functioning of the cannula [64]. The midesophageal bicaval view can help identify the return/outflow port with color Doppler and ensure that flow is directed toward the tricuspid valve. When properly positioned, the amount of recirculation with double lumen ECMO cannula is <2%.

Question 38

Which structure is labeled by the Asterix (Fig. 8.51)?

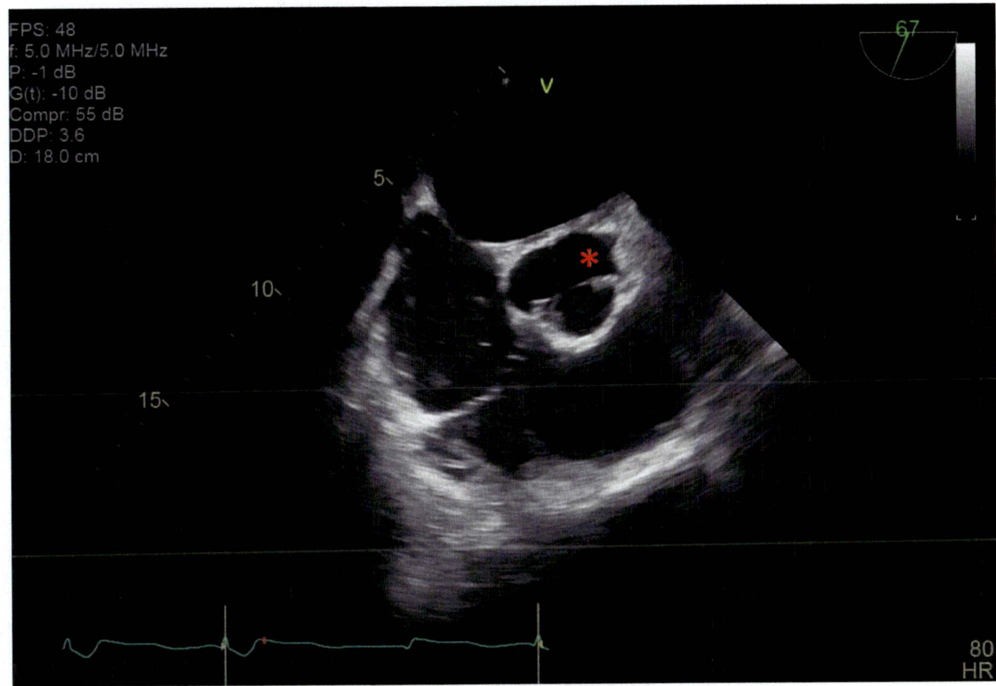

Fig. 8.51 Midesophageal aortic valve short axis view

A. Left coronary cusp
B. Right coronary cusp
C. Noncoronary cusp
D. Anterior coronary cusp

Answer A. The left coronary cusp is indicated by the Asterix.

This is a midesophageal aortic valve short axis view demonstrating all three aortic valve cusps. Note the difference in orientation between transthoracic and transesophageal views. The noncoronary cusp is always adjacent to the interatrial septum. The right coronary cusp is adjacent to the right ventricle. In this image the right coronary cusp is the furthest from the probe. The remaining cusp is the left coronary cusp [1].

In the midesophageal long axis view, the coronary cusps can be identified as well. The right coronary cusp is the cusp furthest from the probe. The cusp closest to the probe is either the left or noncoronary cusp. In the midesophageal aortic valve short axis view, imagine drawing a line directly from the probe downward through the center of the aortic valve. This line represents the orthogonal view—the midesophageal long axis view. Notice how the line bisects the right coronary cusp. This identifies the cusp furthest from the probe as the right coronary cusp in both the midesophageal long axis and aortic valve short axis views.

Question 39

A 33-year-old female with a history of morbid obesity, asthma, and rheumatoid arthritis is admitted to the medical intensive care unit with shortness of breath, hypotension, and tachycardia. She is intubated due to respiratory distress. Her lactate is 3.8 mmol/L. Two liters of lactated ringer are administered as blood cultures are drawn and empiric antibiotics are started. Despite fluid resuscitation, her blood pressure continues to fall and a norepinephrine infusion is required. Due to poor TTE windows, a TEE probe is placed (Figs. 8.52 and 8.53).

What would be the most likely finding on TEE in the setting of cardiac tamponade in this patient?

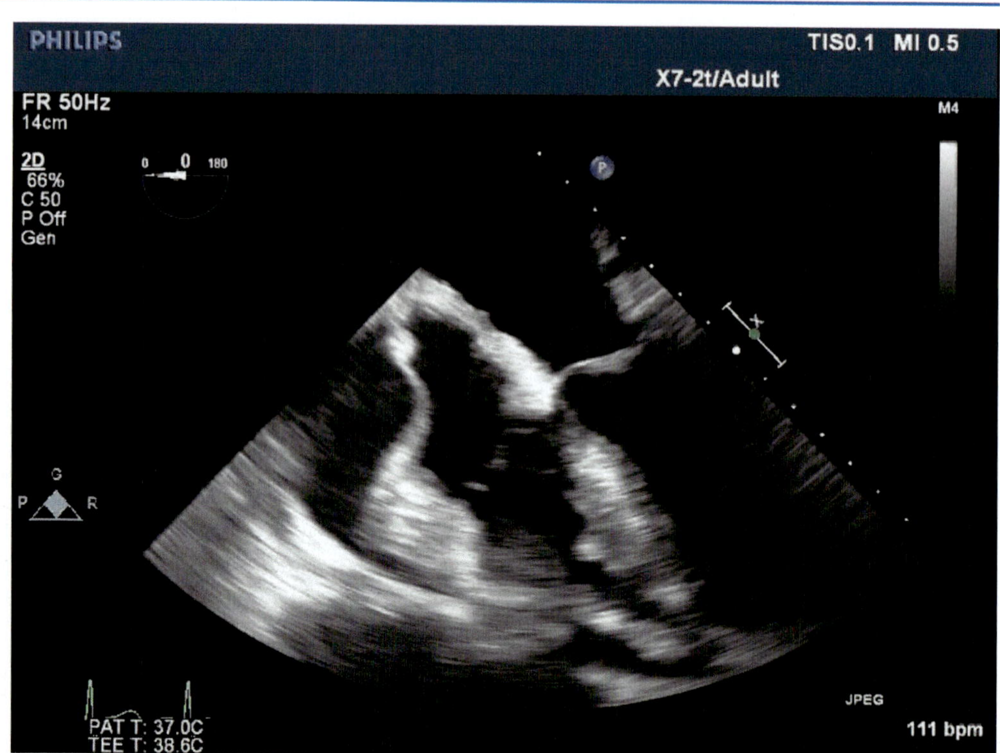

Fig. 8.52 Midesophageal four-chamber view

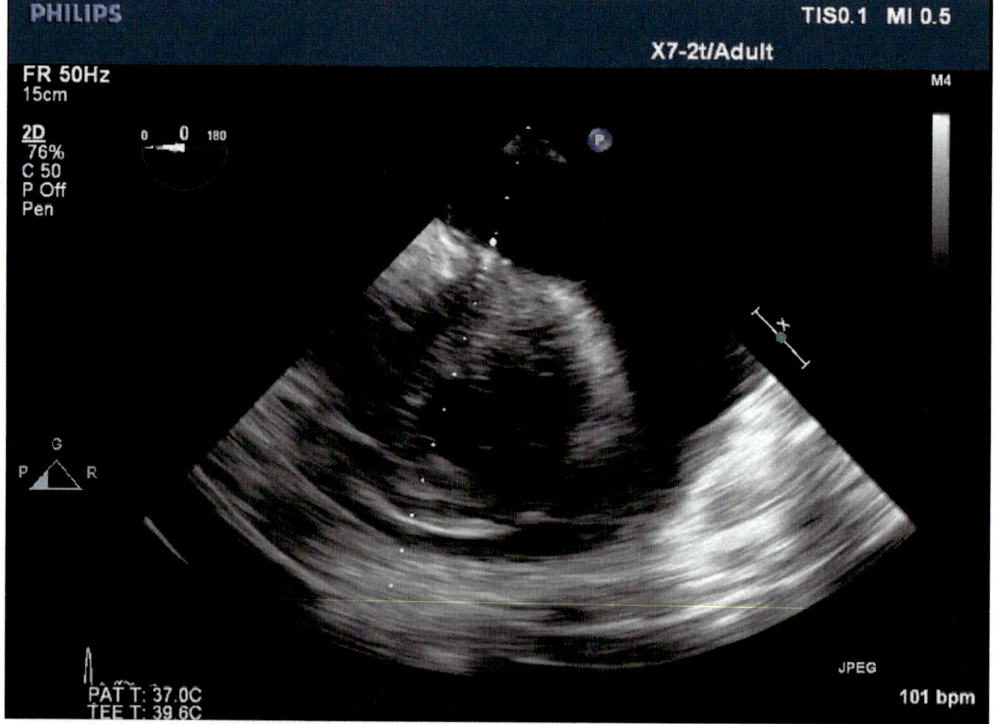

Fig. 8.53 Transgastric short axis view

A. Systolic right atrial collapse
B. Systolic right ventricular collapse
C. Respiratory variation in mitral inflow velocities >45%
D. Respiratory variation in tricuspid inflow velocities >650%

Answer A. Systolic right atrial collapse is a sensitive sign of cardiac tamponade.

In circumferential cardiac tamponade, the intracardiac fluid and pericardial fluid volume become fixed resulting in compression of the cardiac chambers and exaggerated ventricular interdependence. Due to the increased pericardial pressures, cardiac chambers will be compressed most significantly when their pressures are at their lowest during the cardiac cycle. Right atrial pressures are typically lowest during late diastole and systole and as a result, late diastolic or systolic compression of the right atrium is a sensitive echocardiographic sign of cardiac tamponade (Video 8.6) [65]. The right atrial inversion time index is a ratio of the duration of inversion to the entire cardiac cycle. Values greater than 0.34 have high specificity for the diagnosis of cardiac tamponade. Right ventricular collapse occurs during early to mid-diastole in patients with cardiac tamponade.

Exaggerated ventricular interdependence also occurs during cardiac tamponade resulting in increased blood flow to the right heart and increased blood flow to the left heart during inspiration with the reverse occurring during expiration [66]. The opposite occurs during mechanical ventilation. Utilizing Doppler echocardiography, tricuspid and mitral inflow velocities and their variation can be measured during the respiratory cycle. Tricuspid inflow velocity variation of 45% and mitral velocity variation of 25% is considered significant ventricular interdependence. This exaggerated ventricular interdependence is blunted during mechanical ventilation and therefore less accurately measured with TEE.

Question 40

A TEE image of the descending thoracic aorta is displayed (Fig. 8.54). What is the severity grade of aortic atherosclerosis?

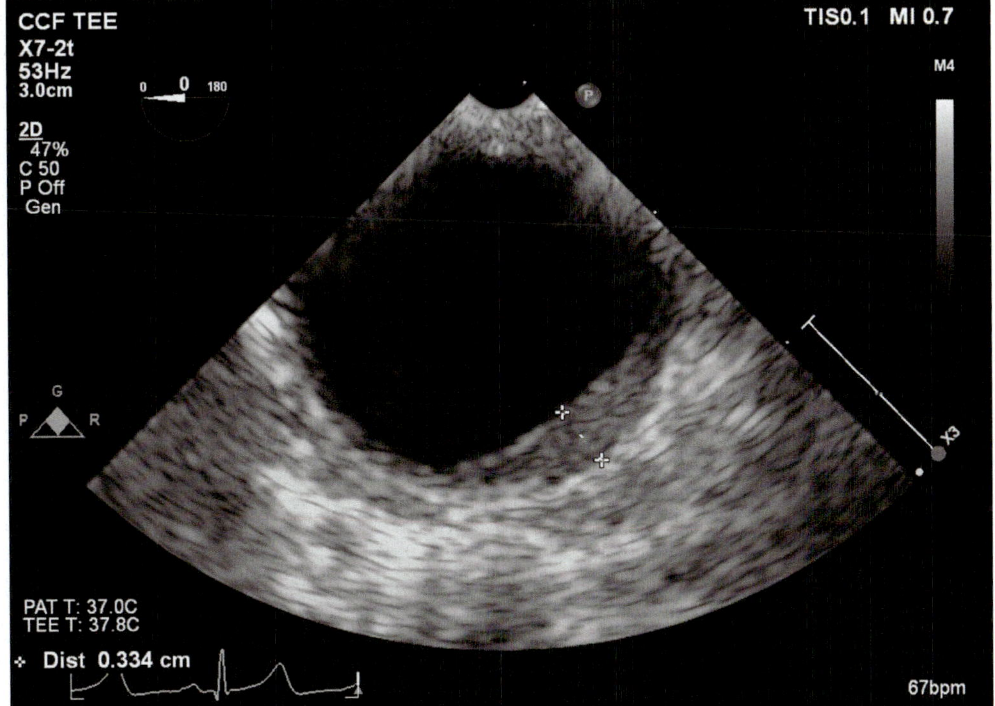

Fig. 8.54 Descending thoracic aorta short axis view demonstrating aortic atherosclerosis

A. Grade 1
B. Grade 2
C. Grade 3
D. Grade 4
E. Grade 5

Answer C. Grade 3.

According to American Society of Echocardiography guidelines, atherosclerotic plaques of the descending aorta are graded from grade 1 to grade 5 depending on the severity [67]. Grade 1 is normal, with an intimal thickness <2 mm. Grade 2 is mild, with an intimal thickness of 2–3 mm. Grade 3 is moderate, with an intimal thickness of 3–5 mm. Grade 4 is severe, with an intimal thickness >5 mm with no mobile components. Grade 5 represents complex atheroma and is composed of grades 2 through 4 with a mobile or ulcerated component.

Aortic atheromas have been associated with an increased risk of cerebral and systemic embolic events. Plaque features that represent and increased risk for embolization are a plaque thickness greater than 4 mm often with an irregular surface, ulceration, or a mobile component.

Question 41

Which of the following views is presented below (Fig. 8.55)?

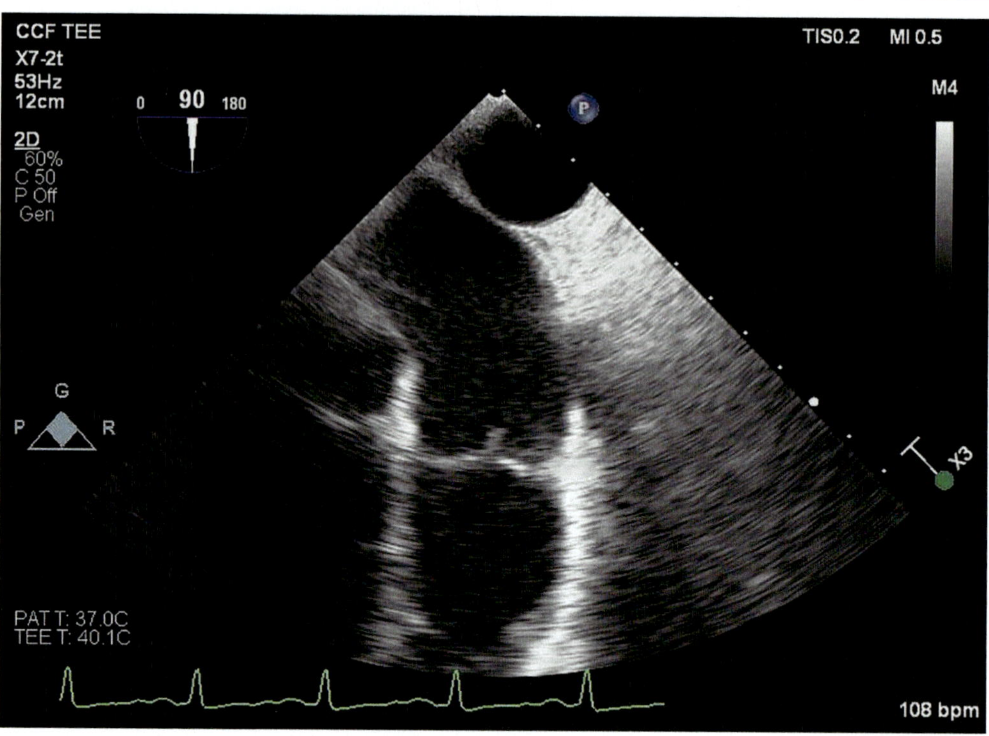

Fig. 8.55 TEE view

A. Upper esophageal aortic arch short axis
B. Upper esophageal aortic arch long axis
C. Upper esophageal pulmonary artery long axis
D. Upper esophageal pulmonic valve long axis

Answer A. This is the upper esophageal aortic arch short axis view.

After imaging the descending aorta, follow the aorta up to the left subclavian artery. Just proximal to the left subclavian artery (at an omniplane of zero degrees) turn the probe to the right (clockwise) to image the aortic arch long axis view. This should appear as a long axis view of the aorta from the center of the display near the probe and extending to the left of the screen. From this view, increase the depth and rotate the omniplane forward toward 90°. This should bring the pulmonary artery and pulmonic valve into view as well as the short axis of the aortic arch [1]. This view is useful for measuring the right ventricular outflow tract diameter as well as for using Doppler to evaluate the pulmonic valve [68]. This view is difficult to attain in many patients and may be impossible to attain in some.

References

1. Hahn RT, Abraham T, Adams MS, Bruce CJ, Glas KE, Lang RM, Reeves ST, Shanewise JS, Siu SC, Stewart W, Picard MH. Guidelines for performing a comprehensive transesophageal echocardiographic examination: recommendations from the American Society of Echocardiography and the Society of Cardiovascular Anesthesiologists. J Am Soc Echocardiogr. 2013;26(9):921–64.
2. Cote G, Denault A. Transesophageal echocardiography-related complications. Can J Anaesth. 2008;55(9):622–47.
3. Seo YS. Prevention and management of gastroesophageal varices. Clin Mol Hepatol. 2018;24(1):20–42.
4. Nigatu A, Yap JE, Lee Chuy K, Go B, Doukky R. Bleeding risk of transesophageal echocardiography in patients with esophageal varices. J Am Soc Echocardiogr. 2019;32(5):674–6 e2.
5. Kelava M, Koprivanac M, Alfirevic A, Geube M, Hargrave J. Safety of transesophageal echocardiography for cardiac surgery in patients with histories of bariatric surgery. J Am Soc Echocardiogr. 2020;33(1):130–2.
6. Hilberath JN, Oakes DA, Shernan SK, Bulwer BE, D'Ambra MN, Eltzschig HK. Safety of transesophageal echocardiography. J Am Soc Echocardiogr. 2010;23(11):1115–27; quiz 220–1, 1127.
7. Bosch NA, Cimini J, Walkey AJ. Atrial fibrillation in the ICU. Chest. 2018;154(6):1424–34.
8. January CT, Wann LS, Alpert JS, Calkins H, Cigarroa JE, Cleveland JC Jr, Conti JB, Ellinor PT, Ezekowitz MD, Field ME, Murray KT, Sacco RL, Stevenson WG, Tchou PJ, Tracy CM, Yancy CW, American College of Cardiology/American Heart Association Task Force on Practice G. 2014 AHA/ACC/HRS guideline for the management of patients with atrial fibrillation: a report of the American College of Cardiology/American Heart Association task force on practice guidelines and the Heart Rhythm Society. J Am Coll Cardiol. 2014;64(21):e1–76.
9. January CT, Wann LS, Calkins H, Chen LY, Cigarroa JE, Cleveland JC Jr, Ellinor PT, Ezekowitz MD, Field ME, Furie KL, Heidenreich PA, Murray KT, Shea JB, Tracy CM, Yancy CW. 2019 AHA/ACC/HRS focused update of the 2014 AHA/ACC/HRS guideline for the Management of Patients with Atrial Fibrillation: a report of the American College of Cardiology/American Heart Association task force on clinical practice guidelines and the Heart Rhythm Society. J Am Coll Cardiol. 2019;74(1):104–32.
10. Kapoor PM, Muralidhar K, Nanda NC, Mehta Y, Shastry N, Irpachi K, Baloria A. An update on transesophageal echocardiog-

raphy views 2016: 2D versus 3D tee views. Ann Card Anaesth. 2016;19(Supplement):S56–72.
11. Morrissey C. Echo for diastology. Ann Card Anaesth. 2016;19(Supplement):S12–S8.
12. Chao TH, Tsai LM, Tsai WC, Li YH, Lin LJ, Chen JH. Effect of atrial fibrillation on pulmonary venous flow patterns assessed by Doppler transesophageal echocardiography. Chest. 2000;117(6):1546–50.
13. Agmon Y, Khandheria BK, Gentile F, Seward JB. Echocardiographic assessment of the left atrial appendage. J Am Coll Cardiol. 1999;34(7):1867–77.
14. Beigel R, Wunderlich NC, Ho SY, Arsanjani R, Siegel RJ. The left atrial appendage: anatomy, function, and noninvasive evaluation. JACC Cardiovasc Imaging. 2014;7(12):1251–65.
15. Owais K, Mahmood F, Montealegre-Gallegos M, Khabbaz KR, Matyal R. Left atrial appendage, intraoperative echocardiography, and the anesthesiologist. J Cardiothorac Vasc Anesth. 2015;29(6):1651–62.
16. Slama M, Tribouilloy C, Maizel J. Left ventricular outflow tract obstruction in ICU patients. Curr Opin Crit Care. 2016;22(3):260–6.
17. Manabe S, Kasegawa H, Arai H, Takanashi S. Management of systolic anterior motion of the mitral valve: a mechanism-based approach. Gen Thorac Cardiovasc Surg. 2018;66(7):379–89.
18. Anavekar NS, Oh JK. Doppler echocardiography: a contemporary review. J Cardiol. 2009;54(3):347–58.
19. Nampiaparampil RG, Swistel DG, Schlame M, Saric M, Sherrid MV. Intraoperative two- and three-dimensional transesophageal echocardiography in combined myectomy-mitral operations for hypertrophic cardiomyopathy. J Am Soc Echocardiogr. 2018;31(3):275–88.
20. Hiltrop N, Bennett J, Desmet W. Circumflex coronary artery injury after mitral valve surgery: a report of four cases and comprehensive review of the literature. Catheter Cardiovasc Interv. 2017;89(1):78–92.
21. Lang RM, Badano LP, Mor-Avi V, Afilalo J, Armstrong A, Ernande L, Flachskampf FA, Foster E, Goldstein SA, Kuznetsova T, Lancellotti P, Muraru D, Picard MH, Rietzschel ER, Rudski L, Spencer KT, Tsang W, Voigt JU. Recommendations for cardiac chamber quantification by echocardiography in adults: an update from the American Society of Echocardiography and the European Association of Cardiovascular Imaging. Eur Heart J Cardiovasc Imaging. 2015;16(3):233–70.
22. Cartwright BL, Jackson A, Cooper J. Intraoperative pulmonary vein examination by transesophageal echocardiography: an anatomic update and review of utility. J Cardiothorac Vasc Anesth. 2013;27(1):111–20.
23. Fuehner T, Kuehn C, Welte T, Gottlieb J. ICU care before and after lung transplantation. Chest. 2016;150(2):442–50.
24. Evans A, Dwarakanath S, Hogue C, Brady M, Poppers J, Miller S, Weiner MM. Intraoperative echocardiography for patients undergoing lung transplantation. Anesth Analg. 2014;118(4):725–30.
25. MacKnight BM, Maldonado Y, Augoustides JG, Cardenas RA, Patel PA, Ghadimi K, Gutsche JT, Ramakrishna H. Advances in imaging for the management of acute aortic syndromes: focus on transesophageal echocardiography and type-A aortic dissection for the perioperative echocardiographer. J Cardiothorac Vasc Anesth. 2016;30(4):1129–41.
26. Mussa FF, Horton JD, Moridzadeh R, Nicholson J, Trimarchi S, Eagle KA. Acute aortic dissection and intramural hematoma: a systematic review. JAMA. 2016;316(7):754–63.
27. Elsayed RS, Cohen RG, Fleischman F, Bowdish ME. Acute type a aortic dissection. Cardiol Clin. 2017;35(3):331–45.
28. Evangelista A, Maldonado G, Gruosso D, Gutierrez L, Granato C, Villalva N, Galian L, Gonzalez-Alujas T, Teixido G, Rodriguez-Palomares J. The current role of echocardiography in acute aortic syndrome. Echo Res Pract. 2019;6(2):R53–63.
29. Patil TA, Ambli SK. Transesophageal echocardiography evaluation of the aortic arch branches. Ann Card Anaesth. 2018;21(1):53–6.
30. Kawahito K, Adachi H, Murata S, Yamaguchi A, Ino T. Coronary malperfusion due to type a aortic dissection: mechanism and surgical management. Ann Thorac Surg. 2003;76(5):1471–6; discussion 6, 1476.
31. Neri E, Toscano T, Papalia U, Frati G, Massetti M, Capannini G, Tucci E, Buklas D, Muzzi L, Oricchio L, Sassi C. Proximal aortic dissection with coronary malperfusion: presentation, management, and outcome. J Thorac Cardiovasc Surg. 2001;121(3):552–60.
32. Loukas M, Sharma A, Blaak C, Sorenson E, Mian A. The clinical anatomy of the coronary arteries. J Cardiovasc Transl Res. 2013;6(2):197–207.
33. Crowley J, Cronin B, Essandoh M, D'Alessandro D, Shelton K, Dalia AA. Transesophageal echocardiography for Impella placement and management. J Cardiothorac Vasc Anesth. 2019;33(10):2663–8.
34. Patel KM, Sherwani SS, Baudo AM, Salvacion A, Herborn J, Soong W, Kendall MC. Echo rounds: the use of transesophageal echocardiography for confirmation of appropriate Impella 5.0 device placement. Anesth Analg. 2012;114(1):82–5.
35. Pratt AK, Shah NS, Boyce SW. Left ventricular assist device management in the ICU. Crit Care Med. 2014;42(1):158–68.
36. Flores AS, Essandoh M, Yerington GC, Bhatt AM, Iyer MH, Perez W, Davila VR, Tripathi RS, Turner K, Dimitrova G, Andritsos MJ. Echocardiographic assessment for ventricular assist device placement. J Thorac Dis. 2015;7(12):2139–50.
37. Hahn RT. State-of-the-art review of echocardiographic imaging in the evaluation and treatment of functional tricuspid regurgitation. Circ Cardiovasc Imaging. 2016;9(12):e005332.
38. Nguyen TQ, Hansen KL, Bechsgaard T, Lonn L, Jensen JA, Nielsen MB. Non-invasive assessment of intravascular pressure gradients: a review of current and proposed novel methods. Diagnostics (Basel). 2018;9(1):5.
39. Tan CO, Harley I. Perioperative transesophageal echocardiographic assessment of the right heart and associated structures: a comprehensive update and technical report. J Cardiothorac Vasc Anesth. 2014;28(4):1100–21.
40. Flo Forner A, Hasheminejad E, Sabate S, Ackermann MA, Turton EW, Ender J. Agreement of tricuspid annular systolic excursion measurement between transthoracic and transesophageal echocardiography in the perioperative setting. Int J Cardiovasc Imaging. 2017;33(9):1385–94.
41. Capper SJ, Ross JJ, Sandstrom E, Braidley PC, Morgan-Hughes NJ. Transoesophageal echocardiography for the detection and quantification of pleural fluid in cardiac surgical patients. Br J Anaesth. 2007;98(4):442–6.
42. Cavayas YA, Girard M, Desjardins G, Denault AY. Transesophageal lung ultrasonography: a novel technique for investigating hypoxemia. Can J Anaesth. 2016;63(11):1266–76.
43. Orihashi K, Matsuura Y, Hamanaka Y, Sueda T, Shikata H, Hayashi S, Nomimura T. Retained intracardiac air in open heart operations examined by transesophageal echocardiography. Ann Thorac Surg. 1993;55(6):1467–71.
44. Lamm G, Auer J, Punzengruber C, Ng CK, Eber B. Intracoronary air embolism in open heart surgery—an uncommon source of myocardial ischaemia. Int J Cardiol. 2006;112(3):e85–6.
45. Carmona P, Mateo E, Casanovas I, Pena JJ, Llagunes J, Aguar F, De Andres J, Errando C. Management of cardiac tamponade after cardiac surgery. J Cardiothorac Vasc Anesth. 2012;26(2):302–11.
46. Grumann A, Baretto L, Dugard A, Morera P, Cornu E, Amiel JB, Vignon PP. Localized cardiac tamponade after open-heart surgery. Ann Thorac Cardiovasc Surg. 2012;18(6):524–9.
47. Canadyova J, Zmeko D, Mokracek A. Re-exploration for bleeding or tamponade after cardiac operation. Interact Cardiovasc Thorac Surg. 2012;14(6):704–7.
48. Lui JK, Banauch GI. Diagnostic bedside ultrasonography for acute respiratory failure and severe hypoxemia in the medical intensive care unit: basics and comprehensive approaches. J Intensive Care Med. 2017;32(6):355–72.

49. Hoole SP, Falter F. Evaluation of hypoxemic patients with transesophageal echocardiography. Crit Care Med. 2007;35(8 Suppl):S408–13.
50. Mojadidi MK, Ruiz JC, Chertoff J, Zaman MO, Elgendy IY, Mahmoud AN, Al-Ani M, Elgendy AY, Patel NK, Shantha G, Tobis JM, Meier B. Patent foramen ovale and hypoxemia. Cardiol Rev. 2019;27(1):34–40.
51. Batouty NM, Sobh DM, Gadelhak B, Sobh HM, Mahmoud W, Tawfik AM. Left superior vena cava: cross-sectional imaging overview. Radiol Med. 2019;125:237–46.
52. Podolsky LA, Jacobs LE, Schwartz M, Kotler MN, Ioli A. Transesophageal echocardiography in the diagnosis of the persistent left superior vena cava. J Am Soc Echocardiogr. 1992;5(2):159–62.
53. Klein M, Wang A. Infective endocarditis. J Intensive Care Med. 2016;31(3):151–63.
54. Baddour LM, Wilson WR, Bayer AS, Fowler VG Jr, Tleyjeh IM, Rybak MJ, Barsic B, Lockhart PB, Gewitz MH, Levison ME, Bolger AF, Steckelberg JM, Baltimore RS, Fink AM, O'Gara P, Taubert KA, American Heart Association Committee on Rheumatic Fever E, Kawasaki Disease of the Council on Cardiovascular Disease in the Young CoCCCoCS, Anesthesia, Stroke C. Infective Endocarditis in Adults: Diagnosis, Antimicrobial Therapy, and Management of Complications: A Scientific Statement for Healthcare Professionals from the American Heart Association. Circulation. 2015;132(15):1435–86.
55. Vincent LL, Otto CM. Infective endocarditis: update on epidemiology, outcomes, and management. Curr Cardiol Rep. 2018;20(10):86.
56. Lester SJ, Wilansky S. Endocarditis and associated complications. Crit Care Med. 2007;35(8 Suppl):S384–91.
57. Afonso L, Kottam A, Reddy V, Penumetcha A. Echocardiography in infective endocarditis: state of the art. Curr Cardiol Rep. 2017;19(12):127.
58. Nishimura RA, Otto CM, Bonow RO, Carabello BA, Erwin JP 3rd, Fleisher LA, Jneid H, Mack MJ, McLeod CJ, O'Gara PT, Rigolin VH, Sundt TM 3rd, Thompson A. AHA/ACC focused update of the 2014 AHA/ACC guideline for the Management of Patients with Valvular Heart Disease: a report of the American College of Cardiology/American Heart Association task force on clinical practice guidelines. J Am Coll Cardiol. 2017;70(2):252–89.
59. Nishimura RA, Otto CM, Bonow RO, Carabello BA, Erwin JP III, Guyton RA, O'Gara PT, Ruiz CE, Skubas NJ, Sorajja P, Sundt TM III, Thomas JD, Anderson JL, Halperin JL, Albert NM, Bozkurt B, Brindis RG, Creager MA, Curtis LH, DeMets D, Guyton RA, Hochman JS, Kovacs RJ, Ohman EM, Pressler SJ, Sellke FW, Shen WK, Stevenson WG, Yancy CW, American College of C, American College of Cardiology/American Heart A, American Heart A. 2014 AHA/ACC guideline for the management of patients with valvular heart disease: a report of the American College of Cardiology/American Heart Association Task Force on Practice Guidelines. J Thorac Cardiovasc Surg. 2014;148(1):e1–e132.
60. Nadkarni A, Oldham MA, Howard M, Berenbaum I. Drug-drug interactions between warfarin and psychotropics: updated review of the literature. Pharmacotherapy. 2012;32(10):932–42.
61. Zoghbi WA, Chambers JB, Dumesnil JG, Foster E, Gottdiener JS, Grayburn PA, Khandheria BK, Levine RA, Marx GR, Miller FA Jr, Nakatani S, Quinones MA, Rakowski H, Rodriguez LL, Swaminathan M, Waggoner AD, Weissman NJ, Zabalgoitia M, American Society of Echocardiography's G, Standards C, Task Force on Prosthetic V, American College of Cardiology Cardiovascular Imaging C, Cardiac Imaging Committee of the American Heart A, European Association of E, European Society of C, Japanese Society of E, Canadian Society of E, American College of Cardiology F, American Heart A, European Association of E, European Society of C, Japanese Society of E, Canadian Society of E. Recommendations for evaluation of prosthetic valves with echocardiography and doppler ultrasound: a report From the American Society of Echocardiography's Guidelines and Standards Committee and the Task Force on Prosthetic Valves, developed in conjunction with the American College of Cardiology Cardiovascular Imaging Committee, Cardiac Imaging Committee of the American Heart Association, the European Association of Echocardiography, a registered branch of the European Society of Cardiology, the Japanese Society of Echocardiography and the Canadian Society of Echocardiography, endorsed by the American College of Cardiology Foundation, American Heart Association, European Association of Echocardiography, a registered branch of the European Society of Cardiology, the Japanese Society of Echocardiography, and Canadian Society of Echocardiography. J Am Soc Echocardiogr. 2009;22(9):975–1014; quiz 82–4.
62. Sordelli C, Severino S, Ascione L, Coppolino P, Caso P. Echocardiographic assessment of heart valve prostheses. J Cardiovasc Echogr. 2014;24(4):103–13.
63. Chambers JB. The echocardiography of replacement heart valves. Echo Res Pract. 2016;3(3):R35–43.
64. Griffee MJ, Tonna JE, McKellar SH, Zimmerman JM. Echocardiographic guidance and troubleshooting for venovenous extracorporeal membrane oxygenation using the dual-lumen bicaval cannula. J Cardiothorac Vasc Anesth. 2018;32(1):370–8.
65. McCanny P, Colreavy F. Echocardiographic approach to cardiac tamponade in critically ill patients. J Crit Care. 2017;39:271–7.
66. Kearns MJ, Walley KR. Tamponade: hemodynamic and echocardiographic diagnosis. Chest. 2018;153(5):1266–75.
67. Goldstein SA, Evangelista A, Abbara S, Arai A, Asch FM, Badano LP, Bolen MA, Connolly HM, Cuellar-Calabria H, Czerny M, Devereux RB, Erbel RA, Fattori R, Isselbacher EM, Lindsay JM, McCulloch M, Michelena HI, Nienaber CA, Oh JK, Pepi M, Taylor AJ, Weinsaft JW, Zamorano JL, Dietz H, Eagle K, Elefteriades J, Jondeau G, Rousseau H, Schepens M. Multimodality imaging of diseases of the thoracic aorta in adults: from the American Society of Echocardiography and the European Association of Cardiovascular Imaging: endorsed by the Society of Cardiovascular Computed Tomography and Society for Cardiovascular Magnetic Resonance. J Am Soc Echocardiogr. 2015;28(2):119–82.
68. Shillcutt SK, Tavazzi G, Shapiro BP, Diaz-Gomez J. Pulmonic regurgitation in the adult cardiac surgery patient. J Cardiothorac Vasc Anesth. 2017;31(1):215–28.

Valvular Assessment: Mitral and Aortic Valves

9

Brett J. Wakefield, Kristen Holler, and Carlos E. Trombetta

Question 1
The aortic root is composed of which of the following elements?

A. Left ventricular outflow tract, aortic annulus, aortic valve leaflets, sinus of Valsalva, sinotubular junction
B. Left ventricular outflow tract, aortic annulus, aortic valve leaflets, sinus of Valsalva, sinotubular junction, proximal ascending aorta
C. Aortic annulus, aortic valve leaflets, sinus of Valsalva, sinotubular junction
D. Aortic annulus, aortic valve leaflets, sinus of Valsalva

Answer C.
Key Point. The aortic root is composed of the aortic annulus, aortic valve leaflets, the sinus of Valsalva, and the sinotubular junction.

The aortic root extends from the basal attachments of the aortic valve cusps, which is referred to as the aortic annulus, to the sinotubular junction [1]. The left ventricular outflow tract and the ascending aorta are not considered to be elements of the aortic root. It is important to note that the aortic annulus is not a distinct anatomic ring, but a virtual ring formed by at the basal connections of the aortic valve cusps. The distal attachments of the aortic valve cusps form the shape of a crown [2].

The annulus should be measured in the parasternal long axis view in mid-systole [3]. Normal annulus measurements are 2.6 ± 0.3 cm in men and 2.3 ± 0.3 cm in women. The sinus of Valsalva and the sinotubular junction should be measured at end-diastole. Normal values for the sinus of Valsalva are 3.4 ± 0.3 cm in men and 3.0 ± 0.3 cm in women. Normal values for the sinotubular junction are 2.9 ± 0.3 cm in men and 2.6 ± 0.3 cm in women.

Question 2
Which of the following structures is identified with the red Asterix? (Fig. 9.1)

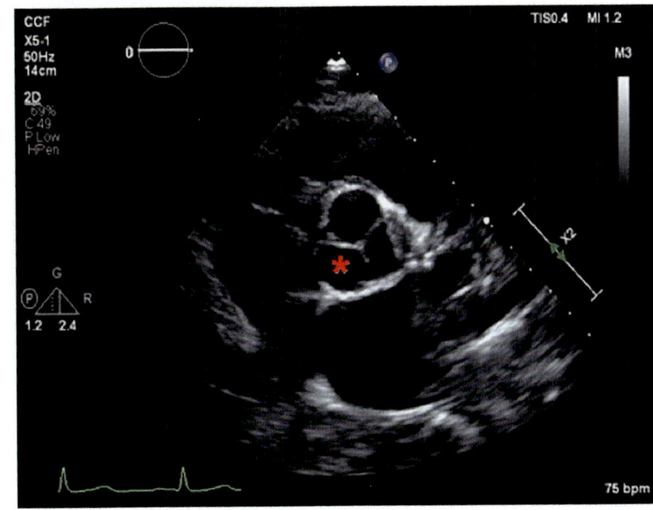

Fig. 9.1 parasternal short axis view of the base of the heart. The aortic valve is seen in the center of the image

Supplementary Information The online version contains supplementary material available at https://doi.org/10.1007/978-3-031-45731-9_9.

B. J. Wakefield (✉) · K. Holler · C. E. Trombetta
Department of Cardiothoracic Anesthesiology, Cleveland Clinic, Cleveland, OH, USA
e-mail: wakefib@ccf.org; hollerk@ccf.org; trombec@ccf.org

R. Sreedharan et al. (eds.), *Critical Care Echocardiography*, https://doi.org/10.1007/978-3-031-45731-9_9

A. Left coronary cusp
B. Right coronary cusp
C. Noncoronary cusp
D. Anterior coronary cusp

Answer C.

Key Point. The noncoronary cusp is adjacent to the interatrial septum.

This view is a parasternal short axis view with a focus on the aortic valve [4]. All three aortic valve leaflets can be seen, the right, left, and noncoronary cusps. These cusps can be identified based on the neighboring anatomy [2]. The noncoronary cusp is adjacent to the interatrial septum. The right coronary cusp is adjacent to the right ventricle. The left coronary cusp is adjacent to the left ventricular free wall.

Question 3

Which of the following structures is identified by the arrow? (Fig. 9.2)

A. Right coronary cusp
B. Left coronary cusp
C. Noncoronary cusp
D. Anterior coronary cusp

Answer A.

Key Point. The right coronary cusp is the positioned anterior to the other coronary cusps.

The parasternal long axis view allows a longitudinal view of the aortic valve [4]. This offers information on the pliability of the aortic valve leaflets and may indicate the presence of aortic stenosis or aortic insufficiency [2]. The aortic valve cusp closest to the probe (most anterior cusp) is the right coronary cusp. The distal cusp in this view is either the left or noncoronary cusp.

Question 4

Which of the following is **MOST likely correct** regarding the aorta in patients with a bicuspid aortic valve?

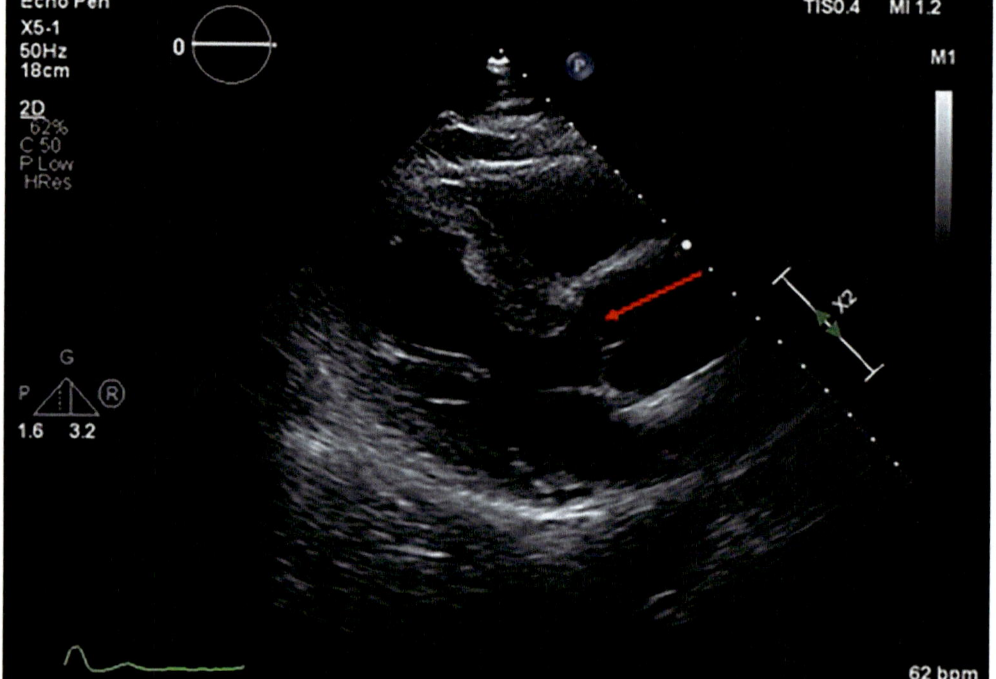

Fig. 9.2 Parasternal long axis view

A. The aortic root is rarely properly assessed by transthoracic echocardiography
B. The degree of aortic dilatation consistently correlates with the severity of the aortic stenosis
C. The risk of aneurysm and dissection is lower that of the general population
D. Bicuspid aortic valve is associated with coarctation of the aorta

Answer D.

Key Point. Bicuspid aortic valve is associated with coarctation of the aorta.

A bicuspid aortic valve is one of the most common congenital cardiac anomalies and is found in up to 2% of the population with a male predominance (3:1) [5]. The bicuspid valve is typically composed of two unequal leaflets, the larger of which has a central raphe representing the fusion of two leaflets. Most commonly, the left and right coronary cusps are fused [6].

In patients with suspected ascending aorta pathology, the parasternal long axis view allows for proper assessment of the aortic root, measurements should be made at the level of the aortic annulus, sinus, sinotubular junction and mid ascending aorta. The severity of vascular complications occurs independently of the degree of severity of aortic stenosis in patients with a bicuspid aortic valve. Compared with the general population, the risk of aortic aneurysms and aortic dissection is higher in this patient population [7]. In addition, coarctation of the aorta is more common in patients with bicuspid aortic valve [8]..

Question 5

In patients with calcific aortic stenosis, which of the following **BEST** describes the natural history of the disease?

A. Aortic sclerosis is a late stage of the process, with severe limitation of flow through the valve orifice.
B. Early calcium deposits occur at cusp attachments and along the line of cusp coaptation.
C. Involvement of leaflets happens simultaneously.
D. Commissural fusion is an early sign of severe disease.

Answer B.

Key Point. In calcific aortic stenosis, calcium deposits occur at cusp attachments and along the cusp coaptation; as opposed to rheumatic aortic stenosis where calcification occurs at the commissures.

Calcific aortic stenosis is the most prevalent cardiac disorder among patients in developed countries [9]. It is characterized by fibrosis and calcifications of the aortic valve leaflets and evolves over years or decades. Initially calcium deposits are seen at cusp attachments and along the coaptation line. Multiple areas of focal calcifications progressively appear. Aortic sclerosis occurs prior to the onset of aortic stenosis and thus, there is no compromise of flow through the orifice. As calcium deposits invade the leaflets, the leaflets lose their mobility and become more rigid, which limits blood flow through the orifice. This process affects each leaflet separately and asymmetrically. In contrast to calcific aortic stenosis, rheumatic aortic stenosis is characterized by commissural fusion.

Question 6

An 82-year-old female presents to the emergency department with an intertrochanteric femur fracture after a fall. Bedside transthoracic echocardiography (TTE) is performed. What is the **BEST** TTE view in order to evaluate gradients through the aortic valve?

A. Parasternal long axis view
B. Apical four-chamber view
C. Apical five-chamber view
D. Subcostal four-chamber view

Answer C.

Key Point. Gradients through the aortic valve can be measures from the apical five-chamber and apical long axis views.

The measurement of gradients through any valve relies on the principles of the Doppler echocardiography [10]. In order to gain accurate values, the beam of the ultrasound probe must align parallel with the flow of blood through the region of interest. For the aortic valve, the views which allow a parallel ultrasound beam through the aortic valve are the apical five-chamber view and the apical long axis view. The jet will be maximal at an incident angle of zero degrees and any angle greater than zero degrees will underestimate the measured value. Thus, the highest measurement attained should be reported.

The apical five-chamber view is obtained starting from the apical four-chamber view [4]. The probe is directed anteriorly until the left ventricular outflow tract and the aortic valve come into view. Color-Doppler can be applied to identify any turbulence or regurgitation. From the apical four-chamber view the probe is rotated counterclockwise 120 degrees (through the apical two-chamber at 60 degrees of rotation) to obtain the apical long axis view. The left ventricular outflow tract and aortic valve should come into view on the right side of the screen with optimal alignment allowing Doppler interrogation.

Question 7

The following continuous wave Doppler waveform is obtained. Given the peak velocity of 4.83 m/s, what is the peak gradient? (Fig. 9.3)

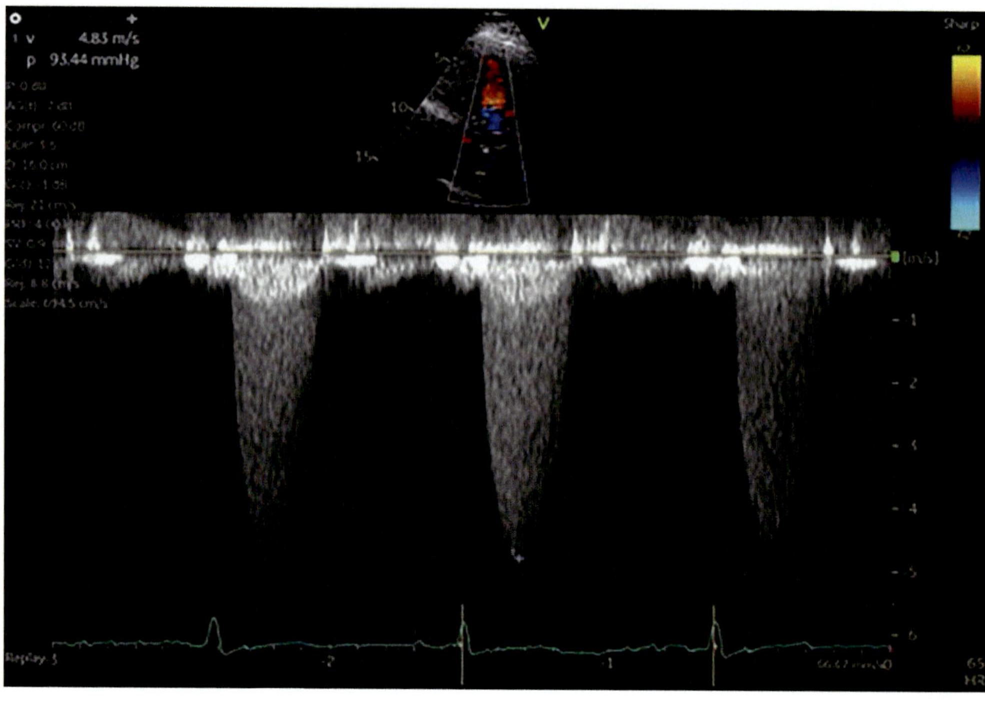

Fig. 9.3 Continuous wave Doppler envelope through the aortic valve. Aortic valve peak velocity = 4.83 m/s

A. 19 mmHg
B. 23 mmHg
C. 70 mmHg
D. 93 mmHg

Answer D.

Key Point. The simplified Bernoulli equation can be used to calculate the peak gradient through the aortic valve.

The Bernoulli equation relies on the law of conservation of energy to transform velocities through regions of the heart into gradients [11]. Clinical use of the Bernoulli equation has been condensed to the use of the modified Bernoulli equation and the simplified Bernoulli equation. The simplified Bernoulli equation assumes a low proximal velocity to the area of high velocity in question. This allows estimation of pressure gradients across stenotic valves.

Simplified Bernoulli equation: $\Delta P = 4\ V^2$

ΔP = pressure gradient, V = peak velocity on spectral Doppler envelope

The peak gradient is $4 * (4.83^2) = 93$ mmHg.

The modified Bernoulli equation needs to be used when the proximal velocity cannot be ignored [12]. Typically, proximal velocities greater than 1.5 cm/s require the use of the modified Bernoulli equation

Modified Bernoulli equation: $\Delta P = 4(V_2^2 - V_1^2)$.

ΔP = pressure gradient, V_2 = distal peak velocity, V_1 = proximal peak velocity.

Question 8

In a patient with severe aortic stenosis, the following parameters were identified: left ventricular outflow tract (LVOT) velocity time integral (VTI), stenotic aortic valve jet VTI, and aortic valve planimetry. Which additional parameter is needed to assess the patient's aortic valve area through the continuity equation?

A. LVOT cross sectional area
B. Mitral valve flow VTI
C. Pulmonic valve flow VTI
D. LVOT mean gradient

Answer A.

Key Points. Using the continuity equation, the aortic valve area can be estimated from the LVOT cross sectional area, LVOT VTI, and aortic valve VTI.

The continuity equation relies on the law of conservation of mass to estimate cardiac values [13]. The law of conservation of mass states that the flow through one orifice (LVOT) should equal the flow through another orifice (aortic valve) in the absence of a shunt. This is primarily used to estimate the aortic valve area. When applying the continuity equation to the aortic valve, the flow through the left ventricular outflow tract should equal the flow through the aortic valve. In addition, the stroke volume through the left ventricular outflow tract should equal the stroke volume through the aortic valve.

$$\text{Stroke Volume}_{\text{LVOT}} = \text{Stroke Volume}_{\text{Aortic Valve}}$$

$$\text{Stroke Volume} = \text{LVOT area}^{*}\ \text{LVOT VTI} = \pi(\text{LVOT diameter}/2)^{2*}\ \text{LVOT VTI}$$

$$\text{LVOT area}^{*}\ \text{LVOT VTI} = \text{Aortic valve area}^{*}\ \text{Aortic valve VTI}$$

Stroke volume can be measured using the diameter of the LVOT and the velocity time integral (VTI) through the LVOT [10]. The LVOT diameter can be measured in the parasternal long axis view. Considering the radius (or diameter/2) is squared in the stroke volume equation, error can be magnified by incorrect measurements. The VTI can be measured using spectral Doppler. In the apical long axis or apical five-chamber views, the pulsed-wave Doppler sample volume is placed in the LVOT. The characteristic waveform is traced producing a value, the VTI (centimeters). The VTI can be thought of as "stroke distance," or how far the blood travels during a given time period. The aortic valve VTI can be measured by using continuous wave Doppler through the aortic valve and tracing the waveform. The continuity equation can be rearranged to solve for the aortic valve area:

$$\text{Aortic valve area} = \left(\text{LVOT area}^{*}\ \text{LVOT VTI}\right) / \left(\text{Aortic valve VTI}\right)$$

Question 9
The following echocardiographic values were obtained with TTE. The dimensionless index of this patient is associated with what degree of aortic stenosis?

LVOT VTI (cm)	15.6
LVOT Diameter (cm)	2.2
LVOT Peak Velocity (cm/s)	64.3
AV VTI (cm)	104
AV Peak Gradient (mmHg)	56
AV Mean Gradient (mmHg)	38
AV Peak Velocity (cm/s)	374

A. Not associated with aortic stenosis
B. Mild
C. Moderate
D. Severe

Answer D.
Key Point. The dimensionless index is the ratio of the VTI through the LVOT to the VTI of the aortic valve. Values of less than 0.25 correlates with severe aortic stenosis.

The dimensionless index (DI), also known as the velocity time integral (VTI) ratio or the velocity ratio, is the ratio of the LVOT VTI to the aortic valve VTI [10]. This measurement reduces error by excluding the LVOT diameter. Patients with no aortic stenosis will have a ratio approaching 1. As aortic stenosis develops, this ratio drops (Table 9.1).

$$\text{Dimensionless Index} = \text{VTI}_{\text{LVOT}} / \text{VTI}_{\text{Aortic Valve}}$$

The dimensionless index in this patient is 0.15 (15.6/104).

Table 9.1 Aortic valve severity based on dimensionless index

	Mild	Moderate	Severe
DI	>0.5	0.25–0.50	<0.25

Question 10
Which of the following values indicates severe aortic stenosis?

Table 9.2 Severity grading of aortic stenosis

	Mild	Moderate	Severe
Peak velocity (m/s)	2.6–2.9	3.0–4.0	>4.0
Mean gradient (mmHg)	<20	20–40	>40
AVA (cm^2)	>1.5	1.0–1.5	<1.0
Indexed AVA (cm^2/m^2)	>0.85	0.60–0.85	<0.6
Dimensionless Index	>0.5	0.25–0.5	<0.25

A. Peak velocity 3.5 m/s
B. Aortic valve area 1.1 cm^2
C. Indexed aortic valve area 0.66 cm^2/m^2
D. Mean gradient 45 mmHg

Answer D.
Key Point. A mean gradient greater than or equal to 40 mmHg is indicative of severe aortic stenosis.

The American Society of Echocardiography issued an update on assessment of the aortic valve in 2017 [10]. According to this new document, the primary hemodynamic parameters used to assess the severity of aortic stenosis are peak jet velocity, mean pressure gradient, and aortic valve area by continuity equation (Level 1 Recommendation). Each of these measures requires optimal alignment of blood flow and the ultrasound beam. Peak jet velocity and the mean pressure gradient are both flow dependent and may underestimate the severity in states of low flow or low cardiac output. The aortic valve area by continuity equation is relatively flow independent; however, measurement error is more likely. Alternative measures of stenosis severity include aortic valve area by planimetry, and the dimensionless index. Values associated with aortic stenosis grading are shown below (Table 9.2).

Question 11
A 65-year-old patient with asymptomatic severe aortic stenosis should be considered for surgery if the following is present.

A. Increased aortic stenosis jet velocity more than 0.3 m/s per year.
B. LVEF > 50%
C. LV hypertrophy
D. Maximum aortic stenosis jet velocity 4.0–4.9 m/s

Answer A.
Key Point. Asymptomatic patients with aortic stenosis can be considered for aortic valve replacement under certain circumstances.

Asymptomatic patients with severe aortic stenosis should be considered for surgery if any of the following are present [14]:

- Left ventricular ejection fraction (LVEF) <50%, elevated brain natriuretic peptide, pulmonary hypertension
- Patients that develop symptoms during exercise testing
- Increased mean pressure gradient by exercise by >20 mmHg
- Peak velocity progression >0.3 m/s per year
- Very severe AS: peak velocity > 5.5 m/s, AVA < 0.6 cm^2
- Patients going for concomitant heart surgery

Question 12
A 75-year-old female with severe chronic obstructive pulmonary disease (COPD) presents to the medical intensive care unit with an acute COPD exacerbation. Due to undifferentiated hypotension, transthoracic echocardiography is performed and the following values were ascertained:

AVA by continuity equation (cm^2)	0.9
Mean aortic pressure gradient (mmHg)	30
LV ejection fraction	35%
Indexed stroke volume (mL/m^2)	25

Once recovered from her acute illness, what is the next **BEST** step in management?

A. Transcatheter aortic valve replacement
B. Surgical aortic valve replacement
C. Dobutamine stress echocardiography
D. Cardiac MRI

Answer C.
Key Point. Dobutamine stress echocardiography is indicated in patients with a low ejection fraction and measurements consistent with aortic stenosis in order to evaluate for low-flow low-gradient aortic stenosis.

In patients with left ventricular systolic dysfunction or a reduced stroke volume, the aortic valve gradients and velocities may be normal or low despite the presence of aortic stenosis [15]. This process is termed low-flow low-gradient aortic stenosis and presents a diagnostic challenge. The definition of low-flow low-gradient aortic stenosis involves the presence of the following four characteristics: [10]

1. Aortic valve area < 1.0 cm^2
2. Left ventricular ejection fraction <50%
3. Mean aortic valve gradient <40 mmHg
4. Stroke volume index <35 mL/m^2

Dobutamine stress echocardiography allows differentiation of true aortic stenosis and pseudosevere aortic stenosis. In true aortic stenosis, the mean aortic valve gradient and velocity will increase above severe levels while the aortic valve area remains below 1.0 cm^2. In true aortic stenosis the left ventricular dysfunction is typically a consequence of the aortic stenosis and may improve after valve replacement. In pseudosevere aortic stenosis, the pressure gradient and velocities will likely increase; however, the aortic valve area will increase above 1.0 cm^2 indicating non-severe aortic stenosis. In these patients the left ventricular dysfunction is typically due to another cause, such as ischemic or dilated cardiomyopathy, and thus, the ejection fraction will likely not improve with aortic valve replacement.

Question 13
A 79-year-old female patient with dyspnea on exertion and syncope is found to have an aortic valve area of 0.8 cm^2, mean gradient of 32 mmHg, stroke volume index <35 mL/m^2 and a left ventricular ejection fraction of 55% on transthoracic echocardiography. These findings are consistent with a diagnosis of:

A. High grade Aortic Stenosis
B. Paradoxical low flow low gradient Aortic Stenosis
C. Normal flow low gradient Aortic Stenosis
D. Low flow low gradient Aortic Stenosis

Answer B.
Key Point. Paradoxical low-flow low-gradient aortic stenosis is characterized by a small aortic valve area (<1.0 cm^2), a low gradient (<40 mmHg), low flow (stroke volume index <35 mL/m^2) and a preserved left ventricular ejection fraction (>55%).

Echocardiographic assessment of paradoxical low-flow, low-gradient severe aortic stenosis is complex and is related to left ventricular outflow. Characteristically, it includes a small aortic valve area (<1.0 cm^2), low gradient (<40 mmHg), low flow (stroke volume index <35 mL/m^2) and preserved left ventricular ejection fraction (>55%) [10]. These patients have exaggerated left ventricular concentric remodeling with fibrosis in combination with reduced filling and left ventricular compliance. Although the ejection fraction may be normal, their left ventricular function shows a dramatic reduction in longitudinal strain [15].

Commonly this is suspected in patients with inaccurate LVOT and Doppler measurements. As a result, accurate measurements are of paramount importance. Due to the continuity equation, overestimation of the LVOT diameter would cause overestimation of the aortic valve area, not underestimation. Both exercise and dobutamine stress echocardiography can be useful in assessing the response of the aortic valve area and the gradients to increased flows. This condition increases the risk of operative mortality.

Question 14
Which of the following hemodynamic goals is **LEAST likely** to benefit patients with aortic stenosis?

A. Maintain sinus rhythm
B. Avoid myocardial depression
C. Maintain low systemic vascular resistance
D. Avoid tachycardia

Answer C.
Key Point. Low systemic vascular resistance should be avoided in patients with aortic stenosis.

The goals of management for patients with aortic stenosis include maintaining sinus rhythm, a low to normal heart rate, optimal cardiac output, normal systemic vascular resistance, and adequate preload [16]. The loss of sinus rhythm will decrease left ventricular filling which can reduce stroke volume and cardiac output. The ideal heart rate is likely between 60–80 beats per minute. Due to the fixed orifice of the aortic valve, it may be difficult for the heart to increase stroke volume, and thus, cardiac output is more reliant on the heart rate. As a result, bradycardia can result in profound reductions in cardiac output. On the other hand, tachycardia will reduce diastolic filling time and systolic ejection time as well as increase myocardial oxygen demand. These factors can quickly lead to reductions in cardiac output and myocardial ischemia. Systemic vascular resistance is important to maintain in these patients as well [17]. Acute drops in systemic vascular resistance (which may occur with induction of anesthesia) can produce marked decrease in perfusion due to the hearts reduced ability for a compensatory increase stroke volume. In addition, due to the left ventricular hypertrophy present in these patients, higher systemic blood pressure and thus coronary perfusion pressures may be required to optimize oxygen delivery.

Question 15
A patient with a subaortic membrane and aortic stenosis presents for surgical resection. Bedside TTE is performed and the following spectral Doppler waveforms are obtained. What is the transvalvular gradient through the aortic valve? (Figs. 9.4 and 9.5)

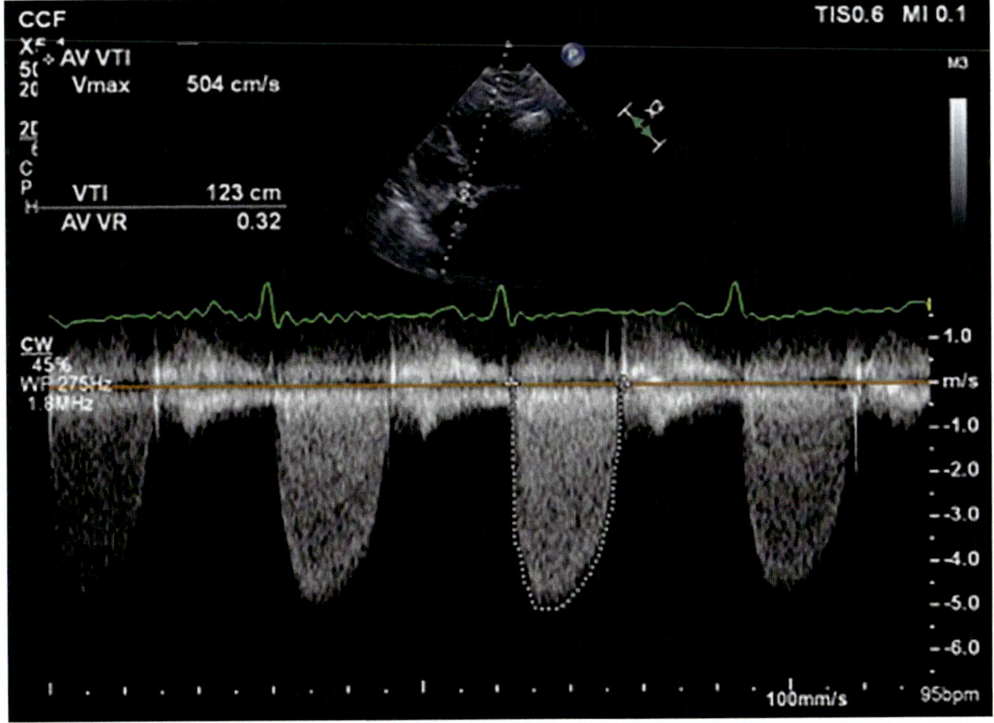

Fig. 9.4 Continuous wave Doppler envelope through the aortic valve. *V*max (aortic valve) = 504 cm/s

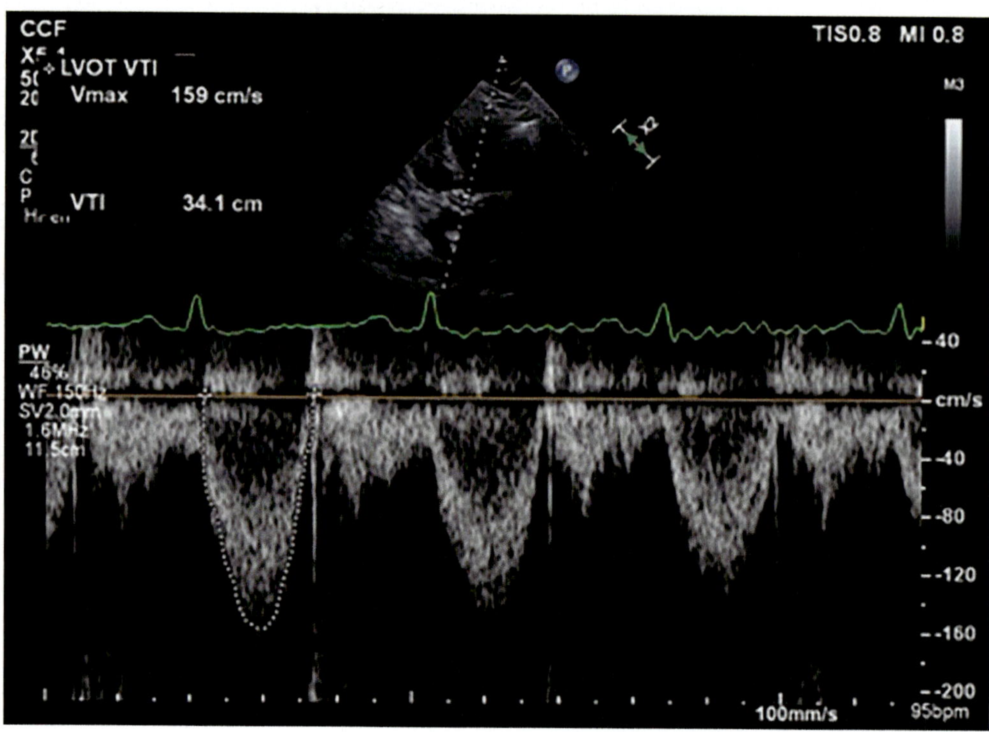

Fig. 9.5 Pulsed wave Doppler envelope through the left ventricular outflow tract. *V*max (LVOT) = 159 cm/s

A. 112.6 mmHg
B. 101.6 mmHg
C. 91.6 mmHg
D. 47.6 mmHg

Answer C.

Key Point. The modified Bernoulli equation should be used when proximal velocities exceed 1.5 m/s.

As detailed in an earlier question, the Bernoulli equation relies on the law of conservation of energy to transform velocities through regions of the heart into gradients [11]. Clinical use of the Bernoulli equation has been condensed to the use of the modified Bernoulli equation and the simplified Bernoulli equation. The simplified Bernoulli equation assumes a low proximal velocity to the area of high velocity in question. This allows estimation of pressure gradients across stenotic valves.

Simplified Bernoulli equation: $\Delta P = 4\ V^2$

ΔP = pressure gradient, V = peak velocity on spectral Doppler envelope

The modified Bernoulli equation needs to be used when the proximal velocity cannot be ignored [12]. Typically, proximal velocities greater than 1.5 cm/s require the use of the modified Bernoulli equation. This occurs in patients with a subaortic membrane, hypertrophic cardiomyopathy, or other forms of left ventricular outflow tract obstruction. This may also occur in high flow or hyperdynamic states. In this patient, the presence of a subaortic membrane results in increased left ventricular outflow tract velocities which need to be incorporated into the modified Bernoulli equation, rather than the simplified Bernoulli equation, to calculate the transvalvular gradient.

Modified Bernoulli equation: $\Delta P = 4(V_2^2 - V_1^2)$

ΔP = pressure gradient, V_2 = distal peak velocity, V_1 = proximal peak velocity

According to the modified Bernoulli equation, the peak transvalvular gradient through the aortic valve is $4 * (5.04^2 - 1.59^2) = 91.6$ mmHg.

Question 16

The accompanying video and figures, highlight a congenital abnormality. Which cardiac condition is **MOST** likely associated with the highlighted congenital abnormality (Video 9.1 and Figs. 9.6 and 9.7)?

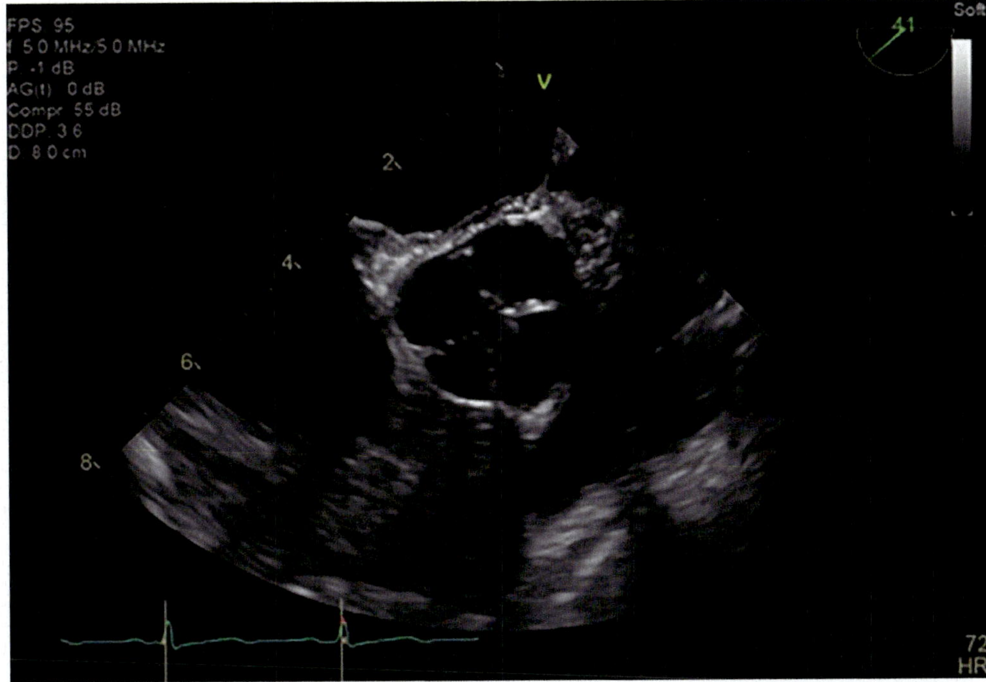

Fig. 9.6 Midesophageal aortic valve short axis view during diastole

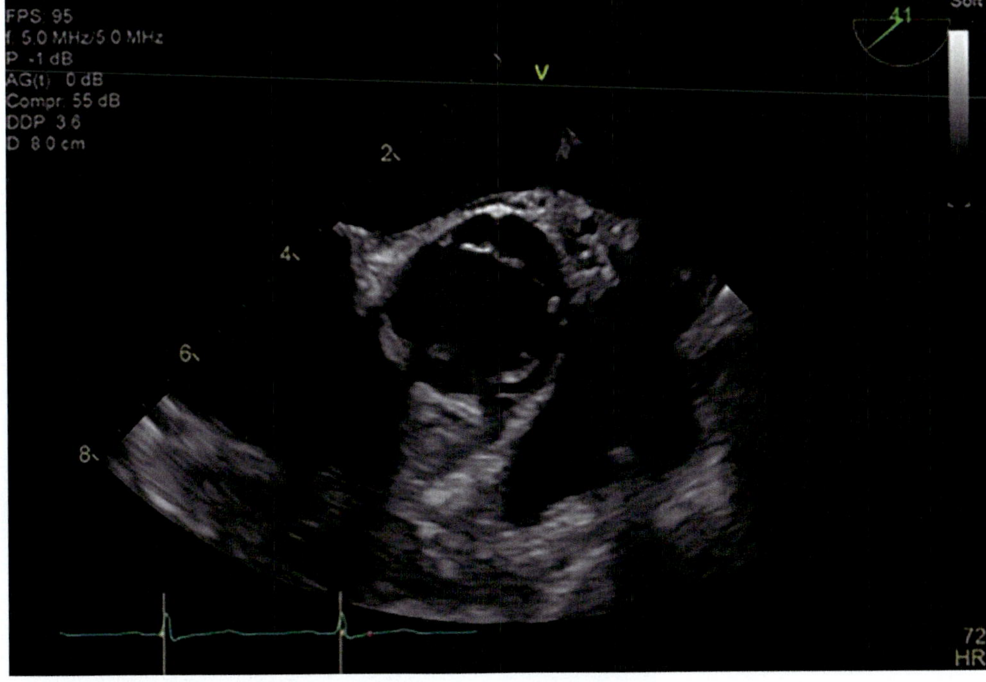

Fig. 9.7 Midesophageal aortic valve short axis view during systole

A. Coronary artery anomalies
B. Atrial septal defect
C. Ventricular septal defect
D. Coarctation of the aorta

Answer A.

Key Point. A quadricuspid aortic valve is associated with coronary artery anomalies.

A quadricuspid aortic valve is a rare congenital anomaly that occurs in 0.05 to 0.1% of patients [18]. This type of valve has four distinct commissures with four valve leaflets. The fourth leaflet is given the name "supernumerary cusp." The most common associated anomalies are coronary artery and coronary ostium abnormalities [19]. Many patients may never require surgery; however, those that do typically present in their fifth or sixth decade with aortic regurgitation.

Question 17

Which of the following asymptomatic patients with severe aortic insufficiency should undergo surgical aortic valve replacement?

A. LVEF 55%
B. LVEF 45%
C. LV end-systolic diameter 45 mm
D. LV end-diastolic diameter 60 mm

Answer B.

Key Point. Patients with asymptomatic severe aortic insufficiency and an LVEF <50% should undergo aortic valve replacement.

Asymptomatic Severe Aortic Regurgitation – Surgical Qualifications [20].

- LVEF < 50%
- LV ESD > 50 mm
- LV EDD > 65 mm (and low surgical risk)

LVEF left ventricular ejection fraction, *LV ESD* left ventricular end-systolic diameter, *LV EDD* left ventricular end-diastolic diameter.

Guidelines for the management of patients with valvular heart disease were published by the American Heart Association and American College of Cardiology in 2014. These guidelines detailed the management of patients with aortic regurgitation and highlight which patients should be referred for surgery. Patients with symptomatic severe aortic regurgitation should be referred for surgery regardless of left ventricular function. This is a class I indication for aortic valve surgery. Patients with asymptomatic severe (class I) or moderate (Class IIa) aortic regurgitation can undergo aortic valve surgery when undergoing cardiac surgery for another reason. Patients with asymptomatic severe aortic regurgitation who are not undergoing cardiac surgery for a separate reason are less straightforward. These patients may be offered surgery depending of their left ventricular function. Patients with a LVEF less than 50% (class I), a LV ESD greater than 50 mm (Class IIa), or a LV EDD greater than 65 mm (with low surgical risk, IIb) may be referred for aortic valve surgery.

Question 18

A 56-year-old male with a long-standing history of uncontrolled hypertension presents to the emergency department with shortness of breath. Due to poor TTE views, TEE is performed and the resulting images are presented below (Figs. 9.8, 9.9 and 9.10). What classification of aortic regurgitation is demonstrated?

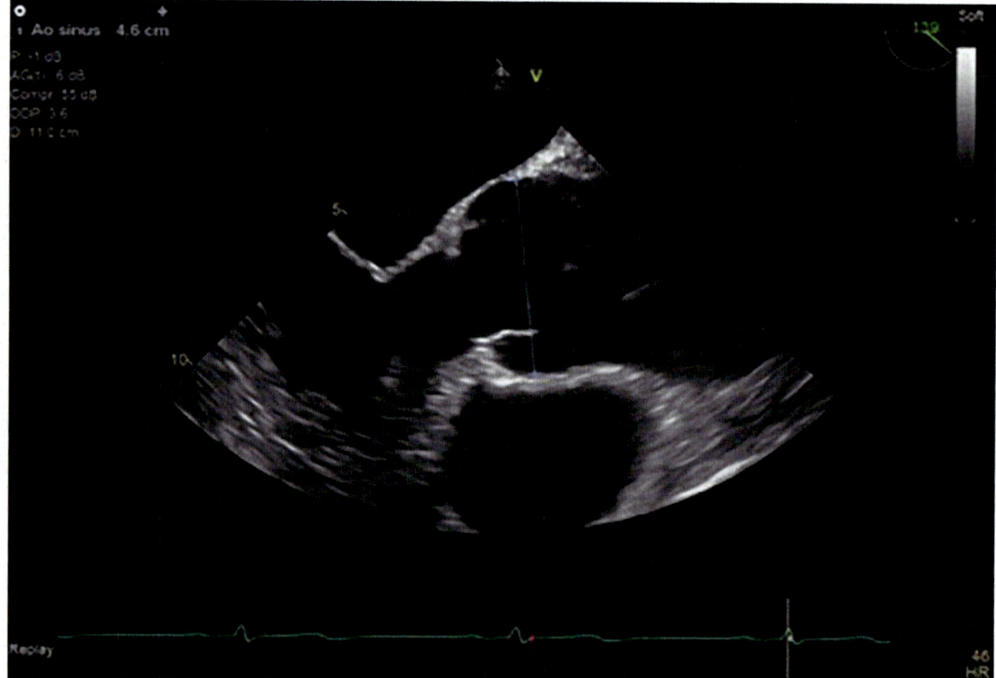

Fig. 9.8 Midesophageal view of the aortic valve. Sinus of Valsalva diameter = 4.6 cm

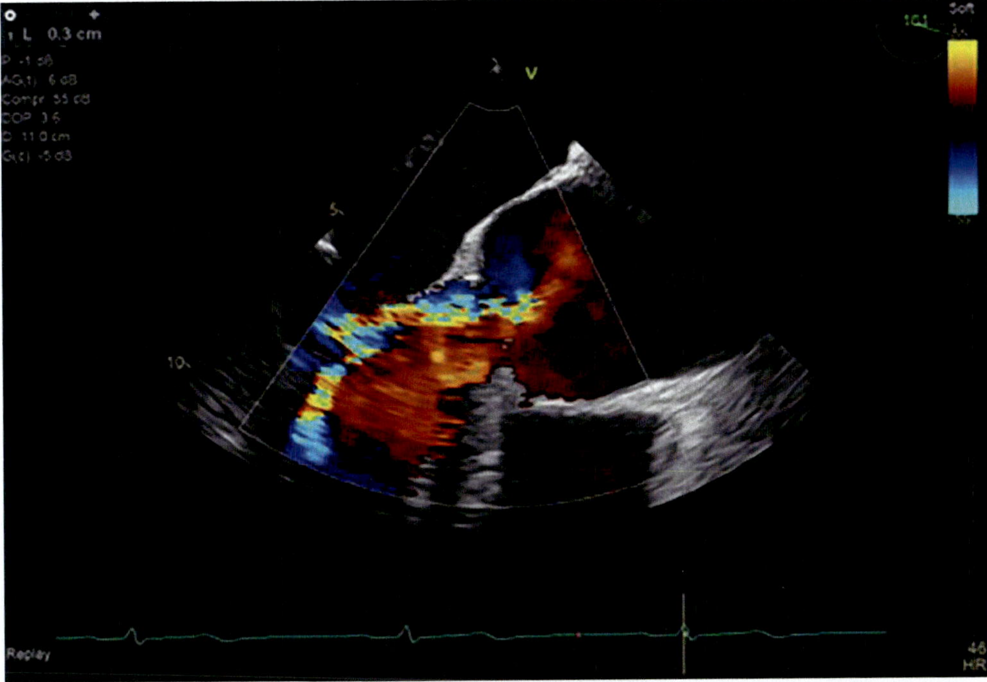

Fig. 9.9 Midesophageal view of the aortic valve during diastole with color flow Doppler imaging

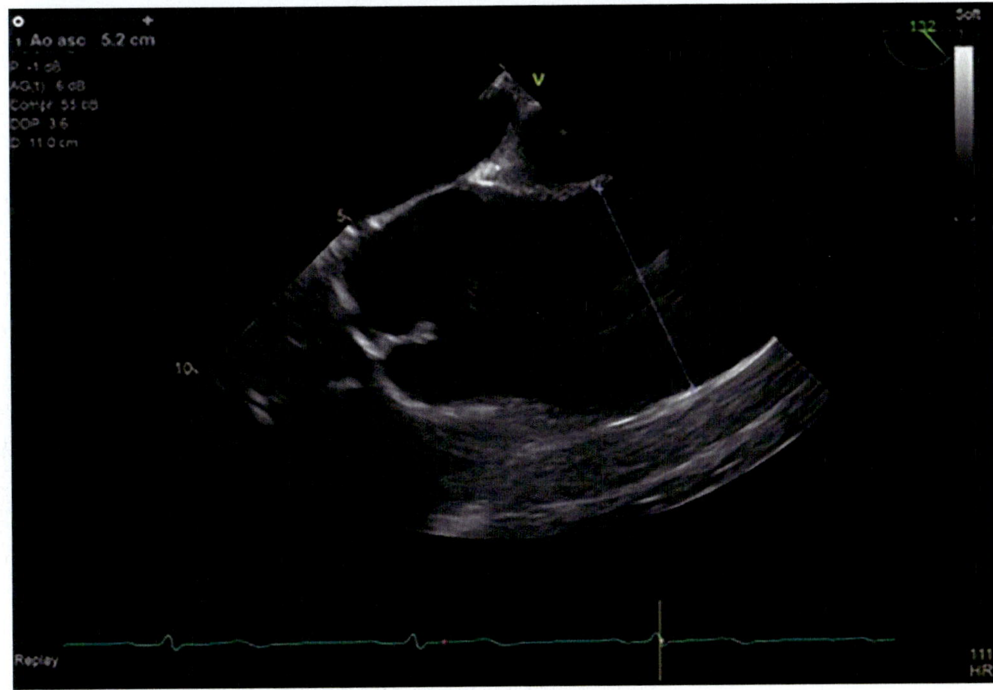

Fig. 9.10 Midesophageal view of the ascending aorta. Ascending aorta diameter = 5.2 cm

A. Type 1b
B. Type 1d
C. Type 2
D. Type 3

Answer A.

Key Point. Aneurysmal dilation of the sinus of Valsalva, sinotubular junction, and the ascending aorta is consistent with a type 1b aortic regurgitation according to the El Khoury classification scheme.

The El Khoury classification system is used to classify the etiology of aortic regurgitation (Table 9.3) [21]. This system mirrors the Carpentier classification system for mitral regurgitation [22]. Type I indicates normal aortic cusp motion. This can be further classified based on the leaflet and aortic root morphology. Type II indicates cusp prolapse and type III indicates cusp restriction. Type Ia, Ib, and Ic aortic regurgitation will typically have a central regurgitant jet while type Id will have a variable jet depending on the location and severity of the perforation. The jet of type II aortic regurgitation, cusp prolapse, will typically be eccentrically directed away from the prolapsing cusp. Type III aortic regurgitation, cusp restriction, will have a variable jet depending on the number of leaflets involved and the severity of restriction. In the case of one restricted leaflet, the jet will typically be eccentrically directed toward the abnormal cusp.

Table 9.3 El Khoury classification of aortic regurgitation

Classification	Description
Type I	Normal cusp motion
Type Ia	Dilation of sinotubular junction and ascending aorta
Type Ib	Dilation of sinus of Valsalva and sinotubular junction
Type Ic	Dilation of the aortic annulus
Type Id	Cusp perforation or fenestration
Type II	Cusp prolapse
Type III	Cusp restriction

Question 19

Further TEE evaluation generates the following spectral Doppler waveform. What is indicated by this envelope? (Fig. 9.11)

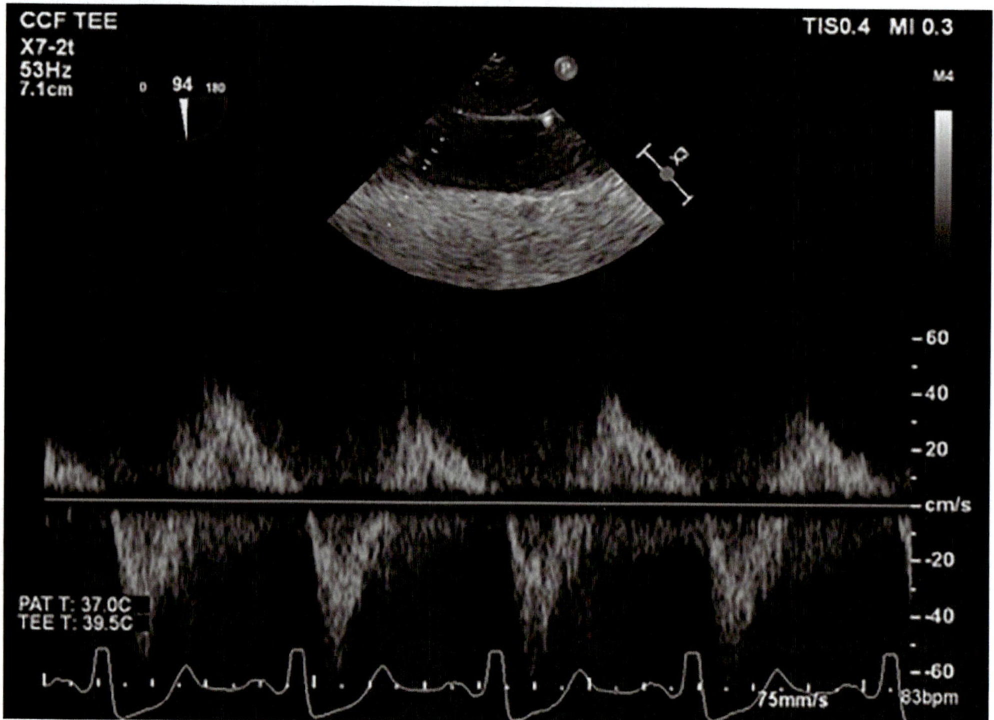

Fig. 9.11 Spectral Doppler envelope

A. Hepatic vein systolic reversal
B. Normal hepatic venous flow
C. Holodiastolic aortic flow reversal
D. Normal aortic flow

Answer C.

Key Point. The pulsed wave Doppler sample volume is placed in the distal descending thoracic aorta. The spectral Doppler envelope indicates reversal of aortic flow during diastole consistent with severe aortic regurgitation.

Holodiastolic flow reversal in the descending thoracic aorta or abdominal aorta is a supportive sign of severe aortic regurgitation [22]. Early diastolic flow reversal is normal and seen in patients without aortic regurgitation; however, severe aortic regurgitation can allow considerable reversal of flow from the aorta into the left ventricle during diastole. This sign becomes more specific for severe aortic regurgitation the further distal in the aorta this phenomenon is evaluated (flow reversal in abdominal aorta is more specific than flow reversal in proximal descending aorta) [23]. It is important to note that several conditions can cause holodiastolic flow reversal without evidence of aortic regurgitation. Any fistulous communication between the aorta and another cardiac chamber (such as a ruptured sinus of Valsalva) or upper extremity arteriovenous fistulae can all cause this echocardiographic sign [24] (Fig. 9.12).

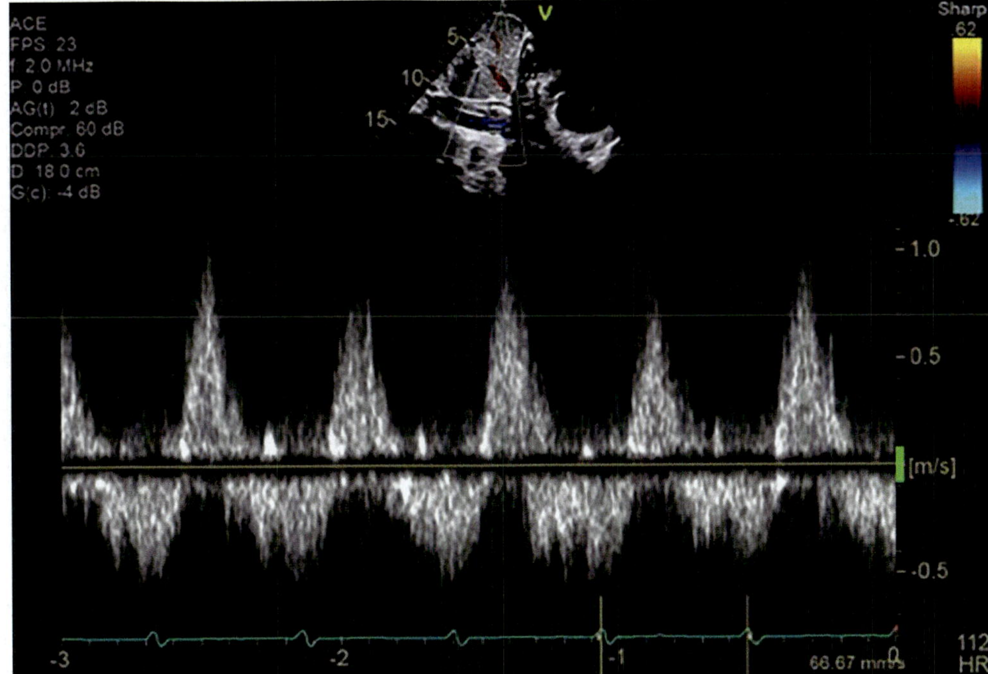

Fig. 9.12 TTE view demonstrating a spectral Doppler envelope of the descending aorta. Note the holodiastolic blood flow reversal

Question 20

A 78-year-old male presents to the ICU following exploratory laparotomy with hypotension and evidence of pulmonary edema. A TEE probe is placed. Based on the TEE image below, how severe is this patient's aortic regurgitation? (Fig. 9.13)

A. No aortic regurgitation
B. Mild aortic regurgitation
C. Moderate aortic regurgitation
D. Severe aortic regurgitation

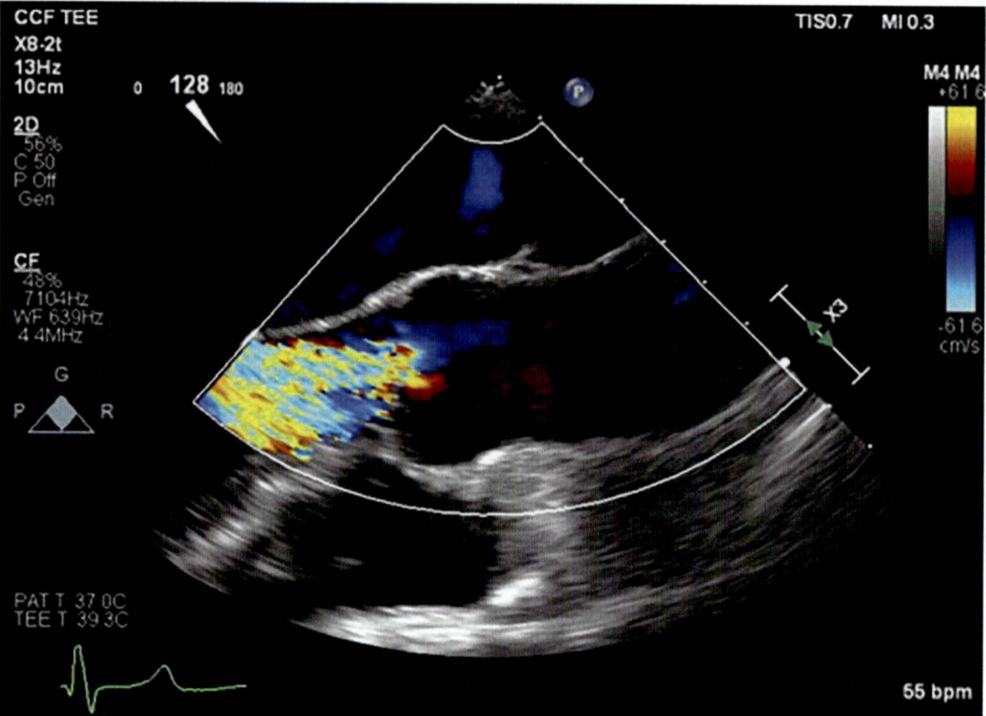

Fig. 9.13 Midesophageal view of the aortic valve

Answer D.

Key Point. The ratio of the jet width to the diameter of the left ventricular outflow tract can be used to grade the severity of aortic regurgitation. Values ≥65% are consistent with severe aortic regurgitation.

The jet width to LVOT diameter ratio can be used to help categorize the severity of aortic regurgitation [22]. In the parasternal long axis view (TTE) or the midesophageal long axis view (TEE) color-flow Doppler is utilized to image the aortic regurgitation jet. The optimal imaging plane and alignment will demonstrate the jet's flow convergence, vena contracta, and regurgitant jet. The vena contracta represents the narrowest portion of the jet as in passes through the aortic valve. This typically occurs just apical to the coaptation of the aortic valve leaflets. The zoom feature should be utilized to maximize the image and improve quantification [25]. The jet area and LVOT diameter should be measured 1 centimeter from the vena contracta. This method may underestimate the amount of aortic regurgitation in eccentric jets and is more accurate with central jets. A value less than 25% represents mild aortic regurgitation, 25–64% for moderate aortic regurgitation, and ≥ 65% for severe aortic regurgitation. In this patient example, the regurgitant jet takes up almost the entire LVOT diameter and is consistent with severe aortic regurgitation.

Question 21

Further evaluation of the aortic valve yields a proximal isovelocity surface area (PISA) radius of 0.82 cm with an aliasing velocity of 40 cm/s. What is needed to calculate the effective regurgitant orifice area?

A. Aortic regurgitation VTI
B. Aortic regurgitation peak velocity
C. Aortic regurgitation mean velocity
D. Aortic regurgitation pressure half time

Answer B.

Key Point. The PISA radius, aliasing velocity, and aortic regurgitation peak velocity are required to calculate the effective regurgitant orifice area with the proximal isovelocity surface area (PISA) method.

The PISA or flow convergence method can be used to estimate the effective orifice area of a valve [22]. It can be used in mitral regurgitation, mitral stenosis, tricuspid regurgitation, aortic regurgitation, and intracardiac shunts. This method relies on the principle of continuity. As blood flows or converges toward a narrow orifice (blood from aorta entering the left ventricle via a small regurgitant orifice area of the aortic valve), the blood forms concentric hemispheres of increasing velocity (velocity is highest at the orifice) and decreasing surface area (smallest surface area closest to the orifice). This flow convergence can be observed with TTE or TEE color-flow Doppler as a half-circle on the aortic side of the aortic valve.

The principle of continuity is based on the law of conservation of mass. The law of conservation of mass states that the flow through one orifice should equal the flow through another orifice in the absence of a shunt. If flow equals area multiplied by velocity, then:

$$A_1 \times V_1 = A_2 \times V_2$$

In this case, the two orifices are the regurgitant orifice and one of the hemispheres of flow convergence. Using this principle, the flow through the hemisphere at a particular radius will be equal to the flow through the regurgitant orifice. The equation then becomes:

$$A_{\text{hemisphere}} \times V_{\text{hemisphere}} = A_{\text{valve orifice}} \times V_{\text{valve orifice}}$$

In order to find the area and the velocity of the hemisphere, color Doppler must be applied to the aortic valve [26]. The only way to know exactly what the velocity is at one area using color flow Doppler involves using the scale or aliasing velocity, also known as the Nyquist limit. In standard color flow Doppler echocardiography, the color red indicates flow toward the probe while the color blue indicates color away from the probe. If blood flow toward the probe exceeds the aliasing velocity (velocity set on the color flow scale), the color aliases and turns to red. At that exact point (the point of aliasing), the velocity of blood is known (the velocity of blood is the aliasing velocity). Therefore is we measure the distance from the orifice or vena contracta to the point of aliasing we can use the radius to find the area of the hemisphere ($A_{\text{hemisphere}} = 2\pi r^2$) and we can estimate the effective regurgitant orifice area (EROA) using the continuity equation.

$$2\pi r^2 \times \text{Aliasing velocity} = V_{\text{max through valve}} \times \text{EROA}$$

$$\text{EROA} = 2\pi r^2 (\text{Aliasing velocity}) / (V_{\text{max}})$$

Question 22

In addition to the value in Question 19, what additional information is needed for the regurgitant volume?

A. Aortic insufficiency VTI
B. Aortic insufficiency peak velocity
C. Aortic insufficiency mean velocity
D. Aortic insufficiency pressure half time

Answer A.

Key Point. The aortic insufficiency velocity time integral (VTI) is required to calculate the regurgitant volume.

The regurgitant volume is calculated as the effective regurgitant orifice area multiplied by the velocity time integral (VTI) of the aortic regurgitation jet [22]. This is akin to calculating the stroke volume by multiplying the orifice area of the left ventricular outflow tract by the VTI through the LVOT.

$$\text{Regurgitant volume} = \text{Effective regurgitant orifice area} \times \text{VTI}_{\text{regurgitant jet}}$$

The regurgitant fraction can also be calculated as the regurgitant volume divided by the stroke volume through the regurgitant valve [26]. In the setting of aortic regurgitation, the regurgitant fraction would be the regurgitant volume divided by the stroke volume through the aortic valve (or the LVOT, which is easier to measure).

Question 23
Which of the following echocardiographic values indicates severe aortic insufficiency?

A. Vena contracta 0.5 cm
B. Pressure half time 520 ms
C. Effective regurgitant orifice area 0.35 cm^2
D. Cross sectional area jet area/area of LVOT 55%

Answer C.

Key Point. Effective regurgitant orifice area greater than 0.3 cm^2 indicates severe aortic insufficiency.

Many parameters can be used to interrogate the severity of aortic regurgitation. In 2017, the American Society of Echocardiography published guidelines on the evaluation of valvular regurgitation [22]. It is highly recommended to read these guidelines prior to the exam. Table 9.4 shows the grading recommendations based on echocardiographic findings

Table 9.4 Severity grading of aortic regurgitation

Parameters	Mild	Moderate	Severe
Qualitative			
Jet density	Faint	Dense	Dense
Aortic diastolic flow reversal	Brief, early diastolic	Intermediate	Prominent holodiastolic
Semiquantitative			
Pressure half-time (ms)	>500	200–500	<200
Vena contracta (cm)	<0.3	0.3–0.6	>0.6
Jet width/LVOT diameter (%)	<25	25–64	≥65
Jet CSA/LVOT CSA (%)	<5	5–59	≥60
Quantitative			
EROA (cm^2)	<0.10	0.10–0.29	≥0.30
Regurgitant volume (mL)	<30	30–59	≥60
Regurgitant fraction (%)	<30	30–49	≥50

LVOT left ventricular outflow tract, *CSA* cross-sectional area, *EROA* effective regurgitant orifice area

Question 24
A 19-year-old male with a history of intravenous heroin abuse presents to the emergency department in respiratory distress. CXR demonstrates diffuse pulmonary edema. Following an uneventful intubation he is transferred to the ICU. His blood pressure is 140/90 with a heart rate of 110. The following images are found on bedside TTE (Videos 9.2 and 9.3 and Figs. 9.14 and 9.15). What is the **BEST** next step in management?

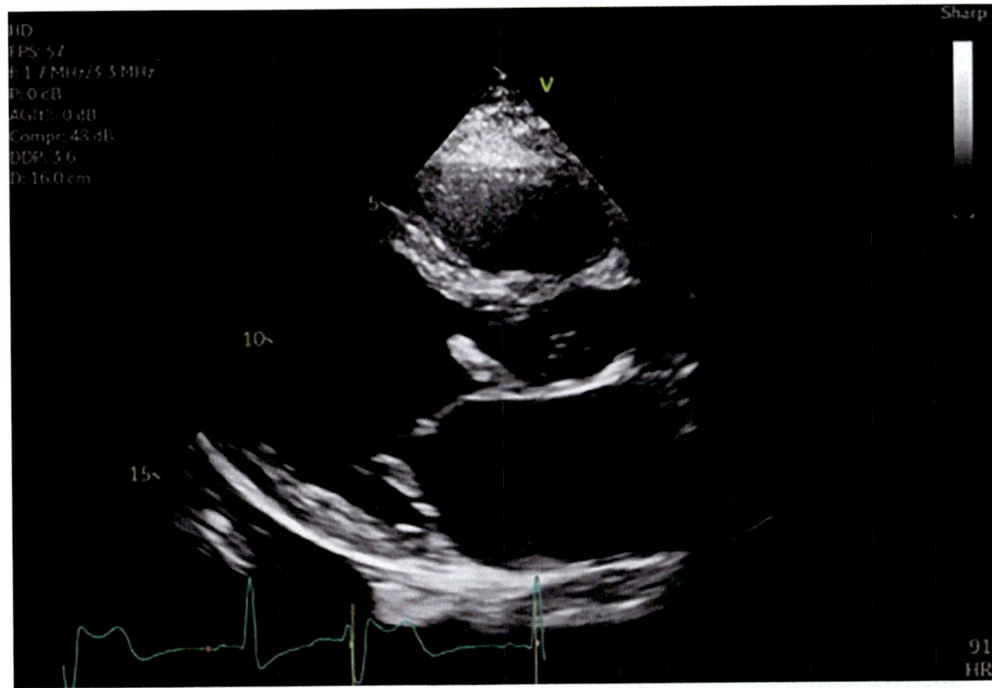

Fig. 9.14 Parasternal long axis view

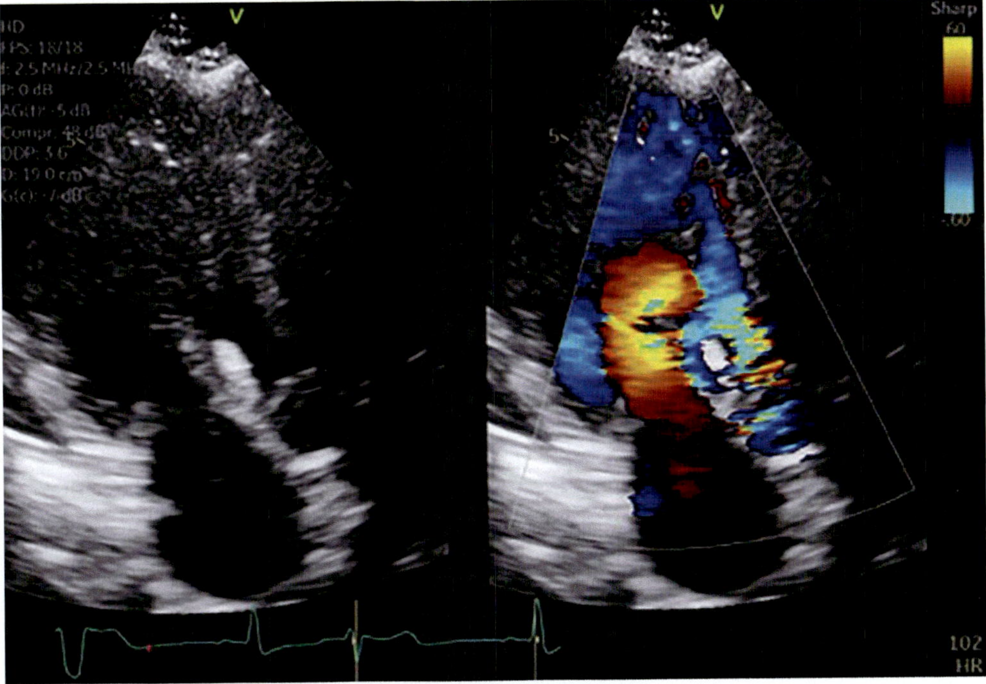

Fig. 9.15 Apical long axis view with and without color flow Doppler

A. Intra-aortic balloon pump mechanical circulatory support
B. Sodium nitroprusside infusion
C. Labetalol infusion
D. Epinephrine infusion

Answer B.

Key Point. Patients with normal or increased blood pressure and severe acute aortic regurgitation benefit from afterload reduction with nitroprusside.

Patient with severe acute aortic regurgitation require emergent aortic valve surgery particularly is there is evidence of cardiogenic shock or pulmonary edema [27]. This patient will require aortic valve replacement; however, medical management with afterload reduction can be instituted while awaiting surgery. Medical therapy will differ depending on the hemodynamic status of the patient. Normal to low systemic vascular resistance is helpful to promote forward flow and afterload reduction can be accomplished with vasodilators such as nitroprusside, nitroglycerin, nicardipine, and clevidipine [28]. Patients with aortic regurgitation require normal to higher than normal heart rates to promote forward flow and reduce diastolic time and thus regurgitant volume. As a result, beta-blockers are not typically used in patients with acute severe aortic regurgitation unless a concomitant aortic dissection is present. Intra-aortic balloon pumps are contraindicated in patients with moderate to severe aortic regurgitation due to the increased diastolic pressure and increased regurgitant volume. Epinephrine may be useful in patients with acute aortic regurgitation and cardiogenic shock; however, this patient has a normal to slightly elevated blood pressure and thus would benefit more from afterload reduction.

Question 25

Which of the following echocardiographic measurements is more accurate in patients with acute aortic regurgitation when compared to chronic aortic regurgitation.

A. Vena contracta
B. Effective regurgitant orifice area
C. Jet area to LVOT area ratio
D. Pressure half time

Answer D.

Key Point. The pressure half time is more accurate in acute aortic regurgitation and may underestimate the severity of chronic aortic stenosis due to ventricular remodeling (Fig. 9.16).

The pressure half-time is the amount of time required for the pressure gradient to decrease by half. This can be measured with continuous wave Doppler evaluation of the aortic regurgitant jet. A typical spectral waveform of a regurgitant jet will have a steep upslope at the onset of diastole and regurgitation which then tapers down linearly throughout the remainder of diastole. Using an echocardiographic software package, a line can be drawn along this deceleration and a pressure half-time can be calculated by the machine. A half-time greater than 500 ms suggests mild aortic regurgitation while a half-time less than 200 ms indicates severe aortic regurgitation [22].

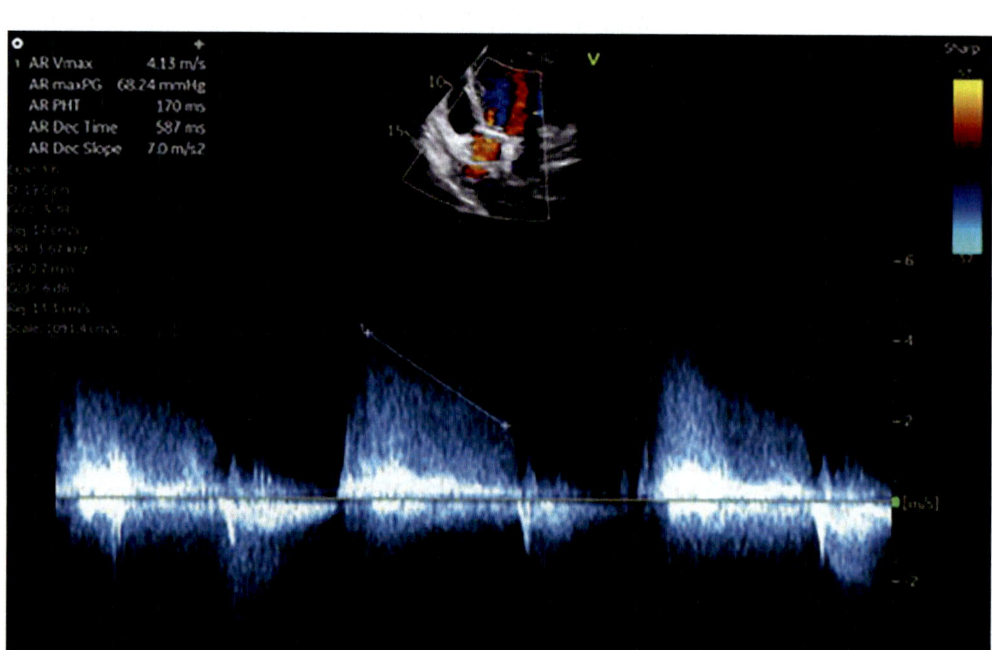

Fig. 9.16 Apical five-chamber view with a continuous wave Doppler envelope through the aortic valve. Note the steep decline in the waveform consistent with a short pressure half time (170 ms in this image) and severe aortic regurgitation

The pressure half-time correlates with the amount of time required for equilibration of pressures between the left ventricle and the aorta in diastole and as a result, the pressure half time is influenced by left ventricular compliance [29]. Patients with mild aortic regurgitation and severe diastolic dysfunction may have a short pressure half time because the diastolic pressures between the aorta and left ventricle equilibrate quickly (increased left ventricular diastolic pressures due to severe diastolic dysfunction). In addition, chronic aortic regurgitation allows for left ventricular remodeling and compensation. As a result, left ventricular end diastolic pressures may not be elevated (allowing longer time for equilibration of pressures) and the pressure half-time may be in the mild or moderate range despite severe aortic regurgitation.

Question 26

A previously healthy 34-year-old female patient presents to the intensive care unit after surgical repair of an open femur fracture following a motor vehicle accident. Bedside echo is performed to guide ongoing volume resuscitation. In this parasternal long axis view, which of the following mitral valve segments appears to prolapse (red arrow)? (Fig. 9.17).

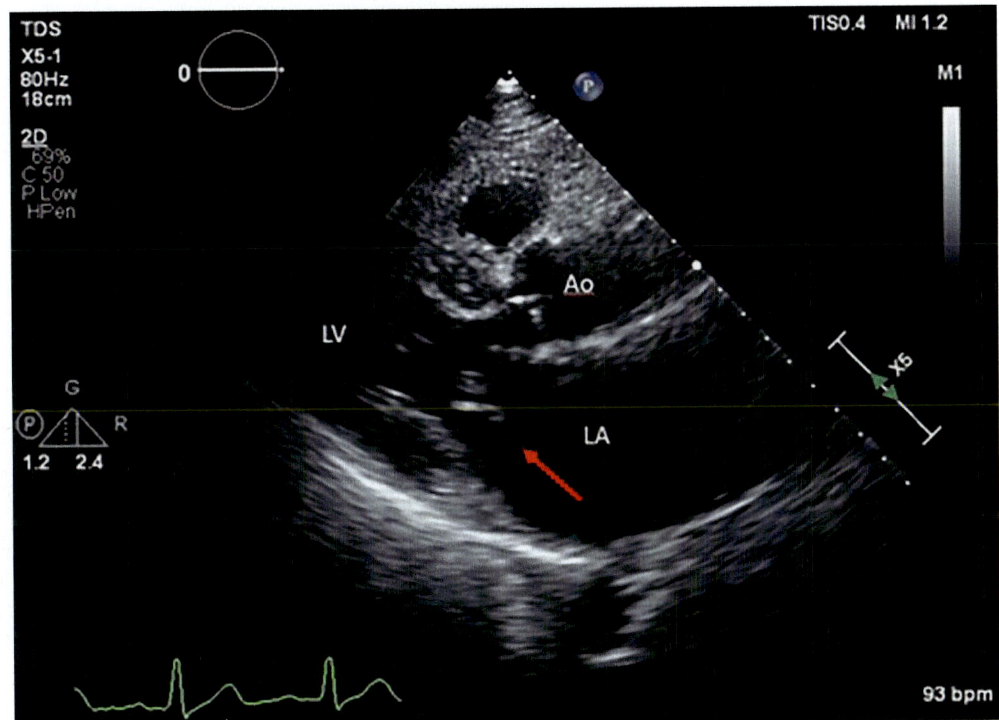

Fig. 9.17 Parasternal long axis view. Left ventricle (LV), Left atrium (LA), Aorta (Ao)

A. A2
B. A3
C. P1
D. P2

Answer D.

Key Point. In the parasternal long axis view the visualized mitral valve segments are A2 and P2.

In the parasternal long axis view the anterior mitral leaflet is in close proximity to the aortic valve. This view cuts across the AP diameter of the valve in the middle of the commissure resulting in a view of the A2 and P2 leaflet segments [30].

Question 27

A 3-Dimensional surgeon's view of the mitral valve is shown below. Which segment of the mitral valve is the cause of the patient's mitral regurgitation? (Fig. 9.18)

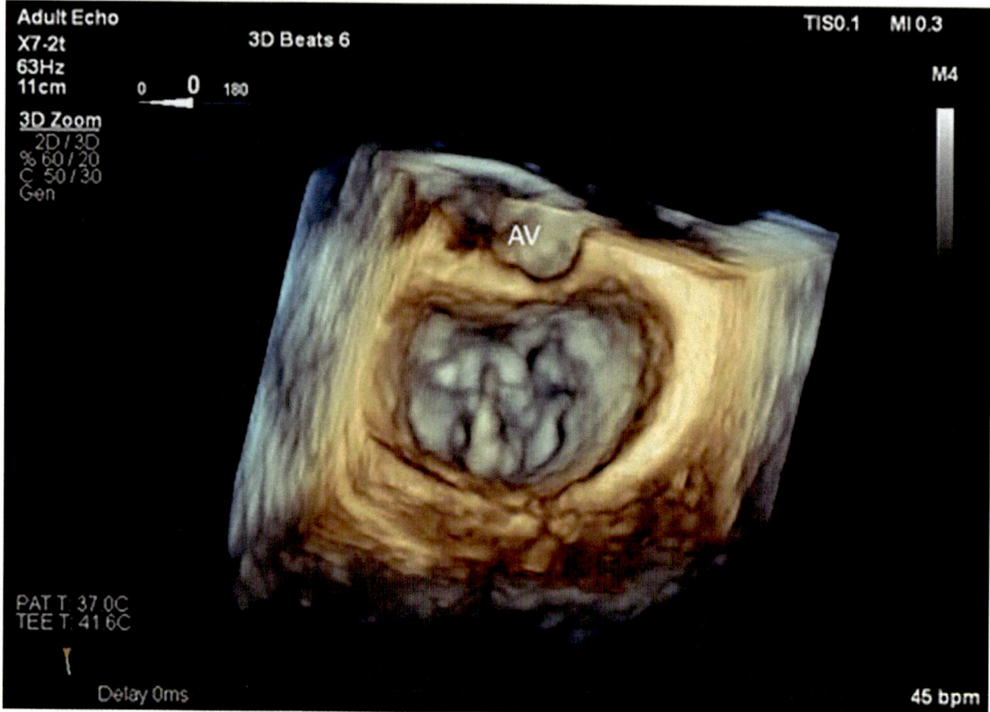

Fig. 9.18 3-Dimensional reconstruction of the mitral valve in the surgeon's en face view. AV, aortic valve

A. A1
B. A2
C. P2
D. P3

Answer C.

Key Point. In the surgeon's view of the mitral valve the valve is oriented with the aortic valve superiorly lateral commissure to the left and medial commissure to the right.

Carpentier's description of mitral valve anatomy names the posterior leaflet segments P1, P2 and P3 from lateral to medial. The anterior leaflet is divided into three regions, A1 A2 and A3, corresponding to the posterior leaflet segments [30].

Question 28

Which of the following is **MOST Likely correct** regarding anatomy of the mitral valve?

A. The largest diameter of the mitral valve can be seen in the parasternal long axis view
B. The posterior mitral leaflet comprises less of the annular circumference than the anterior leaflet
C. The anterior leaflet is in fibrous continuity with the left and non-coronary cusps of the aortic valve
D. The anterior leaflet has anatomic scallops while the posterior leaflet is divided into three regions based on their corresponding anterior leaflet

Answer C.

Key Point. The anterior leaflet is in fibrous continuity with the left and non-coronary cusps of the aortic valve.

The mitral valve is often described as saddle shaped. The parasternal long axis view provides an AP diameter of the valve. This is the high axis of the valve and is smaller than the commissural diameter also referred to as the mediolateral or low axis of the valve. The posterior leaflet is narrow and extends around approximately 2/3 of the annulus while the anterior leaflet is much broader and attaches to the remaining 1/3 of the annulus. The anterior leaflet is in continuity with the interannular fibrosa and is associated with the left and non-coronary cusps [30]. The posterior leaflet has distinct indentations or scallops, P1 P2 and P3 from lateral to medial, while the anterior leaflet is arbitrarily divided into three segments based on the relationship to the corresponding posterior scallop, A1 A2 A3 [31]. The anterolateral and posteromedial papillary muscles support the mitral valve leaflets. Three orders of chordae attach the valve to the papillary muscles.

Question 29

Identify the structure indicated by the red arrow. (Fig. 9.19)

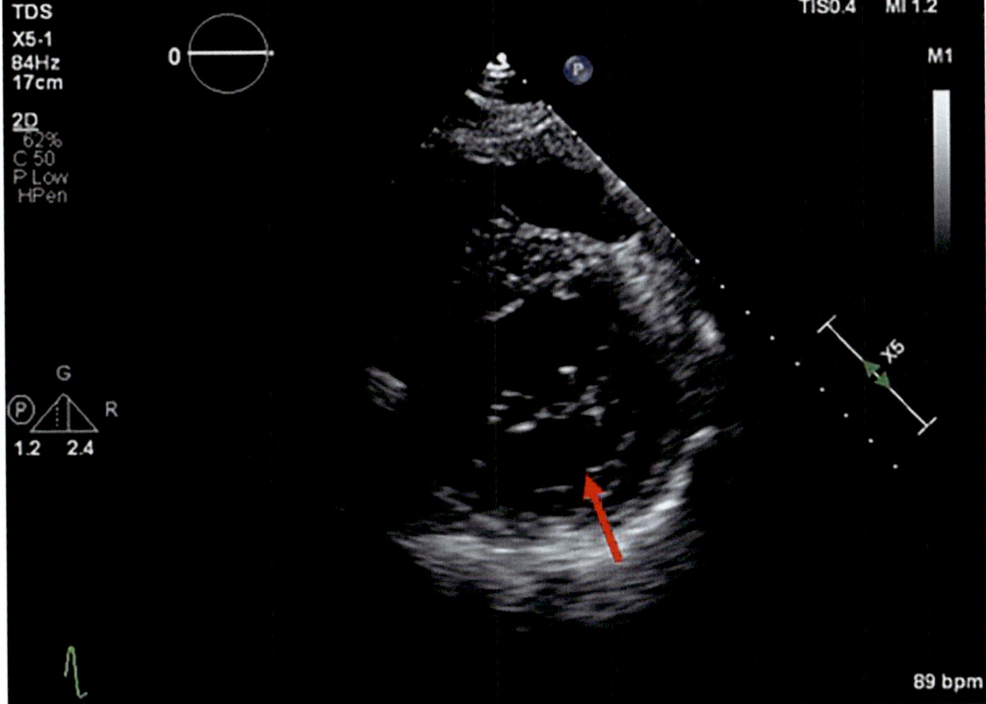

Fig. 9.19 Basal parasternal short axis view

A. Anterior mitral valve leaflet
B. Posterior mitral valve leaflet
C. Anterolateral papillary muscle
D. Posteromedial papillary muscle

Answer B.

Key Point. Parasternal long axis, parasternal short axis, apical four chamber and apical long axis views can be utilized to assess different regions of the valve for pathology.

Transthoracic echocardiography is the main tool to assess the mitral valve for pathology. In the basal parasternal short axis view the two leaflets and commissures can be seen [32]. The valve can be assessed for restriction, lack of coaptation in systole, as well as mitral valve area by planimetry in diastole in this view. The anterior mitral valve leaflet will appear more superior or closer to the ultrasound probe while the posterior leaflet will appear more inferior or farther from the ultrasound probe. The papillary muscles are not visible in the basal short axis view but can easily be seen by moving the view more caudally to the midventricular level.

Question 30

A 56-year-old male presents to the emergency room with a 72-h history of chest pain. He is diagnosed with acute myocardial infarction with ST segment elevations in leads II, III and AVF. A holosystolic murmur is auscultated at the apex. Bedside TTE is performed. Ischemia of which of the labelled structures is most likely to be the cause of the patient's murmur? (Fig. 9.20)

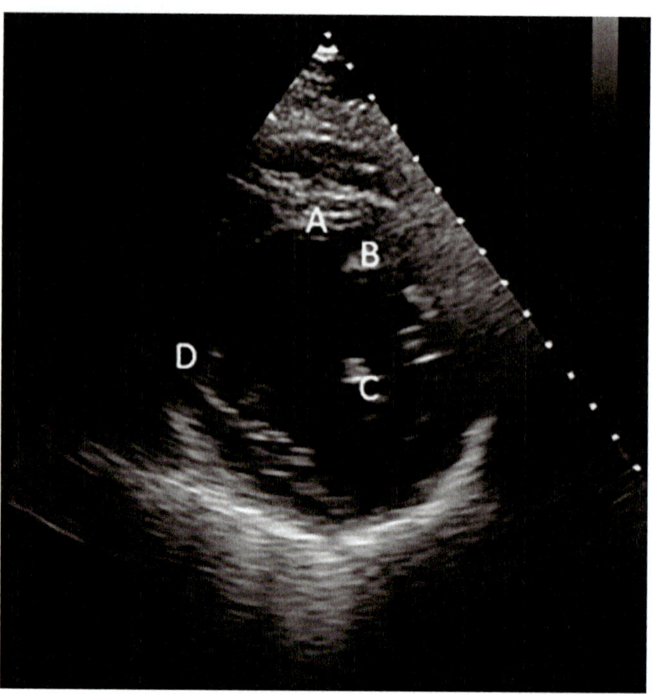

Fig. 9.20 Transthoracic echocardiographic view

A. A
B. B
C. C
D. D

Answer C.

Key Point. Posteromedial papillary muscle rupture is more common than anterolateral papillary muscle rupture due to its single blood supply from the posterior descending coronary artery (PDA).

Papillary muscle rupture after myocardial infarction (MI) typically occurs 2–7 days post ischemic event [33]. It is more common in ST elevation MI but can occur in non-ST elevation MI. It is a rare complication (1–5%) but has a high mortality rate without emergent surgical intervention, up to 50% in 24 hours. Posteromedial papillary muscle rupture is much more common (6–12×) than anterolateral papillary muscle rupture due to its single blood supply from the PDA. Diagnosis should be considered in patients following the first week post myocardial infarction with sudden acute onset heart failure symptoms.

Question 31

Which coronary artery or arteries are most likely to have caused ischemia of the structure in the Question 30?

A. Left circumflex artery or right coronary artery
B. Right coronary artery
C. Left anterior descending artery or left circumflex artery
D. Cannot be determined based on the information provided

Answer A.

Key Point. The posteromedial papillary muscle is higher risk for ischemia due to its single blood supply from the posterior descending coronary artery (PDA).

The posteromedial papillary muscle is higher risk for ischemia due to its single blood supply from the PDA [33]. Coronary artery dominance is defined by which vessel gives rise to the PDA which supplies the inferior 1/3 of the interventricular septum. Most individuals (80–85%) are right dominant where the PDA is supplied by the right coronary artery. The remainder are left or codominant. In left dominant coronary circulation the PDA is supplied by the circumflex coronary artery.

Question 32

Which of the following echocardiographic findings in this patient's parasternal long axis view is most indicative of their disease process? (Fig. 9.21)

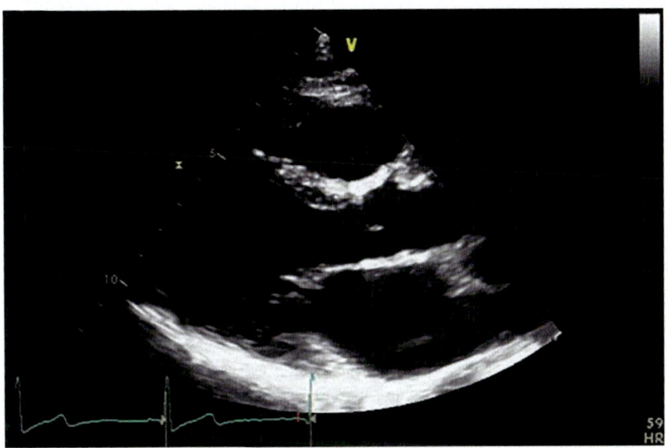

Fig. 9.21 Transthoracic parasternal long axis view

A. Hockey stick appearance of the anterior mitral leaflet.
B. Redundant anterior mitral leaflet tissue.
C. Severe calcification of the aortic valve leaflets.
D. Severe right ventricular hypertrophy.

Answer A.

Key Point. In a transthoracic echo of a patient with mitral stenosis the parasternal long-axis view demonstrates characteristic hockey-stick appearance of the anterior mitral leaflet, decreased mobility of the posterior mitral leaflet, and markedly enlarged left atrium.

In a transthoracic echo of a patient with mitral stenosis the parasternal long-axis view demonstrates characteristic hockey-stick appearance of the anterior mitral leaflet, decreased mobility of the posterior mitral leaflet, and markedly enlarged left atrium [34]. Other findings include commissural fusion resulting in a "fish mouth" appearance of the mitral valve in a parasternal short axis view, and chordal thickening and fusion in apical views. Flow acceleration and the formation of proximal isovelocity surface area (PISA) across the mitral valve in diastole are commonly seen with color flow Doppler interrogation. Although commonly found concomitantly in rheumatic heart disease, there is no evidence of aortic stenosis or right ventricular hypertrophy in the above image.

Question 33

Which of the following statements is **MOST likely correct** regarding the etiology of mitral stenosis?

A. Rheumatic heart disease is the most common cause of mitral stenosis in developing countries but calcific degeneration is the most common cause in developed countries
B. The mechanism of mitral stenosis in rheumatic heart disease is typically annular calcification while the mechanism of degenerative mitral stenosis is typically commissural fusion
C. Valve thickening more often affects the bases of the leaflets in rheumatic heart disease while the tips are more often affected in degenerative calcification
D. Calcification of the mitral annulus more frequently causes mitral regurgitation than mitral stenosis

Answer D.

Key Point. Rheumatic heart disease is the most common cause of mitral stenosis worldwide and has associated characteristic echocardiographic findings.

Rheumatic heart disease is the most common cause of mitral stenosis worldwide, including in developed countries. The main mechanism of stenosis in rheumatic heart disease is commissural fusion [35]. Leaflet thickening tends to affect primarily the leaflet tips in rheumatic disease which the annulus and leaflet bases are affected in degenerative calcification. Calcification of the mitral annulus in degenerative valvular disease often has few or no hemodynamic consequences and more often results in mitral regurgitation.

Question 34

In a patient with mitral stenosis, which of the following is **MOST likely correct** in regards to disease severity?

A. Mitral valve area measured by planimetry of 1.8 cm^2 corresponds to moderate disease
B. PHT of 110 ms corresponds to severe disease
C. Mean pressure gradient of 9 mmHg corresponds to moderate disease
D. Deceleration time of the mitral E wave of 380 ms corresponds to severe disease

Answer C.

Key Point. A mean gradient from 5 to 10 mmHg is consistent with moderate mitral stenosis.

A normal mitral valve area (MVA) in an adult is approximately 4–6 cm^2 [35]. Severe stenosis is defined as a MVA less than 1 cm^2, moderate is between 1.0 and 1.5 cm^2 and mild is greater than 1.5 cm^2. There are multiple methods to calculate or measure MVA. Planimetry of the valve orifice can be performed in a parasternal short axis basal view. Pressure half time (PHT) is the length of time required for the maximum diastolic velocity to reach half its value. A longer PHT means that it takes longer for the pressures between the left atrium and left ventricle to equilibrate, meaning a smaller valve area. The formula for deriving MVA from PHT is: MVA = 220/PHT.

Mean gradient through the mitral valve can be used to assess severity as well. A mean gradient less than 5 mmHg is mild stenosis while a mean gradient greater than 10 mmHg is severe stenosis. A mean gradient from 5 to 10 mmHg is consistent with moderate mitral stenosis.

The mitral valve deceleration time corresponds to the length of time from the peak velocity of the E wave to the end of the antegrade flow. The formula used to calculate the mitral valve area from this parameter is the following: MVA = 759/DT.

Question 35

A 68 year old female patient presents to the ICU with worsening shortness of breath, pedal edema and palpitations. Bedside TTE is performed and an apical four-chamber view is obtained. Which of the following is MOST likely correct regarding this patient's mitral inflow gradient? (Fig. 9.22)

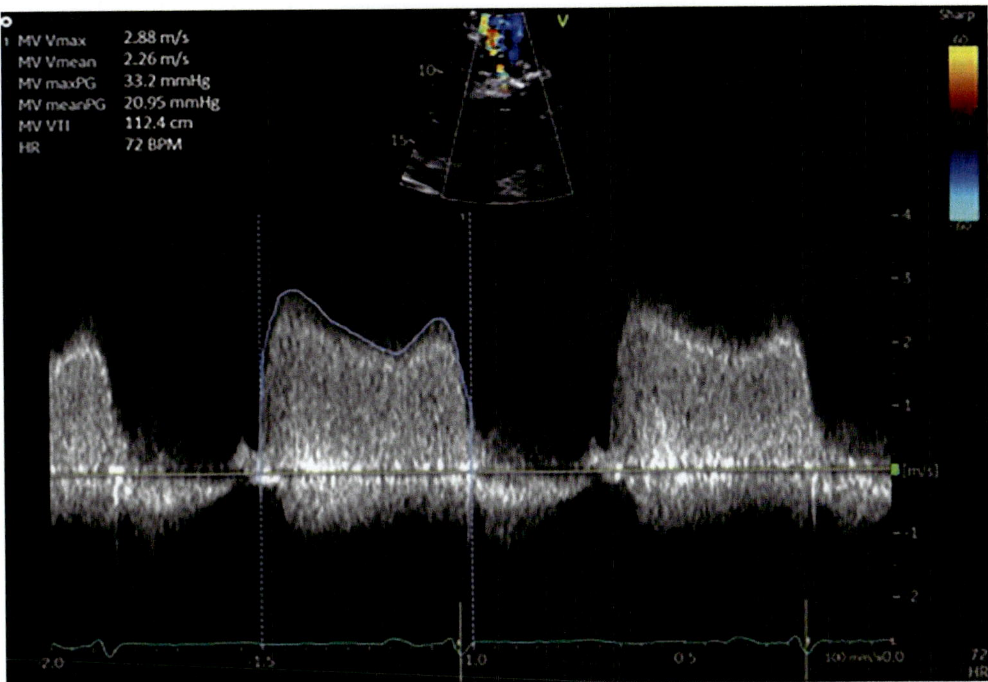

Fig. 9.22 Continuous wave Doppler spectral envelope through the mitral valve in the apical four-chamber view

A. The patient has severe mitral stenosis based on the mean gradient through the valve
B. The patient has severe mitral stenosis based on the peak gradient through the valve
C. The patient has severe mitral stenosis based on the maximum velocity of flow through the valve
D. The severity of mitral stenosis cannot be determined based on the information provided

Answer A.

Key Point. Quantification of valvular stenosis severity is based on mean gradient.

Quantification of valvular stenosis severity is based on mean gradient [35]. Maximal gradient is dependent on peak mitral velocity which in turn is affected by left atrial pressure and left ventricular diastolic function. As such it is not useful in quantifying stenosis severity. There are multiple parameters with which to quantify mitral stenosis severity, mean gradient is one parameter. A mean gradient <5 mmHg is mild, 5–10 mmHg is moderate and > 10 mmHg is severe. Of note, heart rate should be reported and should be between 60–80 bpm as heart rate will affect transmitral flow. Additionally, in patients in atrial fibrillation mean gradient should be averaged over 5 cycles.

Question 36

The use of pressure half time (PHT) for grading severity of mitral stenosis is not valid when which of the following is present?

A. Left ventricular dysfunction
B. Mild aortic valve insufficiency
C. Right ventricular dysfunction
D. Severe left atrial hypertrophy

Answer A.

Key Point. Multiple factors influence transmitral flow and can affect the validity of using pressure half time (PHT) to calculate mitral valve area.

Pressure half time (PHT) is the time it takes to decrease to half of the peak mitral inflow velocity [34, 36]. Use of PHT has several limitations. Estimates are not accurate in the following circumstances: left ventricular hypertrophy, left ventricular wall motion abnormalities, left ventricular diastolic dysfunction, recent commissurotomy and greater than mild aortic insufficiency [35].

Question 37

The following mitral valve inflow spectral Doppler tracing was obtained in the apical 4-chamber view. Based on the measured pressure half time (PHT) what is the mitral valve area (MVA)? (Fig. 9.23)

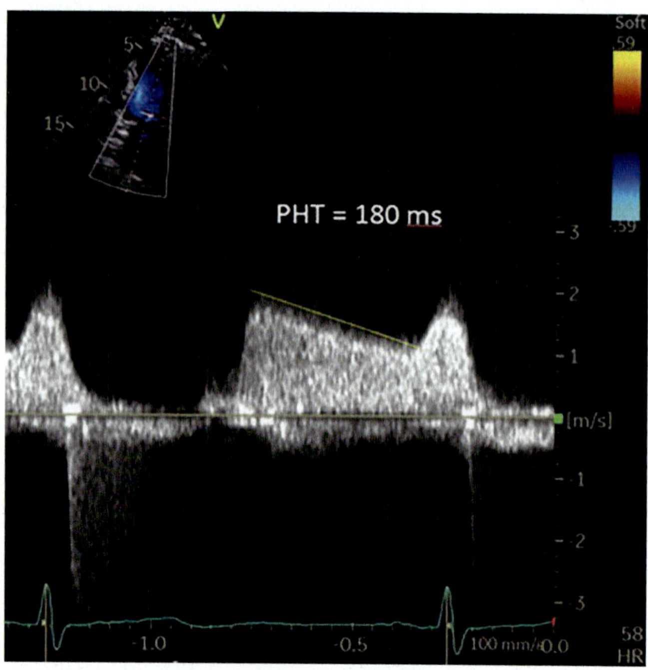

Fig. 9.23 Continuous wave Doppler spectral envelope through the mitral valve in the apical four-chamber view

A. 1.1 cm²
B. 1.2 cm²
C. 1.3 cm²
D. 1.4 cm²

Answer B.

Key Point. Pressure half time is widely used to calculate mitral valve area as it is easy to perform, but it has several limitations.

Pressure half time (PHT) is the length of time required for the maximum diastolic velocity to reach half its value [35, 36]. A longer PHT means that it takes longer for the pressures between the left atrium and left ventricle to equilibrate, meaning a smaller valve area. The formula for deriving MVA from PHT is: MVA = 220/PHT.

See explanation for question 36 for limitations regarding the use of pressure half time.

Question 38

What is the severity of mitral stenosis based on the calculated MVA from Question 37?

A. Mild
B. Moderate
C. Severe
D. Cannot be determined based on the information provided

Answer B.

Key Point. Mitral valve area can be calculated using the pressure half time equation.

Mitral valve area can be calculated using the pressure half time equation: MVA = 220/PHT [35]. A normal mitral valve area (MVA) in an adult is approximately 4 to 6 cm². Severe stenosis is defined as a mitral valve area less than 1 cm², moderate is between 1.0 and 1.5 cm² and mild is greater than 1.5 cm².

Question 39

Calculate the mitral valve area (MVA) based on the following TTE images (Figs. 9.24, 9.25 and 9.26)

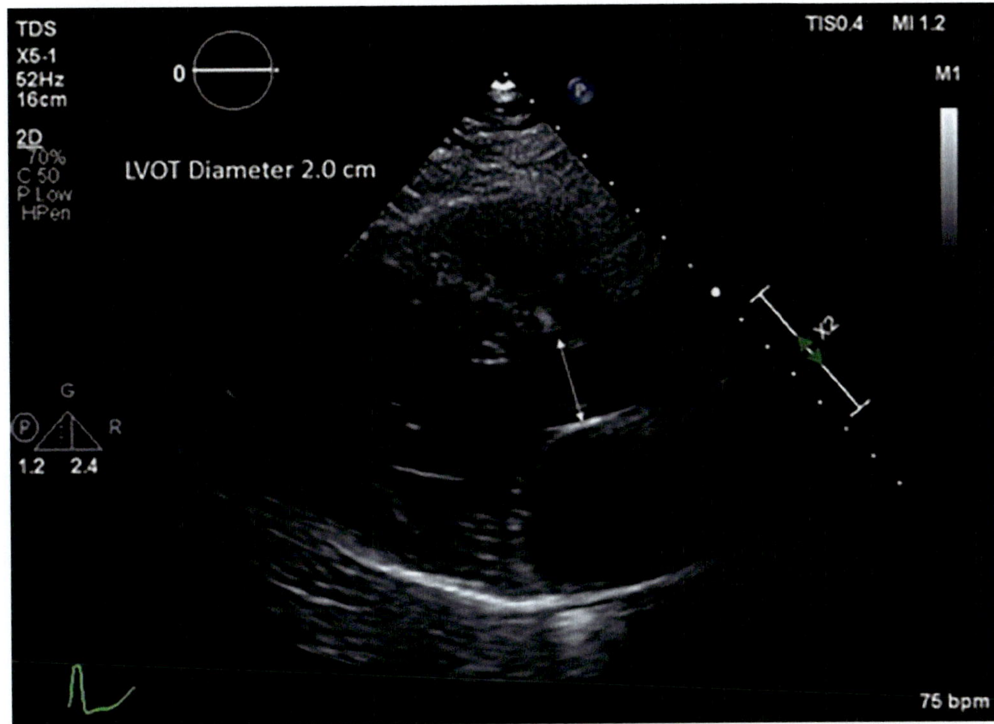

Fig. 9.24 Transthoracic parasternal long axis view. LVOT diameter 2.0 cm

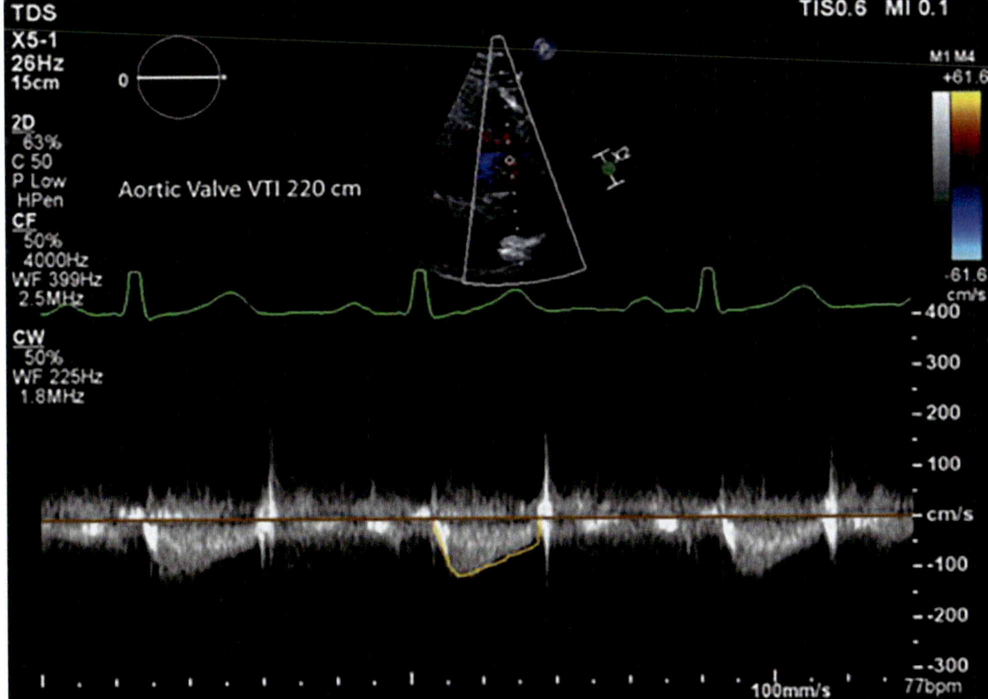

Fig. 9.25 Continuous wave Doppler envelope through the aortic valve. Aortic valve VTI 220 cm

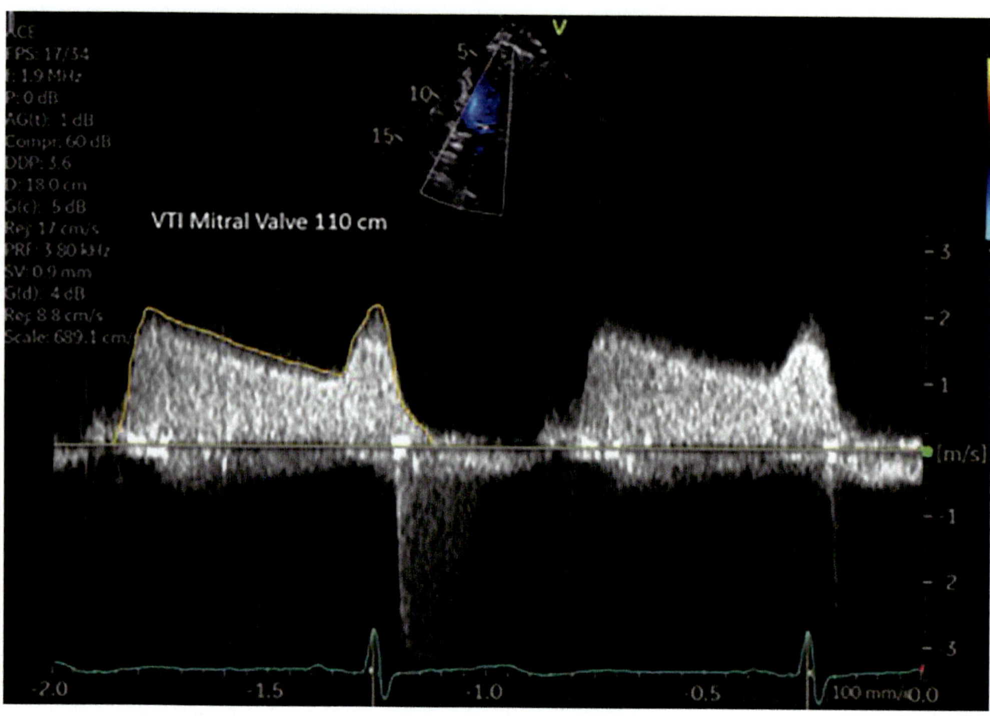

Fig. 9.26 Continuous wave Doppler envelope through the mitral valve. Mitral valve VTI 110 cm

A. 3.2 cm^2
B. 6.3 cm^2
C. 12.5 cm^2
D. Cannot be determined based on the information provided

Answer B.

Key Point. Mitral valve area can be calculated using the continuity equation.

As when calculating aortic valve area using the continuity equation, [35] mitral valve area can similarly be calculated using the following formula:

$$MVA = \pi^{*} r^{2*} \left(VTI_{Aortic} / VTI_{Mitral}\right)$$

In the above example MVA = $\pi * (1)^2 * (220/110) =$ 6.3 cm^2

Where r^2 is the radius of the left ventricular outflow tract as measured in parasternal long axis, VTI_{Aortic} is the VTI of blood outflow through the aortic valve measured in the apical four chamber view and VTIMitral is the VTI of mitral inflow also measured in the apical four chamber view in centimeters. The blood flow through the mitral valve is equal to the blood flow through the LVOT and thus can be used to calculate mitral valve area in the absence of significant mitral or aortic regurgitation.

Question 40

Which of the following is **MOST likely correct** regarding the mechanism of mitral regurgitation in different etiologies?

A. In rheumatic heart disease the mechanism is leaflet thickening and scarring
B. In endocarditis the mechanism is usually scarring of the leaflets around the infected areas
C. In Barlow disease there is restriction in motion of the leaflets
D. In radiation related disease there is perforation of the leaflets

Answer A.

Key Point. Determining the mechanism of mitral regurgitation is important in distinguishing the etiology of the lesion.

Mitral regurgitation (MR) is divided into two categories: Primary MR, which is an abnormality of the leaflets and secondary MR, which results from ventricular remodeling and a distortion of the mitral valve apparatus [22]. The above etiologies are all examples of etiologies of primary MR. The most common cause of primary MR is myxomatous degeneration causing mitral valve prolapse. It has a wide range of disease presentations from a focal abnormality to diffuse involvement of multiple segments of both leaflets.

In Barlow's disease there are multiple areas affected within the leaflets, and is a result of abnormal accumulation of mucopolysaccharides in the leaflets and chordae [37]. Over time this results in redundant, billowing leaflets, elongated chordae, and prolapse of the leaflets.

In endocarditis there is leaflet thickening, vegetation disruption of the coaptation line, and destruction of leaflet tissue resulting in perforation of the involved leaflets. In rheumatic disease the leaflets are thickened and scarred, restricting their motion and preventing their coaptation. In radiation heart disease there is early onset thickening and calcification of the leaflets.

Question 41

When assessing the Continuous Wave Doppler (CW) spectral envelope of a patient with mitral regurgitation (MR), which of the following is **MOST likely correct** regarding disease severity?

A. The MR Doppler signal is denser in severe MR
B. The jet in severe MR lasts only during the first half of systole
C. In mild MR the contour of the signal can be triangular
D. Both central and eccentric jets can be effectively assessed by continuous wave doppler

Answer A.

Key Point. Characteristics of the doppler spectral envelope can aid in determining severity of mitral regurgitation.

The Doppler signal represents the speed of flow of red blood cells against time. The velocity of a typical MR jet is high (4–6 m/s) due to the large pressure gradient between the left ventricle and left atrium in systole [22]. In severe regurgitation the spectral envelope appears dense, corresponding to more red blood cells in motion and is a qualitative method to assess MR severity. Severe mitral regurgitant flow happens throughout systole as the pressure in the left ventricle exceeds the pressure in the left atrium for the majority of systole. In severe MR, the jet can appear to be triangular in shape or peak early due to prominent regurgitant flow. Ideally the cursor should be aligned with the vena contracta and the body of the mitral regurgitation jet to accurately capture the full regurgitant flow velocity. Eccentric jets may be difficult to align thus making this modality inaccurate when assessing severity of eccentric jets.

Question 42

A 20-year-old female presents with a holosystolic murmur. She recently relocated to the United States from Madagascar in order to attend college. A still image from her bedside echocardiogram is shown below. Which of the following is the most likely etiology of her valvular heart disease? (Fig. 9.27)

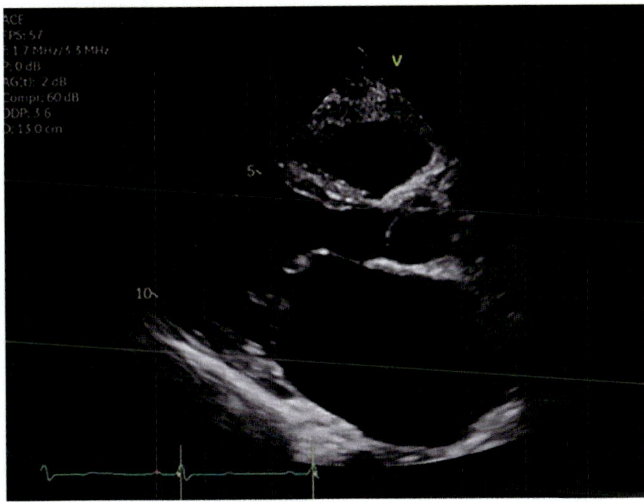

Fig. 9.27 Parasternal long axis view

A. Papillary muscle rupture due to ischemic heart disease
B. Rheumatic valve disease after an isolated episode of acute rheumatic fever
C. Mitral valve prolapse with a systolic valve excursion into the left atrium ≥2 cm beyond the annulus
D. Bi-leaflet prolapse secondary to a dilated LV due to ischemic heart disease

Answer B.

Key Point. Rheumatic valvular disease can occur even after a single isolated episode of rheumatic fever.

Young female patients from underdeveloped countries can present with severe rheumatic mitral regurgitation. This can occur after an isolated infection or multiple episode of rheumatic fever. The mitral valve is most commonly affected followed by the aortic and tricuspid valves less commonly. While rheumatic heart disease is the most common cause of mitral stenosis worldwide, it more often presents with mitral regurgitation [38].

Papillary muscle rupture secondary to ischemic heart disease can cause severe, acute mitral regurgitation. Usually occurring 2–7 days following an ischemic event. It is less likely in this age group.

Patients with degenerative mitral valve disease will have associate mitral valve prolapse, showing an abnormal leaflet motion into the left atrium ≥2 mm beyond the mitral annulus [22].

Ischemic mitral regurgitation (secondary mitral regurgitation) results from ventricular remodeling, apical displacement, and restriction and tethering of the mitral leaflets.

Question 43

A 67 year old male patient presents to the intensive care unit with symptoms of acutely decompensated heart failure. He is urgently intubated due to hypoxia. A TEE is performed due to the severity of his symptoms with the following TEE image obtained. Which of the following is the mechanism of his valvular disease? (Fig. 9.28)

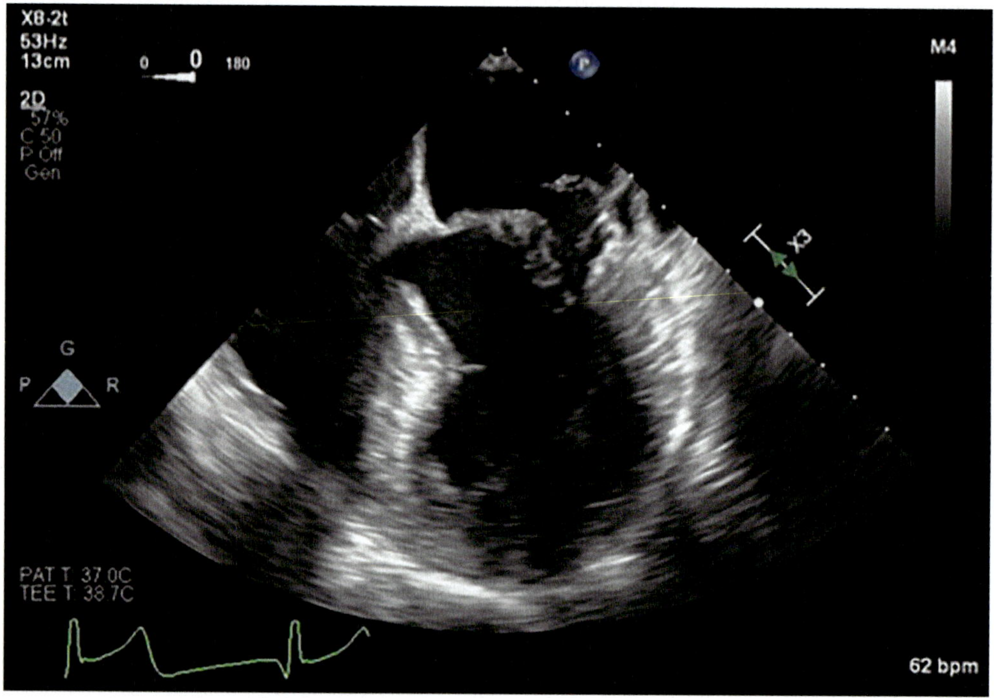

Fig. 9.28 TEE midesophageal four-chamber view

A. Carpentier Type I
B. Carpentier Type II
C. Carpentier Type IIIa
D. Carpentier Type IIIb

Answer B.

Key Point. The Carpentier classification of mitral regurgitation is divided into three main categories based on leaflet motion characteristics.

Carpentier's classification for mitral valve regurgitation is based on the characteristics of leaflet motion [39, 40]. Type I is normal leaflet motion, with the mechanism for the regurgitation being annular dilatation or leaflet perforation. Type II is excessive leaflet motion, with portions of the leaflet prolapsing or flailing the level of the valve annulus. Type III is restricted leaflet motion and is further subdivided into IIIa: restriction in both systole and diastole and IIIb: restricted in systole only.

Question 44

Which of the following is **MOST likely correct** regarding the degree of severity of mitral regurgitation in the patient in Question 45?

A. A calculated Effective Regurgitant Orifice Area (EROA) ≥ 0.4 cm^2 corresponds to mild disease
B. A regurgitant volume ≥ 60 ml corresponds to severe disease
C. A regurgitant fraction ≤45% corresponds to severe disease
D. A vena contracta ≥0.7 cm corresponds to moderate disease

Answer B.

Key Point. There are multiple indices with which to assess the severity of mitral regurgitation.

According to the current guidelines, a vena contracta ≥0.7 cm, an EROA ≥0.4 cm^2, regurgitant volume ≥ 60 mL, and regurgitant fraction ≥50% constitute severe mitral regurgitation [22, 41].

Question 45

When using the simplified PISA method to assess the severity of mitral gurgitation, which of the following is **MOST likely correct**?

A. The MR jet's velocity is assumed to have a velocity of 4 m/s
B. The baseline shift of the aliasing velocity (Nyquist) should be set to 40 cm/s
C. The effective regurgitant orifice area (EROA) corresponds to aliasing radius divided by two
D. An aliasing radius ≥ 0.5 cm corresponds to severe disease

Answer B.

Key Point. The PISA method of calculating effective regurgitant orifice area (EROA) can be simplified to increase its ease of use in clinical settings.

The simplified PISA method of calculating the EROA assumes a pressure difference of 100 mm Hg between the left atrium and left ventricle, when setting the aliasing velocity to 40 cm/s, it simplifies the EROA calculation formula from:

$$\text{EROA} = 2\ \pi \times \text{aliasing radius}^2 \times \text{velocity}_{\text{ALIASING}} / \text{velocity}_{\text{REGURGITANT JET}}$$

To: $\text{EROA} = \text{aliasing radius}^2/2$

This simplified method reduced the time needed to calculate EROA and increases its ease of use in clinical settings [42].

Question 46

Which of the following findings is **MOST likely correct** regarding the severity of mitral regurgitation?

A. Using the mitral regurgitant jet's area to determine severity is load independent
B. Pulmonary venous flow reversal during diastole is a sensitive indicator of severity
C. Left atrial volume reliable correlates with severity of regurgitation
D. When assessing mitral valve flow, a low E velocity and A wave dominance excludes severe MR

Answer D.

Key Point. There are multiple methods to assess the severity of MR, each with its own limitations.

Pulsed Wave Doppler tracing of the mitral valve inflow can be useful in assessing the severity of a patient's MR. [41] The E wave will have an increased velocity in patients with severe MR corresponding to a dominant early filling pattern. A pattern similar to that seen in patients with impaired relaxation, low E wave and dominant A wave velocity, excludes severe MR.

Mitral regurgitant jet area is dependent on the patient's hemodynamics, including blood pressure and filling conditions. Pulmonary flow reversal during systole is an indicator of severity of regurgitation. There is a progressive decrease in the systolic velocity with an eventual reversal of systolic flow in severe disease. Evidence of this in more than one vein is a more reliable marker of severity. Left atrial volume is a non-specific finding that occurs in multiple disease states with elevated left atrial pressure, it does not directly correlate with severity of regurgitation.

Question 47

Which of the following is **MOST likely correct** regarding secondary mitral regurgitation (MR)?

A. The most common mechanism is symmetrical apical displacement of leaflets, resulting in a central MR jet
B. Leaflet tethering is often asymmetrical in ischemic cardiomyopathy, causing an eccentric regurgitant jet
C. Tenting area is useful in determining severity as it measures area from leaflet tips to the annular plane during diastole
D. Tenting height does not correlate with the severity of MR

Answer B.

Key Point. In secondary MR the leaflets are anatomically normal but are restricted due to apical tethering or ventricular dilation and remodeling.

In secondary MR the leaflets are morphologically normal, they are pulled apically into the LV as papillary muscles get displaced with the dilating LV chamber [43]. The leaflet tethering is often asymmetrical, with the P3 scallop tethered more than the P1.

The tenting area is measured from the leaflet tips to the annular plane performed during mid-systole [44]. The coaptation height is the maximal distance from leaflet tips to annular plane correlating well with the severity of disease.

Using 3D the tenting volume has been calculated, by measuring the tethering distance from the papillary muscle tip to the mitral annulus plane.

Question 48

A 79 year old female patient with a history of coronary artery disease presents to the emergency room with a complaint of worsening shortness of breath over the past several months. An apical 4 chamber view from the patient's bedside echocardiogram is shown. In this patient with severe secondary mitral regurgitation, which of the following is **MOST likely correct** regarding the color flow Doppler image of her mitral regurgitant (MR) jet? (Fig. 9.29)

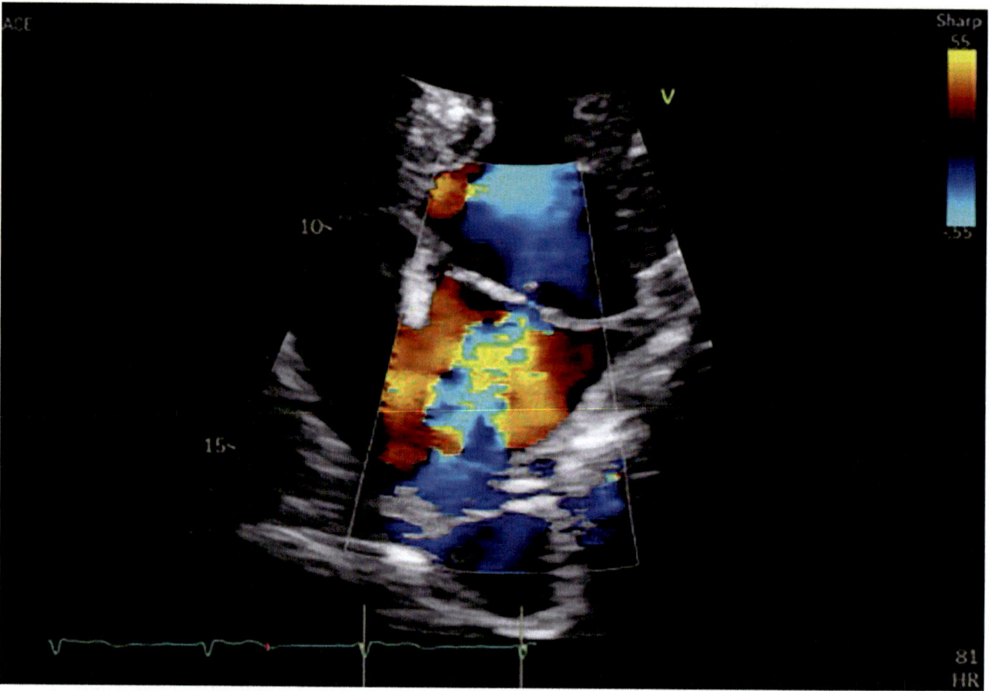

Fig. 9.29 Apical four-chamber view with color flow Doppler

A. The MR jet area is a reliable method for grading the severity of MR
B. The patient's blood pressure has no effect on the observed jet area
C. In the case of eccentric jets, the jet area can underestimate the severity of the MR
D. Jets observed in the two chamber view correlate with severity of the MR

Answer C.

Key Point. MR jet area is influenced by multiple hemodynamic factors.

The absence of an MR jet is useful for excluding MR. However, its size is not always reliable for determining the severity of regurgitation.

MR jet areas are dependent on multiple hemodynamic factors, independent of the severity of the MR. [41] These include patient hemodynamic factors (blood pressure, heart rate and filling pressures), compliance of the left atrium, and eccentricity of the jet. In eccentric or wall-hugging jets the energy of the jet spreads along the wall and loses energy, showing a smaller jet area [45]. Slit like orifices can overestimate the severity of the jet when examined in two chamber views, as color flow Doppler will show the regurgitation along the line of MV coaptation, and not a cross section of the effective orifice.

Question 49

In a patient with severe mitral regurgitation, which of the following is **MOST likely correct** regarding vena contracta?

A. It is best measured in the parasternal long axis zoomed view, perpendicular to mitral leaflet closure
B. It effectively estimates the severity of MR in holosystolic jets
C. It is not a valid method to estimate MR with eccentric jets
D. A value ≥0.4 cm corresponds to severe regurgitation

Answer A.

Key Point. The vena contracta is the narrowest high velocity region of flow between the proximal flow convergence area and the jet as it moves into the left atrium and can be used to assess severity of regurgitation.

The vena contracta is the narrowest high velocity region of flow between the proximal flow convergence area and the jet as it moves into the left atrium [22]. Ideally it is assessed in a zoomed parasternal long axis view, where the flow is perpendicular to the mitral leaflet closure. Cutoff values for vena contracta (VC) correspond to mild MR in patients with VC ≤ 0.3 cm, and severe when the VC is ≥0.7 cm [46]. It can be used reliably to assess both central and eccentric jets.

The vena contracta can overestimate the severity of jets that are not holosystolic, especially those that occur during late systolic prolapse.

Question 50

Calculate the regurgitant volume based on the following information:

LVOT Diameter = 2 cm
MV Diameter = 4 cm
LVOT VTI = 60 cm
MV VTI = 30 cm

A. 94.2 mL
B. 188.4 mL
C. 376.8 mL
D. Cannot be determined based on the information provided

Answer B.

Key Point. Regurgitant volume can be calculated by subtracting the stroke volume through the LVOT from the stroke volume through the mitral valve.

Regurgitant volume can be calculated when both the total mitral inflow and left ventricular stroke volume are known. In this manner $SV_{LVOT} = SV_{MV}\text{-}R_{Vol}$ where SV_{LVO} is left ventricular stroke volume, SV_{MV} is total mitral inflow volume and R_{Vol} is regurgitant volume. Rearranging this equation to solve for regurgitant volume results in the following:

$$R_{Vol} = SV_{MV} - SV_{LVOT}$$

$$SV_{LVOT} = CSA_{LVOT}{}^{*}\ VTI_{LVOT}$$
$$CSA_{LVOT} = \pi^{*}\ r^{2}$$

$$SV_{MV} = CSA_{MV}{}^{*}\ VTI_{MV}$$

$$CSA_{MV} = \pi^{*}\ r^{2}$$

LVOT diameter is measured in systole at the level of the annulus in the same location that LVOT VTI is measured with pulsed wave doppler in an apical four chamber view. MV diameter is measured in mid diastole in the apical 4 chamber view with mitral valve VTI measured with pulsed wave doppler at the level of the mitral valve annulus.

Solving for regurgitant volume based on the above values yields.

$$CSA_{LVOT} = \pi^{*}\ (1)^{2} = 3.14\,\text{cm}^{2}$$

$$CSA_{MV} = \pi^{*}\ (2)^{2} = 12.56\,\text{cm}^{2}$$

$$SV_{LVOT} = CSA_{LVOT}{}^{*}\ VTI_{LVOT} = 3.14^{*}\ 60 = 188.4\,\text{mL}$$

$$SV_{MV} = CSA_{MV}{}^{*} VTI_{MV} = 12.56^{*} 30 = 376.8\,mL$$

$$R_{Vol} = SV_{MV} - SV_{LVOT} = 376.8 - 188.4 = 188.4\,mL$$

A regurgitant volume of 188.4 mL classifies this mitral regurgitation as severe. Cutoff values for mitral regurgitation severity based on regurgitant volume are: mild <30 mL, moderate 30–59 mL and severe >60 mL [22].

References

1. Loukas M, Bilinsky E, Bilinsky S, Blaak C, Tubbs RS, Anderson RH. The anatomy of the aortic root. Clin Anat. 2014;27(5):748–56.
2. Kunihara T. Anatomy of the aortic root: implications for aortic root reconstruction. Gen Thorac Cardiovasc Surg. 2017;65(9):488–99.
3. Lang RM, Badano LP, Mor-Avi V, Afilalo J, Armstrong A, Ernande L, Flachskampf FA, Foster E, Goldstein SA, Kuznetsova T, Lancellotti P, Muraru D, Picard MH, Rietzschel ER, Rudski L, Spencer KT, Tsang W, Voigt JU. Recommendations for cardiac chamber quantification by echocardiography in adults: an update from the American Society of Echocardiography and the European Association of Cardiovascular Imaging. Eur Heart J Cardiovasc Imaging. 2015;16(3):233–70.
4. Mitchell C, Rahko PS, Blauwet LA, Canaday B, Finstuen JA, Foster MC, Horton K, Ogunyankin KO, Palma RA, Velazquez EJ. Guidelines for performing a comprehensive transthoracic echocardiographic examination in adults: recommendations from the american society of echocardiography. J Am Soc Echocardiogr. 2019;32(1):1–64.
5. Shah SY, Higgins A, Desai MY. Bicuspid aortic valve: basics and beyond. Cleve Clin J Med. 2018;85(10):779–84.
6. Siu SC, Silversides CK. Bicuspid aortic valve disease. J Am Coll Cardiol. 2010;55(25):2789–800.
7. Michelena HI, Khanna AD, Mahoney D, Margaryan E, Topilsky Y, Suri RM, Eidem B, Edwards WD, Sundt TM 3rd, Enriquez-Sarano M. Incidence of aortic complications in patients with bicuspid aortic valves. JAMA. 2011;306(10):1104–12.
8. Sinning C, Zengin E, Kozlik-Feldmann R, Blankenberg S, Rickers C, von Kodolitsch Y, Girdauskas E. Bicuspid aortic valve and aortic coarctation in congenital heart disease-important aspects for treatment with focus on aortic vasculopathy. Cardiovasc Diagn Ther. 2018;8(6):780–8.
9. Lindman BR, Clavel MA, Mathieu P, Iung B, Lancellotti P, Otto CM, Pibarot P. Calcific aortic stenosis. Nat Rev Dis Primers. 2016;2:16006.
10. Baumgartner H, Hung J, Bermejo J, Chambers JB, Edvardsen T, Goldstein S, Lancellotti P, LeFevre M, Miller F Jr, Otto CM. Recommendations on the Echocardiographic Assessment of Aortic Valve Stenosis: A Focused Update from the European Association of Cardiovascular Imaging and the American Society of Echocardiography. J Am Soc Echocardiogr. 2017;30(4):372–92.
11. Nguyen TQ, Hansen KL, Bechsgaard T, Lonn L, Jensen JA, Nielsen MB. Non-invasive assessment of intravascular pressure gradients: a review of current and proposed novel methods. Diagnostics (Basel). 2018;9:1.
12. Markin NW, Desjardins G. Subaortic membrane and the "unsimplified" Bernoulli equation. Anesth Analg. 2014;119(1):30–4.
13. Hui S, Mahmood F, Matyal R. Aortic valve area-technical communication: continuity and Gorlin equations revisited. J Cardiothorac Vasc Anesth. 2018;32(6):2599–606.
14. Bonow RO, Carabello BA, Chatterjee K, de Leon AC Jr, Faxon DP, Freed MD, Gaasch WH, Lytle BW, Nishimura RA, O'Gara PT, O'Rourke RA, Otto CM, Shah PM, Shanewise JS, American College of Cardiology/American Heart Association Task Force on Practice G. 2008 focused update incorporated into the ACC/AHA 2006 guidelines for the management of patients with valvular heart disease: a report of the American College of Cardiology/American Heart Association Task Force on Practice Guidelines (Writing Committee to revise the 1998 guidelines for the management of patients with valvular heart disease). Endorsed by the Society of Cardiovascular Anesthesiologists, Society for Cardiovascular Angiography and Interventions, and Society of Thoracic Surgeons. J Am Coll Cardiol. 2008;52(13):e1-142.
15. Sherwood MW, Kiefer TL. Challenges in aortic valve stenosis: low-flow states diagnosis, management, and a review of the current literature. Curr Cardiol Rep. 2017;19(12):130.
16. Mittnacht AJ, Fanshawe M, Konstadt S. Anesthetic considerations in the patient with valvular heart disease undergoing noncardiac surgery. Semin Cardiothorac Vasc Anesth. 2008;12(1):33–59.
17. Frogel J, Galusca D. Anesthetic considerations for patients with advanced valvular heart disease undergoing noncardiac surgery. Anesthesiol Clin. 2010;28(1):67–85.
18. Yuan SM. Quadricuspid aortic valve: a comprehensive review. Braz J Cardiovasc Surg. 2016;31(6):454–60.
19. Suraci N, Horvath SA, Urina D, Rosen G, Santana O. Quadricuspid aortic valve: case series and review of literature. Echocardiography. 2019;36(2):406–10.
20. Nishimura RA, Otto CM, Bonow RO, Carabello BA, Erwin JP 3rd, Guyton RA, O'Gara PT, Ruiz CE, Skubas NJ, Sorajja P, Sundt TM 3rd, Thomas JD, Anderson JL, Halperin JL, Albert NM, Bozkurt B, Brindis RG, Creager MA, Curtis LH, DeMets D, Guyton RA, Hochman JS, Kovacs RJ, Ohman EM, Pressler SJ, Sellke FW, Shen WK, Stevenson WG, Yancy CW, American College of C, American College of Cardiology/American Heart A, American Heart A. 2014 AHA/ACC guideline for the management of patients with valvular heart disease: a report of the American College of Cardiology/American Heart Association Task Force on Practice Guidelines. J Thorac Cardiovasc Surg. 2014;148(1):e1–e132.
21. El Khoury G, Glineur D, Rubay J, Verhelst R, d'Acoz Y, Poncelet A, Astarci P, Noirhomme P, van Dyck M. Functional classification of aortic root/valve abnormalities and their correlation with etiologies and surgical procedures. Curr Opin Cardiol. 2005;20(2):115–21.
22. Zoghbi WA, Adams D, Bonow RO, Enriquez-Sarano M, Foster E, Grayburn PA, Hahn RT, Han Y, Hung J, Lang RM, Little SH, Shah DJ, Shernan S, Thavendiranathan P, Thomas JD, Weissman NJ. Recommendations for noninvasive evaluation of native valvular regurgitation: a report from the American Society of Echocardiography Developed in Collaboration with the Society for Cardiovascular Magnetic Resonance. J Am Soc Echocardiogr. 2017;30(4):303–71.
23. Maurer G. Aortic regurgitation. Heart. 2006;92(7):994–1000.
24. Sutton DC, Kluger R, Ahmed SU, Reimold SC, Mark JB. Flow reversal in the descending aorta: a guide to intraoperative assessment of aortic regurgitation with transesophageal echocardiography. J Thorac Cardiovasc Surg. 1994;108(3):576–82.
25. Evangelista A, del Castillo HG, Calvo F, Permanyer-Miralda G, Brotons C, Angel J, Gonzalez-Alujas T, Tornos P, Soler-Soler J. Strategy for optimal aortic regurgitation quantification by Doppler echocardiography: agreement among different methods. Am Heart J. 2000;139(5):773–81.
26. Lambert AS. Proximal isovelocity surface area should be routinely measured in evaluating mitral regurgitation: a core review. Anesth Analg. 2007;105(4):940–3.

27. Nishimura RA, Otto CM, Bonow RO, Carabello BA, Erwin JP 3rd, Guyton RA, O'Gara PT, Ruiz CE, Skubas NJ, Sorajja P, Sundt TM 3rd, Thomas JD, Members AATF. 2014 AHA/ACC guideline for the management of patients with valvular heart disease: a report of the American College of Cardiology/American Heart Association Task Force on Practice Guidelines. Circulation. 2014;129(23):e521-643.
28. Akinseye OA, Pathak A, Ibebuogu UN. Aortic valve regurgitation: a comprehensive review. Curr Probl Cardiol. 2018;43(8):315–34.
29. Samstad SO, Hegrenaes L, Skjaerpe T, Hatle L. Half time of the diastolic aortoventricular pressure difference by continuous wave Doppler ultrasound: a measure of the severity of aortic regurgitation? Br Heart J. 1989;61(4):336–43.
30. McCarthy KP, Ring L, Rana BS. Anatomy of the mitral valve: understanding the mitral valve complex in mitral regurgitation. Eur J Echocardiogr. 2010;11(10):i3-9.
31. Troianos CA, Konstadt S. Evaluation of mitral regurgitation. Semin Cardiothorac Vasc Anesth. 2006;10(1):67–71.
32. Dal-Bianco JP, Levine RA. Anatomy of the mitral valve apparatus: role of 2D and 3D echocardiography. Cardiol Clin. 2013;31(2):151–64.
33. Harari R, Bansal P, Yatskar L, Rubinstein D, Silbiger JJ. Papillary muscle rupture following acute myocardial infarction: anatomic, echocardiographic, and surgical insights. Echocardiography. 2017;34(11):1702–7.
34. Wunderlich NC, Beigel R, Siegel RJ. Management of mitral stenosis using 2D and 3D echo-Doppler imaging. JACC Cardiovasc Imaging. 2013;6(11):1191–205.
35. Baumgartner H, Hung J, Bermejo J, Chambers JB, Evangelista A, Griffin BP, Iung B, Otto CM, Pellikka PA, Quinones M, American Society of E, European Association of E. Echocardiographic assessment of valve stenosis: EAE/ASE recommendations for clinical practice. J Am Soc Echocardiogr. 2009;22(1):1–23. quiz 101-2
36. Hatle L, Angelsen B, Tromsdal A. Noninvasive assessment of atrioventricular pressure half-time by Doppler ultrasound. Circulation. 1979;60(5):1096–104.
37. Anyanwu AC, Adams DH. Etiologic classification of degenerative mitral valve disease: Barlow's disease and fibroelastic deficiency. Semin Thorac Cardiovasc Surg. 2007;19(2):90–6.
38. Marijon E, Mirabel M, Celermajer DS, Jouven X. Rheumatic heart disease. Lancet. 2012;379(9819):953–64.
39. Carpentier A. Cardiac valve surgery—the "French correction". J Thorac Cardiovasc Surg. 1983;86(3):323–37.
40. Sidebotham DA, Allen SJ, Gerber IL, Fayers T. Intraoperative transesophageal echocardiography for surgical repair of mitral regurgitation. J Am Soc Echocardiogr. 2014;27(4):345–66.
41. Lancellotti P, Moura L, Pierard LA, Agricola E, Popescu BA, Tribouilloy C, Hagendorff A, Monin JL, Badano L, Zamorano JL, European Association, of E. European Association of Echocardiography recommendations for the assessment of valvular regurgitation. Part 2: mitral and tricuspid regurgitation (native valve disease). Eur J Echocardiogr. 2010;11(4):307–32.
42. Pu M, Prior DL, Fan X, Asher CR, Vasquez C, Griffin BP, Thomas JD. Calculation of mitral regurgitant orifice area with use of a simplified proximal convergence method: initial clinical application. J Am Soc Echocardiogr. 2001;14(3):180–5.
43. Kwan J, Shiota T, Agler DA, Popovic ZB, Qin JX, Gillinov MA, Stewart WJ, Cosgrove DM, McCarthy PM, Thomas JD. Real-time three-dimensional echocardiography s. Geometric differences of the mitral apparatus between ischemic and dilated cardiomyopathy with significant mitral regurgitation: real-time three-dimensional echocardiography study. Circulation. 2003;107(8):1135–40.
44. Golba K, Mokrzycki K, Drozdz J, Cherniavsky A, Wrobel K, Roberts BJ, Haddad H, Maurer G, Yii M, Asch FM, Handschumacher MD, Holly TA, Przybylski R, Kron I, Schaff H, Aston S, Horton J, Lee KL, Velazquez EJ, Grayburn PA, Investigators STS. Mechanisms of functional mitral regurgitation in ischemic cardiomyopathy determined by transesophageal echocardiography (from the Surgical Treatment for Ischemic Heart Failure Trial). Am J Cardiol. 2013;112(11):1812–8.
45. Chen CG, Thomas JD, Anconina J, Harrigan P, Mueller L, Picard MH, Levine RA, Weyman AE. Impact of impinging wall jet on color Doppler quantification of mitral regurgitation. Circulation. 1991;84(2):712–20.
46. Grayburn PA, Peshock RM. Noninvasive quantification of valvular regurgitation. Getting to the core of the matter. Circulation. 1996;94(2):119–21.

Tricuspid and Pulmonic Valve

10

Sahar Ahmad and Ibrahim El husseini

Abbreviations

AICD	Automated implantable cardioverter defibrillator
CIED	Cardiac implantable electronic devices
COPD	Chronic obstructive pulmonary disease
CT	Computed tomography
CWD	Continuous wave Doppler
EMS	Emergency Medical Services
ER	Emergency room
IVC	Inferior vena cava
PA	Pulmonary artery
PAH	Pulmonary arterial hypertension
PASP	Pulmonary artery systolic pressure
PISA	Proximal isovelocity surface area
RA	Right atrium
RAP	Right atrial pressure
RV	Right ventricle
RVOT	Right ventricular outflow tract
RVSP	Right ventricular systolic pressure
TEE	Trans-eosophageal echocardiography
TR	Tricuspid regurgitation
TTE	Transthoracic echocardiography

Supplementary Information The online version contains supplementary material available at https://doi.org/10.1007/978-3-031-45731-9_10.

S. Ahmad (✉)
Division of Pulmonary, Critical Care and Sleep Medicine, Stony Brook University Hospital, Stony Brook, NY, USA
e-mail: Sahar.Ahmad@stonybrookmedicine.edu

I. El husseini
Department of Medicine, Division of Pulmonary and Critical Care Medicine, Rutgers University, Robert Wood Johnson Medical School, New Brunswick, NJ, USA
e-mail: ie81@rwjms.rutgers.edu

Question 1
What is the most common cause of pathologic tricuspid regurgitation?

A. Infective endocarditis
B. Rheumatic heart disease
C. Connective tissue disorders
D. Right heart remodeling

Correct answer: D. Right heart remodeling.

Explanation: Secondary tricuspid regurgitation is the most common form of TR, mainly due to RV or RA dilatation resulting in loss of coaptation at the tricuspid leaflets. Known causes of RV dilation include left sided disease especially mitral stenosis as well as primary RV dilation due to RV failure. RV enlargement is seen commonly in pulmonary hypertension.

Although infective endocarditis, rheumatic heart disease, connective tissue disease, cardiac carcinoid and congenital anatomical disorders such as Ebstein anomaly can all cause tricuspid regurgitation (TR) and are considered as a primary cause of TR, the most common cause of TR is secondary to right ventricular remodeling leading to dilatation of the RV cavity or of the tricuspid annulus apparatus [1, 2].

Question 2
A 35 year old female patient with known pulmonary arterial hypertension (PAH) presents to the hospital for worsening lower extremity edema. She has a known history of long standing PAH with noncompliance to her home regimen that resulted in severe tricuspid regurgitation. Which one of the following echocardiographic features is least likely to be present in this patient?

A. Proximal isovelocity surface area (PISA) radius less than 0.9 cm
B. Vena contracta width greater than 0.7 cm
C. Hepatic vein systolic reversal
D. Dilated right atrium and right ventricle.

R. Sreedharan et al. (eds.), *Critical Care Echocardiography*, https://doi.org/10.1007/978-3-031-45731-9_10

Answer: A. Proximal isovelocity surface area (PISA) radius less than 0.9 cm.

Explanation: Evaluation of the severity of tricuspid regurgitation should be done using an integrative approach (using multiple data points to evaluate severity instead of a single echocardiographic finding). With severe tricuspid regurgitation there are multiple expected findings which include the following [1, 3]:

- Enlarged RV, RA and IVC size.
- Vena contracta width greater than 0.9 cm.
- Pisa radius ***greater*** than 0.9 cm.
- hepatic vein flow systolic reversal.
- A dense and triangular jet density and contour (Continuous wave Doppler) with early peaking.
- Jet area more than 10 cm^2.

Question 3
In the absence of pulmonic valve stenosis and with an estimated right atrial pressure of 8 cmH2O, what is the estimated pulmonary artery systolic pressure in a patient with peak TR jet velocity using continuous wave Doppler (CWD) of 2.8 m/s?:

A. 39.3 mmHg
B. 22.4 m/s mmHg
C. 31.3 m/s mmHg
D. 19.2 m/s mmHg

Answer: A. 39.3 mmHg.

Explanation: In the absence of pulmonic valve stenosis and adequate tricuspid regurgitation jet, the pulmonary artery systolic pressure (PASP) can be estimated using the Simplified Bernoulli equation:

Simplified Bernoulli. Pressure (mmHg): $4 \times V^2$ (where V = velocity in m/s).

The pressure gradient is equal to the difference between the right ventricular systolic pressure (RVSP) and the right atrial pressure (RAP) which gives the following equation:

Pressure gradient = RVSP − RAP = $4 \times V^2$, which leads to the following equation:

$$\text{RVSP} = 4\left(\text{V}^2\right) + \text{RAP}$$

Right atrial pressure can be estimated by examining the IVC, although this method was not validated in mechanically ventilated patients. In the absence of pulmonic or subpulmonic stenosis RVSP equals PASP [2, 4].

Question 4 (Part I)
A 34 year old female patient admitted to the intensive care unit for sepsis secondary to pyelonephritis. On admission the resident notes a soft opening snap and a mid-diastolic rumble with presystolic accentuation on auscultation. The patient recalls that she was told she had "a heart murmur" in the past. A transthoracic echocardiography (TTE) was ordered and confirmed the diagnosis of mitral stenosis and tricuspid stenosis with commissural fusion and diastolic bowing.

What is the most common likely cause of tricuspid stenosis in this patient?:

A. Infective endocarditis
B. Carcinoid heart disease
C. Right atrial tumor
D. Rheumatic heart disease.

Answer: D. Rheumatic heart disease.

Explanation: Tricuspid stenosis is uncommon in adults, and the majority of the cases seen in the adult population is due to rheumatic heart disease and is usually associated with mitral valve stenosis. Tricuspid stenosis is rarely seen given the fact that the tricuspid valve is the largest of the cardiac valves.

Other less common causes of tricuspid stenosis include tricuspid valve tumor, congenital tricuspid atresia, carcinoid heart disease [2, 5].

Question 5 (Part II)
Which of the following parameters is an indicator of severe stenosis on TTE in this patient?:

A. Valve area less than 2.0 cm^2
B. mean pressure gradient >2 mmHg
C. pressure half-time ≥ 190 ms (T ½ ≥190 ms)
D. Commissural fusion.

Answer: C. pressure half-time ≥ 190 ms (*T* ½ ≥190 ms).

Explanation: Tricuspid stenosis is a rare disease in adults and almost universally seen with rheumatic heart disease (such as this patient). The 2014 American Heart Association/American College of Cardiology Valvular Heart Disease guidelines define the severe tricuspid valve stenosis using the following parameters:

- Mean pressure gradient >5 mmHg
- Pressure half-time ≥ 190 ms
- Valve area ≤ 1.0 cm^2

Of note, Tricuspid valve area in cm^2 may be estimated as 190 divided by the pressure half-time.

The presence of severe tricuspid stenosis leads to the development of RA enlargement and is associated with a TTE finding of Thickened, distorted, calcified leaflets [6, 7].

Question 6 (Part I)
A 24 year old male patient presents to the hospital for shortness of breath and weakness. He is a poor historian. In the ER, he undergoes a computed tomography (CT) of the chest to rule out a pulmonary embolism that shows evidence of

right lower lobe and left upper lobe pneumonia with an incidental finding of an enlarged main pulmonary artery, there was no evidence of pulmonary embolism. The patient is admitted to the intensive care unit and was started on high flow nasal cannula and appropriate antibiotic coverage.

A goal directed echocardiography showed evidence of right ventricular hypertrophy and thickening of the pulmonic valve suggestive of pulmonic valve stenosis.

Which of the following is the most common cause of pulmonic valve stenosis?

A. Congenital heart disease
B. Infective endocarditis
C. Iatrogenic (PA catheter insertion)
D. Malignancy

Answer: A. Congenital heart disease.

Explanation: Pulmonary valve stenosis is almost always congenital and it can be tricuspid (similar to the normal valve), bicuspid, unicuspid or dysplastic. Dilatation of the pulmonary artery beyond the valve is occasionally seen and does not correlate with the degree of stenosis.

In contrast, acquired pulmonic valve stenosis is extremely rare. Even in the presence of rheumatic heart disease, pulmonic valve stenosis is rare (even when the valve is affected by the rheumatic process). Some rare tumors may compress the RV outflow tract leading to functional pulmonary stenosis [5, 8].

Question 7 (Part II)
Which of the following TTE views is used to evaluate the presence of pulmonic valve stenosis?

A. Subcostal view
B. Parasternal short axis view at the level of the aortic valve
C. Apical four chamber view
D. Apical fiver chamber view

Answer: B. Parasternal short axis view.

Explanation: Initial evaluation of pulmonic valve function is achieved by obtaining a parasternal short axis view at the level of the aortic valve. This will allow the sonographer to evaluate valve anatomy (i.e. thickness) and allows for detection / quantification of pulmonic stenosis using color flow doppler (placed over RVOT) and continuous and pulse wave doppler. Further imaging using M-mode echocardiography and trans-esophageal echocardiography (TEE) can be obtained to further evaluate pulmonic valve disease [5, 9].

Question 8 (Part III)
Which of the following parameters is consistent with the presence of severe pulmonic valve stenosis?

A. Left ventricular hypertrophy
B. Peak jet velocity equal to 4.5 m/s
C. Peak gradient equal to 32 mmHg
D. Concomitant aortic regurgitation

Answer: B. Peak jet velocity equal to 4.5 m/s.

Explanation: Grading pulmonary valve stenosis is done using transthoracic echocardiography (TTE). according to the 2006 American College of Cardiology/ American Heart Association (ACC/AHA) guidelines on the management of valvular heart disease, severe pulmonic valve stenosis is defined by a peak velocity greater than 4 m/s (which corresponds to a peak gradient greater than 64 mmHg, using the simplified Bernoulli equation) and is usually associated with indirect findings suggestive of the severity of the disease such as right ventricular hypertrophy (defined as thickness greater than 5 mm),right ventricular dilatation and tricuspid regurgitation [5, 10, 11].

Question 9 (Part I)
A 28 year old male patient with a history of drug abuse was brought to the ED by EMS for altered mental status and fever. Upon admission the patient was noted to be febrile, altered and hypoxic. He was intubated for airway protection and a subclavian approach central line was placed for venous access.

Patient was admitted to the intensive care unit and was started on broad spectrum antibiotic therapy. The following image was taken during goal directed echocardiography in the intensive care unit to evaluate a new heart murmur from an apical 4 chamber view (Fig. 10.1).

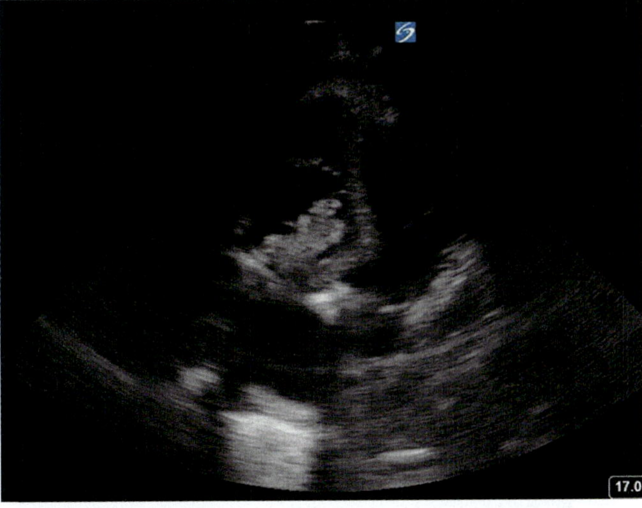

Fig. 10.1 Apical 4 chamber view with echogenic mass seen on tricuspid valve

What is the most likely diagnosis?

A. Angiosarcoma
B. RA thrombus in transit
C. Infective endocarditis
D. Lipomatous hypertrophy of the inter- atrial septum

Answer: C. Infective endocarditis.

Explanation:

The clinical presentation and echocardiographic findings are highly suggestive of infective endocarditis with a tricuspid valve vegetation.

The history of drug abuse, fevers and multiple pulmonary nodules with a basal / peripheral predominance is suggestive of bacteremia with septic emboli. The presence of a tricuspid vegetation further confirms the diagnosis [12, 13] (Fig. 10.2).

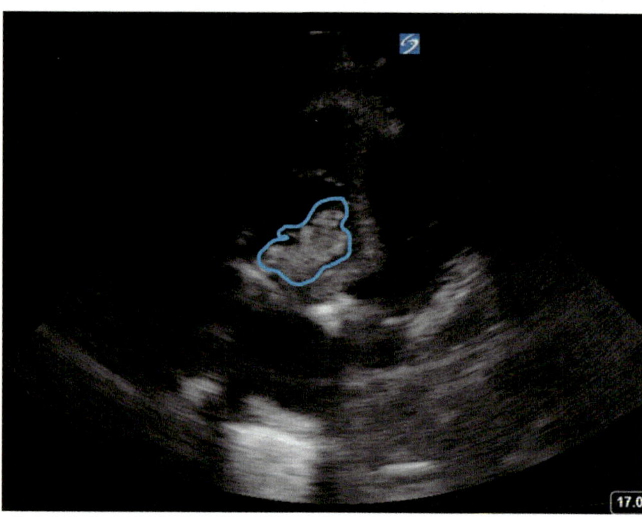

Fig. 10.2 Apical 4 chamber view with tricuspid regurgitation

Question 10 (Part II)

A 28 year old male patient with history of drug abuse was brought to the ED by EMS for altered mental status and fevers. Upon admission the patient was noted to be febrile, altered and hypoxic. He was intubated for airway protection a subclavian approach central line was placed for venous access.

Patient was admitted to the intensive care unit and was started on broad spectrum antibiotic therapy. To further delineate a murmur noted on physical exam, goal directed echocardiography in the intensive care unit was performed. Apical 4 Chamber view is shown.

What is this finding consistent with? (Video 10.1).

A. Normal inflow through tricuspid valve with severe tricuspid regurgitation due to impingement of tricuspid leaflet by catheter.
B. Obstructed turbulent inflow through the tricuspid valve with mild tricuspid regurgitation
C. Obstructed turbulent inflow through the tricuspid valve with severe tricuspid regurgitation.
D. Normal flow through the tricuspid valve

Answer: B. Obstructed turbulent inflow with mild tricuspid regurgitation.

Explanation: Color doppler flow analysis is showing evidence of turbulent inflow at the level of the tricuspid valve vegetation with the presence of mild tricuspid regurgitation (as evidenced by the small "blue" flow on color doppler) [14–16] (Fig. 10.3, Video 10.1).

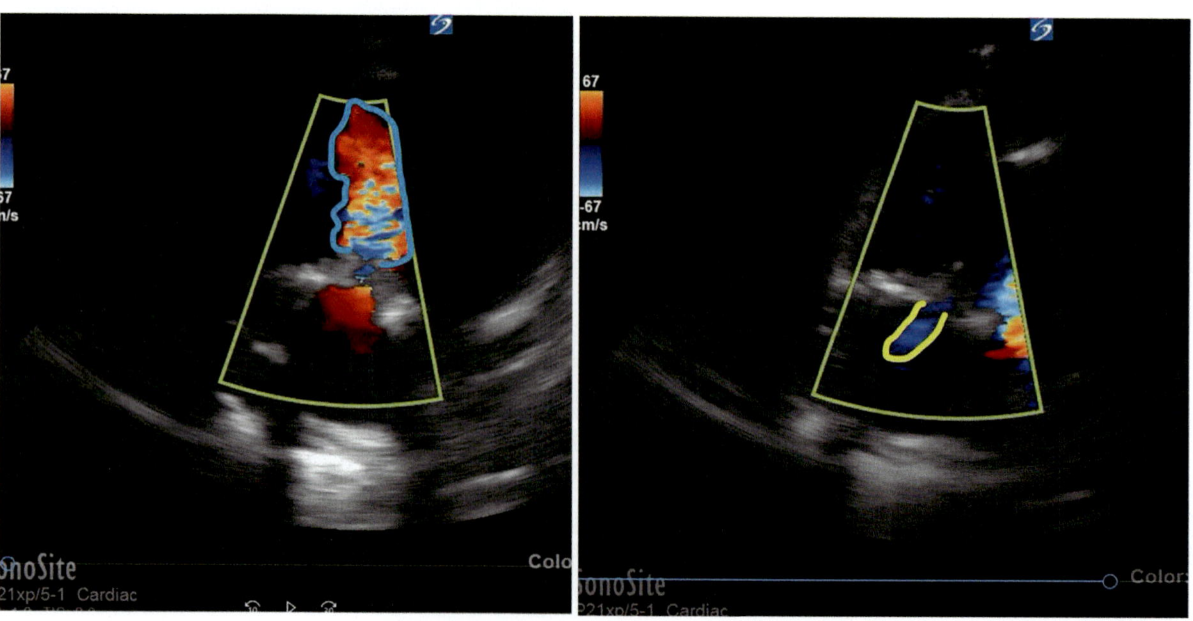

Fig. 10.3 Apical 4 chamber view with annotated echogenic mass seen on tricuspid valve

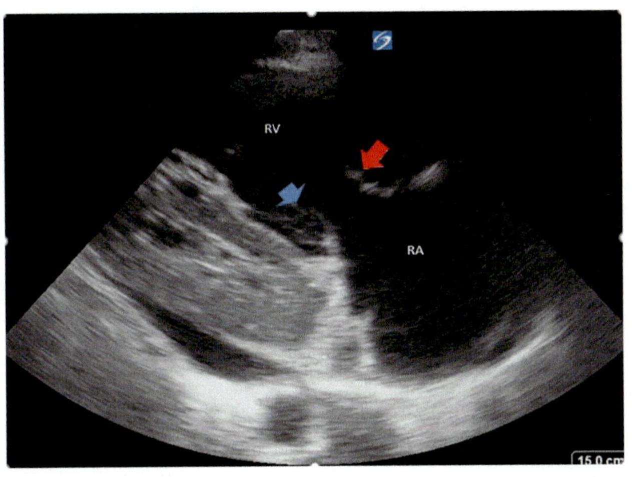

Fig. 10.4 Right ventricular inflow tract view, showing the right atrium (RA), right ventricle (RV) and tricuspid valve leaflets (blue and red arrow)

Question 11 (Part I)
What view is displayed in the transthoracic echocardiogram (TTE) showing (Video 10.2)?

A. Parasternal short axis view at the level of the mitral valve
B. right ventricular inflow tract view
C. right ventricular outflow tract view
D. Parasternal short axis view at the level of the aortic valve.

Answer: B. right ventricular inflow tract view.

Explanation: The preceding video is showing a parasternal long axis view with a right ventricular inflow tract view. The tricuspid valve's anterior leaflet and septal leaflet are well visualized (Fig. 10.4). The red arrow corresponds to the anterior leaflet and the blue arrow corresponds to the septal leaflet [17, 18].

Question 12 (Part II)
How is this view obtained from a parasternal long axis view (Video 10.2)?

A. Slight clockwise rotation of the probe and angling the transducer toward the patient's right hip
B. Slight clockwise rotation of the probe and angling the transducer toward the patient's left hip
C. Slight counterclockwise rotation of the probe and angling the transducer toward the patient's right hip.
D. Slight counterclockwise rotation of the probe and angling the transducer toward the patient's left hip.

Answer: A. slight clockwise rotation of the probe and angling the transducer toward the patient's right hip.

Explanation: To obtain the longitudinal view of the right ventricular inflow tract, rotate the probe slightly in a clockwise direction from the longitudinal parasternal view of the left ventricle and tilt it so that the ultrasound beam is directed slightly downwardly. The anterior cusp of the tricuspid valve is visualized in front and the posterior cusp is visualized at the back. This view is suitable for observation of the tricuspid valve, right ventricle, and the right atrium and to estimate the right ventricular systolic pressure from tricuspid regurgitation [17, 18].

Question 13 (Part III)
Assuming that the right atrial pressure is 5 mmHg and no significant pulmonic stenosis is present what is the right ventricular systolic pressure? (Fig. 10.5, Video 10.3).

A. 13.8 mmHg
B. 24.2 mmHg
C. 19.2 mmHg
D. 14.2 mmHg

Answer: B. 24.2 mmHg.

Explanation: Using the simplified Bernoulli equation:

$$\text{RVSP} = 4\left(\text{V}^2\right) + \text{RAP}$$

$$\text{RVSP} = 4 \times 2.19^2 + 5\,\text{mmHg} = 24.18\,\text{mmHg}$$

It is important to evaluate tricuspid regurgitation jet and estimate right atrial pressure prior to the calculation of the right ventricular systolic pressure in any patient, given that inadequate jet/inadequate placement of the continuous wave doppler might lead to underestimation of the jet maximal velocity and falsely decrease the right ventricular systolic pressure. Evaluation of the tricuspid jet can be done using color doppler mode, and occasionally this can be done in the parasternal long axis view/right ventricular inflow tract view in cases of inadequate apical four chamber [14, 19].

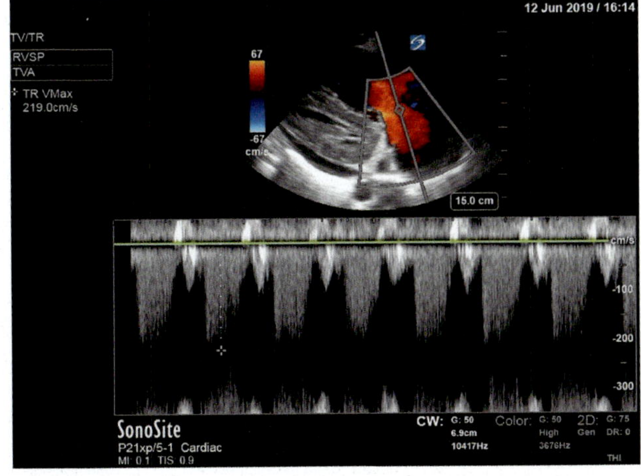

Fig. 10.5 Continuous Wave Doppler at the level of the tricuspid valve

Question 14
A 44 year old male patient with no chronic medical conditions is admitted to the surgical intensive care unit status post motor vehicle accident resulting in right lower extremity femoral fracture and minor bruising in the right upper extremity. His Glasgow coma score on admission was 15. Of note, toxicology was positive for cocaine. He had an episode of hypotension on admission attributed to blood loss. As part of the whole body ultrasound approach, you perform a bedside echocardiography that shows a normal biventricular size and function with no regional wall motion abnormalities and no pericardial effusion. There is mild tricuspid regurgitation (1+).

What is the significance of this echocardiographic finding?

A. Acceleration-deceleration cardiac injury leading to dehiscence of the tricuspid annular ring
B. Cor pulmonale with RV dilation and tricuspid regurgitation due to annulus tenting
C. Myocardial infarct leading to right ventricular dysfunction and functional tricuspid regurgitation
D. Physiologic tricuspid regurgitation without clinical significance.

Answer: D. Mild tricuspid regurgitation is found in up to 80–90% of healthy patients and is rarely of clinical importance.

Explanation: Mild tricuspid regurgitation is a common finding on echocardiography in the setting of normal underlying cardiac function, and the intensivist should be aware of this common abnormality. The majority of these patients are usually asymptomatic and the mild TR has no significant hemodynamic consequences. This abnormality is detected in up to 90% of patients and is usually used (if the jet is adequate) to estimate the right ventricular systolic pressure using the simplified Bernoulli equation [19, 20].

Typically physiologic regurgitation has the following characteristics on echocardiography:

- spatially restricted to area immediately adjacent to valve closure.
- short in duration.
- represents only a small regurgitant volume.

Question 15
Which valve leaflets are shown in the following clip? This image is obtained from a parasternal long axis view with slight angulation of the probe towards the patient's right hip (Video 10.2).

A. Pulmonic valve anterior cusp and right cusp
B. Pulmonic valve anterior cusp and left cusp
C. Tricuspid valve septal and posterior leaflets.
D. Tricuspid valve anterior and septal leaflets.

Answer: D. Tricuspid valve anterior and septal leaflets.

Explanation: The preceding clip is showing a right ventricular inflow tract view from a parasternal long axis view. The tricuspid valve anterior and septal leaflets are seen on this view. In Fig. 10.4 the red arrow corresponds to the anterior leaflet and the blue arrow corresponds to the posterior leaflet [17, 18].

Question 16
A 52 year old male patient with a past medical history of end stage renal disease status-post kidney transplant is admitted to the intensive care unit overnight for septic shock secondary to gram negative bacteremia. While conducting morning rounds, you open the patient's critical care echocardiography images and observe this finding (Video 10.4).

You decide to obtain further echocardiographic images to further investigate this finding.

Which of the following assessments would you obtain next? (Video 10.4).

A. Right ventricular function and size
B. Right atrial volume
C. Inferior vena cava diameter
D. Right ventricular systolic pressure using continuous wave doppler
E. All of the above.

Answer: E. All of the above.

Explanation: When evaluating for tricuspid regurgitation (TR), if the initial color wave doppler is suggestive of significant TR it is imperative to obtain further imaging to further classify the severity and etiology of the TR. These additional imaging include: Right ventricular function and size, Right atrial volume, Inferior vena cava diameter, RVSP using continuous wave doppler.

Significant TR is frequently seen with an enlarged right ventricle, hence the need to assess the RV size and function. Chronic isolated tricuspid regurgitation is usually associated with an increased right atrial size, but in the setting of an acute TR the right atrial size is usually within normal limits. The inferior vena cava might show evidence of systolic expansion during systole in severe TR [3, 6].

Question 17 (Part I)
A 37 year old male patient with history of non-ischemic biventricular dilated cardiomyopathy with an ejection fraction of 20% presents to the hospital for shortness of breath, worsening lower extremity edema and increased abdominal girth. You note that the patient has worsening liver function tests on initial laboratory work-up. A comprehensive bedside

ultrasound exam shows the following findings in the portal vein on Doppler analysis (Fig. 10.6):

What does this finding represent?

A. Normal biphasic/pulsatile flow
B. Non pulsatile/Non phasic flow in the hepatic vein
C. Abnormal biphasic/pulsatile flow
D. Artifact due to measurement error

Answer: C. Abnormal biphasic pulsatile flow in the portal vein (Figs. 10.6, 10.7 and 10.8).

Explanation: Normal portal vein flow is non pulsatile/monophasic in the majority of healthy subjects. The measurement is obtained by visualizing the main portal vein on 2D echo, followed by confirmatory color doppler flow (as seen in Fig. 10.8, the red color is showing flow going towards the probe). The pulsed wave Doppler is then used to further examine the flow, which in this case showed a biphasic / pulsatile appearance (abnormal, in contrast to Fig. 10.7 where the flow is monophasic). This is mainly due to regurgitant flow from the inferior vena cava (IVC) into the portal vein (which is a valve-less vein) [21, 22].

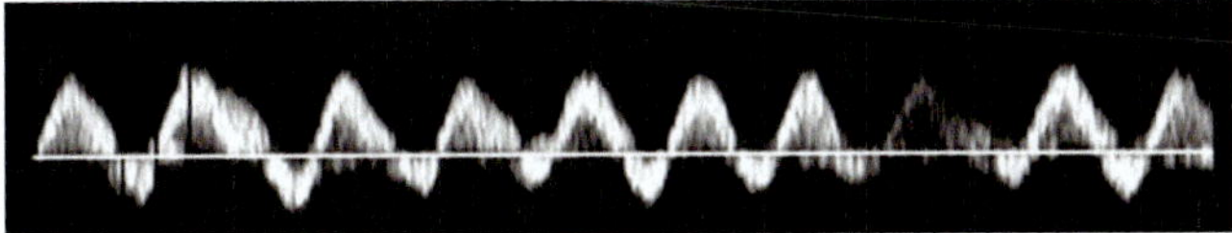

Fig. 10.6 Pulsed Wave Doppler of the main portal vein

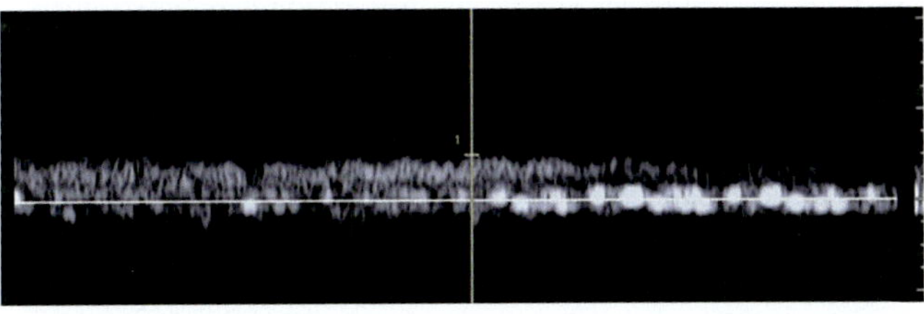

Fig. 10.7 Non pulsatile flow in the portal vein of a patient with compensated heart failure

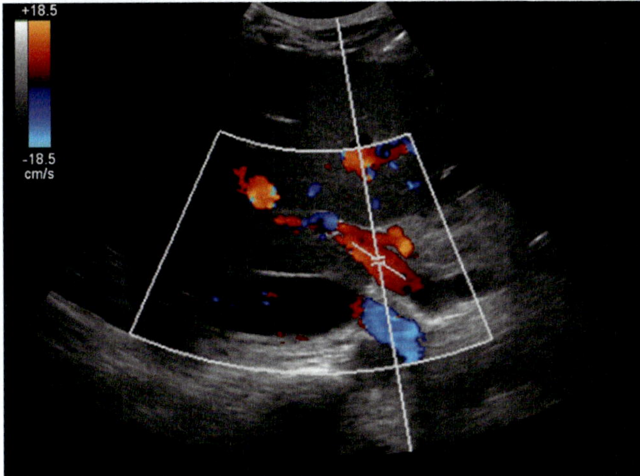

Fig. 10.8 Color doppler flow of portal vein flow

Question 18 (Part II)

A 37 year old male patient with history of non-ischemic dilated cardiomyopathy (biventricular disease, with an ejection fraction of 20%) presents to the hospital for shortness of breath, worsening lower extremity edema and increased abdominal girth. You note that the patient has worsening liver function tests on initial laboratory work-up. A comprehensive bedside ultrasound exam shows the following findings in the main portal vein on Doppler analysis (Fig. 10.7):

Which of the following conditions is NOT usually associated with this finding?

A. Tricuspid regurgitation
B. Cirrhosis with vascular arterio-portal shunting
C. Right heart failure
D. Compensated left heart failure

Answer: D. compensated left heart failure.

Explanation: As mentioned earlier, the normal portal venous waveform is described as phasic, therefore a pulsatile flow is a pathologic finding. Pulsatile portal venous flow occurs when there is a large difference between flow velocity at peak systole and at end diastole. The model for understanding processes that can increase pulsatility involves remembering that the hepatic sinusoids connect the portal veins with the hepatic arteries and veins. In the normal state, the arteries do not contribute significantly to pulsatility (in contrast, the hepatic veins do contribute). Anything that abnormally transmits pressure to the sinusoids will result in a pulsatile portal venous waveform. On the hepatic venous side, tricuspid regurgitation and right-sided heart failure transmit pressure and increase pulsatility. On the arterial side, arteriovenous shunting (as seen in severe cirrhosis) or arteriovenous fistulas (as seen in hereditary hemorrhagic telangiectasia) may have this effect [21, 22].

Question 19

Which of the following echocardiographic features rules out severe tricuspid valve stenosis.

A. Thickened leaflets with limited mobility
B. Reduced pressure half-time (T1/2) through the tricuspid valve during diastole.
C. Right atrial(RA) dilatation
D. Inferior vena cava(IVC) dilatation

Answer: B.

Explanation: Tricuspid valve stenosis is seen in the setting of rheumatic heart disease, congenital heart disease, carcinoid and prosthetic valve malfunction. In patients with severe tricuspid stenosis there is typically an enlarged right atrium and IVC (usually with a normal sized RV, unless there is other concomitant pathology) and the valve leaflets could be thickened with limited mobility.

The Doppler measurements will show a prolonged pressure half-time through the tricuspid valve during diastole with high velocity turbulent diastolic flow. The pressure half-time is typically >190 ms [6].

Question 20

Which of the following tricuspid valve leaflets are shown in the following Fig. 10.9.

A. Red arrow: Anterior leaflet, Blue arrow: Septal leaflet
B. Red arrow: septal leaflet, Blue arrow: posterior leaflet
C. Red arrow: septal leaflet, Blue arrow: anterior leaflet
D. Red arrow: posterior leaflet, Blue arrow: anterior leaflet

Answer: C. Red arrow septal leaflet, Blue arrow: anterior leaflet.

Explanation: The subcostal window can give important information regarding the anatomy of the 4 cardiac chambers (size / function) and also helps identify the different leaflets of both the mitral valve and tricuspid valve. As seen in this image, from a subcostal window, the anterior leaflet (closest to the probe, blue arrow) and the septal leaflet (associated to the septum, red arrow) can be identified [17, 18] (Fig. 10.9).

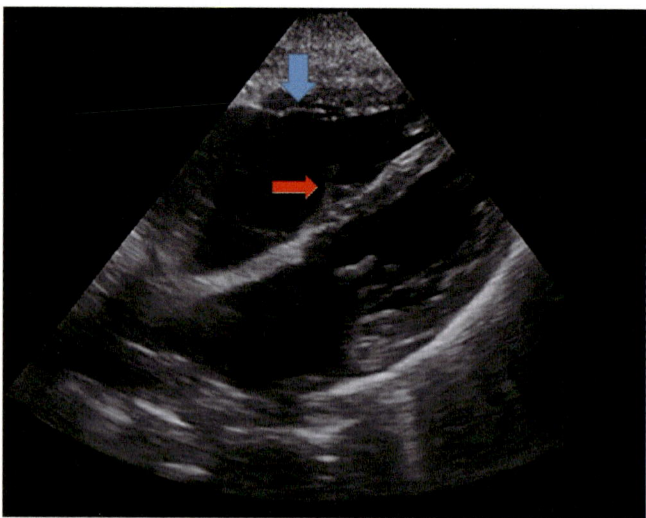

Fig. 10.9 Subcostal view showing the right atrium (RA), right ventricle (RV) and tricuspid valve leaflets (blue and red arrow)

Question 21 (Part I)

A 68 year old male patient with a known history of systolic heart failure and a recent pacemaker placement 3 weeks ago presents to the hospital for a significantly worsened lower extremity edema and increased abdominal girth. Patient states that he is compliant with his medical therapy and fluid/salt restriction. A bedside ultrasound is obtained to assess cardiac function and shows the following (Videos 10.5 and 10.6):

What is the most likely abnormality show in the Fig. 10.10?

A. Normal tricuspid valve flow
B. Tricuspid valve stenosis
C. Tricuspid valve regurgitation
D. Hepatic vein flow reversal

Answer: C. Tricuspid valve regurgitation.

Explanation: The doppler image shown in Fig. 10.10 is consistent with evidence of regurgitation at the level of the tricuspid valve (as evidenced by the retrograde flow). In the setting of a new cardiac implantable electronic devices (CIED) and findings suggestive of heart failure/valvular dysfunction to investigate for any potential valvular abnormality, systolic dysfunction or pericardial effusions. CIED can cause multiple complications (such as valvular dysfunction, pericardial effusion or pneumothorax) and should be considered a differential diagnosis for this patient population [23] (Videos 10.5 and 10.6).

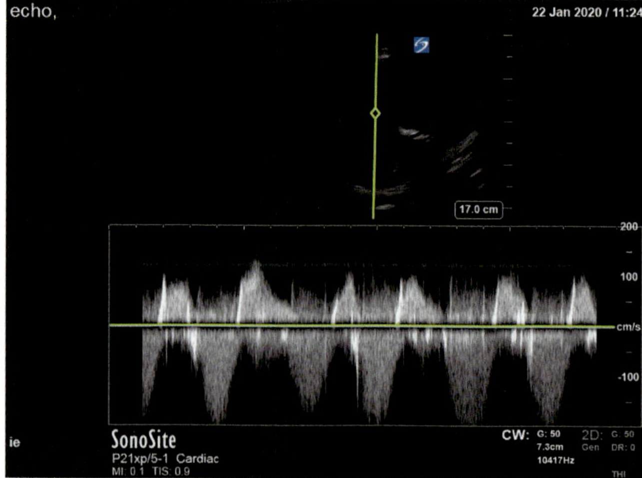

Fig. 10.10 Continuous wave Doppler at the level of the tricuspid valve

Question 22 (Part II)
A 68 year old male patient with a known history of biventricular failure and a recent pacemaker/AICD placement 3 weeks ago presents to the hospital for a significantly worsened lower extremity edema. Patient states that he is compliant with his medical therapy and fluid / salt restriction. A bedside ultrasound is obtained to assess cardiac function with doppler of the tricuspid valve showing tricuspid valve regurgitation.

An EKG and troponins were not suggestive of any ischemic event, blood cultures are negative. What is the most likely cause of the worsening tricuspid regurgitation in this patient?

A. Endocarditis
B. Pulmonary embolism and a clot in transit
C. Iatrogenic from recent pacemaker placement
D. Silent myocardial infarction.

Answer: C. Iatrogenic from recent pacemaker placement.

Explanation: Tricuspid valve dysfunction following Cardiac implantable electronic devices (CIED) implantation can manifest clinically as right-sided heart failure secondary to TR (or less often to tricuspid stenosis) or as left-sided heart failure when RV volume overload impairs LV filling by direct ventricular interaction through the interventricular septum.

Damage to TV leaflets or subvalvular structures during lead implantation or manipulation can occur due to:

- leaflet perforation.
- leaflet laceration,
- leaflet avulsion (primarily during lead extraction).
- transection of papillary muscles or chordae tendineae.

The diagnosis of the CIED related tricuspid regurgitation is similar to any other TR cause, using 2D imaging and doppler studies (which might be attenuated by the echoic leads) [23].

Question 23
Which of the following statement is true regarding using tricuspid jet to right systolic ventricular pressure(RVSP) and pulmonary artery systolic pressure(PASP) in patients with severe tricuspid regurgitation:

A. RVSP tends to be overestimated using doppler measurements.
B. RVSP correlates to PASP in the presence of pulmonic valve stenosis
C. Right atrial pressure estimation is optional for the estimation of PASP.
D. RVSP tends to be underestimated using doppler measurements.

Answer: D. RVSP tends to be underestimated using doppler measurements.

Explanation: The estimation of systolic PAP is based on the peak tricuspid regurgitation velocity (TRV) taking into account right atrial pressure (RAP) as described by the simplified Bernoulli equation.

In patients with severe tricuspid regurgitation (TR), RVSP using doppler measurements can underestimate true PASP (the severity of the regurgitant jet is "too fast" for the doppler signal to register). Also, the TR jet should be optimized (if inadequate TR jet envelope was examined, this would lead to underestimation of the RVSP) [24].

Question 24
A 68 year old male patient with PMH of COPD (group D) with severe emphysema on home oxygen (4 L at rest), presents to the hospital for increased abdominal girth/lower extremity edema for the past few weeks. A bedside abdominal ultrasound was done with Doppler of the main portal vein that showed the following (Fig. 10.6):

Of these echocardiographic findings, which one does NOT correlate with this patient's history and portal vein Doppler:

A. Normal sized right atrium, right ventricle
B. Moderate to severe tricuspid regurgitation
C. Dilated right ventricle
D. Dilated right atrium

Answer: A. Normal sized right atrium, right ventricle.

Explanation: In patients with risk factor for pulmonary hypertension due to chronic lung disease (such as emphysema) the finding of lower extremity edema should be correlated with the possibility of right sided heart dysfunction (right ventricle, tricuspid valve). In patients with cor pulmonale and decompensation (as evidenced by this patient with worsening lower extremity edema) the portal vein doppler signal shows a biphasic signal. When this is present, and in the correct clinical context, it correlates with right sided heart disease and / or portal hypertension from cirrhosis [3, 21, 22].

Question 25
Of the echocardiographic findings visualizable in this subcostal view, which is not expected in the setting of acute severe tricuspid regurgitation (TR)? (Fig. 10.9).

A. Enlarged Right atrium
B. Hepatic vein flow reversal
C. Portal vein flow reversal
D. Normal sized right atrium

Answer: A. Enlarged right atrium.

Explanation: In acute severe TR, the right atrium (RA) is often normal. In chronic severe TR, the RA is classically dilated. Portal vein and hepatic veins will often show flow reversal [1, 25].

Question 26

A 45 year old male patient is currently admitted to the hospital prior to cardiac surgery for correction of a severe tricuspid regurgitation. He was noted to have an elevated creatinine compared to baseline (1.4 compared to 0.7 3 months ago. The resident decides to perform a bedside echocardiogram with a subcostal view/inferior vena cava (IVC) assessment to determine volume status.

In the presence of significant tricuspid regurgitation, what is the expected IVC caliber and degree of respiratory variation compared to healthy subjects? (Figs. 10.11 and 10.12).

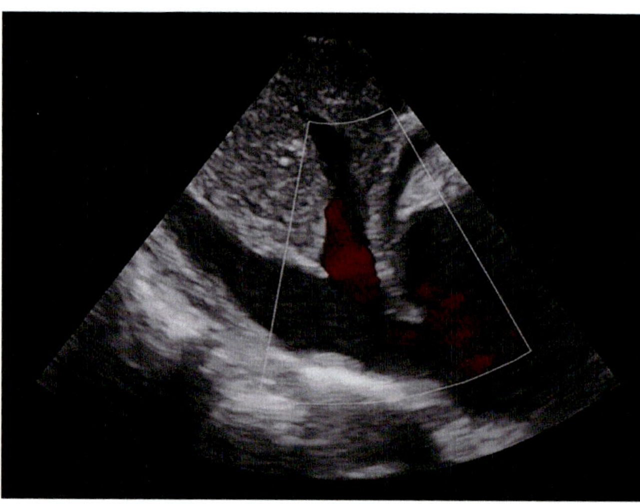

Fig. 10.11 Subcostal view showing the IVC and hepatic vein, showing a plethoric IVC

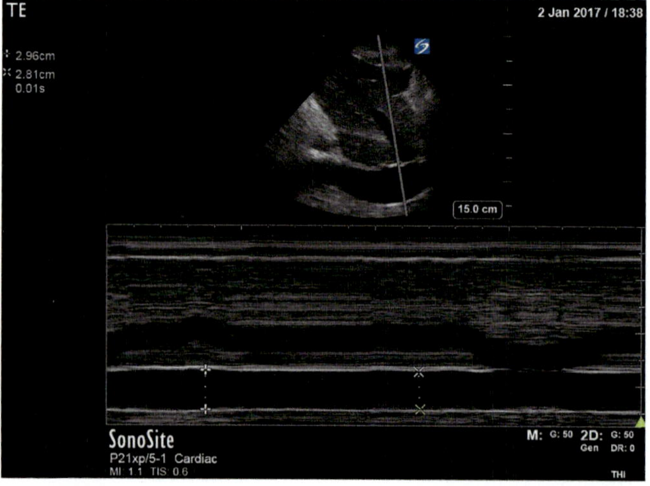

Fig. 10.12 Subcostal M mode through the IVC showing minimal respirophasic changes

A. Unchanged caliber and excess variation.
B. Reduced caliber IVC with excess variation
C. Increased caliber IVC with blunted variation
D. Unchanged caliber unchanged degree of variation

Answer: C. Increased caliber IVC with blunted variation.

Explanation: In the presence of severe tricuspid regurgitation, evaluation of the inferior vena cava size to determine an estimation central venous pressure (CVP) should be approached with caution. With severe TR, the IVC is typically found to be plethoric with evidence of retrograde flow (occasionally seen in patients with severe TR and right heart failure on computed tomography with intravenous contrast). As previously mentioned, IVC size is an indirect indicator of the severity of TR [1, 3]:

- Enlarged RV, RA and IVC size
- Vena contracta width greater than 0.9 cm
- Pisa radius greater than 0.9 cm
- hepatic vein flow systolic reversal.
- A dense and triangular jet density and contour (Continuous wave Doppler) with early peaking
- Jet area more than 10 cm^2

Question 27 (Part I)

You are asked to estimate the right ventricular systolic pressure and the pulmonary artery systolic pressure in a patient with a history of moderate pulmonic stenosis.

You obtain multiple hemodynamic measures using Doppler and obtain the current values:

Tricuspid regurgitation Vmax: 285 cm/s.
Estimated right atrial pressure of 5 mmHg.
Mean pressure gradient across the pulmonic valve of 10 mmHg.

What is the estimated right ventricular systolic pressure in this patient?

A. 37.49 mmHg
B. 32.49 mmHg
C. 47.49 mmHg
D. 27.49 mmHg

Answer: A. 37.49 mmHg.

Explanation: The right ventricular systolic pressure estimation using the bernoulli equation remains valid even in the presence of pulmonic valve stenosis:

$$\text{RVSP} = 4(\text{V}^2) + \text{RAP} \ \left(\text{where } V = \text{velocity in m/s}\right)$$

In this case the following calculation is done: 4 × 2.85 × 2.85 = 32.49. Adding the right atrial pressure (which is equal to 5 in this scenario) would result in a right ventricular systolic pressure of 37.49 [19, 26].

Question 28 (Part II)

You are asked to estimate the right ventricular systolic pressure and the pulmonary artery systolic pressure in a patient with a history of moderate pulmonic stenosis.

You obtain multiple hemodynamic measures using doppler and obtain the current values:

Tricuspid regurgitation Vmax: 285 cm/s.
Estimated right atrial pressure of 5 mmHg.
Mean pressure gradient across the pulmonic valve of 10 mmHg.

What is the estimated pulmonary artery systolic pressure?

a) 37.49 mmHg
b) 32.49 mmHg
c) 47.49 mmHg
d) 27.49 mmHg

Answer: D. 27.49 mmHg.

Explanation: The presence of pulmonic valve stenosis will affect the estimation of pulmonary artery systolic pressure from the right ventricular systolic pressure. In order to account for the effect of the pulmonic stenosis on RVSP and PASP measurements the following formula is used:

$$\text{PASP} = \text{RVSP} - \text{Pressure gradient}(\text{pulmonic valve})$$

In this situation RVSP was equal to 37.49 mmHg and the pressure gradient across the pulmonic valve was equal to 10 mmHg. So PASP = 37.49–10 = 27.49 [19, 26].

Question 29

From the following trans-esophageal echocardiography (TEE) views, which one is NOT considered appropriate for evaluation of tricuspid valve anatomy and function:

A. Midesophageal four chamber view,
B. Midesophageal RV inflow–outflow view
C. Transgastric short axis view
D. Midesophageal two chamber view

Answer: D. Midesophageal two chamber view.

Explanation: TEE is gaining popularity among intensive care physicians due to the ease of use in patients who are mechanically ventilated and the valuable information it can provide in the setting of hemodynamic decompensation. Multiple views can be obtained using a TEE probe, and in order to best evaluate the tricuspid valve the following views are suggested:

Midesophageal four chamber view, midesophageal RV inflow–outflow view, midesophageal modified bicaval view, transgastric short axis view, and transgastric RV inflow view [27, 28].

Question 30

A 24 year old male patient with no known past medical history presents to the hospital after a motor vehicle accident (MVA) with blunt trauma to the chest that resulted in fractured ribs, hip, femur and tibia. On physical examination a new systolic murmur was noted (3/6 in intensity). Hours after admission the patient was noted to be tachycardic, hypotensive. A goal directed echocardiography showed evidence of severe tricuspid regurgitation but with a normal right ventricular size and right atrium size.

What is the most likely cause of the patient's tricuspid regurgitation?

A. Trauma
B. Infective endocarditis
C. Fat embolism causing increase in pulmonary artery pressures and right ventricular overload
D. Congenital tricuspid regurgitation accentuated by loss of intravascular volume.

Answer: A. Trauma.

Explanation: Traumatic tricuspid valve rupture has been known to cause few acute hemodynamic consequences and can frequently be overlooked. Suspicion of this diagnosis is important especially in the setting of a new murmur on auscultation. It is important for the intensivist to accurately diagnose this condition, as it can be due to a flail leaflet / muscle rupture and might require urgent surgical intervention to prevent further hemodynamic decompensation [29].

Question 31

A 29 year old female with some congenital heart disease presents to ICU for severe shortness of breath and lower extremity edema and worsening AKI, The vitals are stable, however serum potassium is 8 Mq/dl. The team decides to perform dialysis catheter insertion for urgent dialysis. The internal jugular vessel was large with smoke sign, POCUS examination of right side of heart is performed? Based on the Video, what is the diagnosis? (Video 10.7).

A. Ebstein's anomaly
B. Arrhythmogenic right ventricular cardiomyopathy
C. Repaired tetralogy of fallot
D. Congenital corrected transposition of great vessel

Answer: A. Ebstein's anomaly.

Explanation: This is an apical four chamber view with visualization of the right sided heart chambers. The condition is characterized by failed delamination (separation of the valve tissue from the myocardium). The displacement of hinge points of septal and posterior toward the apex is the hallmark finding. In echocardiogram, the leaflet appears "sail-like" and associated with severe tricuspid regurgitation and right ventricular failure. The other options may lead to progressive RV dilation and failure but do not lead to a "sail-like" appearance of the tricuspid valve.

Question 32 (Part I)

A patient with dilated cardiomyopathy has an end diastolic pulmonary regurgitation (PR) velocity of 2.5 m/s and an estimated right atrial pressure is 10 mmHg.

Which of following is a correct statement:

A. Pulmonary artery (PA) pressure is normal
B. Pulmonary diastolic pressure is equal to 35 mmHg
C. Pressures cannot be estimated
D. Pulmonary diastolic pressure is equal to 25 mmHg

Answer: B. Pulmonary diastolic pressure is equal to 35 mmHg.

Explanation: Using the patient's velocity of 2.5 m/s, the calculated pressure gradient at end-diastole between the right ventricle and the pulmonary artery is equal to: $4 \times v^2 = 4 \times (2.5 \times 2.5) = 25$. With the assumption that the right ventricular diastolic pressure is equal to the right atrial pressure then the pulmonary artery diastolic pressure is equal to: 25 + RAP = 25 + 10 = 35 mmHg [19, 26].

Question 33 (Part II)

If the patient in the prior question had valvular pulmonary stenosis with a peak gradient of 30 mmHg, the estimated PA end diastolic pressure would be:

A. 35 mmHg
B. 30 mmHg
C. 15 mmHg
D. 65 mmHg

Answer: A. 35 mmHg.

Explanation: Based on the simplified Bernoulli equation, estimating the end diastolic pressure of the pulmonary artery is NOT affected by systolic pressure gradient.

The only two determinants pulmonary artery end diastolic pressure are the pulmonary artery—right ventricle end diastolic gradient and the RV end diastolic pressure, which is assumed to be equal to the right atrial pressure (RAP) [19, 26].

Question 34

What is the abnormality visualized in the following video? (Video 10.8).

A. mild tricuspid regurgitation
B. moderate tricuspid regurgitation
C. severe tricuspid regurgitation
D. no tricuspid regurgitation

Answer: C. Severe tricuspid regurgitation.

Explanation: The following image is suggestive of the presence of severe tricuspid regurgitation based on color Doppler analysis. The following are signs of severe TR based on color flow Doppler analysis: Central jet that occupies ≥50% right atrial area, eccentric jet impinging the RA wall of variable size and color flow jet area occupying >10 cm^2 [1, 2].

Question 35

What is the severity of the tricuspid regurgitation based on the above measurement? (Fig. 10.13).

A. Mild tricuspid regurgitation
B. Severe tricuspid regurgitation
C. Moderate tricuspid regurgitation
D. No tricuspid regurgitation is present

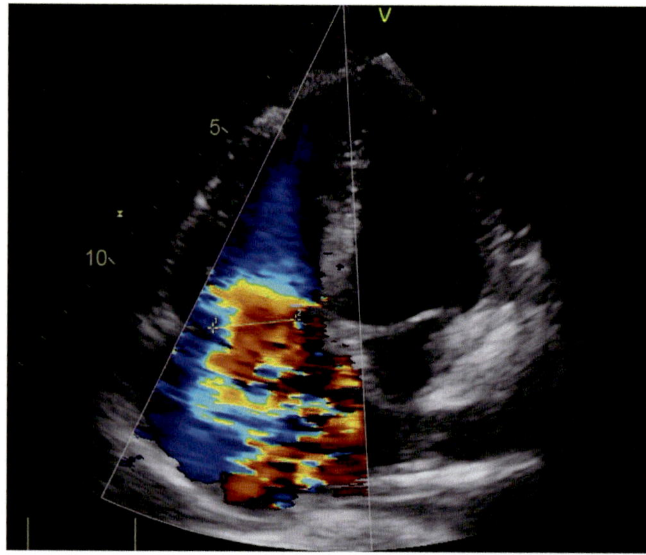

Fig. 10.13 Measurement of vena-contracta

Answer: B. severe tricuspid regurgitation.

Explanation: Vena contracta represents the cross-sectional area of the blood column as it leaves the regurgitant orifice; it thus reflects the regurgitant orifice area. The vena contracta of the tricuspid regurgitation flow is typically imaged in the apical four-chamber view using a careful probe angulation to optimize the flow image, an adapted Nyquist limit (colour Doppler scale, 40–70 cm/s) to identify with clarity the neck of the jet, and a narrow sector scan coupled with the zoom mode to maximize temporal resolution and measurement accuracy. Averaging measurements over at least 2–3 beats is recommended. Vena contracta width > 6.5 mm is usually associated to severe TR [30, 31].

Question 36

Which of the following valves is the least likely to be involved in infectious endocarditis:

A. Tricuspid valve
B. Mitral valve
C. Aortic valve
D. Pulmonic valve

Answer: D. Pulmonic valve.

Explanation: Infectious endocarditis (IE) can affect any of the 4 valves (mitral, tricuspid, aortic and pulmonic valve) but the pulmonic valve is the least likely to be affected. 10% of total IE cases involve the native right heart valves, of which 90% affect the tricuspid valve and less than 10% affect the pulmonic valve making it the valve that is the least affected by IE [32, 33].

Question 37

A 36 year old obese male patient is admitted to the hospital for shortness of breath and hemoptysis for the past 48 h. Patient endorses generalized malaise and fatigue for the past 4–5 weeks. On physical exam, lungs are clear to auscultation, no discrete cardiac murmurs are appreciated (exam limited by body habitus) and erythema is noted on both lower extremities. Chest X ray shows multiple opacities in bilateral peripheral lung fields.

A bedside echocardiogram is obtained and shows the following (Video 10.9):

What is the likely diagnosis?

A. Right Atrial myxoma
B. Pulmonary embolism with a clot in transit
C. Infective endocarditis with vegetation on the tricuspid valve
D. Tricuspid valve fibroelastoma

Answer: C. infective endocarditis with vegetation on the tricuspid valve.

Explanation: (Video 10.9): The patient is likely suffering from endocarditis, given the prodromal symptoms of malaise/fatigue, lower extremity erythematous rash (which likely represents janeway lesions) and multiple peripheral opacities on chest imaging. The history of shortness of breath and hemoptysis is also consistent with pulmonary septic emboli.

Atrial myxoma is less likely given the systemic symptoms above in addition to chest imaging findings. The echocardiogram does not show any evidence of clot in transit, and the clinical scenario does not suggest a massive pulmonary embolism.

Physical exam can be limited in assessing for new heart murmurs in the setting of infectious endocarditis, especially in patients with obesity.

Primary cardiac tumours are rare but the incidence of papillary fibrolastoma (PFE) may be rising. PFE arise form valves and are more commonly seen at the Aortic or mitral valves, only rarely at the tricuspid. These are nodular shaped tumours usually smaller than 1 cm in diameter and would not usually be associated with the systemic findings described int his case. PFE of the tricuspid are usually found incidentally [32–36].

References

1. Otto CM. Valvular regurgitation. Textbook of clinical echocardiography. 5th ed. Philadelphia, Pa: Saunders; 2013. p. 305–39.
2. Luxford J, Bassin L, D'Ambra M. Echocardiography of the tricuspid valve: acknowledgements. Ann Cardiothorac Surg. 2017;6(3):223–39. https://doi.org/10.21037/acs.2017.05.15.
3. Zoghbi WA, Enriquez-Sarano M, Foster E, Grayburn PA, Kraft CD, Levine RA, Nihoyannopoulos P, Otto CM, Quinones MA, Rakowski H, Stewart WJ, Waggoner A, Weissman NJ. American Society of Echocardiography, recommendations for evaluation of the severity of native valvular regurgitation with two-dimensional and Doppler echocardiography. J Am Soc Echocardiogr. 2003;16:777–802.
4. Narasimhan M, Koenig SJ, Mayo PH. Advanced echocardiography for the critical care physician: part 2. Chest. 2014;145:135–42.
5. Otto CM. Valvular stenosis. Textbook of clinical echocardiography. 5th ed. Philadelphia, Pa: Saunders; 2013. p. 271–304.
6. Nishimura RA, Otto CM, Bonow RO, Carabello BA, Erwin JP, Guyton RA, O'gara PT, Ruiz CE, Skubas NJ, Sorajja P. AHA/ACC guideline for the management of patients with valvular heart disease: a report of the American college of cardiology/American

heart association task force on practice guidelines. J Am Coll Cardiol. 2014;63:E57–e185.
7. Anwar AM, Geleijnse ML, Soliman OI, et al. Evaluation of rheumatic tricuspid valve stenosis by real-time three-dimensional echocardiography. Heart. 2007;93(3):363–4.
8. Baumgartner H, Hung J, Bermejo J, Chambers JB, Evangelista A, Griffin BP, Iung B, Otto CM, Pellikka PA, Quiñones M. Echocardiographic assessment of valve stenosis: EAE/ASE recommendations for clinical practice. J Am Soc Echocardiogr. 2009;22(1):1–23.
9. Jassal DS, Thakrar A, Schaffer SA, et al. Percutaneous balloon valvuloplasty for pulmonic stenosis: the role of multimodality imaging. Echocardiography. 2008;25(2):231–5.
10. Bonow RO, Carabello BA, Chatterjee K, de Leon CC Jr, Faxon DP, Freed MD, et al. ACC/AHA 2006 guidelines for the management of patients with valvular heart disease: a report of the American College of Cardiology/American Heart Association Task Force on Practice Guidelines (writing Committee to Revise the 1998 guidelines for the management of patients with valvular heart disease) developed in collaboration with the Society of Cardiovascular Anesthesiologists endorsed by the Society for Cardiovascular Angiography and Interventions and the Society of Thoracic Surgeons. J Am Coll Cardiol. 2006;48:e1–148.
11. Gupta PN, Velappan P, Thampy MSL, Kunju SM. A prominent 'A' notch in the pulmonary valve M mode-one more cause of the same. BMJ Case Rep. 2015;2015:bcr2014208199. Published 2015 Apr 1. https://doi.org/10.1136/bcr-2014-208199.
12. Chan P, Ogilby JD, Segal B. Tricuspid valve endocarditis. Am Heart J. 1989;117(5):1140–6.
13. Ginzton LE, Siegel RJ, Criley JM. Natural history of tricuspid valve endocarditis: a two dimensional echocardiographic study. Am J Cardiol. 1982;49(8):1853–9.
14. Otto CM. Principles of echocardiographic image acquisition and doppler analysis. Textbook of clinical echocardiography. 5th ed. Philadelphia, Pa: Saunders; 2013. p. 1–30.
15. Otto CM. Normal anatomy and flow patterns on transthoracic echocardiography. Textbook of clinical echocardiography. 5th ed. Philadelphia, Pa: Saunders; 2013. p. 31–64.
16. Manolis AS, Melita H. Echocardiographic and clinical correlates in drug addicts with infective endocarditis: implications of vegetation size. Arch Intern Med. 1988;148(11):2461–5.
17. Stankovic I, Daraban AM, Jasaityte R, et al. Incremental value of the en face view of the tricuspid valve by two-dimensional and three-dimensional echocardiography for accurate identification of tricuspid valve leaflets. J Am Soc Echocardiogr. 2014;27:376.
18. Addetia K, Yamat M, Mediratta A, et al. Comprehensive two-dimensional interrogation of the tricuspid valve using knowledge derived from three-dimensional echocardiography. J Am Soc Echocardiogr. 2016;29:74.
19. Parasuraman S, Walker S, Loudon BL, et al. Assessment of pulmonary artery pressure by echocardiography-a comprehensive review. Int J Cardiol Heart Vasc. 2016;12:45–51. Published 2016 Jul 4. https://doi.org/10.1016/j.ijcha.2016.05.011.
20. Schiller NB. Pulmonary artery pressure estimation by Doppler and two-dimensional echocardiography. Cardiol Clin. 1990;8:277.
21. McNaughton DA, Abu-Yousef MM. Doppler US of the liver made simple. Radiographics. 2011;31(1):161–88.
22. Gayatri Joshi MD, et al. US of right upper quadrant pain in the emergency department: diagnosing beyond gallbladder and biliary disease. Radiographics. 2018;38:766–93.
23. Chang JD, Manning WJ, Ebrille E, Zimetbaum PJ. Tricuspid valve dysfunction following pacemaker or cardioverter-defibrillator implantation. J Am Coll Cardiol. 2017;69(18):2331–41.
24. Galiè N, Humbert M, Vachiery J-L, et al. ESC/ERS guidelines for the diagnosis and treatment of pulmonary hypertension. Eur Heart J. 2015;2015:29.
25. Arsalan M, Walther T, Smith RL, Grayburn PA. Tricuspid regurgitation diagnosis and treatment. Eur Heart J. 2017;38(9):634–8.
26. Bossone E, et al. Echocardiography in pulmonary arterial hypertension: from diagnosis to prognosis. J Am Soc Echocardiogr. 2013;26:1–14.
27. Hahn RT, et al. Guidelines for performing a comprehensive transesophageal echocardiographic examination: recommendations from the American Society of Echocardiography and the Society of Cardiovascular Anesthesiologists. J Am Soc Echocardiogr. 2013;26:921–64.
28. Zaroff JG, Picard MH. Transesophageal echocardiographic (TEE) evaluation of the mitral and tricuspid valves. Cardiol Clin. 2000;18:731.
29. Al Maluli H, DeStephan C, Alvarez R. Acute tricuspid valve regurgitation caused by severe blunt chest trauma. J Am Coll Cardiol. 2015;65(10 Supplement):A580.
30. Luigi P. Badano, Denisa Muraru, Maurice Enriquez-Sarano, assessment of functional tricuspid regurgitation. Eur Heart J. 2013;34(25):1875–85.
31. Tribouilloy C, Enriquez-Sarano M, Bailey K, Tajik A, Seward J. Quantification of tricuspid regurgitation by measuring the width of the vena contracta with Doppler color flow imaging: a clinical study. J Am Coll Cardiol. 2000;36:472–8.
32. Chahoud J, Sharif Yakan A, Saad H, Kanj SS. Right-sided infective endocarditis and pulmonary infiltrates: an update. Cardiol Rev. 2016;24:230.
33. Akinosoglou K, Apostolakis E, Marangos M, Pasvol G. Native valve right sided infective endocarditis. Eur J Intern Med. 2013;24:510.
34. Strecker T, Agaimy A, Marwan M, Zielezinski T. Papillary fibroelastoma of the aortic valve: appearance in echocardiography, computed tomography, and histopathology. Heart Valve Dis. 2010;9:812.
35. Kondruweit M, Schmid M, Strecker T. Papillary fibroelastoma of the mitral valve: appearance in 64-slice spiral computed tomography, magnetic resonance imaging, and echocardiography. Eur Heart J. 2008;9:831.
36. Agaimy A, Strecker T. Left atrial myxoma with papillary fibroelastoma-like features. Int J Clin Exp Pathol. 2011;9:307–11.

Suggested Reading

Hauck AJ, Freeman DP, Ackermann DM, et al. Surgical pathology of the tricuspid valve: a study of 363 cases spanning 25 years. Mayo Clin Proc. 1988;63:851.

Daniels SJ, Mintz GS, Kotler MN. Rheumatic tricuspid valve disease: two-dimensional echocardiographic, hemodynamic, and angiographic correlations. Am J Cardiol. 1983;51:492.

Jai Shankar K, Jaiswal PK, Cherian KM. Rheumatic involvement of all four cardiac valves. Heart. 2005;91(6):e50. https://doi.org/10.1136/hrt.2005.060509.

Seckeler MD, Hoke TR. The worldwide epidemiology of acute rheumatic fever and rheumatic heart disease. Clin Epidemiol. 2011;3:67–84.

Watkins DA, Johnson CO, Colquhoun SM, Karthikeyan G, Beaton A, Bukhman G, Forouzanfar MH, Longenecker CT, Mayosi BM, Mensah GA, Nascimento BR, Ribeiro ALP, Sable CA, Steer AC, Naghavi M, Mokdad AH, Murray CJL, Vos T, Carapetis JR, Roth GA. Global, regional, and National Burden of rheumatic heart disease, 1990-2015. N Engl J Med. 2017;377(8):713–22.

Hemodynamics

11

Sharad Patel, Nitin Puri, Shawana Hussain,
and Michael Kouch

Question 1

75 y/o male history of heart failure with preserved ejection fraction (HFpEF), hypertension (HTN), and Diabetus Mellitus (DM) presents with weakness, lethargy, and altered mental status. He is hypotensive at 75/40 mm Hg with a pulse of 95 bpm with hypotension persisting despite 30 cc/kg of crystalloids. Norepinephrine is started and up titrated to 15 μg/min improving blood pressure (105/55). Labs are pending. Bedside ultrasound performed with images shown below. What is the approximate Cardiac Output given a pulse of 95 bpm?

A. 6.89 L/min
B. 3.55 L/min.
C. 4.53 L/min.
D. 5.08 L/min.

Answer: A. Cardiac output is calculated using Left Ventricular Outflow Tract (LVOT) diameter and LVOT-VTI (LVOT Velocity Time Integral). The LVOT diameter is measured in Parasternal Long view in mid-systole at the insertion of AV leaflets. The LVOT VTI is measured at the same point in Apical 5-chamber view (Figs. 11.1 and 11.2).

$$\text{Stroke Volume} = \text{LVOT volume} \times \text{HR}$$

$$\text{LVOT Volume} = \text{LVOT cross sectional area}\left(\text{CSA}\right) \times \text{Length}\left(\text{Velocity Time Integral}\right)$$

$$\text{LVOT CSA} = \pi r^2$$

$2 = 3.14 \times (1.84/2)^2 = 2.65$ cm^2.

LVOT VTI = Length = 27.3 cm.
SV = 2.65 × 27.3 = 72 cm^3.
CO = SV × HR = 95 beats/min × 72 cm^3 = 6.8 L.

An average of 3–5 cardiac cycles LVOT-VTI is recommended in regular sinus rhythm, while an average of 8–10 cardiac cycles is recommended in irregular heart rhythm. Care should be taken to accurately measure the LVOT diameter as the error will be squared [1, 2] (Fig. 11.3).

Question 2

Given the calculated CO. What type of shock is this most likely (Assuming a normal BSA)?

A. Obstructive
B. Cardiogenic
C. Distributive
D. Hypovolemic

Answer: C. The cardiac output calculation indicates a normal to high cardiac output, which immediately reduces the probability that this is cardiogenic, obstructive, or hypovolemic shock. Patients with relatively normal cardiac function typically exhibit a normal to high cardiac output in distributive shock as the primary reason for hypotension and shock is vasoplegia [1, 3].

Question 3

A 75-year- old female with a history of chronic obstructive lung disease (COPD) and obstructive sleep apnea (OSA), presents with acute kidney injury. A point of care ultrasound (POCUS) is performed to assess for venous congestion. She is saturating 95% on 4L Nasal Cannula (NC). What is the estimated RAP (Right atrial pressure) based on the findings below? (Fig. 11.4a)

A. 0–3 cmH_2O
B. 5–8 cmH_2O
C. 8–12 cmH_2O
D. 15 cmH_2O

Supplementary Information The online version contains supplementary material available at https://doi.org/10.1007/978-3-031-45731-9_11.

S. Patel (✉) · N. Puri · S. Hussain · M. Kouch
Division of Critical Care, Cooper University Hospital,
Camden, PA, USA
e-mail: patel-sharad@cooperhealth.edu;
hussain-shawana@CooperHealth.edu;
Kouch-Michael@CooperHealth.edu

R. Sreedharan et al. (eds.), *Critical Care Echocardiography*, https://doi.org/10.1007/978-3-031-45731-9_11

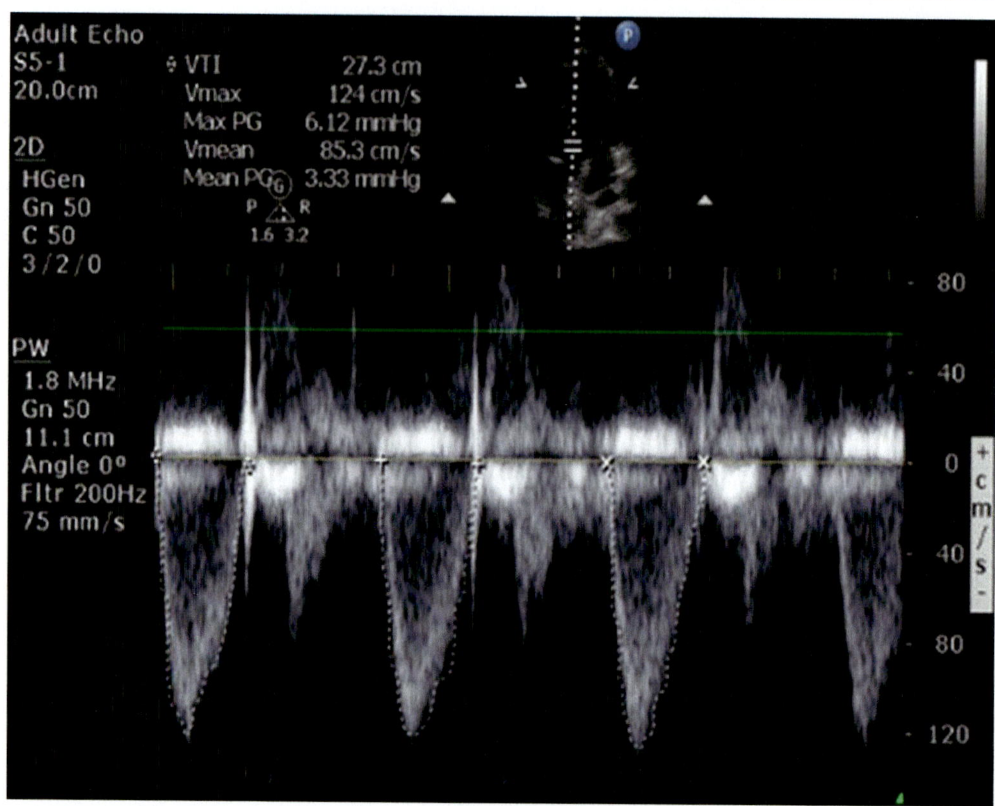

Fig. 11.1 High LVOT VTI

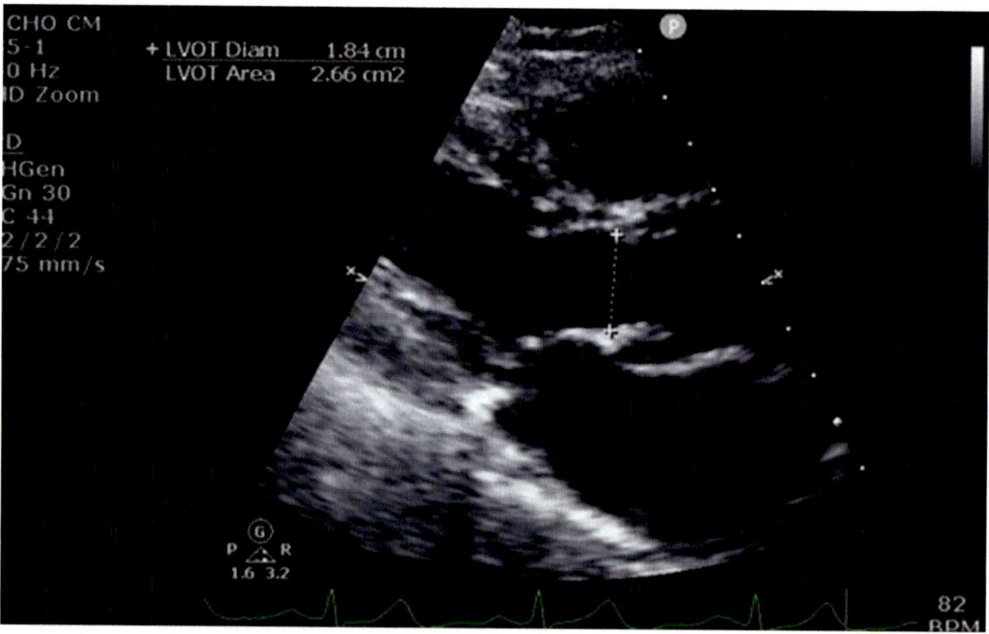

Fig. 11.2 LVOT diameter

Answer: D. The inferior vena cava (IVC) diameter is >2.1 cm with <50% variation. By convention, the RAP is estimated to be equal to or greater than 15 cmH_2O in spontaneously breathing patient. This is considered to be a high RAP [4] (Table 11.1).

Question 4

Which of the following statements is true regarding a spontaneously breathing patient who is hypotensive and has a POCUS that shows his IVC is >2.2 cm with no respiratory variation?

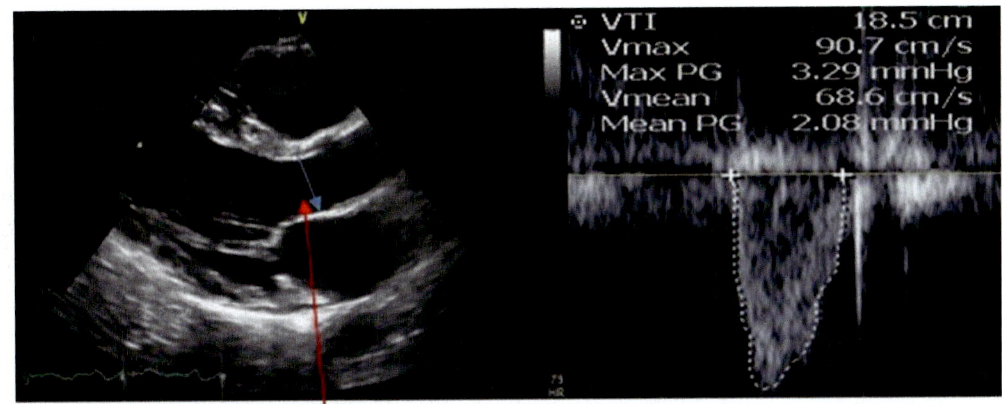

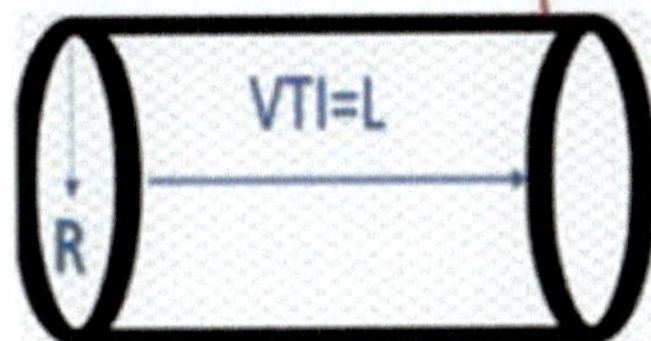

$$LVOT\ Area = \pi r^2$$

Length= VTI

LVOT Area x VTI= Stroke Volume

Stroke Volume x HR= Cardiac Output

Image1-PSLAX with red arrow both identifying the LVOT and pointing out its cylindric geometry. Image 2-Traced VTI. Image 3-Assuming LVOT as a cylinder, VTI is analogous to the length. VTI x LVOT area =Stroke Volume

Fig. 11.3 Stroke volume calculation explanation

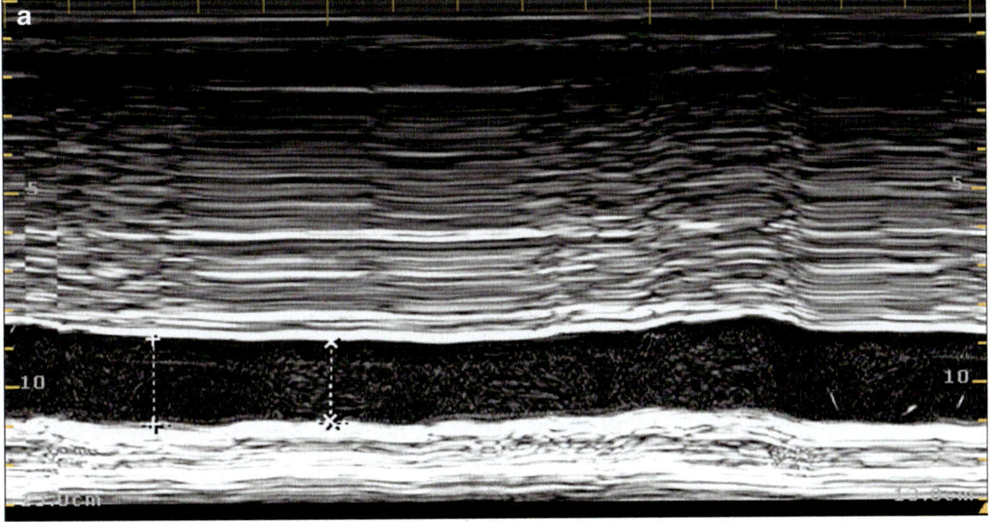

b

RAP	cmH2O	IVC Diameter	IVC Collapse > 50%
Low/Normal	3	< 2.1	> 50%
Intermediate	> 8	> 2.1	> 50%
High	> 15	> 2.1	< 50%

Fig. 11.4 (**a**) IVC size and collapsibility with respiration in spontaneously breathing patient. (**b**) IVC Estimation of CVP

Table 11.1 IVC diameter resiratory variation

IVC diameter inspiration	2.3 cm
IVC diameter expiration	2.2 cm

A. The patient is volume responsive
B. The patient is not volume responsive
C. Volume responsiveness cannot be determined from this isolated data
D. Patient's AKI is due to intravascular depletion

Answer: C. IVC size and variation has been studied extensively in spontaneously breathing patients with conflicting data. In the extremes of ultrasound findings, a fully collapsible or a dilated IVC, there may be a role for the use of the IVC in clinical determination of volume responsiveness, but not as an isolated data point. The determinants of IVC size and variation include cardiac function, intra-abdominal pressure, intrathoracic pressure, and venous return. Therefore, to determine intravascular volume purely from the IVC is overly simplistic. IVC distensibility index is validated for use in patients who are on mechanical ventilation though it was studied with tidal volumes 8–10 cc/kg/IBW. Clinical context should be taken into account when using IVC ultrasound for volume assessment and responsiveness [5–7].

Question 5
Which of the following is a valid clinical scenario for the use of IVC diameter or variation for volume responsiveness?

A. IVC diameter in a spontaneously breathing patient.
B. IVC diameter in a mechanically ventilated patient.
C. IVC distensibility index in a spontaneously breathing patient.
D. IVC distensibility index in a mechanically ventilated patient.
E. IVC distensibility in a patient with intraabdominal hypertension.

Answer: D. The use of IVC for volume responsiveness has been validated in patients who are on passive on mechanical ventilation on 8–10 cc/kg tidal volume and in normal heart rhythm. The M-Mode image of this patient does not demonstrate any respiratory variation (IVC with no respiratory variation). The Distensibility index of the IVC(dIVC) is calculated as (Dmax − Dmin/Dmin). dIVC below 18% predicts a lack of volume responsiveness. IVC measurements have not been conclusively shown to predict volume responsiveness in spontaneously breathing patients. Intrabdominal hypertension may affect IVC size and variability affecting the validity of measurements [7–9].

Question 6
Modified Bernoulli equation is routinely used in echocardiography to estimate

A. Pressure within a chamber.
B. Pressure of the chamber that the flow is going away.
C. Pressure difference between the two chambers.
D. Volume difference between the twochambers.

Answer: C. Doppler echocardiography is used to calculate transvalvular pressure gradients by applying Newton's law of conservation of energy: the total amount of energy within a closed system must stay constant. The components of this equation are described below:

$$\text{Delta}\,P = \frac{1}{2}r\left(v_2^2 - v_1^1\right) + r\grave{o}\,\left(dv/dt\right) \times ds + R\left(m\right)$$

$\frac{1}{2}r\left(v_2^2 - v_1^1\right)$: kinetic energy that results secondary to acceleration in which r is the mass density of blood.

$r\grave{o}\left(dv/dt\right)$: loss of energy due to inertia.
R(m): loss due to viscosity (m) and viscous resistance.

The latter two terms are most often negligible. Therefore, the transvalvular pressure gradient can be simplified to:

$$\text{Delta P} = 4\left(v_2^2 - v_1^2\right)$$

Velocity measurements are squared, as noted in the above equation V_2: is regularly higher than V_1, making the influence of V_1 to be negligible. The equation can be further simplified to Delta P = $4V_2$: The modified Bernoulli equation allows the use of velocity measurements to calculate pressure gradient (i.e., Delta P) across stenotic valves, between cardiac chambers, and across cardiac shunts [10].

Question 7
A 65-year-old female presents with a history of HTN, DM, and COPD is brought in by family due to worsening mental status and weakness. The patient was found to be febrile and hypotensive at 75/40 mmHg. Sepsis protocol was completed, including antibiotics and 30 cc/kg fluid bolus. The patient remains hypotensive and has been started on norepinephrine 5 µg/min. The team performs a bedside pocus to assess for volume responsiveness by performing a passive leg raise and measuring LVOT VTI pre and post. What can be concluded by the imaging?

A. The patient is volume responsive, give more fluids.
B. The patient is not volume responsive, do not give more fluids.

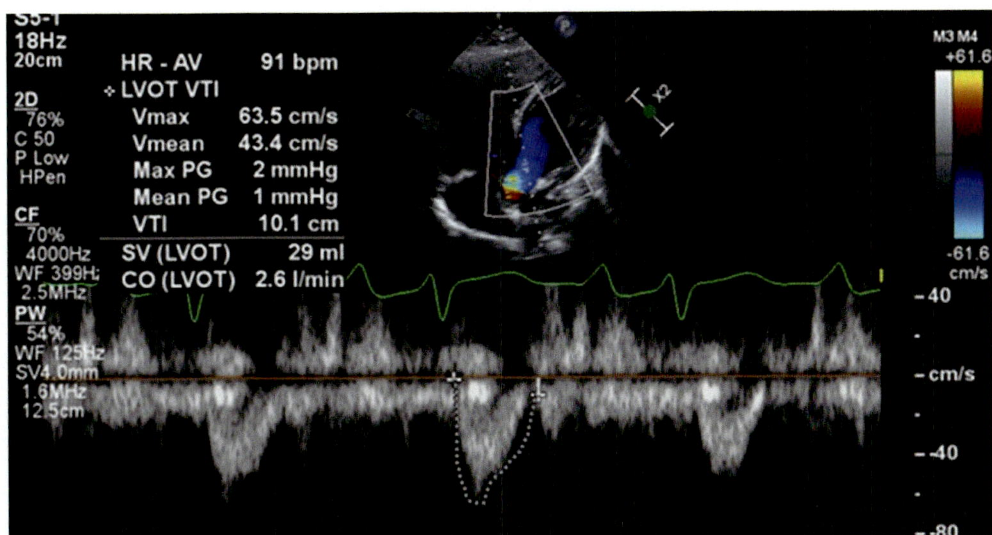

Fig. 11.5 Pre-PLR LVOT VTI

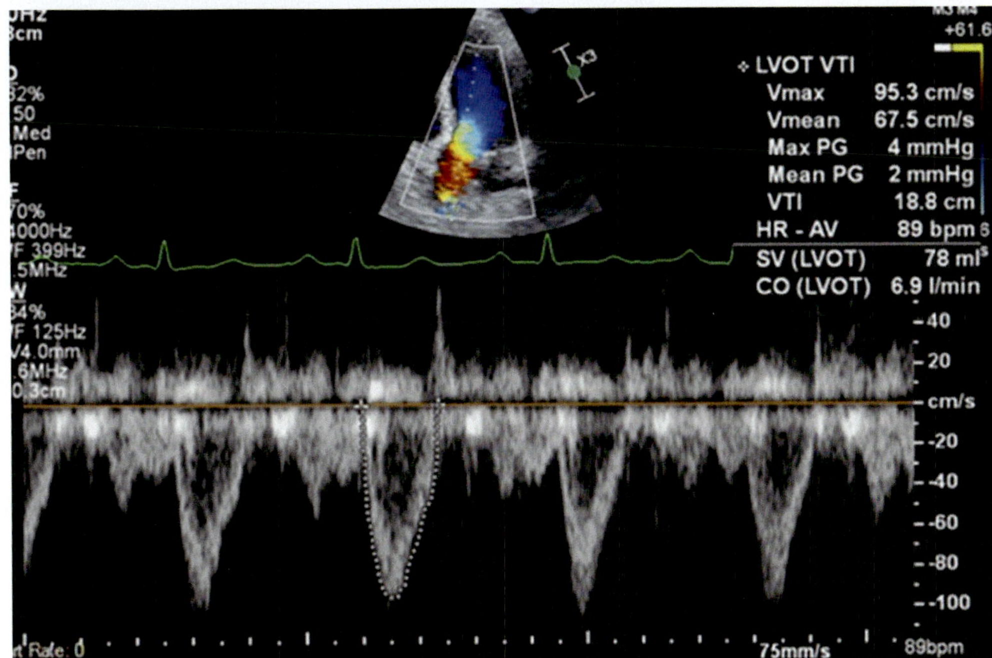

Fig. 11.6 Post-PLR LVOT VTI

C. The PW Doppler angles are markedly different; therefore, this study is inconclusive.
D. LVOT VTI with PLR cannot be used in spontaneously breathing patients.

Answer: C. The PW doppler angle is markedly different in the two images. The Pre-PLR image has a PW angle of interrogation that is >20° as compared to the post- PLR image, which is close to 0°. It is essential to keep the angle and site of interrogation consistent for pre and post-intervention VTI measurements as this error can lead to erroneous conclusions. Volume responsiveness can be assessed by volume administration or passive leg raise with a pre and post VTI measurement. Volume responsiveness is defined by a 10–15% increase in VTI or cardiac output in response to a passive leg raise and fluid bolus respectively. The use of PLR with LVOT VTI has been validated in spontaneously breathing patients [2, 11] (Figs. 11.5 and 11.6).

Question 8

78 year old male with a history of hypertension, Chronic Kidney Disease (CKD) stage IV, DM, and COPD present in respiratory distress requiring intubation. A computerized tomography (CT) of the chest shows evidence of multifocal pneumonia. On day five, he passes his SBT (spontaneous breathing trial), and the team is considering extubation. Echocardiogram performed with results below (PLR results on the next slide). Which statement below is accurate?

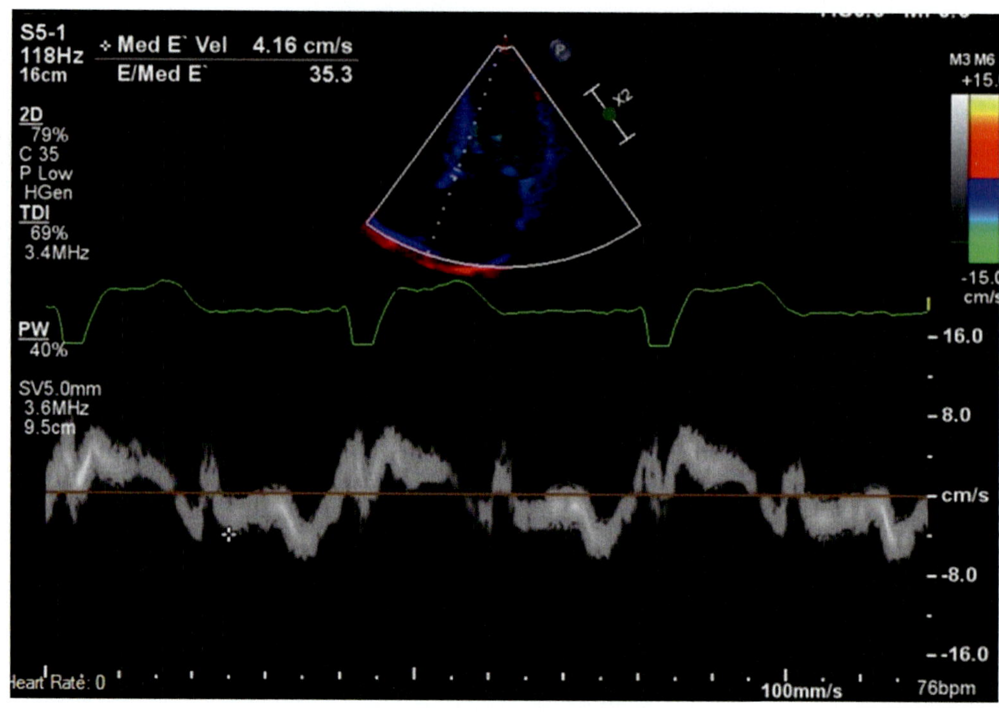

Fig. 11.7 Low medial mitral annulus TDI

A. There are no high-risk features for extubation failure on the ultrasound.
B. The patient is on the steep portion of the Frank-Starling curve with low Left atrial pressure (LAP).
C. The patient is on the flat portion of the Frank-Starling curve with low LAP.
D. There are high-risk features for extubation failure on the ultrasound.

Answer: C. This patient is high risk for extubation failure due to cardiac dysfunction. Based upon the lack of VTI change with PLR, the patient is likely on the flat portion of the Frank-Starling Curve and at risk for elevated pulmonary hydrostatic pressures if Left Ventricle (LV) preload or afterload increases. Removal of positive pressure increases venous return and increases LV afterload, which can contribute to worsened respiratory mechanics upon extubation and predisposing to reintubation. The high E/e′ is persuasive evidence for elevated LAP and has been shown to predict extubation failure. Diuresis may reduce the probability of extubation failure in this clinical scenario. There would have been an increase in VTI with PLR if the patient was on the steep portion of the Frank-Starling Curve [12–14] (Figs. 11.7, 11.8, 11.9 and 11.10).

Question 9

A 65-year-old male with a history of HTN, End Stage Renal Disease (ESRD) presents with cough, fever, and hypotension. The patient remains hypotensive despite 30 cc/kg. Based on the Doppler findings below, what would be the best next step to optimize his hemodynamics?

A. Fluids and Epinephrine.
B. Diuresis and Epinephrine.
C. Fluids and norepinephrine.
D. Fluids and phenylephrine.

Answer: D. Fluids and phenylephrine. The patient's doppler profile has a dagger-shaped profile with late peaking, which is seen with intraventricular obstruction physiology. Patients with LVH without baseline Left Ventricular outflow obstruction (LVOTO) are at risk for developing an LVOTO in hyperadrenergic and or hypovolemic state, as seen in sepsis. Hypotension associated with LVOTO is best managed with vasopressors devoid of inotropy and by increasing preload. The best choice would be phenylephrine and fluids. Epinephrine would be suboptimal given the inotropy/chronotropic effects of it. Using a diuretic and epinephrine would reduce preload and adding inotropy which would be incorrect for this patient. Norepinephrine can be considered, but it has some inotropic effect; therefore, phenylephrine or vasopressin remains superior for this physiology [15, 16] (Fig. 11.11).

Question 10

What is the Systolic Pulmonary Artery Pressure (sPAP) based upon the information in the table (Table 11.2)?

Table 11.2 Tricuspid valve CW velocity/IVC diameter

TV peak velocity	3.0 m/s
IVC diameter	2.4 cm with no respiratory variation

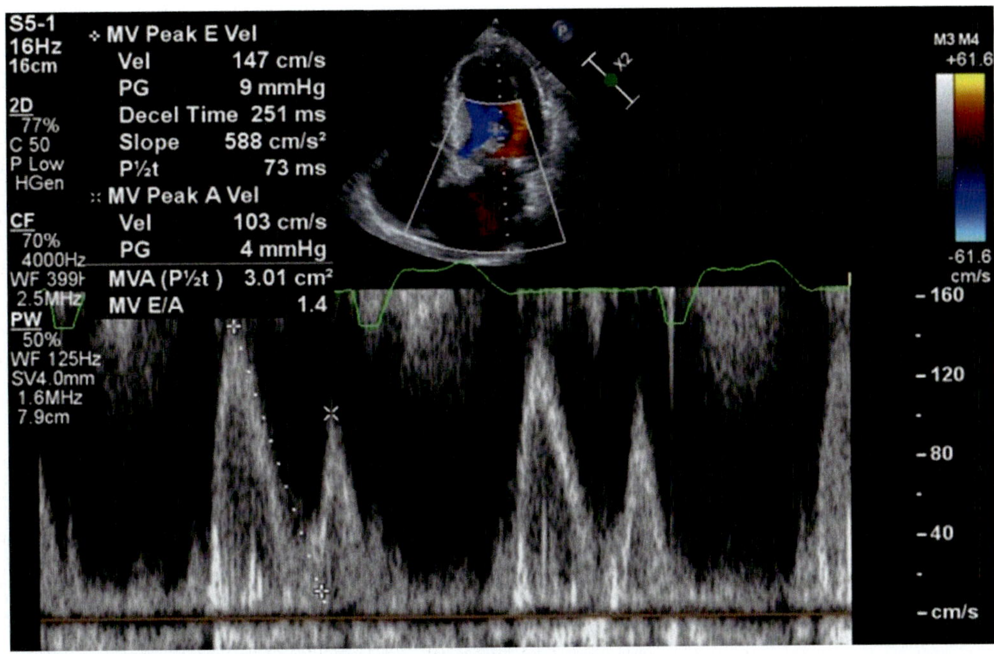

Fig. 11.8 Mitral valve PW Doppler-E/A

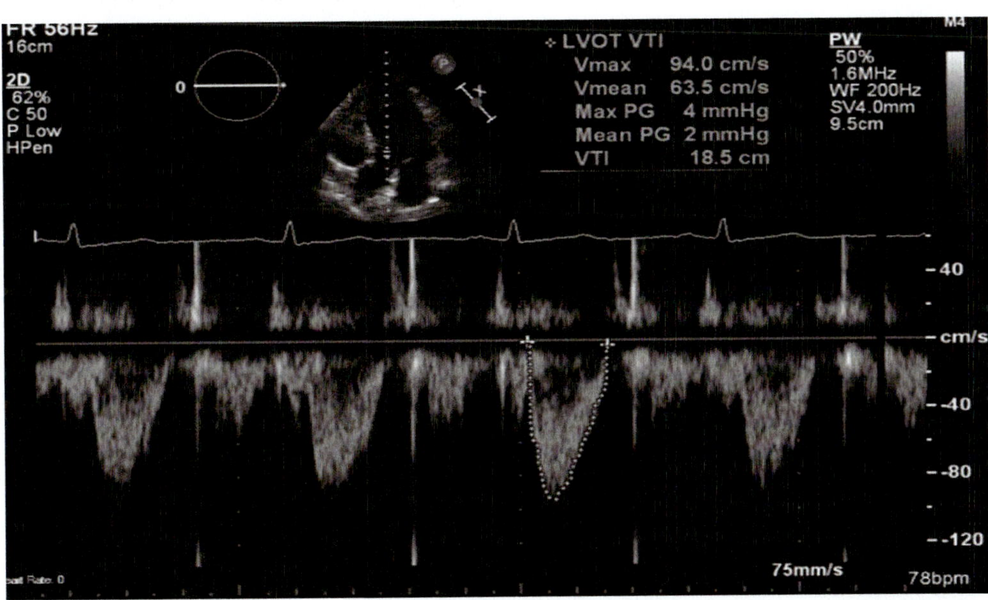

Fig. 11.9 Pre-PLR LVOT VTI

A. 51 mmHg, given that there is no pulmonary artery stenosis.
B. 51 mmHg, given that there is no pulmonary hypertension.
C. 74 mmHg given that there is no pulmonary artery stenosis
D. 74 mmHg, given that there is no pulmonary hypertension.

Answer: A. Calculation of the PASP is done indirectly. Start with the premise that RVSP=PASP with the caveat that there is no pulmonary artery stenosis. We calculate RVSP by first measuring the max Tricuspid Valve regurgitation (TR) velocity with CW, which is then converted to a pressure gradient via the modified Bernoulli equation (see below). The IVC diameter is given at 2.4 cm with no respiratory variation, which equals RAP of greater than 15 mmHg. B. Pulmonary hypertension is not a contraindication to accurate calculation of PASP with the use of the modified Bernoulli equation [4, 17].

$$\text{Right Ventricular Systolic Pressure}\left(\text{RVSP}\right) = (RV\ \text{gradient} - RA\ \text{gradient}) + \text{RAP}$$

$$\begin{aligned}\text{RVSP} = 4\left(V_{TR_{max}}\right)^2 + \text{RAP} &= \text{Pulmonary artery Systolic Pressure}\\ &= 4\left(3\right)^2 + 15\ \text{mmHg}\\ &= 51\ \text{mmHg}\end{aligned}$$

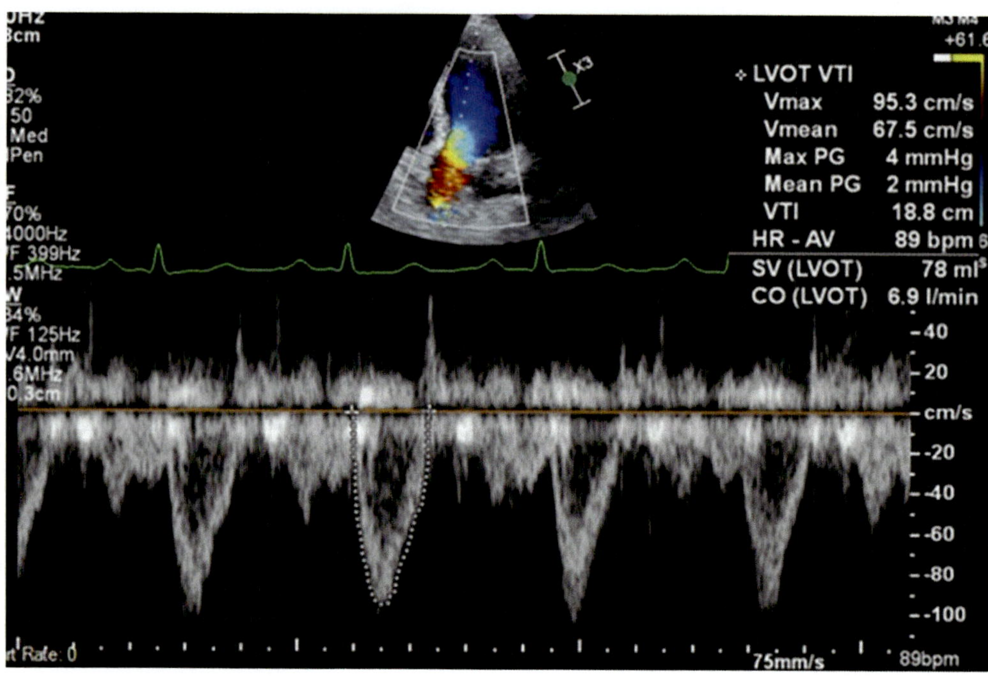

Fig. 11.10 Post-PLR LVOT VTI

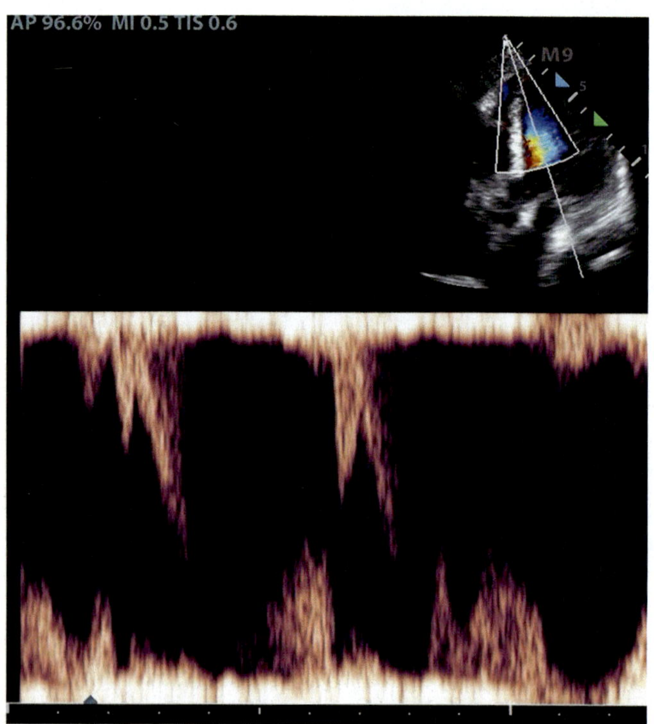

Fig. 11.11 Dagger shaped LVOT VTI-Note mid cavitary position of PW gate

Question 11

72 y/o male with a history of HFpEF, CKD IV, presents with dyspnea on exertion. Lung ultrasound is performed with evidence of a B profile. To further assess the patient's diastolic heart function, his mitral inflow velocity and tissue Doppler are measured at the medial mitral annulus. The results are below. What can be discerned based on the cause of the patient's dyspnea (Table 11.3)?

Table 11.3

Peak E wave velocity	120 cm/s
Medial mitral annular TDI velocity	6 cm/s

A. The patient likely has low left atrial filling pressures, and this is non-cardiogenic pulmonary edema.
B. The patient likely has high LAP filling pressures, and this is non-cardiogenic pulmonary edema.
C. The patient likely has low LAP filling pressures, and this is cardiogenic pulmonary edema
D. The patient likely has high LAP filling pressures, and this patient has cardiogenic pulmonary edema.

Answer: D. The patient has evidence of bilateral pulmonary edema base upon the B profile on lung ultrasound, but it can be challenging to ascertain whether this is cardiogenic or non-cardiogenic. This patient has an E/e > 14, which has been shown to correlate well with an elevated Left Atrial Filling pressure. Based on the high E/e′ of 20, the patient likely has cardiogenic pulmonary edema. An E/e less than 8 correlates well with a low to normal wedge pressure and would likely point towards non-cardiogenic pulmonary edema [18, 19].

Question 12

75 y/o female with a history of ESRD, COPD, Heart failure with reduced Ejection Fraction (HFrEF) (EF 25%), and HTN complains of dyspnea on exertion. Based upon the doppler findings, what can be discerned about the Left atrial pressure (LAP) and Diastolic Dysfunction stage?

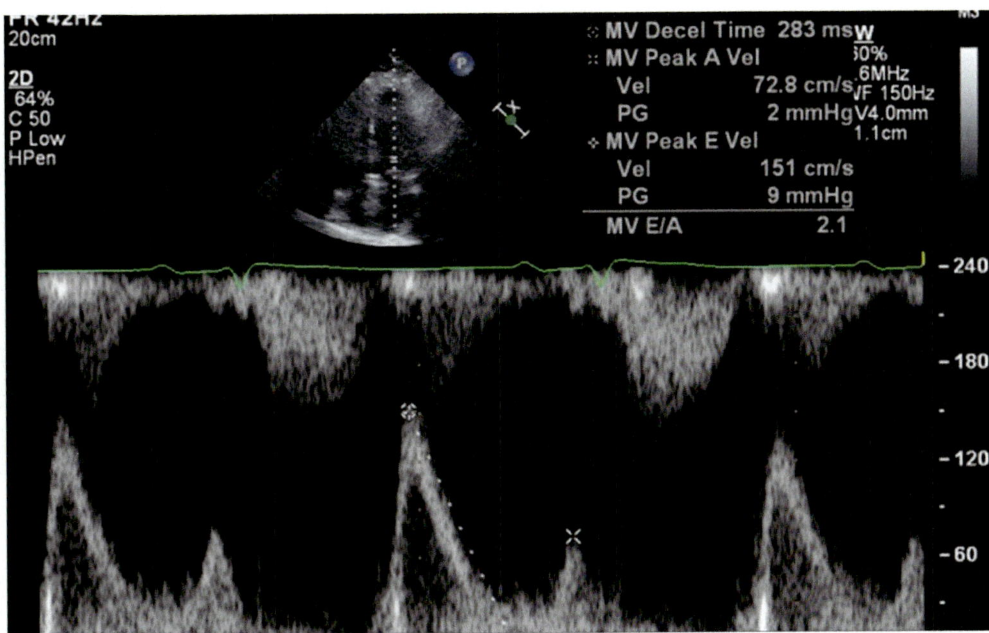

Fig. 11.12 Mitral inflow PW Doppler-E/A ratio >2

A. The patient has elevated LAP and Grade III diastolic dysfunction.
B. The patient has elevated LAP and Grade I diastolic dysfunction.
C. The patient has normal to reduced LAP.
D. The diastolic dysfunction stage cannot be determined without tissue doppler.

Answer: A. In patients with known depressed EF, an E/A ratio >2 is diagnostic for elevated LAP and at least Grade III Diastolic Dysfunction. The dyspnea in this patient may be related to elevated LAP filling pressures, which may be modifiable by diuresis. Grade I Diastolic Dysfunction would demonstrate an E/A ratio <8, which is indicative of low to normal LAP [18, 20] (Fig. 11.12).

Question 13

A 35-year- old male with a history of IVDU presents with complaints fevers and weakness. The patient has intoxicated; therefore, history is limited. He is stable hemodynamically and on 2 L, NC, with oxygen saturation of 95%. The chest radiograph is pending. A bedside echocardiogram is performed. Which are the most accurate conclusions based upon the PW doppler image of the Hepatic Vein shown below (Fig. 11.13)?

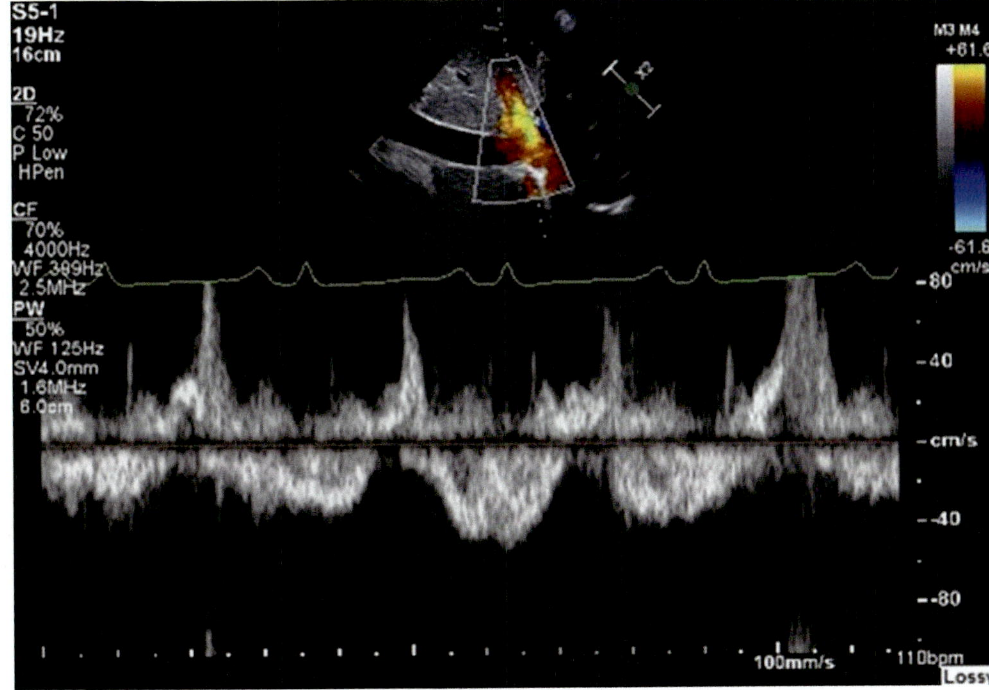

Fig. 11.13 Hepatic vein PW Doppler

A. Low CVP with no TR
B. Normal CVP with mild TR
C. High CVP with severe TR
D. High CVP with mild TR

Answer: C. High CVP with severe TR. The hepatic vein PW doppler image shows evidence of Systolic flow reversal, which is consistent with severe TV regurgitation and likely elevated CVP. In the figures shown below, a normal hepatic vein shows systolic flow predominance, which is eventually lost as the CVP rises and ultimately reversed in the setting of severe TR. The clinical history of the IVDU and fevers are suggestive of endocarditis related Tricuspid valve regurgitation. In answers A and B, Systolic predominance in the hepatic vein PW would be expected. In answer D, an antegrade Diastolic wave but no Systolic wave would exist in the setting of a high CVP and mild TR [21, 22] (Figs. 11.14 and 11.15).

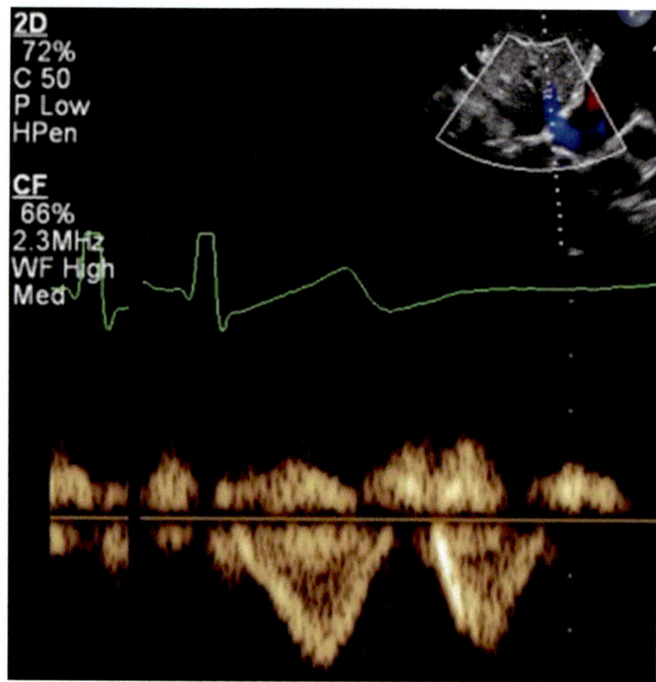

Fig. 11.15 Normal hepatic vein PW

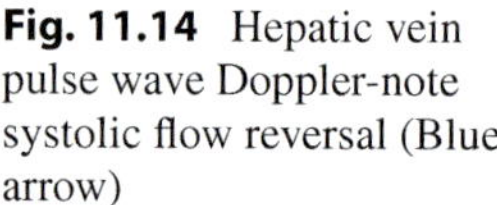

Fig. 11.14 Hepatic vein pulse wave Doppler-note systolic flow reversal (Blue arrow)

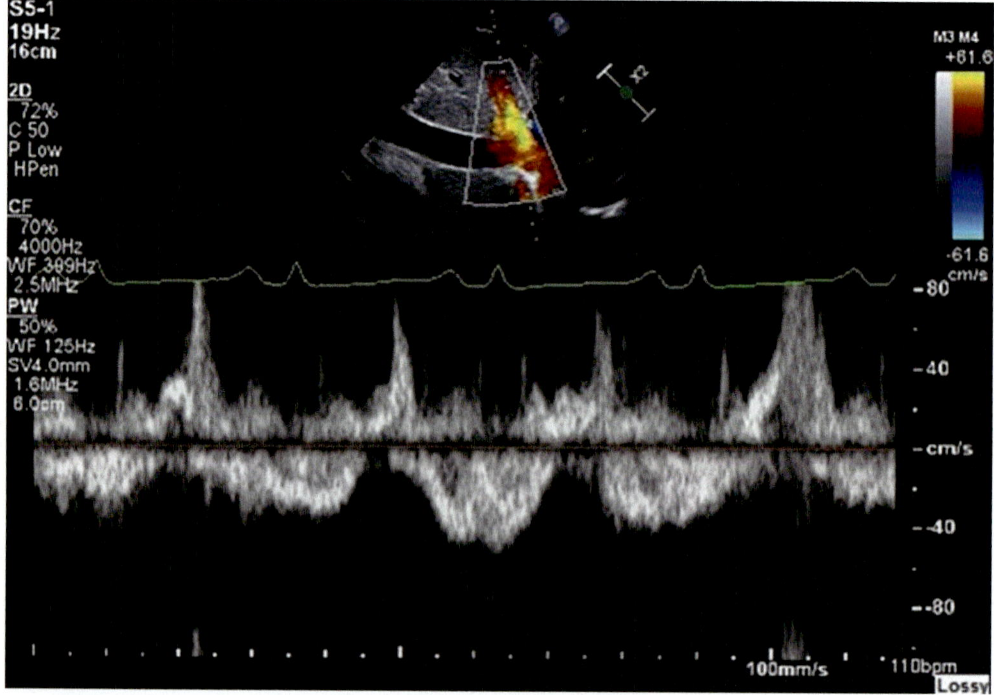

Case: Question 14

A 33-year-old female with a medical history significant for polysubstance abuse, Methacillin Sensitive Staphylococcal Aureus (MSSA) bacteremia who presented with septic shock secondary to bioprosthetic tricuspid endocarditis. She required intubation due to presumed pneumonia, and currently has a P/F ratio of 140. She is sedated and paralyzed. She is on Volume Control, 100 % FiO_2, and 10 of PEEP. She is on 8 cc/kg of ideal body weight. To better characterize her shock, bedside echocardiogram performed below. Describe the pathology (Figs. 11.16, 11.17 and 11.18).

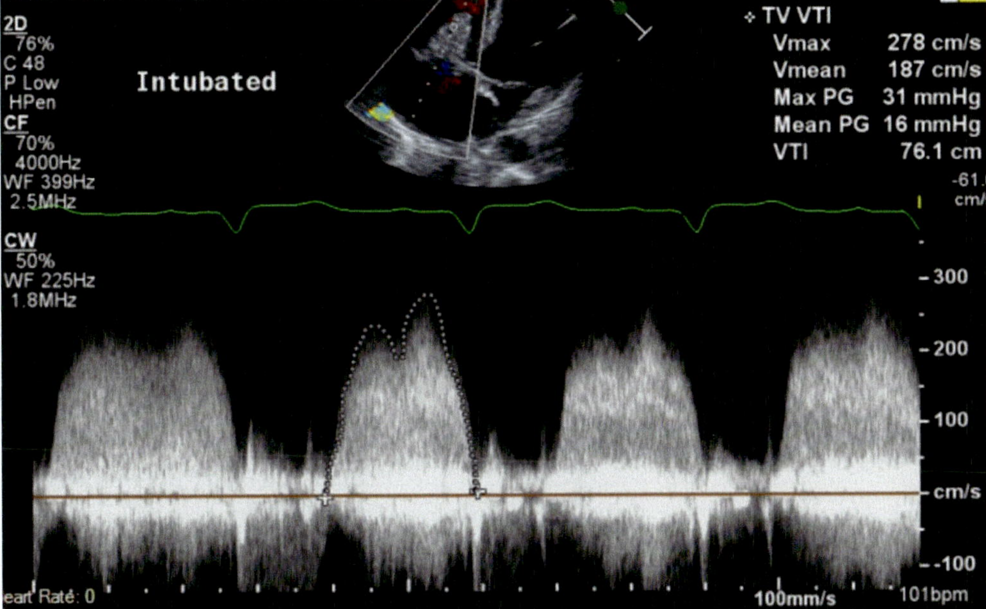

Fig. 11.16 Tricuspid valve CW Doppler

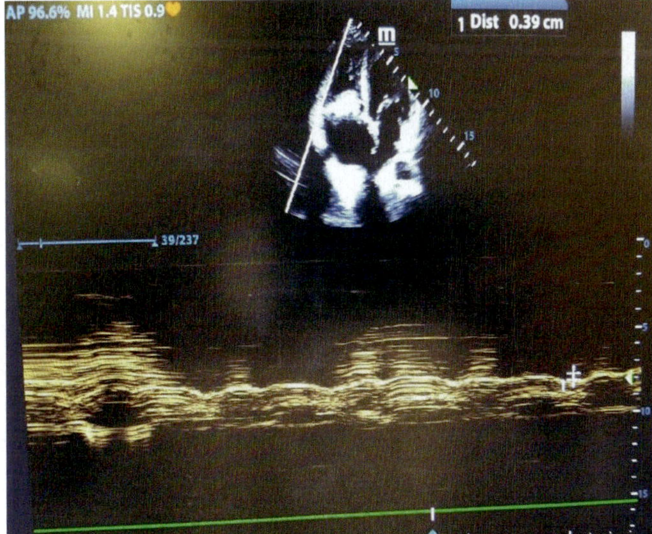

Fig. 11.17 TAPSE

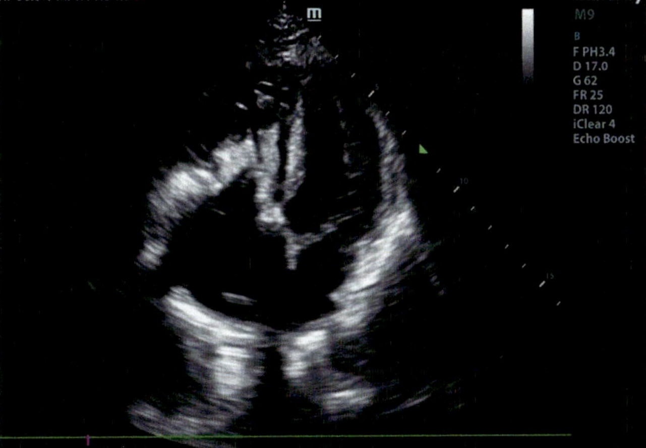

Fig. 11.18 Four-chamber view

A. Tricuspid bioprosthetic valve regurgitation
B. Normal bioprosthetic valve doppler profile
C. Tricuspid bioprosthetic valve Stenosis
D. Need more information

Answer: C. Severe Tricuspid Bioprosthetic Valve Stenosis. The imaging is consistent with thickened leaflets, which are likely related to endocarditis. The doppler profile shows an E wave peak velocity of 2.1 m/s. Peak E wave velocities >1.7 m/s and mean gradient above 6 mmHg are recommended cutoffs to consider tricuspid stenosis in a bioprosthetic valve. Answer A is incorrect due to the antegrade flow on the Doppler profile, which indicates that this is not Tricuspid Regurgitation. Answer B is incorrect since normal bioprosthetic valve peak velocities would fall below 1.7 M/s; therefore, this is not a normal profile. Answer D is incorrect since more information such as Pressure Half Time (PHT) and Mean gradient calculation would be helpful, but there is enough information here to suggest Bioprosthetic valve stenosis [23–25].

Question 15

In patient refered in Questions 14, Volume responsiveness was assessed by performing LVOT VTI variation shown below. Based on the results, what is the appropriate conclusion (Fig. 11.19)?

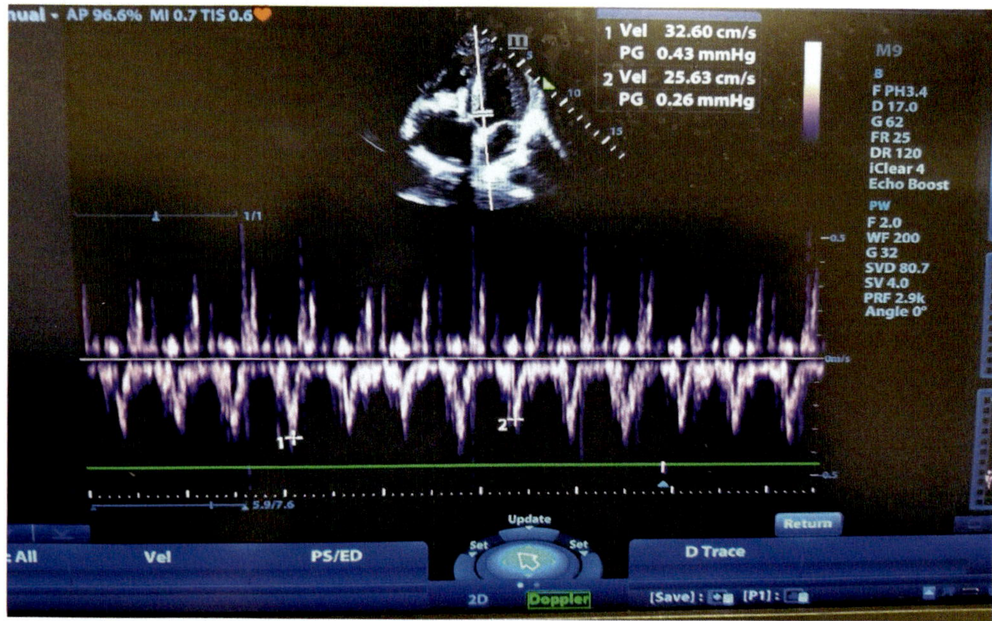

Fig. 11.19 LVOT VTI PW Doppler-note respiratory variation

A. LVOT VTI variation is higher than 14%; therefore, she is fluid responsive.
B. LVOT VTI variation cannot be assessed in paralyzed patients.
C. LVOT VTI variation cutoff is not valid because the Tidal Volume is too high.
D. LVOT VTI variation in patients with RV failure can lead to false positives.

Answer: D. The LVOT VTI variation in this patient on passive mechanical ventilation with appropriate tidal volume is >14%. However, these results should be interpreted with caution as RV failure is associated with false positive LVOT VTI variation. LVOT VTI variation is calculated as (VTImax–VTImin)/ [(VTImax–VTImin)/2] 100%. Prerequisites to use Heart lung interaction method for volume responsiveness assessment are below:

1. Sinus rhythm.
2. No spontaneous breaths.
3. Tidal volumes of 8–10 mL/kg.
4. Normal Intra-abdominal pressure.
5. The patient should not have an open chest.
6. Interpret cautiously in the setting of RV failure.

The patient meets the percent variation cut off, but the RV failure is causing false positive in this patient [26, 27].

Question 16

A 56-year-old female with a past medical history of COPD, intravenous drug user (IVDU) was found down with visible aspiration, requiring intubation prior to arriving at the hospital. Chest imaging reveals bilateral symmetric infiltrates concerning for aspiration. Her MAP is 65 mmHg with the use of levophed and vasopressin. She has received 30 cc/kg crystalloid. You are trying to determine if this patient is volume responsive. She is sedated and paralyzed on 8 cc/kg IBW tidal volume. The image is shown below. What can you determine (Fig. 11.20)?

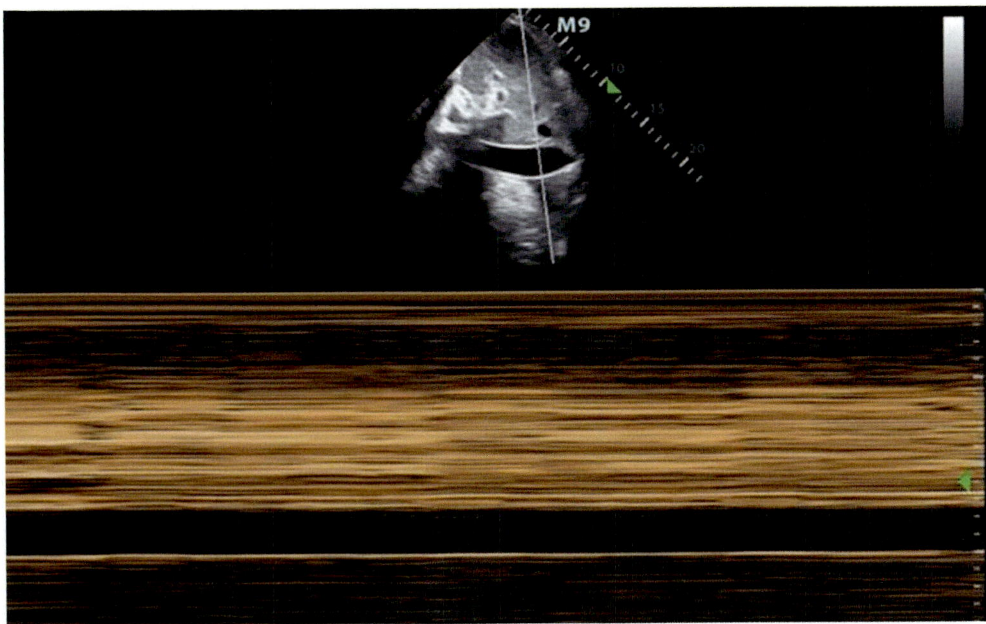

Fig. 11.20 IVC M-mode

A. She is volume responsive
B. She is not volume responsive
C. IVC cannot be used for volume responsiveness
D. It cannot determine in the setting of mechanical ventilation.

Answer: B. The patient is unlikely to be volume responsive, as there is no respiratory variation. IVC distensibility(dIVC) index more than 18% predicts volume responsiveness. The use of IVC for volume responsiveness has been validated for patients who are on mechanical ventilation (caveat is that the patients in this study were on an average of 8.5 cc/kg tidal volume of ideal body weight). The M-Mode image of this patient does not demonstrate any respiratory variation. The Distensibility Index of the IVC(dIVC) should be used if there is variability noted (Dmax-Dmin/Dmin). [7, 8].

Question 17

What is the likely severity of the Tricuspid Regurgitation based upon the images shown below? (Figs. 11.21 and 11.22)

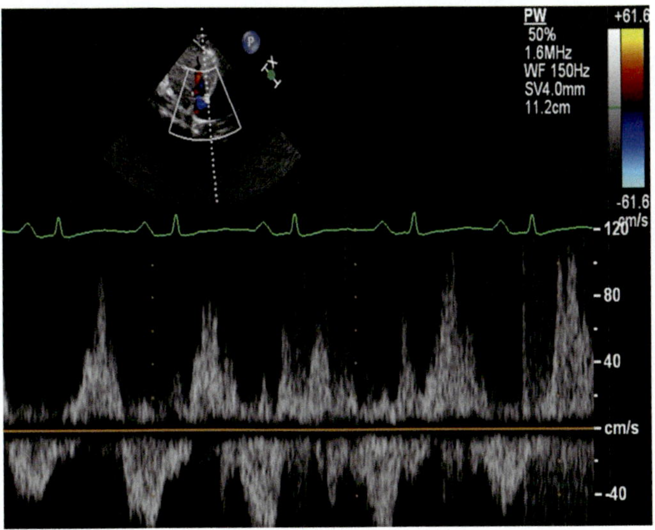

Fig. 11.21 Hepatic vein PW Doppler

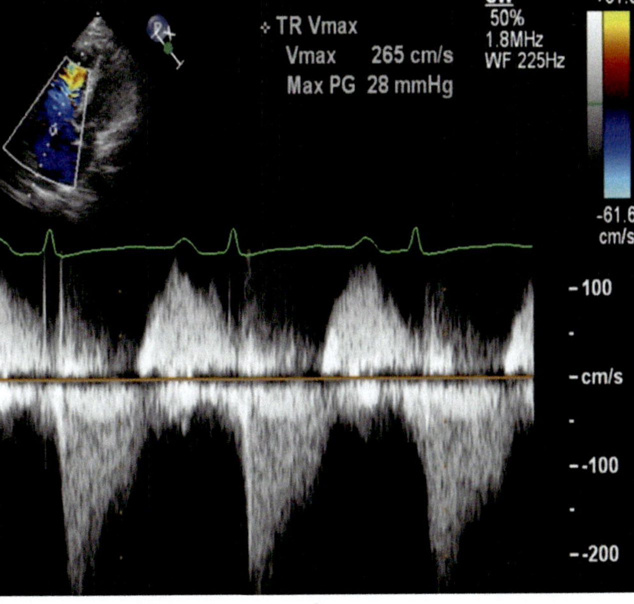

Fig. 11.22 Tricuspid valve CW Doppler

A. Mild TR
B. Moderate TR
C. Severe TR
D. It cannot be determined.

Answer: C. The TR jet is triangular, early peaking, and has a dense signal, all of which are consistent severe TR. The hepatic vein systolic flow reversal fits with severe TR. Mild TR would have a parabolic and less dense signal. Moderate TR CW doppler would be parabolic/triangular, and the hepatic vein would exhibit systolic wave blunting [21] (Figs. 11.23, 11.24 and 11.25).

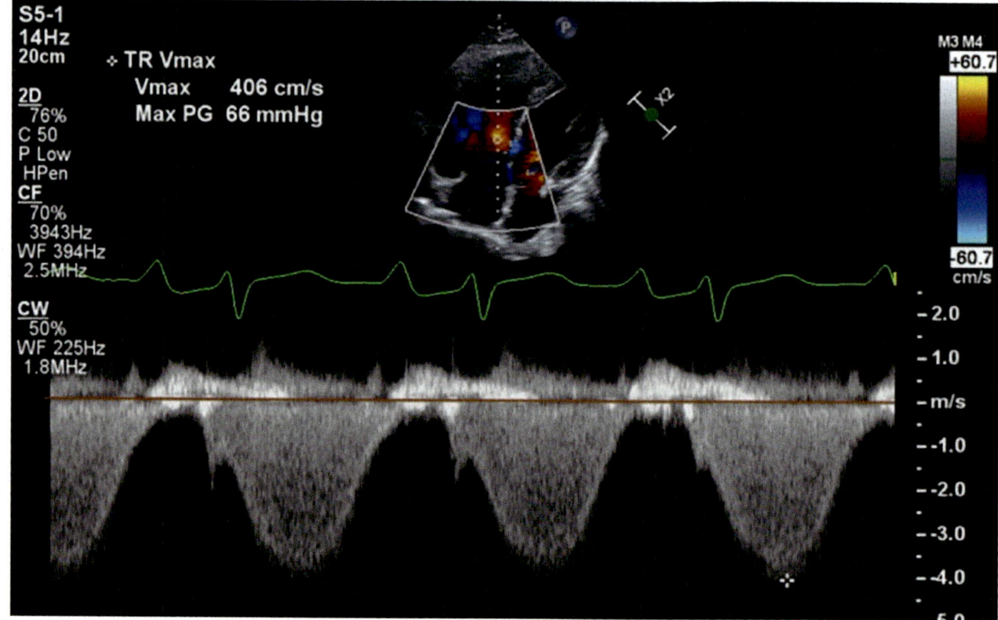

Fig. 11.23 Tricuspid valve CW-moderate severity, note increased triangular shape

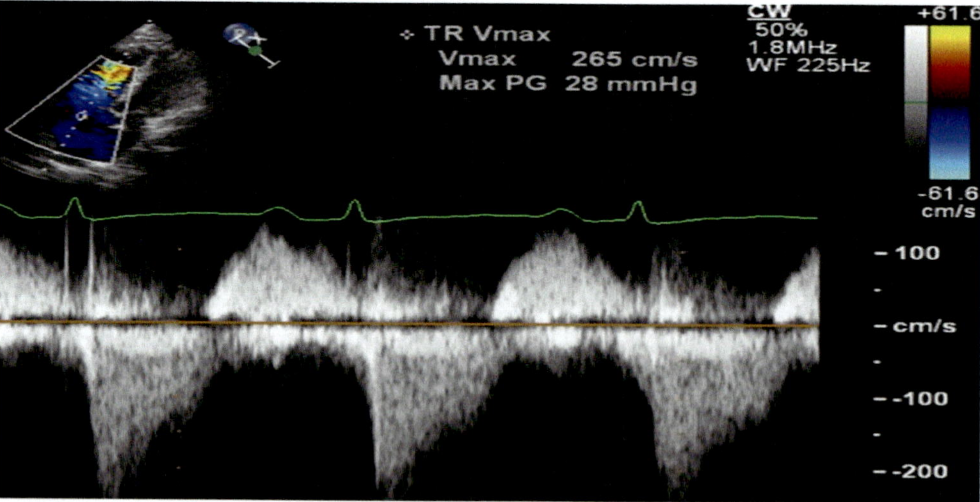

Fig. 11.24 Severe-note increased density compared to antegrade flow. Triangular shape

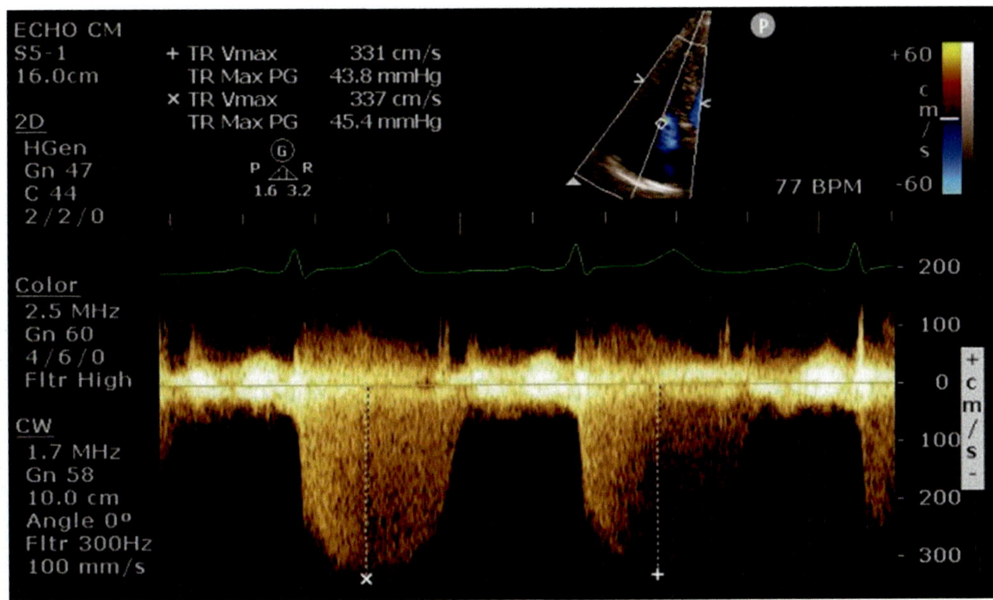

Fig. 11.25 Mild TR-note round shape and low density

Question 18

A 55-year- old male with PMH of COPD and Hypertension presents with dyspnea on exertion, CT-PE protocol did not show pulmonary embolism, but he was found to have dense RLL consolidation. Oxygen saturation (SaO_2) was 80% on maximum support on High Flow Nasal Cannula; therefore, the patient was intubated. Post-intubation SpO_2 dropped to 75% on assist control, FiO_2 100%, and PEEP of 10 cmH_2O. The PEEP was increased to 15 cmH_2O with noted worsening of SpO_2 to 70%. Compliance was 55 mL/cmH_2O (normal range: 50–100 mL/cmH_2O), with no change noted with increase in PEEP. The patient remained hemodynamically stable. The bedside echo is shown below. What is the most likely reason for worsening hypoxia post-intubation (Video 11.1)?

A. Acute Cor pulmonale leading to low cardiac output and reduced mixed venous.
B. Presence of an intracardiac shunt.
C. Presence of an intrapulmonary shunt
D. Alveolar overdistension.

Answer: B. The echocardiogram indicates an intracardiac shunt given the microbubble presence in the L heart within 3–6 beats. The addition of positive pressure ventilation leads to an acute rise in right ventricular pressures. This can lead to an increased right to left shunting if there is a shunt predisposition present (PFO, ASD). The RV/LV ratio is elevated; therefore, acute cor pulmonale is on the differential, but hemodynamics appeared to have remained stable during this time, decreasing the probability that RV dilation is acute in nature. An intrapulmonary shunt would exhibit bubbles in the left heart at 6 bpm and above. The compliance remained stable with the increase in PEEP ; therefore, overdistension is less likely as a cause of the hypoxia [28–30].

Question 19

A 46-year-old male is admitted for chest pain and found to have an STEMI in LAD territory. He is taken for emergent cardiac catheterization and has an drug eluting stent placed. Six days later, he develops dyspnea and hypoxia. On exam, he has a holosystolic murmur best heard at the second intercostal space and the apex. Heart rate is 110 bmp POCUS reveals B-line pattern bilaterally. 2D Echo reveals normal valvular and papillary muscle function. Color doppler shows flow from the left to the right ventricle. Given the information obtained, which of the following is correct (Table 11.4)?

Table 11.4 Diameter and VTI of RVOT/LVOT

	LVOT	RVOT
Diameter	2.0	2.8
VTI	22	17

A. Qp: Qs is 0.67.
B. Flow across the RVOT represents the systemic flow (Qs) in a patient with this type of shunt.
C. Qp: Qs is more than 1.
D. Blood flow entering the pulmonary circulation (Qp) is 7.7 L/min.

Answer: C. This patient is found to have a ventricular septal defect after myocardial infarction. In an acute process in which the pressure is higher within the left ventricle compared to the right, the flow will move in a left to the right direction. This will result in a higher flow through the pulmonary system compared to the systemic circulation. Congestive heart failure and pulmonary edema will likely ensue.

A comparison between pulmonary and systemic blood flow (Qp:Qs) can be used to calculate severity and help guide treatment options. Stroke volume can be calculated independently for both right (pulmonary) and left (systemic) sided systems.

$$Q = CSA \times VTI \times HR$$
$$Q = \left(pr^2\right) \times VTI \times HR$$

$$Qs = Q_{LVOT} = \left(pr^2\right) \times VTI \times HR =$$
$$= \left(p\left(2/2\right)^2\right) \times 22 \times 110 = 7.7L/min$$

$$Qp = Q_{RVOT} = \left(pr^2\right) \times VTI \times HR = 11.5L/min$$
$$= \left(p\left(2.8/2\right)^2\right) \times 17 \times 110 = 11.5L/min$$
$$Qp : Qs = 11.5/7.7 = 1.5$$

Because flow within this intracardiac shunt moves from left to right, flow through the pulmonary system with be higher than the left. Qp:Qs is greater than 1 (Answer C is correct).

If a patient is to have a shunt after the LVOT or RVOT, such as in a patent ductus arteriosus (PDA), the calculation for systemic and pulmonary circulation will change from above. The flow through the PDA will enter the pulmonary system as blood passes into the pulmonary artery. Therefore, the true blood flow to the pulmonary system will include the cardiac output through the RVOT plus the flow through the shunt. Therefore, Qp. Qs will be the amount of flow that leaves through the LVOT minus the shunt fraction. Because all of the systemic flow (Qs) will return to the right side of the heart, the calculated Qs will be calculated as the flow through the RVOT.

Similarly, the true blood flow through the pulmonary system will return to the left heart chambers. True Qp will be measured as the flow through the LVOT. This differs from the calculation above in which the shunt is between ventricles and before LVOT and RVOT. Answer (D) is incorrect. The Qs are calculated at 7.7 L/min [28].

Question 20

65 y/o male with a history of Diverticulosis, COPD, HTN, CKD III brought in by the family for weakness and altered sensorium. BP was 70/30 on presentation with a pulse of 110 and Lactate of 6 mg/dL. BP improved to 90/60 after the 30 cc/kg IBW fluid was given. The patient admits to reduced oral intake. He had some melenic stools. Hgb is 9.5, compared to 11.0 a few months prior. Bedside Echocardiogram doppler studies and PLR performed. What is the type of shock and ideal management course (Fig. 11.26)?

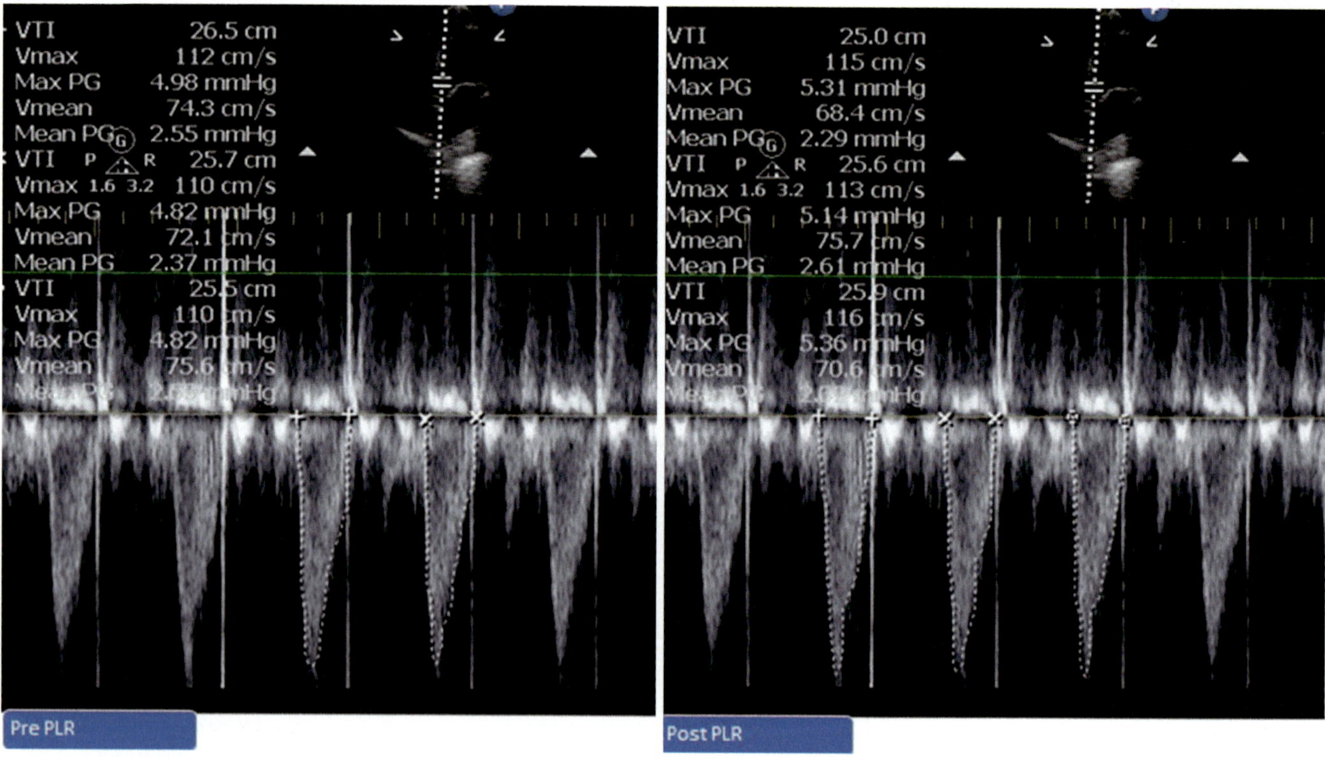

Fig. 11.26 Pre and post PLR LVOT VTI

A. Hypovolemic shock. Would give additional volume.
B. Cardiogenic shock. Would avoid further volume.
C. Distributive Shock Would not give additional volume.
D. Distributive Would give additional volume

Answer: C. Distributive Shock. This patient had a PLR performed with LVOT VTI as the surrogate for stroke volume, and there was minimal change. Given the lack of VTI response with the PLR, the patient is not likely to be volume responsive; therefore, they may not benefit from additional fluids. In hypovolemic shock patient's VTI should significantly respond to PLR. Cardiogenic shock is unlikely as the VTI would likely be low. [1, 31].

Question 21
A 21-year- old female with PMH of IVDU presents with fevers, dyspnea, and chest CT imaging consistent with septic emboli. An echocardiogram shows evidence of pulmonary insufficiency. The CVP measured by the central line is 15. What is the approximate PA diastolic pressure (Fig. 11.27)?

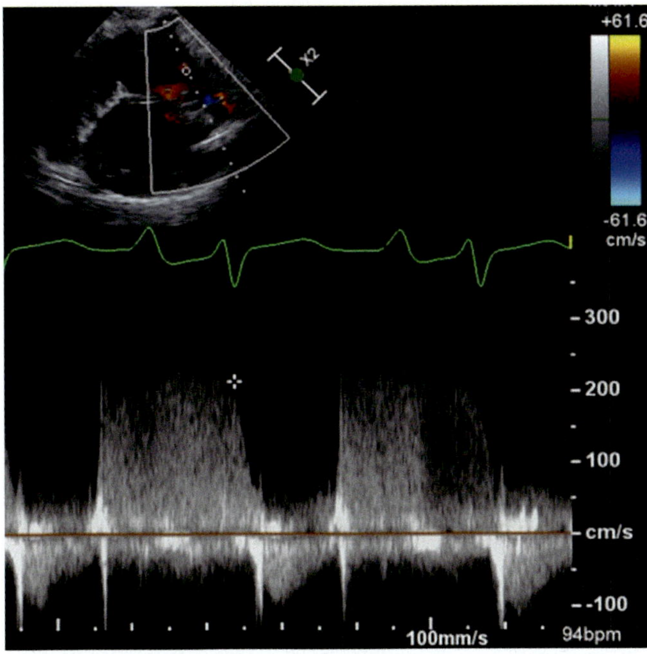

Fig. 11.27 Pulmonary regurgitation CW Doppler

A. 45 mmHg
B. 51 mmHg
C. 31 mmHg
D. 25 mmHg

Answer: C. End-diastolic pulmonary artery pressure (PAEDP) can be measured by first getting pulmonary regurgitation jet velocity at end-diastole with continuous wave. The end-diastolic velocity once inserted into the modified Bernoulli equation ($\Delta P = 4$ V2), which will give us the gradient between PA and the RV at the end of diastole. RVEDP is equal to CVP. Adding the CVP value to the PA–RV gradient leads to the calculation of the PAEDP which, in this case, is 31 mmHg [2, 17].

Question 22
75 yo male with PMH of hypertension, smoking, and hyperlipidemia, presents with progressively worsening dyspnea on exertion. Echocardiography performed. Describe the valvular abnormalities below (Video 11.2).

A. Eccentric AR and Systolic MR only
B. Eccentric AR and Systolic and Diastolic MR
C. Central AR and Systolic MR only
D. Systolic and Diastolic MR with no AR

Answer: B. There is an Eccentric Aortic regurgitation jet with Diastolic MR at the end of diastole, which is followed by Systolic MR. The Aortic regurgitation leads to a rapid rise in LVEDP, which quickly reduces the Left Atrium to Left Ventricle gradient, which leads to Diastolic MR before Systole.

Answer A is incorrect because, eccentric Aortic Regurgitation and Systolic MR are present, but there is an additional Diastolic MR. Answer C is incorrect as the AR jet is eccentric, and there is an additional Diastolic MR. Answer D is incorrect due to AR being present [32, 33].

Question 23
What is the mechanism of the Diastolic MR?

A. Severe Acute AR leading to a rapid rise in LVEDP
B. Chronic elevation of LVEDP
C. Flail Posterior Mitral valve
D. Flail Anterior Mitral Valve

Answer: A. Eccentric AR jet severity can be underestimated, but given the Diastolic MR, it is likely acute and severe. The Diastolic MR occurs due to a rapid rise in LVEDP that causes flow reversal during what should be atrial systole; there is presystolic closure of the mitral valve. This patient may have a chronic elevation of LVEDP, but given the history and simultaneous presence of AR and diastolic MR, acute AR is more likely the cause for the Diastolic MR. C. There is no evidence of posterior mitral valve leaflet restriction in this video. You would expect the mitral valve leaflet tip to point into the Left Atrium during Systole, not seen in this clip. No evidence of a Flail Anterior Mitral valve exists [21, 33].

Question 24

A 67-year-old male with a history of HFpEF, DM, and Coronary Artery Disease (CAD) remains hypotensive with delayed capillary refill and cold extremities. When measuring his cardiac output by Doppler echocardiography, which of the following is TRUE?

A. An angle of 90° between the ultrasound beam and the blood flow will provide the most reliable measurement
B. Blood flow along a curved vessel is uniform at each location within the vessel
C. A 10% underestimation of aortic outflow tract diameter will result in 10% underestimation of cardiac output
D. The laminar flow will result in lower velocity compared to turbulent flow

Answer: D. Doppler echocardiography can measure blood flow by measuring blood velocity and multiplying by cross-sectional area through which blood is traveling. Because blood flow is pulsatile and therefore, not uniform throughout the cardiac cycle, velocity is measured using the velocity time integral (VTI). This is the summation of all velocities during the regular flow period. The doppler equation, DF = $(2fv/c)cos\theta$ shows the importance of the angle of incidence (θ). Because the cosine of 90° is zero, measurements nearest to this value will give a severe underestimation of true velocity. If θ is 0–20°, the cosine of this value will range between 1.0 to 0.92, resulting in only a small underestimation on velocity. Velocity underestimation increases as θ increase more than 20° (answer A is incorrect). Normal flow in the heart is laminar. The flow will be traveling at the same velocity and in the same direction. In curved vessels, the velocity will vary depending on the size of the vessel and flow pattern upon entering the curve. Recorded velocity will depend on the exact location within the vessel (Answer B is incorrect). Cardiac output is measured as stroke volume × heart rate. The calculation of stroke volume is measured as the cross-sectional area × VTI. Because A = πr^2, errors in the measurement of the orifice is "squared" (Answer C is incorrect). Turbulent flow develops at higher velocities or when CSA changes. This will result in higher and more variable flow velocities. The laminar flow will result in a lower velocity with a smoother, thinner flow envelope [2, 34].

Question 25

A 54-year-old male with a history of HFpEF presents with pulmonary edema, hypoxia, and hypertension. He is intubated and mechanically ventilated. His IVC measured 2.2 cm and has no respiratory variation. Below is doppler imaging across his pulmonic valve. Which of the following is TRUE (Fig. 11.28)?

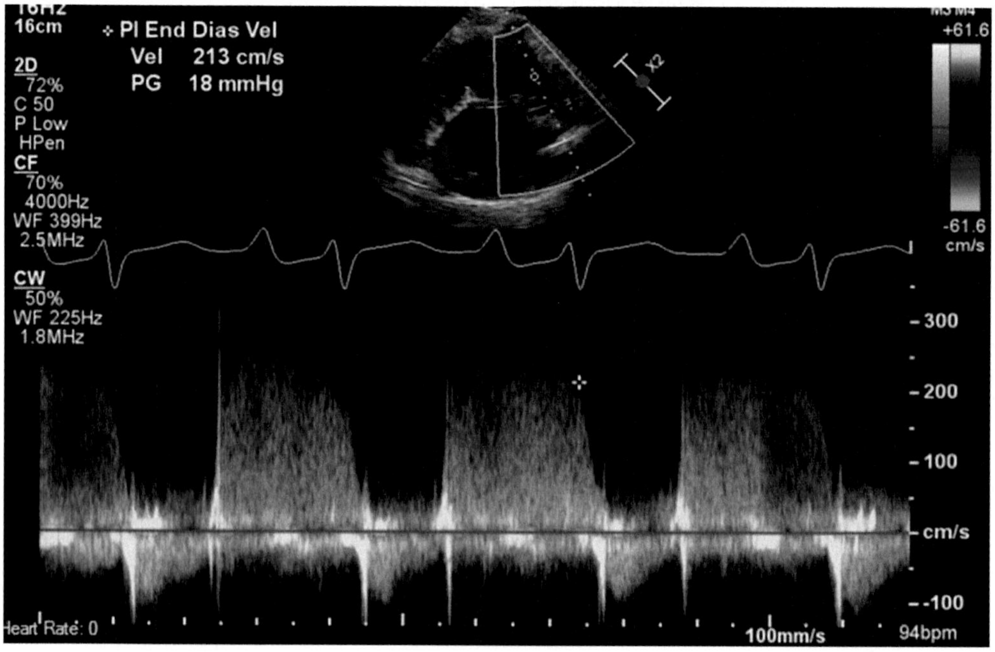

Fig. 11.28 Pulmonary valve regurgitation CW doppler

A. PA diastolic pressure is 18 mmHg
B. Pulmonary artery pressure will be equal to RV pressure in pulmonary stenosis
C. M-mode of the mitral valve may reveal a "B-bump."
D. The gradient between the right ventricle and pulmonary artery is 33 mmHg

Answer: C. The end-diastolic pulmonary regurgitant velocity provides the pressure gradient between the pulmonary artery and the right ventricle at end-diastole. Pulmonary artery diastolic pressure (PADP) can be estimated by adding his pressure gradient to the right atrial pressure (RAP).

$$\text{PADP} = \text{Pulmonary Regurgitant Gradient} + \text{RAP}$$

Using the modified Bernoulli equation:

$$\text{Pulmonary Regurgitant Gradient} = \left[4 \times (2.13)^2\right].$$

The RAP is estimated as 15 mmHg by IVC diameter > 2.1 cm with <50% collapse:

PADP = 18 + 15.
PADP = 33 mmHg.

Answers (A) and (D) are incorrect because the Pulmonary Regurgitant Gradient and PADP are 18 mmHg and 33 mmHg, respectively. In this patient, there is evidence of volume overload with congestive heart failure and no known primary pulmonary hypertension. Given the relative correlation between PADP and Pulmonary artery occlusion pressure, it is likely that this patient has an elevated left ventricular end-diastolic pressure. Classic m-mode finding in this setting is a B-bump. Answer (C) is correct [22]. In the absence of pulmonary artery stenosis, RV systolic pressure (RVSP) is equal to pulmonary artery systolic pressure (PASP). However, in the setting of pulmonary stenosis, RVSP exceeds PASP. Answer (B) is incorrect.

Question 26

A 69-year-old male with a history of HFpEF is being treated for hypoxic respiratory failure requiring mechanical ventilation. Which of the following statements is true (Figs. 11.29 and 11.30)?

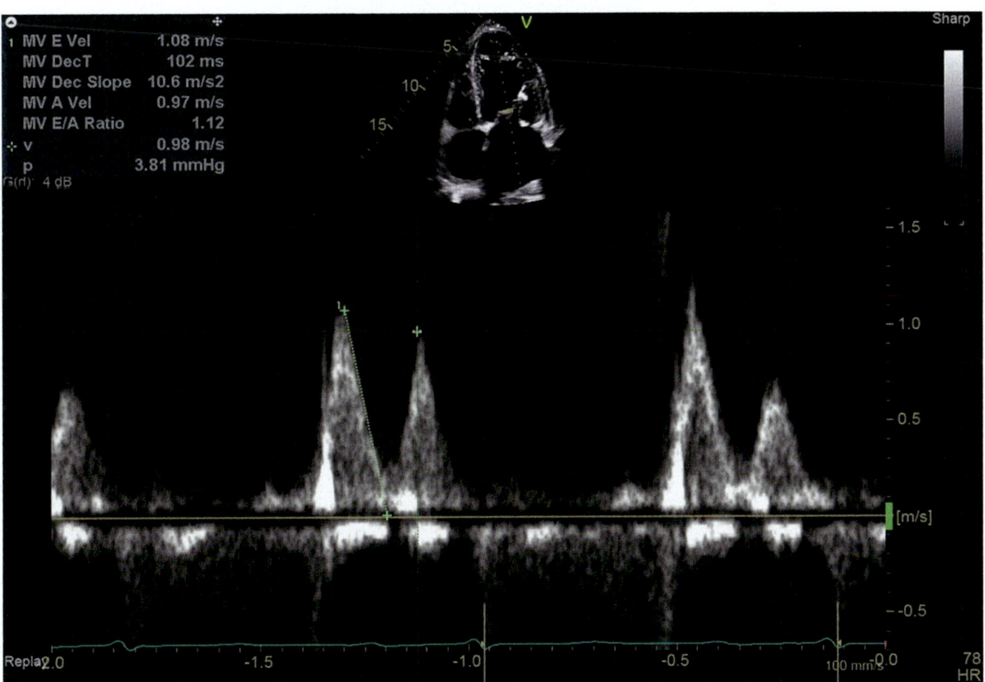

Fig. 11.29 Mitral inflow PW Doppler

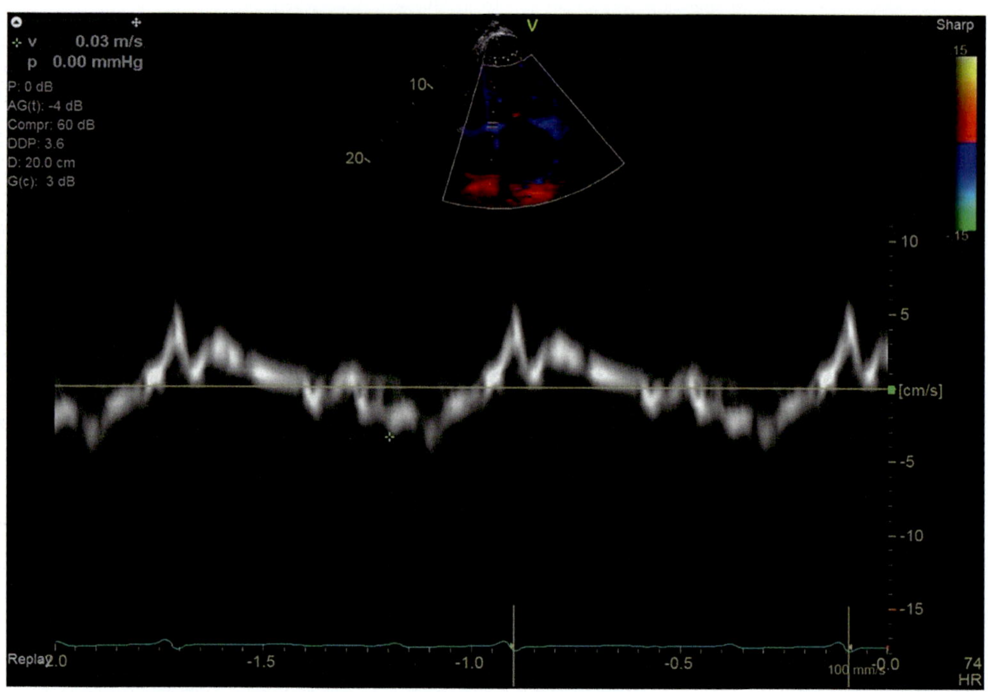

Fig. 11.30 Mitral medial annulus TDI

A. E/e′ ratio would be higher if measured from the lateral mitral valve annulus
B. There is evidence of increased pulmonary capillary wedge pressure
C. Estimation of left atrial pressure is unreliable due to E-A fusion
D. Estimation of left atrial pressure is unreliable due to left bundle branch block

Answer: B. Transmitral inflow velocity (E) correlates with left ventricle filling pressure in heart failure. E values are proportionate to both left atrial pressure (LAP) and relaxation time constant during early diastole. Therefore, as filling pressures increase, there is an associated increase in E wave velocity. The peak velocity of mitral annular tissue Doppler (e′) is related to the LV relaxation time constant and not dependent on load factors in patients with diastolic dysfunction. Therefore, as filling pressures increase, E/e′ ratio will increase. E/e′ ratio >15 is associated with increased LAP and PCWP. Answer (B) is correct. When the diastolic function is normal, e′ values will also increase with higher filling pressure. Answer (C) is incorrect.

E/e′ ratio may be unreliable if one or both doppler measurements are flawed. E wave values are less reliable in severe mitral regurgitation. Tissue doppler (e′) values may be unreliable with severe mitral annular calcification, adjacent wall abnormality due to ischemia, or abnormal septal motion as with left bundle branch block. Answer (D) is incorrect.

E/e′ ratio is usually higher when derived from the septal annulus when compared to the lateral annulus. Answer (A) is incorrect. The septal annulus movement is somewhat limited by tethering by the intervalvular fibrosa resulting in a lower e′ value [18, 35].

Question 27

A 27-year-old male with a past medical history of asthma is admitted with diarrhea and shock for which he is treated with IV fluids and epinephrine. Soon after, he develops tachycardia and hypotension. Continuous-wave Doppler imaging assessment is seen below. What treatment option is best for this patient (Fig. 11.31)?

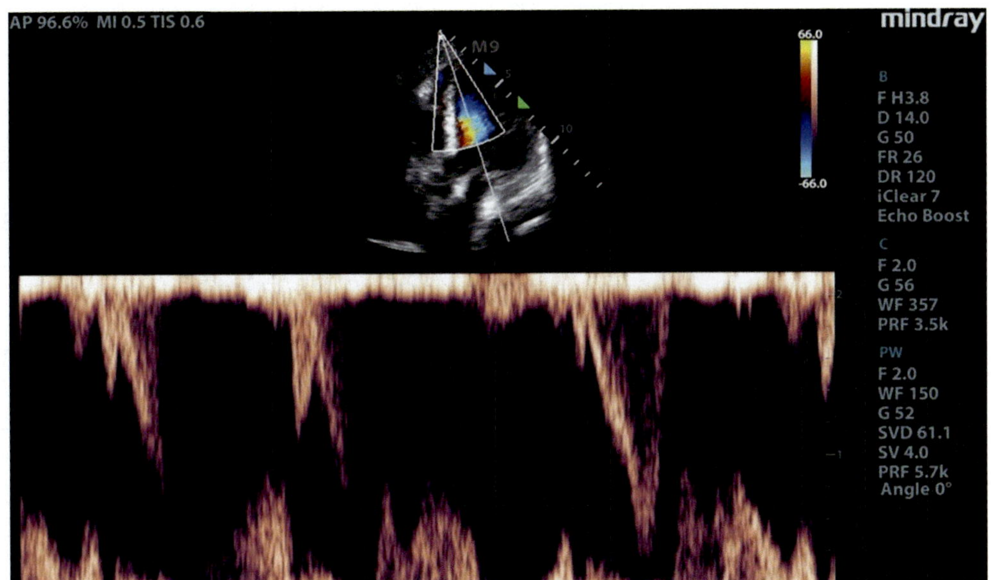

Fig. 11.31 Dagger shaped LVOT VTI-Note mid cavitary PW gate

A. Isoproterenol
B. Dobutamine and loop diuretics
C. Fluids and phenylephrine
D. Nitroglycerine infusion

Answer: C. Doppler imaging reveals late peaking of the maximal gradient consistent with dynamic intraventricular obstruction. This appearance blood flow velocity is often described as "dagger-shaped". The late peaking nature of the velocity differenties it from fixed obstruction such as aortic stenosis, which peaks at mid-systole. Reduction in left ventricular volume, increase in contractility, and decreased in left ventricular outflow resistance will lead to worsening obstruction. Answers A, B, D are incorrect. Treatment options focus on increase left ventricular filling, which can be achieved by additional fluids, use of vasopressors with no inotropic or chronotropic effect and in extreme cases esmolol to reduce heart rate. Answer C is correct [15, 16].

Question 28

A 71-year-old female with hypertension and CHF is treated for heart failure exacerbation. Her blood pressure is 90/48, with a heart rate of 79 beats per minute. Based on the doppler assessment of her aortic regurgitant jet, your estimate left ventricular end-diastolic pressure is (Fig. 11.32)?

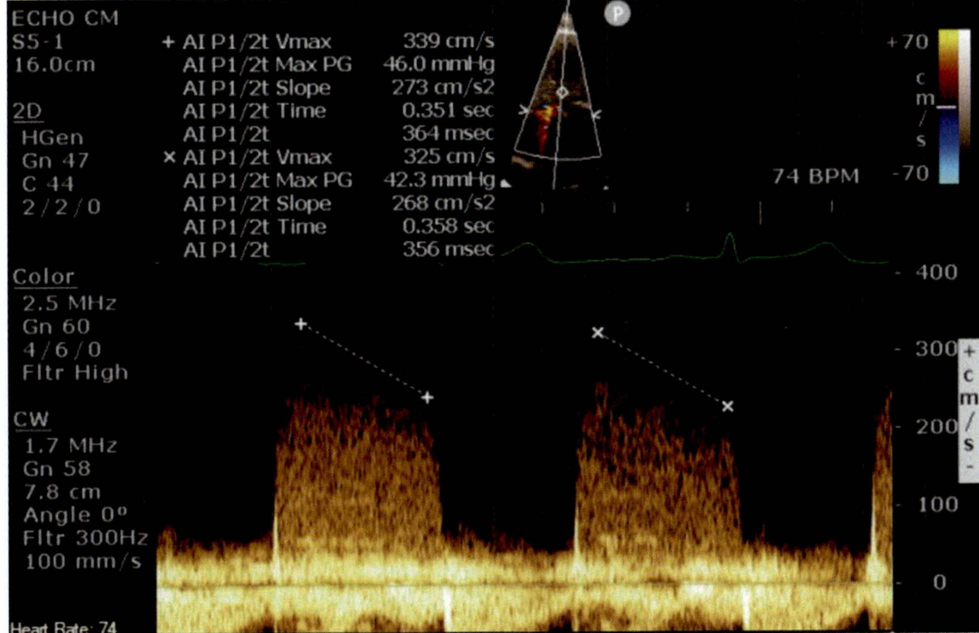

Fig. 11.32 Aortic regurgitation CW Doppler

Early diastolic aortic regurgitant velocity = 3.39 cm/s
End diastolic regurgitant velocity = 2.2 cm/s

A. 28 mmHg
B. 60 mmHg
C. 19 mmHg
D. LVEDP cannot be estimated with aortic regurgitation

Answer: A. Aortic regurgitation can be used to estimate left ventricular end-diastolic pressure (LVEDP). The pressure gradient between diastolic blood pressure (DBP) and LVEDP can be calculated using the modified Bernoulli equation:

$$\text{LVEDP} = DBP - 4{V_{\text{ARMax}}}^{2}$$

$$\text{LVEDP} = 48 - 4(2.2\,\text{m/s})^{2} = 28\ \text{mmHg}$$

It is essential to keep in mind that the estimation of end-diastolic aortic pressure can be difficult with non-invasive measures, and errors can lead to unreliable values when estimating from cuff measurement [2].

Question 29

A 55-year- the old male is being treated for septic shock. Pulse doppler is being used to evaluate fluid responsiveness. Figure A depicts baseline doppler findings. Figure B depicts doppler findings after a 500 cc fluid bolus. Which if the following statements are TRUE regarding these findings (Figs. 11.33 and 11.34)?

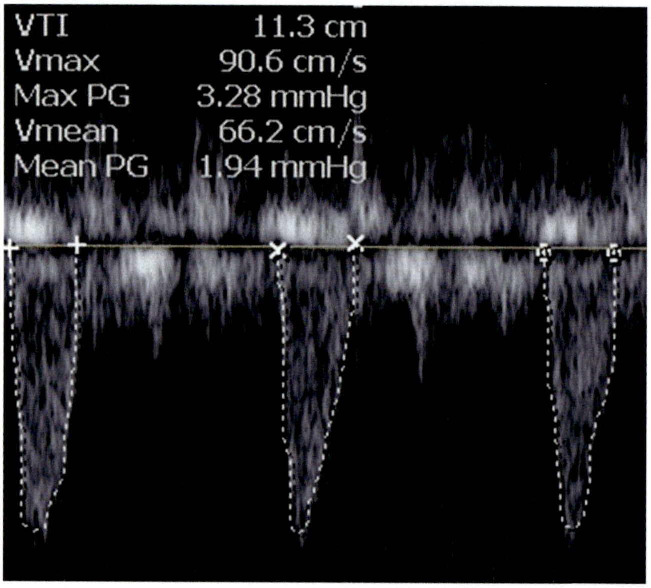

Fig. 11.33 Pre-bolus LVOT VTI

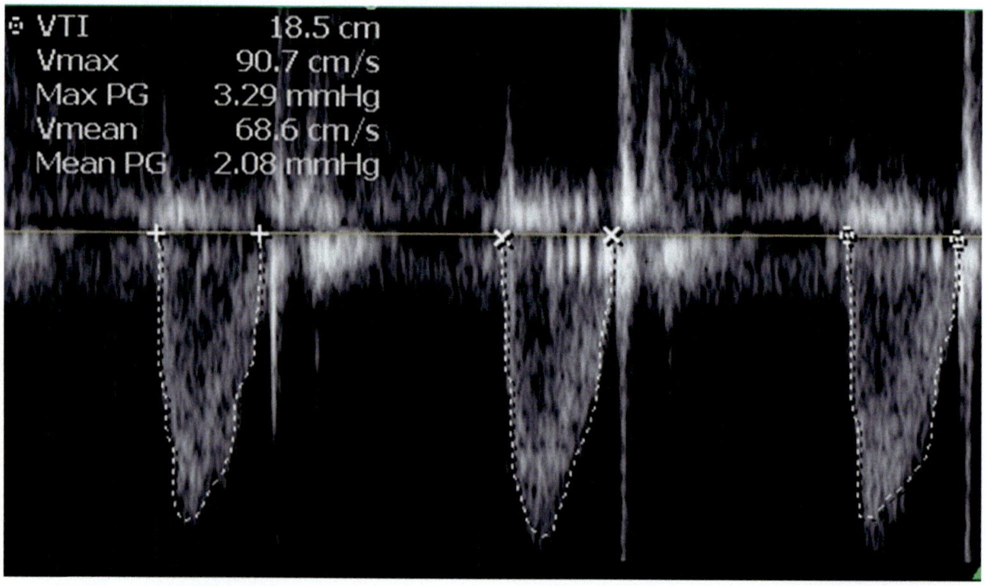

Fig. 11.34 Post-bolus LVOT VTI

A. Static and dynamic parameters for fluid responsiveness are equivocal
B. Left ventricular outflow tract diameter should be measured with each assessment after fluid bolus administration
C. The patient is deemed not fluid responsive if blood pressure does not increase
D. LVOT VTI increase>15% is consistent with fluid responsiveness in this patient

Answer: D. A patient is deemed to be "volume responsive " if the administration of intravenous fluids improves cardiac output by optimizing myocardial function consistent with the Frank-Starling law. Stroke volume will increase with increased venous return until the ventricle is stretched to a specific limit, and further fluids will not improve stroke volume, cardiac output, and oxygen delivery. Mean arterial pressure (MAP) is often used to determine volume responsiveness but is proportional to flow only for a given systemic vascular resistance (SVR). Answer C is incorrect. Preload measures such as central venous pressure (CVP), pulmonary capillary wedge pressure (PCWP), and ventricle volumes influence myocardial contractility depending on the patient's physiologic position on the Frank-Starling curve. However, these static parameters do not reliably predict volume responsiveness (Answer A is incorrect).

Stroke volume (SV) can be measured via the left ventricular outflow tract velocity time integral (VTI) multiplied by the cross-sectional area of the left ventricular outflow tract (LVOT).

$$SV = (LVOTVTI) \times (CSA)$$
$$CSA = pr^2$$

The cross-sectional area of the LVOT does not vary significantly through the respiratory cycle or with changes in preload. Therefore, a single measurement should suffice when calculating changes in stroke volume (Answer B is incorrect). Stroke volume increase greater than 12–15% with 250–500 cc crystalloid or with passive leg raise is associated with volume responsiveness (Answer D is correct) [36, 37].

Question 30

IVC diameter and distensibility is most reliable in which of the following patients?

A. 34 year pregnant old female at 27 weeks gestation
B. 21-year- old college swimmer
C. A 42-year- old male with severe pancreatitis and shock
D. 65-year- old female with pneumonia and shock

Answer: D. The inferior vena cava (IVC) is a compliant vessel whose size varies with changes in CVP and intravascular volume. When the IVC is continuous with the right atrium, CVP is considered equivalent to right atrial pressure (RAP). External factors such as body position, negative intrathoracic pressures, and increased intra-abdominal pressures can influence the size and respiratory variation of the IVC (Answers A and C are incorrect). In young athletes, the IVC often has larger diameters than non-trained counterparts, thus limiting the reliability as a measurement of CVP (Answer B is incorrect). In the absence of these external factors, IVC diameter and respiratory variation or sniff testing can be used to estimate CVP (Answer D is incorrect) [38, 39].

Question 31

Which of the following regarding mean pulmonary artery pressure via doppler echo is TRUE?

A. mPAP can be calculated using a combination of peak pulmonary regurgitant velocity and right atrial pressure
B. The equation for the calculation of mPAP using RVOT acceleration time does not vary with high or low heart rate
C. As PA pressure rises and compliance falls, RVOT acceleration time will increase
D. mPAP calculations are best measured in the apical 4 chamber view

Answer: A. Mean pulmonary arterial pressure (mPAP) can be measured using several doppler parameters: pulmonary regurgitant (PR) jet, RVOT acceleration time, and tricuspid regurgitation velocity time-integral. Peak pressure difference in the setting of pulmonary regurgitation, as measured by the modified Bernoulli equation, is added to right atrial pressure (RAP) to calculate mPAP. This has been validated against pulmonary artery catheter measurements (Answer A is correct).

$$mPAP = 4(PR \text{ peak velocity})^2 + RAP$$

Right ventricular outflow tract (RVOT) acceleration time is measured from the beginning of the flow to the peak flow velocity in the parasternal short-axis view, just proximal to the pulmonary valve (Answer D is incorrect). As pulmonary artery pressure increases, there is a fast equilibration of pressure between the right ventricle and pulmonary artery. Therefore, the peak pressure is reached quickly and RVOT acceleration time is short (Answer C is incorrect).

$$mPAP = 80 \rightarrow (0.5 \times AT_{RVOT})$$

Unfortunately, at heart rates outside of the normal range (i.e., < 60 or 100 bpm); this technique is less reliable for accurate mPAP measurements (Answer B is incorrect) [22, 40].

Question 32
55 male with a history of COPD presents to the emergency department in severe respiratory distress and is intubated for hypoxemic respiratory failure. He has bilateral infiltrates and a P/F ratio of 110. The patient is on two-vasopressors, and the team is trying to determine if more fluids are needed. He is tachycardic but in sinus rhythm. He is on 6 cc/kg of ideal body weight tidal volume and spontaneously breathing. LVOT VTI variation is measured, as shown below. The variation is measured at 21%. Which of the following is correct (Fig. 11.35)?

A. The patient has VTI respiratory variation >14%; therefore, the patient is volume responsive.
B. This test can only be used with a TV of 6 cc/kg of ideal body weight and below. This patient is volume responsive.
C. The cutoff for VTI variation is >25%; therefore, the patient is not volume responsive.
D. This test cannot be accurately used for tidal volumes in spontenously breathing patient.

Answer: D: The patient has to meet the following testing criteria for the test to be accurate

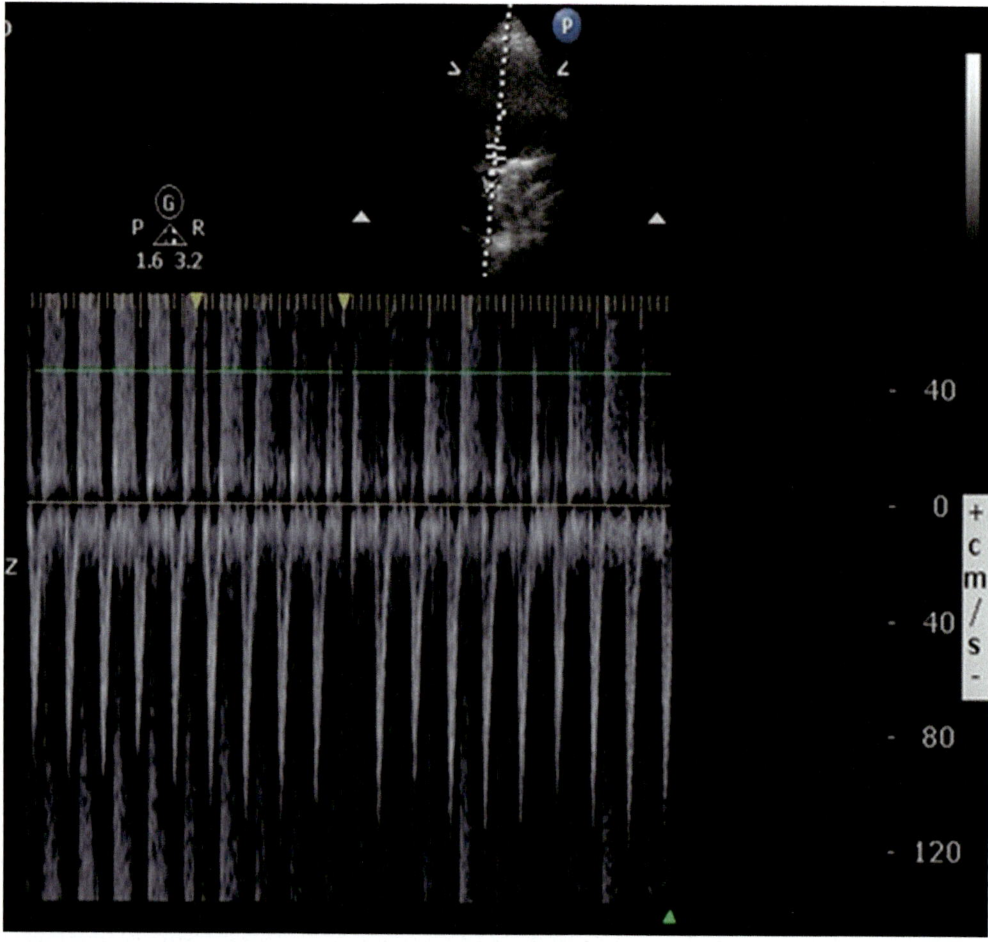

Fig. 11.35 LVOT VTI with respiratory variation

- 8–10 cc/kg of ideal body weight
- Passive on the mechanical ventilator
- Regular rhythm
- No ventricular failure
- normal lung compliance (there needs to be an adequate transmission of the delivered pressure to the intrathoracic space which would be limited severely depressed lung compliance)

The cutoff that has been established is above 15% for this test to predict volume responsiveness [27].

Question 33
A 67-year-old female with a history of advanced COPD is admitted to the ICU with hypoxic respiratory failure and hypotension. The below image shows the doppler assessment across her pulmonary artery. Which of the following is correct regarding the information gathered?

A. There is a strong inverse relationship between pulmonary acceleration time and tricuspid regurgitant jet velocity regarding pulmonary artery pressure calculation.
B. The atrial septal defect would result in an overestimation of PA pressures.
C. Measurement is reliable in the setting of tachycardia.
D. Pulmonary artery acceleration time should not be used in the absence of tricuspid regurgitation.

Answer: A. Pulmonary artery acceleration time (PAT) is measured from the onset of flow across the pulmonary valve to the peak velocity of flow. This value is typical >140 ms in patients without pulmonary artery hypertension. As pulmonary vascular resistance increases, time to peak velocity will occur more quickly, and, therefore, PAT will decrease. A PAT less than 70–90 ms is consistent with severely elevated PA pressures. PAT has been shown to correlate with other ECHO assessments of pulmonary pressures including TRjet maximal velocity (answer A is correct). This estimation is particularly helpful if there is insufficient tricuspid regurgitation to calculate PASP (Answer D is incorrect) (Fig. 11.36).

Several factors can influence this measurement, including doppler angle, heart rate, and the presence of an atrial septal defect, and in severe pulmonary regurgitation. Heart rate should be between 60–100 bpm for reliable measurements (answer C is incorrect). PAT will likely underestimate pulmonary pressures if the right ventricular flow is increased as in the presence of atrial septal defect (answer B is incorrect) [22].

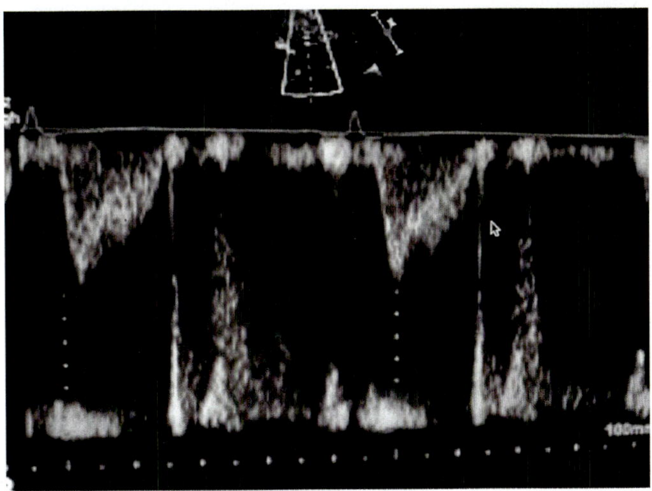

Fig. 11.36 W shaped pulmonary valve PW

Question 34

A 44-year-old male with a history of hypertension, hyperlipidemia, and laparoscopic cholecystectomy 2 months prior is treated in the ICU for hypotension and hypoxic respiratory failure requiring mechanical ventilation. He is noted to have a MAP of 53 mmHg and a heart rate of 112 bpm and is started on vasopressors. He has cold extremities and bilateral rales on the exam. Bedside point of care ultrasound reveals a normal to hyperdynamic LV ejection fraction. You note his LVOT diameter to be 2.1 cm. This clinical scenario is most consistent with what type of shock (Figs. 11.37 and 11.38)?

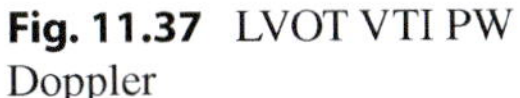

Fig. 11.37 LVOT VTI PW Doppler

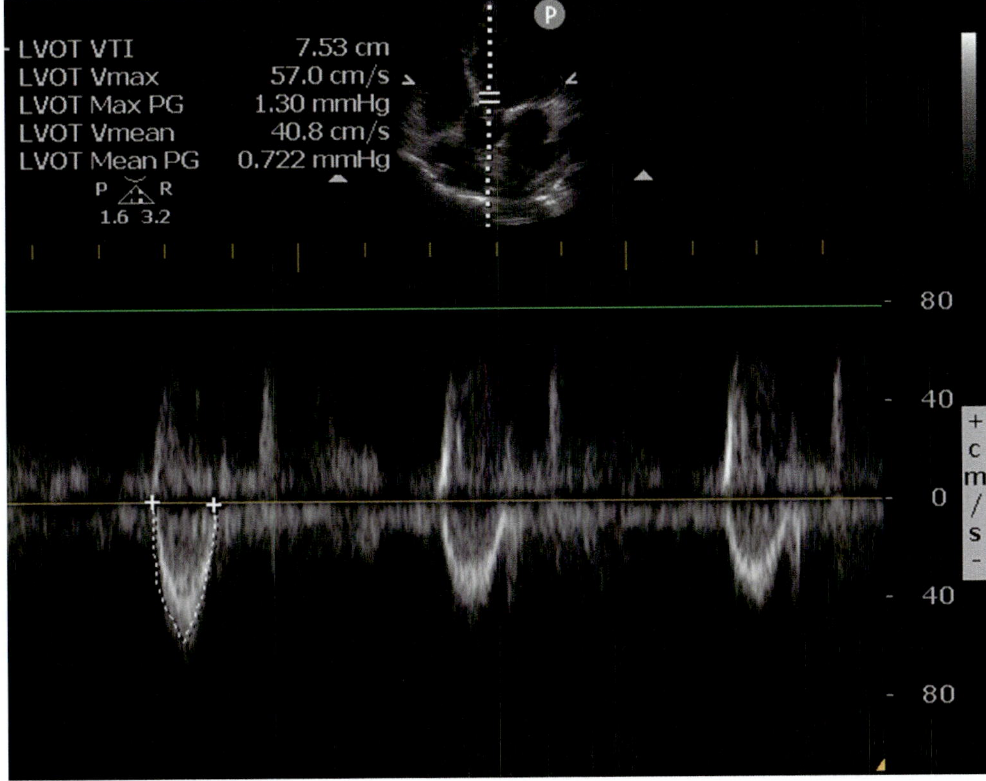

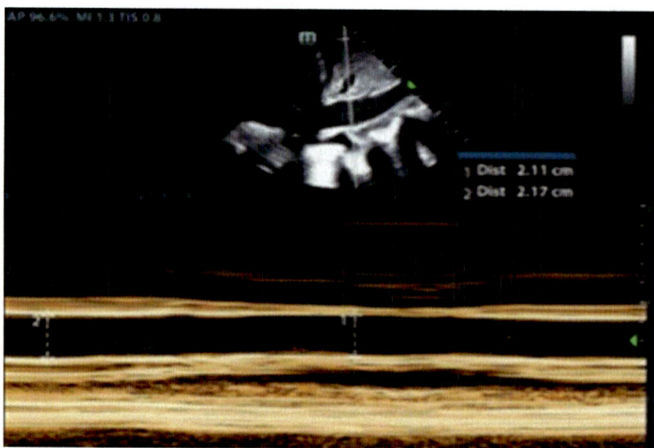

Fig. 11.38 IVC M-mode

A. Cardiogenic
B. Distributive
C. Obstructive
D. Hypovolemic

Answer: C. Rapid assessment with bedside echocardiography can aid in the diagnosis of etiology of shock states. This patient displays evidence of high CVP as noted by IVC diameter >2.1 cm with a minimal respiratory variation. This is evidence leading against hypovolemia (Answer D is incorrect). Visual estimation of ejection fraction is noted to be "normal." However, the cardiac output remains low.

$$CO = \text{stroke volume} \times \text{heart rate}$$
$$SV = CSA_{LV\,OT} \times VTI_{LV\,OT}$$
$$SV = p\, r^2 \times VTI_{LV\,OT}$$
$$SV = p\,(2.1/2)^2 \times (5.39) = 18.67\ \text{mL}$$
$$CO = 18.67 \times 112 = 2.09\ \text{L/min}$$

Shock with low cardiac output makes answers (A) and (C) more likely. In the absence of primary cardiac dysfunction, low cardiac output due to low stroke volume as a result of obstructive pathologies, such as massive pulmonary embolism (PE), is the correct answer (Answer C is correct). Further, high CVP provides some evidence of RV pressure/volume overload in the setting of acute pulmonary hypertension due to massive PE. The resulting physiologic state includes bowing of the intraventricular septum toward the LV cavity, limiting filling, and causing low cardiac output despite normal LV systolic function [41].

Question 35

A 46-year-old male is admitted for chest pain and found to have an ST-elevation myocardial infarction of the left anterior descending artery. He is taken for emergent cardiac catheterization and has a drug-eluting stent placed. 6 days later, he develops dyspnea and hypoxia. On exam, he has a holosystolic murmur best heard at the second intercostal space and the apex. The heart rate is 110 bmp. POCUS reveals a B-line pattern bilaterally. 2D Echo reveals normal valvular and papillary muscle function. Color doppler shows flow from the left to the right ventricle. Given the information obtained, which of the following is TRUE (Table 11.4)?

A. Qp:Qs is measured to be 1.5
B. Flow across the RVOT represents the systemic flow (Qs) in a patient with this type of shunt
C. Qp:Qs is less than 1
D. Blood flow entering the pulmonary circulation (Qp) is 7.7 L/min

Answer: A. This patient is found to have a ventricular septal defect after myocardial infarction. In an acute process in which the pressure is higher within the left ventricle compared to the right, the flow will move in a left to the right direction. This will result in a higher flow through the pulmonary system compared to the systemic circulation. Congestive heart failure and pulmonary edema will likely ensue.

A comparison of shunt fraction can be calculated, and a comparison between pulmonary and systemic blood flow (Qp:Qs) can be used to calculate severity and help guide treatment options.

Flow is calculated as volumetric flow using the equation for cardiac output. Flow should be calculated independently for both right (pulmonary) and left (systemic) sided systems.

$$Q = CSA \times VTI \times HR$$
$$Q = \left(pr^2\right) \times VTI \times HR$$
$$Qs = QLVOT = \left(pr^2\right) \times VTI \times HR = \left(p\left(2/2\right)^2\right) \times 22 \times 110 = 7.7L/\min$$
$$Qp = Q_{RVOT} = \left(pr^2\right) \times VTI \times HR = 11.5L/\min$$
$$= \left(p\left(2.8/2\right)^2\right) \times 17 \times 110 = 11.5L/\min$$
$$Qp : Qs = 7.7/11.5 = 1.5$$

Because flow within this intracardiac shunt moves from left to right, flow through the pulmonary system with be higher than the left. Qp:Qs is greater than 1 (Answer C is incorrect).

If a patient has a shunt present after the LVOT or RVOT, such as in a patent ductus arteriosus (PDA), the calculation for systemic and pulmonary circulation will change from above. Blood will travel from the aorta to the pulmonary artery through the PDA. Therefore, the true blood flow to the pulmonary system will include the cardiac output through the RVOT plus the flow through the shunt. Qs will include the amount of flow that leaves through the LVOT minus the shunt fraction. Because all of the systemic flow (Qs) will return to the right side of the heart, the calculated Qs are calculated as the flow through the RVOT. Similarly, the true blood flow through the pulmonary system will return to the left heart chambers. True Qp is calculated as the flow through the LVOT. This differs from the calculation above in which the shunt is between ventricles and before LVOT and RVOT. Answer (D) is incorrect. The Qs are calculated at 7.7 L/min [42, 43].

Question 36

A 50-year-old with constrictive pericarditis and in atrial fibrillation is suspected of having pulmonary hypertension, and you are trying to decide on how to calculate his pulmonary artery pressure. His vital signs are P: 45 RR: 16 BP:169/70 T:98.6 F Which of the following statements is true?

A. Peak Tricuspid Regurgitation jet will be the most accurate estimate
B. Using peak Pulmonary regurgitation would be inaccurate
C. No method can be accurate due to the patient being in atrial fibrillation
D. Mean pulmonary pressure is calculated using the formula

$90 - (0.62 \times AT_{RVOT})$ would be the most accurate in this patient.

Answer: B In patients with constrictive pericarditis, there is a dissociation of intracardiac from intrathoracic pressure, resulting in early equalization of PA and RV pressures with inspiration. This results in a shorter and steeper PR signal, making the use of PR method inaccurate. The peak tricuspid method could be used with the averaging of six signals. Using the acceleration time of the right ventricle outflow tract is a verified method, but at extremes of heart rate <50 and >100, it can be inaccurate with patients with mean pulmonary artery pressures <25 mmHg [40].

Question 37

A 75-year- old woman with known hypertension comes to your emergency department with chest pain after her dog dies. Due to hypotension, she is started on levophed, but paradoxically she drops her blood pressure. She is hypoxemic, requiring BiPAP, and she is atrial fibrillation with a heart rate of 135 bpm. You make a point of care ultrasound and observe the image below. What should you do next (Fig. 11.39)?

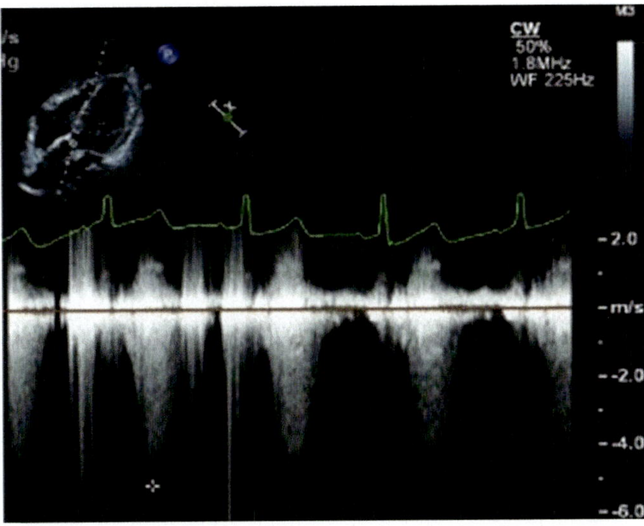

Fig. 11.39 LVOT CW Doppler

A. Stop the levophed and start intravenous fluids
B. Diurese, the patient
C. Do thoracic ultrasound to see if the patient has pneumonia.
D. Start phenylephrine

Answer: D. The patient has obstructive cardiomyopathy likely due to long-standing hypertension, and possibly it is exacerbated now due to Takasubos secondary to the loss of her dog. The Doppler image shows obstructive physiology, and ideal therapy for the patient would be the starting of an alpha-agent to support her blood pressure and reduction of her heart rate. Her respiratory distress is likely due to her cardiac dysfunction and should be evaluated after her obstructive cardiomyopathy is treated [44].

Question 38

A 75-year old male has been on the ventilator with ARDS for 7 days, and his medical team is having difficulty weaning him from the ventilator. His lung ultrasound shows heterogeneous b-lines bilaterally, and prior to giving the patient diuretics to help wean him from the ventilator, a request is made to calculate his left ventricular end-diastolic pressure. Which equation below is correct?

A. Diastolic Blood Pressure + 4(Aortic Regurgitation at end-diastole)^2
B. Systolic Blood Pressure + 4(Aortic Regurgitation at end-systole)^2
C. Diastolic Blood Pressure − 4(Aortic Regurgitation at end-diastole)^2
D. Systolic Blood Pressure − 4(Mitral Regurgitation Maximum)^2

Answer: C. An aortic regurgitant jet is required to perform this calculation. As the aortic regurgitation envelope decays throughout diastole, the end-diastolic velocity is obtained. The aortic end-diastolic velocity is Vmin, and subtracting it from the diastolic blood pressure gives the estimated left ventricular end-diastolic pressure. This is different from the end-diastolic volume which would be an excellent standard for determining if a patient was still volume overloaded. This method to determine LVEDP has clear limitations including the inability to acquire a spectral envelope which may occur in 30% patients and not using the center of the jet when measuring the envelope leading to falsely depressed gradient values causing an overestimation of LVEDP. Answer B is the calculation for Left Ventricular End-Systolic Pressure and answer D is the calculation for left atrial pressure, which can estimate LVEDP in the absence of significant mitral stenosis [45].

Question 39

Which statement is true about the left atrial volume index (LAVI)?

A. It is a measurement of left atrial volume, and it is indexed to ideal body weight
B. If the left atrial volume index is greater than 31 mL/m^2, it is a sign of elevated left atrial pressures
C. A LA volume index >34 mL/m^2 is considered abnormal and represents an independent predictor of mortality, HF, atrial fibrillation and ischemic stroke
D. The left atrial index may stay enlarged even when the LVEDP returns to normal

Answer: C. The left atrial volume is indexed to body surface area. An elevated LAVI is 34 mL/m^2 and is associated with increased mortality, atrial fibrillation, and ischemic stroke. A normal LAVI does not always mean the LVEDP is normal, because the atrium does not immediately dilate when LVEDP is elevated. Also, LVEDP returns to normal LAVI can remain elevated. It is essential to understand what LAVI is and understand its limitations [18, 46].

Question 40

A 25-year-old woman is noted to have atrium secundum on echocardiography. On color Doppler image, a shunt is visualized. What is the shunt flow across ASD?

Data:

Blood Pressure 100/80 mmHg

Heart Rate (HR) 60 beats/min (bpm)

Velocity Time Integral (VTI) across ASD 60 cm Left Ventricular outflow diameter (LVOT)

VTI across Left Ventricular Outflow Tract 20 cm ASD diameter of 1.4 cm

A. 4.2 L/min
B. 5.4 L/min
C. 6.5 L/min
D. 7.4 L/min

Answer: B. To calculate the flow across the ASD, the velocity-time integral is multiplied by the area of the circle.

Flow = Cross-sectional area of orifice (CSA) × VTI × HR

= $(1/2 \times 1.4\ \text{cm})^2 \times 3.14 = 1.54\ \text{cm}^2$

$1.54\ \text{cm}^2 \times 60\ \text{cm} = 92.3$ mL per beat

92.3 mL per beat × 60 bpm = 5.54 L/min

A, C, and D are incorrect calculations [43].

Question 41

A 32-year-old male with a past medical history of obesity and tobacco use is admitted with shortness of breath. Vitals on presentation:

HR 116, RR 22, BP 80/48, saturating 93% on 6 L nasal cannula.

Bedside ultrasound is obtained. Identify the abnormality in the following image (Fig. 11.40):

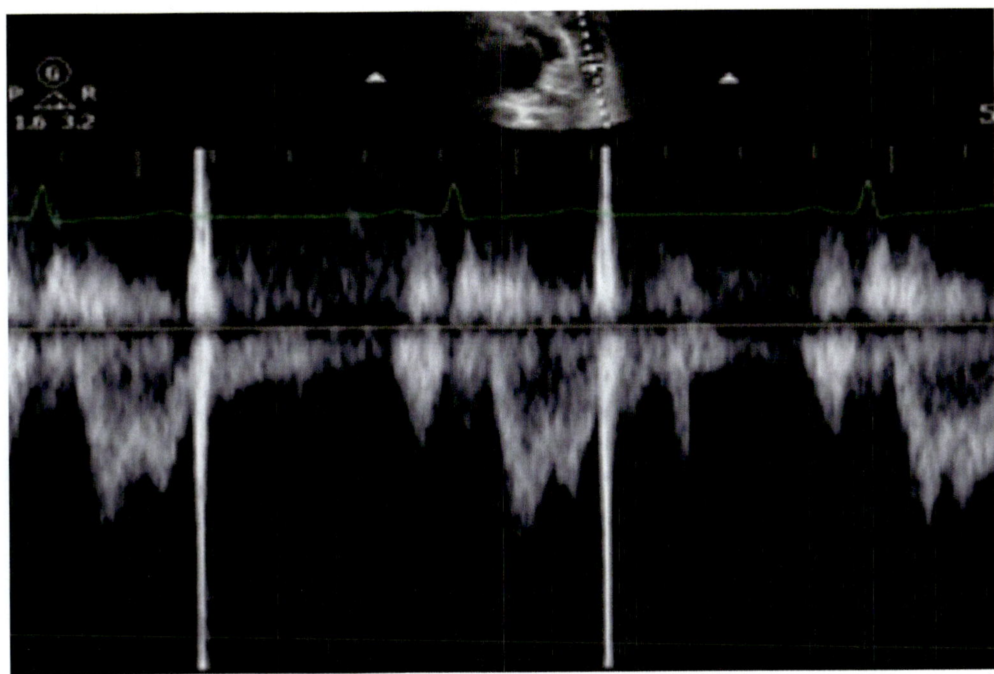

Fig. 11.40 RVOT VTI PW Doppler

A. Pulmonic stenosis
B. Tricuspid regurgitation
C. Increased Pulmonary afterload
D. Pulmonic Regurgitation

Correct Answer: C. This is early systolic notching, which is recognized as an initial spike-wave followed by the more prolonged doppler wave that is more curvilinear or dome-shaped. This finding has a high specificity in patients with massive and submassive pulmonary embolism [47]. A, B, D are incorrect as none of these pathologies are identified in the PW doppler shown.

Question 42

45 year old male admitted to the icu with septic shock and on mechanical ventilation. The patient is being assessed for extubation. He is 6 L positive during his hospital admission so the team performs an echocardiogram to risk stratify for extubation failure. PW doppler at the mitral valve and TDI at the medial mitral annulus performed with results below. What conclusions can you draw about the patient's risk for extubation failure (Figs. 11.41 and 11.42)?

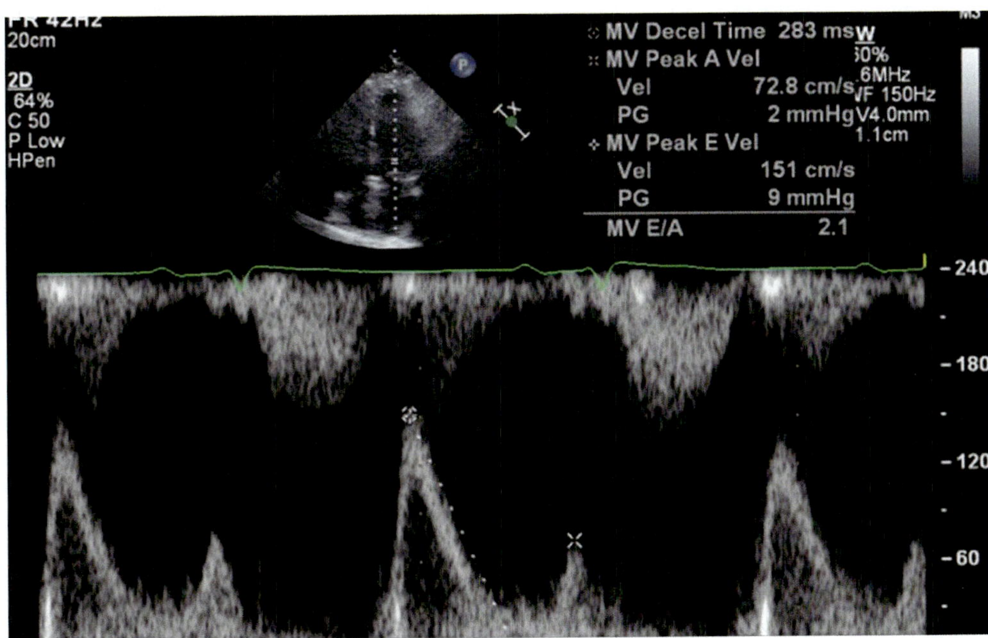

Fig. 11.41 Mitral valve inflow PW Doppler

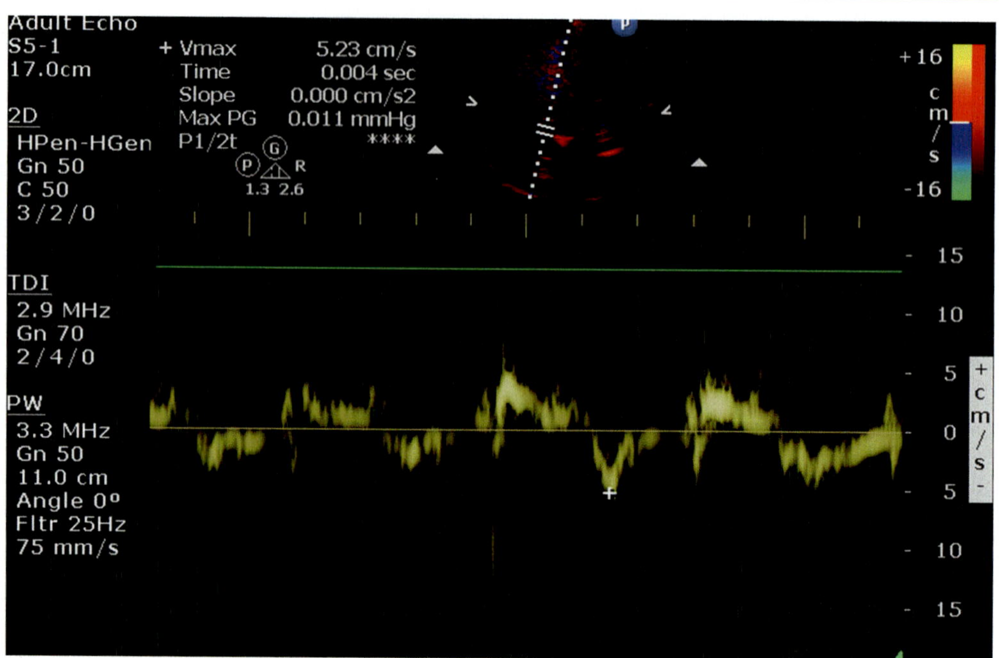

Fig. 11.42 Mitral valve medial annulus TDI

A. Extubate given evidence of low estimated wedge pressure.
B. Extubate the patient as the parameters checked in the echo has not been validated to predict extubation failure.
C. Keep the patient intubated as he has a high risk of extubation failure based on the echo parameters checked.
D. Keep the patient intubated given low estimated wedge pressure because this puts him at high risk for extubation failure.

Answer: C. Keep the patient intubated as the parameters checked put him at high risk for extubation failure. The images show evidence of an elevated E/e′ ratio (based on the TDI of the medial mitral annulus and the Mitral valve PW E wave) which has been shown to predict extubation failure due to congestive heart failure. The removal of positive pressure increases venous return and LV afterload which can lead to extubation failure in patients who already show evidence of increased estimated wedge pressures based on echo. A. Incorrect as the estimated wedge is high. B. Incorrect as this question has been studied and validated. D. Incorrect as the estimated wedge pressure is high and if indeed they were low this would lower the risk for extubation failure [14, 18] point septal separation is seen with M-Mode of the Mitral valve in patients with reduced Systolic Function [48].

Question 43

A 67-year-old male with a past medical history of hypertension, COPD, and a dual-chamber pacemaker is admitted to the ICU with BP of 60/40, HR 110, and oxygen saturation of 88% on non-rebreather. The patient was recently diagnosed with cellulitis of the lower extremity treated with Keflex. What is the etiology of shock in this patient?

The following clip was obtained on TEE with the following hemodynamic parameters (Video 11.3).

LVOT diameter = 2.5 cm
LVOT VTI = 19.1 cm
HR = 110 BPM

A. Obstructive shock from migrating clot in transit
B. Distributive shock
C. Hypovolemic shock
D. None of the above

Answer: B. The video shows right atrium pacemaker lead with mobile, fibrinous vegetation. This is an example of septic shock from pacemaker lead infection.

Given the history of an intracardiac device ,recent infection, and high cardiac output by doppler VTI method choices A , C, and D are incorrect (Figs. 11.43 and 11.44).

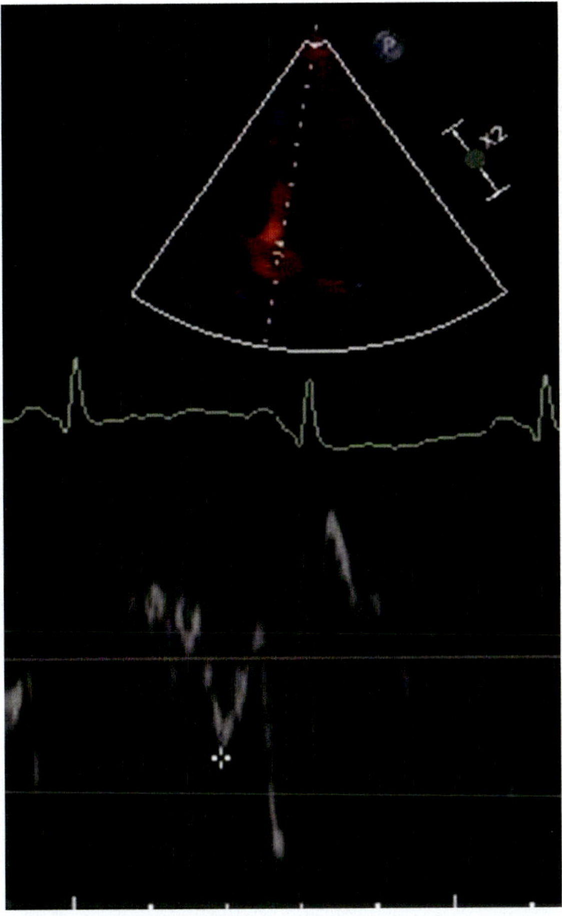

Fig. 11.43 Mitral valve medial annulus TDI

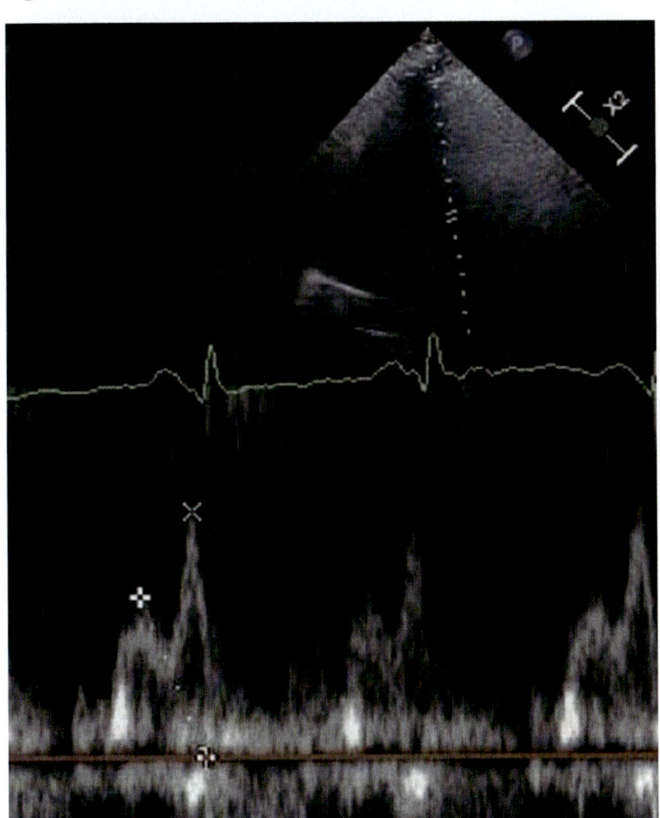

Fig. 11.44 Mitral valve inflow PW Doppler

The doppler VTI method in estimating stroke volume and cardiac output correlates well with results of concurrent thermodilution cardiac output determinations [1]

SV = âĎij * LVOT/2 * LVOT VTI
CO = SV * HR/1000
Normal SV = 60–120 mL
Normal CO = 4–8 L/min

This patient's calculated SV is 94 mL, and CO is 10.3 L/min, which would is high. This would not be expected in other forms of shock listed [2, 49].

Question 44

A 65-year-old male with a past medical history of HTN is admitted with streptococcus pneumonia. His inpatient course was complicated by hypoxic respiratory failure requiring intubation. On hospital day 5, the patient's FiO_2 requirement is significantly lower, and he was placed on the pressure support trial. The patient becomes tachypneic 1 h after being on pressure support. Bedside echocardiography shows the following:

MV E vol = 61 cm/s
MV peak A vel = 93.6 cm/s
Med E′ Vel = 7.25 cm/s

Which of the following statements is true regarding this patient's diastolic function?

A. Grade II diastolic dysfunction is present
B. The patient must have Grade II–III diastolic dysfunction and elevated LAP
C. Grade II diastolic dysfunction but LAP is likely normal
D. Grade I diastolic dysfunction

Answer: D. This patient has Grade I diastolic dysfunction. MV E vol = 61 cm/s MV peak A vel 93.6 cm/s – E/A = 0.7, Med E′ Vel = 7.25 cm/s. E/Med E = 8.4. Grade I diastolic dysfunction is usually present and physiological for age 60 and above ; there is impaired relaxation, and LAP is normal. A, B, C. Grade II diastolic dysfunction would exhibit a pseudo-normalization pattern with an E that is greater than A (as you would see in normal physiology) and typically has an elevated LAP. Any method to reduce venous return would revert the E > A pattern back to an E < A pattern similar to grade I diastolic dysfunction [18].

Question 45

32-year-old previously healthy female with recent right ankle fracture admitted with shortness of breath and hypoxia. She is saturating 88% on 4 L NC. Bedside echocardiography shows the following: IVC diameter 1.5 cm with respiratory variation as shown. Which of the following statements is true (Figs. 11.45 and 11.46)?

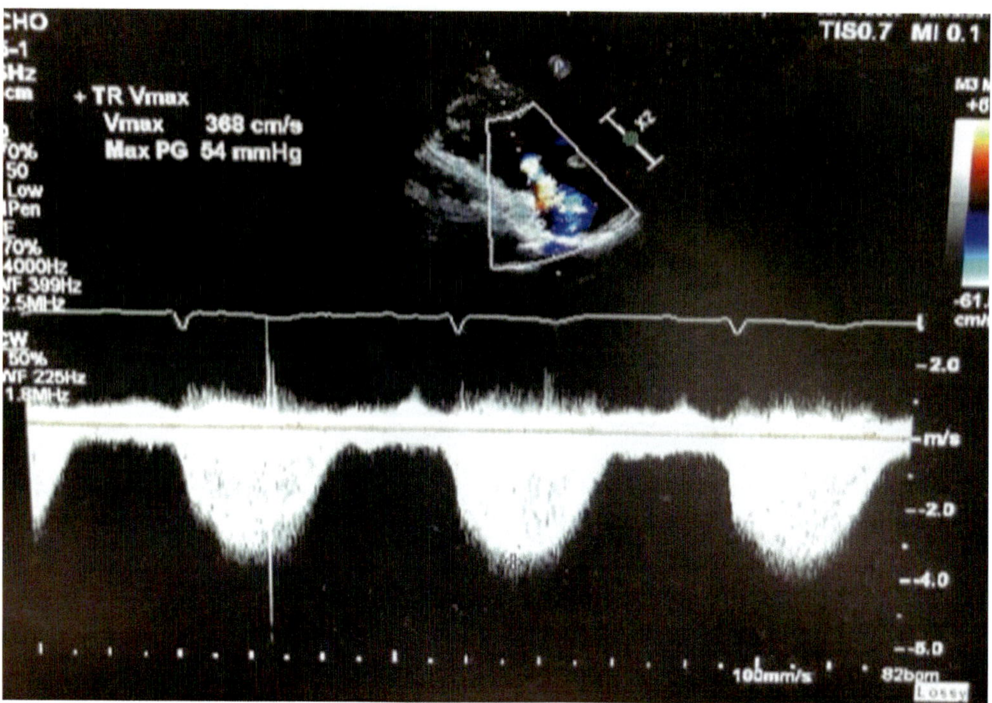

Fig. 11.45 Tricuspid valve CW Doppler

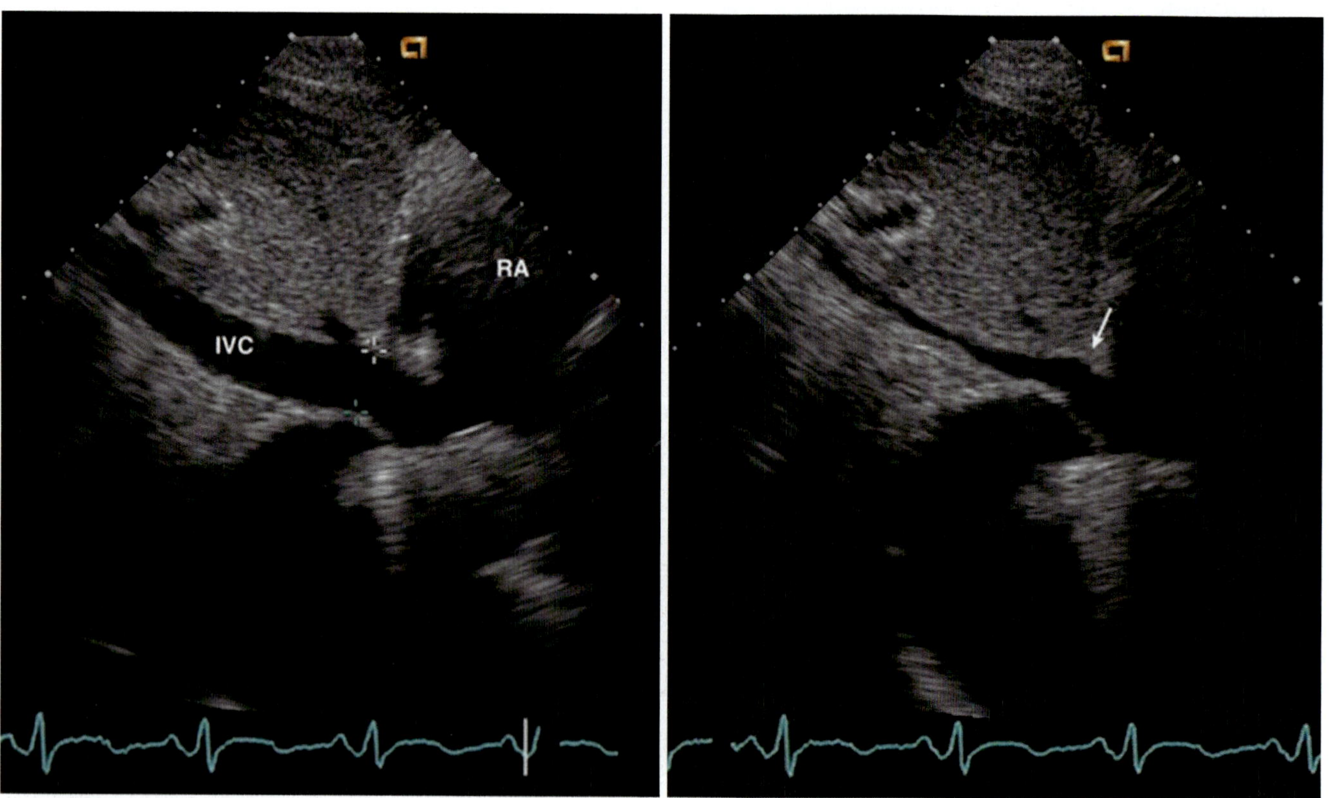

Fig. 11.46 Subcostal IVC-pre and post Sniff

A. RV wall thickness is expected to be higher than 1 cm on subcostal view
B. Her PAP suggests chronic pulmonary hypertension
C. The patient should be given IV fluids for volume resuscitation followed by intubation
D. Her Pulmonary artery acceleration time is likely less than 60

Answer: D. Acute pulmonary HTN. The patient was found to have an acute pulmonary embolism. This question tests knowledge about signs of acute pulmonary embolism. The 60/60 sign requires an RV acceleration time of less than or equal to 60 ms in the presence of tricuspid insufficiency pressure gradient less than or equal to 60 mmHg, but higher than 30 mmHg.

Multiple studies have shown a strong correlation between the presence of acute pulmonary embolism in patients found to have a 60/60 sign [1]. According to another report, a severely disturbed RV ejection pattern (acceleration time <60 ms) in the setting of only moderate elevation of pulmonary arterial systolic pressure, as assessed by trans-tricuspid systolic gradient <60 mmHg, was 98% specific although only 48% sensitive for acute PE among 86 patients with various causes of pulmonary hypertension [2, 50].

Question 46

A 56-year-old male with PMH of HTN, hyperlipidemia, DM type-II admitted to the intensive care unit with hypotension, tachycardia, and respiratory failure.

BP 86/50, HR 120, Temp 35.6, saturating 90% on 100% FiO_2 MR velocity during isovolumetric contraction is shown (Fig. 11.47).

What is the cause of his shock?

A. Distributive shock
B. Obstructive shock
C. Decreased cardiac output
D. High output heart failure

Answer: C. LV contractility dP/dt is estimated by using the time interval between 1 and 3 m/s on MR CW spectral doppler. It is a measure of Left Ventricular Systolic Function. Intuitively the dP/dT is normal when pressure generation by the cardiac muscle occurs in a short time interval, whereas a weak heart will take longer to generate the same amount of pressure (Calculation shown below).

DP/dt = 32/Time
Normal > 1200 mmHg

In this example, dP/dt = 267 suggesting decreased cardiac output In other forms of shock LV dP/dt is typically normal to high (choices A, B, D are incorrect) [51].

Question 47

75 y/o gentleman with chronic history hypertension, CKD IV, and peripheral vascular disease presents to the ER with dyspnea on exertion. The patient is hypoxic and has increased work of breathing. Bedside Echocardiogram performed with the results below. Which of the following statements is true regarding this patient's LVEDP (Fig. 11.48)?

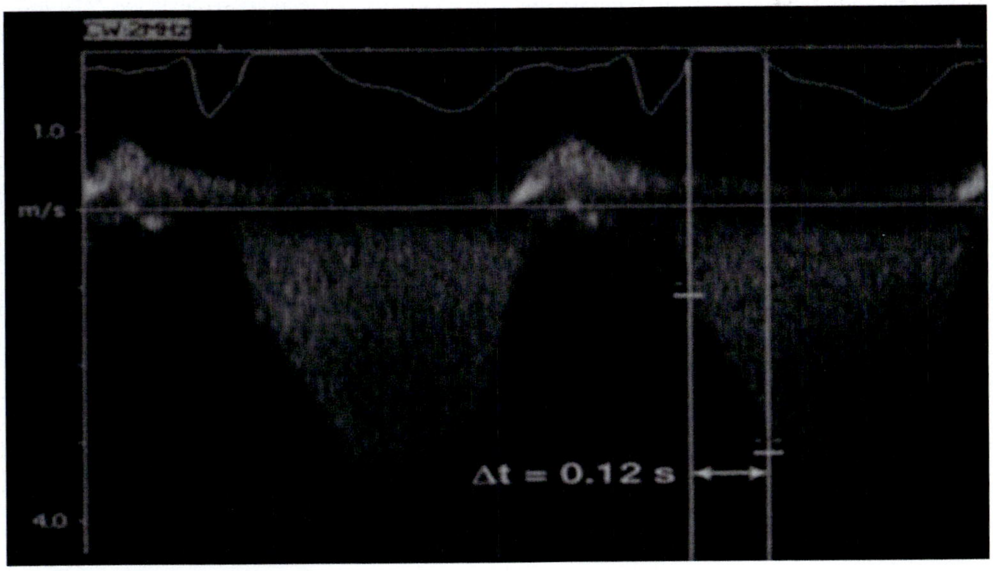

Fig. 11.47 Mitral regurgitation dP/dT

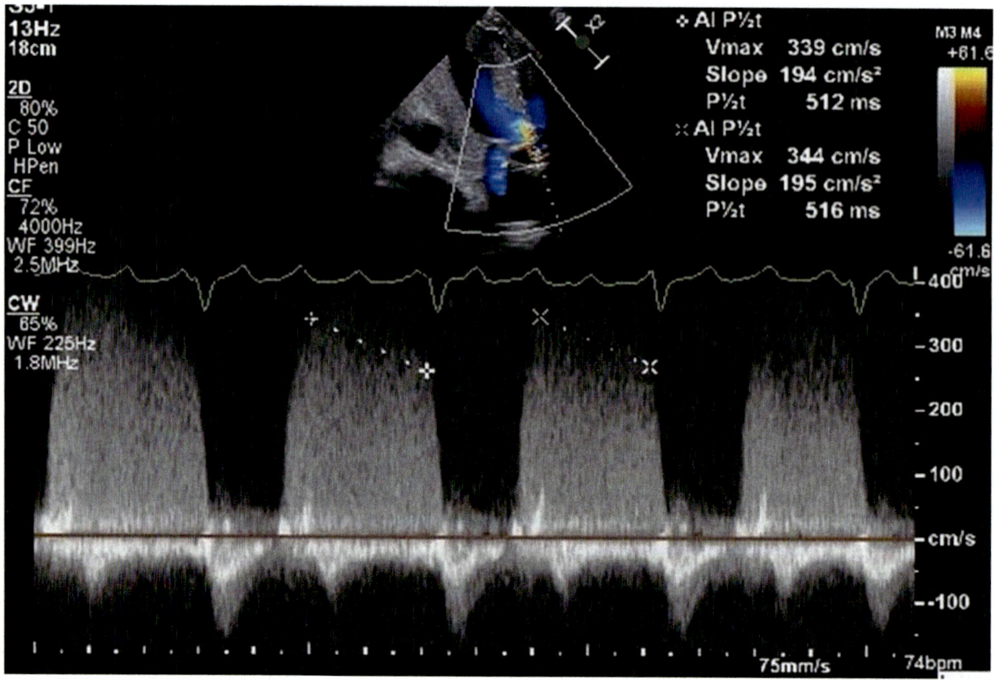

Fig. 11.48 Aortic valve CW Doppler

BP = 120/65, HR 75

A. This patient's LVEDP is high
B. LVEDP can not be calculated with the above information
C. His LVEDP is 10 mmHg
D. Ejection fraction is needed to calculate an accurate LVEDP

Answer: A. LVEDP calculation with the use of a CW AR jet can be calculated in the following way:

$$\text{LV end} - \text{diastolic pressure} = \text{diastolic BP}$$
$$- \text{End Diastolic AR gradient}(\text{AR Vmin})$$

Normal value is 15 mmHg ± 5.

Vmin represents the gradient across the aortic valve at the end of the diastole. Subtracting the gradient from diastolic BP will yield the LVEDP.

$$\text{Pressure gradient} = \text{DBP} - \text{LVEDP} = 4\text{V}^2$$

Rearranging this equation, LVEDP can be calculated in the following manner:

$$\text{LVEDP} = \text{DBP} - 4 \times \text{V}^2$$

65 mmHg – 4 $(2.5\ \text{m/s})^2$ = 40 mmHg therefore A is the correct answer. The patient's dyspnea is likely related to the elevated LVEDP due to the AR [21].

Question 48

Which clinical condition would be most likely compatible with these doppler images? (Figs. 11.49 and 11.50)

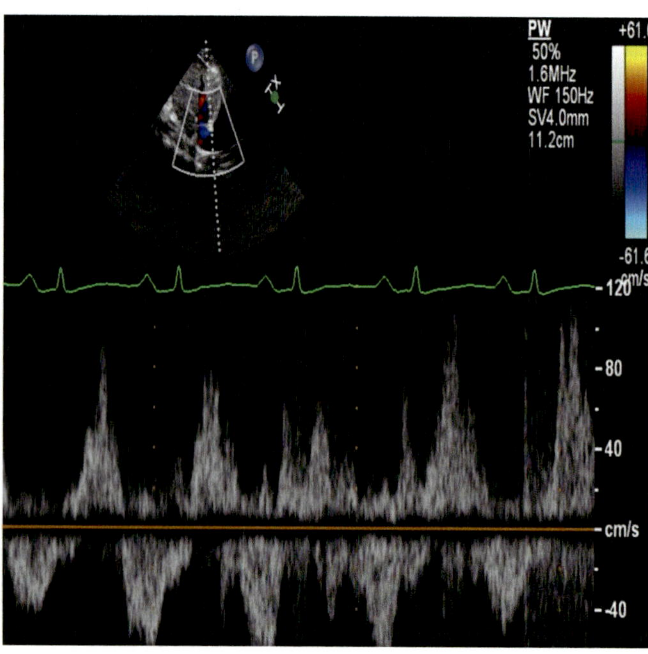

Fig. 11.49 Hepatic vein PW Doppler

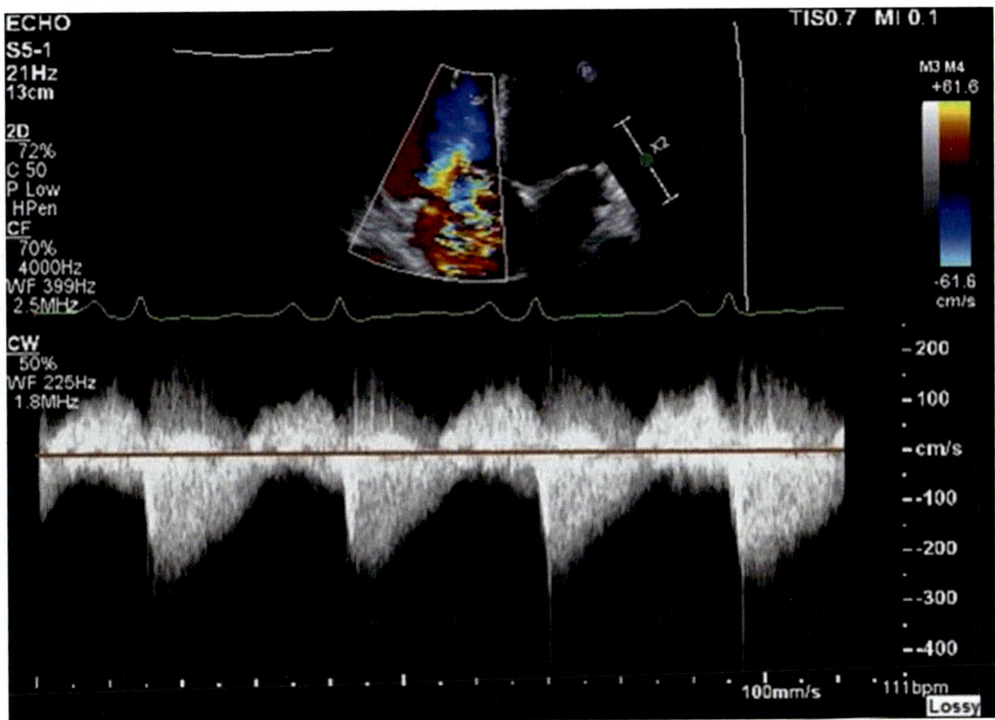

Fig. 11.50 Tricuspid valve CW Doppler

A. Acute Tricupsid Endocarditis
B. Mild to Moderate Left Ventricular Dysfunction
C. Submassive Pulmonary Embolism with no RV dysfunction
D. Mild Mitral Stenosis

Answer: A. These doppler images are most consistent with acute tricuspid regurgitation, with the dense triangular doppler signal during systole and hepatic vein reversal. No single Doppler and echocardiographic measurements or parameters are precise enough to quantify TR severity. The integration of multiple parameters is required. Left ventricular dysfunction can cause tricuspid regurgitation, but usually, it would have to be more than mild. Submassive pulmonary embolism again could cause RV dilatation and hepatic vein systolic reversal, but more likely severe tricuspid endocarditis would cause these doppler findings. Significant mitral stenosis would cause an increase in left atrial pressures and left atrial dilation and could cause pulmonary hypertension, cause tricuspid regurgitation, but mild mitral stenosis would not be the most plausible reason for these doppler findings [21] (Figs. 11.51, 11.52 and 11.53).

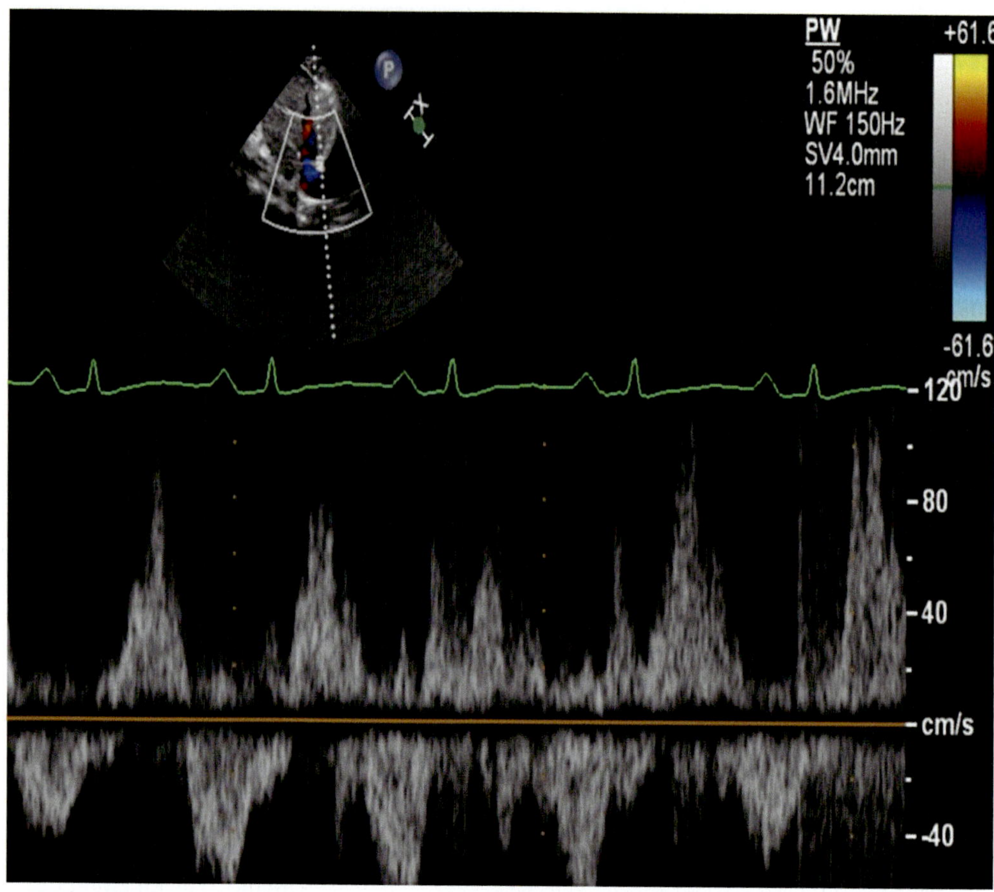

Fig. 11.51 Hepatic vein PW Doppler

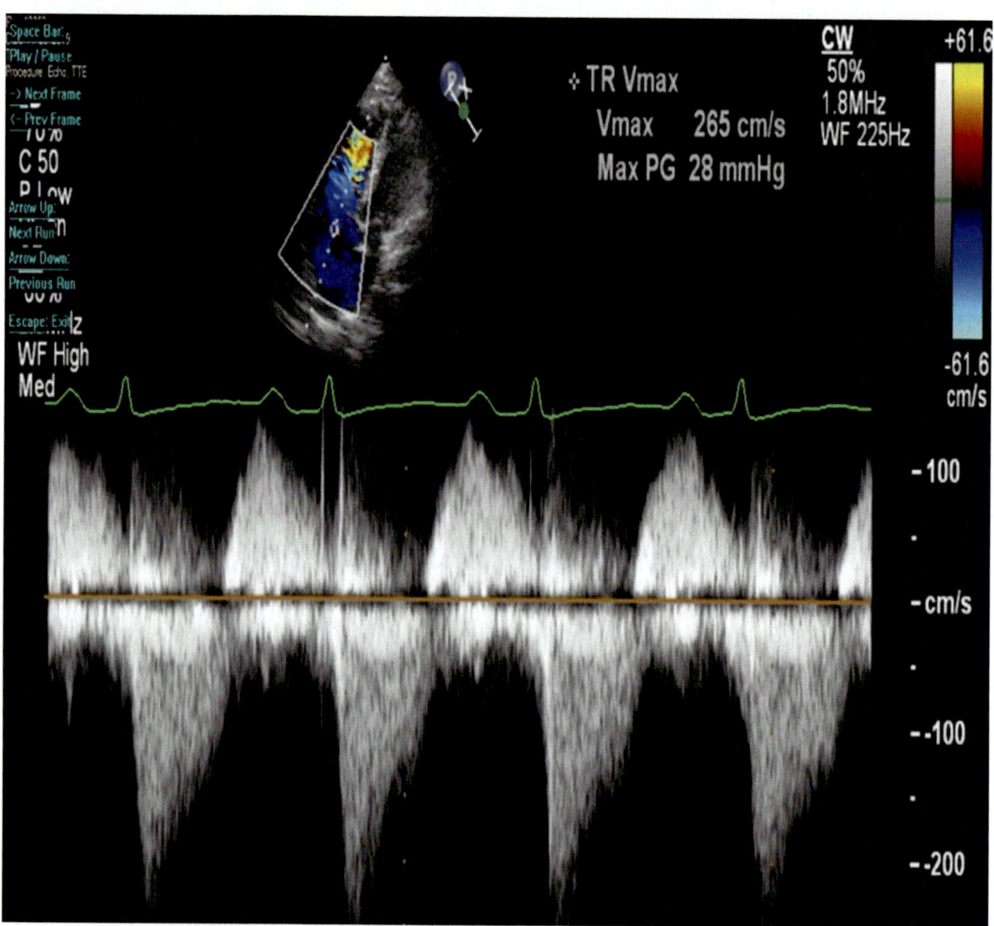

Fig. 11.52 Tricuspid valve CW Doppler

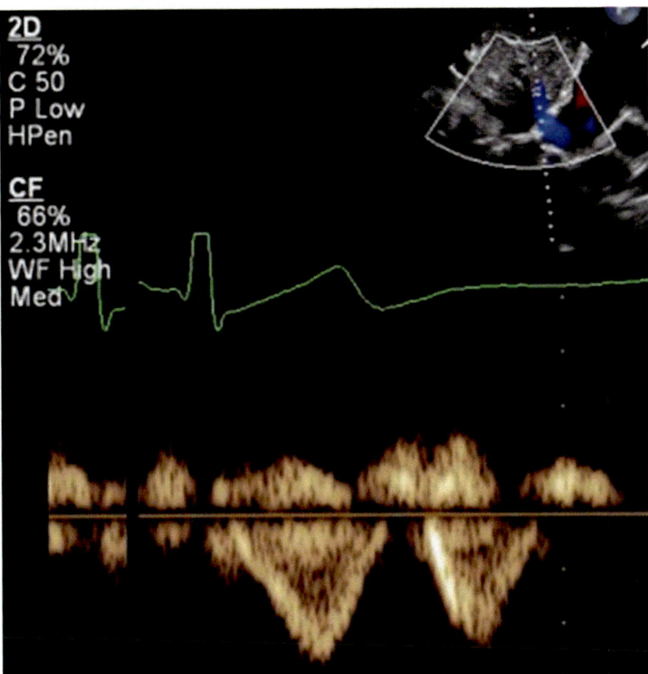

Fig. 11.53 Hepatic vein PW Doppler

Question 49

52 y/o male with a history of EtOH cirrhosis presents with worsening mental status, found to have acute on chronic EtOH hepatitis. Antibiotics started, and sepsis bolus is given. He is admitted to the ICU for airway watch and hypotension, requiring levophed Blood pressure is 80/45. Labs notable for AKI (baseline cr .5 now 2.2). The abdomen is distended with fluid wave present(gets monthly paracentesis, but missed the last session). Bladder pressure is 13 mmHg. Urine sodium is <20 meq/L. The patient's IVC video/image shown below. Estimate the patient's CVP (Video 11.4).

A. CVP is high as there is a diameter greater than 2.1 and a variation of <50%.
B. CVP is low/normal as the diameter is less than 2.1 and >50% diameter.
C. CVP via the IVC cannot be accurately assessed in a spontaneously breathing patient.
D. CVP via the IVC cannot accurately be assessed in a patient in a patient with intraabdominal hypertension.

Answer: D. CVP via the IVC cannot accurately be assessed in a patient with intraabdominal hypertension. Answer B is incorrect since, in appearance, the IVC is small in diameter and has greater than 50% variation which without elevated intraabdominal pressures would indicate a low/normal CVP. The IVC collapses once the IVC intraluminal pressures are lower than the intrabdominal pressures (normal 0-5) which usually occurs in a spontaneously breathing patient. Answer A is incorrect as the IVC is not dilated and there is > 50% variation. Elevated CVP values would lead to a distended IVC with minimal variation but if the intrabdominal pressure rises above the CVP value, you will get a collapsing CVP which can lead to erroneous physiologic conclusions about the CVP. Answer C is incorrect, as CVP estimations are accurate in spontaneously breathing patients [9].

Question 50

A 55-year-old female with a past medical history of poorly controlled diabetes, HTN, tobacco use is admitted to the intensive care unit with hypotension. Her vitals on presentation: HR 100 and regular, BP 85/50, RR of 24, Oxygen saturation is 88% on 6 L of oxygen. Her labs are notable for Cr of 4.5, Lactic acid of 8. She has 3 + pitting edema of the peripheries. PA catheter is inserted, and her wedge pressure is 30. Point of care echocardiography consistent with B profile of the lung and the following clip is shown: Which of the following mitral flow velocity profile is likely in this patient (Video 11.5)?

A. MV E wave velocity = 61 cm/s MV peak A vel 93.6 cm/s Med e′ Vel = 7.25 cm/s.
B. MV E wave velocity = 45 cm/s, Medial e′ vel = 6 cm/s.
C. MV E wave velocity = 150cm/s, Medial e′ vel = 6 cm/s
D. MV E wave velocity varies between 80 cm/s to 100 cm/s, Medial e′ = 6 cm/s

Answer: C. The video clip shows a severely depressed LV, which given the patient's B profile and hemodynamics points towards Cardiogenic Shock with likely elevated LAP. Using E/e′ ratio, we can estimate the mean pulmonary artery wedge pressure (PAWP) where:

$$PAWP = 4 + E / e' (mmHg)$$

4 + 150/6 = 31 mmHg, which corresponds closely to this patient's obtained wedge through Swan- Ganz catheter.

PAWP is standard in the first example representing Grade I diastolic dysfunction(choice A is incorrect).

PAWP is 11 in choice B; however this does not correlate with this patient's wedge pressure [18, 19]. (Choice B is incorrect).

Question 51

A 55-year-old male with a past medical history of obstructive sleep apnea, noncompliance with home BiPAP, COPD, and tobacco use is admitted to the ICU with hypoxic and hypercarbia a respiratory failure requiring intubation and mechanical ventilation. He is on peep of 5, TV 8 cc/kg/ideal body weight, Rate of 12, FiO_2 of 100%, and is saturating only 88%. MAP is above 65 and currently not on pressors.

Bedside point of care ultrasound reveals B- profile of lungs, estimated RAP of 15 mmHg based on IVC evaluation. The following images are also obtained (Figs. 11.54 and 11.55):

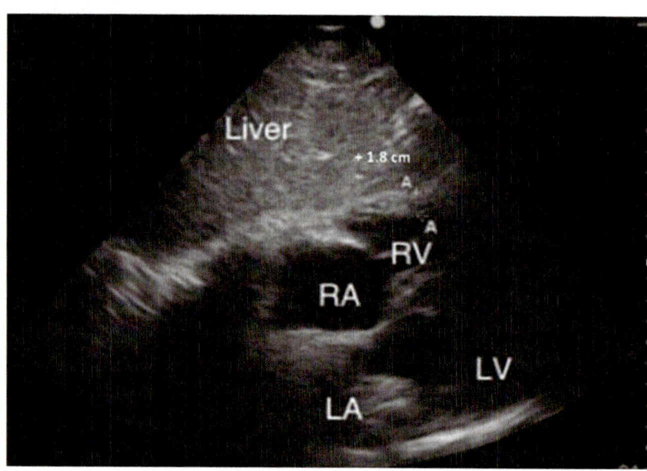

Fig. 11.54 Subcostal four chamber view

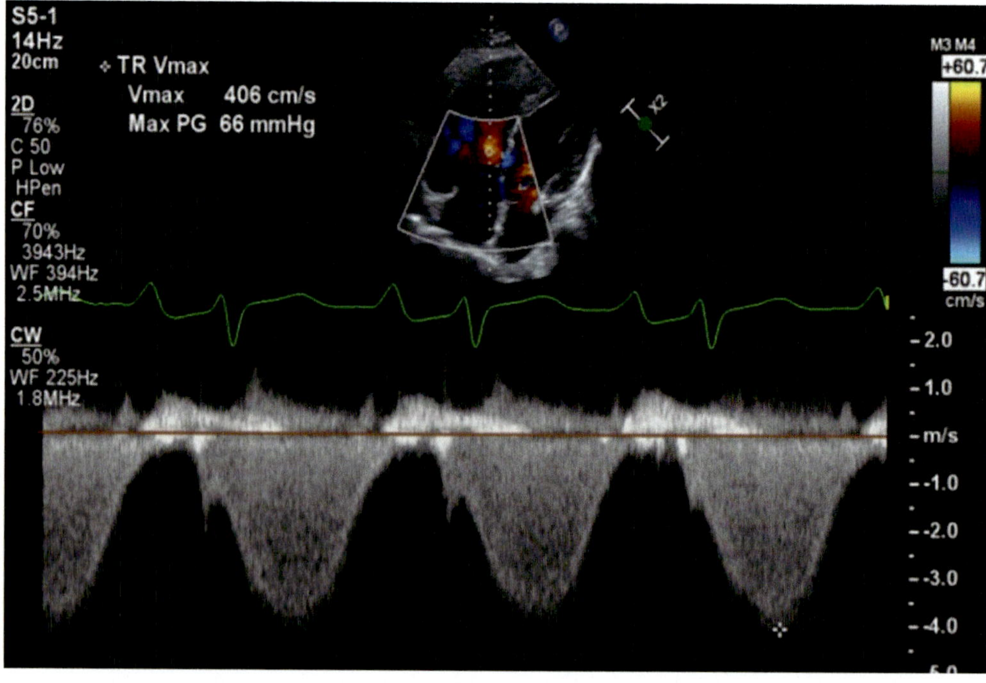

Fig. 11.55 Tricuspid valve CW Doppler

What is the next step in management?

A. Anticoagulation for pulmonary embolism
B. Increase PEEP
C. Bolus 1 liter of Lactate Ringers
D. Initiate diuresis

Choice D is correct. This patient has a thickened RV (maximum normal = 5 mm) given the RV free wall thickness of 18 mm and PASP 79 mmHg, both of which point towards chronic pulmonary hypertension rather than an acute cause such as pulmonary embolism (Choice A is incorrect). Reducing preload by diuretic may decongest the RV and improve the pulmonary edema. Increasing PEEP may provide increased oxygenation if the lung is recruitable, but care must be taken given pulmonary hypertension as an increase in PEEP will lead to increased RV afterload, potentially worsening hemodynamics. C. In the setting of pulmonary hypertension with elevated R sided pressures and pulmonary edema further fluid administration may exacerbate both conditions [52].

Question 52

A 58-year-old male with a history of scleroderma, a known group I pulmonary hypertension that was not improved on oral medication, is admitted to the ICU for initiation of IV epoprostenol.

You are interested in calculating the patient's PVR at the time of initiation of therapy. Bedside echo is obtained with the following results:

LVOT VTI = 27 cm
PV VTI = 9 cm
IVC = 2.5 cm without respiratory variation
TRV = 3 m/sec

What is the patient's PVR?

A. 2.4 WU
B. 3.4 WU
C. 27 WU
D. 8.3 WU

The Correct Answer is B.

PRV can be calculated using the following equation:

$$PVR = TRV/TVI \times 10 + 0.16$$
$$PVR = 3/9 \times 10 + 0.16 = 3.4 \text{ Woods Unit}$$

In the example, the pulmonary artery systolic pressure estimated from the tricuspid regurgitation jet would be 51 mmHg. This high pressure, along with the low pulmonary valve flow, indicated by the TVIot, is consistent with elevated pulmonary vascular resistance.

Echocardiography is useful for the screening of patients with pulmonary hypertension and PVR > 2 WU [2]. However, data to support use as a replacement of invasive hemodynamic monitoring to guide therapy is scant [53].

Question 53

A 43-year-old male with a past medical history of recent MRSA skin infection admitted with acute left limb ischemia, hypotension, and respiratory failure. Vital signs: pulse rate 111/min, BP 90/55 mmHg, RR 23/min, saturating 90% on 100% FiO_2. Bedside Lung ultrasound shows diffuse bilaterally B lines. Cardiac ultrasound shows the following:

LVOT diameter = 2.0 cm
LVOT VTI = 12 cm

What is the next step in managing this patient?

A. Diuretics to lower LV end diastolic pressure
B. Phenylephrine and dobutamine to improve blood pressure
C. Insertion of Intra-aortic balloon pump
D. Surgical repair

Answer: In acute aortic regurgitation, ventricular size remains normal. There is an increase in end-diastolic pressure relative to the regurgitant volume. Impaired forward stroke volume yields decreased systolic pressure and narrow pulse pressure. Although there is some degree of compensation by a Frank-Starling mechanism, the ventricle is functioning on a steep pressure-volume curve because of the lack of chamber dilation. Although there is a marked increase in end-diastolic pressure relative to the regurgitant volume. There is also impaired forward stroke volume. Diuresis, in this case, may worsen ventricular filling and decrease stroke volume further. (choice A is incorrect) Dobutamine may be helpful given evidence of heart failure to improve cardiac output; however, phenylephrine will increase afterload and worsen effective stroke volume. Intra-aortic balloon pump use is contraindicated in acute aortic regurgitation because balloon inflation during diastole is detrimental to left ventricular hemodynamics. This patient has infective endocarditis (IE) involving Aortic valve. He also has features of heart failure, cardiogenic shock (low dP/dT, Low LVOT VTI), and pulmonary edema. The main indication for emergent surgery in Infective endocarditis is heart failure with refractory pulmonary edema or cardiogenic shock [21].

Question 54

A 53-year-old male with a past medical history of hypertension is admitted to the intensive care unit with 3 days of profuse watery diarrhea and hypotension. Vital signs include pulse rate 111/min, BP 70/50 mmHg , respiratory rate of 12/min, saturating 95% on 2 L oxygen.

Bedside point of care ultrasound is performed and the following information is obtained (Fig. 11.56):

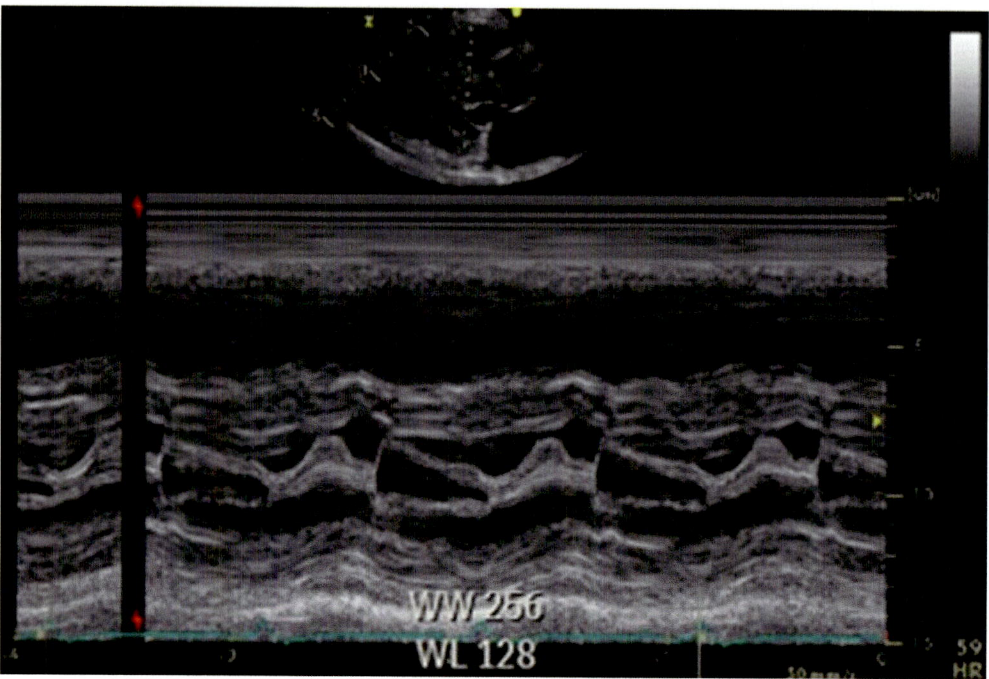

Fig. 11.56 Mitral valve M-mode

MV Peak A vel = 58 cm/s, MV Peak E vel 98 cm/s, Med e′ Vel = 7.25 cm/s

LV posterior wall = 10 mm, LV septal wall = 15 mm

On M-mode of the mitral valve following is seen:

What is the next step in managing this patient's condition?

A. Epinephrine and diuresis.
B. Blocker and diuresis.
C. Epinephrine and fluids
D. Beta-blocker, fluids, and phenylephrine.

Answer: D. This patient has Hypertrophic obstructive cardiomyopathy exacerbated by low intravascular volume due to GI illness, thereby increasing pressure gradient across the LVOT. There are several clues within the question that point towards the diagnosis, such as the presence of systolic anterior motion of the mitral valve (SAM), LV septal wall to LV posterior wall ratio of >1.3. In an acute setting, fluid, phenylephrine, and possibly a negative inotrope such as a β blocker are indicated. Epinephrine and diuresis would likely exacerbate the SAM and should be avoided [16].

Question 55

45 year old with septic shock with LVEF of 52% and lateral mitral annulus E/e′ 20 was noted to have diffuse b-lines noted on lung ultrasonography. The patient has recently been weaned off vasopressors and is given diuretic to wean her from the mechanical ventilator. Which of the below statement is correct?

A. If the ratio decreases and b-lines disappear with diuretic therapy, the patient has diastolic dysfunction.
B. If the ratio increases and b-lines disappear, the patient has diastolic dysfunction, and the diuretic treatment worked
C. E/e′ has not been studied in septic shock
D. E′ reflects the rate of LV contraction during systole

Answer: A. Diastolic dysfunction has been studied in septic shock and has been associated with increased mortality. The E wave measures velocity of flow from left atrium during early passive ventricular filling. The e′ is a reflection of the rate of LV relaxation during diastole. The ratio E/e′ when it is >14 is a sign of elevated left ventricular filling pressure in non- elderly patients. In patients with normal ejection fraction, the ratio should decrease with diuretics and may help with decreasing pulmonary edema, which may facilitate ventilator weaning [18].

References

1. Mercado P, Maizel J, Beyls C, Titeca-Beauport D, Joris M, Kontar L, et al. Transthoracic echocardiography: an accurate and precise method for estimating cardiac output in the critically ill patient. Crit Care. 2017;21(1):136.
2. Quinones MA, Otto CM, Stoddard M, Waggoner A, Zoghbi WA. Recommendations for quantification of Doppler echocardiography: a report from the Doppler quantification task force of the Nomenclature and Standards Committee of the American Society of Echocardiography. J Am Soc Echocardiogr. 2002;15(2):167–84.
3. Blanco P, Aguiar FM, Blaivas M. Rapid ultrasound in shock (RUSH) velocity-time integral: a proposal to expand the RUSH protocol. J Ultrasound Med. 2015;34(9):1691–700.
4. Porter TR, Shillcutt SK, Adams MS, Desjardins G, Glas KE, Olson JJ, et al. Guidelines for the use of echocardiography as a monitor for therapeutic intervention in adults: a report from the American Society of Echocardiography. J Am Soc Echocardiogr. 2015;28(1):40–56.
5. Si X, Xu H, Liu Z, Wu J, Cao D, Chen J, et al. Does respiratory variation in inferior vena cava diameter predict fluid responsiveness in mechanically ventilated patients? A systematic review and meta-analysis. Anesth Analg. 2018;127(5):1157–64.
6. Marik PE, Baram M, Vahid B. Does central venous pressure predict fluid responsiveness? A systematic review of the literature and the tale of seven mares. Chest. 2008;134(1):172–8.
7. Orso D, Paoli I, Piani T, Cilenti FL, Cristiani L, Guglielmo N. Accuracy of ultrasonographic measurements of inferior vena cava to determine fluid responsiveness: a systematic review and meta-analysis. J Intensive Care Med. 2018;35:354–63.
8. Barbier C, Loubieres Y, Schmit C, Hayon J, Ricome JL, Jardin F, et al. Respiratory changes in inferior vena cava diameter are helpful in predicting fluid responsiveness in ventilated septic patients. Intensive Care Med. 2004;30(9):1740–6.
9. Bauman Z, Coba V, Gassner M, Amponsah D, Gallien J, Blyden D, et al. Inferior vena cava collapsibility loses correlation with internal jugular vein collapsibility during increased thoracic or intra-abdominal pressure. J Ultrasound. 2015;18(4):343–8.
10. Heys JJ, Holyoak N, Calleja AM, Belohlavek M, Chaliki HP. Revisiting the simplified bernoulli equation. Open Biomed Eng J. 2010;4:123–8.
11. Cherpanath TG, Hirsch A, Geerts BF, Lagrand WK, Leeflang MM, Schultz MJ, et al. Predicting fluid responsiveness by passive leg raising: a systematic review and meta-analysis of 23 clinical trials. Crit Care Med. 2016;44(5):981–91.
12. Mayo P, Volpicelli G, Lerolle N, Schreiber A, Doelken P, Vieillard-Baron A. Ultrasonography evaluation during the weaning process: the heart, the diaphragm, the pleura and the lung. Intensive Care Med. 2016;42(7):1107–17.
13. Dres M, Teboul JL, Anguel N, Guerin L, Richard C, Monnet X. Passive leg raising performed before a spontaneous breathing trial predicts weaning-induced cardiac dysfunction. Intensive Care Med. 2015;41(3):487–94.
14. Papanikolaou J, Makris D, Saranteas T, Karakitsos D, Zintzaras E, Karabinis A, et al. New insights into weaning from mechanical ventilation: left ventricular diastolic dysfunction is a key player. Intensive Care Med. 2011;37(12):1976–85.
15. Chauvet JL, El-Dash S, Delastre O, Bouffandeau B, Jusserand D, Michot JB, et al. Early dynamic left intraventricular obstruction is associated with hypovolemia and high mortality in septic shock patients. Crit Care. 2015;19:262.
16. Caselli S, Martino A, Genuini I, Santini D, Carbone I, Agati L, et al. Pathophysiology of dynamic left ventricular outflow tract obstruction in a critically ill patient. Echocardiography. 2010;27(10):E122–4.
17. Currie PJ, Seward JB, Chan KL, Fyfe DA, Hagler DJ, Mair DD, et al. Continuous wave Doppler determination of right ventricular pressure: a simultaneous Doppler-catheterization study in 127 patients. J Am Coll Cardiol. 1985;6(4):750–6.
18. Nagueh SF, Smiseth OA, Appleton CP, Byrd BF 3rd, Dokainish H, Edvardsen T, et al. Recommendations for the evaluation of left ventricular diastolic function by echocardiography: an update

from the American Society of Echocardiography and the European Association of Cardiovascular Imaging. Eur Heart J Cardiovasc Imaging. 2016;17(12):1321–60.

19. Lichtenstein DA. BLUE-protocol and FALLS-protocol: two applications of lung ultrasound in the critically ill. Chest. 2015;147(6):1659–70.
20. Vignon P, Repesse X, Vieillard-Baron A, Maury E. Critical care ultrasonography in acute respiratory failure. Crit Care. 2016;20(1):228.
21. Zoghbi WA, Adams D, Bonow RO, Enriquez-Sarano M, Foster E, Grayburn PA, et al. Recommendations for noninvasive evaluation of native valvular regurgitation: a report from the American Society of Echocardiography developed in collaboration with the Society for Cardiovascular Magnetic Resonance. J Am Soc Echocardiogr. 2017;30(4):303–71.
22. Rudski LG, Lai WW, Afilalo J, Hua L, Handschumacher MD, Chandrasekaran K, et al. Guidelines for the echocardiographic assessment of the right heart in adults: a report from the American Society of Echocardiography endorsed by the European Association of Echocardiography, a registered branch of the European Society of Cardiology, and the Canadian Society of Echocardiography. J Am Soc Echocardiogr. 2010;23(7):685–713; quiz 86–8.
23. Maragiannis D, Aggeli C, Nagueh SF. Echocardiographic evaluation of tricuspid prosthetic valves: an update. Hellenic J Cardiol (Hellenike kardiologike epitheorese). 2016;57(3):145–51.
24. Zoghbi WA. New recommendations for evaluation of prosthetic valves with echocardiography and doppler ultrasound. Methodist Debakey Cardiovasc J. 2010;6(1):20–6.
25. Hirata K, Tengan T, Wake M, Takahashi T, Ishimine T, Yasumoto H, et al. Bioprosthetic tricuspid valve stenosis: a case series. Eur Heart J Case Rep. 2019;3(3):ytz110.
26. Mahjoub Y, Pila C, Friggeri A, Zogheib E, Lobjoie E, Tinturier F, et al. Assessing fluid responsiveness in critically ill patients: false-positive pulse pressure variation is detected by Doppler echocardiographic evaluation of the right ventricle. Crit Care Med. 2009;37(9):2570–5.
27. Feissel M, Michard F, Mangin I, Ruyer O, Faller JP, Teboul JL. Respiratory changes in aortic blood velocity as an indicator of fluid responsiveness in ventilated patients with septic shock. Chest. 2001;119(3):867–73.
28. Silvestry FE, Cohen MS, Armsby LB, Burkule NJ, Fleishman CE, Hijazi ZM, et al. Guidelines for the echocardiographic assessment of atrial septal defect and patent foramen ovale: from the American Society of Echocardiography and Society for Cardiac Angiography and Interventions. J Am Soc Echocardiogr. 2015;28(8):910–58.
29. Mojadidi MK, Ruiz JC, Chertoff J, Zaman MO, Elgendy IY, Mahmoud AN, et al. Patent foramen ovale and hypoxemia. Cardiol Rev. 2019;27(1):34–40.
30. Boissier F, Katsahian S, Razazi K, Thille AW, Roche-Campo F, Leon R, et al. Prevalence and prognosis of cor pulmonale during protective ventilation for acute respiratory distress syndrome. Intensive Care Med. 2013;39(10):1725–33.
31. Monnet X, Cipriani F, Camous L, Sentenac P, Dres M, Krastinova E, et al. The passive leg raising test to guide fluid removal in critically ill patients. Ann Intensive Care. 2016;6(1):46.
32. Downes TR, Nomeir AM, Hackshaw BT, Kellam LJ, Watts LE, Little WC. Diastolic mitral regurgitation in acute but not chronic aortic regurgitation: implications regarding the mechanism of mitral closure. Am Heart J. 1989;117(5):1106–12.
33. Agmon Y, Freeman WK, Oh JK, Seward JB. Diastolic mitral regurgitation. Circulation. 1999;99(21):e13.
34. Lewis JF, Kuo LC, Nelson JG, Limacher MC, Quinones MA. Pulsed Doppler echocardiographic determination of stroke volume and cardiac output: clinical validation of two new methods using the apical window. Circulation. 1984;70(3):425–31.
35. Park JH, Marwick TH. Use and limitations of E/e' to assess left ventricular filling pressure by echocardiography. J Cardiovasc Ultrasound. 2011;19(4):169–73.
36. Miller A, Mandeville J. Predicting and measuring fluid responsiveness with echocardiography. Echo Res Pract. 2016;3(2):G1–G12.
37. Monnet X, Rienzo M, Osman D, Anguel N, Richard C, Pinsky MR, et al. Passive leg raising predicts fluid responsiveness in the critically ill. Crit Care Med. 2006;34(5):1402–7.
38. Ciozda W, Kedan I, Kehl DW, Zimmer R, Khandwalla R, Kimchi A. The efficacy of sonographic measurement of inferior vena cava diameter as an estimate of central venous pressure. Cardiovasc Ultrasound. 2016;14(1):33.
39. Hedman K, Nylander E, Henriksson J, Bjarnegard N, Brudin L, Tamas E. Echocardiographic characterization of the inferior vena cava in trained and untrained females. Ultrasound Med Biol. 2016;42(12):2794–802.
40. Parasuraman S, Walker S, Loudon BL, Gollop ND, Wilson AM, Lowery C, et al. Assessment of pulmonary artery pressure by echocardiography—a comprehensive review. Int J Cardiol Heart Vasculature. 2016;12:45–51.
41. McLean AS. Echocardiography in shock management. Crit Care. 2016;20:275.
42. Saric M, Armour AC, Arnaout MS, Chaudhry FA, Grimm RA, Kronzon I, et al. Guidelines for the use of echocardiography in the evaluation of a cardiac source of embolism. J Am Soc Echocardiogr. 2016;29(1):1–42.
43. Lopez L, Colan SD, Frommelt PC, Ensing GJ, Kendall K, Younoszai AK, et al. Recommendations for quantification methods during the performance of a pediatric echocardiogram: a report from the pediatric measurements writing Group of the American Society of echocardiography pediatric and congenital heart disease council. J Am Soc Echocardiogr. 2010;23(5):465–95; quiz 576–7.
44. Nalluri N, Asti D, Anugu VR, Ibrahim U, Lafferty JC, Olkovsky Y. Cardiogenic shock secondary to Takotsubo cardiomyopathy in a patient with preexisting hypertrophic obstructive cardiomyopathy. CASE (Phil). 2018;2(3):78–81.
45. Grayburn PA, Handshoe R, Smith MD, Harrison MR, DeMaria AN. Quantitative assessment of the hemodynamic consequences of aortic regurgitation by means of continuous wave Doppler recordings. J Am Coll Cardiol. 1987;10(1):135–41.
46. Abhayaratna WP, Seward JB, Appleton CP, Douglas PS, Oh JK, Tajik AJ, et al. Left atrial size: physiologic determinants and clinical applications. J Am Coll Cardiol. 2006;47(12):2357–63.
47. Kurnicka K, Lichodziejewska B, Goliszek S, Dzikowska-Diduch O, Zdonczyk O, Kozlowska M, et al. Echocardiographic pattern of acute pulmonary embolism: analysis of 511 consecutive patients. J Am Soc Echocardiogr. 2016;29(9):907–13.
48. Feigenbaum H. Role of M-mode technique in today's echocardiography. J Am Soc Echocardiogr. 2010;23(3):240–57; 335–7, 257.
49. Mayo PH, Narasimhan M, Koenig S. Critical care transesophageal echocardiography. Chest. 2015;148(5):1323–32.

50. Torbicki A, Kurzyna M, Ciurzynski M, Pruszczyk P, Pacho R, Kuch-Wocial A, et al. Proximal pulmonary emboli modify right ventricular ejection pattern. Eur Respir J. 1999;13(3):616–21.
51. Chung N, Nishimura RA, Holmes DR Jr, Tajik AJ. Measurement of left ventricular dp/dt by simultaneous Doppler echocardiography and cardiac catheterization. J Am Soc Echocardiogr. 1992;5(2):147–52.
52. Kaestner M, Schranz D, Warnecke G, Apitz C, Hansmann G, Miera O. Pulmonary hypertension in the intensive care unit. Expert consensus statement on the diagnosis and treatment of paediatric pulmonary hypertension. The European Paediatric Pulmonary Vascular Disease Network, endorsed by ISHLT and DGPK. Heart. 2016;102(Suppl 2):ii57–66.
53. Roule V, Labombarda F, Pellissier A, Sabatier R, Lognone T, Gomes S, et al. Echocardiographic assessment of pulmonary vascular resistance in pulmonary arterial hypertension. Cardiovasc Ultrasound. 2010;8:21.

Fluid Responsiveness and Heart Lung Interactions

12

Simon R. Mucha, Tarik Hanane, and Rishik Vashisht

Question 1

A woman in her 50s with history of dermatomyositis, hypertension and schizophrenia presented with complaint of chest pain. On arrival, she was hypoxemic to 80% saturation on room air and was started on supplemental oxygen at 3 L/min. Her electrocardiogram (EKG) showed sinus tachycardia, left anterior fascicular block, abnormal R wave progression and T wave flattening in lateral leads. She had troponin T level of 0.28 ng/mL, creatinine kinase (CK) level was 799 U/L and CK-MB level was 27.2 ng/mL. Chest X-ray did not show any acute abnormality. She was transferred to coronary intensive care unit for acute on chronic heart failure. Overnight her oxygen saturation decreased to 84% on 6 L nasal cannula and she required 100% oxygen by a non-breather mask. Arterial blood gas obtained at this point showed PaO_2 level of 51 mmHg necessitating endotracheal intubation. Her saturation worsened to 76% on intubation with a positive end expiratory pressure (PEEP) of 5 cmH_2O and decreased further to 71% on increasing the PEEP to 10 cmH_2O. A bedside echocardiogram was done to evaluate the cause of hypoxemia as illustrated in Video 12.1. What is the next best step? [1].

A. Deep sedation, paralysis and increase the PEEP
B. Prone position ventilation
C. Echocardiogram with agitated saline contrast
D. Emergent VV ECMO

Supplementary Information The online version contains supplementary material available at https://doi.org/10.1007/978-3-031-45731-9_12.

S. R. Mucha (✉) · T. Hanane
Department of Critical Care Medicine, Respiratory Institute, Cleveland Clinic, Cleveland, OH, USA
e-mail: muchas@ccf.org; hananet@ccf.org

R. Vashisht
Cardiac Surgery Intensive Care Unit, Sentara Norfolk General Hospital, Norfolk, VA, USA
e-mail: rxvashis@sentara.com

Answer: C. Echocardiogram with agitated saline contrast

Explanation: Point-of-care echocardiography is often useful in the assessment of the patient with dyspnea, hypoxemia, or respiratory failure [2]. The echocardiogram shows severely dilated and severely reduced RV systolic function (Video 12.1). There is high concern for right to left shunt to be the cause of refractory hypoxemia in this patient. When a right-to-left shunt is suspected, the use of agitated saline contrast is often diagnostic. Microbubbles are created by vigorously mixing 9 mL sterile saline with 1 mL room air [3]. The solution is injected immediately into a vein, causing opacification of the right-sided cardiac chambers, best seen in the apical or subcostal view. The microbubbles fracture and diffuse into the lungs while passing through the pulmonary circulation, and so do not reach the left-sided cardiac chambers normally. An intra-cardiac right-to-left shunt allows microbubbles to reach the left-sided cardiac chambers within three cardiac cycles of being seen on the right side. A more delayed appearance of left-sided microbubbles (after 5–6 cardiac cycles) suggests the presence of pulmonary arteriovenous shunts.

Question 2

A bedside echocardiogram with agitated saline was performed (Video 12.2). Based on the echocardiogram what is the next best step?

A. Decrease the PEEP, inhaled pulmonary vasodilators
B. Start Phenylephrine
C. Urgent VV ECMO
D. Cardiology/Surgery consult to close the defect

Answer: A. Decrease the PEEP, inhaled pulmonary vasodilators

Explanation: The video shows significant bubbles appearing on the left side of heart, confirming an intra-cardiac shunt

R. Sreedharan et al. (eds.), *Critical Care Echocardiography*, https://doi.org/10.1007/978-3-031-45731-9_12

(Video 12.2). The cause of intra-cardiac shunt is likely a combination of elevated right sided pressure from reduced biventricular systolic function and underlying pulmonary arterial hypertension, which is further exaggerated by addition of positive end expiratory pressure (PEEP). PEEP applied during mechanical ventilation increases RAP. Higher levels of PEEP increases lung volume from functional residual capacity (FRC) to total lung capacity. This increase in FRC leads to an increase in intra thoracic pressure and increased pericardial, myocardial, and pulmonary vascular transmural pressures. The RV afterload is increased due to increased pulmonary vascular resistance. This combination leads to increased RV pressure and RAP, causing the shunting of blood across the PFO [4, 5]. Thus, the PEEP application in patients with PFO can result in systemic hypoxemia. Decreasing PEEP and inhaled pulmonary vasodilators will decrease the RV afterload decreasing the right sided pressures, thereby reducing the right to left shunt across the PFO.

Question 3

A 23-year-old male with past medical history of failed bone marrow transplant for acute myeloid leukemia presented to the ICU with acute hypoxemic respiratory failure and is intubated on arrival. He is diagnosed with ARDS, is deeply sedated, and started on lung protective ventilation. CT chest with IV contrast showed no pulmonary embolism, diffuse ground glass opacities and basilar consolidation. His ventilator settings are: Vt—420 mL (6 mL/kg), PEEP—16, RR—28, FiO_2—100%. Plateau pressure (PP) is 30.

His ABG is as follows—7.20/54/140/22.

His bedside echocardiogram is shown below (Video 12.3). What is the next best step?

A. Administer t-PA, patient has acute PE
B. Increase PEEP
C. Decrease tidal volume to 350 mL
D. Prone positioning ventilation

Answer: D. Prone positioning ventilation

Explanation: Based on the Echocardiogram, the patient is likely in acute cor-pulmonale (ACP). The incidence of ACP in ARDS has been estimated to be around 30% when the PP range between 27 and 35 cmH_2O [6]. There are various factors that contribute to development of ACP in ARDS patients. Application of high PEEP may increase the right ventricle afterload leading to reduced function. Hypercapnia, which ensues because of increased dead space and decreased tidal volume leads to pulmonary vasoconstriction further leading to decreased RV function. Acidosis has been shown to negatively impact RV contractility. In patients with severely impaired lung compliance, the prone position improves oxygenation without increasing PEEP. Lung recruitment in prone position also leads to improved compliance and alveolar ventilation, thereby decreasing plateau pressure and $PaCO_2$ [7]. All these factors help to unload the right ventricle. Thus, routine echocardiography in ARDS patients should be used to identify ACP. Systematic use of echocardiogram has been endorsed by a French consensus on ARDS management.

The following stem applied to the next three questions.

56-year-old male with a history of colorectal cancer on chemotherapy presented to the emergency department with fever and dizziness. On arrival he is tachycardic with a heart rate of 123 beats/min, hypotensive with blood pressure of 80/42 mmHg, and a respiratory rate of 22/min. Chest X-ray is suggestive of multi-lobar pneumonia. Laboratory examination is significant for WBC count of 16,000/dL and elevated lactate of 6. He has received 3 L of lactated ringer's solution and intravenous antibiotics and is transferred to intensive care unit. On arrival to ICU, his BP is 78/50 mmHg, HR of 120 bpm.

Question 4

As a part of the initial assessment, a bedside ultrasound image of IVC is obtained as shown below (Video 12.4). Based on IVC assessment what is your next best step?

A. Patient is fluid responsive. Bolus additional 1 L of lactated ringer solution and reassess.
B. Patient is in cardiogenic shock, start dobutamine.
C. Fluid responsiveness cannot be established, need additional information.
D. Continue fluid resuscitation up until there is no respiratory variation in IVC

Answer: C. Fluid responsiveness cannot be established, need additional information.

Explanation: IVC diameter in a spontaneously breathing patient is a good tool to non-invasively estimate right atrial pressure (RAP). However, RAP is a static parameter of cardiac preload and does not accurately predict response to fluid administration [8, 9]. IVC variability or collapsibility has been validated in multiple studies as measure of fluid responsiveness in spontaneously breathing patients. In one study, IVC variability of >42% was found to suggest fluid responsiveness, which was also not the case here [10].

Question 5

A passive leg raise test is performed. The change of left ventricular outflow tract-velocity time integral (LVOT-VTI) with the PLR maneuver is assessed at 20%. Based on this information what is the next best step?

A. LVOT-VTI change by PLR cannot be used in spontaneously breathing patients. Proceed with invasive cardiac output measurement.
B. Fluid challenge with lactated ringer's and assess the response.

C. Repeat the test with another provider
D. PLR is not a validated tool to assess fluid responsiveness.

Answer: B. Fluid challenge with lactated ringer's and assess the response.

Explanation: The passive leg raise test consists of raising the lower extremities to 45° from a semi-recumbent position of 45°. Cardiac output or surrogates of cardiac output are measured before the maneuver and 1 min after the maneuver. This maneuver mobilizes around 300 mL of blood from the lower extremities to the heart, simulating fluid administration without the need of IV fluid administration. Change in cardiac output can be reliably measured by assessing the change in LVOT-VTI. An increase in LVOT-VTI of 10% with positive leg raise is consistent with increase in cardiac output of 10% and is considered as a positive. Positive response of LVOT-VTI to the passive leg raise maneuver has been validated and is a widely accepted method to assess fluid responsiveness [11, 12]. The PLR is particularly helpful in conditions where respiratory variation of stroke volume is unreliable, such as spontaneous breathing, cardiac arrhythmias, low tidal volume ventilation and low lung compliance [13].

Question 6

Based on the positive PLR test, the patient receives and additional bolus of 500 mL of lactated ringer's solution, but he remains hypotensive. The patient now complains of shortness of breath and is hypoxemic to 86% on RA. Repeat LVOT-VTI with PLR is again suggestive of fluid responsiveness with a change in LVOT-VTI of 11%. Bedside chest US is shown below (Video 12.5). What is the next best step?

A. Continue to assess for fluid responsiveness and give fluids until PLR test is negative
B. Start vasopressors
C. Check CVP and bolus if CVP is low.
D. Consider Lasix challenge.

Answer: B. Start vasopressors

Explanation: There has been an increasing body of evidence pointing to harmful effects of over-resuscitation, giving rise to the concept of "fluid tolerance". Stroke volume/CO assessment combined with a leg-raise maneuver or a mini fluid bolus can reliably assess volume responsiveness. However, the expected clinical benefit of a small and likely transient increase in cardiac output in a patient deemed to be fluid-responsive needs to be weighed against potential harms of over-resuscitation. Capillary leakage of fluid into the interstitial is greatly increased in septic patients [14]. The patient may still be volume responsive, but may be at risk to develop pulmonary edema (as evidenced by the appearance of B-lines on chest ultrasound) and abdominal compartment syndrome [15]. A common practice is to limit fluid administration by appearance of B lines [16].

Question 7

56-year-old female with past medical history of pulmonary sarcoidosis, pulmonary hypertension undergoes bilateral lung transplant. After lung transplant right ventricular failure and cardiogenic develop. She is started on inhaled epoprostenol, norepinephrine and is transferred to the intensive care unit. On arrival her BP is 93/57, HR is 80/min, oxygen saturation in 95% on 40% FiO_2. A bedside echocardiogram is done to evaluate her cardiac function which is shown below. The arterial line tracing showed pulse pressure variation of 15%. Her norepinephrine requirement is increasing and is currently at 20 μg/kg/min. What is the next best step in management of her shock? (Video 12.6)

A. She is fluid responsive as evidenced by PPV of 15%, give a 500 mL bolus of lactated ringers solution
B. Stop inhaled epoprostenol
C. Do a passive leg raise test
D. Increase norepinephrine

Answer: D. Increase norepinephrine

Explanation: Pulse pressure variation is a method of determining fluid responsiveness in intubated patients. It works on the premise of changing stroke volume with insufflation of the lungs. The increase in intrathoracic pressure during inspiration leads to decrease in venous return to the right atrium, thereby leading to reduced right ventricular (RV) preload. Insufflation during inspiration also increases RV afterload because of the increase in transpulmonary pressure during inspiration. As a result, RV stroke volume decreases during inspiration and is minimal at the end-inspiration. The inspiratory decrease in RV stroke volume leads to a decrease in left ventricular (LV) filling after a phase lag of two to four heartbeats due to the blood pulmonary transit time. This generally occurs during expiration. This cyclical change in LV stroke volume because of reduction in RV stroke volume leads to PPV in patients whose right ventricle is pre-load dependent and whose LV is fluid responsive. However, a failing RV is more sensitive to afterload changes than to preload changes. Increased afterload leads to decrease in RV stroke volume which in turn leads to decrease in LV stroke volume. In addition, in cases of severe RV pressure overload, increased RV afterload during mechanical inspiration leads to a leftward shift of the intraventricular septum, further decreasing LV diastolic filling and thus stroke volume. This leads to a significant respirophasic variation of LV stroke volume and PPV. This, however, is "false positive PPV". Other conditions that can lead to false positive PPV are cardiac arrhythmias, intra-abdominal hypertension and vigorous spontaneous breathing especially in patients with obstructive lung disease [17].

Question 8

Which is a true statement about pulse pressure variability as a predictor for fluid responsiveness?

A. PPV cannot be used in patients with low lung compliance
B. PPV can only be used in patients with ventilated with low tidal volumes (4–6 ml/kg) cardiac arrhythmias
C. PPV can only be used in patients with low lung compliance
D. PPV can only be used in spontaneously breathing patients

Answer: A. PPV cannot be used in patients with low lung compliance

Explanation: Pulsed pressure variation is caused by the transmission of airway pressure to the pleural and pericardial spaces, which induces changes in venous return and cardiac preload. Conditions where transmission of airway pressures is limited could lead to false negative PPV. This could be due to use of low tidal volumes or in lungs that have low compliance like in ARDS. Transmission of intrapulmoary pressure to the mediastinum and thus the heart is decreased in conditions with increased lung stiffness (ARDS, pulmnary fibrosis) and further accentuated by increased chest wall stiffness. Therefore, during low tidal volume ventilation in ARDS, even though the driving pressure is high, the transmission of these pressure through the stiff lung is lower which in turn leads to less PPV [18–20].

Question 9

A seventy-one-year-old male gets admitted to the ICU with septic shock. He receives empiric antibiotics and 2 L of lactated ringer's solution prior to arrival. On arrival to the ICU, he is intubated, and is now passive on the ventilator. BP is 76/48 mmHg, HR—120/min in sinus rhythm. A bedside US shows end expiratory IVC diameter of 8 mm. What is the next best step?

A. Start vasopressors
B. Administer fluid bolus
C. Start inotropes
D. None of the above

Answer: B. Administer fluid bolus.

Explanation: Static parameters, such as CVP are poor predictors of fluid responsiveness, and there is only poor correlation between IVC diameter and Right atrial pressure (RAP). However, it has been suggested that end expiratory IVC diameter (IVC) better reflects transmural RAP, and at extreme values may predict fluid responsiveness accurately. An IVC_{ee} of less than 10 mm can identify fluid responsiveness with a specificity of 90%. Similarly, $IVC_{ee} \geq 27$ mm indicated the absence of fluid responsiveness with a specificity of at least 90% [21].

Question 10

A forty-two-year-old male who was admitted 5 days ago for a pelvic fracture after a motor vehicle crash, is now febrile to 39 °C. His heart rate is 120/min, regular rate and rhythm and his BP is 78/40. Over the course of his hospitalization his net fluid balance is 10 L. He is intubated and deeply sedated. His ventilator settings are as follows—tidal volume 420 cc, respiratory rate 22 breaths/min, PEEP is 12 cmH_2O and FiO_2 is 60%. The resident wants to give him a bolus of 1 L of lactated ringer's. What is the next best step?

A. Go ahead and give the fluid bolus
B. Check for fluid responsiveness by PLR and LVOT VTI change
C. Give a 100 mL of LR bolus and assess LVOT VTI change
D. Give a 500 mL of LR bolus and assess LVOT Aortic VTI change

Answer C: Give a 100 mL of LR bolus and assess LVOT VTI change

Explanation: A change of 10% of cardiac output/LVOT-VTI by PLR is a reliable way of assessing fluid responsiveness. However, this method should not be used in patients with any unstable fractures. One study suggested PLR in patients with intra-abdominal hypertension (abdominal pressures >16 mmHg) may leed to false negative results [22]. In patients in whom PLR cannot be reliably performed, a "mini fluid challenge" bolus is another reliable alternative. LVOT-VTI change of >10% after raid injection of 100 mL of crystalloid fluid was associated with fluid responsiveness with a sensitivity and specificity of 95% and 78%, respectively [23]. Another study evaluated change in stroke volume variation (ΔSVV) and change in pulse pressure variability (ΔPPV) in response to a "mini fluid challenge" in patients with circulatory failure and ventilated with low tidal volumes. The ΔSVV and ΔPPV predicted fluid responsiveness with AUCs of 0.91 and 0.92, respectively [24].

Question 11

A 36-year-old male is admitted with septic shock and multifocal pneumonia requiring intubation for hypoxic respiratory failure. After receiving broad spectrum antibiotics and 30 cc/kg of crystalloids IV, he remains hypotensive and was started on vasopressors. The intensivist decided to determine the cardiac output to better assess the patient's hemodynamics. Which of the following is correct regarding the use of TTE is stroke volume and cardiac output assessment?

A. LVOT diameter measurement should be done at the aortic valve cusps in zoomed parasternal long axis view at the end of systole.
B. LVOT VTI is accurately estimated by using low sweep speed and low wall filters.
C. LVOT VTI is accurately estimated by using high sweep speed and reduced gain.
D. LVOT area (A) is: $A = \pi \, x \, LVOT\text{-}diameter^2$
E. Five or seven VTI measurements should be averaged for a patient with atrial fibrillation at different times of the respiratory cycles

Answer C. LVOT VTI is accurately estimated by using high sweep speed and reduced gain.

Explanation: Stroke volume measurement by echocardiography is an essential variable in the assessment of unstable critically ill patients. It is determined by measuring the LV outflow tract diameter and LVOT velocity time integral using the following formula: the following formula: SV = LVOTVTI × πr^2. The LVOT diameter is measured at the aortic valve cusps in zoomed parasternal long axis view in mid-systole. The PW Doppler is set at high speed, low filters and reduced gain for accurate assessment of LVOT-VTI. In patients with atrial fibrillation, five to seven LVOTVTI measurements should be averaged, preferably at the same time of respiratory cycle.

Question 12

Which of the following is correct regarding the performance of passive leg raising (PLR)?

A. PLR can only be used in patients receiving mechanical ventilation
B. Cardiac arrhythmias are not a major limitation of the use of passive leg raising
C. High abdominal pressures do not interfere with PLR results, because it is performed by moving the legs manually to a 45° angle while the patient is in a supine position at baseline.
D. A change in stroke volume 1-min post-PLR with cutoff value of 20% is used to determine fluid responders.

Answer B. Cardiac arrhythmias are not a major limitation of the use of passive leg raising

Explanation: The passive leg raising (PLR) test has been shown to reliably detect preload responsiveness in both spontaneously breathing and mechanically ventilated patients. Contrary to other dynamic parameters, it keeps its diagnostic value in cardiac arrhythmias, but not in patients with high abdominal pressure. A strict protocol should be followed for accurate results. Patients should be transitioned from a semi-recumbent position to a supine position, while which the legs are raised [assively to 45° and the torso is horizontal. Stroke volume is measured 1-min post PLR. The cutoff value the most frequently found to predict fluid responsiveness with good sensitivity and specificity was 10%.

Question 13

Which of the following will most likely interfere with the accuracy of a passive leg raising maneuver as a test of preload responsiveness?

A. Patient is ventilated with assist control/volume control with set rate of 20 bpm and breathing 30 bpm
B. Ventilation with tidal volume set at 6 mL/kg of ideal body weight
C. Patient with severe ARDS with low lung compliance
D. Patient is in atrial fibrillation with rapid ventricular rate
E. Patient with severe necrotizing pancreatitis and IAP >20 mmHg

Answer E. Patient with severe necrotizing pancreatitis and IAP >20 mmHg

Explanation: The great advantage of the PLR test compared to other dynamic parameters, i.e., PPV, SVV, is that it maintains its accuracy in patients with cardiac arrhythmias, low lung compliance and during spontaneous breathing and ventilation with low tidal volume. The most important limitations are inability to measure the cardiac output in "real time" and increased intra-abdominal hypertension.

Question 14

A 75-year-old male with history significant for hypertension with severe LV hypertrophy and COPD is admitted to the ICU with circulatory shock. Current vital signs are blood pressure 88/56 mmHg, heart rate 120 beats/min, spontaneously breathing with respiratory rate 25 breaths/min. His hemoglobin is 8.0 g/dL and lactate are 5 mmol/L. A point of care ultrasound is performed at the bedside. Which of the following echocardiographic parameters have a good specificity for fluid responsiveness?

A. A hyperdynamic left ventricle.
B. An IVC diameter of 1.7 which collapses by 20% during inspiration.
C. Velocity time integral variation of 10% in spontaneously breathing patient.
D. None of the above.

Answer: A. A hyperdynamic left ventricle.

Explanation: Static parameters have poor predictability for fluid responsiveness. A hyperdynamic LV with papillary apposition on PSAX view, a LVEDA of less than 10 cm^2 and small IVC <1 cm with more than 50% collapse are strong echocardiographic markers of reduced filling pressure, but may also occur in setting of reduced afterload. VTI change in spontaneously breathing patients may be a reflection of respiratory efforts rather than fluid responsiveness and thus is not reliable. E-point septal separation (EPSS) has classically been used for estimation of LVEF and cardiac function and is not validated for fluid responsiveness. IVC collapsibility index ≥15% and stroke volume variation ≥17% and greater suggest fluid responsiveness in spontaneously breathing patient.

Question 15

Which of the following is accurate regarding the measurement of left ventricular end-diastolic area (LVEDA)?

A. LVEDA is best measured by tracing the endocardial border at the level of mitral valve level in the parasternal short axis view.

B. There is strong correlation between LVEDA index and the pulmonary artery occlusion pressure.
C. LVEDA of 15 cm^2 is suggestive of severe hypovolemia.
D. LVEDA is best measured by tracing the endocardial border in the mid-papillary trans-gastric short axis view with TEE.
E. LVEDA remains an accurate surrogate of preload status in the setting of severe LV hypertrophy.

Answer D. LVEDA is best measured by tracing the endocardial border in the mid-papillary trans-gastric short axis view with TEE.

Explanation: Left ventricular end-diastolic area is a static parameter used to assess preload status. It is best measured by tracing the endocardial border at the level of the papillary muscles in the parasternal short axis view in TTE and mid-papillary trans-gastric view in TEE. The normal value is 8–12 cm^2. A value of less than 10 cm^2 is suggestive of severe hypovolemia. This may not be true in the case of severe LV hypertrophy. Although it is used a static measurement of preload, several studies showed no correlation with PAOP.

Question 16

A 42-year-old male with no significant past medical history is admitted to the ICU with severe acute respiratory distress syndrome due to influenza A. He is mechanically ventilated and sedated with propofol, fentanyl. Atracurium was started due to severe patient-ventilator dyssynchrony. His settings are assist control/volume control with a respiratory rate of 25 breaths/min, tidal volume 350 mL (5 mL/kg IBW), positive end-expiratory pressure (PEEP) 15 cmH_2O, and fraction of inspired oxygen (FiO_2) 80%, with oxygen saturation as measured by pulse oximetry (SpO_2) 91%. Plateau pressures is 29 cmH_2O. He became hypotensive and bedside TTE is done. Which is accurate regarding the use of flow velocity variation in assessment of fluid responsiveness?

A. The sensitivity and specificity of SVV in mechanically ventilated patients are more than 80% with area under ROC >0.9
B. SVV is not recommended to be used in patients with significant arrhythmia because it leads to minimal stroke volume variation
C. Only the changes in velocity time integral and not aortic peak velocity changes can be used to assess fluid responsiveness.
D. The above ventilatory settings may be responsible of false positive results and thus VTI variation should not be used to assess fluid responsiveness in this patient.
E. A flow variation across the LVOT of 8% is predictive of fluid responsiveness.

Answer A. The sensitivity and specificity of SVV in mechanically ventilated patients are more than 80% with area under ROC >0.9

Explanation: The aortic flow velocity variation parameters have good specificity and sensitivity of more than 80% with area under ROC curve >0.9. A flow variation across the LVOT of >12% is predictive of fluid responsiveness. They are, however, not accurate in the setting of arrhythmias and low tidal volume. Significant variation in VTI may be related to the arrhythmia and low tidal volume ventilation <8 mL/kg IBW may cause small changes in VTI and responsible for false negative results.

Question 17

Which is correct about stroke volume variation (SVV)?

A. Cardiac arrhythmia could be responsible for false negative results
B. Open chest could be responsible for false positive results
C. Very high respiratory rate could be responsible for false negative results
D. Spontaneous breathing could be responsible for false negative results
E. Increased intra-abdominal pressure could be responsible of false negative results

Answer C. Very high respiratory rate could be responsible for false negative results

Explanation: SVV is a well-established echocardiographic parameter for assessing fluid responsiveness in the right settings. However, caution is advised in certain conditions where it is less reliable; Spontaneous breathing, cardiac arrhythmias and increased intra-abdominal pressure cause false positive results, while very high respiratory rate and open chest result in false negative outcomes.

Question 18

In A recent study of 540 mechanical ventilated patients with acute circulatory failure, comparing various echocardiographic indices used to predict fluid responsiveness, found:

A. Respiratory variations of the maximal Doppler velocity in left ventricular outflow tract have the best specificity.
B. Respiratory variations of the superior vena cava diameter had the best sensitivity.
C. Respiratory variations of the inferior vena cava diameter and pulse pressure performed better than respiratory variations of superior vena cava diameter.
D. A Ventilator-induced change in SVC diameter equal to or exceeding 21% had the best sensitivity in predicting fluid responsiveness.
E. Respiratory variations of the maximal Doppler velocity in left ventricular outflow tract had the better overall sensitivity.

Answer E. Respiratory variations of the maximal Doppler velocity in left ventricular outflow tract had the better overall sensitivity.

Explanation: In a multicenter prospective study conducted in France, various echocardiographic parameters used to predict fluid responsiveness were compared. All patients were in acute circulatory failure and passive on mechanical ventilation. Respiratory variations of the maximal Doppler velocity in left ventricular outflow tract (ΔV_{max} Ao >10%) had the best sensitivity and respiratory variations of superior vena cava diameter (ΔSVC >21%) had the best specificity. Both the aforementioned indices fared better than in inferior vena cava diameter changes and pulse pressure variation [25].

Question 19
Which of the following echocardiographic parameters is useful in assessing fluid responsiveness in a patient receiving pressure support mechanical ventilation?

A. LVOT VTI with respiratory variation exceeding 20%
B. IVC distensibility index of more than 18%
C. LVOT VTI increase by more than 10% after "Mini"-fluid challenge (100 mL).
D. IVC variability index of more than 12%
E. LVEDA measure in PSAX view at the papillary muscles of 10 cm^2

Answer C. LVOT VTI increase by more than 10% after "Mini"-fluid challenge (100 mL).
Explanation: A change in LVOT VTI by more than 10% following a 100 mL infusion of a colloid over 1 min, predicted fluid responsiveness with a sensitivity and specificity of 95% and 78% respectively. The VTI was measured with transthoracic echocardiography. All the other parameters are inaccurate in case of spontaneous breathing and cannot be used [23].

Question 20
What is the estimated right atrial pressure (RAP) in a patient spontaneously breathing with an IVC diameter of 1.7 cm with more than 50% collapsibility?

A. Estimated RAP is 15 mmHg
B. Estimated RAP is 8 mmHg
C. Estimated RAP is 3 mmHg
D. RAP cannot be estimated in a spontaneously breathing patient
E. Estimated RAP is >20 mmHg

Answer: C. Estimated RAP is 3 mmHg
Explanation: Right atrial pressure is typically estimated based on IVC diameter and response to a sniff test. The maximum IVC diameter is measured from M-mode or 2D in the subcostal view, 1–2 cm from IVC–RA junction.

IVC diameter (cm)	Collapsibility (%)	Estimated RAP (mmHg)
IVC <2.1	>50	3
IVC >2.1	>50	8
IVC <2.1	≤50	
IVC >2.1	<50	15

Question 21
Appropriate statements about the use of inferior vena cava (IVC) as a predictor of fluid responsiveness include:

A. The IVC can be visualized only with transthoracic echocardiography.
B. During mandatory mechanical ventilation with no respiratory efforts, the IVC collapses during inspiration because of increased intra-thoracic pressure
C. The respiratory variation of the IVC diameter is better that the respiratory variation of SVC in detecting preload responsiveness.
D. In a meta-analysis, the pooled sensitivity and specificity of respiratory variation of the IVC in predicting preload responsiveness are 76% and 86% respectively.
E. The IVC diameter change cannot be used in patients with cardiac arrhythmias.

Answer D. In a meta-analysis, the pooled sensitivity and specificity of respiratory variation of the IVC in predicting preload responsiveness are 76% and 86% respectively.
Explanation: The IVC diameter variation induced by the cyclical changes in intra-thoracic pressure during mechanical ventilation is used to predict preload responsiveness. During controlled mechanical ventilation (no spontaneous breathing), the IVC dilates during inspiration and collapses in expiration. The IVC diameter is measured with transthoracic echocardiography just distal to the hepatic vein, preferably in 2D or in M-mode with the vessel perpendicular to the US beam. The IVC can also be visualized with TEE in bicaval view. In a metanalysis of 8 studies assessing the accuracy of respiratory variation of IVC diameter (ΔIVC) in predicting preload responsiveness, the pooled sensitivity was 0.76 and pooled specificity was 0.86. The ΔIVC performed better in mechanically ventilated than spontaneously breathing patients. The ΔIVC has the same limitation than PPV and SVV, however, it can be used in patients with arrhythmias [26].

Question 22
A 22-year-old man is admitted to the ICU with vaping associated lung injury requiring intubation due to ARDS. He requires 100% O_2 and PEEP of 18. His oxygenation does not improve with paralytics and proning. He is in circulatory shock and requiring 24 μg/min of norepinephrine with MAP 67 mmHg. VV ECMO cannulation is planned (femoro-atrial configuration) and TEE is used to assess cannula placement and volume responsiveness.

At what position would you assess SVC collapsibility and what is the threshold for a positive result?

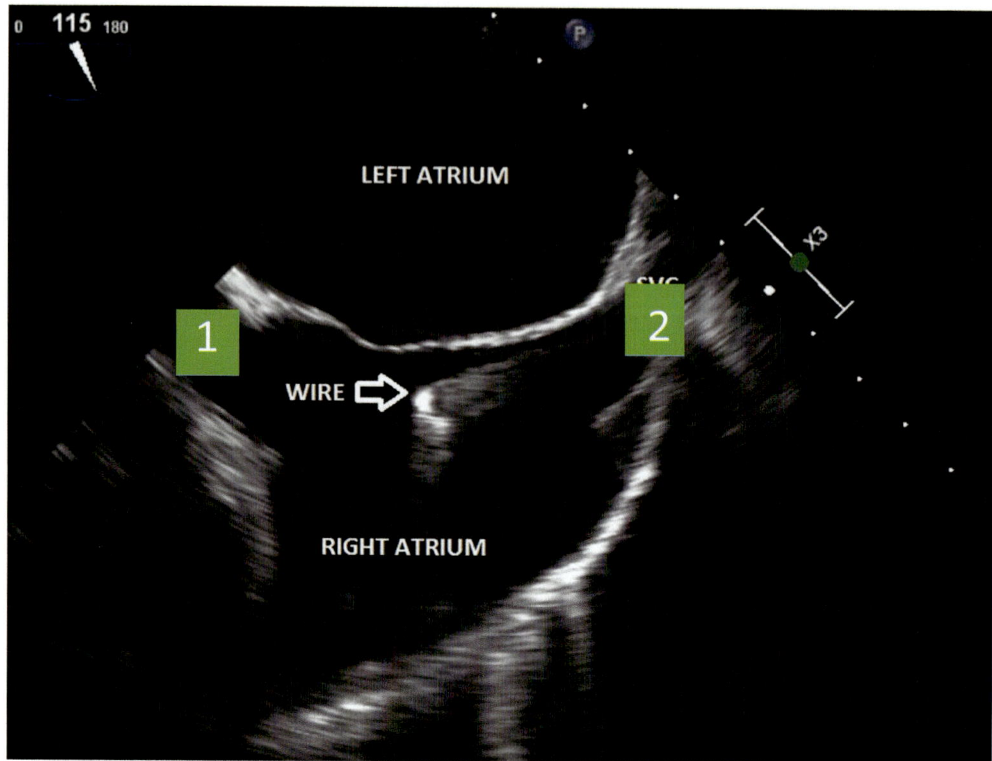

A. Position 1; 18%
B. Position 1; 36%
C. Position 2; 18%
D. Position 2; 36%
E. None of the above

Answer D. Position 2; 36%

Explanation: The ultrasound examination of the SVC collapsibility and fluid responsiveness by TEE is performed by measuring SVC diameter variations in a longitudinal view focused on the mid-esophageal bicaval view. The collapsibility index (CI) = (SVC max − SVC min) × 100/SVC max, of greater than 36% was predictive of preload responsiveness with a sensitivity of 90% and specificity of 100% [27].

Question 23

Which of the following statements is accurate about SVC collapsibility?

A. The maximum diameter is measured during expiration and minimum diameter is measured during inspiration
B. The maximum diameter is measured during inspiration and minimum diameter is measured during expiration
C. SVC collapsibility index can still be reliable in predicting preload responsiveness during spontaneous breathing.
D. SVC collapsibility index is not reliable during cardiac arrhythmias

Answer: A. The maximum diameter is measured during expiration and minimum diameter is measured during inspiration

Explanation: The effects of positive pressure ventilation on SVC diameter are opposite to those on the IVC diameter. In mechanically ventilated patients, the SVC diameter decreases during inspiration and increases during expiration. The SVC collapsibility index is not reliable during spontaneous ventilation, low tidal volume and poor lung compliance but maintains its accuracy during cardiac arrhythmias [25].

Question 24

A previously healthy 27-year-old woman presented to the emergency department after syncope. She is hemodynamically stable and breathing comfortably on room air. Bedside echocardiogram shows no obvious structural pathology. A pulse wave doppler is placed at the following sites:

A. Tricuspid valve
B. Mitral valve
C. Pulmonary valve
D. LVOT

The following measurements were obtained.

peak tricuspid velocity variation is 23%
peak mitral velocity variation is 11%
peak pulmonic valve velocity variation is 9%
peak LVOT velocity variation is 8%

Which of the following statements are most accurate?

A. The respiratory variations of flow suggest tamponade
B. The respiratory variations of flow suggest constrictive cardiomyopathy
C. The respiratory variations of flow require further catheter-based evaluation
D. The respiratory variations of flow are normal respiratory variation

Answer D. The respiratory variations of flow are normal respiratory variation

Explanation: The values show normal respirophasic variation in flow. Under normal circumstances, peak velocity of tricuspid inflow varies by up to 25%, mitral inflow varies by up to 15%. Peak velocity and time velocity integral of aortic and pulmonary flow profiles vary by up to 10% with normal respiration [28–30].

Question 25

Which of the following is true about respiratory variation of the superior vena cava (SVC) and inferior vena cava (IVC) in healthy individuals?

A. In spontaneous breathing the diameter of the SVC decreases during inspiration.
B. In spontaneous breathing, the diameter of the extra thoracic IVC decreases during inspiration.
C. In a passive patient on positive pressure ventilation the SVC diameter increases during inspiration.
D. In a passive patient on positive pressure ventilation, the diameter of the extra thoracic IVC decreases with inspiration.

Answer B. In spontaneous breathing, the diameter of the extra thoracic IVC decreases during inspiration.

Explanation: Respiro-phasic variation of the diameter of the vena cava are related to the changes of transmural pressure (intravascular pressure – extravascular pressure) throughout the respiratory cycle.

Since the SVC is located within the thoracic cavity, a decrease in pleural pressure during active inspiration in spontaneous breathing will increase transmural pressure and increase SVC diameter. During PPV, pleural pressure rises during inspiration leading to decreased transmural pressure and a decrease in SVC diameter.

The transmural pressure of the extrathoracic IVC is determined by the central venous pressure (intravascular pressure) and the abdominal pressure (extravascular pressure). In spontaneous breathing, the pleural pressure and thereby central venous pressures drops during inspiration, while abdominal pressure increases. This leads to a decrease in transmural pressure and a decrease in IVC diameter during inspiration. In PPV, pleural pressure rises during inspiration leading to an increased intravascular pressure. Abdominal pressure may also increase albeit to a lesser extent, leading to a net increase in transmural pressure and an increase in IVC diameter.

It is important to note that the degree of respirophasic variations of vena cava diameter is highly variable depending on fluid status, central venous pressure, respiratory effort, lung compliance and abdominal pressure. In hypovolemia the effect is exaggerated whereas respiratory variations may be blunted or absent in hypervolemia.

Similarly, pleural pressure swings may be less pronounced with positive pressure variation in patients with low lung compliance (interstitial lung disease or ARDS) [29, 31].

Question 26

A 71-year-old woman with diabetes, hypertension, atrial fibrillation, CVA and residual severe aphasia is being treated for aspiration pneumonia. You are asked to assess "volume status". RV and LV appear grossly normal in size and function and there is no obvious valvular pathology. Due to severe aphasia, the patient is unable to perform a sniff test.

During quiet respiration, the maximal IVC diameter is 1.9 cm, the minimal IVC diameter is 1.8 cm.

Which of the following statements is most accurate?

A. Right atrial pressure cannot be assessed because of atrial fibrillation
B. Right atrial pressure cannot be assessed without a sniff test
C. Right atrial pressure is >10 mmHg
D. Right atrial pressure is <10 mmHg

Answer C: Right atrial pressure is >10 mmHg

Explanation: Echocardiographic measurements of the IVC are commonly used to estimate right atrial pressure. Current guidelines recommend size and variability during an inspiratory sniff to estimate RAP—Table. Brennan et al. assessed echocardiographic measures of the IVC to estimate right atrial pressure both during quite breathing and an inspiratory sniff. In quite breathing, a cut-off of 20% in the IVC collapsibility index was able to accurately predict a right atrial pressure over 10 mmHg—answer C is correct. Nine percent of the patients in this study were in atrial fibrillation—answer A is incorrect [32, 33].

IVC diameter	Collapse during sniff (%)	Estimated RAP (mmHg)
<2.1	>50	0–5
>2.1 cm	>50	5–10
>2.1 cm	<50	10–20

Question 27

A 51-year-old woman with myasthenia gravis is admitted to the ICU in myasthenic crisis. Because of worsening respiratory failure, she was placed on BiPAP (iPAP 14 cmH_2O, ePAP 6 cmH_2O 8 cmH_2O) and you are preparing to intubate. Echocardiogram shows an IVC of 2.1 cm without respiratory variation.

Which of the following statements is most accurate?

A. Right atrial pressure is 0–5 mmHg
B. Right atrial pressure is 5–10 mmHg
C. Right atrial pressure is 10–20 mmHg
D. Right atrial pressure is undetermined

Answer D. Right atrial pressure is undetermined.

Explanation: The patient in this scenario is making weak spontaneous efforts while on positive pressure ventilation. Using IVC collapsibility to assess central venous pressure assumes a drop in intra-thoracic pressure with inspiration. In a patient on PPV, it is not possible to estimate the changes in pleural pressure induced by patient effort due to presence of positive pressure throughout the respiratory cycle. Size and variability should not be used to assess right atrial pressure in patients on positive pressure ventilation [32, 34].

Question 28

Which of the following statements is most accurate regarding echocardiographic measurements of flow throughout the respiratory cycle—assuming a healthy patient, sedated and passive on mechanical ventilation?

A. Decrease of pulmonic vein flow during inspiration.
B. Increase of RVOT VTI during inspiration.
C. Decrease of tricuspid valve inflow velocity during expiration.
D. Increase of LVOT VTI during inspiration.

Answer D. Increase of LVOT VTI during inspiration.

Explanation: Effect of PPV on the right ventricle:

- Increased intrathoracic pressure decreases the pressure gradient between mean systemic filling pressure and right atrial pressure, resulting in decreased TR inflow and decreased RV stroke volume.
- Transpulmonary pressure (TPP) is maximal at end inspiration. As TPP rises it can exceed pulmonary venous pressure and pulmonary artery pressure, leading to partial or complete collapse of pulmonary capillaries resulting in an increase in pulmonary vascular resistance and RV afterload—which may lead to decreased stroke volume.

Effect of PPV on the left ventricle

- Rise of TPP during inspiration compresses the pulmonary capillaries and veins, increasing pulmonary venous flow to the left atrium and increasing LV preload at end inspiration.
- As long as the LV is functioning on the ascending limb of the Frank-Starling curve, this transient increase in LV preload leads to increase in LV stroke volume, which is at its maximum at end-inspiration [35].

Questions 29 and 30

You perform a 15 s **expiratory** hold in a healthy patient, who is sedated and passive in mechanical ventilation. Which of the following can most likely be detected using echocardiography?

A. Decrease of LVOT-VTI from baseline
B. Increase of LVOT-VTI from baseline
C. Increase IVC diameter
D. Decrease IVC diameter

You perform a 15 s **inspiratory** hold in a healthy patient, who is sedated and passive in mechanical ventilation. Which of the following can most likely be detected using echocardiography?

A. Decrease of LVOT-VTI from baseline
B. Increase of LVOT-VTI from baseline
C. Increase IVC diameter
D. Decrease IVC diameter

Answers 29—B Increase of LVOT-VTI from baseline; 30—A Decrease of LVOT-VTI from baseline.

Explanation: Compared to the normal respiratory cycle, performing an expiratory hold effectively decreases intrathoracic pressure. This results in a net increase in blood return to the RA and increase in cardiac output, if the patient is "fluid responsive" i.e., on the ascending portion of the Frank Starling curve. An increase in 5% or greater on LVOT-VTI with an expiratory hold has been shown to predict fluid responsiveness.

In contrast, an inspiratory hold, increases intrathoracic pressure, decreasing pre-load and in turn decreasing cardiac output in a pre-load sensitive patient [36].

Questions 31 and 32

A 51-year-old male patient with no known medical history was just admitted with acute hematemesis. You are asked to intubate the patient for airway protection in anticipation of an upper endoscopy. Heart rate 110 bpm, BP 98/51 mmHg, RR 20, SpO_2 99% on RA. A limited bedside echocardiogram shows RV and LV are grossly normal in size and function. Subcostal long axis view of the IVC is shown in below image.

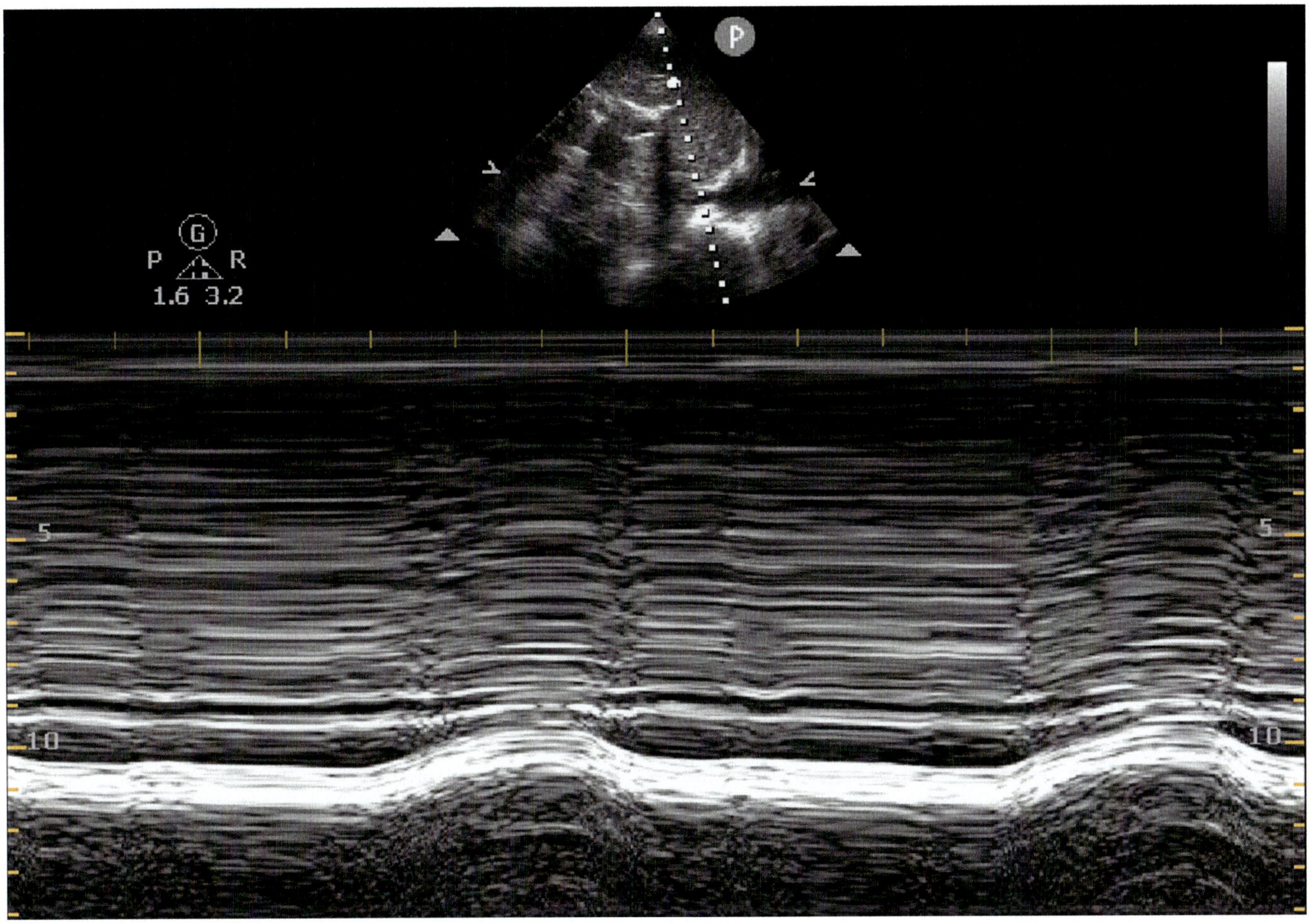

31. Which of the following statements best describes the most likely hemodynamic effects of initiation of positive pressure ventilation (PPV) in the patient above?

A. PPV will reduce LV afterload, increase LV preload and increase cardiac output and blood pressure.
B. PPV will cause a sudden increase of transpulmonary pressure, decreased RV afterload and therefore increase in cardiac output and blood pressure.
C. Initiation of PPV will have minimal hemodynamic effects.
D. PPV will cause a sudden increase of intrathoracic pressure, thereby causing decreased RV preload and a drop in cardiac output and blood pressure.

32. What is the most appropriate next step?

A. Start dobutamine before intubation
B. IV volume resuscitation before intubation
C. Start norepinephrine before intubation
D. Proceed with intubation without additional intervention

Answer 31—D PPV will cause a sudden increase of intrathoracic pressure, thereby causing decreased RV preload and a drop in cardiac output and blood pressure and 32—B IV volume resuscitation before intubation.

Explanation: Based on history and the echocardiographic images provided, the patient in question is hypovolemic. In hypovolemia, a low stressed volume of blood in the venous capacitance vessels leads to a relatively low mean systemic filling pressure (MSFP) and a low pressure-gradient for venous blood return to the right atrium. Even small changes in right atrial pressure will therefore significantly decrease the pressure gradient between MSFP and the right atrium, and thereby dramatically reduce RV preload, leading to a drop in cardiac output. This effect can be minimized volume resuscitation. In the absence of heart or lung disease there is no indication that initiation of PPV would result in significantly elevated TPP or reduce large negative swings in pleural pressure. Therefore, the effect of PPV in RV and LV afterload in this situation would be negligible [29, 37].

Questions 33 and 34

A 38-year-old woman with interstitial lung disease awaiting lung transplant is admitted to your ICU for worsening hypoxic respiratory failure. HR 138 BPM, BP 85/47 mmHg, respiratory rate 34 breaths per minute, SpO_2 86% on 100% FiO_2 High Flow nasal cannula. As the team is getting ready to intubate the patient you perform a limited bedside echo as shown (Videos 12.7 and 12.8):

Echo:

33. What is the most appropriate next step?

A. Give IV metoprolol and diuretics before intubation
B. IV volume resuscitation before intubation
C. Start norepinephrine and prepare inhaled pulmonary vasodilators before intubation
D. Proceed with urgent intubation

34. Which of the following statements best describes the most likely hemodynamic effects of initiation of positive pressure ventilation in the patient above?

A. PPV will reduce LV afterload, increase LV preload and increase cardiac output.
B. PPV will cause an increase in transpulmonary pressure, increased RV afterload and a decrease in cardiac output.
C. Initiation of PPV will have minimal hemodynamic effects.
D. PPV will cause a sudden increase of intrathoracic pressure, a decrease RV preload and a drop in cardiac output.

Answer 33 C, Answer 34 B:

Explanation: Based on history and images provided there is concern the patient has pulmonary hypertension from ILD. The IVC is dilated without respiratory variation suggesting high central venous pressure with a dilated RV with septal flattening suggesting both pressure and volume overload. Given the history of ILD this patient also very likely has poor lung compliance. Initiation of PPV will increase alveolar pressure, with minimal increase in pleural pressure, thus increasing transpulmonary pressure (TPP) and therefore dramatically increasing RV afterload. The increase in TPP will increase RV afterload and decrease cardiac output. To minimize adverse effects of PPV in this patient, the best next step is to stabilize blood pressure with a vasopressor—Norepinephrine, and attempt to reduce PVR with a pulmonary vasodilator.

Question 35

A 74-year-old woman with depression, diabetes, hypertension, hyperlipidemia, COPD and chronic atrial fibrillation is admitted to your unit after being found unresponsive at home. She was intubated on arrival and is now passive on mechanical ventilation. Since intubation tachycardia and hypotension developed. HR 129, BP 85/44 mmHg, SpO_2 91% on FiO_2 of 60%, PEEP of 8, VT 500 mL, RR 24.

Bedside echo is attempted, but limited due to lung interference. Only subcostal long axis view can be obtained, which shows and IVC of 2.4 cm without respiratory variation.

Representative video of lung ultrasound is shown (Video 12.9). Similar ultrasound findings is observed in all lung fields.

What is the most appropriate next step?

A. Bilateral decompression thoracotomy
B. IV fluid bolus
C. D/C cardioversion
D. Check ET-tube position and auto-PEEP

Answer D. Check ET-tube position and auto-PEEP

Explanation: A plethoric IVC without respiratory variability suggest high pressure in the central venous system. Lung ultrasound shows A-line pattern and lung pulse. Bilateral lung pulse rules out tension pneumothorax, but A-lines with decreased lung sliding and inability to obtain cardiac view is suggestive of hyperinflation of the lungs, possibly due to auto PEEP. Therefore the plethoric IVC may be due to high intrathoracic pressure from auto-PEEP in the setting of obstructive lung disease ventilated with high tidal volume and respiratory rate or right main stem intubation [38, 39].

Question 36

A 50 y/o patient without known medical history is examined for syncope. He is asymptomatic, breathing room air at the time of the exam. Based on the image below which of the following statements is most accurate?

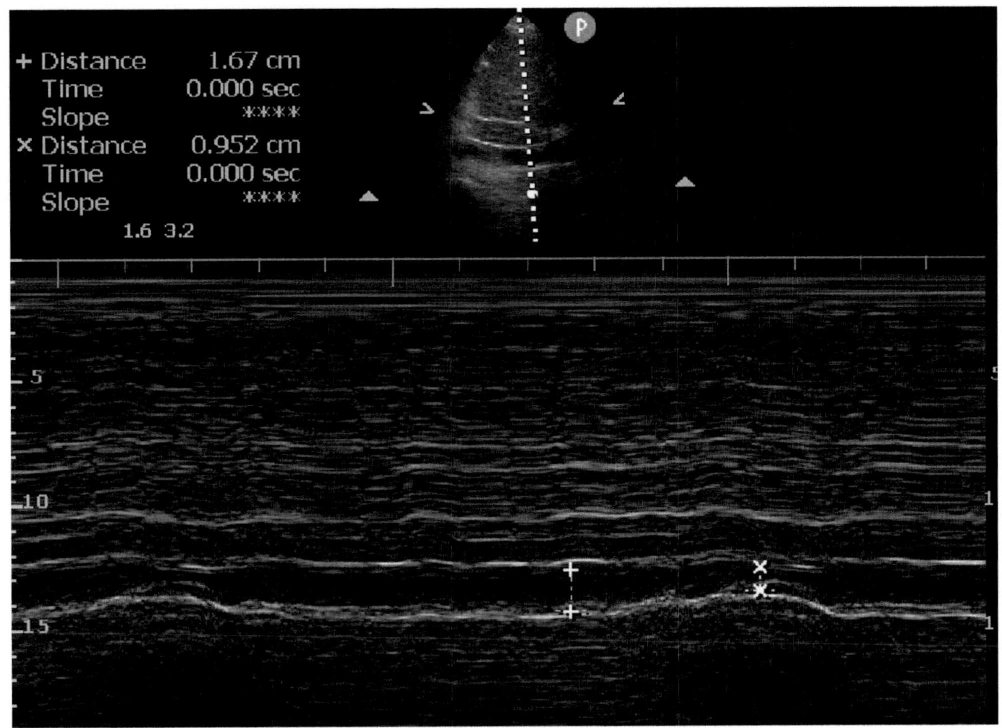

A. The IVC variability index is 43%
B. The IVC collapsibility index in 43%
C. The IVC dispensability index is 43%
D. The IVC variability index is 43%

Answer B. The IVC collapsibility index in 43%

Explanation: Passive Mechanically Ventilated patient.

Variability index (IVCmax – IVCmin)/IVCmean = (IVCmax – IVCmin)/(IVCmax + IVCmin)/2

Distensibility index (IVCmax – IVCmin)/IVCmin

Spontaneously Breathing patient.

Collapsibility index (IVCmax – IVCmin)/IVCmax

Cyclical changes in intrathoracic pressure induce changes in RAP, which alters venous return. In spontaneously breathing patients, intrathoracic pressure decreases during inspiration, leading to IVC collapse. During controlled ventilation, the IVC expands in inspiration because of increased intrathoracic pressure, and thus right atrial pressure. Echocardiographic assessment of IVC variability through the respiratory cycle can be used to predict response to fluid resuscitation. IVC variability can be expressed as variability index or dispensability index in passive mechanically ventilated patient and collapsibility index in spontaneously breathing patient. As the patient is breathing spontaneously on RA, the measurement is collapsibility index.

Question 37

You evaluate a 65-year-old man with ARDS secondary to pneumonia for worsening hemodynamics. HR 101 bpm, BP 98/55 mmHg. He is passive on mechanical ventilation, respiratory rate 22 breaths per minute, PEEP 10, FiO_2 60%, VT 500 mL, plateau pressure 34 cmH_2O, ABG 7.31; pCO_2 47 mmHg, PO_2 81 mmHg.

What is the most appropriate next step?

A. Decrease PEEP
B. Decrease VT
C. Fluid challenge
D. Start diuresis

Answer B. Decrease VT

Explanation: Four parameters have been identified as significant predictors of Right-Ventricular-Dysfunction (RVD) in ARDS: (1) lower respiratory tract infection as a cause of pulmonary ARDS, (2) PaO_2 to FiO_2 ratio <150 mmHg, (3) $PaCO_2$ >48 mmHg, and (4) driving pressure (plateau pressure – total positive end-expiratory pressure) >18 cmH_2O.

High tidal volumes lead to high driving and plateaus pressures. This in turn causes high transpulmonary pressures and overdistention of the alveoli during inspiration. High transpulmonary pressures compresses alveolar vessels and increased pulmonary vascular resistance, contributing to RVD in in ARDS.

In this vignette, both plateau and driving pressures are high and decreasing VT may lead to improvements in both [7, 40, 41].

Questions 38 and 39

A 65 y/o obese man with COPD, diabetes mellitus type 2, hypertension, hyperlipidemia, and peripheral vascular disease was admitted several days ago for hematemesis from a gastric ulcer. He was intubated on admission for airway protection and EGD. He was hypotensive and required several blood transfusions on the day of admission, but has been hemodynamically stable since. A bedside echocardiogram showed mild left ventricular hypertrophy, with normal right and left ventricular systolic function, trace mitral regurgitation. A Spontaneous Breathing Trial (SBT) is started, and the patient develops tachypnea, and tachycardia. HR 105 bpm BP 186/92 mmHg and SpO_2 is 96%.

Repeat Echocardiogram shows unchanged RV/LV size and function, mild mitral regurgitation with an average E/e′ of 15.5.

What is the most appropriate next step?

A. Stop SBT, optimize afterload, diurese and evaluate for ischemia
B. Stop SBT start dobutamine
C. Stop SBT and plan early tracheostomy
D. Start levosimendan

Answer A. Stop SBT, optimize afterload, diurese and evaluate for ischemia

Which of the following is true regarding weaning failure in the patient above?

A. Weaning failure of cardiac origin is unlikely in the absence of structural heart disease.
B. A positive passive leg raise (increase in LVOT-VI >10%) prior to SBT predicts failure to wean.
C. Increase in E′ during weaning is predictive of failure to wean
D. Increased work of breathing during the SBT can unmask previously undetected diastolic dysfunction
E. All of above

Answer E. All of above

Explanation: The patient in this vignette has several risk factors for weaning failure of cardiovascular origin. COPD, obesity and preexisting structural heart disease and diastolic dysfunction have been shown to be risk factors. Weaning from positive pressure ventilation increases left ventricular preload and afterload, it increases work of breathing and increases myocardial oxygen consumption. An SBT is in essence a cardiac stress test and even in the absence of known heart disease can unmask dysfunction and precipitate acute ischemia. Elevated LVEDP as assessed by bedside echocardiography before or during weaning has been shown to correlate with failure to wean or post extubation respiratory failure with high sensitivity and specificity. A negative passive leg raise (failure to increase CO by >10%) prior to SBT can predicted weaning failure due to cardiovascular dysfunction with a sensitivity of 97% and specificity of 81% [42–47].

Question 40

An otherwise healthy 27-year-old man was admitted with anaphylaxis after bee sting to the face. Severe facial and oropharyngeal edema required intubation with a 5.0 endotracheal tube. By day 3 of his ICU stay, he has been hemodynamically stable for over 24 h and the swelling has completely resolved. On a continuous infusion of fentanyl and propofol he is calm and ventilating well on pressure control ventilation (PEEP 5, driving pressure 10). Sedation is discontinued and an SBT is started on CPAP of 5 cmH_2O. Shortly after the patient becomes agitated, is biting on the ET tube and develops tachypnea, tachycardia, and hypoxia. The SBT is terminated, and sedation restarted.

Lung ultrasound shows B-line pattern. Bedside Echo shows grossly normal RV/LV size and function. LVOT diameter 2.1 cm, LVOT VTI 18.5 cm, MV peak E velocity 74 cm/s, MV peak A velocity 51 cm/s, medial mitral annulus e′ velocity 16.1 cm/s, lateral mitral annulus e′ velocity 16.7 cm/s, IVC maximal diameter is 1.5 cm during expiration and a minimal diameter of 0.9 cm during inspiration.

The next day the team plans to repeat the SBT.

Repeat Echocardiogram is essentially unchanged, lung US shows A lines.

On low dose fentanyl infusion, the patient is calm, follows commands and is tolerating pressure control ventilation with PEEP 5 and driving pressure of 8 cmH_2O.

What is the most appropriate next step?

A. Start beta blocker and diuresis
B. Initiate workup for cardiac ischemia
C. Initiate antibiotics ventilator associated pneumonia
D. Extubate the patient

Answer D. Extubate the patient

Explanation: The patient in this scenario likely developed negative pressure pulmonary edema due to strong inspiratory effort against high airway resistance. Profoundly negative swings in intrathoracic pressure (ITP) commonly occur during forced spontaneous inspiratory efforts in patients with airway obstruction, such as biting on a small ET tube, bronchospasm, laryngospasm etc. The fact that the

IVC collapses during inspiration suggests that despite positive pressure ventilation, the patient generates enough inspiratory effort, that the pleural pressure becomes negative.

Highly negative ITP swings also selectively increase LV afterload, which has been shown to contribute to pulmonary edema, even in the absence of underlying heart disease [29].

Question 41

A 65-year-old man with unknown medical history is passive on mechanical ventilation with 6 mL/kg ideal body weight.

Which of the following is most accurately predicts increase in cardiac output by >10% following a fluid bolus?

A. Respiratory variation of stroke volume assessed by LVOT-VTI of 11%
B. IVC distensibility index of 11%
C. CVP <8 mmHg
D. Increase of LVOT-VTI by 11% after passive leg raise

Answer D. Increase of LVOT-VTI by 11% after passive leg raise

Explanation: Static parameters such as CVP or PACWP measure preload but cannot predict a patient's response to increase in preload without knowing the shape of the Frank-Starling curve for this specific patient. Dynamic parameters of fluid responsiveness (stroke volume variation, end-expiratory occlusion test, response to PLR) are all more specific then static parameters. However, each test has specific limitations (see table). There are few contraindications to performing a PLR and it can be used where other methods fail (arrhythmias, ARDS, low tidal volume ventilation, spontaneously breathing). Pooled analysis of 50 trials with over 2000 patients showed that augmentation of cardiac output following a passive leg raise is highly predictive of fluid responsiveness, with a positive LR of 11 and a pooled specificity of >92% [12, 25, 48, 49].

Method	Threshold (%)	Limitations
PPV/SVV	12	Cannot be used in spontaneous breathing, cardiac arrhythmias, low VT, low lung compliance
IVC variation	12	Not in spontaneous breathing, low VT
SVC variation	36	Requires TEE, not in spontaneous breathing
PLR	10	Direct measurement of cardiac output within 1 min
Fluid challenge 500 cc	15	May contribute to fluid overload
End-expiratory occlusion test (EEOT)	5	Requires intubated patient, able to tolerate 15 s inspiratory hold
Combined end-inspiratory/end-expiratory occlusion test	13	Requires intubated patient, able to tolerate inspiratory and expiratory hold

Question 42

An end-expiratory occlusion test is performed in the above patient. Cardiac output assessment based on LVOT-VTI increased from 3.5 to 3.74 L/min. What is the most appropriate next step?

A. The patient is fluid responsive, give fluids
B. The patient is not fluid responsive, place a central line and start norepinephrine
C. Perform both end-expiratory and end-inspiratory occlusion test
D. Echocardiography lacks sensitivity to assess changes in cardiac output in response to end-inspiratory and end-expiratory occlusion tests and alternative measures to assess fluid responsiveness should be used

Answer C. Perform both end-expiratory and end-inspiratory occlusion test

The reported threshold to detect fluid responsiveness with the end-expiratory occlusion test is 5%. This is below the precision threshold reported for cardiac output measurement using TTE. Jozwiak et al. assessed accuracy and reproducibility of various TTE measures in critically ill patients. They concluded 10% to be the least significant change, i.e. the minimum change that can be considered significant and not due to imprecision of the measurement of LVOT-VTI. The change in CO in the question stem is above 5%—which suggests the patient is fluid responsive, but below the 10% least-significant-change threshold of TTE. The same group of authors demonstrated that by combining the sum of absolute values of changes in velocity-time integral during both end-inspiratory and end-expiratory occlusions, fluid responsiveness could be assessed using a threshold of 13%. This threshold is within the precision of transthoracic echocardiography and allowed assessment of fluid responsiveness with both sensitivity and specificity above 90% [36, 50].

Question 43

A 37-year-old woman is admitted for sepsis from pyelonephritis. On presentation she was encephalopathic and febrile. HR was 128 bpm, BP 83/47 mmHg, with lactic acid level of 2.8 mmol/L and serum creatinine of 1.6 from baseline 0.9. She has been started on empiric antibiotics and has received 30 mL/kg of crystalloids and an arterial line is inserted for close monitoring. By the time a Critical Care Echocardiogram is performed the heart rate HR is 98 bpm, BP 105/60 mmHg, repeat lactic acid is 1.8. On exam the patient is alert and oriented, capillary refill is less than 3 seconds and she has made 80 mL of urine in the last hour.

IVC diameter end expiration 1.8 cm, IVC diameter inspiration 1.4 cm.

Pulse pressure variation on the arterial line wave form is 14%.

What is the most appropriate next step?

A. Based on pulse pressure variation, this patient should be given a fluid bolus
B. Start Norepinephrine
C. Based on IVC variability of >20% this patient should receive a fluid bolus
D. Continue antibiotic therapy and monitor clinically

Answer D. Continue antibiotic therapy and monitor clinically

Explanation: The goal for fluid resuscitation in septic shock is to improve organ perfusion and oxygen utilization by increasing cardiac output and oxygen delivery. However, excess fluid is associated with excess risk of death in patients with sepsis. After initial resuscitation, additional fluid resuscitation is only indicated if the patient has both evidence of tissue hypoperfusion and will likely increase cardiac output in response to additional fluid—i.e. is "fluid responsive". Clinically, the patient appears to have restored organ perfusion (normal mentation, decreased lactate, normal capillary refill and improved urine output). Additional administration of IV fluid in this case is unlikely to improve organ function, indeed may lead to iatrogenic fluid overload which is associated with poor outcomes.

Pulse pressure variation, a surrogate of stroke volume variation, accurately predicts response to fluid in patients who are passive on mechanical ventilation. In active breathing it is highly dependent on respiratory effort, therefore highly variable and in-accurate. Should not be used to predict response to fluid loading in spontaneously breathing patients.

Similarly, IVC size and collapsibility has been extensively studied to assess fluid responsiveness in spontaneously breathing patients. Recent meta-analysis of various studies of IV variability have shown IVC size and variability to be relatively poor predictors of response to fluid loading. Only very high variability (cIVC >39–42%) and standardized inspiratory effort have been shown to be accurate in predicting a positive response in cardiac output [51–55].

Question 44

A 47-year-old woman is admitted with septic shock from lobar pneumonia. Empiric antibiotics and 30 mL/kg of crystalloids have been given. She remains tachycardic (HR 103 bpm), tachypneic (RR 28), hypotensive, oliguric and mildly encephalopathic. Lactic acid remains elevated at 4.3 mmol/L.

Echocardiogram shows normal RV size and function, and a small, hyperdynamic LV.

LVOT diameter 1.8 cm, LVOT VTI 26.5 cm, MV peak E velocity 98 cm/s, MV peak A velocity 69 cm/s, medial mitral annulus e′ velocity 15.5 cm/s, lateral e′ velocity 17.3 cm/s, IVC end expiration 2.9 cm, IVC early inspiration 2.7 cm.

What is the most appropriate next step?

A. Start Norepinephrine
B. Assess respiratory variation of LVOT VTI
C. Fluid challenge and repeat LVOT VTI
D. Fluid challenge and re-assess E/e′

Answer A. Start Norepinephrine

Explanation: The patient in this case has normal right and left ventricular function with a high VTI/cardiac output. While IVC variability has overall poor predictive value for fluid responsiveness in spontaneous breathing, an IVC of 2.8 cm and above has a high negative predictive value for fluid responsiveness. Given the already high cardiac output and dilated IVC it is unlikely that additional fluid loading would further increase cardiac output in this patient.

Respiratory variation of stroke volume and peak aortic velocity should not be used to assess fluid responsiveness in spontaneously breathing patients.

Left atrial pressure alone—either measure by PA catheter or estimated using E/e′—is also a poor predictor of response to fluid therapy [53, 56].

Question 45

A 38-year-old man without known medical history is found down in the field. On arrival to your department he is intubated, given empiric antibiotics and 2 L of crystalloids for hypotension. ABG after intubation shows a pH of 6.9, pCO_2 of 38 pO_2 189. Ventilator settings are adjusted to VT 500, RR 38, PEEP 8.

Respirophasic variation of VTI: max VTI 19.4, min VTI 18.9.

The patient remains hypotensive with MAP 62 mmHg and HR 89 bpm.

Which of the following is the most appropriate statement regarding fluid responsiveness based on respiratory variation of VTI in this patient?

A. The patient is fluid responsive
B. Decrease RR to determine fluid responsiveness
C. The patient is not fluid responsive
D. Fluid responsiveness cannot be determined without an accurate measurement of LVOT diameter.

Answer B. Decrease RR to determine fluid responsiveness

Explanation: Respiratory variation of stroke volume depends on the combined effect of PPV on RV and LV preload. During PPV inspiration, there is a simultaneously increase in LV preload from increased pulmonary vein drainage and decrease in RV preload from decreased venous return. This leads to an initial increase in LV stroke volume during inspiration, followed within a few beats to a decrease LV stroke volume. The pulmonary transit time is usually 3–4 beats and is dependent on heart rate. At high respiratory rates, the effect of increased pulmonary venous drainage and decreased RV stroke volume during inspiration may merge, abolishing respiratory variation of stroke volume. De Backer et al. demonstrated that stroke volume variation becomes negligible if the HR to RR ratio decreases below 3.6 [57].

Question 46

A previously healthy 28-year-old man is intubated and sedated in the ICU following a motor vehicle accident. He has external fixation of complex lower extremity fractures and is being monitored for elevated Intra-cranial pressure. Over the past 2 h, his MAP has dropped from 75 to 63 mmHg and his urine output has decreased to 20 mL/h.

He is passively ventilated with a tidal volume of VT 6 mL/kg and is in normal sinus rhythm.

An arterial line, central venous catheter and ICP monitor are in place. CVP is 6 mmHg and ICP is 14 mmHg with a MAP of 63 mmHg with a pulse pressure variation (PPV) of 11%.

Which of the following is the most accurate statement regarding expected cardiac output response to an IV fluid bolus in this patient?

A. Based on pulse pressure variation the patient is not fluid responsive, no fluid should be given
B. Increase of PPV to 18% after a tidal volume challenge suggests fluid responsiveness
C. The patient is fluid responsive, give 500 mL of crystalloid bolus and reassess PPV
D. Fluid responsiveness should be assessed by LVOT–VTI before and after a passive leg raise

Answer B. Increase of PPV to 18% after a tidal volume challenge suggests fluid responsiveness

Explanation: PPV has been extensively studied and can predict fluid responsiveness with high accuracy. Although, there are many limitations that will render PPV invalid, such as low VT ventilation, poor lung compliance as in ARDS, active respiratory effort, and atrial fibrillation. This patient is passive, in sinus rhythm, and has no indication of poor lung compliance or intra-abdominal HTN, so PPV can be used to predict fluid responsiveness. He has a PPV of 11%, which is within a "a grey zone" of indeterminate significance. The predictive value of the PPV can be increased using a "tidal volume challenge". An increase of PPV by >3.5% or an increase in SVV of >2.5% during a brief period of passive ventilation at a higher tidal volume of 8–12 mL/kg has been shown to accurately predict fluid responsiveness. Passive leg raise has repeatedly been shown to accurately predict fluid responsiveness under conditions that render PPV and SVV inaccurate (arrhythmias, low tidal volume ventilation, ARDS, spontaneous breathing). Elevated ICP and lower extremity pathology, such as unstable fractures in this case, however are contraindications to PLR [48, 58, 59].

Question 47

You evaluate a 47-year-old man who just underwent ERCP for cholangitis and gallstone pancreatitis. The patient is passive on mechanical ventilation. VT 6 mL/kg, PEEP 8, FiO_2 30%, RR 20, Pplat 31. Over the past 4 h, his urine output has decreased to <10 mL/h, lactic acid level has increased from 1.8 to 2.8 mmol/L. Norepinephrine was started to maintain MAP >65 mmHg.

On exam, the abdomen is tense, and sedation has recently increased due to abdominal pain.

Bedside echo shows small, hyperdynamic LV with "kissing ventricles" LVOT VTI is 19.8, IVCmax 1.3 cm without respiratory variation.

What is the most appropriate next step?

A. Give 500 cc bolus of crystalloids
B. Start esmolol and phenylephrine
C. Perform a passive leg raise
D. Check bladder pressure

Answer D. Check bladder pressure

Explanation: Intrabdominal hypertension is common in critically ill patients and may render assessment of fluid responsiveness using IVC and passive leg raise yield false negative results.

This patient is at risk for abdominal compartment syndrome. He has low compliance/high driving pressure (Pplat – PEEP of 23) with minimal oxygen requirement suggesting high abdominal pressure. Beurton et al. recently demonstrated that in the presence of intraabdominal hypertension (defined as end-expiratory bladder pressure >12 mmHg), the passive leg raise had a sensitivity and specificity of only 43% and 89% respectively. The authors concluded elevated intraabdominal pressure may lead to decreased venous flow to the RA due to compression of the IVC and reduced capacitance of the splanchnic venous system. In the setting of known or suspected abdominal hypertension, alternatives to the PLR—such as a fluid challenge—may be more suitable to determine fluid responsiveness [21, 22, 60, 61].

Question 48

A 59-year-old woman with advanced breast cancer is admitted with septic shock and respiratory failure from pneumonia. She is on mechanical ventilation FiO_2 50%, Volume control, VT 400 mL, PEEP 10 cmH_2O. She is in sinus rhythm, HR 89 bpm. After initial fluid resuscitation of 3 L crystalloids, she is requiring moderate doses of norepinephrine to maintain MAP >65 mmHg.

Bedside echocardiogram shows a moderate pericardial effusion. IVC 2.4 cm without respiratory variability.

Doppler evaluation of mitral and tricuspid valve inflow velocities through multiple respiratory cycles shows 18% variation of peak mitral valve e-wave velocity and 35% variation of peak tricuspid valve e-wave velocity.

What is the most appropriate next step?

A. Perform pericardiocentesis
B. Continue current therapy
C. Place a pulmonary artery catheter to assess for tamponade physiology
D. Give fluids

Answer C. Place a pulmonary artery catheter to assess for tamponade physiology

Explanation: Classic echocardiographic findings of tamponade physiology are distorted by mechanical ventilation. Respiratory variability of E-wave velocities of the tricuspid and mitral valves are exaggerated in tamponade during spontaneous breathing, but may be absent in mechanical ventilation. Absence of MV or TV E-wave variability should not be used to rule out tamponade physiology in patients on mechanical ventilation [62]. Pulmonary artery catheter showing equalization of the diastolic pressures across all chambers without respiratory variation is highly diagnostic of tamponade physiology.

Question 49

A 57-year-old man with diabetes mellitus, hypertension and end stage renal disease was admitted 72 h ago with ARDS and septic shock from pneumonia. After initial fluid resuscitation and initiation of empiric antibiotics he remains on norepinephrine and mechanical ventilation (PEEP 12 cmH_2O, VT of 6 mL/kg IBW, FiO_2 of 50%). He is currently in normal sinus rhythm with a heart rate of 95 bpm, BP 98/56 mmHg on NE 0.07 μg/kg/min (unchanged in the past 6 h).

Current lactate level is 1.9 mmol/L and central venous SpO_2 is 69%. Due to hypotension, renal replacement therapy has not yet been initiated.

A passive leg raise is performed. LVOT VTI before PLR 18.1 cm, LVOT VTI 1 min after passive leg raise changes to 19.2 cm.

What is the most appropriate next step?

A. Give 100 mL fluid challenge and re-assess VTI
B. Volume resuscitation with 1000 mL of crystalloids
C. Initiate renal replacement therapy
D. Continue current care

Answer C. Initiate renal replacement therapy

Explanation: Cumulative fluid balance is an independent predictor of mortality in sepsis and ARDS. A conservative fluid strategy has been shown to reduce time on mechanical ventilation. Fluid removal has been shown to reduce extrapulmonary lung volume and other volume indices. Concerns over hemodynamic instability may lead to delayed initiation of RRT and fluid removal. Decrease in cardiac output as an adverse effect of excessive fluid removal should occur in the case of preload dependence, i.e. when changes in cardiac preload physiologically result in changes in cardiac output. Changes in cardiac Index induced by passive leg raise have been shown to predict intradialytic hypotension with good sensitivity and specificity. Using a threshold of 9%, PLR has a positive and negative predictive value of 91% and 89% respectively [63, 64].

Question 50

A 78-year-old male with CAD, systolic heart failure with LV systolic function as shown in Video 12.10 comes to the ICU with acute hypoxic respiratory failure likely due to acute pulmonary edema for heart failure exacerbation. He is in visible respiratory distress with a RR of 38/min and appears confused. You want to intubate the patient. BP is 188/98, HR 118/min, Lactate is 4.3.

Which one of the following options is correct for this patient?

A. Immediately after intubation the LV preload will decrease, and LV afterload will decrease
B. After intubation the intrathoracic pressure will abruptly rise causing the LV afterload to increase
C. After intubation the intraventricular septum will abruptly shift causing a drop in CO
D. No change

Answer: A. Immediately after intubation the LV preload will decrease, and LV afterload will decrease

Explanation: Positive pressure ventilation leads to increased intratoracic pressure (ITP), which is transmitted to the right atrium, and RV preload decreases. This drop in RV preload eventually leads to decrease in LV preload too. An increase in ITP decreases LV afterload by decreasing the LV transmural pressure gradient. The impact of these changes on cardiac output is determined by the load dependency of the heart. In preload dependent heart, PPV will cause drop in stroke volume and cardiac output. In an afterload dependent heart, reduction in afterload will improve cardiac output.

Question 51

You are about to perform a PLR in a patient who is intubated but awake, to assess for fluid responsiveness. The patient weighs 300 lb. You should do the following except:

A. Perform a 2 person PLR with you lifting one leg and another person lifting the second leg
B. Carefully suction the bronchial secretions before the test
C. Inform the patient about the move
D. Carefully monitor heart rate during the maneuver

Answer: A. Perform a 2 person PLR with you lifting one leg and another person lifting the second leg

Explanation: Pain, discomfort, cough and awakening during the maneuver can cause sympathetic stimulation leading to tachycardia which can lead to mistaken cardiac output changes. Simple precautions to be taken before the maneuver. Patients should be informed prior to start of the test, PLR must be performed by adjusting the bed and not by manually raising the patient's legs, careful tracheal suctioning prior to the test to avoid coughing and monitoring heart rate before and during the maneuver [49].

Question 52

Which of the following is a reliable marker for assessing fluid responsiveness in mechanically ventilated-patients?

A. Assessing LVOT-VTI change on PLR
B. Assessing LVOT-VTI change on end-expiratory occlusion test
C. Respiratory variations of superior vena cava diameter
D. A and B
E. All the above

Answer: E. All the above

Explanation: All of-Positive pressure causes cyclical changes in the loading conditions of the right and left heart. These cyclical changes cause changes in stroke volume and hence the cardiac output in the preload-dependent heart. A positive response. This test has been widely accepted and validated as a method to assess fluid responsiveness [11]. In a large trial, Respiro phasic superior vena cava (ΔSVC) diameter changes of greater or equal to 21%, as assessed by trans-esophageal echocardiogram had a specificity of 84% in predicting fluid responsiveness [25]. LVOT-VTI increase of 9% on a 12 s end-expiratory occlusion test had a sensitivity and specificity of 89% and 95% respectively [65].

References

1. Vashisht R, Dugar S, Alappan N, Moghekar A. A woman with refractory hypoxemia. Chest. 2019;156(2):e33–5. https://doi.org/10.1016/j.chest.2019.03.044.
2. Vashisht R, Dugar S, Alappan N, Moghekar A. Acute orthodeoxia: evaluation using point-of-care ultrasound imaging. Ann Am Thorac Soc. 2017;14(4):594–6. https://doi.org/10.1513/AnnalsATS.201612-972CC.
3. Silvestry FE, Cohen MS, Armsby LB, Burkule NJ, Fleishman CE, Hijazi ZM, et al. Guidelines for the echocardiographic assessment of atrial septal defect and patent foramen ovale: from the American Society of Echocardiography and Society for Cardiac Angiography and Interventions. J Am Soc Echocardiogr. 2015;28(8):910–58. https://doi.org/10.1016/j.echo.2015.05.015.
4. Granati GT, Teressa G. Worsening hypoxemia in the face of increasing PEEP: a case of large pulmonary embolism in the setting of intracardiac shunt. Am J Case Rep. 2016;17:454–8. https://pubmed.ncbi.nlm.nih.gov/27377010.
5. Luecke T, Pelosi P. Clinical review: positive end-expiratory pressure and cardiac output. Crit Care. 2005;9(6):607–21. https://pubmed.ncbi.nlm.nih.gov/16356246.
6. Jardin F, Vieillard-Baron A. Is there a safe plateau pressure in ARDS? The right heart only knows. Intensive Care Med. 2007;33(3):444–7. https://doi.org/10.1007/s00134-007-0552-z.
7. Vieillard-Baron A, Rabiller A, Chergui K, Peyrouset O, Page B, Beauchet A, et al. Prone position improves mechanics and alveolar ventilation in acute respiratory distress syndrome. Intensive Care Med. 2005;31(2):220–6. https://doi.org/10.1007/s00134-004-2478-z.
8. Kumar A, Anel R, Bunnell E, Habet K, Zanotti S, Marshall S, et al. Pulmonary artery occlusion pressure and central venous pressure fail to predict ventricular filling volume, cardiac performance, or the response to volume infusion in normal subjects. Crit Care Med. 2004;32(3):691–9. https://journals.lww.com/ccmjournal/Fulltext/2004/03000/Pulmonary_artery_occlusion_pressure_and_central.12.aspx.
9. Marik PE, Cavallazzi R. Does the central venous pressure predict fluid responsiveness? An updated meta-analysis and a plea for some common sense. Crit Care Med. 2013;41(7):1774–81. https://journals.lww.com/ccmjournal/Fulltext/2013/07000/Does_the_Central_Venous_Pressure_Predict_Fluid.22.aspx.
10. Lanspa MJ, Grissom CK, Hirshberg EL, Jones JP, Brown SM. Applying dynamic parameters to predict hemodynamic response to volume expansion in spontaneously breathing patients with septic shock. Shock. 2013;39(2):155–60. https://doi.org/10.1097/SHK.0b013e31827f1c6a. PMID: 23324885; PMCID: PMC3580843.
11. Monnet X, Marik P, Teboul J-L. Passive leg raising for predicting fluid responsiveness: a systematic review and meta-analysis. Intensive Care Med. 2016;42(12):1935–47. https://doi.org/10.1007/s00134-015-4134-1.
12. Monnet X, Marik PE, Teboul J-L. Prediction of fluid responsiveness: an update. Ann Intensive Care. 2016;6(1):111. https://doi.org/10.1186/s13613-016-0216-7.
13. Monnet X, Teboul J-L. Assessment of volume responsiveness during mechanical ventilation: recent advances. Crit Care. 2013;17(2):217. https://pubmed.ncbi.nlm.nih.gov/23510457.
14. Hahn RG, Lyons G. The half-life of infusion fluids: an educational review. Eur J Anaesthesiol. 2016;33(7):475–82. https://pubmed.ncbi.nlm.nih.gov/27058509.
15. Martin GS, Eaton S, Mealer M, Moss M. Extravascular lung water in patients with severe sepsis: a prospective cohort study. Crit Care. 2005;9(2):R74–82. https://pubmed.ncbi.nlm.nih.gov/15774053.
16. Lichtenstein D. Fluid administration limited by lung sonography: the place of lung ultrasound in assessment of acute circulatory failure (the FALLS-protocol). Expert Rev Respir Med. 2012;6(2):155–62. https://doi.org/10.1586/ers.12.13.
17. Teboul JL, Monnet X, Chemla D, Michard F. Arterial pulse pressure variation with mechanical ventilation. Am J Respir Crit Care Med. 2019;199(1):22–31.
18. Wiklund CU, Morel DR, Orbring-Wiklund H, Romand J-A, Piriou V, Teboul J-L, et al. Influence of tidal volume on pulse pressure variations in hypovolemic ventilated pigs with acute respiratory distress-like syndrome. Anesthesiol J Am Soc. 2010;113(3):630–8. https://doi.org/10.1097/ALN.0b013e3181e908f6.
19. Muller L, Louart G, Bousquet P-J, Candela D, Zoric L, de La Coussaye J-E, et al. The influence of the airway driving pressure on pulsed pressure variation as a predictor of fluid responsiveness. Intensive Care Med. 2010;36(3):496–503. https://doi.org/10.1007/s00134-009-1686-y.
20. De Backer D, Heenen S, Piagnerelli M, Koch M, Vincent J-L. Pulse pressure variations to predict fluid responsiveness: influence of

tidal volume. Intensive Care Med. 2005;31(4):517–23. https://doi.org/10.1007/s00134-005-2586-4.
21. Vieillard-Baron A, Evrard B, Repessé X, Maizel J, Jacob C, Goudelin M, et al. Limited value of end-expiratory inferior vena cava diameter to predict fluid responsiveness impact of intra-abdominal pressure. Intensive Care Med. 2018;44(2):197–203. https://doi.org/10.1007/s00134-018-5067-2.
22. Mahjoub Y, Touzeau J, Airapetian N, Lorne E, Hijazi M, Zogheib E, et al. The passive leg-raising maneuver cannot accurately predict fluid responsiveness in patients with intra-abdominal hypertension. Crit Care Med. 2010;38(9):1824–9. https://journals.lww.com/ccmjournal/Fulltext/2010/09000/The_passive_leg_raising_maneuver_cannot_accurately.9.aspx.
23. Muller L, Toumi M, Bousquet P-J, Riu-Poulenc B, Louart G, Candela D, et al. An increase in aortic blood flow after an infusion of 100 ml colloid over 1 minute can predict fluid responsiveness: the mini-fluid challenge study. Anesthesiology. 2011;115(3):541–7. https://doi.org/10.1097/ALN.0b013e318229a500.
24. Mallat J, Meddour M, Durville E, Lemyze M, Pepy F, Temime J, et al. Decrease in pulse pressure and stroke volume variations after mini-fluid challenge accurately predicts fluid responsiveness†. Br J Anaesth. 2015;115(3):449–56. https://doi.org/10.1093/bja/aev222.
25. Vignon P, Repessé X, Begot E, Léger J, Jacob C, Bouferrache K, et al. Comparison of echocardiographic indices used to predict fluid responsiveness in ventilated patients. Am J Respir Crit Care Med. 2017;195(8):1022–32.
26. Zhang Z, Xu X, Ye S, Xu L. Ultrasonographic measurement of the respiratory variation in the inferior vena cava diameter is predictive of fluid responsiveness in critically ill patients: systematic review and meta-analysis. Ultrasound Med Biol. 2014;40(5):845–53. https://doi.org/10.1016/j.ultrasmedbio.2013.12.010.
27. Vieillard-Baron A, Chergui K, Rabiller A, Peyrouset O, Page B, Beauchet A, et al. Superior vena caval collapsibility as a gauge of volume status in ventilated septic patients. Intensive Care Med. 2004;30(9):1734–9. https://doi.org/10.1007/s00134-004-2361-y.
28. Magder S. Heart-lung interaction in spontaneous breathing subjects: the basics. Ann Transl Med. 2018;6(18):348. https://pubmed.ncbi.nlm.nih.gov/30370275.
29. Pinsky MR. Cardiopulmonary interactions: physiologic basis and clinical applications. Ann Am Thorac Soc. 2018;15(Suppl 1):S45–8. https://pubmed.ncbi.nlm.nih.gov/28820609.
30. Ginghina C, Beladan C, Iancu M, Calin A, Popescu BA. Respiratory maneuvers in echocardiography: a review of clinical applications. Cardiovasc Ultrasound. 2009;7:42.
31. No Title.
32. Porter TR, Shillcutt SK, Adams MS, Desjardins G, Glas KE, Olson JJ, et al. Guidelines for the use of echocardiography as a monitor for therapeutic intervention in adults: a report from the American Society of Echocardiography. J Am Soc Echocardiogr. 2015;28(1):40–56. https://doi.org/10.1016/j.echo.2014.09.009.
33. Brennan JM, Blair JE, Goonewardena S, Ronan A, Shah D, Vasaiwala S, et al. Reappraisal of the use of inferior vena cava for estimating right atrial pressure. J Am Soc Echocardiogr. 2007;20(7):857–61. https://doi.org/10.1016/j.echo.2007.01.005.
34. Rudski LG, Lai WW, Afilalo J, Hua L, Handschumacher MD, Chandrasekaran K, et al. Guidelines for the echocardiographic assessment of the right heart in adults: a report from the American Society of Echocardiography: endorsed by the European Association of Echocardiography, a registered branch of the European Society of Cardiology, and the Canadian Society of Echocardiography. J Am Soc Echocardiogr. 2010;23(7):685–713. https://doi.org/10.1016/j.echo.2010.05.010.
35. Michard F, Teboul JL. Using heart-lung interactions to assess fluid responsiveness during mechanical ventilation. Crit Care. 2000;4(5):282–9. https://pubmed.ncbi.nlm.nih.gov/11094507.
36. Jozwiak M, Depret F, Teboul J-L, Alphonsine J-E, Lai C, Richard C, et al. Predicting fluid responsiveness in critically ill patients by using combined end-expiratory and end-inspiratory occlusions with echocardiography. Crit Care Med. 2017;45(11):e1131–8. https://journals.lww.com/ccmjournal/Fulltext/2017/11000/Predicting_Fluid_Responsiveness_in_Critically_Ill.34.aspx.
37. Van Den Berg PCM, Jansen JRC, Pinsky MR. Effect of positive pressure on venous return in volume-loaded cardiac surgical patients. J Appl Physiol. 2002;92(3):1223–31. https://doi.org/10.1152/japplphysiol.00487.2001.
38. Narasimhan M, Koenig SJ, Mayo PH. A whole-body approach to point of care ultrasound. Chest. 2016;150(4):772–6. https://doi.org/10.1016/j.chest.2016.07.040.
39. Volpicelli G, Elbarbary M, Blaivas M, Lichtenstein DA, Mathis G, Kirkpatrick AW, et al. International evidence-based recommendations for point-of-care lung ultrasound. Intensive Care Med. 2012;38(4):577–91. https://doi.org/10.1007/s00134-012-2513-4.
40. Zochios V, Parhar K, Tunnicliffe W, Roscoe A, Gao F. The right ventricle in ARDS. Chest. 2017;152(1):181–93. https://doi.org/10.1016/j.chest.2017.02.019.
41. Mekontso Dessap A, Boissier F, Charron C, Bégot E, Repessé X, Legras A, et al. Acute cor pulmonale during protective ventilation for acute respiratory distress syndrome: prevalence, predictors, and clinical impact. Intensive Care Med. 2016;42(5):862–70. https://doi.org/10.1007/s00134-015-4141-2.
42. Vignon P. Cardiovascular failure and weaning. Ann Transl Med. 2018;6(18):354. http://atm.amegroups.com/article/view/19970.
43. Routsi C, Stanopoulos I, Kokkoris S, Sideris A, Zakynthinos S. Weaning failure of cardiovascular origin: how to suspect, detect and treat—a review of the literature. Ann Intensive Care. 2019;9:6.
44. Liu J, Shen F, Teboul J-L, Anguel N, Beurton A, Bezaz N, et al. Cardiac dysfunction induced by weaning from mechanical ventilation: incidence, risk factors, and effects of fluid removal. Crit Care. 2016;20(1):369. https://pubmed.ncbi.nlm.nih.gov/27836002.
45. Dres M, Teboul J-L, Anguel N, Guerin L, Richard C, Monnet X. Passive leg raising performed before a spontaneous breathing trial predicts weaning-induced cardiac dysfunction. Intensive Care Med. 2015;41(3):487–94. https://doi.org/10.1007/s00134-015-3653-0.
46. Moschietto S, Doyen D, Grech L, Dellamonica J, Hyvernat H, Bernardin G. Transthoracic echocardiography with Doppler tissue imaging predicts weaning failure from mechanical ventilation: evolution of the left ventricle relaxation rate during a spontaneous breathing trial is the key factor in weaning outcome. Crit Care. 2012;16(3):R81. https://pubmed.ncbi.nlm.nih.gov/22583512.
47. Lamia B, Maizel J, Ochagavia A, Chemla D, Osman D, Richard C, et al. Echocardiographic diagnosis of pulmonary artery occlusion pressure elevation during weaning from mechanical ventilation. Crit Care Med. 2009;37(5):1696–701. https://journals.lww.com/ccmjournal/Fulltext/2009/05000/Echocardiographic_diagnosis_of_pulmonary_artery.22.aspx.
48. Bentzer P, Griesdale DE, Boyd J, MacLean K, Sirounis D, Ayas NT. Will this hemodynamically unstable patient respond to a bolus of intravenous fluids? JAMA. 2016;316(12):1298–309. https://doi.org/10.1001/jama.2016.12310.
49. Monnet X, Teboul J-L. Passive leg raising: five rules, not a drop of fluid! Crit Care. 2015;19(1):18. https://doi.org/10.1186/s13054-014-0708-5.
50. Jozwiak M, Mercado P, Teboul J-L, Benmalek A, Gimenez J, Dépret F, et al. What is the lowest change in cardiac output that transthoracic echocardiography can detect? Crit Care. 2019;23(1):116. https://doi.org/10.1186/s13054-019-2413-x.
51. Airapetian N, Maizel J, Alyamani O, Mahjoub Y, Lorne E, Levrard M, et al. Does inferior vena cava respiratory variability predict fluid responsiveness in spontaneously breathing patients? Crit Care. 2015;19:400. https://pubmed.ncbi.nlm.nih.gov/26563768.
52. Sakr Y, Rubatto Birri PN, Kotfis K, Nanchal R, Shah B, Kluge S, et al. Higher fluid balance increases the risk of death from sepsis: results from a large international audit. Crit Care Med. 2017;45(3):386–94. https://journals.lww.com/ccmjournal/

Fulltext/2017/03000/Higher_Fluid_Balance_Increases_the_Risk_of_Death.2.aspx.
53. Long E, Oakley E, Duke T, Babl FE, (PREDICT) on behalf of the PR in EDIC. Does respiratory variation in inferior vena cava diameter predict fluid responsiveness: a systematic review and meta-analysis. Shock. 2017;47(5):550–9. https://journals.lww.com/shockjournal/Fulltext/2017/05000/Does_Respiratory_Variation_in_Inferior_Vena_Cava.3.aspx.
54. Orso D, Paoli I, Piani T, Cilenti FL, Cristiani L, Guglielmo N. Accuracy of ultrasonographic measurements of inferior vena cava to determine fluid responsiveness: a systematic review and meta-analysis. J Intensive Care Med. 2018;35(4):354–63. https://doi.org/10.1177/0885066617752308.
55. Bortolotti P, Colling D, Colas V, Voisin B, Dewavrin F, Poissy J, et al. Respiratory changes of the inferior vena cava diameter predict fluid responsiveness in spontaneously breathing patients with cardiac arrhythmias. Ann Intensive Care. 2018;8(1):79. https://pubmed.ncbi.nlm.nih.gov/30073423.
56. De Backer D, Fagnoul D. Intensive care ultrasound: VI. Fluid responsiveness and shock assessment. Ann Am Thorac Soc. 2014;11(1):129–36. https://doi.org/10.1513/AnnalsATS.201309-320OT.
57. De Backer D, Taccone FS, Holsten R, Ibrahimi F, Vincent J-L. Influence of respiratory rate on stroke volume variation in mechanically ventilated patients. Anesthesiology. 2009;110(5):1092–7. https://doi.org/10.1097/ALN.0b013e31819db2a1.
58. Myatra SN, Prabu NR, Divatia JV, Monnet X, Kulkarni AP, Teboul J-L. The changes in pulse pressure variation or stroke volume variation after a "tidal volume challenge" reliably predict fluid responsiveness during low tidal volume ventilation. Crit Care Med. 2017;45(3):415–21. https://journals.lww.com/ccmjournal/Fulltext/2017/03000/The_Changes_in_Pulse_Pressure_Variation_or_Stroke.5.aspx.
59. Cannesson M, Le Manach Y, Hofer CK, Goarin JP, Lehot J-J, Vallet B, et al. Assessing the diagnostic accuracy of pulse pressure variations for the prediction of fluid responsiveness: a "gray zone" approach. Anesthesiology. 2011;115(2):231–41. https://doi.org/10.1097/ALN.0b013e318225b80a.
60. Beurton A, Teboul J-L, Girotto V, Galarza L, Anguel N, Richard C, et al. Intra-abdominal hypertension is responsible for false negatives to the passive leg raising test. Crit Care Med. 2019;47(8):e639–47. https://journals.lww.com/ccmjournal/Fulltext/2019/08000/Intra_Abdominal_Hypertension_Is_Responsible_for.30.aspx.
61. Via G, Tavazzi G, Price S. Ten situations where inferior vena cava ultrasound may fail to accurately predict fluid responsiveness: a physiologically based point of view. Intensive Care Med. 2016;42(7):1164–7. https://doi.org/10.1007/s00134-016-4357-9.
62. Faehnrich JA, Noone RB Jr, White WD, Leone BJ, Hilton AK, Sreeram GM, et al. Effects of positive-pressure ventilation, pericardial effusion, and cardiac tamponade on respiratory variation in transmitral flow velocities. J Cardiothorac Vasc Anesth. 2003;17(1):45–50. https://doi.org/10.1053/jcan.2003.9.
63. Monnet X, Cipriani F, Camous L, Sentenac P, Dres M, Krastinova E, et al. The passive leg raising test to guide fluid removal in critically ill patients. Ann Intensive Care. 2016;6(1):46. https://doi.org/10.1186/s13613-016-0149-1.
64. De Laet I, Deeren D, Schoonheydt K, Van Regenmortel N, Dits H, Malbrain ML. Renal replacement therapy with net fluid removal lowers intra-abdominal pressure and volumetric indices in critically ill patients. Ann Intensive Care. 2012;2 Suppl 1(Suppl 1):S20. https://pubmed.ncbi.nlm.nih.gov/23282287.
65. Georges D, de Courson H, Lanchon R, Sesay M, Nouette-Gaulain K, Biais M. End-expiratory occlusion maneuver to predict fluid responsiveness in the intensive care unit: an echocardiographic study. Crit Care. 2018;22(1):32. https://pubmed.ncbi.nlm.nih.gov/29415773.

13 Lung Ultrasonography

Enrico Boero, Ana Luisa Silveira Vieira, Serena Rovida, and Giovanni Volpicelli

Question 1

A 57-year-old male patient with a history of chronic obstructive pulmonary disease (COPD) and chronic heart failure (CHF) is admitted to the emergency department (ED) complaining of progressive dyspnea and desaturation for 3 days. During the first visit a bedside lung ultrasound is performed. The video 13.1 shows the ultrasound findings detected in the evaluation of all chest areas, bilaterally:

What did the ultrasound image find and its clinical correlation in this patient?

A. A lines + lung sliding; to rule out lung diseases.
B. A lines + lung sliding; compatible with COPD exacerbation.
C. B lines + lung sliding; compatible with decompensated heart failure.
D. B lines + lung sliding; compatible with viral pneumonia.

Supplementary Information The online version contains supplementary material available at https://doi.org/10.1007/978-3-031-45731-9_13.

E. Boero (✉)
Department of Anesthesiology and Intensive Care, San Giovanni Bosco Hospital, Turin, Italy

A. L. Silveira Vieira
Department of Point of Care Ultrasound, Faculty of Medicine of Barbacena, Barbacena, Minas Gerais, Brazil

S. Rovida
Department of Emergency and Trauma Center, Linköping University, Linköping, Sweden

G. Volpicelli
Emergency Medicine, Department of Medical and Surgical Science, Magna Graecia University, Catanzaro, Italy

Answer: **B.**

Key point: A combination of A-lines plus lung sliding diffusely present on both sides is a pattern indicating normal or excessive content of air in the alveolar space.

Rationale: A-lines are horizontal hyperechoic line artifacts that reverberate at fixed intervals from the pleural line. The A-lines appear at the same distance between the probe and the pleural line. The combination "A-lines plus lung sliding" is a sign of normal or excessive content of air in the peripheral alveolar spaces. In situations where these findings are diffuse and bilateral it is compatible with normal lung or hyperinflated lungs as observed in COPD [1].

Question 2

Eighty-two-year-old woman is admitted in the ED complaining of dyspnea, cough and fever. A bedside lung ultrasound is performed. The video 13.2 shows multiple and coalescent B-lines limited to the bases of the right lung.

How are B-lines generated?

A. B-lines are artifacts of reverberation generated by the hyperinflation of the peripheral alveoli.
B. B-lines are generated when there is a great difference in acoustic impedance between pleura and aerated alveoli.
C. B-lines are generated when the acoustic mismatch between the lung and the surrounding tissues are lowered due to air content decrease and increase in lung density.
D. B-lines are generated when the lung becomes consolidated.

Answer: **C.**

Key point: B-lines are generated when there is increase in lung density.

Rationale: B-lines are defined as discrete laser-like vertical hyperechoic reverberation artifacts that arise from the pleural line, extend to the bottom of the screen without fading and move synchronously with lung sliding. When the density of the lung increases due to exudate, transudate,

R. Sreedharan et al. (eds.), *Critical Care Echocardiography*, https://doi.org/10.1007/978-3-031-45731-9_13

collagen, blood, with consequent decrease in the air content, the acoustic mismatch between the lung and the surrounding tissues are lowered and the ultrasound beam is reflected repeatedly, creating this kind of comet-tail artifacts, known as B-lines [2–6].

Question 3
What is the clinical correlation of B-lines?

A. B-lines are only signs of pulmonary congestion due to decompensated heart failure.
B. B-lines are hyperechoic and vertical reverberation artifacts due to decrease in lung density.
C. B-lines are horizontal and hyperechoic signs that represent thickened sub pleural interlobular septa.
D. B-lines are artifacts with high sensitivity but low specificity because they may be found in several lung conditions*.

Answer: **D.**

Key point: B-lines presents high sensitivity for lung diseases but low specificity.

Rationale: B-lines are vertical and hyperechoic artifacts as laser-like that indicate the presence of thickened sub pleural interlobular septa due to accumulation of exudate, transudate, collagen, blood, or others; all these conditions increase the density of the lung due to loss of air content. B-lines present high sensitivity in ruling-out all these conditions, but low specificity because the increment in density of the lung may be observed in a long list of different pulmonary diseases. Matching B-lines with the observed distribution pattern of B-lines on the chest surface and the clinical information increases the diagnostic specificity for lung diseases. Regarding the case reported in this question, a focal distribution of B-lines limited to one lung area (right basis) in the clinical context of acute dyspnea, cough and fever is compatible with the diagnosis of lung infection (bacterial pneumonia).

Question 4
Regarding the ultrasound appearance of B-lines, what other artifacts can be misdiagnosed for B-lines (Video 13.3)?

A. C-lines.
B. Z-lines.
C. A-lines.
D. Lung pulse.

Answer: **B.**

Key point: For operators with low experience, Z-lines can be misdiagnosed as B-lines.

Rationale: Similar to B-lines, Z-lines are vertical and hyperechoic artifacts; however, they do not extend to the bottom of the screen and usually they are fixed and do not move synchronously with respiration. While multiple B-lines have a definite association with clinical pulmonary conditions, Z-lines are usually isolated or few and are devoid of any meaning. For operators with low experience, Z-lines can be misdiagnosed for B-lines.

Question 5
A 72-year-old male patient is admitted to the ED for acute onset of dyspnea. After the physical examination and chest imaging, he was diagnosed with a diffuse interstitial syndrome due to acute decompensated heart failure.

Can B-lines be used as a tool to monitor the effect of the treatment administered to this patient (Video 13.4)?

A. It is not possible as B-lines are a tool for diagnosis, not for monitoring.
B. It is not possible to count B-lines, unless your ultrasound machine is equipped with a software that can automatically perform quantification.
C. Counting B-lines is not clinically useful as they are just artifacts.
D. It is possible to use a simple technique to semi-quantify B-lines and correlate the count with the severity of congestion.

Answer: **D.**

Key point: B-lines are an important tool for diagnosing diffuse interstitial syndrome, but also for monitoring the response to treatment.

Rationale: B-lines are an important tool of monitoring patients with diffuse interstitial syndrome. Some techniques can be used to semi-quantify B-lines. The technique based on the evaluation of 28 intercostal spaces is one of them. The exam is performed in oblique scan, along the intercostal spaces on the chest surface, with the patient in supine or near-to-supine position. The right hemithorax is scanned from the second to the fifth intercostal space, the left hemithorax from the second to the fourth, repeating four times on both sides, along the parasternal, mid-clavicular, anterior axillary and mid axillary lines. In each rib space, B-lines are counted from 0 to 10, or if confluent, it is assessed the percentage of the rib space occupied by B-lines and divided by 10. For instance, 40% of screen with confluent B-lines means 4 B-lines.

Question 6
A young patient is brought in cardiac arrest to the ED. Ultrasound is used to identify possible causes of cardiac

arrest and also to guide endotracheal intubation and confirm bilateral ventilation.

Which ultrasound finding can rule out selective bronchial intubation?

A. Bilateral lung sliding.
B. Bilateral lung pulse.
C. Bilateral lung point.
D. Bilateral A-lines.

Answer: **A.**

Key point: Lung sliding is a sign indicating that the lung is ventilating.

Rationale: Lung sliding is the horizontal movement of the lung against the chest wall (Video 13.5), synchronous with ventilation. After the oral-tracheal intubation, the presence of lung sliding on both sides rules out unilateral bronchial intubation.

Question 7

A 38-year-old female patient presents in shock due to complicated pyelonephritis with severe sepsis. After receiving fluid resuscitation, she needs norepinephrine to maintain a mean arterial pressure of 65 mmHg. The intensivist places a central line guided by ultrasound in the right internal jugular vein and uses ultrasound to rule out a possible post-procedural pneumothorax. Which sign can rule out pneumothorax after the procedure?

A. A-lines.
B. Lung pulse.
C. Lung point.
D. All the previous alternatives are correct.

Answer: **B.**

Key point: Lung pulse means that the parietal and visceral pleural surfaces are in contact with each other.

Rationale: The lung pulse is the rhythmic and vertical movement of the pleura in synchrony with the cardiac beats (Video 13.6). Its presence during lung ultrasound indicates that the parietal and visceral pleura oppose one to the other without interposition of air, thus excluding the possibility of pneumothorax in the area where the probe is placed. Lung pulse may be detected also in other clinical situations, such as selective bronchial intubation [7].

Question 8

A 23 year old male presents to the emergency department (ED) for acute onset of dyspnea. He has stable vital parameters and after a while is evaluated: he reports no medical history and medications. After the physical examination, you perform the lung ultrasound which reveals Video 13.7.

What finding is shown in Video 13.7**?**

A. A sort of lung contour on chest X-ray
B. A dynamic ultrasonographic sign on B-mode showing the lateral margin of intra-pleural air collection
C. A static ultrasonographic sign showing both lung sliding and A-pattern
D. A nonspecific sign of pneumothorax that is shown on ultrasound M-mode

Answer: B—A dynamic ultrasonographic sign on B-mode showing the lateral margin of intra-pleural air collection.

Key point: lung ultrasound has high specificity for pneumothorax and finding a lung point on a hemithorax of a patient allows to recognize the presence of pneumothorax with a very high predictive value.

Rationale: Sudden onset of dyspnea can be due to a considerable range of etiologies, including spontaneous pneumothorax. In young patients, pre-test probability for this diagnosis is more elevated than in older patients. Lung ultrasound scanning of this patient should aim to assess the whole respiratory system, with particular attention to the search for the lung point sign. Lung point, in fact, is a highly specific ultrasound sign of pneumothorax. It arises on the screen when scanning the point where the visceral pleura begins to separate from the parietal pleural, that correspond to the lateral margin of the pneumothorax. As a dynamic sign, it shows an alternation of movement in the central part of the image coupling a normal lung appearance (i.e., lung sliding) and the complete absence of lung signs [8, 9].

Question 9

A 34 year old female presents to ED for acute onset of dyspnea. She has stable vital signs and reports a smoking history (10 pack-years).

After the physical examination, you perform the lung ultrasound shown in Video 13.8.

What is the finding seen in Video 13.8**?**

A. A condition of increased lung stiffness that needs an appropriate elastographic assessment
B. Another name for M-mode sign called "stratosphere sign"
C. A dynamic ultrasonographic sign on B-mode showing the lateral margin of intra-pleural air collection
D. A nonspecific sign of pneumothorax that brings together the absence of lung sliding, lung pulse and B-lines

Answer: D—A nonspecific sign of pneumothorax that brings together the absence of lung sliding, lung pulse and B-lines.

Key point: Still lung provides a strong suspicion of the presence of a pneumothorax but, due to its lower specificity, it is necessary to search for the lung point.

Rationale: Still lung is the short name standing for the situation in which none of the pneumothorax-excluding signs are present. Thus, it is defined by the complete absence of lung sliding, lung pulse and B-lines. It is sonographically explained by the bad interface between chest wall and intrapleural air. It is worthy to note that every pneumothorax shows this sign in the least dependent regions (i.e., anterior chest wall in supine patients) due to the tendency of air to move according to gravity, so that the most lateral projection of the still lung corresponds to the lung point. However, in clinical studies, still lung didn't demonstrate to be as specific as lung point to diagnose pneumothorax. Unfortunately, there can be situations in which an ultrasound examination of a pneumothorax may not find a classic lung point. Pneumothoraces can present without a lung point when they are massive and the lung is too retracted towards the hilum to maintain any contact between the visceral and parietal pleura. Another possibility is that the pleural contact zone is so small and posterior that the operator can't reach it without moving the patient. Whatever the situation, in these cases the physician must rely on the presence of still lung and integrate this sign with clinical judgment.

Question 10

Referring to the clinical cases presented in Questions 8 and 9, could the use of M-mode be of any help in the diagnosis?

What is the M-mode appearance of lung sliding, still lung, and lung point (Fig. 13.1)**?**

A. As ultrasonographic dynamic signs, none of them is visible on M-mode
B. They can appear as barcode, seashore and stratosphere sign, respectively
C. The first presents with a sub-pleural echo-poor region, the second with a hyperechoic sliding line, and the third with the alternative of both.
D. They can appear as two signs called seashore, stratosphere, and the alternation of both, respectively.

Answer: D—They can appear as two signs called seashore, stratosphere, and the alternation of both, respectively.

Key point: M-mode can aid in pneumothorax diagnostic signs recognition, guaranteed that the chest wall and the ultrasound probe remain tightened to avoid any interference on the image.

Rationale: Lung sliding, lung pulse, and lung point are dynamic signs. This means that three out of four signs involved in pneumothorax diagnosis can be visualized only in real-time on the ultrasound machine or as a video clip, but lose their information as still images. M-mode imaging has the property of creating a static image made by the changes over time of a single line of view of the ultrasound beam. This implies that it can capture the dynamic phenomena, showing them with less spatial information.

For this reason, M-mode has emerged as a means to prove and export printed images of lung sliding, lung pulse, and lung point. It can also show the still lung.

On M-mode, normal lung sliding appears as an image where the upper part shows horizontal static and parallel lines and the lower shows a granular and irregular appearance. This pattern has been given the name of "seashore sign", where the parallel lines mimic a smooth sea, and the

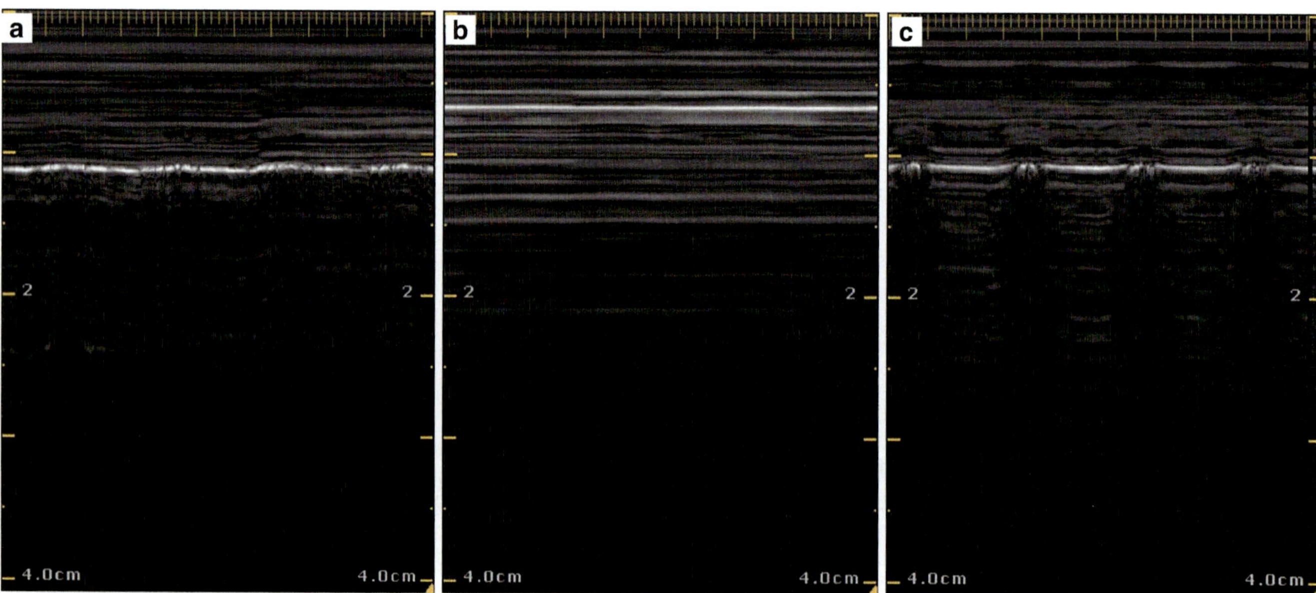

Fig. 13.1 M-mode in pneumothorax. Panel (**a**) seashore sign; panel (**b**) stratosphere sign; panel (**c**) alternation of the two signs when M-mode line is put at the lung point

granular part mimics the sand. It is a necessary condition to every M-mode imaging that the chest wall and the ultrasound probe remain tightened to avoid any interference on the image.

Lung pulse will appear with a lower image part showing a less granular pattern with brief granular vertical insertions, manifested according to heart rhythm.

In the case of pneumothorax, where a still lung is visible on the B-mode, it is expected that M-mode will show horizontal static and parallel lines both in the upper and in the lower part of the image. This pattern has been given the name of "stratosphere sign" or "barcode sign". This arises because the intrapleural air prevents any lung dynamic phenomena to be visible at the pleural level.

Lastly, as the lung point on B-mode shows a movement of to-and-fro given by the alternation of the still lung on one side and lung sliding on the other, putting the M-mode line of view on this will produce an image alternating seashore and stratosphere signs [10, 11].

Question 11

A 25 year old male presented to the ED with shortness of breath and a history of spontaneous pneumothorax. He is clinically stable and needs to be transferred for thoracic surgery evaluation. After your visit, you wonder if this patient has a large or a small air collection.

How do we semi-quantify size of pneumothorax (Fig. 13.2)**?**

A. Searching for the cutaneous projection on the skin we can use lung point position to infer pneumothorax dimension.
B. We can only use common chest X-ray formulas or dichotomous criteria to differentiate between small and large pneumothoraxes.
C. We can semi-quantify pneumothorax dimensions measuring the lung sliding.
D. It is only possible using thoracic CT scan, but it is useless in daily practice and guidelines do no take it into consideration.

Answer: A—The cutaneous projection on the skin referring to the lung point position can be used to infer pneumothorax dimension.

Key point: Lateral projection of lung point gets farther and farther as the air collection increases.

Rationale: As a pneumothorax generates, a certain amount of air enters the pleural cavity, mismatching lung elastic recoil and chest wall elastic forces that generate the negative intrapleural pressure. The deflation tends to bring the lung progressively near the hilum and, in the supine patient, the gravity pushes it toward the posterior part of the chest wall. For this reason, the detachment of the visceral and parietal pleura starts anteriorly, and progress laterally and, then, posteriorly. It is possible to predict a volume less or equal to 15% of the ipsilateral hemithorax if the lung point is found between sternum and mid axillary line, and a volume higher than 15% if it is found beyond the mid axillary line. Since lung point arise at the level of the lateral margin of air collection, it roughly indicates how much air entered the pleural cavity, as supported from US and CT studies, both in human and animal model.

Question 12

A 33 year old traumatic patient is brought into the shock room. He was victim of a car accident, with long on-scene time due to difficult extrication, and arrives drowsy, slightly hypotensive, and was desaturating on room air before an oxygen mask was applied. As soon as you complete your

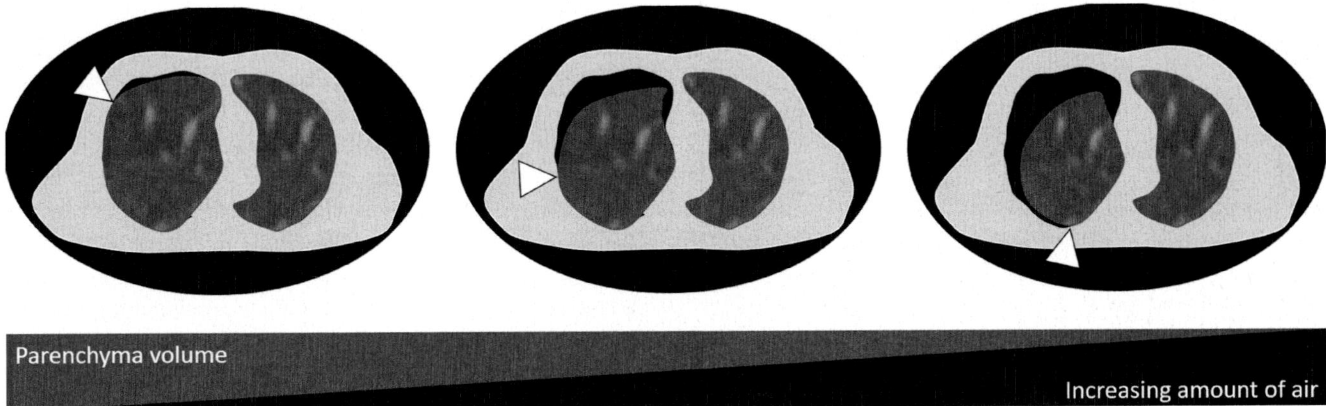

Fig. 13.2 Pneumothorax volume progression scheme. As pneumothorax gets bigger, the lung point projects more lateral, from anterior to posterior

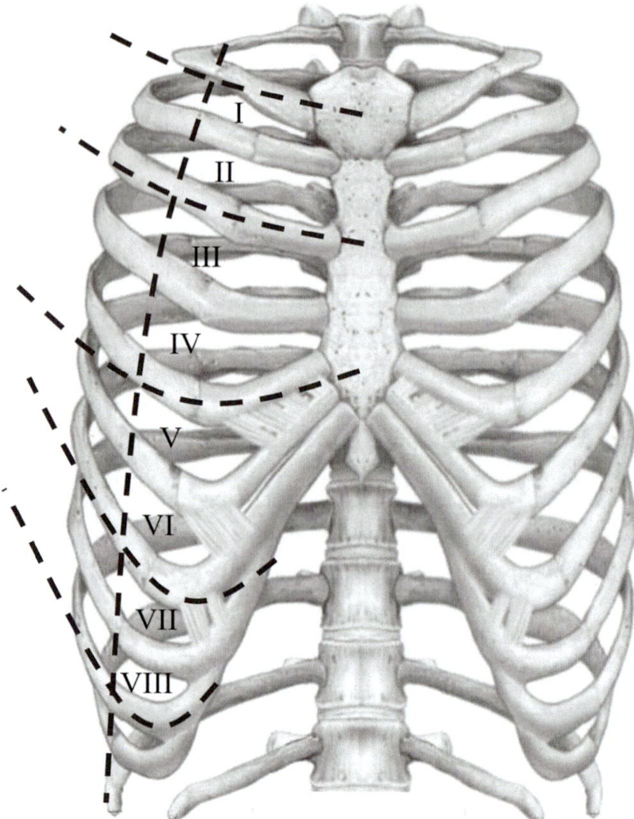

Fig. 13.3 Scheme showing the intercostal spaces and midclavicular line to identify most informative region to look for a pneumothorax in case of suspicion

primary survey you start the extended-focused assessment with sonography for trauma (E-FAST).

Where is the best point to investigate a patient with a suspected pneumothorax (Fig. 13.3)**?**

A. The patient with suspected pneumothorax must be investigated on the whole chest.
B. I scan every intercostal space on the anterior face of the chest wall, eventually removing the immobilization straps.
C. It is the least dependent region of each hemithorax, normally located parasternal and at the lower intercostal spaces.
D. Apical scans are the most sensitive to diagnose pneumothorax both in traumatic and spontaneous cases.

Answer: C—It is the least dependent region of each hemithorax, normally located parasternal and at the lower intercostal spaces.

Key point: In majority, the free air of a pneumothorax is free to collect according to gravity, and, in the supine patients, this means anteriorly and above the inferior half of the lungs.

Rationale: As explained in Question 11 rationale, air collection is typically freely moving inside the pleural cavity. As the anteroposterior diameter of the chest increases from apex to base, when a patient is exactly supine (i.e., with a zero-degree inclination of the bed) the least dependent point of the pleural cavity is also its most caudal. This justifies the finding that most pneumothoraxes are detectable at a parasternal level from the fifth to eighth intercostal spaces or lateral to the midclavicular line at seventh or eighth space. In the case of a patient positioned at 30°, the operator has to do some adjustment, as well as in obstructive patients, and in any chest wall anatomical deformation. Given this preamble, this is the position where the operator should start looking for lung sliding, lung pulse, or B-lines because finding any of them would exclude a pneumothorax with the highest negative predictive value.

Question 13

A 60 year old patient already admitted to the ward for an acute heart failure exacerbation underwent landmark-based thoracentesis due to respiratory impairment. The procedure was carried out without any overt complication.

How do we use lung ultrasound to detect post-procedural pneumothorax?

A. There isn't a protocol to search for pneumothorax after procedures
B. It is impossible to do, since lung ultrasound can only diagnose spontaneous pneumothorax
C. Searching for the lung point between clavicle and trapezius muscle in the sitting patient.
D. Post-procedural pneumothorax diagnosis is carried out as for any other pneumothorax.

Answer: D—Post-procedural pneumothorax diagnosis is carried out as for any other pneumothorax.

Key point: irrespective of the etiology of the pneumothorax, if there is a free air, it will behave the same as other cases of pneumothorax, collecting in the least dependent regions.

Rationale: lung puncture is a well-known complication of thoracentesis and the most frequent cause of post-procedural pneumothorax. It is advised to perform thoracentesis under dynamic ultrasonographic guidance. This means that the needle tip should be in continuous view under the US beam, to avoid any sensitive structure, including the lung.

In the case of a suspected post-procedural pneumothorax patient should be put supine, to induce air eventually present to collect in the least dependent region, allowing the operator to scan the patient according to the standard method. In particular, if the thoracentesis is performed in a sitting position, it is necessary to remember that the least dependent region would be the apex, where the ultrasound scan is less feasible due to clavicle, scapula, and first rib hindrance. However, it is unclear how much time does the air take to eventually move from the apex to the base.

Question 14

A 40 year old traumatic patient is brought into the ED. She was victim of pedestrian run over, and was carried to the hospital by emergency service on immobilization safeguards in clinical stable conditions. The junior doctor performing the evaluation and point of care US tells you that it is unclear whether or not the patient has got a pneumothorax. You ask him to repeat the exam with M-mode and, if still in doubt, will join him at the bedside.

How can M-mode aid in the diagnosis of a pneumothorax?

A. M-mode can aid less experienced operators since it may give a clear alternation of the extreme patterns, the seashore sign and the stratosphere sign.
B. M-mode aids the diagnostic process because it is the preferred modality to perform lung ultrasound
C. M-mode can aid the diagnostic process when used laterally on the chest to evaluate lung excursion.
D. M-mode aids the diagnostic process in every patient suffering from traumatic pneumothorax.

Answer: **A**—M-mode can aid less experienced operators since it may give a clear alternation of the extreme patterns, the seashore sign and the barcode sign.

Key point: M-mode can aid in pneumothorax diagnostic signs recognition when showing a clear alternation of seashore and stratosphere signs.

Rationale: as explained in Question 10 rationale, there is a corresponding M-mode appearance of the B-mode detection of lung sliding, lung pulse, lung point, and still lung. This aids in image collection, storage and easily provides evidence of your findings in the medical records. Furthermore, there is little evidence that M-mode aids less experienced operators to recognize a pneumothorax. While a consensus exists on B-mode, there is not a consensus on M-mode, yet. A relevant limitation to this technique is that it needs a very firm scan of the thorax to enhance a pleural line without any dynamic lung sign, and this may be difficult in the context of a rapid breathing patient, eventually moving due to pain and agitation.

For this reason, it is advisable that the operator performs the best-known technique to find a lung point, reducing any residual doubt about the diagnosis, prior to clinical decisions [12].

Question 15

The 40 year old patients of Question 14 showed a big left sided pneumothorax and a low-grade spleen lesion treated conservatively. A chest drain was inserted in the ED and then she was admitted. A couple of days after, you are asked whether or not this patient should undergo thoracic CT scan to evaluate the pneumothorax resolution.

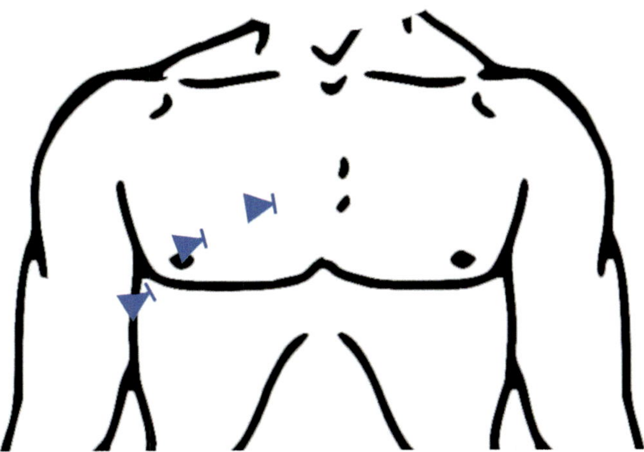

Fig. 13.4 Lung point migration scheme. If marked on the skin during LUS monitoring of pneumothorax dimension lung point (arrowheads pointing a bar) may allow to prove pneumothorax resolution

How do we use lung ultrasound to monitor pneumothorax dimension and resolution (Fig. 13.4)**?**

A. LUS is unreliable in pneumothorax monitoring
B. LUS provides only diagnostic information about pneumothorax, and it is of limited use in sizing it
C. LUS allow to monitor pneumothorax dimension base on the position of B-lines due to re-expansion edema
D. LUS allow to monitor pneumothorax resolution by mapping the migration of the lung point on the patient chest

Answer: **D.**

Key point: Pneumothorax resolution can be monitored with the progression of lung point towards mediastinum after the treatment is established, whether it is conservative, needle aspiration or chest drain.

Rationale: according to the explanations given in Question 11 rationale, a free air collection in the pleural cavity will detach the lung from the chest wall proportionally to its amount. This process happens while the pneumothorax is generating, but also when resolving, either spontaneously or by evacuation of the air.

Question 16

A 63 year old severe thoracic trauma patient is brought to your ED after a motor vehicle crash. He's awake and alert, but dyspneic and desaturating on room air. Patient is now becoming hypotensive.

Which of the following is a pitfall of pneumothorax imaging (Video 13.9)?

A. It is an unreliable technique when multiple B-lines are found aside a big subpleural consolidation.
B. As acoustic impedance changes between soft tissues and air, this may prevent the correct imaging of internal organs.

C. M-mode imaging is of aid only in the diagnosis of traumatic pneumothorax.
D. It is less informative with bilateral cases of pneumothorax.

Answer: B—As acoustic impedance changes between soft tissues and air, this may prevent the correct imaging of internal organs.

Key point: in trauma patients, and often in COVID-19, the presence of subcutaneous emphysema may be a hindrance to the correct examination of the patient.

Rationale: a relevant role in signal attenuation is played by the reflection and the scattering of the ultrasonographic beam, due to changes in acoustic impedance within soft tissues. When the US beam encounters calcific structures or air, the change in impedance is big enough to provoke a complete reflection. An infrequent complication of both trauma and COVID-19 in the development of subcutaneous emphysema, which is characterized by various degrees of air diffusion into the soft tissues of the chest wall. This air may prevent the signal to even reach the pleura and the lung, making the diagnosis of pneumothorax impossible on the basis of the four signs explained in this chapter. However, the thickness of the emphysema, or its distribution, may not be a problem. Keeping a gentle pressure on the soft tissue above the desired window may help moving away some air and, thus, easing the imaging process. Sometimes, vertical artifacts arises from the trapped air bubbles, creating the so-called E-lines (emphysema-lines).

Question 17

A dyspneic 55 year old patient admitted to the medical floors for pneumonia suddenly deteriorates and you are called for an urgent evaluation. Patient is slightly agitated and desaturating, but rapidly recover after oxygen supplementation, and there is no impending respiratory arrest or hemodynamic compromise. A standard POCUS examination with the convex probe seems to be unremarkable. With some remaining doubt about possible pulmonary embolism, you switch to linear probe to enhance your vascular evaluation and to go into detail of pleural artifacts. Thus, you obtain this clip from the right side of the chest (Video 13.10).

Which are the pitfalls of pneumothorax imaging?

A. The presence of pleural effusion impedes the visualization of a lung point and, thus, the diagnosis of pneumothorax.
B. If B-lines are present and coalescent on one side and absent on the opposite, the second one has probably a pneumothorax.
C. Posterior consolidations exclude the possibility of an anterior pneumothorax.
D. It is possible to confuse a pulsating structure lying nearby the pleura with an expression of lung pulse.

Answer: D—It is possible to confuse a pulsating structure lying nearby the pleura with an expression of lung pulse.

Key point: pulsation of intercostal artery and internal mammary artery, in particular, can mimic the lung pulse and suggest the presence of a contact between lung and chest wall. This pitfall should be known and avoided.

Rationale: as properly described in Question 12 rationale, the operator should start scanning both hemithorax from a parasternal area between fifth and eighth intercostal space. As shown, pneumothoraxes will present here with a still lung pattern (i.e., without any sign of lung sliding, lung pulse or B-lines in the scan). However, in these specific zones, a transverse scan may show a cross sectional image of the internal mammary artery (IMA) that is pulsing due to the heartbeat, moving the pleural line, as well as the lung pulse does. Two things must be noted: the first, pulsation tends to be very localized in the artery surroundings, leaving areas of still lung on the right and left side, and there is no such pattern in the lung pulse. Second, pulsation of the artery is clearly directed inward, sometimes physically moving the pleural line, and this is impossible in the case of a normal lung contacting the parietal pleura and moving accordingly to the heartbeat. A similar reasoning may be carried out for intercostal arteries, but it is far more common to encounter the IMA when looking for pneumothorax.

Question 18

A 27-year-old man is involved in a high velocity motor vehicle accident. He is brought to the ED after having been orally intubated. Abdominal and chest ultrasound are performed immediately upon arrival. The focused abdominal sonography in trauma (FAST) exam is negative, but extending the ultrasound evaluation to the lung it is detected an area in the left base showing coalescent and multiple B-lines with irregular pleura (Video 13.12). What is the most probable meaning for B-lines in this case?

A. Bacterial pneumonia.
B. Acute pulmonary congestion.
C. Lung contusion.
D. Lung cancer.

Answer: **C.**

Key point: Multiple B-lines are the sign of interstitial syndrome. Their distribution can be focal or diffuse.

Rationale: Multiple B-lines are the sonographic sign of interstitial syndrome. When B-lines are diffuse and bilateral, some of the possible diagnoses are pulmonary edema from various causes, including cardiogenic edema and ARDS, but also interstitial pneumonia, pneumonitis, and fibrosis. In other situations, the pattern of interstitial syndrome can be focal, that means limited to a focal lung area (Video 13.11). A focal pattern of multiple B-lines can be found in the following conditions: pneumonia, pneumonitis, atelectasis, pulmonary contusion, pulmonary infarction, pleural disease, and lung cancer. It is also proven that in about 20% of hospitalized patients without any lung disease, focal B-lines may be found in the lung bases. The correlation between the distribution of multiple B-lines and the clinical setting is mandatory for correct interpretation and diagnosis.

Question 19

A 74-year-old female patient with a previous diagnosis of asthma and CHF is admitted to the ED complaining of acute dyspnea and sudden onset of chest pain. A bedside cardiac and lung ultrasound are immediately performed. The video below shows lung ultrasound findings present diffusely and bilaterally (Video 13.14). What highly probable diagnosis can be hypothesized in this case?

A. Decompensated asthma.
B. Acute pulmonary edema due to heart failure.
C. COPD exacerbation.
D. Pulmonary embolism.

Answer: **B.**

Key point: Lung ultrasound is a great tool to differentiate acute asthma or exacerbation of COPD from other pathologies in acute respiratory failure.

Rationale: Detection of multiple diffuse B-lines is a highly sensitive sign of interstitial syndrome. B-lines are useful to differentiate pathologies characterized by increase in lung density, such as pulmonary edema, from conditions with increased pulmonary aeration. In hyperinflated lungs, like in decompensated asthma or COPD exacerbation, the lung ultrasound will show predominance of A-lines [13, 14].

Question 20

A critically ill patient with severe sepsis is intubated and ventilated for 10 days in the intensive care unit. He shows consolidations compatible with atelectasis in the lung basis. Is it possible to measure the loss of lung aeration by means of lung ultrasound?

A. Lung ultrasound is not useful to monitor loss of aeration.
B. It is possible to measure the loss of aeration by assigning a score to different lung ultrasound patterns: A-lines, separated B-lines, coalescent B-lines, consolidation.
C. The evaluation of loss of aeration should be performed by scanning only the lateral and anterior chest.
D. The technique of four areas in the anterior chest, two per side, is used to score loss of lung aeration.

Answer: **B.**

Key point: Lung ultrasound is a useful tool to score loss of pulmonary aeration.

Rationale: The rationale for assessing loss of lung aeration is based on the possibility that lung ultrasound may detect different densities of the lungs. Normal aerated lung shows A-lines. Initial loss of aeration shows spaced B-lines. Increases in extravascular lung water increases the number of B-lines until they become coalescent. The extreme loss of air content is detected as consolidation.

Question 21

Regarding the patient described in Question 18, lung ultrasound was performed to assess the degree of aeration. How should a lung ultrasound score be obtained?

A. The 28 rib spaces technique should be applied.
B. 12 posterior, lateral and anterior chest areas must be scanned.
C. Lung ultrasound score for aeration ranges from −32 to +32.
D. To obtain a correct aeration score we need to sum the score of eight anterior-lateral areas.

Answer: **B.**

Key point: Lung ultrasound score for assessing loss of aeration is based on the insonation of 12 chest areas and summing the scores assigned to each one.

Rationale: The measurement of lung aeration is performed in 12 areas of the whole chest. To each region we will assign a score of: 0 point if the pattern is A (regular sliding with absence of significant B-lines and consolidation); 1 point if the pattern is B1 (at least three well-defined and well separated either regularly spaced or irregularly spaced B lines); 2 points if the pattern is B2 (multiple coalescent B-lines); 3 points if the pattern is a consolidation (a subpleural echo-poor region or one with tissue-like echotexture). The range of the aeration score is from 0 (fully aerated) to 36 (total loss of aeration). An increase in aeration score suggest decreased aeration.

Question 22

An end stage renal disease patient arrives to the clinic for his routine dialysis session. However, this time he presents with desaturation, dyspnea, and hypertension. The weight is 2.5 kg above the clinically established dry weight. The patient undergoes hemodialysis and 2.5-L ultrafiltration is obtained. At the end of the session, he has normal saturation at rest in room air, but is still hypertensive and tachypneic. Pulmonary ultrasound is performed. B-lines are visualized diffusely and bilaterally, as it is shown in the clip (Video 13.14).

How to interpret the ultrasound findings in this clinical context?

A. Lung ultrasound findings suggest that this patient needs more fluid removal.
B. Detection of B-lines right after the hemodialysis session has no meaning.
C. B-lines cannot be linked to pulmonary congestion in this case.
D. Auscultation and evaluation of legs edema are more sensitive tools than lung ultrasound to define dry weight.

Answer: **A.**

Key point: Lung ultrasound is a useful tool for assessing pulmonary congestion in dialysis patients.

Rationale: Traditionally, dry weight is defined by using low sensitivity tools, such as pulmonary auscultation and assessment of legs edema. Lung ultrasound is far more sensitive in diagnosing an increase in extravascular pulmonary water. In hemodialysis patients, the presence of significant B-lines after hemodialysis is associated with higher mortality. B-lines should be used as an important tool for the assessment of pulmonary congestion and definition of dry weight in this population.

Question 23

A 58-year-old patient with chronic heart failure and a history of previous pulmonary embolism is admitted to the ED complaining of acute dyspnea. Lung ultrasound is performed at the bedside.

What is the main application of lung ultrasound in the evaluation of a chronic cardiac patient?

A. Lung ultrasound is a useful tool for diagnosing and monitoring congestion in patients with chronic heart failure.
B. Permanence of B-lines can predict future hospitalization and bad prognosis in asymptomatic heart failure patients.
C. The presence of B-lines at discharge in a patient treated for decompensated heart failure is related to a higher risk of readmission in the coming months.
D. All the previous alternatives are correct.

Answer: **D.**

Key point: Lung ultrasound for B-lines is a useful tool for diagnosing and monitoring pulmonary congestion as well as for predicting future hospitalizations in chronic heart failure patients.

Rationale: The conventional technique to evaluate pulmonary congestion at bedside in heart failure patients is based on scanning of 28 intercostal spaces on both sides, anterior and lateral (the right hemithorax is scanned from the second to the fifth intercostal space, the left hemithorax from the second to the fourth, repeating 4 times on both sides, along the parasternal, mid-clavear, the anterior axillary and mid axillary lines). An alternative simplified technique was used based on counting the positivity of eight anterior-lateral areas for multiple B-lines. Lung ultrasound for B-lines is a sensitive tool for diagnosing and monitoring congestion as well as to predict hospitalization in heart failure patients.

Question 24

A correct exam and interpretation of interstitial syndrome by lung ultrasound is crucial to avoid misdiagnoses. It is important to be aware about the possible pitfalls when lung ultrasound is used to diagnose the interstitial syndrome.

Which one of the following situations cannot be considered a source of potential pitfalls?

A. Z-lines can be misdiagnosed for B-lines.
B. B-lines restricted to the lung bases can be detected in normal lungs.
C. One or two B-lines between two ribs in a longitudinal view cannot be considered an abnormal finding.
D. Contemporary visualization of A-lines and B-lines in the same scan cannot be considered a pathologic pattern.

Answer: **D.**

Key point: Not experienced people must be careful to avoid misinterpretations for diagnosing and interpreting interstitial syndrome.

Rationale: A positive scan for interstitial syndrome is sonographically diagnosed when multiple B-lines, i.e. more than three B-lines between two ribs in a longitudinal scan, are visualized in a single scan. The interstitial syndrome can be diffuse when positive scans are detected in at least two chest areas per side, or focal in all the other situations. The contemporary presence of A-lines and B-lines in the same scan is a possibility that never influences the diagnosis as the number of B-lines present in the scan site should be counted as such. Z-lines should be always distinguished from the B-lines by observing the characteristics of the artifacts. A focal presence of multiple B-lines, especially when limited to the lung bases, is compatible with a normal lung.

Question 25

A 84 year old male presents with an ongoing fever and productive cough for 1 week. He is febrile (temp 101.7 °F), tachycardic (pulse 130 bpm) and has leukocytosis (WBC 21K). A bedside lung ultrasound is performed as shown in the video (Video 13.15).

What is the sonographic appearance of a consolidative process?

A. Diffuse bilateral B lines with severe pleural effusion.
B. Isoechoic appearance with the liver in early stage.
C. It can vary from focal interstitial syndrome to lung hepatization.
D. Absence of dynamic bronchogram in a context of lobar hepatization.

Answer: C—it can vary from focal interstitial syndrome to lung hepatization.

Key point: lung ultrasound has high sensitivity for alveolar consolidation but poor specificity, therefore the nature of the sonographic findings has always to be correlated to the clinical setting.

Rationale: This transverse lung view acquired with a convex probe (2.5–5 MHz) demonstrates a focal interstitial syndrome with multiple B lines on the left lung base with a minimal amount of pleural effusion just above the diaphragm with underlying air bronchograms. The increase in fluid in the lung tissue with progressive loss of air content generates comet-tail reverberation artifacts, known as B-lines. Due to their variable extension and position, lung consolidations are not amenable to a standardized scanning protocol. In the case of suspicion of a consolidation process, the entire accessible lung surface should be evaluated, with particular focus to the posterior regions.

Question 26

A 32-year-old pregnant woman presents with worsening shortness of breath since a week. She also reports a 5 day history of fever which is now resolved. A chest X-ray reveals an opaque left lower lobe with possible consolidation, pleural effusion or collapse.

What does the definition of 'lung hepatization' stand for?

A. Presence of scattered bilateral B lines with subpleural consolidation.
B. Appearance of lung parenchyma with triphasic arterial doppler suggestive for necrotic alteration.
C. Alteration of lung tissue such that it resembles liver tissue in a context of lobar consolidation.
D. Presence of dynamic bronchograms that resemble hepatic biliary tract.

Answer: C—alteration of lung tissue such that it resembles liver tissue in a context of lobar consolidation.

Key point: ultrasound can differentiate with high accuracy effusion from consolidation when the chest X-ray is equivocal.

Rationale: This transverse lung view acquired with a convex probe (2.5–5 MHz) demonstrates a dense lower consolidation above the diaphragm (Video 13.16). The lung appears nearly identical to the liver in terms of density as inflammatory cells and fibrinous exudate accumulation give a white-gray appearance to lung tissue. Sonographic air bronchograms appear as multiple hyperechoic millimeter-long, lentil-shaped air inlets or as hyperechoic branching tubular structures within the consolidated lung parenchyma [15].

Question 27

A 8 year old child presents his mother with a 3 days history of coughing. On auscultation, there are crepitations on the right sided lung base. A bedside ultrasound is performed as shown.

What is the shred sign (Fig. 13.5)**?**

A. Artifact created by high impedance between chest wall soft and chest wall muscles.
B. Dynamic sonographic sign present when respiratory variation decreases the distance between the parietal and visceral pleura, when separated by a pleural effusion.
C. Absent lung sliding with the perception of heart activity at the pleural line.
D. Irregular junction between consolidated and aerated lung.

Answer: D—irregular junction between consolidated and aerated lung areas.

Key point: Distinguish shred sign from a loculated pleural effusion.

Rationale: This view acquired with a linear array probe (5–13 MHz) reveals subpleural details of a small consolidation with a shred sign visible at the border between the consolidation and the closer aerated lung that moves together with respiratory efforts [16].

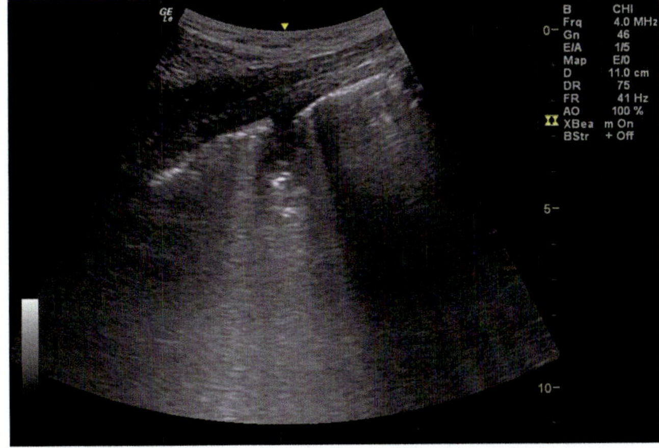

Fig. 13.5 Shred sign

Question 28

A chest X ray of a 37-year-old male presenting with fever and dyspnea revealed a left sided opacity suspicious for an infective process.

What is the role of color-Doppler imaging in lung consolidation (Video 13.17)?

A. Characterize the consolidation vascularity and flow pattern.
B. Quantify the size of lung consolidation.
C. Differentiate focal from diffuse interstitial syndrome.
D. Grade severity of the lung consolidation.

Answer: A—characterize the consolidation vascularity and flow pattern.

Key point: Color Doppler imaging in ultrasound allows performing qualitative and quantitative assessment of lung lesions.

Rationale: This transverse view is acquired with a convex probe (2.5–5 MHz) revealing a triphasic arterial waveform (red in color) and the monophasic bronchial arterial flow (blue in color). When compared to chest radiography, Doppler signal accurately differentiates pleural from pulmonary parenchymal lesions. Color Doppler LUS has also been studied in evaluation of abscess and empyema and to a lesser extent in pneumothorax [17].

Question 29

What are the sonographic findings of a dynamic air bronchogram?

A. Hypoechoic tubular structure seen during inspiration in the context of pneumonia.
B. Bubble of gas seen in pleural effusion.
C. Hypoechoic tubular structure indicating patent airways.
D. Hyperechoic line and dots within a hypoechoic lung area, thought to represent air trapped in small airways.

Answer: D—hyperechoic line and dots within a hypoechoic lung area, thought to represent air trapped in small airways.

Key point: Air bronchogram refers to the phenomenon of air-filled bronchi being made visible by the opacification of surrounding alveoli (Video 13.18).

Rationale: This video acquired with a convex probe (2.5–5 MHz) in a transverse shows the presence of a hypoechoic pulmonary consolidation that contains hyperechoic lines and flecks that move with respiration. Dynamic air bronchograms move centrifugally with respiration and represent fluid mixed with air inside larger bronchi in the context of a consolidation. The specificity and positive predictive value of dynamic air bronchogram in presence of alveolar consolidation to predict pneumonia is 94% and 97% respectively [18].

Question 30

What are the sonographic findings of a static air bronchogram?

A. Hypoechoic tubular structure mimicking the lung vessels in the context of pneumonia.
B. Bubble of gas seen in pleural effusion that moves with respiratory cycles.
C. Hypoechoic tubular structure indicating patent airways.
D. Hyperechoic line and dots within a hypoechoic lung area, which can be seen in both atelectasis and pneumonia.

Answer: D—hyperechoic lines and dots within a hypoechoic lung area, which can be seen in both atelectasis and pneumonia (Video 13.19).

Key point: A static bronchogram remains fixed throughout the respiratory cycle.

Rationale: This video acquired with a convex probe (2.5–5 MHz) in a transverse shows the tubular structures of the static bronchogram. It signified trapped gas bubble in the bronchus isolated from the main bronchus. Although these structures can be seen in pneumonia, they are often detected in the presence of compressive or resorptive lung atelectasis secondary to pleural effusion.

Question 31

What are the clinical findings of a fluid bronchogram?

A. Hypoechoic tubular structure seen during inspiration in the context of pneumonia.
B. Bubble of gas seen in pleural effusion.
C. Anechoic tubular structures representing fluid-clogged bronchi.
D. Hyperechoic line and dots within a hypoechoic lung area, thought to represent air trapped in small airways.

Answer: C—anechoic tubular structures representing fluid-clogged bronchi.

Key point: The absence of Doppler flow in the fluid filled bronchi confirms that these are not vessels but airways (Video 13.20).

Rationale: This video acquired with a convex probe (2.5–5 MHz) in a transverse shows the presence of a consolidation with fluid bronchograms consisting of ramified linear images that correspond to distended bronchi filled with fluid and lack of air over hypoechogenic pulmonary parenchyma. The presence of this sign suggests pulmonary atelectasis due to endobronchial obstruction.

Question 32

A 51 year old female with known metastatic breast cancer and recent drainage of pleural effusion presents with worsening dyspnea. She is tachycardic (pulse 150 bpm) and dyspneic (respiratory rate 40). You want to look for a possible pleural effusion and thus perform a bedside lung ultrasound as shown in the video (Video 13.21).

What is the curtain sign?

A. The point where the visceral pleura begins to separate from the parietal pleural.
B. The pulsation of the lung parenchyma synchronous with the heart beat.
C. The aerated lung dynamically swinging in a cranial-caudal direction over the diaphragm with the respiratory efforts.
D. The transition point between the aerated and consolidated lung visible during expiration.

Answer: C—the aerated lung dynamically swinging in a cranial-caudal direction over the diaphragm with the respiratory efforts.

Key point: The presence of curtain signs rules out even the minimal effusion.

Rationale: This video showing the transverse view acquired with a convex probe (2.5–5 MHz) reveals the curtain sign at the costophrenic recess. Every time a pleural effusion is suspected, the operator should search for free fluid collection in the most dependent region of each hemithorax. Thus, in the supine patient, this means to scan at the level of the posterior axillary line on both sides, crossing an intercostal space typically comprised between sixth and eighth, depending on patient habitus and clinical conditions. It is useful to start scanning from a well-defined organ (e.g., the liver on the right side or the spleen on the left) and then move cranially to be sure to reach the pleural cavity. The finding of a curtain sign in these regions signifies that the examination reached the most inferior aspect of lung and that there is no fluid collection in the pleural cavity [19, 20].

Question 33

A 55 year old female with known metastatic lung cancer presents with worsening dyspnea on minimal efforts. She is tachycardic and dyspneic at rest. A bedside lung ultrasound is performed as shown in figure.

What is the spine sign (Fig. 13.6)**?**

A. The visualization of the vertebral bodies in the thoracic cavity above the diaphragm.
B. The pulsation of the lung parenchyma synchronous with the heart beat.
C. The visualization of the vertebral bodies in the abdominal cavity below the diaphragm
D. The point where the visceral pleura begins to separate from the parietal pleura.

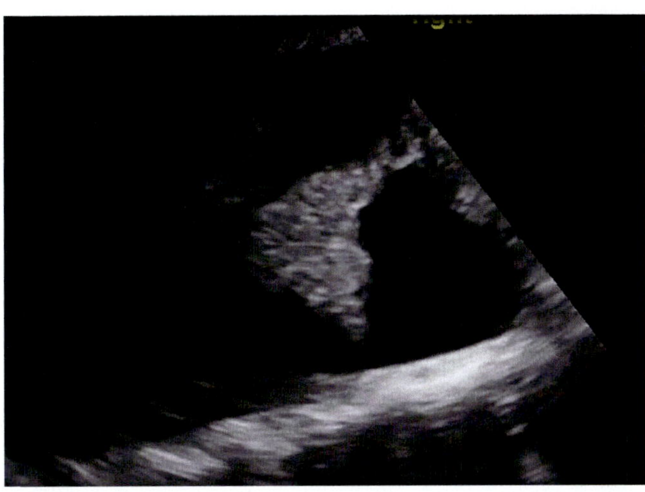

Fig. 13.6 The spine sign. When a pleural effusion is large enough to allow ultrasound beams to pass through it, a scan parallel to the spine will show a bright indented hyperechoic line in the far field of the image

Answer: A—the visualization of the vertebral bodies in the thoracic cavity above the diaphragm.

Key point: The spine sign is an indirect indicator of pleural effusion.

Rationale: This video (Video 13.27) shows the transverse view acquired with a convex probe (2.5–5 MHz) at the right lung base along the posterior axillary line. An anechoic pleural effusion is detected and the spine replaces the usual curtain sign seen in normal condition. The finding of the spine sign is not necessary per se to identify a pleural effusion that is defined by an echo poor region within the pleural cavity but it is a marker of a properly conducted scan in the context of an effusion [21].

Question 34

A 37 year old car driver has been brought in after sustaining a collision with a van. He was tachycardic and hypotensive on arrival with reduced air entry sound on his right side lung. An E-FAST reveals the presence of fluid in the costophrenic recess and abnormality in the lung base.

How does pleural effusion appear on ultrasound?

A. Hyperechoic pleural content with vivid doppler sign.
B. According to its internal echogenicity could be anechoic, complex non-septated, and complex septated.
C. Can not be associated to an inflammatory process.
D. According to the size can be classified as grade 1, 2, 3 or 4.

Answer: B—internal echogenicity could be anechoic, complex non-septated, and complex septated.

Key point: the accuracy of ultrasound allows the detection of even a minimal amount of 50 mL of pleural effusion in the costophrenic space and helps in defining its composition.

Rationale: When looking for free fluid collection within the pleural cavity it is possible to find an anechoic area. This finding, together with the trauma settings in an otherwise healthy patient, is highly suggestive of a hemothorax. It is also possible to have an underlying lung contusion that might be seen as a free-floating lung characterized by a focal interstitial syndrome or lung consolidation.

Question 35

A 67 years old male presents with chest pain and orthopnea. On clinical examination he has right sided reduced breath sounds and a bedside ultrasound is performed as shown in the video (Video 13.22).

What are the sonographic characteristics of a transudate?

A. Simple anechoic fluid collection.
B. Homogeneously or heterogeneously echogenic fluid collection with or without septations.
C. Hyperechoic fluid collection in the pleural space with debris.
D. Anechoic fluid collection with septae and floating fibrin strands.

Answer: A—simple anechoic fluid collection.

Key point: accuracy of ultrasound to distinguish exudate from transudate.

Rationale: This transverse view is acquired with a convex probe (2.5–5 MHz) at the right lung base along the posterior axillary line showing a large echo-free fluid collection immediately superior to the diaphragm highly suggestive for transudative effusion. The fluid distribution inferiorly as well as posterior-anteriorly to the lung itself defines this effusion as large.

Question 36

What is the most appropriate categorization for size of this pleural effusion (Video 13.23)?

A. No pleural effusion is present.
B. Small pleural effusion is present.
C. Large pleural effusion is present.
D. Moderate pleural effusion is present.

Answer: B—Small pleural effusion is present.

Key point: Recognize even the smallest pleural effusion with 100% sensitivity with ultrasound.

Rationale: This transverse view of the left lung base shows a minimal echo free pleural effusion in a context of lung consolidation. Three different formulae are used commonly in clinical practice for effusion size estimation including Balik, Eibenberger and Goecke's formulas. However, effusion size can also be calculated by counting intercostal spaces (ICS) from the costophrenic angle (small-localized to 1 ICS, medium 2–3 ICS, large 4 ICS).

Question 37

What is the most appropriate categorization for size of this pleural effusion (Video 13.24)?

A. No pleural effusion is present.
B. Small pleural effusion is present.
C. Large pleural effusion is present.
D. Moderate pleural effusion is present.

Answer: C—Large pleural effusion is present.

Key point: Recognize large pleural effusion.

Rationale: This video obtained by tilting the probe cranially on the posterior axillary line shows extension of the fluid above four intercostal spaces suggesting large exudate.

Question 38

What is the sinusoid sign (Fig. 13.7)?

A. The dynamic sign present when respiratory variation allows the visualization of the vertebral bodies in the thoracic cavity above the diaphragm.
B. The pulsation of the lung parenchyma synchronous with the heart beat.
C. The dynamic sign present when respiratory variation decreases the distance between the parietal and visceral pleura (lung) when separated by a pleural effusion.
D. The point where the visceral pleura begins to separate from the parietal pleura when air between two layers is present.

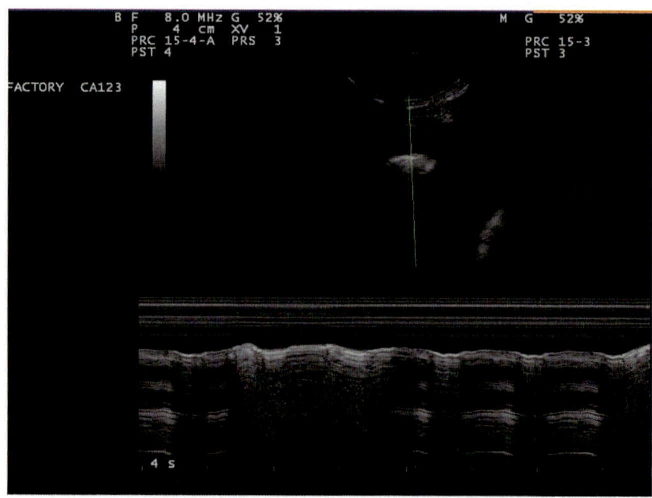

Fig. 13.7 Sinusoid sign on an M-mode track

Answer: C—the dynamic sign present when respiratory variation decreases the distance between the parietal and visceral pleura when separated by a pleural effusion.

Key point: differentiate pleural effusion from subpleural consolidation, both of which may appear anechoic.

Rationale: This video (Video 13.25) acquired in a transverse view along the posterior axillary line shows a pleural effusion and a consolidated lung. The accompanying image depicts a sinusoid sign. During the respiratory cycle the oscillation of the lung line (visceral pleura) toward the parietal pleura can be appreciated. This sonographic sign is highly sensitive and specific for pleural effusion as this sign will not be generated by alveolar consolidation, which behaves like a solid lesion.

Question 39

A 50 year old male with a history of HIV presents with chest pain, ongoing fever and significant weight loss for 2 months. On clinical examination he has R-sided crepitations and a chest X-ray shows the presence of parapneumonic fluid on the left lung base.

What are the sonographic findings for empyema?

A. Unilateral, complex effusion with echogenic speckled appearance and often loculated.
B. Unilateral, simple anechoic large effusion often associated with lung consolidation.
C. Parapneumonic, bilateral complex pleural effusion in acutely decompensated heart failure.
D. Unilateral, complex effusion with presence of doppler sign synchronous to the respiratory cycle.

Answer: A—unilateral, complex effusion with echogenic speckled appearance and often loculated.

Key point: differentiate between complex septated pleural effusion and empyema.

Rationale: **In empyema,** the presence of highly echogenic swirling fluid within a pleural effusion may be seen, as well as a certain amount of septations may be noted. Differential diagnosis from a complex pleural effusion relies on two futures: empyema creates an obtuse angle with the chest wall and they have a lenticular shape, whereas pleural effusions are crescentic in shape.

Question 40

A 3-year-old boy was referred to the clinic with complaints of dry cough and fever for 5 days. A chest X-ray showed an opacification with gas-fluid-levels in the right hemithorax.

Which are the sonographic findings of a lung abscess?

A. Irregular wall width, a blurred outer margin, an oval or round shape.
B. Sharp lenticular margin, positive pleural separation.
C. Anechoic fluid content with a thick well-defined wall.
D. Unilateral fluid collection in the context only detectable at the lung base.

Answer: A—irregular wall width, a blurred outer margin, an oval or round shape.

Key point: separation of the parietal pleura from the visceral pleura may help to differentiate between pleural empyema from lung abscess sitting on the outer side of the lung.

Rationale: Correct differentiation between lung abscess and empyema is important; however technical limitations in ultrasound scanning and image resolution make it difficult to reliably differentiate on the basis of the collection's shape or wall thickness.

Question 41

A patient is admitted for surgical treatment of appendicitis. Three days after surgery, a chest X-ray shows opacity at the base of the right lung. Lung ultrasound is performed (Video 13.26). The video below shows the preview image.

What is the best interpretation for this image?

A. Consolidation plus pleural effusion*.
B. Isolated large pleural effusion.
C. Consolidation without pleural effusion.
D. Pulmonary consolidation associated with multiple B-lines.

Answer: **A.**

Key point: Lung ultrasound has high sensitivity for diagnosing consolidation and pleural effusion. The differential diagnosis between consolidation and fluid can be immediate and easy to perform by lung ultrasound.

Rationale: The sonographic sign of lung consolidation is a subpleural echo-poor region or one with tissue-like echotexture. Pleural effusion is usually an anechoic space between the parietal and visceral pleura, indicating the presence of fluid. In case of complex effusion, some echogenic foci can be detected inside the fluid.

Question 42

A dyspneic patient presents with a large pleural effusion diagnosed by lung ultrasound.

How can chest ultrasound aid thoracentesis (Fig. 13.8)**?**

A. Lung ultrasound can differentiate the area of pleural effusion from the abdominal organs.
B. Lung ultrasound can guide the procedure in real time by visualizing the needle and the effusion.
C. Lung ultrasound can be useful to assess the amount of pleural effusion and evaluate the risks of thoracentesis.
D. All the previous alternatives are correct*.

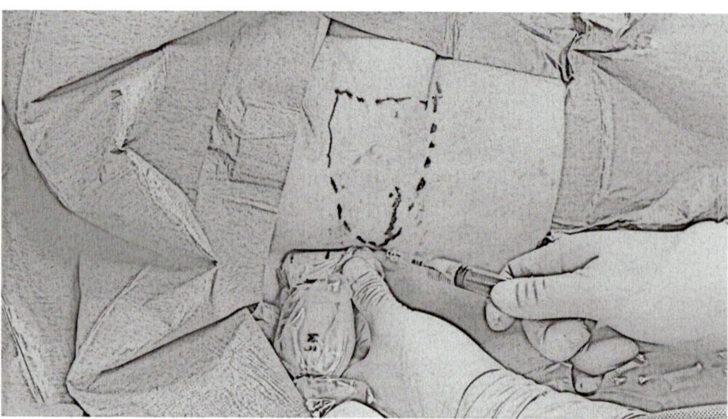

Fig. 13.8 Ultrasound guided thoracentesis performed pointing to a right sided pleural effusion and in close proximity to the safety triangle delineated by pectoralis major, latissimus dorsi and fifth intercostal space. Patient head on the left side of the image

Answer: **D.**

Key point: Ultrasound is a useful and practical bedside tool to evaluate the amount of pleural effusion and to guide thoracentesis.

Rationale: The use of lung ultrasound in thoracentesis reduces the rate of complications, including pneumothorax, and increases the success of fluid removal when compared to conventional methods. Lung ultrasound is especially useful when the pleural effusion is small or loculated [22, 23].

Question 43

You arrive at scene with multiple trauma victims. You recognize that two of the victims need prompt endotracheal intubation for impending respiratory arrest. After intubating victim A, her peripheral oxygen saturation stabilize at 88% and do not increase further, while blood pressure remains stable and you move your attention to the second critical patient.

Is ultrasound useful for the detection of endotracheal intubation?

A. Yes, because it clearly allows to visualize the tube below the glottis in the trachea.
B. Yes, because it allows visualization of vocal cords and the interference produced by the tube passing between them.
C. No, because, as stated by the name, the airway is filled with air, that block US propagation.
D. Yes, but only in the case of an airway filled with fluids (secretions, water, blood, or something else).

Answer: B—Yes, because it allows visualization of vocal cords and the interference it produces by the tube passing between them.

Key point: Ultrasonographic support to endotracheal intubation is a recognized application of POCUS in airway management. A method to verify the procedure success is to see the tube passing through the trachea at the vocal cords level.

Rationale: During endotracheal intubation, transverse scan at the level of vocal cords provides an acceptable window to evaluate the passage of the endotracheal tube. In the sonographic real-time check, a rapid sliding of a hyperechoic surface just below the vocal cords indicates the passage of the tube cuff, which is the largest point of the tube itself, while the tube body will present a double-arch image with its convex face directed inward. However, any air eventually present between the tube and the larynx or trachea may severely limit this kind of visualization. Another drawback of the technique is that it requires an extra operator, who maintain the ultrasound probe fixed on the patient neck while the rest of the team is performing a procedure.

Question 44 (Case Continuation)

After intubating victim B, her peripheral oxygen saturation lowers and tachycardia worsen. Suspecting an inadvertent esophageal intubation you perform the procedure once again, correctly positioning the endotracheal tube, with final improvement in the vital parameters.

After a while, a second medical team reaches the scene, bringing also a portable US machine, and the second physician suggests to complete patient A and patient B evaluations with POCUS.

Is ultrasound useful for the detection of esophageal intubation?

A. No, esophagus is posterior to trachea and, thus, unreachable by ultrasound.
B. Yes, and it is done by the same operator who performs orotracheal intubation.
C. Yes, because it allows visualization of esophageal lumen when the tube in inserted in it.
D. Yes, as it is the standard of care to verify correct endotracheal tube placement.

Answer: C—Yes, because it allows visualization of esophageal lumen when the tube in inserted in it.

Key point: ultrasonographic support to endotracheal intubation is a recognized application of POCUS to the airway management and its easiest application is to verify endotracheal tube not passing into the esophagus lumen.

Rationale: as explained in Question 44 rationale, US can assist during endotracheal intubation. A second way to manage the check of correct intubation is to look for an easier phenomenon, scanning a more US-friendly target as neck soft tissues are. In particular, esophagus can be easily found posterior to trachea and its virtual lumen can be identified in the healthy volunteer asking for a normal water swallowing. In the case of an inadvertent tube passage into the esophagus lumen two things happens: the lumen enlargement and the manifestation of the so-called "double-lumen sign". This sign will indicate the tube body with a double-arch image, having its convex face directed inward and a posterior black shadow due to US beam reflection from the tube itself. This method to verify correct endotracheal intubation may seem more indirect, but is easier to carry out and provide the necessary information.

Question 45 (Case Continuation)

Back to victim A, you register vital signs are unchanged and peripheral oxygen saturation still 88%. The lung ultrasound evaluation shows a lack of sliding on the left side. In doubt for possible pneumothorax, you look for lung pulse, finding it on both sides. Then, after a gentle retraction of the endotracheal tube lung sliding appear on left side and oxygen saturation increases.

Is ultrasound useful for the detection of endobronchial intubation (Fig. 13.9)**?**

A. Yes, if an abolished lung sliding is accompanied by lung pulse it indicates a normal but not ventilated lung.
B. No, bronchi are filled with air and too deep into the chest and behind the lungs to be visible.
C. Yes, as it is possible to use differential lung ultrasound score to correctly assess which lung is being ventilated.
D. Yes, in fact it is possible to find a lung point on the non-ventilated side.

Answer: A—Yes, if an abolished lung sliding is accompanied by lung pulse it indicates a normal but not ventilated lung.

Key point: lung sliding is the sign indicating a ventilated lung, absence of lung sliding with presence of lung pulse may indicated mainstem intubation on the contra-lateral side.

Rationale: Once a patient has been correctly intubated in the tracheal lumen, it may be possible that the tube is placed too deep, typically in the right main bronchus, or that it passively moves during other maneuvers, producing an inadvertent selective intubation. It is common practice to check immediately after intubation for a possible wrong positioning of the tube with auscultation. However, auscultation alone has a low sensitivity, and capnography cannot differentiate between endotracheal and endobronchial intubation. When selectively intubated, the ventilated lung will behave as usual. On the contrary, the other lung will be initially inflated and not ventilated, showing an abolished lung sliding and a present lung pulse. Then it will progressively deflate while developing atelectasis, which shows as a progression toward increasing number of B-lines and then consolidation (i.e., increasing it LUS score). The finding of a lung with pulse and without sliding should always prompt the suspicion of apnea, irrespective of the cause. In the case of inadvertent endotracheal intubation, LUS is able to allow the diagnosis and demonstrate the resolution of the problem.

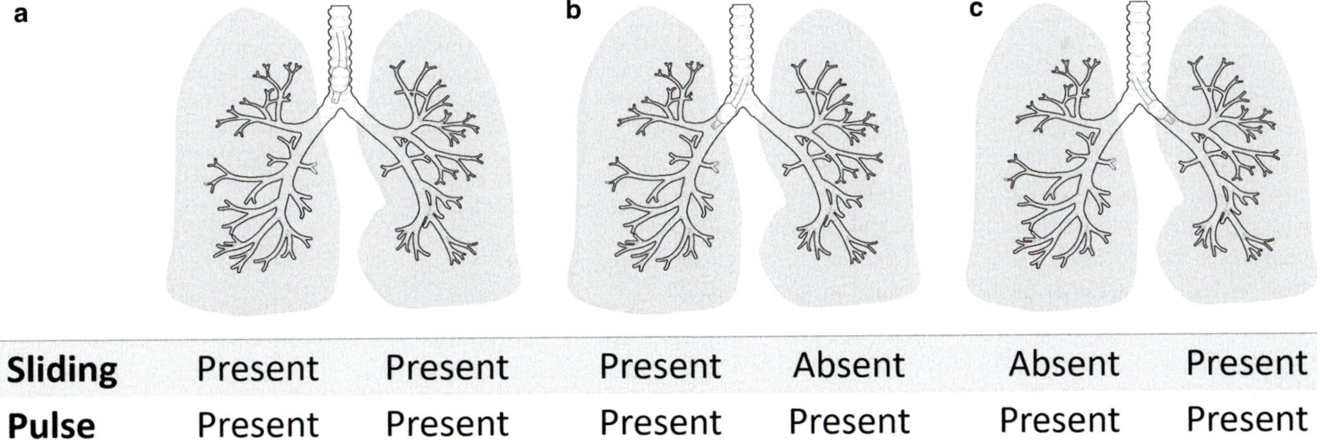

	a		b		c	
Sliding	Present	Present	Present	Absent	Absent	Present
Pulse	Present	Present	Present	Present	Present	Present

Fig. 13.9 Endobronchial intubation detection by means of lung ultrasound. Panel (**a**) shows endotracheal intubation. Panel (**b**) shows right main stem intubation. Panel (**c**) shows left main stem intubation. Lung pulse remains always visible if there is no associated pneumothorax; lung sliding remains only on the ventilated side

Question 46

A 55-year old male patient with severe respiratory distress is brought to the ED by the ambulance. He was found at home sitting, pale, desaturating on room air, and with wheezing on auscultation. He was administered bronchodilators without clinical improvement. On arrival in the ED, the patient becomes hypotensive and shows peripheral cyanosis.

What is the role of lung ultrasound in outpatient respiratory failure (Fig. 13.10)**?**

A. There is no role for LUS in this case, because most respiratory impairment of acute patients is due to heart and vascular problems
B. LUS is able to detect lung involvement of different medical conditions and can differentiate cardiogenic pulmonary edema, ARDS and diseases without lung involvement
C. LUS is able to diagnose lung involvement of acute conditions, such as heart failure but is useless for airway diseases
D. There is no role for LUS in this patient management diagnosis, since asthma and COPD are not amenable of sonographic evaluation

Answer: B—LUS is able to detect lung involvement of different medical conditions and can differentiate cardiogenic pulmonary edema, ARDS and diseases without lung involvement.

Key point: most of respiratory and many cardiac acute conditions have a primary or secondary pulmonary involvement.

Rationale: as already detailed in Questions 18 and 19 rationale, LUS has proven able in detecting different pathologies such as pneumothorax, pleural effusion, as well as detecting sign of pulmonary congestion and loss of aeration, whatever is the process causing them. Every process that can show as the unilateral or bilateral increase in lung density, the appearance of lung consolidations or the presence of a pleural pathology is susceptible of detection on a LUS scan. Moreover, the exclusion of such process is also informative, because it narrows the range of possible differential diagnosis that may be causing the clinical picture, thus giving clues also on a possible acute asthma attack or on an acute-decompensated COPD. In the case of the non-critical acute-ED patients, a scanning protocol characterized by four scanning zones (two anterior, two lateral) on both sides, has proven enough to provide the physician with the relevant information [24–26].

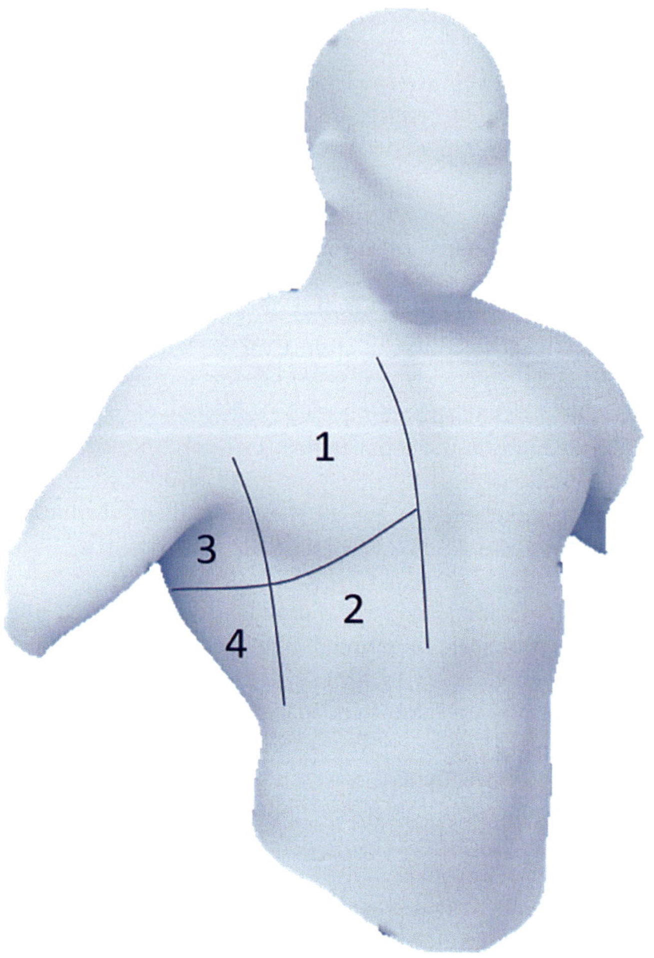

Fig. 13.10 Four-scanning zones for the non-critical patients. When evaluating a patient for dyspnea a simplified scanning scheme with eight zones is suggested to detect interstitial syndrome. Anterior zones are medially delimitated by the parasternal line and by anterior axillary line, laterally. Lateral scans are delimitated posteriorly by the posterior axillary line. Both anterior and posterior scan are divided in the upper and lower half of the lung

Question 47

A 67-year old female patient admitted to ICU for acute necrotizing pancreatitis suddenly develops peripheral oxygen desaturation and impending respiratory failure.

What is the role of lung ultrasound in the critical patient respiratory failure?

A. There is no role for LUS in this case, because most respiratory failure cases are due to cardiac causes
B. There is no role for LUS in this case, because there is no evidence on LUS effectiveness in ARDS patients
C. LUS is able to differentiate the underlying condition of the ICU patients due its narrower differential diagnosis spectrum causing respiratory failure
D. LUS is useless for airway diseases, that are the most frequent cause of respiratory failure in the ICU

Answer: C—LUS is able to differentiate the underlying condition of the ICU patients due its narrower differential diagnosis spectrum causing respiratory failure.

Key point: Most cases of acute respiratory failure in critical care patients can be diagnosed accurately with the use of lung ultrasound.

Rationale: in the particular setting of critical care patient the only validated diagnostic protocol is the BLUE protocol of Lichtenstein. It involves the scanning of three point (called BLUE-points), searching first for lung sliding, then combining it with the presence or absence of B-lines, and eventually with the finding of a lung point, deep vein thrombosis or postero-lateral-alveolar-pleural syndrome. The resulting algorithm allows to differentiate between pulmonary edema, pulmonary embolism, pneumonia, pneumothorax, COPD/asthma as the most likely cause of the acute respiratory failure with an accuracy of 90% [27–33].

Question 48

A 65 year old ICU patient with a significant smoking history (35 pack-year) has been admitted for a necrotic-hemorrhagic acute pancreatitis and septic shock. Chest X-ray is requested for sudden development of respiratory distress. CXR shows a diffuse opacity, worst on the right side, with patchy bilateral parenchymal infiltrates.

What is the difference in accuracy for pneumothorax diagnosis (Table 13.1)**?**

A. There is no known difference in accuracy between LUS and CXR

Table 13.1 Sensitivity and specificity comparison of lung ultrasound and chest X-ray in three systematic reviews and meta-analysis

	LUS sens	LUS spec	CXR sens	CXR spec
Ding et al. [34]	0.88	0.99	0.52	1.00
Alrajhi et al. [35]	0.91	0.98	0.50	0.99
Alrajab et al. [36]	0.79	0.98	0.40	0.99

B. LUS is very specific for pneumothorax diagnosis, but has a higher sensitivity than CXR

C. LUS is very specific for pneumothorax diagnosis, but CXR has higher sensitivity

D. LUS is very sensitive for pneumothorax diagnosis, but CXR has higher specificity

Answer: B—LUS is a very specific means for pneumothorax diagnosis, but has a higher sensitivity of CXR.

Key point: whenever suspecting a pneumothorax, if an ultrasound machine is available, lung US should be done as soon as possible, since it brings the highest amount of information with the lowest resource consumption.

Rationale: Both CXr and Ultrasound are available bedside, requires dedicated machinery and cost less than a thoracic CT scan, but while US requires only a brief training, CXR necessitates a dedicated technician. US is the only one without ionizing radiation.

Four systematic reviews with meta-analysis have addressed the question of CXr vs. Ultrasound and report the finding that Ultrasound sensitivity and specificity are 87% and 99% respectively, while CXR are 46% and 100% respectively [34–37].

Question 49

A 23 year old male reaches your ED complaining of new onset of respiratory discomfort. He has got stable vital parameters and physical examination is unremarkable. Chest X-ray is performed in upright position, showing a right-sided pneumothorax with a horizontal interpleural distance of 2 cm at hilum level. One colleague suggests to drain it with a small-bore chest drain, while junior doctor point out that maybe this situation could be managed better after a different evaluation with ultrasound.

What is the difference in accuracy for pneumothorax quantification (Fig. 13.11)**?**

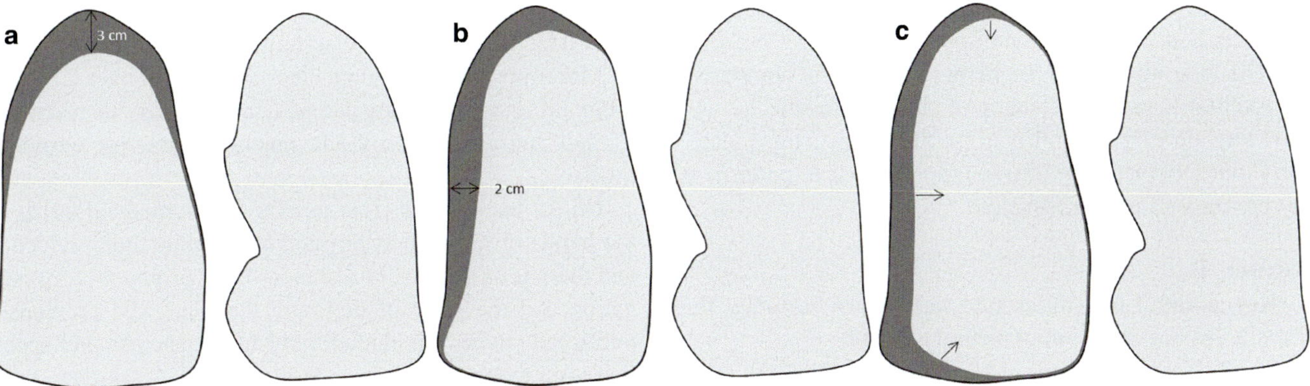

Fig. 13.11 Scheme of CXR-based measures used to differentiate between small and large pneumothorax. Panel (**a**) American College of Chest Physicians criterion; panel (**b**) British Thoracic Society criterion; panel (**c**) Belgian Society of Pulmonology criterion

A. LUS is very specific in quantifying pneumothorax dimension, but has a lower sensitivity than CXR.
B. As LUS is a very specific means for pneumothorax diagnosis, it is also better in pneumothorax quantification.
C. CXR has confirmed to have a better prediction of small and large pneumothoraxes.
D. There is no concluding evidence on differences in accuracy between LUS and CXR in estimating pneumothorax dimensions.

Answer: D—There is no concluding evidence on differences in accuracy between LUS and CXR in estimating pneumothorax dimensions.

Key point: lung ultrasound is capable of differentiating small and large pneumothoraces.

Rationale: three widespread criteria are used to define a "large" pneumothorax: an interpleural distance at the apex of at least 3 cm, according to the American College of Chest Physicians; an interpleural distance at the level of hilum of 2 cm, according to British Thoracic Society; a complete detachment from apex to base of the 2 pleurae, according to Belgian Society of Pulmonology.

As detailed in Question 11 rationale, LUS has demonstrated the ability to quantify different amount of intrapleural air collection both in the animal model and in the human. However, even though this finding is consistent within the studies, larger studies on human are still needed. On the other hand, chest X-ray based size prediction of pneumothorax has demonstrated to be an unreliable means to carry out pneumothorax quantification. Thus, there is a lack a conclusive method to be used bedside, avoiding unnecessary radiation exposure of CT scan.

Question 50

A 62-year-old patient with chronic heart failure is admitted to the ED complaining of dyspnea and fever. Chest X-ray and lung ultrasound are performed at bedside.

How to interpret the result of the two exams?

A. Lung ultrasound has a lower accuracy in comparison to chest X-ray for detection of pleural effusion.
B. The lung ultrasound has higher accuracy in comparison to chest X-ray for detection of pleural effusion.
C. Lung ultrasound confirmed the fluid to be a transudate.
D. Color Doppler lung ultrasound is needed to confirm the presence of pleural effusion.

Answer: **B.**

Key point: Lung ultrasound has higher accuracy than chest X-ray for detection of pleural effusion.

Rationale: The accuracy of chest ultrasound to detect pleural effusion is higher in comparison to a chest X-ray. Regarding the nature of the fluid, when the image is completely anechoic, lung ultrasound is not enough to differentiate transudate and exudate. In this situation, thoracentesis is recommended. On the other hand, when internal echoes are seen by lung ultrasound it is highly suggestive of exudate or hemothorax. Color Doppler has been utilized to aid in the diagnosis of lung abscess, atelectasis but not to determine the nature of pleural effusion [38].

Question 51

A 77 year old female presents to the ED with fever and productive cough since 1 week. She is febrile, slightly desaturating on room air (SpO_2 91%), tachycardic, and laboratory exams show leukocytosis (WBC 17,000). On auscultation crackles are audible on front right side.

What is the accuracy of lung ultrasound in detecting pneumonia (Fig. 13.12)**?**

A. Very low, in fact ultrasounds can't reach the dept of such an inflammatory process
B. Low, CXR has a superior sensitivity to pulmonary infiltrates
C. Good, literature shows an uncertain level of accuracy, but low-quality studies suggest a good level
D. Very good, there is a certain amount of evidence showing both sensitivity and specificity reaching above 90%

Answer: D—Very good, there is a certain amount of evidence showing both sensitivity and specificity reaching above 90%.

Key point: most of pneumonic processes provoke loss of pulmonary aeration and eventually produce a visible consolidation reaching the pleural surface. Thus, LUS is a valid alternative for the diagnosis of pneumonia.

Rationale: LUS performs well both as a rule-in and rule-out test for pneumonia in adults admitted to EDs and medical wards, both critically-ill and non-critically-ill. Even in patients with acute dyspnea, where the differential diagnosis is broad, LUS has a good discrimination.

Moreover, LUS has some clear advantages over CXR for pregnant and bedridden patients, as well as, in resource-limited settings where CXR machines are not currently available.

On the backside, its role in EDs and in medical wards in the hands of non-expert physicians requires more evidence and there is still a lack of a standardized protocol of investigation. All the relevant literature that reviewed previously published studies concluded that LUS sensitivity and specificity can reach values above 90% [39, 40].

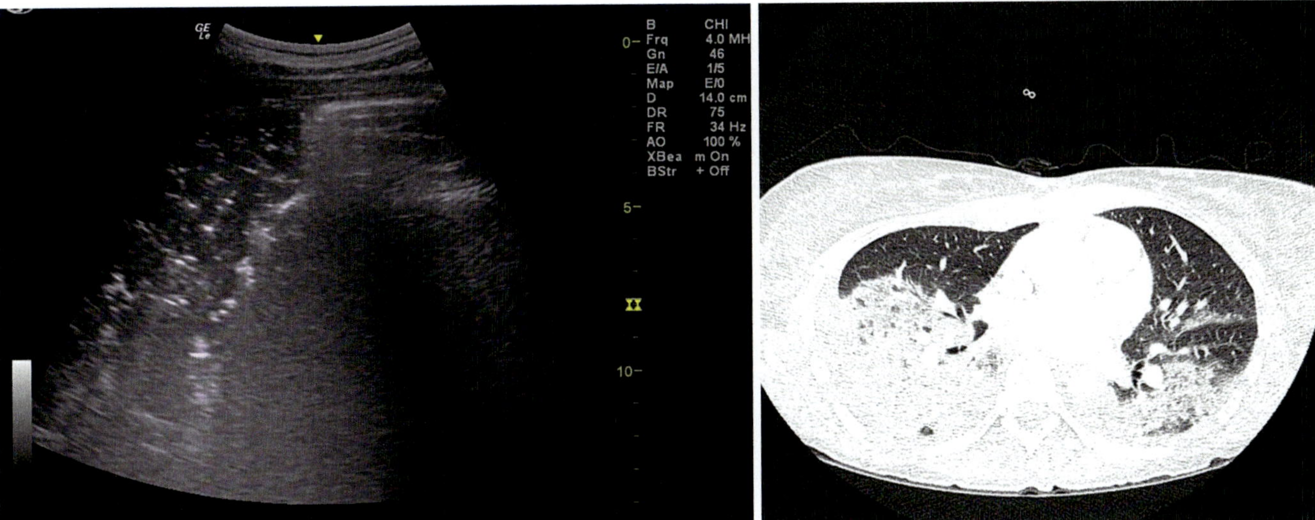

Fig. 13.12 LUS and CT comparison

Question 52

A 47-year-old male patient is admitted in the emergency department complaining of cough and fever for 3 days. The oxygen saturation is 87%. Blood exam showed leukocytosis. Chest X-ray is negative for infection. Lung ultrasound was performed at bedside showing (Video 13.13).

How should it be interpreted?

A. The lung ultrasound image is characteristic of pneumonia.
B. Chest X-ray has similar accuracy to lung ultrasound to differentiate causes of consolidation.
C. Chest X-ray has lower sensitivity but higher specificity than lung ultrasound for differential diagnosis of consolidations.
D. The correlation between lung ultrasound findings and the clinical setting is mandatory to a correct diagnosis.

Answer: **D.**

Key point: Lung ultrasound presents good accuracy in diagnosing and differentiating consolidations comparing to chest X-ray.

Rationale: Lung consolidation is visualized as an echo-poor or tissue like image, depending on the extent of air loss and fluid predominance. Lung consolidations may have a variety of causes including infection, pulmonary embolism, lung cancer and metastases, compression atelectasis, obstructive atelectasis, and lung contusion. For the correct differential diagnosis of consolidations the correlation between image and clinical setting is mandatory. Furthermore, some sonographic features of the lesion can be of help to differentiate the cause of the consolidation: the quality of the deep margins of the consolidation, the presence of comet-tail reverberation artifacts at the far-field margin, the presence of dynamic air bronchogram, the presence of fluid bronchogram and the vascular pattern within the consolidation. In contrast to community and hospital-acquire pneumonia, it is still difficult to report a precise accuracy of LUS on undifferentiated lung consolidations [41].

Question 53

It's the beginning of a night shift in the emergency room, when a 38 year old male is brought in by the emergency medical services for a severe case of dyspnea. There is no hemodynamic impairment, but respiratory rate is above 30, and peripheral oxygen saturation below 70% on room air and 86% on reservoir mask. The patient has no other signs of disease, but a 5 days history of cough and crackles on auscultation. He has no past medical history, and is only exposed to frequent air travel due to work reasons.

What is the role of lung ultrasound in COVID-19 diagnosis?

A. There is no role for LUS in this diagnosis, since COVID-19 pneumonia has mainly an interstitial involvement
B. There is no role for LUS in this diagnosis, because most respiratory impairment of COVID-19 is due to microvascular phenomena that are not amenable of ultrasonographic assessment
C. LUS is able to early detect lung involvement also in asymptomatic patients, and can both aid in excluding suspected case and in keeping a high suspicion over a negative RT-PCR test
D. LUS is able to diagnose COVID-19 associated pneumonia thanks to its ability in detecting the typical small consolidations that are the most frequent encountered lesions

Answer: C—LUS is able to early detect lung involvement also in asymptomatic patients, and can both aid in excluding suspected case and in keeping a high suspicion over a negative RT-PCR test.

Key point: LUS has shown to provide a good estimation of lung involvement in COVID-19 patients, and should be integrated in the clinical workup to diagnose COVID-19 pneumonia.

Rationale: Patients suffering of COVID-19 may develop COVID associated pneumonia. As already described, LUS has shown to improve the diagnostic accuracy in patients presenting with acute respiratory symptoms, and is more accurate than chest X-ray in these diagnoses. In COVID-19 patients, both physical examination and chest X-ray showed poor correlation with the pneumonia diagnosis. LUS permits COVID-19 pneumonia to be diagnosed even in patients with normal vital signs. Moreover, there is a strong correlation between CT and LUS scans in COVID-19 patients and this supports the preferential use of LUS over CT in scenarios where CT is inappropriate (e.g., pregnancy) or difficult to perform. In particular two facts sustain the role of LUS in this diagnosis. First, interstitial lung involvement is already known to be depicted by the B-pattern, and is the most common and consistent finding in COVID-19 patients. Second, the "light beam" is a newly described LUS sign that corresponds to the early appearance of "ground-glass" opacity on a CT scan, and it is highly represented in COVID-19 pneumonia patients (Video 13.29). Referring this to its clinical application, when the pre-test probability of COVID-19 is low, a LUS bilateral A-pattern with sliding suggests that COVID-19 pneumonia is unlikely, with a high negative predictive value. On the contrary, the presence of bilateral B-lines, irregular pleural line, and sub-pleural consolidations increase the probability of COVID-19 pneumonia in patient with high pretest probability. In the case of an intermediate probability patient (i.e., with other co- or pre-existing pulmonary conditions), LUS predictiveness decrease, and a third test should be use in unclear situations [42–44].

Question 54 (Case Continuation)

After starting the NIV support, his dyspnea reduces as respiratory rate decrease to 24, and oxygen saturation reaches 93%. On arterial blood gas-analysis partial oxygen pressure is 64 mmHg and P/F ratio is 80. After completing the basic workup and case re-evaluation NIV trial seems to be failing and patient is sedated and intubated before transfer to the ICU.

What is the role of lung ultrasound in COVID-19 prognostication (Fig. 13. 13)**?**

A. Lung ultrasound plays a role as an indicator of disease severity, predicting the disease progression, and LUS score is the most studied instrument for this purpose.
B. Lung ultrasound is a very sensitive means for carrying out the COVID-19 diagnosis, but has greater limitation when applied to patient stratification.
C. Lung ultrasound provides the clinicians with valuable clinical information only when finding big posterior consolidations.
D. Lung ultrasound has no role in COVID-19 prognostication since it is subject to the unpredictable effect of other organ involvement.

Answer: A.

Key point: a high overall LUS score, multifocal and bilateral pleural and lung abnormalities, can be used for the early assessment of COVID-19 severity in the ED and at ICU admission.

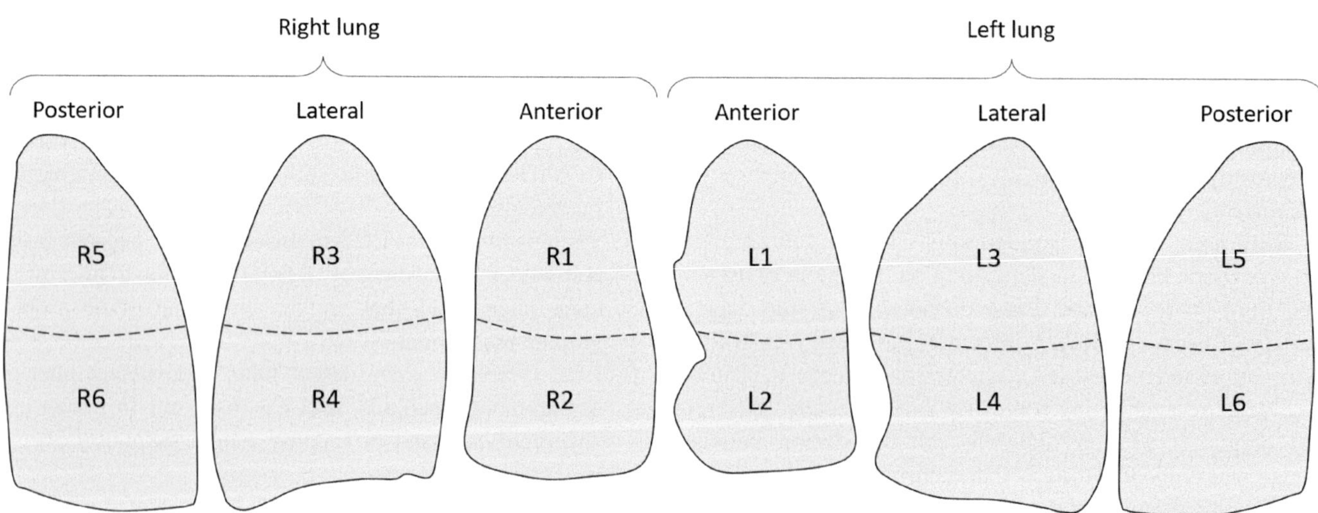

Fig. 13.13 12-zones scanning scheme used in determining LUS-score. Each hemithorax is divided into anterior, lateral, and posterior faces. Each face is divided into superior and inferior halves. Labelling of the zones starts from anterior-superior (Right 1) and ends at the posterior-inferior (Right 6) on both sides

Rationale: COVID-19 prognostication may reflect different focus on several steps of patient's history. In particular, the need for hospital admission, the need for escalating respiratory support, the need for intensive care treatment, and the risk of death.

A certain amount of evidence has been produced on this topic, founding a significant correlation between LUS findings and poor outcomes, such as the ones above mentioned. All these studies referred to the LUS score as the means to stratify patients. It was observed that a moderate loss of aeration on LUS is associated with a higher need for NIV, whereas a severe loss of lung aeration is associated with an increased likelihood of ICU admission, NIV failure and mortality.

Question 55 (Case Continuation)
On day 1, patient worsening conditions prompt the execution of ARDS rescue maneuvers, and he is positioned prone, with a significant response. On day 2–4, cyclic prone-positioning allows a partial recover and P/F ratio raise to 135. On day 5 a newly onset of fever, white blood cells increase and worsening respiratory function halts this improvement. Patient is put on antibiotic therapy for a week. On day 10 he successfully pass a spontaneous breathing trial and gets extubated.

What is the role of lung ultrasound in COVID-19 monitoring?

A. LUS is able to detect the typical small consolidations, but can't follow the disease progression.
B. There is no role for LUS in COVID-19 monitoring because most respiratory impairment of COVID-19 is due to bronchial inflammation and internal phenomena that aren't reached by ultrasound.
C. There is no role for LUS in this monitoring since COVID-19 pneumonia has mainly an interstitial involvement.
D. LUS can be utilized as a monitoring tool in management of COVID-19 Pneumonia.

Answer: D.

Key point: LUS is a good means to follow lung density changes and evolution of lung pathologies; being repeatable, cheap and bedside, it represents the ideal imaging monitoring method for respiratory patients such as in COVID-19 pneumonia.

Rationale: In patients treated on a low intensity level (i.e., home-based, nursing homes, general wards) LUS may contribute to assess disease progression with changes in LUS score. Moreover, in medium intensity patients, it could aid to predict non-invasive ventilation outcome. In invasive mechanical ventilation, LUS may aid the assessment of disease progression and the response to treatments in COVID-19 patients.

References

1. Lichtenstein DA, Menu Y. A bedside ultrasound sign ruling out pneumothorax in the critically ill. Lung sliding. Chest. 1995;108(5):1345–8.
2. Jambrik Z, Monti S, Coppola V, et al. Usefulness of ultrasound lung comets as a nonradiologic sign of extravascular lung water. Am J Cardiol. 2004;93(10):1265–70. https://doi.org/10.1016/j.amjcard.2004.02.012.
3. Dietrich CF, Mathis G, Blaivas M, et al. Lung B-line artefacts and their use. J Thorac Dis. 2016;8(6):1356–65. https://doi.org/10.21037/jtd.2016.04.55.
4. Lichtenstein DA, Mezière GA, Lagoueyte JF, Biderman P, Goldstein I, Gepner A. A-lines and B-lines: lung ultrasound as a bedside tool for predicting pulmonary artery occlusion pressure in the critically ill. Chest. 2009;136(4):1014–20. https://doi.org/10.1378/chest.09-0001.
5. Agricola E, Bove T, Oppizzi M, et al. "Ultrasound comet-tail images": a marker of pulmonary edema: a comparative study with wedge pressure and extravascular lung water. Chest. 2005;127(5):1690–5. https://doi.org/10.1378/chest.127.5.1690.
6. Reissig A, Kroegel C. Transthoracic sonography of diffuse parenchymal lung disease: the role of comet tail artifacts. J Ultrasound Med. 2003;22(2):173–80.
7. Lichtenstein DA, Lascols N, Prin S, Mezière G. The "lung pulse": an early ultrasound sign of complete atelectasis. Intensive Care Med. 2003;29(12):2187–92. https://doi.org/10.1007/s00134-003-1930-9.
8. Lichtenstein D, Mezière G, Biderman P, Gepner A. The "lung point": an ultrasound sign specific to pneumothorax. Intensive Care Med. 2000;26(10):1434–40.
9. Aspler A, Pivetta E, Stone MB. Double-lung point sign in traumatic pneumothorax. Am J Emerg Med. 2014;32(7):819.e1–2. https://doi.org/10.1016/j.ajem.2013.12.059.
10. Shriki J. Ultrasound physics. Crit Care Clin. 2014;30(1):1–24, v. https://doi.org/10.1016/j.ccc.2013.08.004.
11. Hedrick WR, Hykes DL, Starchman DE. Ultrasound physics and instrumentation. Amsterdam: Elsevier Mosby; 2005.
12. Prada G, Vieillard-Baron A, Martin AK, et al. Echocardiographic applications of M-mode ultrasonography in anesthesiology and critical care. J Cardiothorac Vasc Anesth. 2019;33(6):1559–83. https://doi.org/10.1053/j.jvca.2018.06.019.
13. Copetti R, Soldati G, Copetti P. Chest sonography: a useful tool to differentiate acute cardiogenic pulmonary edema from acute respiratory distress syndrome. Cardiovasc Ultrasound. 2008;6:16. https://doi.org/10.1186/1476-7120-6-16.
14. Nazerian P, Vanni S, Volpicelli G, et al. Accuracy of point-of-care multiorgan ultrasonography for the diagnosis of pulmonary embolism. Chest. 2014;145(5):950–7. https://doi.org/10.1378/chest.13-1087.
15. Reissig A, Copetti R, Mathis G, et al. Lung ultrasound in the diagnosis and follow-up of community-acquired pneumonia: a prospective, multicenter, diagnostic accuracy study. Chest. 2012;142(4):965–72. https://doi.org/10.1378/chest.12-0364.
16. Mongodi S, Via G, Girard M, et al. Lung ultrasound for early diagnosis of ventilator-associated pneumonia. Chest. 2016;149(4):969–80. https://doi.org/10.1016/j.chest.2015.12.012.
17. Yang PC, Luh KT, Chang DB, Yu CJ, Kuo SH, Wu HD. Ultrasonographic evaluation of pulmonary consolidation. Am Rev Respir Dis. 1992;146(3):757–62. https://doi.org/10.1164/ajrccm/146.3.757.
18. Lichtenstein D, Mezière G, Seitz J. The dynamic air bronchogram. A lung ultrasound sign of alveolar consolidation ruling out atelectasis. Chest. 2009;135(6):1421–5. https://doi.org/10.1378/chest.08-2281.

19. Joyner CR, Herman RJ, Reid JM. Reflected ultrasound in the detection and localization of pleural effusion. JAMA. 1967;200(5):399–402.
20. Evans PT, Zhang RS, Cao Y, et al. The use of thoracic ultrasound to predict transudative and exudative pleural effusion. POCUS J. 2021;6(2):97–102. https://doi.org/10.24908/pocus.v6i2.15193.
21. Dickman E, Terentiev V, Likourezos A, Derman A, Haines L. Extension of the thoracic spine sign. J Ultrasound Med. 2015;34(9):1555–61. https://doi.org/10.7863/ultra.15.14.06013.
22. Lichtenstein D, Hulot JS, Rabiller A, Tostivint I, Mezière G. Feasibility and safety of ultrasound-aided thoracentesis in mechanically ventilated patients. Intensive Care Med. 1999;25(9):955–8.
23. Mayo PH, Goltz HR, Tafreshi M, Doelken P. Safety of ultrasound-guided thoracentesis in patients receiving mechanical ventilation. Chest. 2004;125(3):1059–62.
24. Gargani L, Volpicelli G. How I do it: lung ultrasound. Cardiovasc Ultrasound. 2014;12:25. https://doi.org/10.1186/1476-7120-12-25.
25. Dexheimer Neto FL, de Andrade JMS, Raupp ACT, et al. Diagnostic accuracy of the bedside lung ultrasound in emergency protocol for the diagnosis of acute respiratory failure in spontaneously breathing patients. J Bras Pneumol. 2015;41(1):58–64. https://doi.org/10.1590/S1806-37132015000100008.
26. Daabis R, Banawan L, Rabea A, Elnakedy A, Sadek A. Relevance of chest sonography in the diagnosis of acute respiratory failure: comparison with current diagnostic tools in intensive care units. Egypt J Chest Dis Tuberc. 2014;63(4):979–85. https://doi.org/10.1016/j.ejcdt.2014.05.005.
27. Lichtenstein DA, Mezière GA. Relevance of lung ultrasound in the diagnosis of acute respiratory failure: the BLUE protocol. Chest. 2008;134(1):117–25. https://doi.org/10.1378/chest.07-2800.
28. Bouhemad B, Mongodi S, Via G, Rouquette I. Ultrasound for "lung monitoring" of ventilated patients. Anesthesiology. 2015;122(2):437–47. https://doi.org/10.1097/ALN.0000000000000558.
29. Lichtenstein D, Goldstein I, Mourgeon E, Cluzel P, Grenier P, Rouby JJ. Comparative diagnostic performances of auscultation, chest radiography, and lung ultrasonography in acute respiratory distress syndrome. Anesthesiology. 2004;100(1):9–15.
30. Lichtenstein DA. Lung ultrasound in the critically ill: the BLUE protocol. Berlin: Springer; 2015.
31. Lichtenstein DA. Whole body ultrasonography in the critically ill. Berlin: Springer-Verlag; 2010. www.springer.com/us/book/9783642053276. Accessed 8 Sep 2018.
32. Chichra A, Makaryus M, Chaudhri P, Narasimhan M. Ultrasound for the pulmonary consultant. Clin Med Insights Circ Respir Pulm Med. 2016;10:1–9. https://doi.org/10.4137/CCRPM.S33382.
33. Smit JM, Haaksma ME, Winkler MH, et al. Lung ultrasound in a tertiary intensive care unit population: a diagnostic accuracy study. Crit Care. 2021;25(1):339. https://doi.org/10.1186/s13054-021-03759-3.
34. Ding W, Shen Y, Yang J, et al. Diagnosis of pneumothorax by radiography and ultrasonography: a meta-analysis. Chest. 2011;140(4):859–66.
35. Alrajhi K, Woo MY, Vaillancourt C. Test characteristics of ultrasonography for the detection of pneumothorax: a systematic review and meta-analysis. Chest. 2011;141(3):703–8.
36. Alrajab S, Youssef AM, Akkus NI, Caldito G. Pleural ultrasonography versus chest radiography for the diagnosis of pneumothorax: review of the literature and meta-analysis. Crit Care. 2013;17(5):R208.
37. Lichtenstein DA, Mezière G, Lascols N, et al. Ultrasound diagnosis of occult pneumothorax. Crit Care Med. 2005;33(6):1231–8.
38. Dancel R, Schnobrich D, Puri N, et al. Recommendations on the use of ultrasound guidance for adult thoracentesis: a position statement of the Society of Hospital Medicine. J Hosp Med. 2018;13(2):126–35. https://doi.org/10.12788/jhm.2940.
39. Xirouchaki N, Magkanas E, Vaporidi K, et al. Lung ultrasound in critically ill patients: comparison with bedside chest radiography. Intensive Care Med. 2011;37(9):1488–93. https://doi.org/10.1007/s00134-011-2317-y.
40. Ye X, Xiao H, Chen B, Zhang S. Accuracy of lung ultrasonography versus chest radiography for the diagnosis of adult community-acquired pneumonia: review of the literature and meta-analysis. PLoS One. 2015;10(6):e0130066. https://doi.org/10.1371/journal.pone.0130066.
41. Lichtenstein DA, Lascols N, Mezière G, Gepner A. Ultrasound diagnosis of alveolar consolidation in the critically ill. Intensive Care Med. 2004;30(2):276–81. https://doi.org/10.1007/s00134-003-2075-6.
42. Fox S, Dugar S. Point-of-care ultrasound and COVID-19. Cleve Clin J Med. Published online May 14, 2020. https://doi.org/10.3949/ccjm.87a.ccc019.
43. Moazedi-Fuerst FC, Kielhauser S, Brickmann K, et al. Sonographic assessment of interstitial lung disease in patients with rheumatoid arthritis, systemic sclerosis and systemic lupus erythematosus. Clin Exp Rheumatol. 2015;33(4 Suppl 91):S87–91.
44. Volpicelli G, Gargani L. Sonographic signs and patterns of COVID-19 pneumonia. Ultrasound J. 2020;12(1):22. https://doi.org/10.1186/s13089-020-00171-w.

Pulmonary Hypertension, Pulmonary Embolism and ARDS

14

Neal F. Chaisson, Steven Fox, and Matthew T. Siuba

Question 1

A 45 year old female with no prior medical history presents with acute onset dyspnea on exertion and poor exercise tolerance. HR 112, BP 110/80, SpO2 88% on room air. Echo reveals a small left ventricle (LV) with normal systolic function, septal flattening in systole and diastole, right ventricle (RV) diastolic diameter greater than LV diastolic diameter, RV free wall thickness of 11 mm in the subcostal view and moderator band hypertrophy . Tricuspid regurgitant (TR) jet velocity is 4.4 m/s. Which of the following is the best answer regarding these echocardiographic findings?

A. This patient has an acute pulmonary embolism.
B. This suggests acute cor pulmonale.
C. One cannot determine if acute RV failure is present
D. This suggests left ventricular diastolic dysfunction.

Correct Answer: C. Explanation: Chronic cor pulmonale leads to right ventricular remodeling and hypertrophy, characterized by increased RV free wall thickness. This is best measured in the subcostal 4 chamber view at end diastole, taking care to avoid trabeculations. RV free wall thickness 5 mm or less is considered normal. Free wall thickness > 10 mm is highly suggestive of chronic cor pulmonale.

The findings, in this case, are consistent with a chronic process (choice C) rather than an acute process (choice B). Several echocardiographic parameters are suggestive of the chronicity of RV dysfunction. Key among them is the presence of RV hypertrophy. When evaluating a patient with signs of chronic cor pulmonale, it is important to recognize that the same findings may be seen despite an acute on chronic insult to the RV. Therefore, diagnosing an acute pulmonary embolism in this patient based on echo alone is not feasible (choice A). While left ventricular diastolic dysfunction can cause cor pulmonale, the findings here are not exclusive to patients with left ventricular diastolic dysfunction (choice D).

Supplementary Information The online version contains supplementary material available at https://doi.org/10.1007/978-3-031-45731-9_14.

N. F. Chaisson (✉) · S. Fox · M. T. Siuba
Cleveland Clinic, Respiratory Institute, Cleveland, OH, USA
e-mail: chaissn@ccf.org; siubam@ccf.org

Question 2

A 45 year old male with no prior medical history presents with acute onset dyspnea on exertion. HR 112, BP 110/80, SpO2 88% on room air. Echo reveals a normal sized LV with hyperdynamic systolic function, septal flattening in systole and diastole, RV diastolic diameter greater than LV diastolic diameter, RV free wall diameter 4 mm in parasternal short axis, tricuspid annular plane systolic excursion (TAPSE) 1.3, and preserved movement of the RV apex. The RV free wall is hypokinetic. Right ventricular systolic pressure (RVSP) is 45 mmHg and TR acceleration time is 50 milliseconds. Which of the following is the best choice?

A. This suggests idiopathic pulmonary arterial hypertension.
B. This suggests acute cor pulmonale, without chronic pulmonary hypertension
C. This suggests the presence of chronic thromboembolic pulmonary hypertension (CTEPH)
D. This suggests left ventricular diastolic dysfunction.

Correct Answer: B. Explanation: This echo demonstrates several signs of acute cor pulmonale (choice B). Among these signs are the defining features of McConnell's sign; preserved apical RV motion with reduced transverse motion of the RV free wall. McConnell's sign is highly specific for acute pulmonary embolism in patients with signs and symptoms consistent with acute pulmonary embolism. The 60/60 sign is defined by TR gradient <60 mmHg and TR acceleration time < 60 milliseconds. The RV pressure peaks earlier and with less amplitude in acute cor pulmonale, since the RV has not had time to remodel in a way that allows for a prolonged contraction time and a higher pressure. The 60/60 sign has been shown to have a 94% specificity for diagnosis of PE.

R. Sreedharan et al. (eds.), *Critical Care Echocardiography*, https://doi.org/10.1007/978-3-031-45731-9_14

There are no features here to suggest either idiopathic pulmonary arterial hypertension or CTEPH (answer choice A and C) as both represent processes that occur in a subacute or chronic fashion and neither can be conclusively diagnosed by echocardiography alone. In addition, an RV free wall <5 mm suggests an acute process rather than chronic RV hypertrophy. There are no findings here to suggest left ventricular diastolic dysfunction (answer choice D).

Question 3

When measuring RV diameter and Fractional area change (FAC), which of the following views, as depicted in the images, will provide you with the highest intra-rater and inter-rater accuracy? (Figs. 14.1, 14.2 and 14.3).

A. Image 1
B. Image 2
C. Image 3

Correct Answer: A. Explanation: Variability of axis can lead to variation and error in right ventricular linear and area measurements. Thus a standardized approach is important. The American Society of Echocardiography recommends RV-focused view as the preferred view to obtain RV linear dimensions (Image 1). The RV-focused view is obtained by lateral displacement of the transducer from the conventional A4C view position together with a probe rotation to obtain the largest RV dimension in its long axis. The RV-focused view enhances RV cavity and free wall visualization without foreshortening. The visualization of the entire RV both during systole and diastole further improves accuracy. Use of an off-axis view as depicted by Image 2 (choice B) and Image 3 (choice C) could lead to an underestimation of RV diameter. An oblique or foreshortened view can lead to an overestimation of the RV diameter.

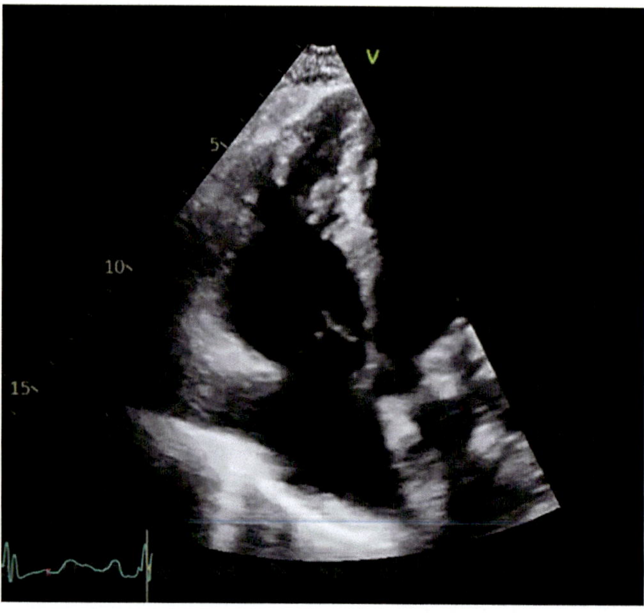

Fig. 14.1 RV focused apical apical 4-chamber view

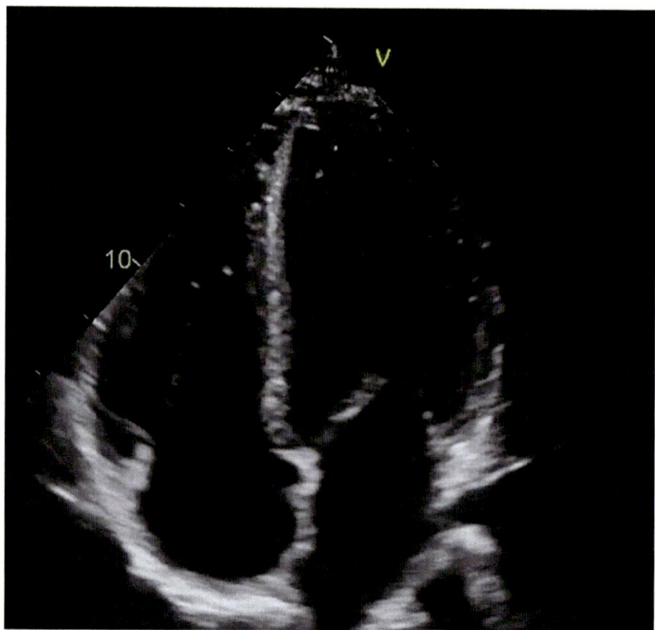

Fig. 14.2 Conventional apical 4-chamber view

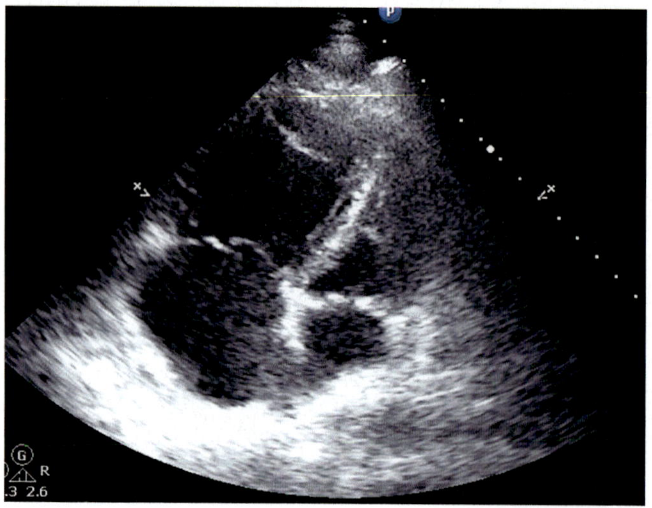

Fig. 14.3 RV modified view

Question 4
Which of the following lung ultrasound findings is *least* consistent with pulmonary embolism?

A. A lines in all lung fields
B. B lines in all lung fields
C. Subpleural consolidation
D. Pleural effusion

Correct Answer: B. Key Point: Common lung ultrasound findings in patients with pulmonary embolism include an A-line pattern, subpleural consolidation (due to pulmonary infarct), and pleural effusion.

Explanation: B-line pattern in all lung fields is not routinely observed in acute pulmonary embolism (choice B). While focal areas of pulmonary edema can be seen, B-lines in all lung fields is more commonly seen in patients with congestive heart failure, acute respiratory distress syndrome (ARDS), or interstitial fibrosis where diffuse parenchymal edema or interstitial thickening is present. Pulmonary embolism (PE) is most commonly associated with a predominant A line pattern (choice A) due to lack of interstitial edema. Patients with PE can also develop subpleural consolidations (choice C) and pleural effusions (choice D). The typical subpleural consolidation is triangular or round in shape, and 0.5–3 cm in diameter. These are most commonly found in the inferior/posterior lung zones. Subpleural consolidation in patients with suspected pulmonary embolism is 75% sensitive and 95% specific for acute pulmonary embolism when evaluated using a protocol. Multiorgan ultrasound, including cardiac, lung, and DVT study can further aid in this assessment and may improve both sensitivity and specificity for detecting acute PE in the appropriate patient.

Question 5
A 44 year old male with history of lower extremity DVT, not currently on anticoagulation, presents from home with new onset of cough and left sided pleuritic chest pain. Temperature 100.3 HR 102, BP 130/90, RR 22, SpO2 90% on 2 L nasal cannula. Lungs are clear to auscultation. There is bilateral 1+ lower extremity edema. Point of care ultrasound of the lung is shown below. Which of the following choices is most accurate? (Fig. 14.4).

A. These findings are consistent with pleural effusion
B. These findings are consistent with acute pulmonary embolism
C. These findings are consistent with pulmonary edema
D. These findings are consistent with pneumothorax

Correct Answer: B. Explanation: The images in this question show subpleural consolidation at the region of chest pain. The remainder of the lung fields show A-lines on lung ultrasound. Subpleural consolidation is a common finding in pulmonary embolism (choice B), most often due to peripheral lung infarct. In prospective studY of patients with suspected PE, a lung ultrasound protocol which assessed patients for the presence of subpleural consolidation (0.5–3 cm in diameter, triangular or round shaped) or pleural effusion found that the findings demonstrated a 74% sensitivity and 94% specificity for the diagnosis of PE. However, it should be noted that subpleural consolidations also occur in many other processes. Therefore, this finding in isolation is insufficient to make a diagnosis of PE. A confirmatory diagnosis of acute PE still requires CT angiogram of the chest. These images do not show a pleural effusion (choice A). Pulmonary edema would be likely if the image showed predominant B-lines (choice C). While the presence of A-lines can be seen in patients with pneumothorax, a definitive diagnosis of pneumothorax can only be made when a lung point is noted. The region of interest shows an area of consolidation which is not consistent with pneumothorax (choice D).

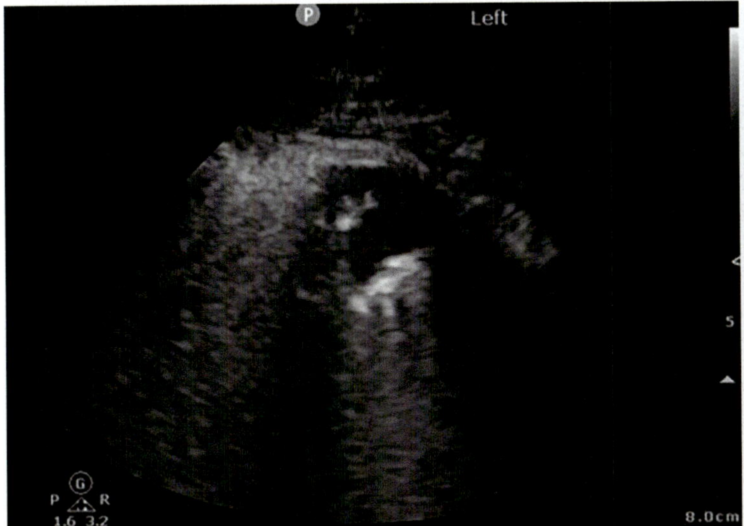

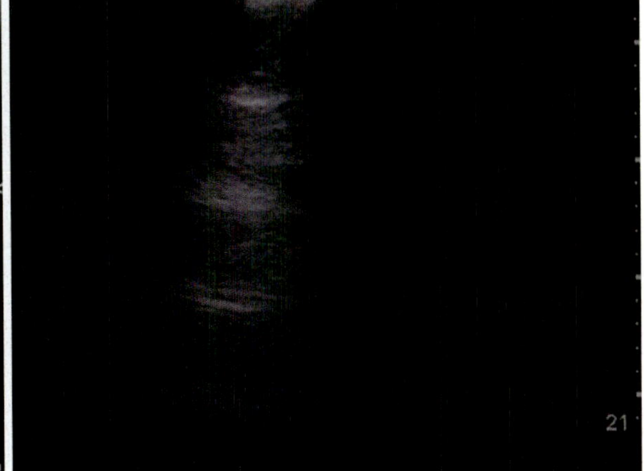

Fig. 14.4 Left image: Left lateral lung at site of pleuritic chest pain. Right image: All other lung segments

Question 6

In normotensive patients, which of the following choices is the strongest echocardiographic predictor of mortality in acute pulmonary embolism?

A. Tricuspid regurgitant jet acceleration time
B. RVSP
C. TAPSE
D. RV/LV diastolic diameter ratio
E. Subjective evaluation of hypokinesis

Correct Answer: C. Explanation: TAPSE (choice C) has been shown to highly predictive of mortality in patient with hemodynamically stable pulmonary embolism in comparison to RV/LV diastolic diameter ratio (choice D) (on echo or on multidetector CT) or RVSP (choice B) or tricuspid regurgitant acceleration time (choice A). A 2015 study demonstrated that TAPSE <15 mm was associated with a 45% chance of mortality, while all patients with TAPSE >18 mm survived. The authors concluded that low TAPSE (<15 mm) should prompt ICU admission due to high risk for deterioration. A larger study (630 patients) found similar results, with TAPSE <15 mm conferring an odds ratio of 25 for death, greater than that for RV end diastolic diameter, RV:LV ratio, and subjective evaluation of hypokinesis (choice E).

Question 7

An 80 year old female is brought to the Emergency Department with shortness of breath and pleuritic chest pain. She is on hemodialysis three times weekly via a catheter placed in her internal jugular vein. Vitals are as follows: HR 80, BP 124/84, RR 12, SpO_2 92% on 2 L nasal cannula. CT angiogram of the chest reveals clots in the bilateral main pulmonary arteries. The following clip is obtained at the bedside. Which of the following is the best approach to management? (Video 14.1).

A. Systemic TPA should be administered.
B. The optimum management is controversial. Multidisciplinary discussion should be initiated urgently.
C. Systemic anticoagulation alone should be administered.
D. Blood cultures should be collected, antibiotics initiated, and anticoagulation held.

Correct Answer: B. Explanation: With growing use of point of care ultrasound, thrombi in the right atrium and ventricle are increasingly being identified, either unexpectedly or in the context of a known pulmonary embolism.

Although nearly 100% of right heart thrombi are associated with PE, this statistic may be influenced by selection bias.

Clot in transit is associated with a high mortality rate among patients with PE. In patients with evidence of hypotension, guidelines recommend thrombolytic therapy in absence of contraindications. For normotensive patients, data remains controversial. No randomized trials exist and retrospective studies have found conflicting results regarding mortality by treatment type, likely limited by numerous confounders. As a result, management of this condition remains subject to expert opinion and should be treated based on the consensus of a multidisciplinary group of experts when available (choice B). Administering thrombolytic therapy without consideration for contraindications (choice A) or relying on systemic anticoagulation alone (choice C) in all cases is not an ideal approach.

It can be difficult to distinguish a vegetation (infective endocarditis) from an intracardiac thrombus (clot in transit). Given the clinical setting here (known PE without other signs of infection), as well as the appearance of the echodensity (mobile and not attached to the tricuspid valve), this is almost certainly clot in transit rather than infective endocarditis (choice D).

Question 8

A 25 year old male was admitted 7 days ago with influenza A, complicated by severe ARDS. Neuromuscular blockade and proning have been initiated. Ventilator settings are as follows: FiO_2 100%, positive end expiratory pressure (PEEP) 18 cm H_2O, RR 28 Tidal volume (Vt) 300 mL (6 mL/kg ideal body weight (IBW)). Plateau pressure is 42 cm H_2O. Arterial blood gas shows a pH 7.10, pCO_2 60 mmHg, pO_2 50 mmHg. He had an echo on admission which revealed a hyperdynamic LV and RV. Both were normal size, shape, and function. He is now requiring high doses of norepinephrine to maintain adequate blood pressures. He is net positive 2 L since admission. He is too unstable to go for CT angiography of the chest to evaluate for PE. You repeat an echo, which reveals a severely dilated right ventricle with RVSP of 70 mm Hg. Which of the following would most likely lead to improvement in RV function?

A. Systemic alteplase
B. Venovenous ECMO
C. Increasing the PEEP
D. IV fluid administration

Correct Answer: B. Key Point: ARDS and aggressive ventilator strategies (high Vt, high PEEP) may lead to RV dysfunction. ECMO may improve RV dysfunction in patient with severe ARDS.

Explanation: With the clinical history provided, the most likely etiology for this patient's RV failure is a combination of ARDS, high tidal volumes and high PEEP strategy. Approximately 27% of patients with ARDS develop acute cor pulmonale. Several mechanisms are likely responsible for this. Interstitial thickening in ARDS can lead to intra-alveolar vascular compression with subsequent increase in pulmonary vascular resistance. High PEEP and high tidal volumes can elevate RV afterload from mechanical compression of intra-alveolar vessels. Hypoxia mediated vasoconstriction also plays a role in increasing pulmonary vascular resistance (PVR).

In patients with severe ARDS, ECMO has been shown to improve RV dysfunction (choice B). Venovenous or veno-arterial ECMO enables one to reduce pulmonary vascular resistance caused by hypoxia, and reduce high PEEP or large tidal volumes. While pulmonary vascular resistance is unlikely to normalize, improvements in tissue oxygenation, acidosis, and intraalveolar capillary compression may yield improved RV function and cardiac output.

While pulmonary embolism cannot be ruled out in this patient, it is less likely the main cause of this patient's RV dysfunction. Thus, systemic alteplase would not be recommended unless the diagnosis of PE is confirmed with other modalities (choice A). Neither increasing PEEP, nor administering IV fluids would improve RV function (choice C and D).

Question 9

A 55 year old male was admitted 7 days ago with influenza A, complicated by severe ARDS. Ventilator settings as follows: FiO2 100%, PEEP 24 cm H_2O, RR 28, Vt 400 mL (8 mg/kg IBW). Arterial blood gas pH is 7.25, pCO_2 55 mmHg, and pO2 50 mmHg. Neuromuscular blockade and proning have been initiated. He is now requiring high doses of norepinephrine to maintain perfusion. He is net positive 8 liters since admission. Echocardiogram reveals a moderately dilated right ventricle, RV free wall thickness of 1.0 cm, TAPSE of 1.8 cm, RVSP of 65 mmHg, with RV acceleration time of 70 ms. There is no McConnell's sign. He has never had a prior echocardiogram. Based on this echocardiogram, which of the following statements best reflect the chronicity of his RV dysfunction?

A. This patient has features of chronic RV dysfunction.
B. His echo is consistent with acute cor pulmonale
C. His echo findings do not provide enough information to determine if his RV dysfunction is acute or chronic.
D. His echo suggests normal RV function.

Correct Answer: C. Explanation: This patient has a thickened right ventricular free wall (>5 mm) consistent with chronic right ventricular hypertrophy. However, what is described as a "chronic" change may actually develop within 48–72 h in patients with ARDS and elevated RV afterload. This patient has been in the hospital with severe ARDS for 7 days. Therefore, one might expect to see features associated with chronic RV dysfunction, such as RV free wall hypertrophy on this patient's echocardiogram. Thus, the presence of RV hypertrophy in this patient may have developed during this hospital stay or may have been present for a long period of time (choice C). We cannot conclude with high likelihood that he has acute RV dysfunction (choice B) or chronic right heart disease that was present prior to this admission (Choices A and B). Several features on this echo suggest RV dysfunction, so choice D is incorrect.

Question 10

A 40 year old female, 20 weeks pregnant, is presenting to the emergency department with dyspnea and pleuritic chest pain. She takes no home medications other than prenatal vitamins. Vitals are as follows: HR 92, BP 145/90, RR 22, SpO2 90% on room air. Exam reveals left calf tenderness and increased diameter of the left calf compared to the right. Chest radiograph is clear. EKG shows normal sinus rhythm with no ST or T wave changes. Troponin and BNP are normal. Pulmonary embolism is suspected. Transthoracic echocardiogram is performed at the bedside while CT angiography (CTA) of the chest is being ordered. Which of the following findings on point of care ultrasound would eliminate the need for CTA?

A. RV with normal size, shape, TAPSE and RVSP
B. Lung ultrasound revealing a left lower lobe subpleural consolidation
C. Severely dilated and thickened right ventricle, with RVSP of 70 mmHg
D. Mildly dilated right ventricle, with TAPSE of 1.5 cm, RVSP of 40 mmHg and acceleration time of 40 milliseconds
E. Non-compressible left popliteal vein and a grossly normal RV

Correct Answer: E. Explanation: Noncompressible veins on ultrasonography of the lower extremities can indicate the presence of acute DVT (specificity 97%, positive likelihood ratio 30), in patients with moderate or high pre-test probability for acute pulmonary embolism. Finding a proximal DVT would prompt immediate initiation of anticoagulation. In a patient at low-risk for in-hospital or 30-day mortality (normal vital signs, no signs of right heart strain), CTA would not change management, and could be avoided in this pregnant patient in order to minimize radiation exposure. This approach is supported by guidelines from the American Thoracic Society/Society of Thoracic Radiology.

Point of care ultrasound cannot rule out PE. Therefore, normal findings on ultrasound (choice A) should not preclude further diagnostic imaging with CTA. Sub pleural consolidation on lung ultrasound (choice B) in this patient could be consistent with pulmonary infarct due to PE, but it is not specific for this diagnosis and can be seen in other clinical conditions such as pneumonia. In a patient with this finding, CTA would still be necessary to confirm the presence of PE. Answer choice C represents findings in chronic pulmonary hypertension. However, an acute component cannot be excluded in a patient with these findings. With this clinical presentation, CTA would still be necessary. Answer choice D represents findings in acute cor pulmonale. These would be highly concerning for right heart strain due to acute PE, but do not confirm the presence of pulmonary embolism. In this case, CT would still be indicated.

Question 11

Which of the following images demonstrates the most appropriately placed cursor for standardized measurement of TAPSE?

A. See Fig. 14.5
B. See Fig. 14.6
C. See Fig. 14.7
D. See Fig. 14.8

Correct Answer: C. Explanation: TAPSE is measured using M-mode echocardiography with the cursor aligned along the tricuspid lateral annulus in the apical 4 chamber view (choice C). The contraction of longitudinally oriented RV muscle fiber results in systolic displacement of the tricuspid annulus toward the RV apex. TAPSE measures the distance of this excursion at peak systole. The cursor should follow the direction of RV longitudinal excursion (passing near or through the RV apex). The cursor axis in answer choice A does not pass near the RV apex. The cursor in answer choice B passes too lateral (beyond the tricuspid valve annulus) and is not through the RV apex. Answer choice D shows a subxiphoid view. Subcostal echocardiographic assessment of tricuspid annular kick (SEATAK) or subcostal TAPSE (sTAPSE) has recently been proposed as an alternative to conventional TAPSE in critically ill patients.

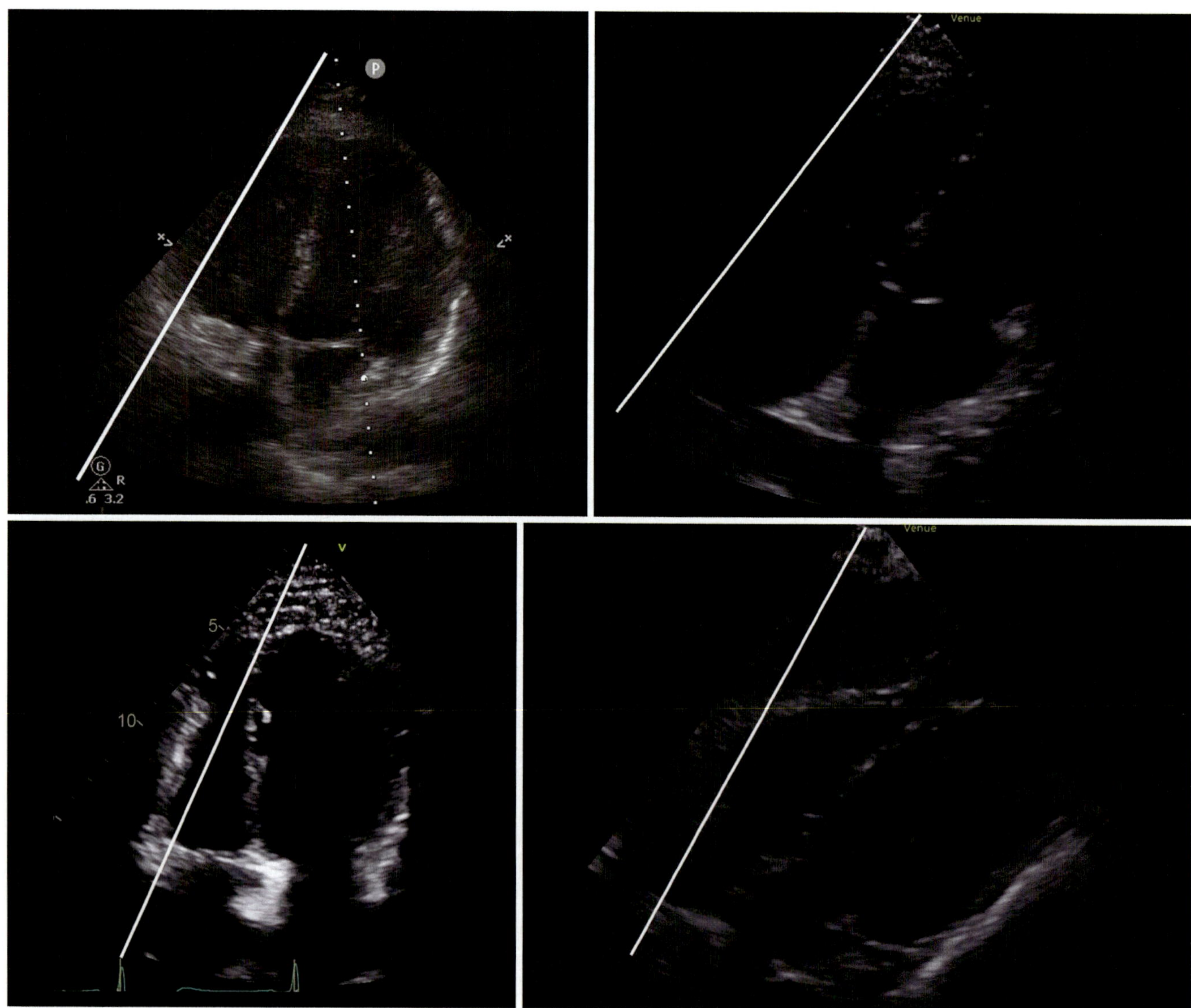

Figs. 14.5–14.8 Apical 4 chamber view

Question 12

Which of the following is a normal measurement or set of measurements regarding right ventricular size or function?

A. Tricuspid annular tissue doppler velocity (RV S′) 18.4 cm/s
B. Tricuspid valve regurgitant jet velocity: 374 cm/s
C. Right ventricle basal diameter 4.4 cm
D. Pulmonary artery diameter 3.92 cm

Correct Answer: A. Explanation: Answer choice A describes the peak velocity at the tricuspid annulus using tissue Doppler imaging (RV S′). A normal value for RV S′ is greater than 9.5 cm/s, as shown here. Answer choice B describes a tricuspid regurgitant velocity of 374 cm/s. In patients with a TR jet velocity greater than 340 cm/s, presence of pulmonary hypertension should be suspected, regardless of other findings. Answer choice C describes the RV basal end diastolic diameter. Abnormal values for this are greater than 4.2 cm. Note that mid-RV diameter above 3.5 cm is considered abnormal. Answer choice D describes the pulmonary artery diameter. This should be obtained in the parasternal long axis view. A pulmonary artery diameter of greater than 2.5 cm is considered abnormal. A diameter greater than 3.3 cm should prompt further evaluation for the presence of pulmonary hypertension.

Question 13

In a patient with interstitial edema, what finding on lung ultrasound is most consistent with cardiogenic pulmonary edema?

A. Confluent B lines throughout both lungs
B. Irregular pleural surface in both lungs
C. Subpleural consolidations
D. Intermittent B lines with areas of lung sparing
E. Reduced lung sliding

Correct Answer: A. Explanation: Lung ultrasound can help to distinguish cardiogenic from non-cardiogenic pulmonary edema. Features of lung ultrasound that suggest non-cardiogenic etiology of pulmonary edema include presence of pleural irregularity (choice B), reduced or absent lung sliding (choice E), presence of consolidations (choice C) and presence of spared areas of the lung (choice D). These features occur more commonly when an inflammatory component (ie: ARDS) is responsible for the presence of edema. It is important to note that cardiogenic and non-cardiogenic pulmonary edema can present simultaneously, so observing these signs does not exclude the possibility of concomitant cardiogenic pulmonary edema.

Confluent B lines (choice A) can occur in either cardiogenic or non-cardiogenic pulmonary edema. Of the choices listed, this is the most consistent with cardiogenic pulmonary edema.

Question 14

55 year-old woman with no prior cardiopulmonary disease is hospitalized after an episode of clostridium difficile colitis requiring total colectomy. On postoperative day 10 she develops new signs and symptoms concerning for pulmonary embolism. Which of the following echocardiographic findings would be most specific for pulmonary embolism?

A. Systolic flattening of the right ventricle
B. Tricuspid regurgitant velocity of 5 m/s and acceleration time of 70 milliseconds
C. Tricuspid regurgitant velocity of 3 m/s and acceleration time of 50 milliseconds
D. Tricuspid regurgitant velocity of 4 m/s in the absence of RV hypertrophy
E. RV:LV diastolic dimension >1

Correct Answer: C. Explanation: The 60/60 sign is defined as a tricuspid valve insufficiency gradient of less than 60 mmHg, in combination with an acceleration time of <60 milliseconds. The tricuspid valve insufficiency gradient is calculated by the Modified Bernoulli Eq. ($4 \times V^2$) where V is equal to the TR jet velocity. Answer choice C meets this criteria, with a tricuspid valve insufficiency gradient of 36 mmHg (4×3 m/s^2) and acceleration time of 50 ms. The 60/60 sign has been prospectively validated and its specificity is excellent. The specificity of McConnell's sign, 60/60 sign, and RV overload criteria were 100%, 94%, and 45% respectively. RV overload criteria were defined as 1 or more of: systolic flattening of the right ventricle (choice A), right sided cardiac thrombus, RV: LV diastolic dimension >1 (choice E), RV parasternal diastolic dimension >30 mm, systolic flattening of the interventricular septum, acceleration time < 90 ms, and tricuspid insufficiency pressure gradient >30 mm Hg in absence of RV hypertrophy (choice D). In patients without known previous cardiorespiratory disease, the specificity of McConnell's sign, 60/60 sign, and RV overload criteria were 100%, 100%, and 78% respectively. Thus, 60/60 sign and McConnell's sign have been shown to be more specific for pulmonary embolism than the other signs listed.

Question 15

65 y/o female with idiopathic pulmonary arterial hypertension (mean PA pressure 53 mmHg) on oral sildenafil presents to the emergency department with altered mental status. Temp 101.4 F., BP 85/50 mmHg, HR 110, 92% on 2 L nasal cannula (baseline), RR 22. Urinalysis revealed 4+ WBCs, 4+ bacteria, 1+ blood and 1+ protein. She is started on antibiotics and admitted to the ICU with a diagnosis of septic shock.

Chest X ray is clear. Ultrasound reveals the following M-mode image of the IVC in long axis with relaxed spontaneous breathing. What is the most appropriate choice regarding IVC ultrasound and its influence on volume management? Fig. 14.9.

A. The IVC M-mode image shown should not influence fluid administration decisions
B. The IVC M-mode image shown indicates that diuretics should be administered
C. The IVC M-mode image shown indicates that IV fluids should be administered
D. The pulsatile findings in this image suggest it is an image of the abdominal aorta

Correct Answer: A. Explanation: A dilated IVC is common in patients with pulmonary hypertension due to chronically elevated right atrial pressures. In patients with pulmonary hypertension, a dilated and non-collapsible IVC does not help to clarify decisions regarding volume management (choice A). IVC collapsibility is a reasonable predictor of right atrial pressure, but over-reliance on this interpretation can lead to errors in determining whether or not a patient would benefit from IV fluids or diuresis. There are numerous other factors in spontaneously breathing patients than can confound interpretation of IVC measurements, including heavy breathing, variable patient effort on a ventilator, intra-abdominal hypertension, and cirrhosis. Therefore, IVC measurement in isolation should not be used to guide fluid administration (choice B) or the need for diuresis (choice C), but rather should be integrated as part of the clinical picture. Adjunctive methods of volume responsiveness assessment should be employed to help guide decision-making.

The IVC can be mistaken for the abdominal aorta, leading to measurement error (choice D). Confirmation that the image is indeed the IVC can be done by observing the hepatic vein draining into it, and by observing subsequent entry into the right atrium. IVC may appear pulsatile in patient with severe tricuspid regurgitation, a common finding in advance pulmonary hypertension, making this an unhelpful distinction.

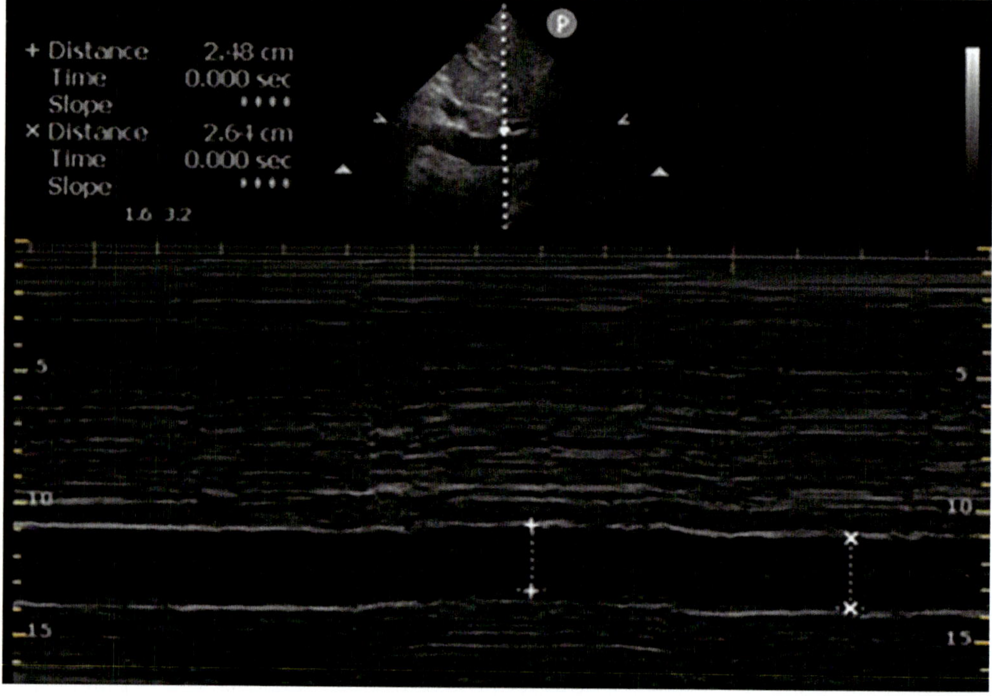

Fig. 14.9 M-mode imaging of the inferior vena cava

Question 16
Which of the following is true regarding the presence of a pericardial effusion in patients with pulmonary arterial hypertension (PAH)?

A. Pericardial effusion is not associated with PAH.
B. Left atrial or left ventricular collapse, even without right atrial or right ventricular collapse, may indicate tamponade physiology
C. Variation in tricuspid and mitral inflow velocities is unhelpful in tamponade assessment in patients with PAH
D. Presence of a large tricuspid regurgitant jet velocity makes tamponade unlikely due to equalization of RA and RV pressures

Correct Answer: B. Explanation: The occurrence of pericardial effusion in PAH is a poor prognostic sign (choice A). Patients with small or moderate pericardial effusion and PAH have up to three-fold higher 1-year mortality than those with trace or no pericardial effusion. Pericardial effusion typically occurs due to elevated right atrial pressure, which probably results in impaired lymphatic and venous drainage to the right atrium. The size of the effusion is related to right atrial pressure and to the severity of tricuspid regurgitation, and inversely related to cardiac index. Patients with PAH and pericardial effusion can develop atypical cardiac tamponade characterized by isolated left ventricle or left atrial compression. Right sided collapse and pulsus paradoxus may be absent in severe PAH as right sided pressure may be higher than pericardial pressure preventing its collapse. (choice B).

Question 17
Which of the following is most accurate regarding RV fractional area change (FAC)

A. FAC of <55% is considered abnormal
B. FAC is equal to RV end systolic area divided by RV end diastolic area
C. The tracing for RV area should include RV trabeculations (Figs. 14.10 and 14.11).
D. Reduced FAC is specific for acute cor pulmonale

Correct Answer: C. Explanation: RVFAC is defined as RV end diastolic area (RV EDA) minus RV end-systolic area (RV ESA), all divided by RV EDA (choice B). FAC = (RVEDA-RVESA)/RVEDA. An RVFAC less than 35% is considered abnormal (choice A). The tracing for RV area should include RV trabeculations (tracing should be deep to the trabeculations) (choice C). Reduced FAC may be seen in acute or chronic RV failure, and is not specific to acute cor pulmonale (choice D).

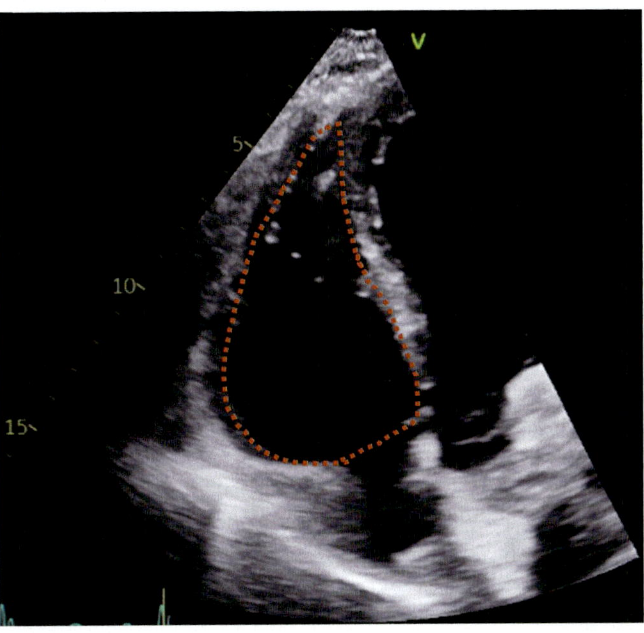

Fig. 14.10 Tracing for RV fractional area change measurement during diastole

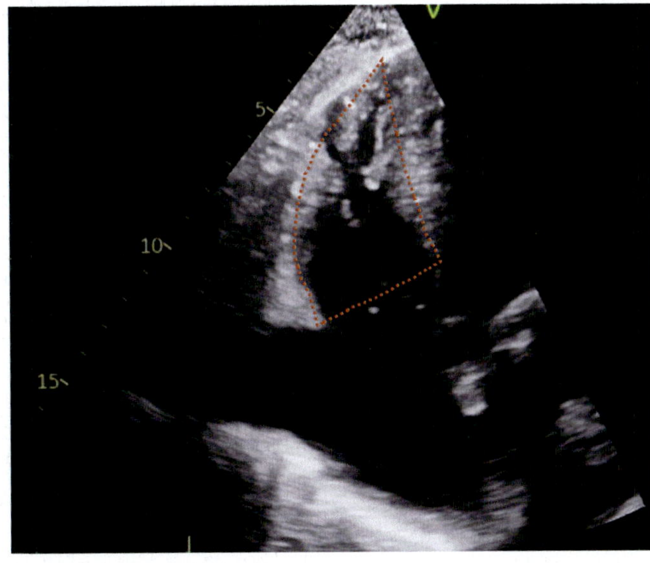

Fig. 14.11 Tracing for RV fractional area change measurement during systole

Question 18
A 74-year old male with a past medical history of diabetes and hypertension presents to the ICU with hypotension and tachycardia. You assess the patient and identify a basal end diastolic diameter of 45 mm. The best view for obtaining this measurement is:

A. Apical 5-chamber view
B. Subcostal view
C. Standard apical 4-chamber view
D. RV focused apical 4-chamber view

Correct Answer: D. Explanation: Obtaining one-dimensional views of the right ventricle can be challenging due to its complex geometry. The American Society of Echocardiography (ASE) recommends that transverse RV (free wall—septum) dimensions be measured using the RV focused apical 4-chamber view (choice D) at the base of the RV or at the level of the papillary muscles (approximately half-way between the apex and the RV base). The rationale for using the RV focused apical 4-chamber view instead of the *standard* apical 4-chamber view (choice C) is to minimize the potential for angular variation when measuring RV basal diameter. Angular variation occurs easily in the *standard* apical 4-chamber view following small rotational changes of the ultrasound probe. The subcostal (choice B) and apical 5-chamber (choice A) views are not recommended for measuring RV basal diameter as they either foreshorten or do not reliably visualize the RV septum and free wall at its maximal diameter.

Question 19

A 57 year old male is in the ICU with influenza related pneumonia and ARDS. A point of care ultrasound reveals a TAPSE of 1.0 cm. In critically ill patients with ARDS, this finding is associated with:

A. increased mortality
B. acute pulmonary embolism
C. increased risk of extubation failure
D. right coronary infarct

Correct Answer: A. Explanation: In patients with ARDS, the finding of a low TAPSE is associated with RV dysfunction and an increased risk of mortality (choice A). A small study (n = 38) evaluating echocardiographic parameters in patients with ARDS showed that patients who died within 30 days of their TTE had an average TAPSE of <1.7 cm compared to survivors whose TAPSE were higher. This finding has been corroborated by larger studies which suggest that a TAPSE of <1.7 cm is highly specific (but not sensitive) for RV dysfunction. In patients with ARDS, TAPSE can be depressed even in the absence of pulmonary embolism (choice B) or right coronary infarct (choice D). In addition, while patients with RV failure often demonstrate poor tolerance to positive pressure ventilation, TAPSE is not associated with increased risk of extubation failure (choice C).

Question 20

Your patient with pulmonary hypertension is undergoing echocardiography. Which of the following can lead to an erroneous TAPSE measurement?

A. Septal deviation
B. Apical longitudinal rotation
C. Dilated right atrium
D. Pericardial effusion

Correct Answer: B. Explanation: TAPSE is calculated by measuring the longitudinal displacement of the lateral tricuspid annulus toward the apex in an apical 4-chamber view. Because the majority of RV systolic contraction occurs in the longitudinal plane, greater longitudinal displacement is generally consistent with better RV function. This measure makes several assumptions. Among these is the assumption that the apex is fairly immobile throughout the cardiac cycle. In Apical longitudinal rotation, an abnormal clockwise rotation of the apex occurs during systole. This phenomenon is more commonly observed in patients with LV dysfunction, but has been described in patients with PAH as well. The reason apical rotation may occur in PAH patients is unclear. When present, apical longitudinal rotation can alter TAPSE and create a falsely normal TAPSE value (choice B). Although TAPSE is angle and load dependent, the presence of septal deviation (choice A), right atrial dilation (choice C), or pericardial effusion (choice D) would not lead to an erroneous TAPSE measurement. Those conditions would however have a significant impact on the validity of TAPSE as a surrogate measure of RV function.

Question 21

You are performing an echocardiogram on a patient in your emergency room who presents with hypotension. Which of the following is present on this image? (Fig. 14.12).

A. Flying "W" Sign (Mid-systolic notch)
B. 60/60 Sign
C. McConnell's Sign
D. Septal "D"Sign

Correct Answer: A. Explanation: This image demonstrates the flying "W" sign, also known as mid-systolic notching (choice A). Midsystolic notching is indicative of decreased compliance in the pulmonary circulation. In patients with poorly compliant pulmonary circulation, pressure waves reflecting off arterial branch points propagate backwards at a higher velocity than normal. If these waves travel fast enough, they will return to the pulmonic valve during systole. In this situation, deceleration of the pulmonary artery flow velocity occurs, forming a "notched" appearance within the pulmonic outflow Doppler tracing. This finding is called the flying "W" sign and is often seen in patients with pulmonary hypertension. As PH severity increases and pulmonary arterial compliance decreases, the midsystolic notch occurs earlier in systole. The 60/60 sign (choice B) is a marker of acute pulmonary embolism. This sign involves identifying a tricuspid insufficiency pressure gradient <60 mmHg and a

PA acceleration time < 60 ms. While one could measure PA acceleration time in this image, tricuspid regurgitation cannot be assessed here. McConnell's Sign (choice C) is seen when RV free wall hypokinesis or akinesis occurs but the apex is spared. This finding is specific for acute pulmonary embolism and is seen in the apical 4-chamber view. The septal D sign (choice D) occurs when RV volume or pressure overload occurs, causing septal shift into the left ventricle. It is most clearly identified in the parasternal short axis view at the papillary level (Fig. 14.13).

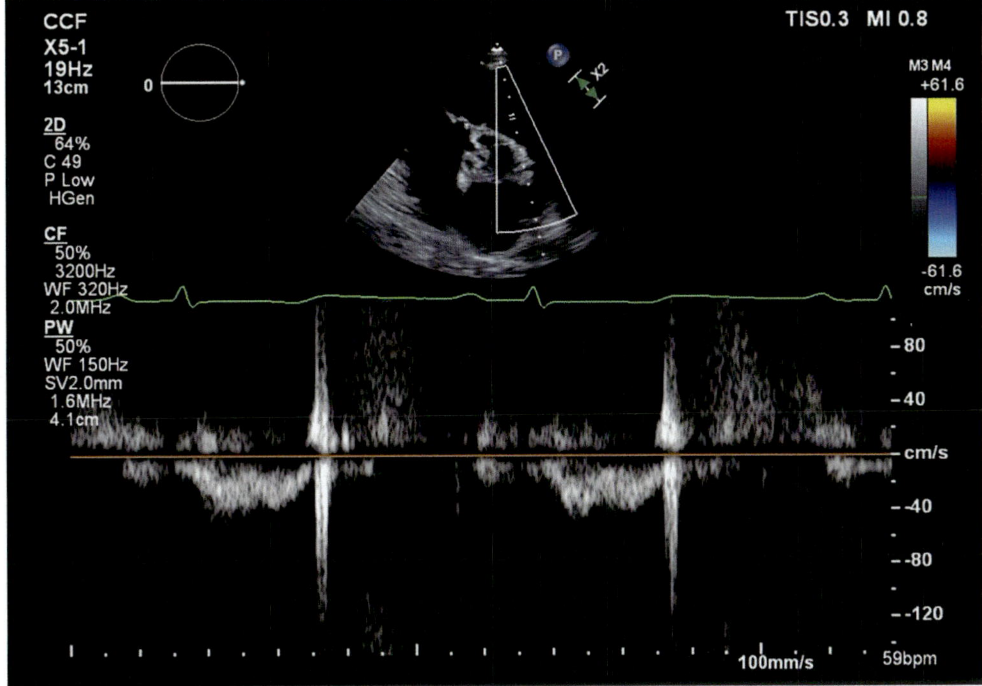

Fig. 14.12 Doppler imaging of flow across the pulmonic valve

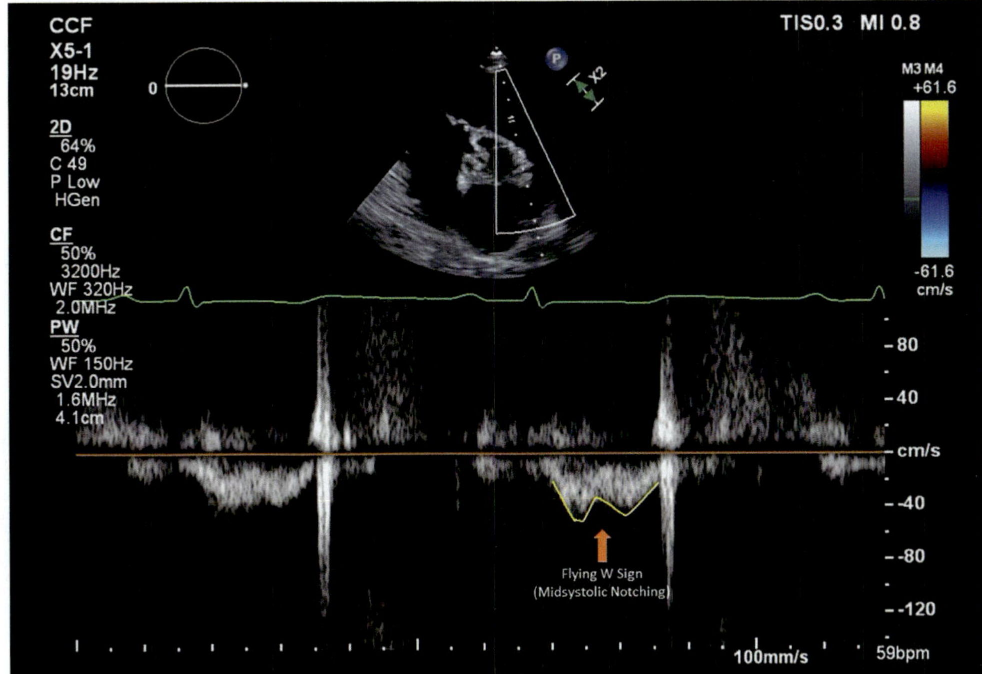

Fig. 14.13 Depiction of midsystolic notching across the pulmonic valve

Question 22

A 54 year old male is admitted to the ICU with acute respiratory failure. The patient is receiving mechanical ventilation with ventilator setting of volume control ventilation, Vt 500 (8 mL/kg), PEEP 20 cmH_2O, FiO_2 85%. The right ventricular end diastolic diameter (RVEDD) at the base is 48 mm. The most likely explanation for this finding is:

A. Atrial fibrillation.
B. Elevated PEEP.
C. High FIO_2.
D. Pulmonary arterial hypertension.

Correct Answer: B. Explanation: In patients who are receiving positive pressure ventilation, increased airway pressure, either from high PEEP (choice B) or large tidal volumes can lead to compression of intra-alveolar pulmonary vessels. In this setting, patients often experience signs of increased RV afterload including RV dilation and systolic dysfunction. When measuring the linear dimensions of the RV, a basal diameter greater than 41 mm from free wall to septum suggests a dilated ventricle. The complex, concentric shape of the RV and the lack of good landmarks within the ventricle can make it challenging to assess. Care must be taken to ensure that the RV is not foreshortened and the RV is imaged at an angle where the maximal basal diameter can be obtained. The preferred view to perform this measurement is the RV focused view. While patients with pulmonary arterial hypertension (choice D) often have an increased RVEDD, this finding is not diagnostic for pulmonary arterial hypertension and nothing in the question stem suggests that this patient has a history of pulmonary arterial hypertension. Increased inspired oxygen (choice C) and atrial fibrillation (choice A) do not cause RV dilation on their own.

Images/Videos

Question 23

A 35 year old male presents to your ICU from the regular nursing floor with hypotension. The patient was hospitalized 3 days ago for an emergency appendectomy. The surgery was complicated by bowel perforation. The patient's vital signs are HR 59, BP 88/35, SaO_2 94% on 2 L by nasal cannula. You perform a bedside echocardiogram. Based on the image, which of the following is the most likely? (Figs. 14.14 and 14.15).

A. The patient has a pulmonary embolism
B. The patient has moderate tricuspid regurgitation
C. The patient has moderate pulmonic valve regurgitation
D. The patient has normal RV function.

Correct Answer: D. Explanation: The image above shows a pulsed tissue Doppler signal measured at the lateral annulus of the tricuspid valve (RV S′). Measurement of the peak systolic RV S′ is a simple and reliable way to assess RV function. In critically ill patients. Validation studies comparing pulsed RVS' or TASV with radionuclide angiograph have shown good correlation and excellent discriminative ability of TASV to differentiate normal and abnormal RV systolic function. RV S′ less than 9.5 cm/s suggests RV systolic dysfunction. RVS' value above 9.5 cm/sec is highly suggestive of normal RV systolic function (choice D). RV S′ is neither sensitive nor specific for diagnosing acute pulmonary embolism (choice A). Valvular regurgitation can be assessed by continuous Doppler imaging through the tricuspid or pulmonic valve. The Doppler imaging shown in this image is tissue Doppler imaging of tricuspid annulus and does not provide information about valvular regurgitation (choices B and C).

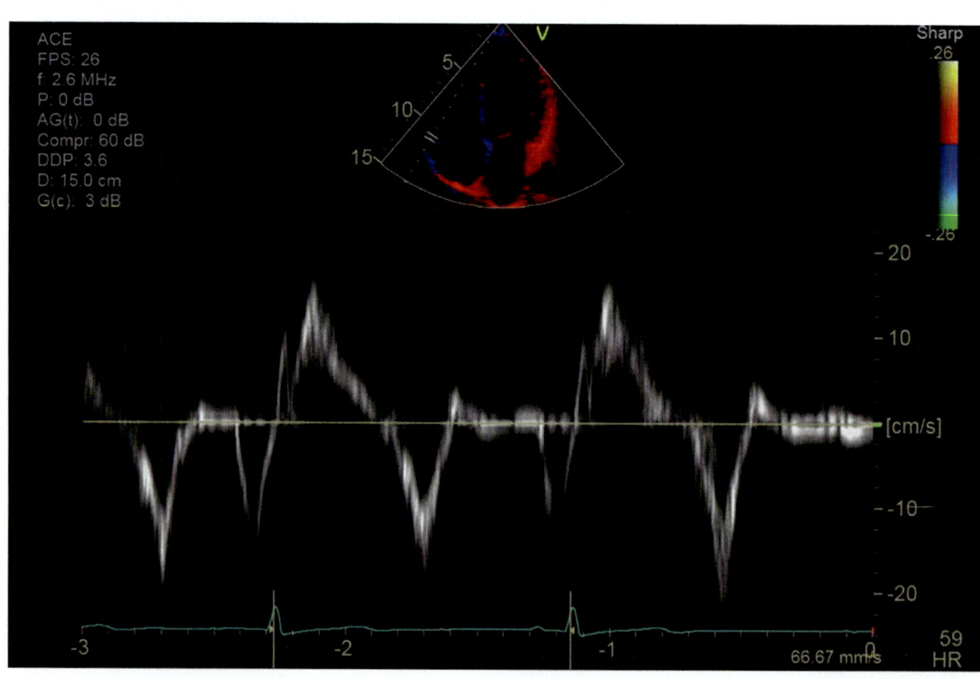

Fig. 14.14 Tissue doppler imaging in the apical four chamber view

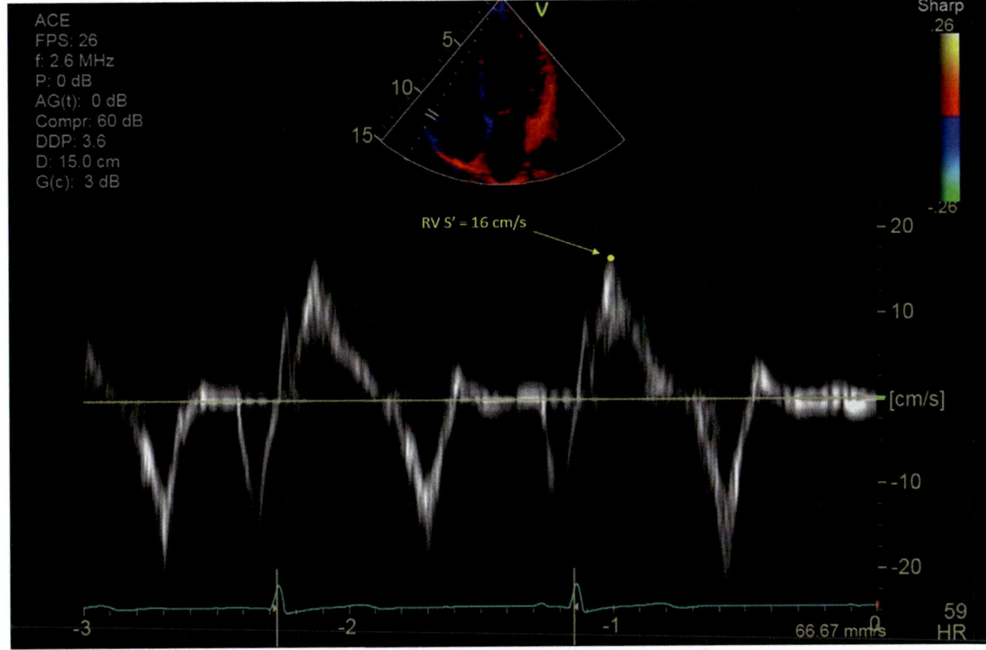

Fig. 14.15 RV S' identified as the point of maximal tissue velocity during RV contraction

Question 24

A 56 year old female presents to the ER with syncope 5 days after undergoing a total knee replacement. He is not on anticoagulation. In addition to a positive McConnell's sign, which of the following signs is the most specific for identifying an acute pulmonary embolism?

A. Low TAPSE
B. Elevated RVSP
C. Presence of paradoxical septal motion
D. Increased RV end diastolic diameter

Correct Answer: C. Explanation: There have been several studies evaluating the value of echocardiography to predict acute pulmonary embolism. In a large meta-analysis of 24 studies, the authors reported that the most specific signs of acute pulmonary embolism included McConnell's sign (97% specific), presence of a right heart thrombus (99% specific), and presence of paradoxical septal motion (choice C) (95% specific). TAPSE (choice A), RVSP (choice B), and RV end diastolic diameter (choice D) demonstrated a specificity less than 80%. In addition, the authors of the meta-analysis concluded that there are no echocardiographic findings which are highly sensitive for ruling out an acute pulmonary embolism.

Question 25

A patient in your ICU is receiving mechanical ventilation for acute respiratory failure with ARDS. They are mildly hypotensive. You perform an echocardiogram to evaluate for presence of PH. The inferior vena cava is 2.5 cm and does not vary with respiration. The maximal regurgitant velocity through the tricuspid valve is 320 cm/s. Which of the following is true?

A. The patient should be examined for tension pneumothorax
B. The patient does not have PH
C. A determination of right atrial pressure cannot be made
D. Systolic pressure gradient across the tricuspid valve should not be used to assess for PH in this patient.

Correct Answer: C. Explanation: Echocardiographic PA pressure estimates can be used when screening for the presence of PH in critically ill patients. The modified Bernoulli equation is the most common calculation for estimating PA pressure. This equation is dependent on both estimation of maximal tricuspid regurgitant jet (TR jet) velocity and estimation of right atrial pressure. Right atrial pressure is normally estimated by assessing the IVC diameter and degree of respirophasic collapse. In patients who are spontaneously breathing, the IVC diameter (>2.1 cm) and absence of collapse during inspiration would suggest an elevated right atrial pressure of ~15 mmHg. But, in patients who are receiving positive pressure ventilation, the physiologic effects of both PEEP and driving pressure preclude one from accurately estimating right atrial pressure (choice C). Fortunately, current guidelines only suggest calculating the systolic pressure gradient across the tricuspid valve when assessing for PH (choice D). The physiologic impact of positive pressure ventilation does not have the same effect on the measurement of systolic pressure gradient across the tricuspid valve. Guidelines suggest that a TR jet <280 cm/s, without other signs of RV dysfunction, makes the diagnosis of PH less likely (choice B). While patients with tension pneumothorax may have echocardiographic signs of PH, these signs are neither sensitive nor specific for pneumothorax (choice A).

Question 26

A 47 year old patient with pulmonary arterial hypertension presents to the ICU with acute decompensated RV failure. Tissue Doppler imaging of the RV free wall is performed. What is the best explanation for the peaks identified by the arrows? (Fig. 14.16).

A. Signifies isovolumic contraction
B. Signifies pulmonic regurgitation
C. Signifies diastolic relaxation
D. Signifies peak tricuspid systolic velocity

Correct Answer: A. Explanation: The figure above shows tissue Doppler imaging of the lateral tricuspid annulus. The arrows point to a brief upstroke in the velocity of RV free wall contraction which occurs during isovolumic contraction in early systole (choice A). In this patient, the isovolumic contraction is accentuated and prolonged due to the patient's severe PH and RV dysfunction. RV diastolic relaxation (choice C) occurs later, after completion of systolic contraction in this image. Pulmonic regurgitation (choice B) is identified using color Doppler imaging. The positive wave succeeding isovolumic contraction signifies peak tricuspid systolic velocity (TASV or RV S′) (Choice D) and occurs at the end of QRS complex as noted here. A careful assessment is needed to delieniate RVS' from Isovolumetric contraction waveform for accurate RV systolic assessment (Fig. 14.17)

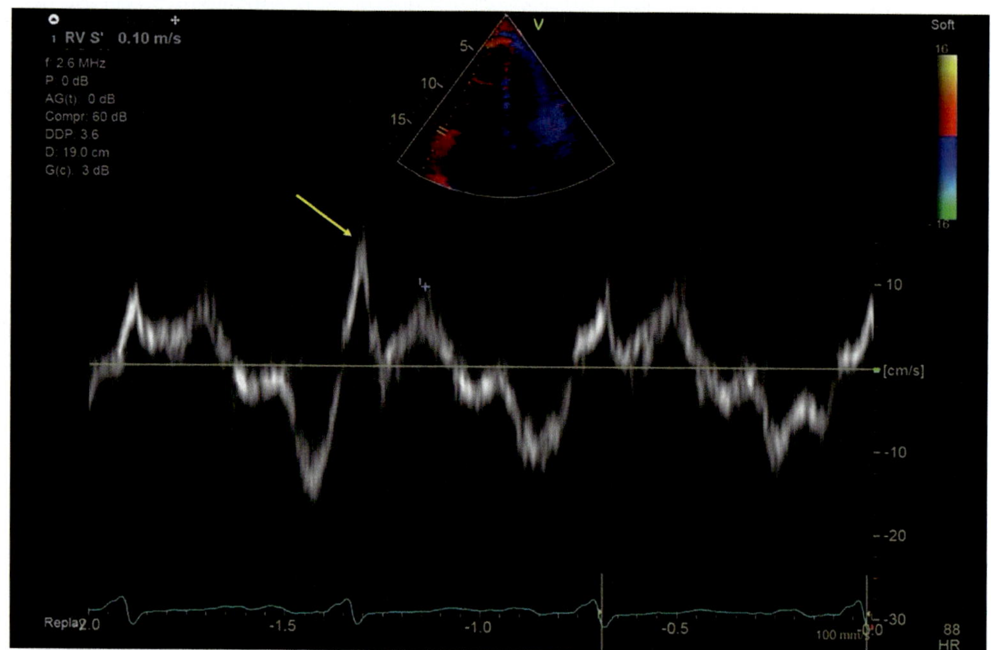

Fig. 14.16 Tissue Doppler imaging in the apical four chamber view

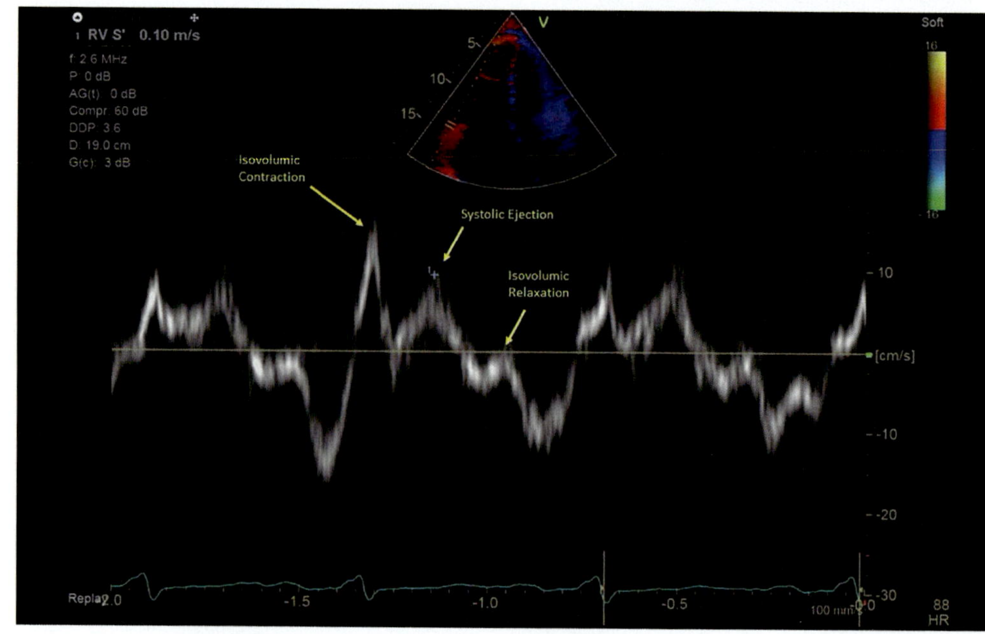

Fig. 14.17 Correlation between tissue Doppler imaging and phases of the cardiac cycle

Question 27

A 28 year old patient with a past medical history of repaired Tetralogy of Fallot presents to the hospital with signs of volume overload and acute RV failure. The patient has a respiratory rate of 14, blood pressure of 92/60, and a heart rate of 130. You are evaluating the patient's RV. When measured at end expiration, the RV E/A ratio is 0.6. Which of the following situations will most likely contribute to an erroneous assessment of diastolic dysfunction in this patient?

A. Measurement of E/A at end expiration.
B. Heart rate of 120.
C. The patient's young age.
D. Absent tricuspid regurgitation.

Correct Answer: B. Explanation: RV diastolic dysfunction is increasingly being recognized in patients with RV pressure or volume overload. An E/A ratio < 0.8 is highly suggestive of impaired RV relaxation. Tachycardia can adversely affect the accuracy of E/A ratio when evaluating for diastolic dysfunction (choice B). When tachycardia occurs, the shorter cardiac cycle causes the time spent in active RV filling (A wave) to increase relative to time spent in passive filling (E wave) making this measure less accurate. E/A ratio should be measured at end expiration (choice A). Inspiration causes increased venous return to the right atrium and a subsequent increase in the E wave relative to the A wave. As patients age, the normative E/A ratio decreases by approximately 0.1 per decade. This should be considered in patients who are elderly (choice C). Because the presence of tricuspid regurgitation can alter diastolic filling patterns, patients with moderate or severe tricuspid regurgitation have been excluded from most studies looking at RV diastolic dysfunction. The absence of tricuspid regurgitation should not influence this patient's assessment (choice D).

Question 28

A 63 year old patient is transferred to your ICU with acute respiratory failure and hypotension 3 days after receiving a partial bowel resection for a colon mass. The patient was intubated during a rapid response on the regular nursing floor just prior to transfer. Current vital signs show a systemic blood pressure of 90/49 mmHg (mean 63 mmHg), saturation 91%, respiratory rate 22 and a heart rate of 102. Chest X-ray shows new bilateral peripheral infiltrates. The patient's ventilator is set at a tidal volume of 470 mL (6 mL/kg), PEEP 14 cmH_2O, and FIO_2 0.7. An arterial blood gas shows a pH 7.20, pCO_2 56, pO_2 65. You assess the patient with point of care echocardiogram. The RV is dilated and there is paradoxical septal motion towards the LV at the end of systole. What is the next best step?

A. Recruitment maneuver.
B. Evaluate the patient for acute pulmonary embolism.
C. Increase the PEEP on the ventilator.
D. Decrease the tidal volume on the ventilator.

Correct Answer: B. Explanation: The presence of acute cor pulmonale can be detected on echocardiography by dilation of the RV and the presence of paradoxical septal motion at the end of systole (septal dyskinesia). In patients with RV pressure overload, the systolic contraction of the RV is often prolonged relative to LV systole. Under these conditions, the septum may "bounce" towards the LV as the RV continues to contract and the LV begins diastole. Acute cor pulmonale can occur for many reasons in critical illness, including ARDS, acute PE, or from the effects of positive pressure ventilation. This patient has several features concerning for PE including a history of malignancy, peripheral infiltrates on X-ray, and acute decompensation following surgery. In these situations evaluation for PE is warranted (choice B) Recruitment maneuver (choice A) is unlikely to be of benefit as it will increase trans-alveolar pressure and hence RV afterload in an RV that is already dilated and dysfunctional due to increased RV afterload. Ventilator settings should also be optimized in all patients with acute cor pulmonale to minimize RV afterload and preserve venous return to the RV. Increasing PEEP would increase RV afterload (choice C). Since the current pO_2 and arterial saturation are reasonable, this would not be advisable at this time. Changes to the tidal volume (choice D) would decrease RV afterload. But given the arterial blood gas values, this change would be expected to lower pH and is unlikely to be well tolerated.

Question 29

A patient presents to the Emergency Department with massive pulmonary embolism and hypotension. Echocardiography reveals a dilated RV with severe RV systolic dysfunction. Systemic thrombolytic therapy is administered. Which of the following is recommended as a method of reassessing RV function following therapeutic intervention for acute pulmonary embolism?

A. Documented absence of thrombus in the right atrium.
B. Increase in RV ejection fraction.
C. Improved RV E/E'.
D. Improved RV fractional area of change (FAC).

Correct Answer: D. Explanation: In patients who present with acute pulmonary embolism, hypotension, elevated troponin levels and echocardiographic signs of RV dysfunction or strain are associated with increased mortality. In these cases, thrombolytic therapy may be warranted. The American Society of Echocardiography recommends serial evaluation and monitoring of RV FAC (choice D), RV systolic pressure, right atrial pressure and RV size as key determinants of the effect of therapeutic interventions on RV function and strain in patients treated for acute pulmonary embolism. While the presence of thrombus in the RA is nearly 100% specific for acute pulmonary embolism, the absence of such finding (choice A) does not provide useful information regarding the effect of thrombolysis. Because of the complex geometry of the RV, RV ejection fraction (choice B) does not correlate well with other markers of RV function and should not be used in the serial assessment of RV function. RV E/E' (choice C) is a marker of diastolic dysfunction and has not been assessed as monitoring parameter to assess response to thrombolytic.

Question 30

Compared to TAPSE, which of the following advantages does RV global longitudinal strain by speckle tracking echo (STE) have in the assessment of patients with PH?

A. Strain imaging has significantly better prognostic value than TAPSE.
B. Speckle tracking is not angle dependent.
C. Strain imaging is easily reproducible compared to TAPSE.
D. Strain imaging only assesses septal motion.

Correct Answer: B. Explanation: RV global longitudinal strain imaging is an emerging method of assessing RV function. Adapted from the left ventricle, strain imaging carries promise in accurately assessing RV function in patients. Although both TAPSE and global longitudinal strain (GLS) imaging carry very good prognostic significance in pulmonary hypertension (choice A), there are some advantages of GLS over other conventional markers of RV function. The first is that GLS can measure RV function in an angle independent fashion (choice B) when speckle tracking capabilities are employed. Second, GLS integrates multiple regions of the RV into the calculation, including both the RV free wall and septum (choice D). TAPSE only utilizes a single point on the RV free wall when assessing RV function. Thus, TAPSE is subject to inaccuracies if regional variation of systolic function exists within the RV. Finally, strain imaging may offer a better assessment of intrinsic myocardial activity than TAPSE as it is a relatively load independent measure of RV function. TAPSE is easy to perform, highly reproducible and offers excellent interobserver variability (choice C).

Question 31

You are evaluating a patient who presents with pulmonary hypertension and decompensated RV failure in your ICU. You perform an echocardiogram and note that the RV index of myocardial performance (RIMP), performed by tissue Doppler imaging, is 0.37. You also note that the IVC is distended at 2.5 cm and does not vary with respiration. What influence does this patient's IVC findings have on the RIMP?

A. It shortens the isovolumic relaxation time.
B. It increases the isovolumic relaxation time.
C. It increases the ejection time.
D. It decreases the ejection time.

Correct Answer: A. Explanation: RV index of myocardial performance (RIMP) is a method of assessing RV myocardial function. While most 2-D assessments of RV function only measure systolic displacement of the RV myocardium, the advantage of measuring RIMP is that it offers both systolic and diastolic information about the RV. It is calculated by dividing the sum of the isovolumic contraction and relaxation time in a single cardiac cycle by the time spent ejecting blood through the pulmonic valve. It can be measured either by tissue Doppler imaging of the RV free wall at the level of the tricuspid annulus (as in this case) or by combining data obtained from pulsed wave Doppler through the pulmonic valve in the parasternal short axis view and the apical 4-chamber view through the tricuspid valve. In patients with pulmonary hypertension, RIMP is prognostic. A major limitation of RIMP is that it's correlation with RV function is poor in patients with elevated right atrial pressure. This is due to rapid equalization of the RV and RA pressures during diastole, with subsequent decrease in the isovolumic relaxation time (choice A). This patient has elevated right atrial pressure based on the dilated and non-collapsing IVC. Elevated right atrial pressure does not affect the ejection time (choice C and D).

Question 32

You are evaluating a patient who presents to the ICU with hypotension. You perform an echocardiogram and note that the RVSP is elevated (44 mmHg). In addition, the RV is moderately dilated. CT is negative for pulmonary embolism. The RV dp/dt is 490 mmHg/s. Which of the following is true.

A. This patient's dp/dt suggests normal RV function.
B. This patient has an increased risk of death.
C. This patient has pulmonary arterial hypertension.
D. This patient's dp/dt suggests RV diastolic dysfunction.

Correct Answer: A. Explanation: It is possible to evaluate RV systolic function by measuring dp/dt. This is done by measuring the time required (in seconds) for the tricuspid regurgitant jet velocity to increase by a known amount; typically from 1 cm/s to 2 cm/s. While robust data on normal values of dp/dt are lacking, guidelines suggest that a dp/dt < 400 mmHg/s is associated with RV dysfunction. In patients with pulmonary hypertension, a dp/dt <410 mmHg/s was associated with an increased risk of mortality. Because this patient has a dp/dt above these thresholds, there is no clear evidence of RV systolic dysfunction (choice A) or increased risk of mortality (choice B). None of the data provided in the stem, including the dp/dt, provides evidence of diastolic dysfunction (choice D). Finally, while the patient has elevated RVSP and dilated RV, right heart catheterization is required to make a diagnosis of pulmonary arterial hypertension. Since this diagnosis cannot be made by echocardiography alone, choice C is incorrect.

Question 33

A 78 year old male from South Africa presents to the emergency room with acute onset exertional dyspnea and lightheadedness 1 day after a 15 hour trans-continental flight to the United States. In the emergency room, his vital signs are stable. A CT scan reveals bilateral pulmonary emboli. An echocardiogram is performed. The RV end-diastolic diameter to LV end-diastolic diameter ratio (RVEDD: LVEDD) is 0.5. Based on this clinical presentation and echo finding, which of the following is true?

A. The patient has RV dysfunction.
B. The patient should receive thrombolytic therapy.
C. The patient has pulmonary hypertension.
D. The patient should be started on systemic anticoagulation.

Correct Answer: D. Key Point: In patients with acute pulmonary embolism, RVEDD: LVEDD ratio greater than 0.9 suggests RV dysfunction and is associated with increased in-hospital mortality.

Explanation: Echocardiography is an insensitive tool for diagnosis of PE but is useful in identifying patients with RV dysfunction and increased risk of death. In a study of 1416 patients admitted with a diagnosis of acute PE, a right ventricular end-diastolic diameter to left ventricular end-diastolic diameter ratio (RVEDD:LVEDD) >0.9 was associated with RV dysfunction and an increased risk of in-hospital mortality. In these patients, the use of thrombolytic therapy remains controversial as the risk of bleeding after thrombolysis is high, especially in patients over 75 years old. This patient's RVEDD: LVEDD is only 0.5, thus there is no evidence of RV dysfunction (choice A). Since this patient does not have evidence of RV dysfunction and is not hemodynamically unstable, thrombolytic therapy is not indicated (choice B). The patient should receive systemic anticoagulation for his acute pulmonary embolism (choice D). The RVEDD: LVEDD is often increased in patients with pulmonary hypertension, but this finding does not confirm the presence of pulmonary hypertension (choice C).

Question 34

Which of the following echo parameters is the best predictor of RV: PA uncoupling in patients with pulmonary arterial hypertension?

A. TAPSE.
B. TAPSE/RV systolic pressure (RVSP).
C. RV global longitudinal strain.
D. RV index of myocardial performance (RIMP).

Correct Answer: B. Explanation: RV: PA interactions can be accurately assessed by measuring the relationship between RV end systolic elastance (Ees) and pulmonary arterial elastance (Ea). In patients with pulmonary hypertension, clinical decompensation occurs when RV:PA interactions become uncoupled and the Ees:Ea ratio decreases. Measuring the Ees:Ea ratio is difficult to do as there are several challenges associated with measurement of RV volumes. To overcome these challenges, echocardiographic surrogates to predict Ees:Ea relationship and RV:PA uncoupling have been proposed. These parameters include TAPSE/RV systolic pressure, TAPSE/PA acceleration time, fractional area of change/mean PA pressure, RV area change/end-systolic area and stroke volume/end-systolic area. In a study of 52 patients, these echo parameters were validated against invasive pressure/volume loop analysis. A diminished TAPSE/RV systolic pressure ratio was predictive of RV: PA uncoupling (choice B). This parameter also demonstrated prognostic relevance in patients with pulmonary arterial hypertension. In this study, there was no correlation between RV: PA coupling and TAPSE (choice A). Neither RV global longitudinal strain nor RIMP have been validated against pressure volume loop analysis to determine their value in predicting RV: PA coupling in pulmonary arterial hypertension patients (Choice C and D).

Question 35

A 44 year old man with no known past medical history is admitted to the intensive care unit after being intubated in the emergency department for hypoxemic respiratory failure. Ventilator settings are as follows: FiO_2 0.90, PEEP 10 cm H_2O, RR 28 Vt 400 mL (6 mL/kg IBW). Plateau pressure is 24 cm H_2O. Bedside echo shows grossly preserved LV and RV systolic function. Lung ultrasound images are shown below. In addition to images shown, lung sliding is reduced in certain locations. What is the most likely diagnosis based on the data and imaging shown? (Fig. 14.18)

A. Cardiogenic pulmonary edema
B. Acute respiratory distress syndrome (ARDS)
C. Pulmonary embolism
D. Pneumothorax

Correct Answer: B. Explanation: Given the clinical history, lung imaging, and normal cardiac function, ARDS is the most likely diagnosis. According to published guidelines, lung ultrasound findings associated with ARDS (vs. cardiogenic pulmonary edema) include "absence or reduction of lung sliding, 'spared areas' of normal parenchyma, pleural line abnormalities (irregular thickened fragmented pleural line), and nonhomogeneous distribution of B-lines.". In contrast, cardiogenic pulmonary edema is associated with symmetric distribution of B-lines as well as normal, brisk lung sliding (choice A).

Subpleural consolidation can be seen in patients with pulmonary embolism. But this finding alone is not suffcient to make a diagnosis of PE. The absence of lung sliding is found in pneumothorax, but is not diagnostic (choice D). In order to diagnose pneumothorax, persence of lung point is necessary.

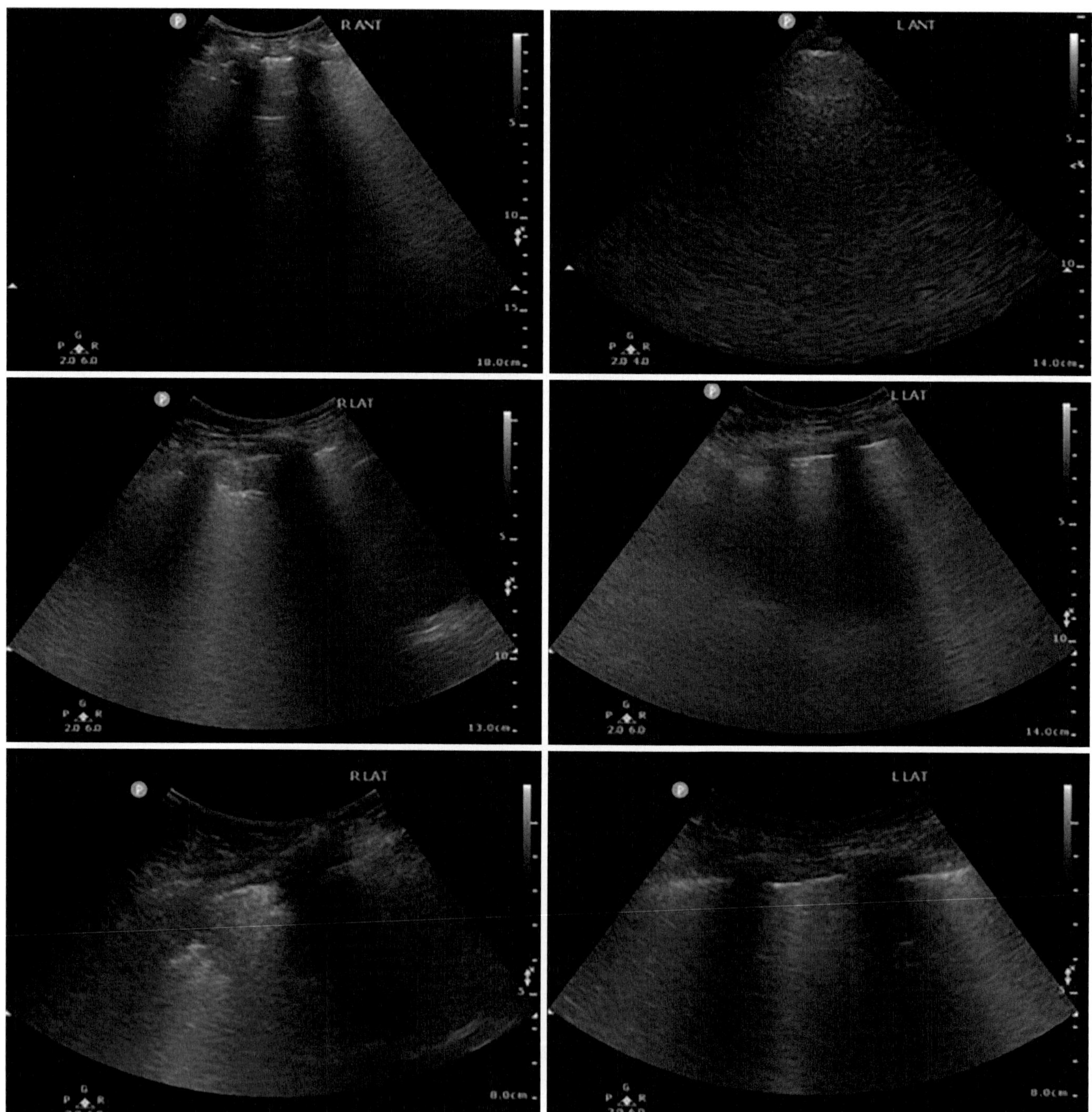

Fig. 14.18 Lung ultrasound images: Images on left represent left lung, Images on right represent right lung. Top images represent anterior, apical images. Middle and bottom images represent lateral views of lung fields

Question 36

Which of the following markers used in clinical trials is most commonly associated with RV dysfunction from lung injury or mechanical ventilation.

A. Presence of a lung point
B. Depressed ejection fraction with apical ballooning
C. A-lines seen throughout lung ultrasound field
D. RVEDA:LVEDA >0.6 + septal dyskinesia

Correct Answer: D. Explanation: Acute cor pulmonale occurs in approximately 22% of moderate-to-severe ARDS patients and is associated with increased mortality risk. In most trials it is defined as RVEDA: LVEDA >0.6 + septal dyskinesia (choice D). The presence of a lung point (choice A) is associated with pneumothorax and is not diagnostic of ARDS. The presence of depressed ejection fraction with apical ballooning (choice B) is indicative of Takotsubo cardiomyopathy, in most cases associated with cardiogenic pulmonary edema. The presence of A-lines (choice C) can be seen in patients with ARDS, but it is uncommon to see this uniformly throughout lung fields in patients with ARDS. More commonly, patients with ARDS demonstrate B-lines with areas of sparing as well as areas of patchy consolidation throughout the lung fields.

Question 37

A 20 year old woman is admitted to the ICU and treated for ARDS. Vitals are remarkable for HR 112, MAP 74, SpO_2 89%. Ventilator settings are as follows: FiO_2 0.90, PEEP 8 cm H_2O, RR 28 Vt 380 mL (6 mL/kg IBW). Plateau pressure is 22 cm H_20. Initial bedside echo shows grossly normal LV and RV systolic function. Lung ultrasound is notable for patchy B-lines throughout 75% of the lung fields. Given the above findings, the PEEP is increased incrementally to 16 cm H_2O, with plateau pressure 26. FiO_2 is able to be reduced to 0.50 with a subsequent PaO_2 70 mmHg on arterial blood gas analysis. Vitals are otherwise unchanged. Post-PEEP titration images show increased proportion of A-lines bilaterally. In areas where there is diminished lung sliding, a lung pulse is noted. What is the next best step in management?

A. Tube thoracostomy
B. Decrease PEEP
C. Decrease FiO_2
D. Continue current management

Correct Answer: D. Explanation: In this vignette the patient demonstrates ARDS with insufficient lung recruitment based on the initial lung ultrasound findings. After increasing PEEP, lung recruitment improved as demonstrated by increased proportion of images with A-lines and lung sliding. The presence of a lung pulse or lung sliding rules out pneumothorax in that location, so tube thoracotomy is not needed (choice A). There were no adverse hemodynamic changes associated with these changes to suggest the PEEP level set is too high (choice B) or that the PEEP is causing acute cor pulmonale. The PaO_2 (70 mmHg) is within the acceptable PaO_2 range for ARDS management according to current guidelines. Lowering the FIO_2 (choice C) is not necessary.

Question 38

A 62 year old woman is admitted to the ICU and treated for ARDS. Vitals are remarkable for HR 98, MAP 72, SpO_2 93%. On arterial blood gas, pH is 7.35 and PaO_2 is 75. Ventilator settings are as follows: FiO_2 0.60, PEEP 16 cm H_2O, RR 28 Vt 350 mL (6 mL/kg IBW). Plateau pressure is 28 cm H_2O. Bedside echo shows RVEDA: LVEDA ratio of 0.4 and TAPSE 2.0 cm. Lung ultrasound is notable for patchy B-lines in 25% of the lung fields. Which intervention should be performed at this time to optimize the patient?

A. Continue current ventilator settings
B. Increase PEEP
C. Venovenous ECMO
D. Increase FiO_2

Correct Answer: A. Explanation: In patients with ARDS, RV dysfunction can occur. Echocardiographic signs associated with RV dysfunction include an RVEDA: LVEDA ratio > 0.6, TAPSE <1.7 cm, presence of septal dyskinesia at end-systole. None of these features are present in this patient's echocardiogram. The patient's FiO_2 and PEEP are within the parameters suggested by current ARDS guidelines and there is no mention of impaired hemodynamics on the current settings. Therefore, no adjustments to the ventilator are needed (choice A). Choice B may raise the plateau further and could lead to acute cor pulmonale. VV ECMO (choice C) is unnecessary given the ability to manage the patient using conventional ventilator therapy. There is no benefit to increasing FiO_2 in this patient given the current O_2 saturation and PaO_2.

Question 39

A 24 year old woman is admitted to the ICU and treated for ARDS. Vitals are remarkable for HR 124, MAP 63, SpO_2 92%. Ventilator settings are as follows: FiO_2 0.70, PEEP 12 cm H_2O, RR 22, Vt 350 mL (6 mL/kg IBW). Plateau pressure is 24 cm H_2O. Initial bedside echo shows grossly preserved LV and RV systolic function. Lung ultrasound is notable for patchy B-lines throughout 50% of the lung fields. Arterial blood gas results demonstrate pH 7.21 with $PaCO_2$ 68, PaO_2 110, and HCO3 23. Given the blood gas result, the RR is increased to 36 breaths per minute. Several minutes later the patient develops progressive hypotension and hypoxemia. Lung ultrasound images are notable for >75% A-line pattern, areas of diminished and absent lung sliding with no lung point and scattered subpleural consolidation. What is the next best step in management?

A. Increase FiO_2
B. Tube thoracostomy
C. Disconnect from the ventilator and decrease set respiratory rate
D. Begin vasopressor infusion

Correct Answer: C. Explanation: This patient is experiencing dynamic hyperinflation as a result of an increased ventilator respiratory rate. In patients with ARDS and concomitant underlying obstructive airways pathology, a rapid respiratory rate, can lead to insufficient expiratory time between breaths and dynamic hyperinflation. When dynamic hyperinflation occurs, transpulmonary pressures increase. This can cause decreased venous return as well as increased RV afterload from intraparenchymal compression of pulmonary vasculature. In these cases, the best choice may be to briefly disconnect the patient from the ventilator to allow exhalation and subsequent improvement in both RV preload and afterload. The patient should then be reconnected to the ventilator at a lower respiratory rate. The absence of lung sliding is not diagnostic for pneumothorax. This patient's diminished lung sliding is likely a result of over distention. Pneumothorax can only definitely be diagnosed by the presence of a lung point. Therefore, tube thoracotomy is not indicated (choice B). Increasing FiO_2 or adding vasopressors (Choice A and D) would have had no effect on this patient's condition as they do not address the underlying pathology causing the patient's hypotension.

Question 40

Which of the following findings on lung ultrasound is most suggestive of cardiogenic pulmonary edema rather than ARDS?

A. Irregular pleural line
B. Decreased lung sliding
C. Normal lung sliding
D. Subpleural consolidations

Correct Answer: C. Explanation: There are several features which can be used to distinguish ARDS from cardiogenic pulmonary edema. Current guidelines suggest that areas of absent or reduced lung sliding (choice B), areas of normal lung parenchyma adjacent to regions with B-lines, presence of irregular pleural borders (choice A), and regions of pleural thickening or irregularities on lung ultrasound imaging (choice D) are suggestive of ARDS as opposed to cardiogenic pulmonary edema. In contrast, lung ultrasound findings associated with cardiogenic pulmonary edema includes symmetric distribution of B-lines as well as normal, brisk lung sliding (choice C).

Question 41

A 32 year old man is admitted to the ICU and treated for ARDS. Vitals are remarkable for HR 132, MAP 62, SpO_2 86%. He is on moderate dose norepinephrine. Ventilator settings are as follows: FiO_2 1.0, PEEP 20 cm H_2O, RR 28 Vt 400 mL (6 mL/kg IBW). Plateau pressure is 33 cm H_2O. The arterial blood gas shows the following results: pH 7.18, $PaCO_2$ 62, PaO_2 54, HCO3 18. Lung ultrasound images show B-lines in 50% of lung zones. Echo images are shown. What is the most appropriate next intervention? (Fig. 14.19).

A. Decrease PEEP
B. Increase PEEP
C. Fluid bolus
D. Venovenous extracorporeal membrane oxygenation (ECMO)

Correct Answer: D. Explanation: This patient with ARDS is being ventilated with low tidal volume, high FIO_2 and high PEEP pressures. The presence of significant B lines suggests inadequate lung recruitment on lung ultrasound images. In patients such as these, the effects of high airway pressures on RV preload and afterload can contribute to hemodynamic instability and RV failure. In this patient, the echocardiography image shows an increased RVEDA: LVEDA >1 and depressed RV FAC < 35%, consistent with acute cor-pulmonale. RVFAC is defined as RV end diastolic area (RV EDA) minus RV end-systolic area (RV ESA), all divided by RV EDA (FAC = (RVEDA-RVESA)/RVEDA). Risk factors for acute cor pulmonale include PaO_2:FiO_2 ratio less than 150, $PaCO_2$ greater than or equal to 48, driving pressure (defined as the difference between plateau pressure and PEEP) greater than or equal to 18. Decreasing PEEP (choice A) may help to improve the patient's hypotension, but will likely worsen their hypoxemia. Increasing PEEP (choice B) would likely worsen the RV afterload by raising the mean airway pressure. A fluid bolus (choice C) is unlikely to improve hypotension in this patient since the most likely cause of hypotension is RV dysfunction in the setting of acute cor pulmonale. In this patient, VV ECMO is indicated to provide adequate ventilation while allowing for lower airway pressures and improved RV afterload (Fig. 14.20).

Images/Videos:

Figs. 14.19 and 14.20.

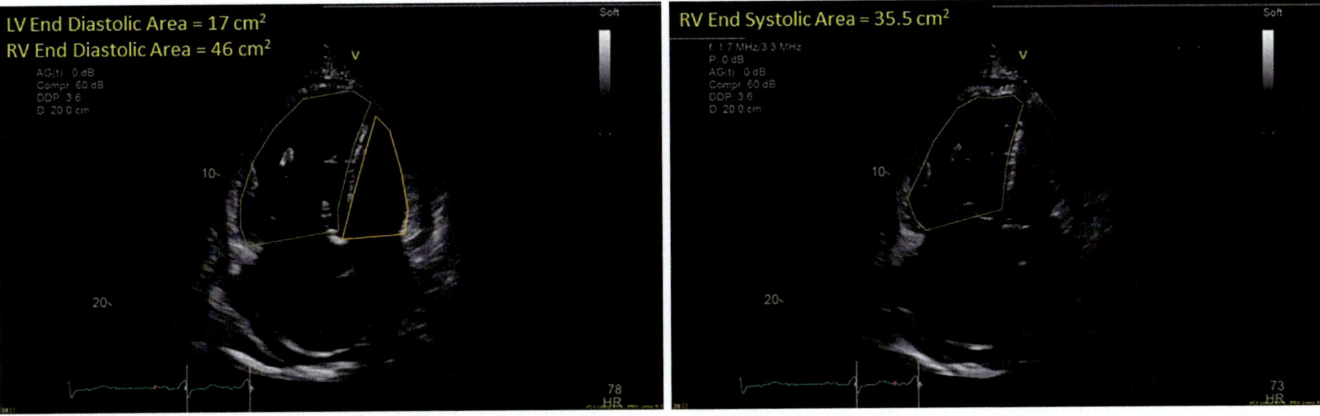

Fig. 14.19 Apical 4-chamber view with ventricular chamber sizes in systole and diastole

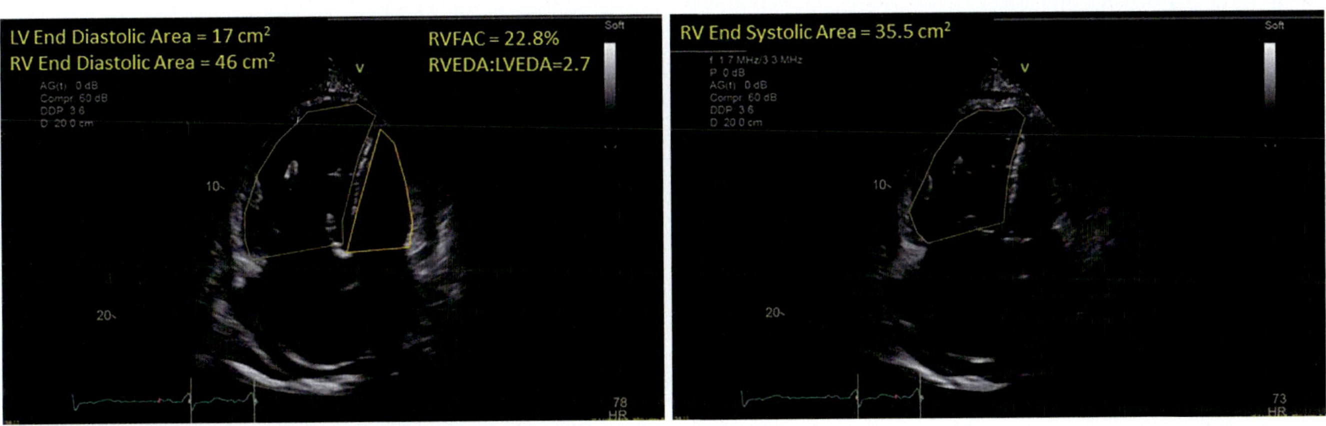

Fig. 14.20 Calculation of RVEDA: LVEDA and RVFAC in apical 4-chamber view

Question 42

A 72 year old woman is admitted to the ICU and treated for ARDS. Vitals are remarkable for an irregular rhythm consistent with atrial fibrillation, HR 98, MAP 82, SpO_2 92%. Ventilator settings are as follows: FiO_2 0.50, PEEP 12 cm H_2O, RR 28 Vt 350 mL (6 mL/kg IBW). Plateau pressure is 24 cm H_2O. Point of care ultrasonography shows moderately depressed left ventricular ejection fraction, TAPSE 2.0 cm, as well as dense symmetric B-lines throughout all lung fields. Lung sliding is present. Which statement represents the most likely diagnosis for this patient?

A. This patient has acute cor pulmonale
B. This patient has an acute PE
C. The lung ultrasound findings are consistent with ARDS.
D. This patient has cardiogenic pulmonary edema.

Correct Answer: D. Explanation: This patient has LV dysfunction and symmetric B-lines with preserved lung sliding. This constellation of findings is consistent with cardiogenic pulmonary edema (choice D). Findings consistent with ARDS (choice C) include areas of absent or reduced lung sliding, areas of normal lung parenchyma adjacent to lung zones demonstrating B-lines, presence of irregular pleural borders, and regions of pleural thickening or irregular pleural imaging on lung ultrasound. There is no evidence of acute cor pulmonale in this patient given normal RV systolic function and size (choice A). Additionally, there are no ultrasound findings consistent with pulmonary embolism (choice B).

Question 43

A 44 year old man with no known past medical history is admitted to the intensive care unit after being intubated in the emergency department for hypoxemic respiratory failure. Vitals are remarkable for HR 112, MAP 74, SpO_2 89%. Ventilator settings are as follows: FiO_2 0.90, PEEP 10 cm H_2O, RR 28, Vt 400 mL (6 mL/kg IBW). Plateau pressure is 24 cm H_2O. Bedside echo shows grossly preserved LV and RV systolic function. Lung ultrasound images reveal a B pattern in all most zones, with a few areas of A-pattern, some areas with decreased lung sliding, and several areas of subpleural consolidation. Based on these images, what intervention might be beneficial to improve oxygenation?

A. Decrease PEEP
B. Decrease tidal volume
C. Increase PEEP
D. Increase FiO_2

Correct Answer: C. Explanation: This patient's lung ultrasound images are consistent with ARDS and include multiple lung regions demonstrating B-lines, pleural irregularities and patchy regions of lung consolidation. In addition, the patient does not have any echocardiographic findings consistent with LV dysfunction. In this setting, increasing PEEP (choice c) may improve alveolar recruitment. Measuring lung recruitment as PEEP is titrated can be achieved using point of care lung ultrasound. Decreasing PEEP (choice A) or tidal volume (choice B) would lower mean airway pressure and would most likely worsen alveolar recruitment. The result would be a decrement in this patient's oxygen saturation. Increasing the FiO_2 would not be expected to change oxygenation in a meaningful way (choice D).

Question 44
An 82 year old man with ARDS secondary to influenza is intubated and admitted to the ICU. His set PEEP is 18. Which of the following signs is suggestive of decreased pulmonary arterial compliance?

A. Midsystolic notching of the RV outflow tract (RVOT) envelope
B. TAPSE less than 1.6 cm
C. IVC diameter greater than 2.1 cm with <50% collapse
D. RV fractional area change less than 35%

Correct Answer: A. Explanation: Mid-systolic notching (choice A) is an indicator of decreased compliance in the pulmonary circulation. In this case, mid-systolic notching can occur when patients are subjected to high levels of PEEP or when the severity of ARDS itself causes decreased pulmonary arterial compliance. In patients with poorly compliant pulmonary circulation, pressure waves reflecting off arterial branch points propagate backwards at a higher velocity than normal. If these waves travel fast enough, they will return to the pulmonic valve during systole. In this situation, deceleration of the pulmonary artery flow velocity occurs, forming a "notched" appearance within the pulmonic outflow doppler tracing. Choices B and D reflect measures of RV systolic dysfunction. Although decreased pulmonary artery compliance often leads to RV systolic dysfunction, the findings themselves do not necessarily indicate the presence of increased PVR. Finally, choice C represents a measure of right atrial pressure. This measure is not a measure of pulmonary artery compliance.

Question 45
A 19 year old male with progressive hypoxemia due to influenza is intubated for respiratory failure. After intubation, his hypoxia worsens. He receives bag-valve mask ventilation for several minutes with moderate success at improving her oxygenation. He is subsequently hooked back up to the ventilator, but begins to desaturate within minutes. The current vent settings are FiO_2 1.0, PEEP 20 cm H_2O, RR 28, Vt 600 mL (9 mL/kg IBW). Lung ultrasound images are obtained (See Video 14.2). What is the next best step in management?

A. Decrease PEEP
B. Resume bag mask ventilation
C. Tube thoracostomy
D. Prone position ventilation.

Correct Answer: C. Explanation: The ultrasound images of the right anterior chest demonstrate a lung point, indicating the presence of a pneumothorax in this patient. This patient likely developed pneumothorax from barotrauma associated with aggressive bag mask ventilation and large tidal volumes. The incidence of pneumothorax in ARDS has decreased in the era of lung protective ventilation but can still occur at a rate of up to 10–15%. Aggressive bag mask ventilation is a particular area of risk as large tidal volumes and high airway pressures are often delivered inadvertently when using these devices. Given the presence of a pneumothorax, the most appropriate treatment is tube thoracotomy. Changing the level of PEEP, resuming bag mask ventilation, or employing prone positioning (choices B-D) would not address this patient's pneumothorax.

Question 46
A 44 year old man is admitted to the ICU and treated for ARDS. Vitals are remarkable for HR 112, MAP 74, SpO_2 89%. Ventilator settings are as follows: FiO_2 0.90, PEEP 10 cm H_2O, RR 28 Vt 400 mL (6 mL/kg IBW). Plateau pressure is 24 cm H_2O. Initial bedside echo shows grossly preserved LV and RV systolic function. Lung ultrasound is notable for patchy B-lines throughout 75% of the lung fields. Given the above findings, the PEEP is increased to 16 cm H_2O, with a new plateau pressure of 34 cm H_2O. The saturation improves to 94% but the patient's MAP drops to 58 mmHg. Post-PEEP titration sonography reveals 75% A-lines, and echocardiography shows RVEDA: LVEDA ratio of 0.8. Which intervention below is most likely to improve the hemodynamics?

A. Prone position ventilation
B. Increase PEEP further
C. Fluid bolus
D. Neuromuscular blockade

Correct Answer: A. Explanation: This patient has ARDS pathology and initially demonstrates ultrasound findings consistent with insufficient lung recruitment. By increasing PEEP, the lung recruitment improved as demonstrated by the predominance of A-lines with associate lung sliding. However, in this patient, over distention of recruited lungs likely occurred. This is demonstrated by an increase in driving pressure (Plateau - PEEP pressure) following PEEP titration. The physiologic impact of over distended lungs is increased RV afterload. This occurs from compression of intra-parenchymal pulmonary vessels when lung is over distended and can cause hemodynamic instability as well as echocardiographic findings consistent with RV dysfunction and acute cor-pulmonale. In this case, the patient's RVEDA:LVEDA ratio was >0.6; a finding suggestive of cor-pulmonale. Prone positioning (choice A) has been shown to unload the right ventricle in patients with ARDS. This is likely due to the improvement in alveolar recruitment of basilar lung parenchyma. This leads to decreased levels of over-distention and subsequent decrease in pulmonary vascular compression. Increasing PEEP (choice B) may worsen the acute cor pulmonale by further raising the driving pressure and pulmonary vascular compression. Neither fluid bolus (Choice C) nor neuromuscular blockade (choice D) have shown any benefit in improving acute cor pulmonale in patients with ARDS.

Question 47

A 38 year old man treated for severe ARDS and related acute cor pulmonale has been extubated and is off vasopressors. His vitals are unremarkable and he is spontaneously breathing on nasal cannula. Which measurement below would be consistent with persistent RV systolic dysfunction?

A. RV fractional area change (FAC) 25%
B. TAPSE 1.9 cm
C. RV S′ 11 cm/s
D. IVC diameter of 2.0 cm with less than 50% collapse on inspiration

Correct Answer: A. Explanation: RV FAC less than 35% is considered abnormal (choice A). According to published guidelines, other parameters which suggest RV systolic dysfunction include TAPSE <1.6 cm (choice B) and RV S′ < 10 cm/s (choice C). IVC diameter (choice D) provides an estimated right atrial pressure in patients who are spontaneously breathing. It is not a marker of RV systolic function.

Question 48

A 24 year old woman is admitted to the ICU and treated for ARDS. Vitals are remarkable for HR 124, MAP 80, SpO_2 92%. Ventilator settings are as follows: FiO_2 0.70, PEEP 12 cm H_2O, RR 22, Vt 350 mL (6 mL/kg IBW). Plateau pressure is 24 cm H_2O. Lung ultrasound is notable for patchy B-lines throughout 50% of the lung fields. The medical team is considering diuresis and wishes to assess right atrial pressure first. Which of the findings below would be associated with elevated right atrial pressure (i.e. greater than 8 mmHg) in this patient?

A. IVC of 1.8 cm that collapses >50% with respiration
B. IVC of 1.8 cm that collapses <50% with respiration
C. IVC of 2.4 cm that collapses <50% with respiration
D. Right atrial pressure cannot be estimated in this patient

Correct Answer: D. Explanation: Right atrial pressure is estimated by assessing the IVC diameter and degree of respirophasic collapse during passive, spontaneous tidal breathing. In patients who are receiving positive pressure ventilation, a proportion of both PEEP and driving pressure is reflected through the lung parenchyma into the pleural space. This raises pleural pressure. Increased pleural pressure causes decreased venous return to the RA as well as dilation of the inferior vena cava. These changes preclude one from accurately estimating right atrial pressure under these circumstances (choice D).

Question 49

A 44 year old man is admitted to the ICU and treated for ARDS. Vitals are remarkable for HR 112, MAP 74, SpO_2 89%. Ventilator settings are as follows: FiO_2 0.90, PEEP 10 cm H_2O, RR 28 Vt 400 mL (6 mL/kg IBW). Plateau pressure is 24 cm H_2O. Initial bedside echo shows grossly preserved LV and RV systolic function. Lung ultrasound is notable for patchy B-lines throughout 75% of the lung fields. Given the above findings, the PEEP is increased to 16 cm H_2O, with plateau pressure 34 cm H_2O. FiO_2 is reduced to 0.60. The RV free wall thickness is 4 mm in diameter. The patient's MAP has decreased to 58. Post-PEEP titration reveals 75% A lines and an RV FAC of 20%. Lung sliding is present. What is the explanation for the hemodynamic change?

A. Pneumothorax
B. LV dysfunction
C. Pulmonary embolism
D. Overdistention of the lung

Correct Answer: D. Explanation: This patient has ARDS pathology and initially demonstrates ultrasound findings consistent with insufficient lung recruitment. By increasing PEEP, his lung recruitment likely occurred, as demonstrated by a shift on lung ultrasound to a predominant pattern of A-lines. Since sliding is present, it is unlikely that this patient's hypotension is a result of pneumothorax (choice A).

The echocardiographic finding of a depressed RV FAC of <35% and normal RV free wall thickness of <5 mm, suggests acute RV dysfunction. Although acute pulmonary embolism (choice C) could cause similar echocardiographic features of acute cor pulmonale the most likely reason for RV dysfunction in this patient is overdistention of the lungs (choice D). This is demonstrated by an increase in driving pressure (Plateau - PEEP pressure) following PEEP titration in concert with a predominant A-line pattern on lung ultrasound. Risk factors for acute cor pulmonale in patients with ARDS include PaO_2:FiO_2 ratio less than 150, $PaCO_2$ greater than or equal to 48, and driving pressure greater than or equal to 18. There is no evidence to suggest that this patient has LV dysfunction (choice B) from the information provided.

Question 50

A 44 year old man with no known past medical history is admitted to the intensive care unit after being intubated in the emergency department for hypoxemic respiratory failure. Ventilator settings are as follows: FiO_2 0.70, PEEP 10 cm H_2O, RR 28 Vt 400 mL (6 mL/kg IBW). Plateau pressure is 22 cm H_2O. Bedside echo shows grossly preserved LV and RV systolic function. Lung ultrasound is notable for symmetric, dense B-lines throughout four lung zones bilaterally. Lung sliding is present throughout the four lung zones. What is the most likely diagnosis based on the data and imaging shown?

A. Cardiogenic pulmonary edema
B. Acute respiratory distress syndrome (ARDS)
C. Pulmonary embolism
D. Lung contusion

Correct Answer: A. Key Point: Sonographic findings associated with cardiogenic pulmonary edema include a symmetric, uniform distribution of B-lines with normal lung sliding. Preserved systolic function does not rule out cardiogenic pulmonary edema.

Explanation: Given the clinical history and lung imaging, cardiogenic pulmonary edema is the most likely diagnosis (choice A). While the LV systolic function was normal, this does not rule out cardiogenic pulmonary edema due to other causes (e.g. diastolic dysfunction, acute valvulopathy). According to published guidelines, lung ultrasound findings associated with ARDS (choice B) include areas of absent or reduced lung sliding, areas of normal lung parenchyma adjacent to lung zones demonstrating B-lines, presence of irregular pleural borders, and regions of pleural thickening or irregular pleural imaging on lung ultrasound. The ultrasound images described to not suggest a pulmonary embolism (choice C). The expected lung ultrasound finding for pulmonary contusion is normal lung parenchyma (A-lines) with a region of focal B-line pattern at the area of contusion (choice D).

Clinical Pearls

1. Sonographic findings indicating RV failure in critically ill patients include S′ > 9.5 cm/s, TAPSE <16 mm, RV fractional area change <35%, dp/dt < 400 mmHg/s, RVEDD:LVEDD ratio greater than 0.9, McConnell's sign, and abnormal/paradoxical septal motion.
2. Sonographic findings indicating chronic right ventricular remodeling include RV free wall thickness greater than 5 mm, moderator band hypertrophy, and high RVSP. It is impossible to distinguish acute-on-chronic RV failure from chronic RV failure alone on echocardiography. In patients with ARDS, echocardiographic changes consistent with chronic right ventricular hypertrophy can develop within 48–72 h of disease onset.
3. Causes for acute cor pulmonale in an ICU patient include severe ARDS, acute pulmonary embolism, and high transpulmonary pressures from positive pressure ventilation.
4. Sonographic features favoring ARDS over cardiogenic pulmonary edema include subpleural consolidations, spared areas of normal lung (A-lines), reduced lung sliding, and pleural irregularity
5. Common lung ultrasound findings in pulmonary embolism include an A-line pattern, focal subpleural consolidation (due to pulmonary infarct), and pleural effusion.
6. TAPSE 16 mm or less has been strongly associated with poor prognosis in patients with pulmonary hypertension, and in patients with pulmonary embolism. TAPSE should be measured with the M-mode cursor passing through the apex and the tricuspid lateral annulus
7. IVC diameter and collapsibility has minimal utility in estimating right atrial pressure or volume responsiveness in a patient who is active on the ventilator.
8. ARDS and aggressive ventilator strategies may lead to RV dysfunction. RV protective ventilation strategies including low tidal volume ventilation and PEEP optimization may improve ventilator associated RV dysfunction. Prone positioning and ECMO also can reduce pulmonary vascular resistance and improve RV function in patients with severe ARDS.
9. The 60/60 sign, defined as tricuspid regurgitant pressure gradient less than 60 mmHg and tricuspid regurgitant acceleration time less than 60 milliseconds, is highly specific for acute pulmonary embolism.
10. Left sided chamber collapse may be seen before right sided chamber collapse in patients with severe pulmonary hypertension and pericardial effusion.
11. The flying "W" sign (midsystolic notching) may occur in patients with pulmonary hypertension and other diseases where decreased pulmonary arterial compliance occurs.

12. Serial assessment of RV FAC is recommended following thrombolysis of acute massive pulmonary embolism.
13. Measuring RV function by RV global longitudinal strain with speckle tracking allows angle independent, load independent, global assessment of RV myocardial function.

Further Reading

Ameloot K, Palmers P-J, Vande Bruaene A, et al. Clinical value of echocardiographic Doppler-derived right ventricular dp/dt in patients with pulmonary arterial hypertension. Eur Heart J Cardiovasc Imaging. 2014;15(12):1411–9. https://doi.org/10.1093/ehjci/jeu134.

Arkles JS, Opotowsky AR, Ojeda J, et al. Shape of the right ventricular Doppler envelope predicts hemodynamics and right heart function in pulmonary hypertension. Am J Respir Crit Care Med. 2011;183(2):268–76. https://doi.org/10.1164/rccm.201004-0601OC.

Barthélémy R, Roy X, Javanainen T, Mebazaa A, Chousterman BG. Comparison of echocardiographic indices of right ventricular systolic function and ejection fraction obtained with continuous thermodilution in critically ill patients. Crit Care. 2019;23(1):312. https://doi.org/10.1186/s13054-019-2582-7.

Boissier F, Katsahian S, Razazi K, Thille AW, Roche-Campo F, Leon R, et al. Prevalence and prognosis of cor pulmonale during protective ventilation for acute respiratory distress syndrome. Intensive Care Med. 2013;39(10):1725–33.

Bouhemad B, Brisson H, Le-Guen M, Arbelot C, Lu Q, Rouby J-J. Bedside ultrasound assessment of positive end-expiratory pressure-induced lung recruitment. Am J Respir Crit Care Med. 2011;183(3):341–7.

Bouhemad B, Mongodi S, Via G, Rouquette I. Ultrasound for "lung monitoring" of ventilated patients. Anesthesiol J Am Soc Anesthesiol. 2015;122(2):437–47. https://doi.org/10.1097/ALN.0000000000000558.

Chaisson NF, Mathai SC, Hassoun PM. Assessment of tricuspid annular plane systolic excursion (TAPSE) by 2d and m-mode echocardiography in pulmonary arterial hypertension patients. In: B64. Right ventricle in pulmonary vascular disease. New York, NY: American Thoracic Society; 2012. p. A3459.

Collier P, Xu B, Kusunose K, et al. Impact of abnormal longitudinal rotation on the assessment of right ventricular systolic function in patients with severe pulmonary hypertension. J Thorac Dis. 2018;10(8):4694–704. https://doi.org/10.21037/jtd.2018.07.118.

Copetti R, Soldati G, Copetti P. Chest sonography: a useful tool to differentiate acute cardiogenic pulmonary edema from acute respiratory distress syndrome. Cardiovasc Ultrasound. 2008;6(April):16.

Edwards PD et al. "CT Measurement of main pulmonary artery diameter. - PubMed - NCBI." n.d.. Accessed 9 Dec 2019. https://www.ncbi.nlm.nih.gov/pubmed/10211060.

Fields JM, Davis J, Girson L, et al. Transthoracic echocardiography for diagnosing pulmonary embolism: a systematic review and meta-analysis. J Am Soc Echocardiogr. 2017;30(7):714–723.e4. https://doi.org/10.1016/j.echo.2017.03.004.

Filopei J, Kory P, Ramesh N, Astua A, Steiger D. A clot in transit: life threatening diagnosis or incidental finding? Chest. 2016;150(4):1147A.

Frémont B, Pacouret G, Jacobi D, Puglisi R, Charbonnier B, de Labriolle A. Prognostic value of echocardiographic right/left ventricular end-diastolic diameter ratio in patients with acute pulmonary embolism: results from a monocenter registry of 1,416 patients. Chest. 2008;133(2):358–62. https://doi.org/10.1378/chest.07-1231.

Galiè N, Humbert M, Vachiery JL, et al. 2015 ESC/ERS Guidelines for the diagnosis and treatment of pulmonary hypertension: The Joint Task Force for the Diagnosis and Treatment of Pulmonary Hypertension of the European Society of Cardiology (ESC) and the European Respiratory Society (ERS): Endorsed by: Association for European Paediatric and Congenital Cardiology (AEPC), International Society for Heart and Lung Transplantation (ISHLT). Eur Heart J. 2016a;37(1):67–119. https://doi.org/10.1093/eurheartj/ehv317.

Galiè N, Humbert M, Vachiery J-L, et al. 2015 ESC/ERS Guidelines for the diagnosis and treatment of pulmonary hypertension: The Joint Task Force for the Diagnosis and Treatment of Pulmonary Hypertension of the European Society of Cardiology (ESC) and the European Respiratory Society (ERS): Endorsed by: Association for European Paediatric and Congenital Cardiology (AEPC), International Society for Heart and Lung Transplantation (ISHLT). Eur Heart J. 2016b;37(1):67–119. https://doi.org/10.1093/eurheartj/ehv317.

Jaff MR, McMurtry MS, Archer SL, et al. Management of massive and submassive pulmonary embolism, iliofemoral deep vein thrombosis, and chronic thromboembolic pulmonary hypertension: a scientific statement from the American Heart Association. Circulation. 2011;123(16):1788–830. https://doi.org/10.1161/CIR.0b013e318214914f.

Jardin F, Vieillard-Baron A. Acute cor pulmonale. Curr Opin Crit Care. 2009;15(1):67–70.

Joshi H, Dugar S, Panitchote A, Moghekar A, Duggal A. 1099: Acute respiratory distress syndrome and persistent right ventricular dysfunction. Crit Care Med. 2019;47(January):526.

Kossaify A. Echocardiographic assessment of the right ventricle, from the conventional approach to speckle tracking and three-dimensional imaging, and insights into the "right way" to explore the forgotten chamber. Clin Med Insights Cardiol. 2015;9:65–75. https://doi.org/10.4137/CMC.S27462.

Kurzyna M, Torbicki A, Pruszczyk P, Burakowska B, Fijałkowska A, Kober J, Oniszh K, et al. Disturbed right ventricular ejection pattern as a new doppler echocardiographic sign of acute pulmonary embolism. Am J Cardiol. 2002;90(5):507–11.

Lang RM. et al. "Recommendations for cardiac chamber quantification by echocardiography in adults: an update from the American Society of Echocardiography and the E... - PubMed - NCBI." n.d.. Accessed 8 Dec 2019. https://www.ncbi.nlm.nih.gov/pubmed/25559473.

Lazzeri C, Cianchi G, Bonizzoli M, Batacchi S, Peris A, Gensini GF. The potential role and limitations of echocardiography in acute respiratory distress syndrome. Ther Adv Respir Dis. 2016;10(2):136–48. https://doi.org/10.1177/1753465815621251.

Lee J-H, Park J-H. Strain analysis of the right ventricle using two-dimensional echocardiography. J Cardiovasc Imaging. 2018;26(3):111–24. https://doi.org/10.4250/jcvi.2018.26.e11.

Leung AN, Bull TM, Jaeschke R, Lockwood CJ, Boiselle PM, Hurwitz LM, James AH, et al. An official American Thoracic Society/Society of Thoracic Radiology clinical practice guideline: evaluation of suspected pulmonary embolism in pregnancy. Am J Respir Crit Care Med. 2011;184(10):1200–8.

Lichtenstein DA, Mezière G, Lascols N, et al. Ultrasound diagnosis of occult pneumothorax. Crit Care Med. 2005;33(6):1231–8. https://doi.org/10.1097/01.ccm.0000164542.86954.b4.

Lobo JL, Sobradillo P, Obieta-Fresnedo I, Rivas A, Valle R, Navarro C, Jimenez D. TAPSE as a prognostic factor in hemodynamically stable pulmonary embolism. Eur Respir J. 2011;38(Suppl 55):2347. https://erj.ersjournals.com/content/38/Suppl_55/p2347.abstract.

Luecke T, Pelosi P. Clinical review: positive end-expiratory pressure and cardiac output. Crit Care. 2005;9(6):607.

Mathis G, Blank W, Reissig A, Lechleitner P, Reuss J, Schuler A, Beckh S. Thoracic ultrasound for diagnosing pulmonary embolism: a prospective multicenter study of 352 patients. Chest. 2005;128(3):1531–8.

Matsukubo H, Matsuura T, Endo N, Asayama J, Watanabe T. Echocardiographic measurement of right ventricular wall thickness. A new application of subxiphoid echocardiography. Circulation. 1977;56(2):278–84.

Mekontso Dessap A, Boissier F, Charron C, Bégot E, Repessé X, Legras A, et al. Acute cor pulmonale during protective ventilation for acute respiratory distress syndrome: prevalence, predictors, and clinical impact. Intensive Care Med. 2016;42(5):862–70.

Miranda DR, van Thiel R, Brodie D, Bakker J. Right ventricular unloading after initiation of venovenous extracorporeal membrane oxygenation. Am J Respir Crit Care Med. 2015;191(3):346–8.

Motoji Y, Tanaka H, Fukuda Y, et al. Association of apical longitudinal rotation with right ventricular performance in patients with pulmonary hypertension: insights into overestimation of tricuspid annular plane systolic excursion. Echocardiography. 2016;33(2):207–15. https://doi.org/10.1111/echo.13036.

Nazerian P, Volpicelli G, Gigli C, Lamorte A, Grifoni S, Vanni S. Diagnostic accuracy of focused cardiac and venous ultrasound examinations in patients with shock and suspected pulmonary embolism. Intern Emerg Med. 2018;13(4):567–74.

Paczyńska M, Sobieraj P, Burzyński Ł, Kostrubiec M, Wiśniewska M, Bienias P, Kurnicka K, Lichodziejewska B, Pruszczyk P, Ciurzyński M. Tricuspid annulus plane systolic excursion (tapse) has superior predictive value compared to right ventricular to left ventricular ratio in normotensive patients with acute pulmonary embolism. Arch Med Sci. 2016;12(5):1008.

Pomero et al. "accuracy of emergency physician-performed ultrasonography in the diagnosis of deep-vein thrombosis: a systematic review and meta-analysis.—PubMed—NCBI." n.d.. Accessed 4 Dec 2019. https://www.ncbi.nlm.nih.gov/pubmed/23138420.

Porter TR, Shillcutt SK, Adams MS, et al. Guidelines for the use of echocardiography as a monitor for therapeutic intervention in adults: a report from the American Society of Echocardiography. J Am Soc Echocardiogr. 2015;28(1):40–56. https://doi.org/10.1016/j.echo.2014.09.009.

Rose PS et al. "Treatment of right heart thromboemboli—PubMed—NCBI." n.d.. Accessed 4 Dec 2019. https://www.ncbi.nlm.nih.gov/pubmed/11888964.

Rudski LG, Lai WW, Afilalo J, Hua L, Handschumacher MD, Chandrasekaran K, Solomon SD, Louie EK, Schiller NB. Guidelines for the Echocardiographic Assessment of the Right Heart in Adults: A Report from the American Society of Echocardiography Endorsed by the European Association of Echocardiography, a Registered Branch of the European Society of Cardiology, and the Canadian Society of Echocardiography. J Am Soc Echocardiogr. 2010;23(7):685–713; quiz 786–88.

Sahay S, Tonelli AR. Pericardial effusion in pulmonary arterial hypertension. Pulm Circ. 2013;3(3):467.

Shah TG, Wadia SK, Kovach J, Fogg L, Tandon R. Echocardiographic parameters of right ventricular function predict mortality in acute respiratory distress syndrome: a pilot study. Pulm Circ. 2016;6(2):155–60. https://doi.org/10.1086/685549.

Soni NJ, Arntfield R, Kory P. Point of Care Ultrasound. Elsevier; 2019.

Squizzato A, Galli L, Gerdes VEA. Point-of-care ultrasound in the diagnosis of pulmonary embolism. Crit Ultrasound J. 2015;7:7.

Tamborini G, Pepi M, Galli CA, et al. Feasibility and accuracy of a routine echocardiographic assessment of right ventricular function. Int J Cardiol. 2007;115(1):86–9. https://doi.org/10.1016/j.ijcard.2006.01.017.

Tello K, Wan J, Dalmer A, et al. Validation of the tricuspid annular plane systolic excursion/systolic pulmonary artery pressure ratio for the assessment of right ventricular-arterial coupling in severe pulmonary hypertension. Circ Cardiovasc Imaging. 2019;12(9):e009047. https://doi.org/10.1161/CIRCIMAGING.119.009047.

Vieillard-Baron A, Price LC, Matthay MA. Acute cor pulmonale in ARDS. Intensive Care Med. 2013;39(10):1836–8.

Vieillard-Baron A, Prin S, Chergui K, Dubourg O, Jardin F. Echo–doppler demonstration of acute cor pulmonale at the bedside in the medical intensive care unit. Am J Respir Crit Care Med. 2002;166(10):1310–9.

Volpicelli G, Elbarbary M, Blaivas M, Lichtenstein DA, Mathis G, Kirkpatrick AW, et al. International evidence-based recommendations for point-of-care lung ultrasound. Intensive Care Med. 2012;38(4):577–91.

Pericardial Diseases

15

Jason Phillips, Ariel Vinas, Thamer Alaifan, and Nilam J. Soni

For Questions 1–5, assess the volume of pericardial fluid present in each echocardiographic image.

Question 1
What is the most appropriate categorization for size of this pericardial effusion (Fig. 15.1, Video 15.1)?

A. No pericardial effusion is present.
B. Trivial pericardial effusion is present.
C. Small pericardial effusion is present.
D. Moderate pericardial effusion is present.
E. Large pericardial effusion is present.

Answer: A—No pericardial effusion is present.

Key point: Ascites and pleural effusions must be differentiated from pericardial effusions.

Rationale: This subcostal 4-chamber view demonstrates a large volume of ascites and a glimpse of a right pleural effusion (far field, screen left). Pericardial effusions may be circumferential (surrounding the heart) or loculated (localized to one particular region of the heart) [1]. There is no pericardial effusion surrounding this heart. In the near field, the falciform ligament is seen (screen center), along with an echogenic, cirrhotic liver (screen left).

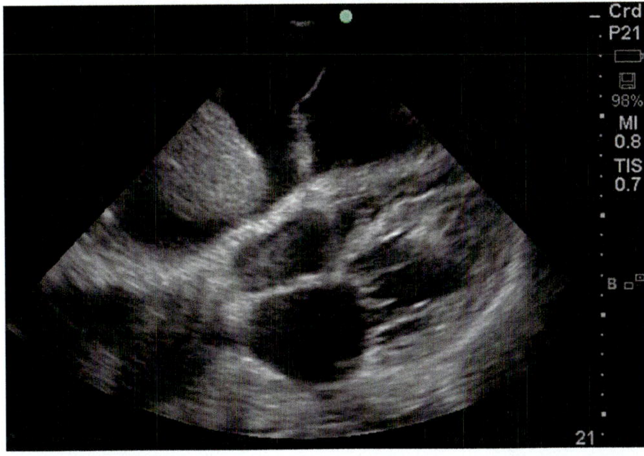

Fig. 15.1 Large ascites is seen in a subcostal 4-chamber view. Note the right pleural effusion in the far field and absence of a pericardial effusion

Supplementary Information The online version contains supplementary material available at https://doi.org/10.1007/978-3-031-45731-9_15.

J. Phillips (✉) · A. Vinas
Division of Cardiology, Department of Medicine, University of Texas Health San Antonio, San Antonio, TX, USA
e-mail: phillipsj3@uthscsa.edu; vinas@uthscsa.edu

T. Alaifan
Division of Critical Care Medicine, Department of Medicine, London Health Sciences Centre, Western University, London, ON, Canada

N. J. Soni
Division of Pulmonary Diseases & Critical Care Medicine/ Division of Hospital Medicine, Department of Medicine, University of Texas Health San Antonio, San Antonio, TX, USA
e-mail: sonin@uthscsa.edu

R. Sreedharan et al. (eds.), *Critical Care Echocardiography*, https://doi.org/10.1007/978-3-031-45731-9_15

Question 2

What is the most appropriate categorization for size of this pericardial effusion (Fig. 15.2, Video 15.2)?

A. No pericardial effusion is present.
B. Trivial pericardial effusion is present.
C. Small pericardial effusion is present.
D. Moderate pericardial effusion is present.
E. Large pericardial effusion is present.

Answer: E—Large pericardial effusion is present.

Key point: Recognize that large pericardial effusions have >2 cm depth.

Rationale: This parasternal long-axis view shows a large pericardial effusion that is primarily seen in the near field. Pericardial effusions >2 cm in depth are categorized as large [2]. Note the serpentine movement of the right ventricular free wall and diastolic right ventricular collapse which are consistent with tamponade physiology by echocardiography. This patient has right ventricular hypertrophy most likely due to chronically elevated pulmonary artery pressure which can explain why the right ventricular collapse is seen in mid–/late-diastole rather than early diastole.

Question 3

What is the most appropriate categorization for size of this pericardial effusion (Fig. 15.3, Video 15.3)?

A. No pericardial effusion is present.
B. Trivial pericardial effusion is present.
C. Small pericardial effusion is present.
D. Moderate pericardial effusion is present.
E. Large pericardial effusion is present.

Answer: C—Small pericardial effusion is present.

Key point: Recognize a small pericardial effusion and differentiate it from a left pleural effusion.

Rationale: This parasternal long-axis view shows a small pericardial effusion and left pleural effusion. Separation of the pericardial and pleural effusion is best appreciated in the far field. The pericardial effusion is seen tracking anterior to the descending thoracic aorta and is adjacent to the left ventricle and atrium. Based on this image alone, the most appropriate quantification of this patient's pericardial effusion is small since the pericardial separation is <1 cm at end-diastole. Trivial pericardial effusions are defined as being <1 cm but only visualized in systole while small pericardial effusions are <1 cm but seen in both systole and diastole. Moderate pericardial effusions are 1–2 cm and large pericardial effusions are >2 cm [2].

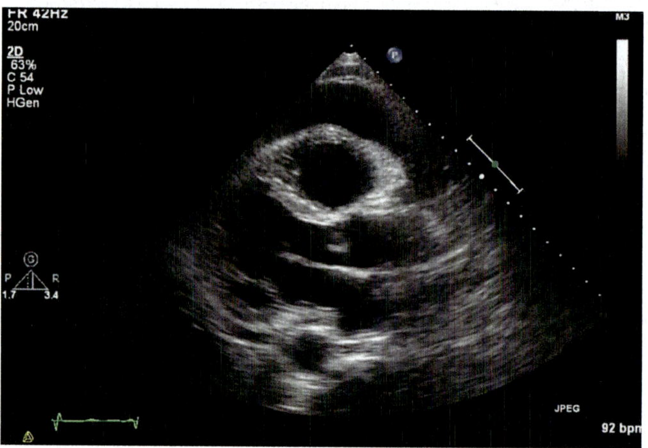

Fig. 15.2 Large pericardial effusion is seen in a parasternal long-axis view. Note the serpentine movement of the right ventricular free wall and diastolic right ventricular collapse which are consistent with tamponade physiology

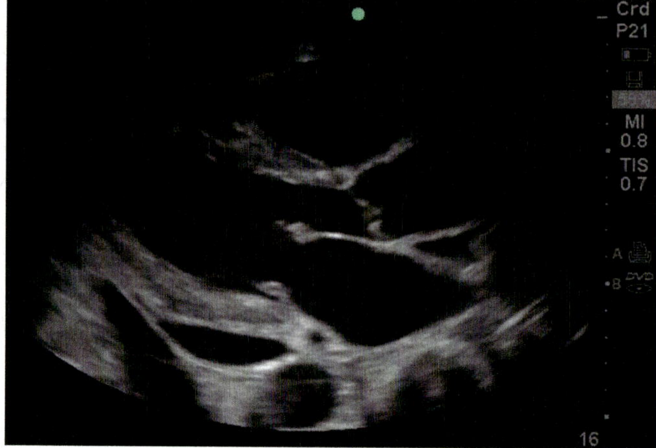

Fig. 15.3 Small posterior pericardial effusion and left pleural effusion are seen in a parasternal long-axis view

Question 4

What is the most appropriate categorization for size of this pericardial effusion (Fig. 15.4, Video 15.4)?

A. No pericardial effusion is present.
B. Trivial pericardial effusion is present.
C. Small pericardial effusion is present.
D. Moderate pericardial effusion is present.
E. Large pericardial effusion is present.

Answer: E—Large pericardial effusion is present.

Key point: Appreciate the variability of depth of a large circumferential pericardial effusion.

Rationale: This parasternal short-axis view demonstrates a large circumferential pericardial effusion. The variability in depth of the pericardial effusion underscores the importance of obtaining multiple views when assessing the size of an effusion. From a parasternal long-axis view, the imaging plane bisects the anteroseptal and inferolateral left ventricular walls, and this effusion may appear to be small or moderate in size. Note the prominent septal bounce due to elevated right ventricular volume.

Question 5

What is the most appropriate categorization for size of this pericardial effusion (Fig. 15.5, Video 15.5)?

A. No pericardial effusion is present.
B. Trivial pericardial effusion is present.
C. Small pericardial effusion is present.
D. Moderate pericardial effusion is present.
E. Large pericardial effusion is present.

Answer: B—Trivial pericardial effusion is present.

Key point: Recognize a trivial pericardial effusion.

Rationale: A sliver of anechoic space is seen in the far field deep to the inferoseptal left ventricular wall during systole and is most consistent with a trivial pericardial effusion. Trivial pericardial effusions are <1 cm and only seen during systole, whereas small pericardial effusions are <1 cm and visualized during both systole and diastole [2].

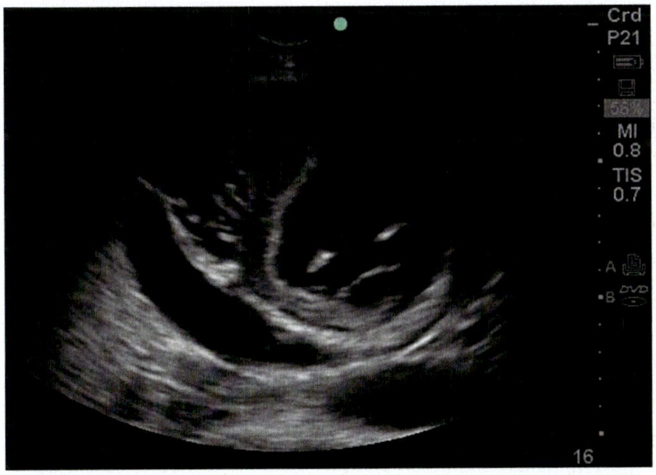

Fig. 15.4 Large pericardial effusion is seen in a parasternal short-axis view

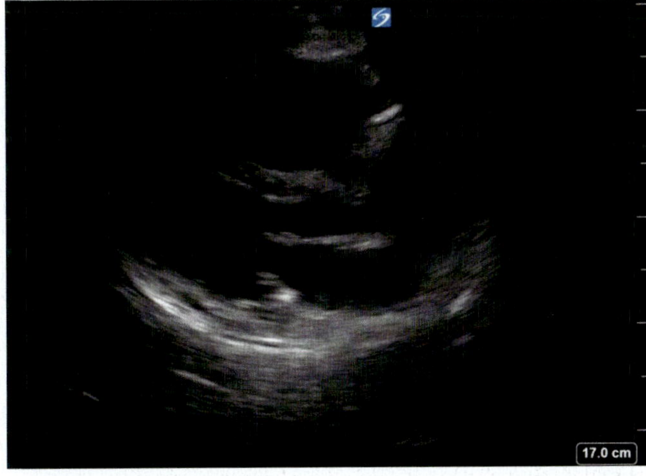

Fig. 15.5 Trivial posterior pericardial effusion is seen in a parasternal long axis view

Question 6

A 48 year-old man with stage IV metastatic squamous cell carcinoma of the lung and recent hospitalization for right axillary deep venous thrombosis presents with increasing shortness of breath, early satiety, and fatigue. He is febrile (temp 101.7 °F), tachycardic (pulse 115 bpm) and has a leukocytosis (WBC 17.8 K). A bedside echocardiogram is performed. The parasternal long-axis views are shown in Fig. 15.6. What is the most appropriate quantification of the size of his pericardial effusion based on the images shown?

A. No pericardial effusion is present.
B. Trivial pericardial effusion is present.
C. Small pericardial effusion is present.
D. Moderate pericardial effusion is present.
E. Large pericardial effusion is present.

Answer: C—Small pericardial effusion is present.

Key point: Understand when in the cardiac cycle to assess the size of a pericardial effusion.

Rationale: Pericardial effusion size is estimated by measuring the echo-free space between the visceral and parietal pericardium at end-diastole. Only Fig. 15.6a shows a still image in end-diastole. Using the scale on the right side of the image, the echolucent space is clearly smaller than 1 cm but still visible throughout the cardiac cycle suggesting a small effusion. Trivial pericardial effusions would only be seen in systole, but not in diastole. Moderate pericardial effusions are estimated between 1–2 cm and large ones are >2 cm [2].

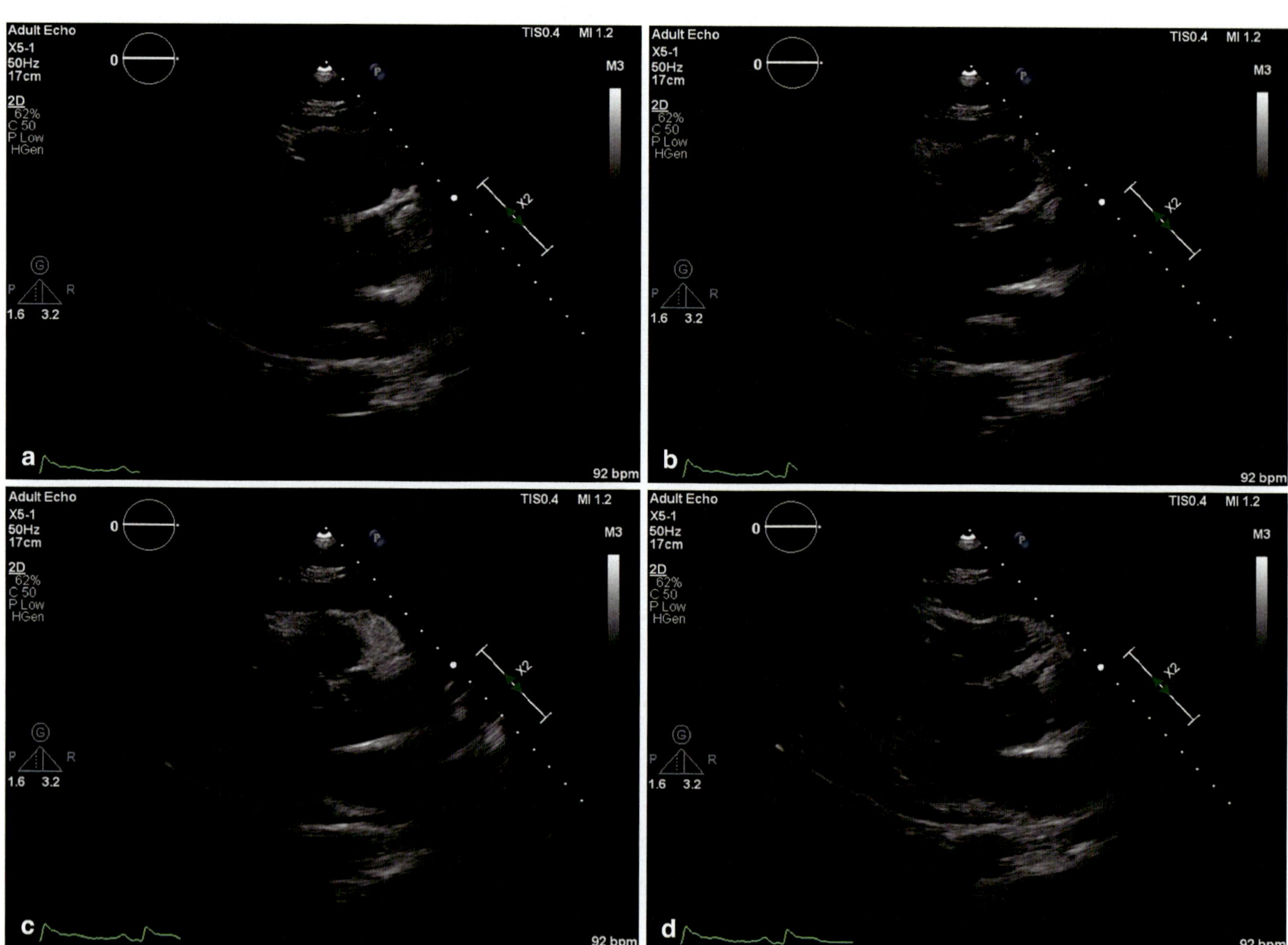

Fig. 15.6 (**a**) Pericardial effusion during *end-diastole* from a parasternal long-axis view. (**b**) Pericardial effusion during *early systole* from a parasternal long-axis view. (**c**) Pericardial effusion during *end-systole* from a parasternal long-axis view. (**d**) Pericardial effusion during *mid-diastole* from a parasternal long-axis view

Question 7

A 74 year-old woman presented to the emergency department with progressive shortness of breath and cough. A bedside echocardiogram was performed. What finding is indicated by the arrow (Fig. 15.7)?

A. Thoracic aortic aneurysm with pericardial effusion.
B. Pericardial mass with pericardial effusion.
C. Chest wall mass with pleural effusion.
D. Atelectatic lung with pleural effusion.

Answer: D—Atelectatic lung with pleural effusion.

Key point: Differentiate pleural and pericardial effusion.

Rationale: A large circumferential pericardial effusion and pleural effusion can be appreciated from this parasternal long-axis view. The pericardium is seen deep to the inferolateral left ventricular wall (screen center) separating the anechoic pericardial fluid from pleural fluid. From a parasternal long-axis view, pericardial fluid is seen confined between the left heart and descending thoracic aorta, tracking anterior to the descending thoracic aorta. In contrast, pleural fluid extends deep to the descending thoracic aorta but does not cross anterior to the descending thoracic aorta. A chest wall mass is not seen, and the descending thoracic aorta is grossly normal from this view.

For questions 8 and 9, refer to Fig. 15.8 and Video 15.6.

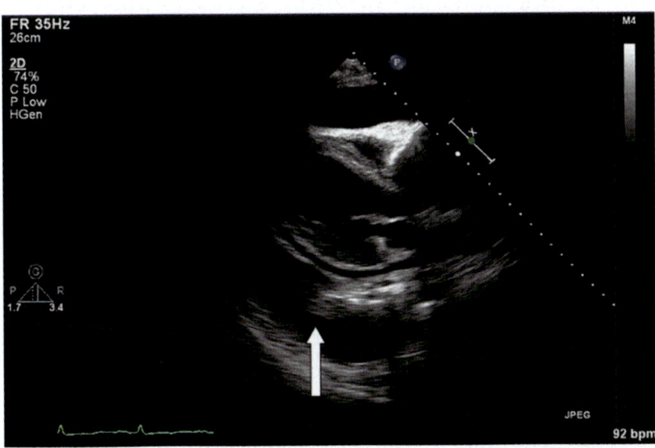

Fig. 15.7 Circumferential pericardial effusion with left pleural effusion and atelectatic lung is seen from a parasternal long-axis view. It is important to note a left pleural effusion will extend deep to the descending thoracic aorta but not cross anterior to the descending thoracic aorta. A cardiac mirror image could be mistaken for a left pleural effusion, but usually movement of the left ventricle and mitral valve distinguish a mirror image

Question 8

An 81 year-old man awoke complaining to his wife of chest and back pain. Shortly afterwards, he suffered a syncopal episode, fell, and hit his head. The emergency medical service was contacted and the patient was taken to the closest emergency department. A bedside echocardiogram was performed (Fig. 15.8, Video 15.6).

Which of the following findings is demonstrated by this patient's echocardiogram?

A. Small pericardial effusion with an epicardial fat pad.
B. Small complex pericardial effusion.
C. Large pericardial effusion with pericardial tumor.
D. Large pericardial effusion with organized thrombus.

Answer: D—Large pericardial effusion with organized thrombus.

Key point: Differentiate epicardial fat, blood coagulum, and pericardial tumor.

Rationale: Sudden loss of consciousness in the setting of chest and back pain in an elderly man raises concern for a cardiovascular emergency. In this case, a large pericardial effusion is seen on bedside echocardiogram with a mobile echodense structure that is most consistent with a thrombus. While epicardial fat pads are commonly located over the right ventricle, they are not freely mobile within the pericardial space. A complex pericardial effusion can be considered once life-threatening conditions are ruled out, but the acute onset of the patient's symptoms requires urgent evaluation. A pericardial tumor would appear adherent to the pericardium and not float freely as the thrombus in the video.

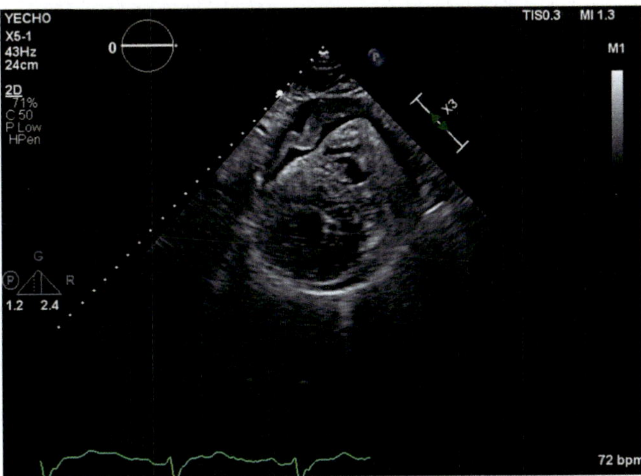

Fig. 15.8 Large pericardial effusion with organized thrombus is seen

Question 9

What is the most appropriate next step in the management of the patient described in question 8 (Fig. 15.8, Video 15.6)?

A. Order a STAT CT scan of the head to evaluate for acute stroke.
B. Obtain a comprehensive transthoracic echocardiogram to evaluate for signs of effusive constrictive pericarditis.
C. Perform emergent pericardiocentesis at the bedside.
D. Order a STAT CT scan of the chest to evaluate for acute aortic dissection.

Answer: D—Order a STAT CT scan of the chest to evaluate for acute aortic dissection.

Key point: Recognize an acute ascending aortic dissection and its management.

Rationale: This elderly man's history of sudden loss of consciousness associated with chest and back pain is highly suggestive of acute aortic dissection, and the most appropriate next step is to obtain a contrast-enhanced CT scan, preferably a CT angiogram, of the chest and abdomen. Although transesophageal echocardiography is an excellent test to evaluate the thoracic aorta and may be the preferred initial test at some institutions, it requires sedation to perform and does not allow visualization of the distal extent of the dissection to the abdominal aorta. It is important to note that emergent surgical intervention is indicated and pericardiocentesis should be avoided in the setting of hemopericardium due to aortic dissection. A STAT CT scan of the head is not indicated as the patient's history, especially chest and back pain, is not suggestive of acute stroke. The emergent nature of the patient's condition does not allow sufficient time to obtain a comprehensive transthoracic echocardiogram [3].

Question 10

A 63-year-old man on mechanical ventilation for acute respiratory failure due to influenza A and community acquired pneumonia is in the intensive care unit. He has been hemodynamically stable and is gradually weaning from mechanical ventilation. On his fourth hospital day, he becomes hypotensive and requires 2 vasopressor agents to maintain his systolic blood pressure in the 80's mmHg and a mean arterial blood pressure of 65 mmHg. A bedside echocardiogram is performed to evaluate his hypotension (Figs. 15.9, 15.10 and 15.11; Videos 15.7, 15.8 and 15.9. Which of the following is the most appropriate next step in his management?

A. Perform an urgent ultrasound-guided pericardiocentesis.
B. Start dobutamine infusion as an inotropic agent.
C. Order a comprehensive transthoracic echocardiogram.
D. Insert a left-sided chest tube.

Answer: A—Perform an urgent ultrasound-guided pericardiocentesis.

Key point: Recognize clinical signs and echocardiographic findings of cardiac tamponade in patient with a large pericardial effusion with chamber compression.

Rationale: The key echocardiographic signs of cardiac tamponade that can be rapidly detected include presence of a pericardial effusion, small cardiac chambers, and a plethoric inferior vena cava. In this case, the patient has hemodynamic compromise requiring vasopressor support, a large pericardial effusion, plethoric IVC without respiratory variation, and left-sided chamber compression which is consistent with cardiac tamponade that requires urgent pericardiocentesis. There are other echocardiographic findings of tamponade related to increased pericardial pressure (right-sided chamber collapse) and increased ventricular interdependence (respiratory variation of ventricular dimensions and transvalvular velocities) that are supportive of cardiac tamponade but not necessarily required when a clinical diagnosis has been made. The most appropriate next step in management is pericardiocentesis which should not be delayed to obtain a comprehensive transthoracic echocardiogram. Intravenous fluid resuscitation and vasopressor support can temporarily augment cardiac output while setting up for an ultrasound-guided pericardiocentesis. There was no pleural effusion seen on imaging which obviates the need for insertion of a left-sided chest tube.

For questions 11 and 12, refer to Fig. 15.12a, b.

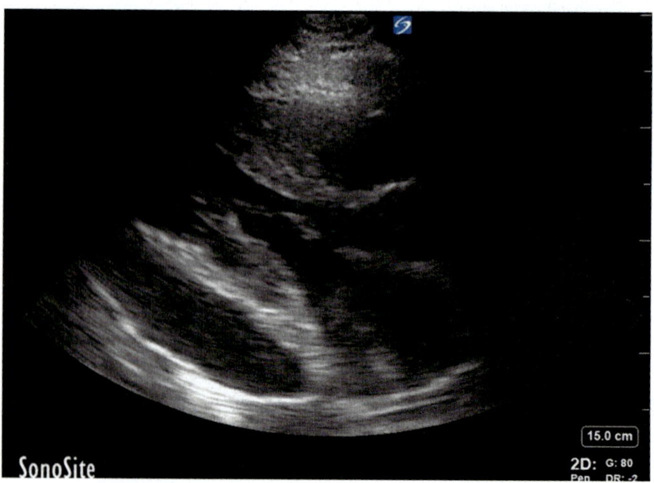

Fig. 15.9 Large posterior pericardial effusion with left ventricular chamber collapse is seen in a parasternal long-axis view

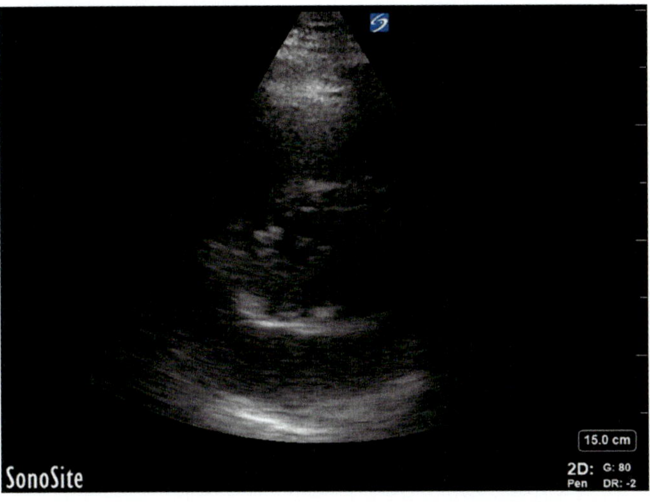

Fig. 15.10 Large pericardial effusion is seen in a parasternal short-axis view

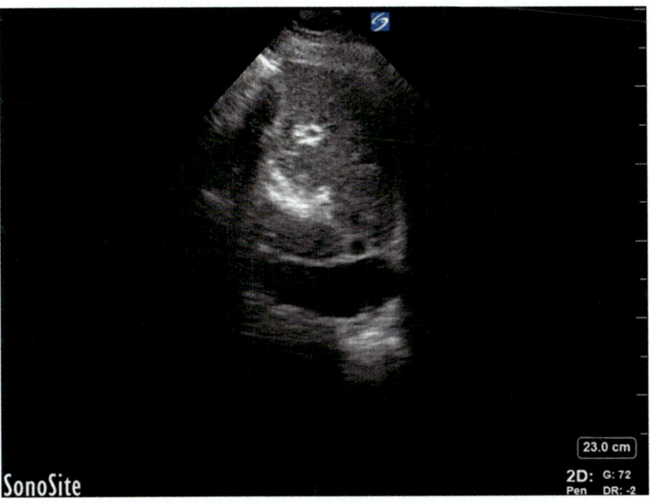

Fig. 15.11 Dilated and plethoric inferior vena cava is seen from a subcostal view

Question 11

A 57 year-old woman presents with increasing shortness of breath for the past several weeks. On exam, her BP is 94/46, heart sounds are distant, lungs are clear, and her jugular venous pulse appears elevated. A bedside echocardiogram is performed and reveals a large pericardial effusion. What is the respiratory variation of her tricuspid valve (TV) and mitral valve (MV) inflow based on the images below (Fig. 15.12a, b)?

A. TV 44%→MV 81%
B. TV 44%→MV 45%
C. TV 80%→MV 81%
D. TV 80%→MV 45%

Answer: D—TV 80% →MV 45%

Key point: Calculate variation of mitral and tricuspid valve inflow.

Rationale: Respirometers are routinely used to evaluate heart lung interaction during phases of respiratory cycle. In spontaneously breathing individuals, Doppler peak velocities in the tricuspid valve increase during inspiration, while they decrease in the mitral valve. A physiological variation in trans-valvular flow exists with normal respiratory cycle. In the presence of pericardial tamponade, peak velocities across both will be exaggerated with respiratory cycle.

To calculate respiratory variation for both the TV and MV, the reader uses the peak inflow velocity that occurs on the first beat during expiration and the first beat during inspiration. Then, use the equation (expiration—inspiration)/expiration to calculate the respiratory variation. Note that for TV this will result in a negative percent value.

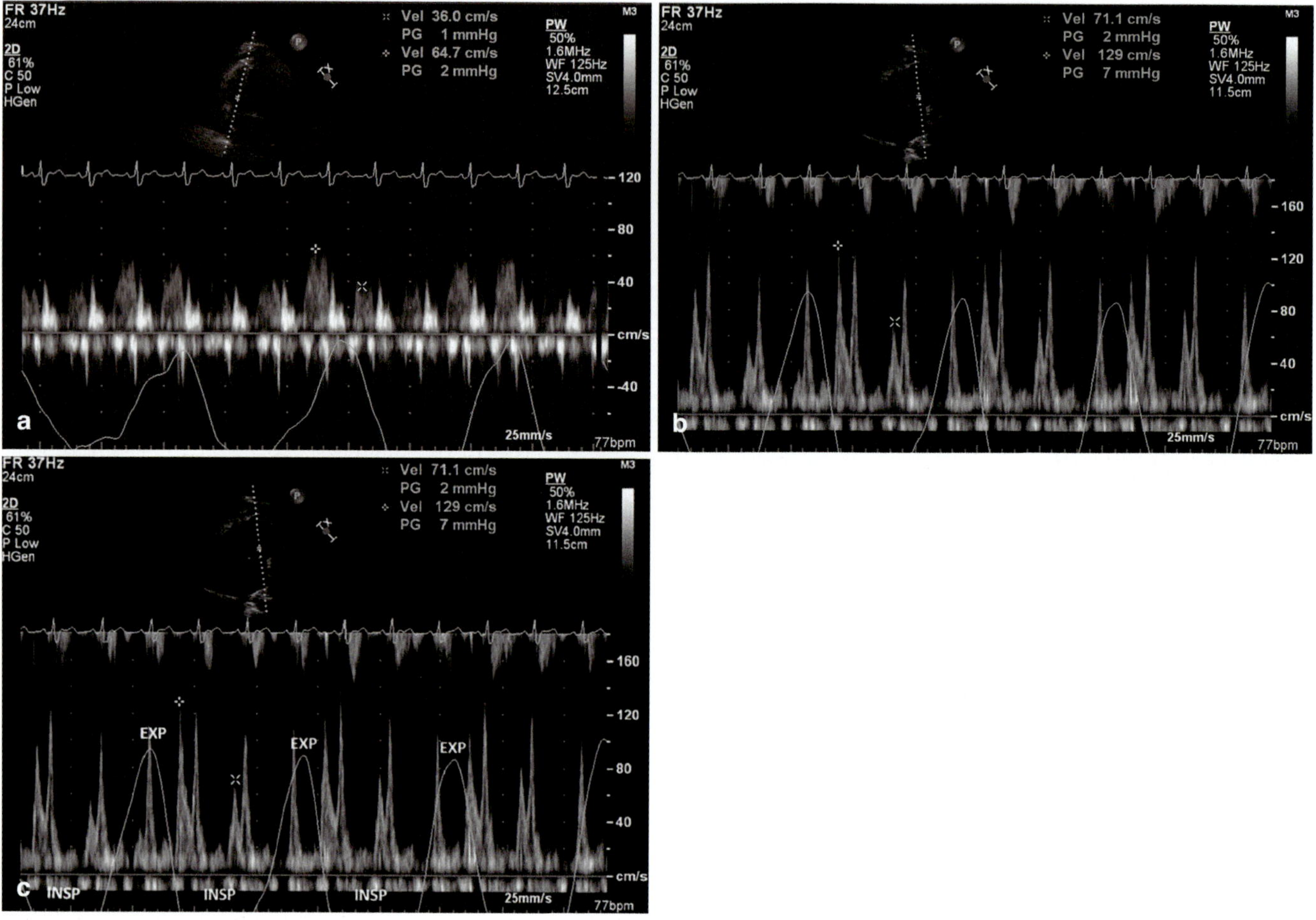

Fig. 15.12 (**a**) Tricuspid inflow variation measured using spectral Doppler from a modified apical 4-chamber view. (**b**) Mitral inflow variation measured using spectral Doppler from a modified apical 4-chamber view. (**c**) Clearly labels expiration and inspiration

Question 12

Based on the respiratory variation of the mitral and tricuspid valve inflows (Fig. 15.12a, b), does this patient have echocardiographic evidence of cardiac tamponade physiology?

A. No—respiratory variation consistent with tamponade (TV > 60% and MV > 30%) is not seen.
B. No—respiratory variation consistent with tamponade (TV > 30% and MV > 60%) is not seen.
C. Yes—respiratory variation consistent with tamponade (TV > 60% and MV > 30%) is seen.
D. Yes—respiratory variation consistent with tamponade (TV > 30% and MV > 60%) is seen.

Answer: C—Yes—respiratory variation consistent with tamponade (TV > 60% and MV > 30%) is seen.

Key point: Diagnose cardiac tamponade using respiratory variation of mitral and tricuspid valve inflow.

Rationale: Cardiac tamponade is a clinical diagnosis that is confirmed by echocardiographic findings of hemodynamic compromise. In addition to other echocardiographic findings, respiratory variation >60% for TV and > 30% for MV is considered significant and supportive of a diagnosis of cardiac tamponade [2].

Question 13

Which of the following echocardiographic findings approaches 100% sensitivity and specificity for a diagnosis of cardiac tamponade?

A. RA collapse for at least 1/3 of the cardiac cycle.
B. Early RV diastolic collapse.
C. MV respiratory variation >30%.
D. Dilated IVC with decreased respiratory variation.

Answer: A—RA collapse for at least 1/3 of the cardiac cycle.

Key point: Appreciate the sensitivity and specificity of different echocardiographic signs of tamponade.

Rationale: RV diastolic collapse begins to appear as pericardial pressure increases above the diastolic filling pressure. The higher the pericardial pressure, the longer the duration of RV diastolic collapse. Therefore, *early* RV diastolic collapse is not the best finding for diagnosing cardiac tamponade. Other conditions can cause exaggerated respiratory variation across both the tricuspid and mitral valves (e.g. COPD, constriction, acute PE, RV infarction, positive pressure ventilation) neither should be used as criteria for cardiac tamponade without other supportive findings. One such supportive finding is a dilated IVC with decreased respiratory variation, but again this is a finding that can be seen with other cardiac pathologies (e.g. acute decompensated congestive heart failure, right ventricular failure, Mechanical ventilation). Only the duration of collapse of the RA, when more than 1/3 of the cardiac cycle, has been shown to be 94% sensitive and 100% specific for the diagnosis of cardiac tamponade physiology [2, 4, 5].

Question 14

A 67 year-old man with history of COPD, HTN, hyperlipidemia, and DM is brought to the emergency department by ambulance. He complained of shortness of breath prior to losing consciousness. CPR was started en route to the hospital with return of spontaneous circulation after approximately 5 min of compressions. Vital signs: temperature 99 °F, pulse 93 bpm, BP 92/54 mmHg, respiratory rate of 14 breathes/min, oxygen saturation 98% on mechanical ventilation, height 172 cm, weight 123 kg. The patient is admitted to the medical ICU on a norepinephrine drip. A bedside echocardiogram is performed to evaluate his hypotension. Which of the following conditions can be diagnosed based on image shown (Fig. 15.13, Video 15.10)?

A. Pericardial effusion.
B. Epicardial fat pad.
C. Organized hemocoagulum.
D. Pericardial tumor.

Answer: B—Epicardial fat pad.

Key point: Differentiate pericardial fluid from other anechoic or hypoechoic structures in the pericardial space.

Rationale: Epicardial fat typically appears as a relatively anechoic space overlying the right ventricle, but can appear hyperechoic when more than 15 mm thick. Epicardial fat pads often appear to move with the heart throughout systole and diastole, unlike the anechoic space of a pericardial effusion. Organized hemocoagulum typically appears as a freely mobile echogenic structure within a pericardial effusion. A pericardial tumor would appear as a hypoechoic solid mass [6].

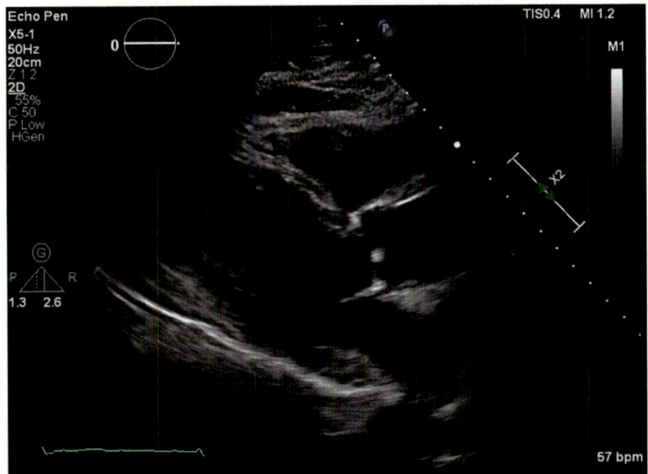

Fig. 15.13 Epicardial fat pad is seen in the near field, anterior to the right ventricle, in a parasternal long-axis view

Question 15

62 year-old male with history of metastatic squamous cell carcinoma extending to thoracic spine undergoes surgical decompression for spinal cord compression. Post-operatively he is transferred to the medical ICU on mechanical ventilation. For patients receiving mechanical ventilation, which of the following echocardiographic findings has a low sensitivity for diagnosis of a hemodynamically significant pericardial effusion?

A. Right atrial systolic collapse.
B. Right ventricular diastolic collapse.
C. Dilated IVC without respiratory variation.
D. Swinging heart in a large pericardial effusion.

Answer: C—Dilated IVC without respiratory variation.

Key point: Appreciate the changes of echocardiographic signs of cardiac tamponade with mechanical ventilation.

Rationale: Positive pressure ventilation, especially with high levels of positive end-expiratory pressure, causes elevation in central venous pressure which decreases the sensitivity of a dilated plethoric IVC to diagnose a hemodynamically significant pericardial effusion. The sensitivity of the other echocardiographic findings listed is not as affected by mechanical ventilation as the inferior vena cava [7].

Question 16

A 27 year-old woman with no significant past medical history presents to her primary care provider complaining of worsening shortness of breath with exertion and chest pain. Chest X-ray is unremarkable except for an enlarged cardiac silhouette. A bedside echocardiogram is performed and the subcostal 4-chamber view is shown (Fig. 15.14**,** Video 15.11).

Which of the following conditions is the most likely diagnosis based on the echocardiogram?

A. Epicardial fat.
B. Blood coagulum.
C. Pericardial tumor.
D. Right ventricular thrombus.

Answer: C—Pericardial tumor.

Key point: Differentiate epicardial fat, blood coagulum, and pericardial tumor.

Rationale: There is a large, multi-lobed, immobile echo dense structure adjacent to the right ventricle that is most consistent with a pericardial tumor. In this case, tissue obtained by CT-guided biopsy was consistent with a synovial sarcoma. Epicardial fat pads are commonly located over the right ventricle, have uniform thickness (not multi-lobed), and would not compress the RV chamber. Organized blood coagulum would appear as a gelatinous, mobile, echodense structure [2, 6]. Both Fig. 15.14 and Video 15.11 show an extracardiac mass adjacent to the right ventricle, and there is no evidence of an intracavitary thrombus.

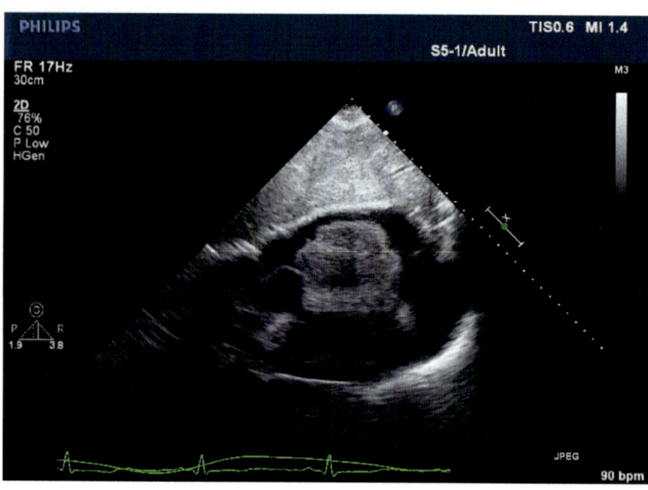

Fig. 15.14 Large echodense mass and pericardial effusion are seen adjacent to the right ventricle from a subcostal view

Question 17

All of the following are typically seen with both tamponade and constrictive pericarditis except ________________ .

A. Ventricular interdependence.
B. Increased central venous pressure.
C. Early diastolic filling.
D. Increased respiratory variation with ventricular filling.

Answer: C—Early diastolic filling.

Key point: Cardiac tamponade and constrictive pericarditis share many features in common and understanding the specific differences is important in diagnosis.

Rationale: Both cardiac tamponade and constrictive pericarditis limit the ability of the heart to fill with blood. During spontaneous breathing, inspiration decreases intrathoracic pressure and increases flow into the right ventricle. In both cardiac tamponade and constrictive pericarditis, the limited ability of the ventricles to expand outward results in a shift of the interventricular septum from right to left as the right ventricle fills (ventricular interdependence). This interdependence increases the normal respiratory variation pattern, although to a lesser degree with constriction than tamponade. Finally, the impaired filling of the ventricles causes central venous pressure to increase. One distinguishing finding of these two conditions is diastolic filling. In constrictive pericarditis, early diastolic filling (rapid y-descent) is rapid but quickly increases and results in the commonly referenced "square root" sign on hemodynamic tracings. Tamponade on the other hand, has decreased filling in diastole due to the increased pressure from the pericardial space (blunted y-descent) [2, 8].

Question 18

A 72 year-old woman with primary pulmonary hypertension was admitted to an outside hospital for recurrent syncope. She was found to have bilateral pleural effusions and approximately 1 L of pleural fluid was drained from each side by thoracentesis. Despite fluid removal, she was persistently hypotensive and norepinephrine was given to maintain adequate perfusion. A bedside echocardiogram was ordered with the following findings (Videos 15.12 and 15.13, Fig. 15.15). Which of the following findings is most consistent with his patient's echocardiographic images?

A. RV diastolic collapse.
B. LV diastolic collapse.
C. LV systolic failure.
D. Acute pulmonary embolism.

Answer: B—LV diastolic collapse.

Key Point: Patients with elevated pulmonary artery pressure may not have RV diastolic collapse despite being in tamponade.

Rationale: As seen in the videos, the RV is severely dilated and hypertrophied with a prominent moderator band suggestive of chronic pulmonary hypertension. There is no evidence of right ventricular diastolic collapse. An acute pulmonary embolism would not cause such severe right ventricular hypertrophy and dilatation. While the LV is small and underfilled, the mid-cavity is obliterated in systole, suggesting a left ventricular ejection fraction >70%. There is a moderate circumferential pericardial effusion, and the M-mode image and videos demonstrate collapse of the LV in early diastole [9].

For Questions 19–23, Match Each of the Conditions Listed Below with Their Effect on Pulsus Paradoxus in Patients with or Without Cardiac Tamponade. Select Either A or B for Each Question

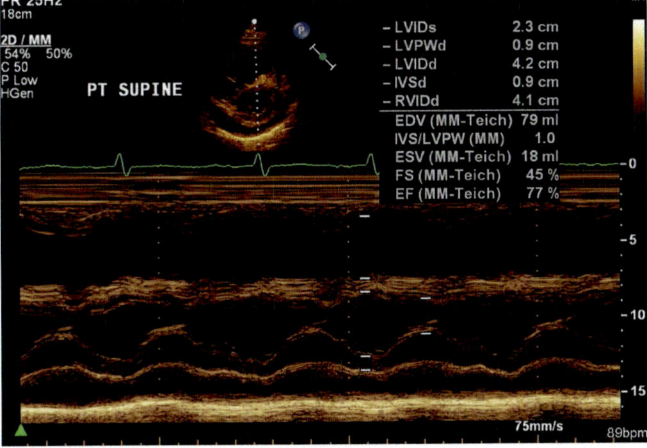

Fig. 15.15 M-mode image demonstrating collapse of the left ventricle in early diastole

A. Presence of Pulsus Paradoxus in Absence of Cardiac Tamponade.
B. Absence of Pulsus Paradoxus in Presence of Cardiac Tamponade.

Question 19: High left ventricular filling pressure ____.
Question 20: Marked dyspnea ____.
Question 21: Chronic obstructive pulmonary disease ____.
Question 22: Positive pressure ventilation ____.
Answer: 19—B; 20—A; 21—A; 22—B.

Key point: Recognize medical conditions that can either cause or mask pulsus paradoxus and Doppler signs of cardiac tamponade.

Rationale: Pulsus paradoxus and increased respiratory variation of TV and MV inflow velocities are not specific to cardiac tamponade. Pulsus paradoxus and increased ventricular interdependence can also be seen with constrictive pericarditis, pulmonary embolism, marked dyspnea, and chronic obstructive pulmonary disease. On the contrary, certain conditions can mask pulsus paradoxus in the setting of cardiac tamponade including positive pressure ventilation, aortic insufficiency, atrial septal defect, and high left ventricular filling pressure.

Question 23

54-year-old woman is admitted to the cardiovascular surgical intensive care unit post-valve sparing aortic root reconstruction after presenting with acute aortic dissection. Overnight her chest tube output and urine output decrease significantly. Her vital signs are a temperature of 37.1 degrees Celsius, heart rate of 102 bpm, oxygen saturation 95% on pressure assist control with FiO_2 50%. She requires increasing doses of vasopressors to maintain a mean arterial pressure of 65 mmHg. Transthoracic echocardiography was attempted but views were inadequate, and a point-of-care transesophageal echocardiogram is performed (Fig. 15.16, Videos 15.14 and 15.15). Based on the constellation of findings, what is the most likely diagnosis in this patient?

A. Obstructive shock due to massive pulmonary embolism.
B. Cardiac tamponade due to posterior pericardial effusion with thrombus.
C. Cardiogenic shock due to myocardial ischemia.
D. Graft failure due to a large abscess.

Answer: B—Cardiac tamponade due to posterior pericardial effusion with thrombus.

Key point: Recognize regional cardiac tamponade as a complication of cardiac surgical procedures that can cause hemodynamic deterioration.

Rationale: Approximately 1–2% of post-cardiac surgery patients develop a pericardial effusion [10]. Regional cardiac tamponade can occur from formation of loculated, eccentric pericardial effusions or localized hematomas. When regional cardiac tamponade is suspected, transesophageal echocardiography is often needed because optimal windows may not be obtained by transthoracic echocardiography due to the posterior location of an effusion, surgical dressings, patients positioning, or chest tubes [11]. In this patient, a large loculated pericardial effusion with thrombus is seen compressing both the right atrium and ventricle from the mid-esophageal 4-chamber view (Video 15.14). The loculated pericardial effusion with thrombus measured 4.7 × 7.6 cm (Fig. 15.17). Since the patient is <24 h post-surgery, it was too early for development of an infection or abscess. The images are not consistent with cardiogenic shock since the left ventricle was hyperdynamic and underfilled due to compromised forward flow from the right ventricle. The right ventricle was compressed and not dilated making a massive pulmonary embolism unlikely.

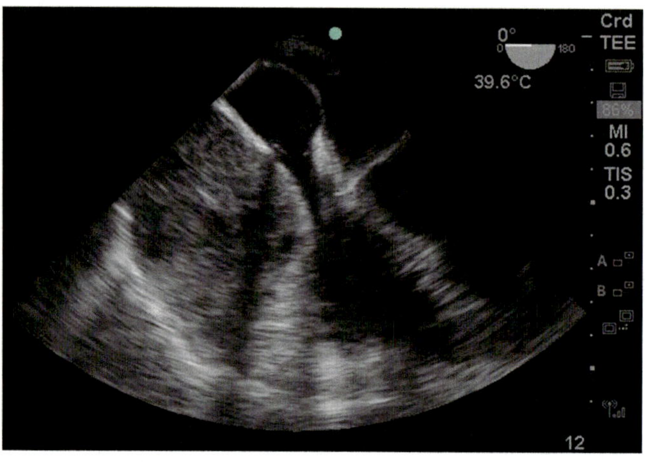

Fig. 15.16 Mid-esophageal 4-chamber view by transesophageal echocardiography demonstrating a large thrombus posteriorly (screen left) compressing the right atrium and ventricle

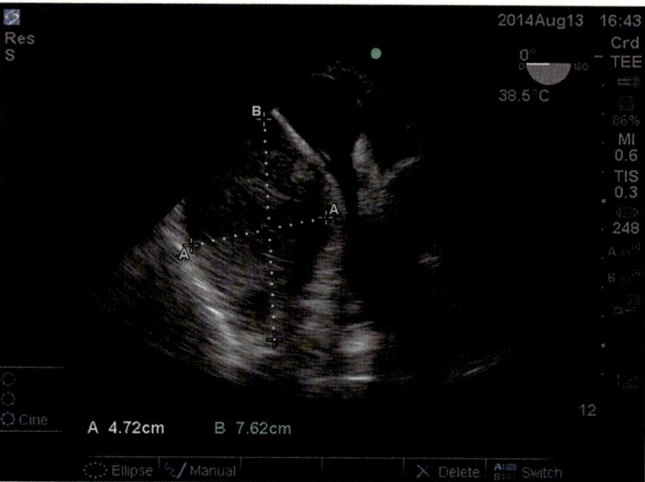

Fig. 15.17 A large thrombus measuring 4.7 cm × 7.6 cm is seen compressing the right atrium and ventricle from a mid-esophageal 4-chamber view using transesophageal echocardiography

Question 24

A 73 year-old man with pulmonary fibrosis, hypothyroidism, hypertension, and kidney stones is admitted overnight with cough and shortness of breath. He is diagnosed with a left lower lobe pneumonia with pleural effusion by chest X-ray and is started on vancomycin + piperacillin and tazobactam (Fig. 15.18). The following morning he is persistently tachycardic with a pulse of 116, hypotension with a BP of 90/50 and is still complaining of shortness of breath. An ultrasound exam is performed along the left posterior axillary line to evaluate the pleural effusion for thoracentesis (Videos 15.16). Which of the following findings is demonstrated in this patient's ultrasound images?

A. Pleural effusion.
B. Pleural effusion and ascites.
C. Pleural effusion and pericardial effusion.
D. Pericardial effusion and ascites.
E. Pleural effusion, pericardial effusion, and ascites.

Answer: C—Pleural effusion and pericardial effusion.

Key point: Differentiate a pericardial effusion, pleural effusion, and ascites.

Rationale: This patient's ultrasound exam reveals a large left-sided pleural effusion and a large pericardial effusion that was not previously suspected. A short-axis view of the left ventricle at the mitral valve level is seen as well as a large circumferential pericardial effusion. Paradoxical motion of the diaphragm is seen but ascites is not seen in the subdiaphragmatic space (screen right, Video 15.16).

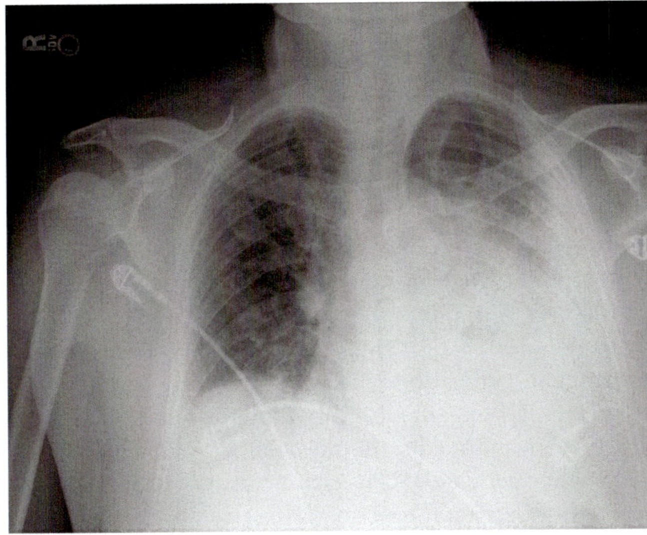

Fig. 15.18 Obscured left lower lobe suspected to be a left-sided pleural effusion is seen from a portable chest X-ray

Question 25

After performing the initial ultrasound examination of the patient in Question 24, additional views are obtained from the left anterior chest (Videos 15.17, 15.18, 15.19, and 15.20). Which of the following is the most appropriate next step in the management of this patient?

A. Continue vancomycin + piperacillin and tazobactam and observe the patient.
B. Administer intravenous furosemide.
C. Perform diagnostic thoracentesis.
D. Perform pericardiocentesis.

Answer: D—Perform pericardiocentesis.

Key point: Recognize cardiac tamponade and appropriate next steps in management.

Rationale: This patient's bedside echocardiogram demonstrates a tachycardic heart swinging within a large pericardial effusion and a dilated plethoric inferior vena cava. Although the corresponding EKG is not provided, the patient appears to have right atrial collapse in late diastole. These echocardiographic findings combined with his clinical findings of shortness of breath, hypotension, and tachycardia are consistent with early cardiac tamponade, and consultation with cardiology for pericardial drainage is the most appropriate next step. Given the concern for cardiac tamponade, the patient's preload must be maintained, and administration of intravenous fluids, rather than furosemide, may be needed until pericardiocentesis can be performed. Though emergent bedside pericardiocentesis may be considered, it is not clinically indicated at this time. Observing the patient without any intervention, and performing a diagnostic thoracentesis are incorrect because the primary culprit, the large pericardial effusion, must be addressed first.

Question 26

A 55 year-old man with a history of diabetes mellitus, hypertension, and myocardial infarction with multivessel disease underwent a 3-vessel coronary artery bypass surgery. His post-operative course is complicated by a right-sided pleural effusion and cellulitis of his left leg where the vein graft was removed. Cultures of the seropurulent drainage from the infected site are positive for methicillin-resistant *Staphylococcus aureus* (MRSA). He is discharged to a rehabilitation facility with IV antibiotics on post-operative day seven. He is readmitted to the hospital 2 weeks after discharge complaining of orthopnea, scrotal edema, and lower extremity edema. His jugular venous pulse is elevated on exam. A bedside echocardiogram is performed (Fig. 15.19, Videos 15.21 and 15.22). His IVC is dilated, and the lateral

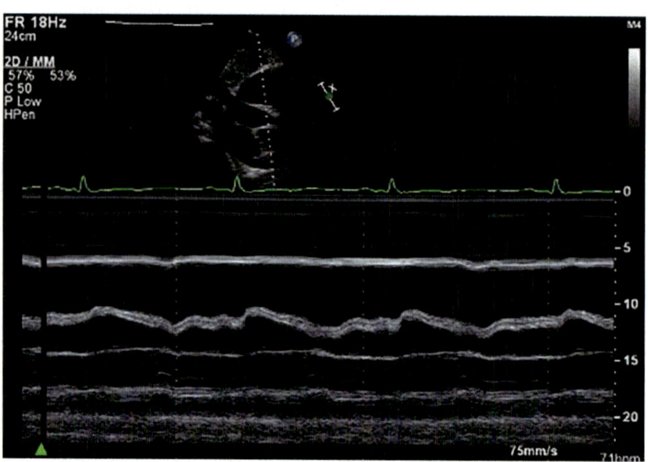

Fig. 15.19 M-mode image demonstrating a large posterior pericardial effusion that is causing right ventricular diastolic collapse

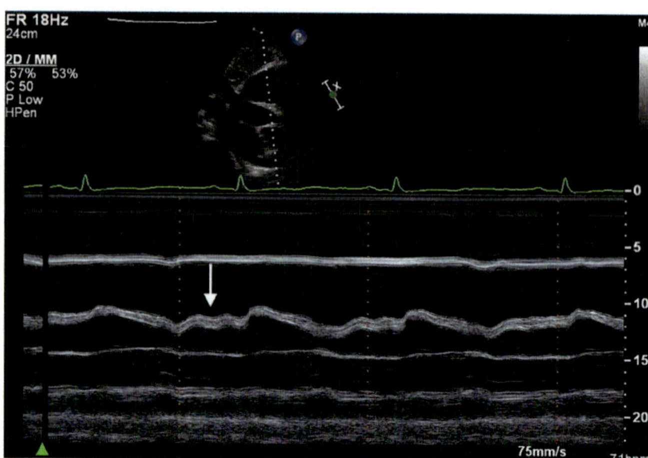

Fig. 15.20 M-mode image with an arrow depicting right ventricular diastolic collapse

E' is 11.4 cm/s and medial E' is 9.07 cm/s. Based on his echocardiographic findings, what is the most likely diagnosis?

A. Cardiac tamponade due to a loculated pericardial effusion.
B. Endocarditis due to MRSA bacteremia.
C. Acute heart failure due to coronary artery bypass graft failure.
D. Effusive-constrictive pericarditis due to recent cardiac surgery.

Answer: A—Cardiac tamponade due to a loculated pericardial effusion.

Key point: Recognize regional cardiac tamponade in the post-operative setting.

Rationale: A loculated pericardial effusion is seen adjacent to the right atrium and right ventricle. On M-mode, right ventricular diastolic collapse is suggestive of cardiac tamponade (**arrow,** Fig. 15.20). Given the clinical presentation, this patient was taken to the operating room and 250 mL of fluid was drained from the pericardial space. Additionally, 900 mL was drained from the right pleural space and 1.1 L from the left pleural space. The patient reported immediate improvement in his shortness of breath post-operatively. Although endocarditis cannot be ruled out based on the images provided, there are no gross valvular lesions seen. Suspicion of early graft failure should be in the differential diagnosis, but visualization of a large pericardial effusion compressing the right heart chambers would be the leading diagnosis and most immediate cause of hemodynamic compromise. Effusive-constrictive pericarditis, while uncommon, is in the differential diagnosis. The medial and lateral tissue velocities by Doppler are not reversed (*annulus reversus*) which makes this diagnosis unlikely.

Question 28

75 year-old man with a history of hypertension, gout and GERD presents with subacute exertional shortness of breath over the past 2–3 weeks. He denies any prior history of viral syndrome, chest radiation, or cardiac surgeries. A CT angiogram performed in the emergency department is negative for pulmonary embolism or consolidation, but notes some mild pericardial enhancement. On examination, heart rate is 110 bpm, BP is 110/70, oxygen saturation is 88-90% on room air. Transthoracic echocardiogram is performed (Figs. 15.21, 15.22, 15.23 and 15.24). Based on the clinical presentation and echocardiographic findings, which of the following is the most likely diagnosis?

A. Shunt.
B. Restrictive cardiomyopathy.
C. Constrictive pericarditis.
D. Pneumonia.

Answer: C—Constrictive pericarditis.

Key point: Recognize the echocardiographic features of constrictive pericarditis.

Rationale: This patient has two findings consistent with constrictive pericarditis: "annulus reversus" and "annulus paradoxus." First, the lateral mitral annular velocity is higher than the medial mitral annular velocity normally; however, in pericardial constriction, there is tethering of lateral left ventricular wall to the pericardium resulting in reversal of the mitral annular velocities (medial > lateral velocity) which is termed "annulus reversus" (Figs. 15.21 and 15.22). Second, the ratio of peak mitral inflow velocity / tissue velocity (E/e') is normal in this patient although left ventricular filling pressure is likely elevated. Normally, elevated left ventricular filling pressure increases the E/e' ratio.

However, in constriction, the ratio of E/e' is normal because left ventricular filling occurs almost exclusively through longitudinal expansion of the LV since lateral expansion of the heart is limited by pericardial constriction. Therefore, mitral annular longitudinal motion is preserved (or accentuated) maintaining the ratio of E/e' as "normal" despite usually elevated LV filling pressure. This phenomenon is termed "annulus paradoxus." Additionally, even though a respirometer was not used, expiratory diastolic flow reversal of hepatic vein flow and decreased forward flow can be appreciated (**arrow,** Fig. 15.25). As a reference, a ratio of expiratory diastolic flow reversal / diastolic forward flow greater than or equal to 0.8 is highly suggestive of constriction [12]. Finally, though not specific for constriction, a dilated plethoric IVC (Fig. 15.24) supports a diagnosis of constrictive pericarditis.

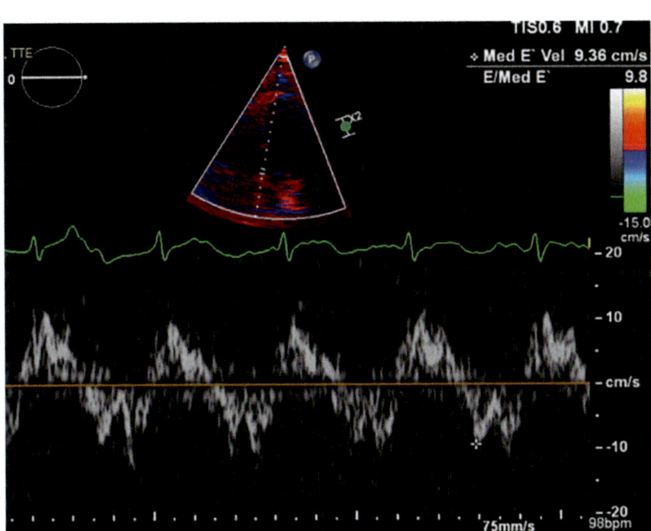

Fig. 15.21 Septal tissue Doppler velocity (E') measuring 9.36 cm/s

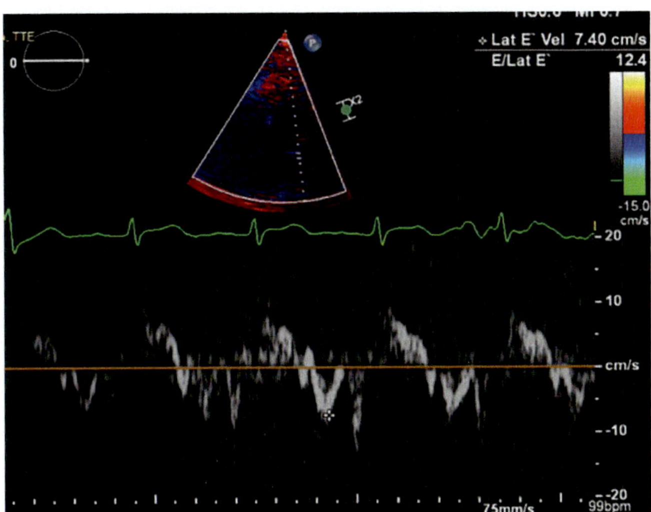

Fig. 15.22 Lateral tissue Doppler velocity (E') measuring 7.40 cm/s

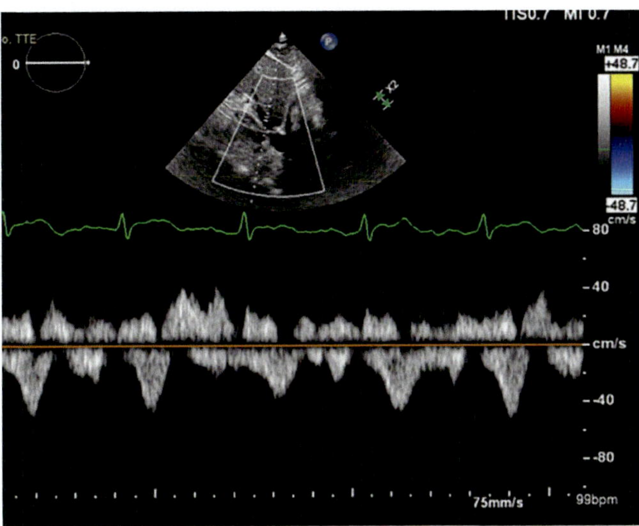

Fig. 15.23 Expiratory diastolic flow reversal and decreased forward flow is seen by pulsed-wave Doppler interrogation of the hepatic vein

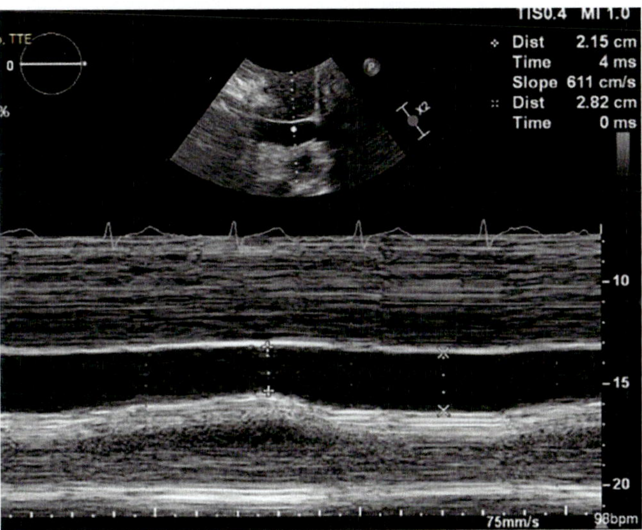

Fig. 15.24 Dilated, plethoric inferior vena cava is seen by M-mode

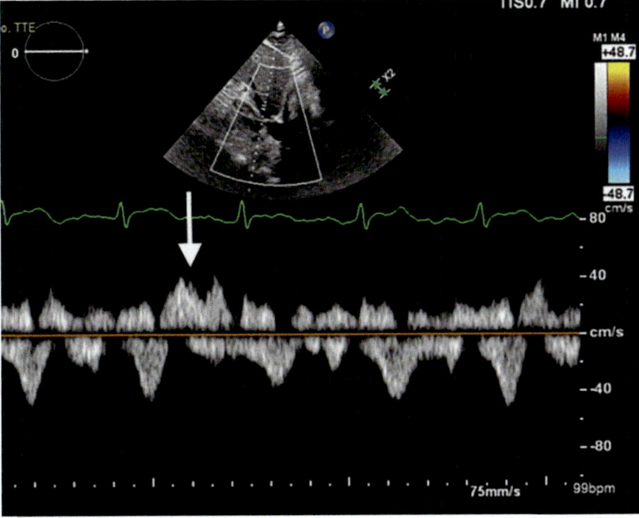

Fig. 15.25 Expiratory diastolic flow reversal of the hepatic vein is depicted by the arrow

Question 29

69-year-old woman with history of mechanical mitral and aortic valve replacement for rheumatic heart disease presents with shortness of breath. She denies fever, chills, or symptoms of an upper respiratory tract infection, and she has been compliant with her anticoagulation (warfarin). Here vital signs are temperature of 37.2 degrees Celsius, pulse of 105, blood pressure of 100/50, and oxygen saturation of 91% on room air. A portable chest X-ray shows complete opacification of the left lung. Labs are notable for a white cell count of 10,000, hemoglobin of 9 mg/dL, platelets of 180, 000, INR of 7, lactate of 4 mmol/L, and creatinine of 2.04 mg/dL. A lung ultrasound exam shows a large complex septated effusion (Fig. 15.26, Video 15.23). A chest tube is inserted and 450 mL of serosanguinous pleural fluid is drained. She is given fluid resuscitation, broad-spectrum antibiotics, and fresh frozen plasma to reverse her anticoagulation. She continues to be hypotensive and a bedside echocardiogram is performed (Fig. 15.27, Videos 15.24 and 15.25). Which of the following is the most appropriate next step in her management?

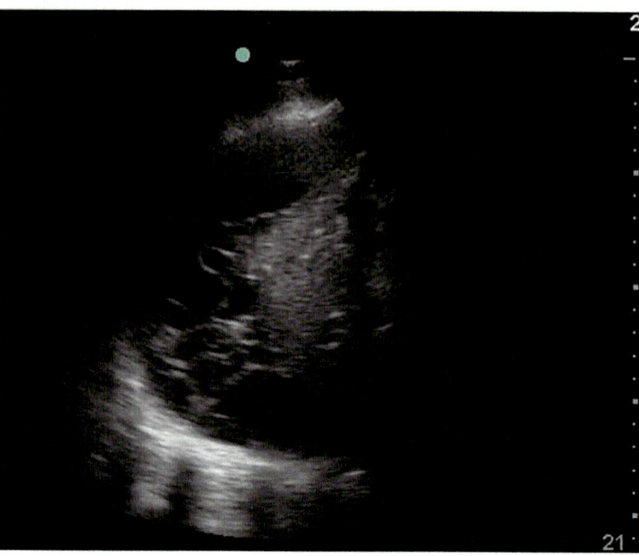

Fig. 15.26 Large, complex septated left pleural effusion is seen from the lateral chest wall. Note the shadows from the vertebral bodies in the far field

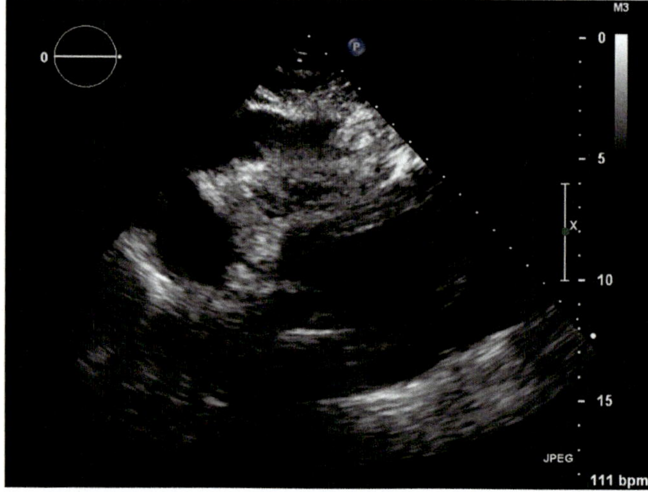

Fig. 15.27 Large pericardial effusion with right ventricular collapse is seen from a subcostal 4-chamber view

A. Perform emergent bedside pericardiocentesis.
B. Obtain a comprehensive transthoracic echocardiogram.
C. Consult cardiothoracic surgery for consideration of a pericardial window.
D. Insert of a second chest tube.

Answer: C—Consult cardiothoracic surgery for consideration of a pericardial window.

Key point: Identification and management of a large septated pericardial effusion due to hemorrhage.

Rationale: The bedside transthoracic echocardiography images show a moderate to large circumferential pericardial effusion. In the setting of anticoagulation with a supratherapeutic INR, a new pericardial effusion raises concern for pericardial hemorrhage. The large echogenic densities and multiple septations suggest thrombus formation with loculations. Given the septations on imaging, history of previous cardiac surgery, and recent anticoagulation, the pericardial effusion is unlikely to drain adequately with placement of a percutaneous drain. Surgical drainage via a pericardial window is the preferred management strategy [11, 13]. Emergent pericardiocentesis is not indicated at this time but may be considered as a temporizing measure if the patient becomes hemodynamically unstable while awaiting surgery. In some cases, pre-operative pericardiocentesis may reduce the risk of hemodynamic collapse during induction of anesthesia. Requesting a comprehensive transthoracic echocardiogram will delay the most appropriate course of action. Inserting an additional chest tube will not address the complex pericardial effusion.

Question 30

Which of the following statements is *FALSE* about the different approaches to perform pericardiocentesis?

A. Parasternal approach carries risk of injury to the internal mammary arteries.
B. Apical approach has relatively higher risk of pneumothorax than cardiac injury.
C. Apical approach has relatively lower risk to coronary arteries.
D. Subcostal approach requires a shorter length needle to reach the pericardial space.
E. Subcostal approach has relatively higher risk of right atrial injury.

Answer: D—Subcostal approach requires a shorter length needle to reach the pericardial space.

Key point: Understand the advantages and disadvantages of the different approaches for pericardiocentesis.

Rationale: Selection of a site for pericardiocentesis is based on the characteristics of the pericardial effusion (location, size and presence of loculations) and the advantages and disadvantages of the different echocardiographic windows (subcostal, parasternal and apical windows). The subcostal or subxiphoid approach requires a longer length needle to reach the pericardial space, usually 7–9 cm in adults. The subcostal or subxiphoid approach has the lowest risk for pneumothorax, but there is relatively higher risk of right atrial and liver injury. In some cases the liver lobe might be traversed intentionally if an alternative site is not available.

An advantage of the apical approach include relatively low risk of injury to the small apical coronary arteries. The risk of pneumothorax is relatively higher than cardiac injury with the apical approach. The parasternal approach is frequently used, especially under echocardiographic guidance that provides great visualization of the pericardial structures, but it carries the risk of pneumothorax and injury to the internal mammary vessels [11, 14, 15].

Question 31

A 24 year-old woman with no prior history is involved in a motor vehicle collision. She suffers a left chest laceration, small left-sided pneumothorax with bilateral pulmonary contusions, and a splenic laceration. Her wounds were cleaned and dressed, and she was monitored for two days in the hospital. She recovered well and was discharged in stable condition. Six days after discharge she presents with nausea and vomiting. Her vital signs in the emergency department are temperature 99.6 °F, heart rate 144 bpm, blood pressure 120/54 mmHg, respiratory rate 16 breaths/min, and oxygen saturation 100% on room air. An EKG is obtained (Fig. 15.28). Pulsus paradoxus was measured at 8 mmHg. A focused bedside echocardiogram is performed (Video 15.26, Figs. 15.29 and 15.30).

Based on this constellation of findings presented, what is the most likely diagnosis in this patient?

A. Constrictive pericarditis.
B. Cardiac tamponade.
C. ST-elevation myocardial infarction.
D. Acute pulmonary embolism.

Answer: A—Constrictive pericarditis.

Key point: Recognize the echocardiographic differences between constrictive pericarditis and cardiac tamponade.

Rationale: The patient's EKG shows diffuse ST elevation not conforming to any specific coronary distribution which is suggestive of pericarditis, rather than ST-elevation myocardial infarction. In acute pulmonary embolism, the RV may show stunning of the free wall with sparing of the apex (McConnell's sign). Although this patient has a pericardial effusion, no right ventricular collapse is seen; however, a septal bounce is seen which is due to ventricular interdependence. Fibrinous stranding within the fluid adjacent to the RV is suggestive of a subacute or chronic effusion. The findings of pericarditis on EKG, pericardial effusion with fibrinous stranding, and septal bounce are concerning for effusive constrictive pericarditis. The tissue Doppler shows "annulus reversus," defined as a medial mitral annular tissue Doppler of >7 cm/s and higher than the lateral annular tissue Doppler velocity which is the reverse of what normally occurs, further supporting a diagnosis of constrictive pericarditis [2].

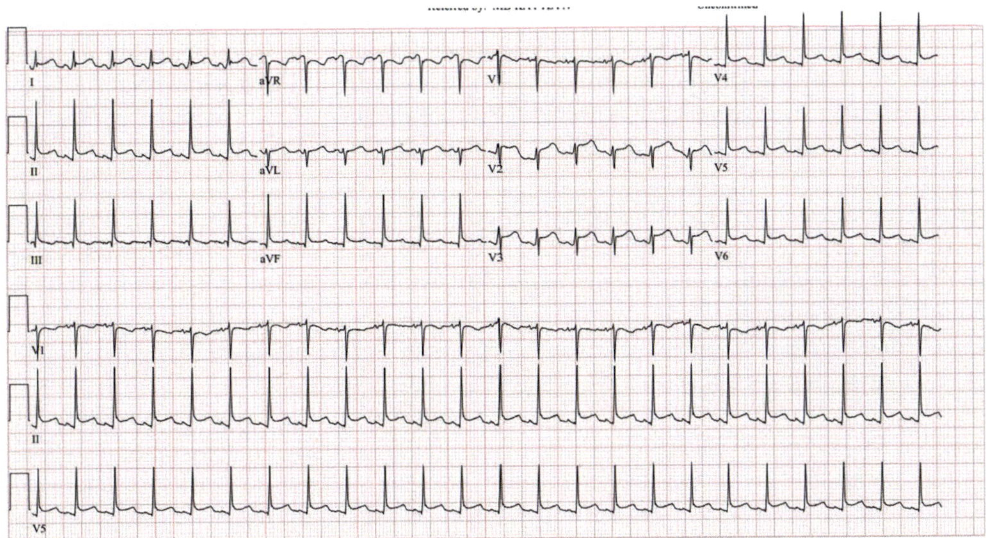

Fig. 15.28 Electrocardiogram demonstrates diffuse ST elevation with PR depression consistent with pericarditis

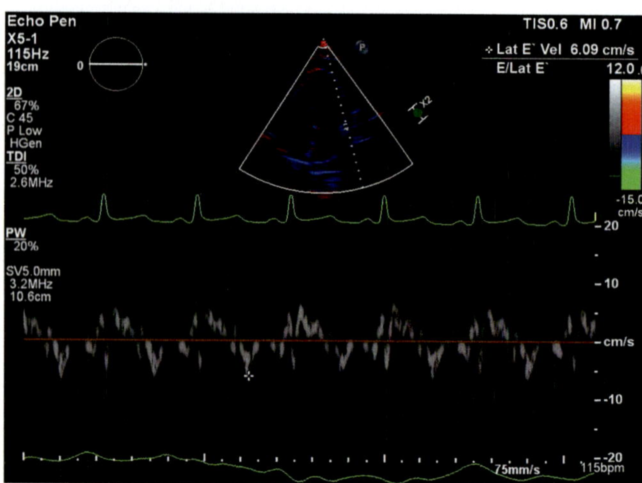

Fig. 15.29 Lateral tissue Doppler velocity (E') is 6.09 cm/s

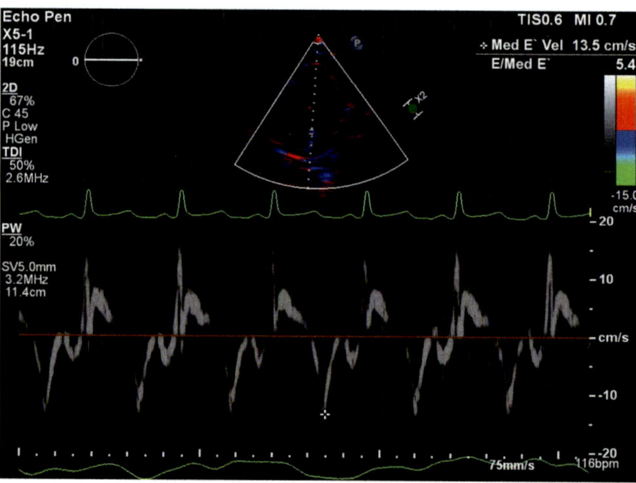

Fig. 15.30 Septal tissue Doppler velocity (E') is 13.5 cm/s

Question 32

A 42 year-old woman with severe pulmonary hypertension with RVSP of 90 mm Hg was admitted to ICU with worsening leg swelling and hypotension. A bedside echocardiogram was ordered with the following findings (Videos 15.27). Which of the following findings can confirm diagnosis of tamponade based on the patient's echocardiographic images?

A. RV diastolic collapse.
B. RA systolic collapse.
C. TV flow variation.
D. Left atrial diastolic collapse.

Answer: D—Left atrial collapse.

Key Point: Patients with elevated pulmonary artery pressure may not have right sided chamber collapse despite being in tamponade. LA chamber inversion/collapse may be signs of tamponade in severe pulmonary hypertension.

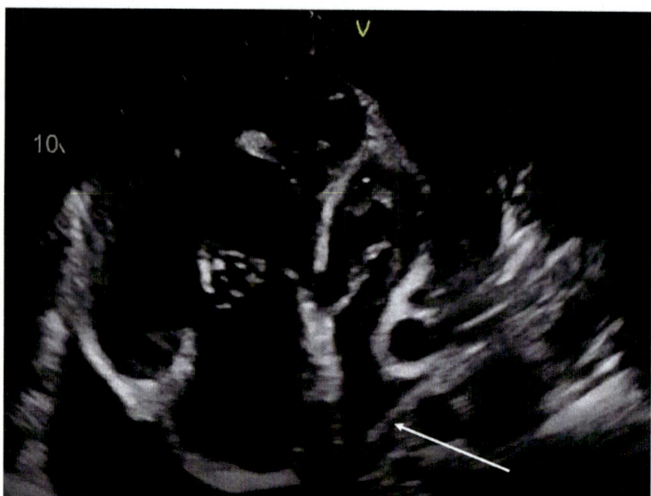

Fig. 15.31 Apical 4 chamber view with annotation showing LA free wall inversion

Rationale: As seen in the videos, the RV is severely dilated and hypertrophied suggestive of chronic pulmonary hypertension. There is no evidence of right atrial or right ventricular diastolic collapse. LA being the cardiac chamber with lowest pressure in setting of severe pulmonary hypertension, may collapse during diastole as observed in these case (Fig. 15.31). Other modalities may be required to confirm the diagnosis. If fluid is evenly distributed in the pericardial space, the increase in the intra-cavitary pressure is uniform. Right heart catheterization will show "equalization, defined as difference of no more than 5 mm Hg" of the right atrial pressure, right ventricular end-diastolic pressure, and pulmonary artery wedge pressure (which approximates mean left atrial pressure).

Question 33

A 65 year-old male with ESRD on hemodialysis is admitted to floor for inability to tolerate outpatient dialysis session due to hypotension. Chest X ray performed on admission shows increase cardiac silhouette. The tunneled dialysis catheter insertion site appears clean. The patient is afebrile with WBC count of 10.8 K. Another session of dialysis is attempted during hospitalization and is associated with significant hypotension, tachycardia and alteration in mental status. Which of the following may be the cause for patient decline based on echocardiographic images (Videos 15.28 and 15.29)?

A. Catheter associated blood stream infection.
B. Dialysis disequilibrium syndrome.
C. Low pressure tamponade physiology.
D. Dynamic LVOT obstruction.

Answer: C—Low pressure tamponade physiology.

Key Point: Tamponade physiology occurs when pericardial pressure in presence of pericardial fluid exceeds pressure in cardiac chamber causing compression and limiting venous return.

Rationale: Low-pressure cardiac tamponade is a form of cardiac tamponade in which a relatively low pericardial pressure cause cardiac chamber collapse because of low pressure within the cardiac chamber in presence of concomitant hypovolemia. The echocardiographic images show RA free wall inversion and RV diastolic collapse along with small IVC with significant respiratory variation suggesting a relatively low RA pressure. The onset of shock during dialysis occurred from fluid removal inducing decrease in chamber pressure and ensuing chamber collapse. No signs of catheter site infection was present. The dynamic LVOT obstruction occurs in presence of systolic anterior motion of mitral leaflet and usually observed in hyperdynamic circulation, which is not the case here.

Clinical Pearls

1. Trivial pericardial effusions are <1 cm but only visualized in systole. Small (<1 cm), moderate (1–2 cm), and large (>2 cm) pericardial effusions are seen in both systole and diastole.
2. Pericardial effusions must be differentiated from epicardial fat (echolucent, adherent to the heart), blood coagulum (echodense, freely mobile), and pericardial tumors (echodense, adherent to the pericardium).
3. Pericardial effusions must be differentiated from ascites and pleural effusions from the most common cardiac views. Ascites is seen in the near field from a subcostal 4-chamber view, a right pleural effusion can be seen in the far field (screen left) from a subcostal 4-chamber view, and a left pleural effusion can be seen deep to the descending thoracic aorta from a parasternal long-axis view or adjacent to the left ventricle from an apical 4-chamber view.
4. Epicardial fat appears relatively hypoechoic or anechoic, overlies the right ventricle, and moves with cardiac contractions, unlike pericardial effusions. In a parasternal long-axis view, epicardial fat is typically seen superficial to the right ventricle in the near field, whereas pericardial effusions are seen in both the near field and far field anterior to the descending thoracic aorta.
5. Organized hemocoagulum typically appears as a freely mobile echogenic structure within a pericardial effusion. A pericardial tumor would appear as a hypoechoic solid mass [6].
6. Cardiac tamponade is a clinical diagnosis that is confirmed by echocardiographic findings. The following findings are considered significant and supportive of a diagnosis of cardiac tamponade in patients with a pericardial effusion: right atrial collapse >1/3 of the cardiac cycle, right ventricular diastolic collapse, respiratory variation >60% for tricuspid valve inflow and > 30% for mitral valve inflow, ventricular interdependence, and a dilated plethoric inferior vena cava.
7. Pulsus paradoxus and increased respiratory variation of TV and MV inflow velocities are not specific to cardiac tamponade and can be seen with constrictive pericarditis, pulmonary embolism, marked dyspnea, and chronic obstructive pulmonary disease. On the contrary, pulsus paradoxus may not be seen with cardiac tamponade in the setting of positive pressure ventilation, aortic insufficiency, atrial septal defect, and high left ventricular filling pressure.
8. In unstable patients with clinical and echocardiographic findings consistent with cardiac tamponade, preparation should be made to perform ultrasound-guided pericardiocentesis either at the bedside or in the cardiac catheterization laboratory without further delay to obtain additional imaging.
9. In patients with hemopericardium, thrombus will appear as a mobile echodense structure within pericardial fluid. If the hemopericardium is suspected to be due to acute aortic dissection, then emergent surgical intervention is indicated and pericardiocentesis should generally be avoided.
10. In post-cardiac surgery patients with clinical signs of tamponade, consider a loculated pericardial effusion. An isolated posterior pericardial effusions often requires transesophageal echocardiography for diagnosis.
11. Both cardiac tamponade and constrictive pericarditis share many echocardiographic abnormalities in common. A few key findings can help differentiate these conditions. Reversal of the medial and lateral mitral valve tissue velocities (annulus reversus) is an important finding of constrictive pericarditis. Furthermore, mitral annular longitudinal motion is preserved in constrictive pericarditis and the ratio of E/e' is "normal" despite usually elevated LV filling pressure (annulus paradoxus).
12. In patients with severe chronic pulmonary hypertension, the right ventricle is dilated, hypertrophied, and less likely collapse with increasing pericardial pressure, and in the setting of cardiac tamponade, left ventricular diastolic collapse may occur before right ventricular diastolic collapse.

References

1. Ivens EL, Munt BI, Moss RR. Pericardial disease: what the general cardiologist needs to know. Heart. 2007;93(8):993–1000.
2. Klein AL, Abbara S, Agler DA, Appleton CP, Asher CR, Hoit B, et al. American Society of Echocardiography clinical recommendations for multimodality cardiovascular imaging of patients with pericardial disease: endorsed by the Society

for Cardiovascular Magnetic Resonance and Society of Cardiovascular Computed Tomography. J Am Soc Echocardiogr. 2013;26(9):965–1012 e15.

3. Hiratzka LF, Bakris GL, Beckman JA, Bersin RM, Carr VF, Casey DE Jr, et al. 2010 ACCF/AHA/AATS/ACR/ASA/SCA/SCAI/SIR/STS/SVM guidelines for the diagnosis and management of patients with Thoracic Aortic Disease: a report of the American College of Cardiology Foundation/American Heart Association Task Force on Practice Guidelines, American Association for Thoracic Surgery, American College of Radiology, American Stroke Association, Society of Cardiovascular Anesthesiologists, Society for Cardiovascular Angiography and Interventions, Society of Interventional Radiology, Society of Thoracic Surgeons, and Society for Vascular Medicine. Circulation. 2010;121(13):e266–369.
4. Gillam LD, Guyer DE, Gibson TC, King ME, Marshall JE, Weyman AE. Hydrodynamic compression of the right atrium: a new echocardiographic sign of cardiac tamponade. Circulation. 1983;68(2):294–301.
5. Ginghina C, Beladan CC, Iancu M, Calin A, Popescu BA. Respiratory maneuvers in echocardiography: a review of clinical applications. Cardiovasc Ultrasound. 2009;7:42.
6. Iacobellis G, Willens HJ. Echocardiographic epicardial fat: a review of research and clinical applications. J Am Soc Echocardiogr. 2009;22(12):1311–9; quiz 417-8.
7. Carmona P, Mateo E, Casanovas I, Pena JJ, Llagunes J, Aguar F, et al. Management of cardiac tamponade after cardiac surgery. J Cardiothorac Vasc Anesth. 2012;26(2):302–11.
8. Shabetai R, Fowler NO, Guntheroth WG. The hemodynamics of cardiac tamponade and constrictive pericarditis. Am J Cardiol. 1970;26(5):480–9.
9. Aqel RA, Aljaroudi W, Hage FG, Tallaj J, Rayburn B, Nanda NC. Left ventricular collapse secondary to pericardial effusion treated with pericardicentesis and percutaneous pericardiotomy in severe pulmonary hypertension. Echocardiography. 2008;25(6):658–61.
10. Ashikhmina EA, Schaff HV, Sinak LJ, Li Z, Dearani JA, Suri RM, et al. Pericardial effusion after cardiac surgery: risk factors, patient profiles, and contemporary management. Ann Thorac Surg. 2010;89(1):112–8.
11. Adler Y, Charron P, Imazio M, Badano L, Baron-Esquivias G, Bogaert J, et al. 2015 ESC Guidelines for the diagnosis and management of pericardial diseases: The Task Force for the Diagnosis and Management of Pericardial Diseases of the European Society of Cardiology (ESC)Endorsed by: The European Association for Cardio-Thoracic Surgery (EACTS). Eur Heart J. 2015;36(42):2921–64.
12. Syed FF, Schaff HV, Oh JK. Constrictive pericarditis—a curable diastolic heart failure. Nat Rev Cardiol. 2014;11(9):530–44.
13. Gumrukcuoglu HA, Odabasi D, Akdag S, Ekim H. Management of cardiac tamponade: a comperative study between echo-guided pericardiocentesis and surgery-a report of 100 patients. Cardiol Res Pract. 2011;2011:197838.
14. Chiara de Carlini CMS. Pericardiocentesis in cardiac tamponade: indications and practical aspects. Cardiol Pract. 2017:15.
15. Fitch MT, Nicks BA, Pariyadath M, McGinnis HD, Manthey DE. Emergency Pericardiocentesis. N Engl J Med. 2012;366(12):e17.

Adult Congenital Heart Disease

16

Tom Kai Ming Wang and Patrick Collier

Question 1
Which of the following congenital heart conditions has the highest prevalence in the general population?

A. Bicuspid aortic valve
B. Atrial septal defect
C. Ventricular septal defect
D. Patent ductus arteriosus
E. Patent foramen ovale

Answer: E. Patent foramen ovale. Bicuspid aortic valve is one of the commonest congenital anomaly occurring in about 1% of the population. Atrial septal defect although accounting for 10–15% of congenital heart disease has a prevalence of about 0.1–0.2%. Ventricular septal defect is slightly more common at 0.4%. Patent ductus arteriosus is the rarest on the list occurring in approximately 0.03% of births. Patent foramen ovale is the commonest at about 25% of the population.

Question 2
Which of the following is not a type of atrial septal defect (ASD)?

A. Ostium primum defect
B. Ostium secundum defect
C. Perimembranous defect
D. Sinus venosus defect
E. Coronary sinus defect

Answer: C. Perimembranous defect. The four main types of ASDs in order of decreasing frequencies are ostium secundum defect, ostium primum defect, sinus venosus defect and coronary sinus defects. Some classify patent foramen ovale as a type of ASD which would make it the commonest. Perimembranous defect is a type of ventricular septal defect.

Supplementary Information The online version contains supplementary material available at https://doi.org/10.1007/978-3-031-45731-9_16.

T. K. M. Wang · P. Collier (✉)
Robert and Suzanne Tomsich Department of Cardiovascular Medicine, Sydell and Arnold Miller Family Heart and Vascular Institute, The Cleveland Clinic Foundation, Cleveland, OH, USA
e-mail: WANGT2@ccf.org; colliep@ccf.org

R. Sreedharan et al. (eds.), *Critical Care Echocardiography*, https://doi.org/10.1007/978-3-031-45731-9_16

Question 3

Which of the following is not an indication for surgical repair of the congenital anomaly shown in Fig. 16.1, an apical 4-chamber view on transthoracic echocardiography?

A. Worsening exercise capacity
B. Desaturation from right-to-left atrial shunting
C. Left ventricular systolic dysfunction
D. Right ventricular systolic dysfunction
E. Atrial tachyarrhythmias

Answer: C. Left ventricular systolic dysfunction. Figure 16.1 shows Ebstein's anomaly. The current American Heart Association/American College of Cardiology guidelines for adult congenital heart disease 2018 recommends that surgical repair or replacement be performed in this condition with significant tricuspid regurgitation if there is one or more of heart failure symptoms, worsening exercise capacity and progressive right ventricular systolic dysfunction. Surgery may also be considered if there is systemic desaturation from right-to-left atrial shunting, paradoxical embolism and atrial tachyarrhythmias.

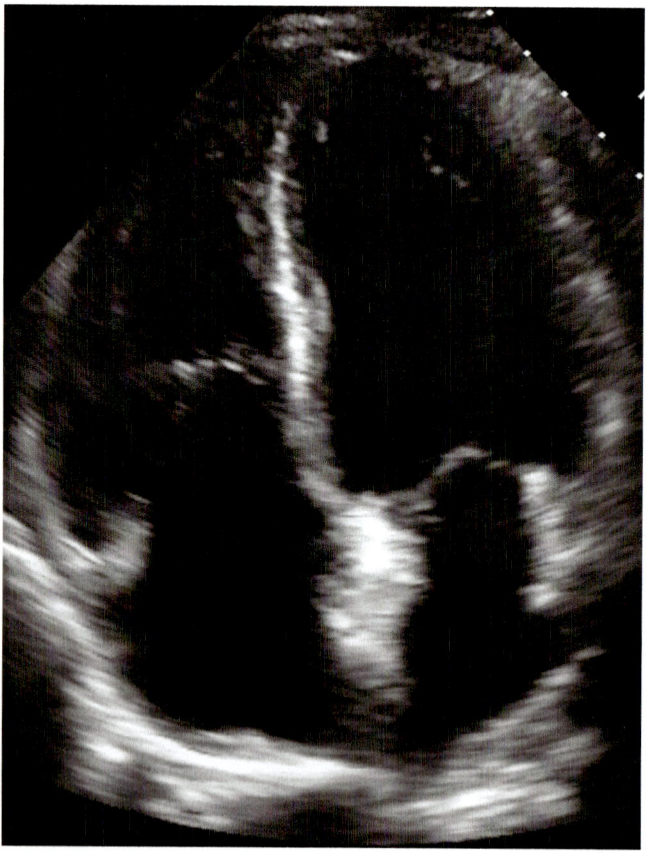

Fig. 16.1 Apical 4-chamber view

Question 4

Echocardiography was used to evaluate the shunt fraction of a patient with a ventricular septal defect, in the absence of other shunts and valvular lesions. The left (LVOT) and right (RVOT) ventricular outflow tract diameters were 2.4 and 2.2 cm, while the LVOT and RVOT tract velocity-time-integrals (VTI) were 15 and 25 cm respectively. What is the shunt fraction (pulmonary flow: systemic flow)?

A. 1.2
B. 1.4
C. 1.6
D. 1.8
E. 2.0

Answer: B. 1.4. Stroke volume can be estimated by the cross-sectional area × VTI = $\pi \times (\text{diameter}/2)^2 \times$ VTI. Therefore the LVOT stroke volume is $3.14 \times (2.4/2)^2 \times 15 = 68$ cm^3, while RVOT stroke volume is $3.14 \times (2.2/2)^2 \times 25 = 95$ cm^3. From this, the shunt fraction can be determined as 95/68 = 1.4.

Question 5

Which of the following does not cause the abnormality demonstrated in Fig. 16.2 (white arrow), a deep esophageal view on transesophageal echocardiography?

A. Patent ductus arteriosus
B. Left-sided superior vena cava
C. Anomalous pulmonary venous return
D. Coronary arterio-venous fistula
E. None of the above

Answer A: Patent ductus arteriosus. Figure 16.2 illustrates a large coronary sinus emptying into the right atrium. This is usually a result of a large volume of blood that drains into the right heart via the coronary sinus. Left-sided superior vena cava, anomalous pulmonary venous return to the coronary sinus and coronary arterio-venous fistula are examples of this. Patent ductus arteriosus is a left-to-right shunt at the level of the left pulmonary artery and aorta, and therefore does not affect the coronary sinus and its size.

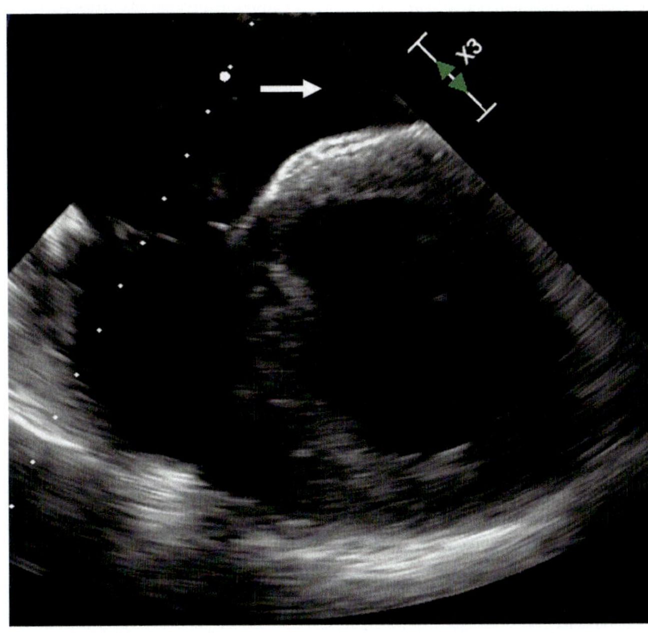

Fig. 16.2 Deep esophageal view on transesophageal echocardiography

Question 6
Which of the following transesophageal echocardiography (TEE) views is preferred to characterize a secundum atrial septal defect (ASD)?

A. Mid-esophageal 4-chamber view
B. Mid-esophageal 2-chamber view
C. Mid-esophageal aortic valve short axis view
D. Mid-esophageal bicaval view
E. Deep transgastric 5-chamber view

Answer: D. Mid-esophageal bicaval view. The optimal view for a cardiac structure to be visualized on echocardiography is for it to be perpendicular to the ultrasound interrogation beam to maximize resolution. On TEE this would be the bicaval view, whereby the interatrial septum runs horizontally across the screen, and perpendicular to the ultrasound beam. This is the preferred view to evaluate the size by two and dimensional echocardiography and flow by color and continuous wave Doppler of ASDs. As the interatrial septum is often a thin structure, there can be drop-out especially on other views that may be mistaken as an ASD. For transthoracic echocardiography, the subcostal 4-chamber view is the best to characterize ASDs.

Question 7
Which of the following congenital heart conditions does not cause Eisenmenger's syndrome?

A. Atrial septal defect
B. Ventricular septal defect
C. Patent ductus arteriosus
D. Aortic coarctation
E. None of the above

Answer: D. Aortic coarctation. Eisenmenger's syndrome is a cardiovascular syndrome whereby long-standing left-to-right shunting leads to pulmonary hypertension and eventually cyanosis because of reversal of this shunt to becoming right-to-left. A necessary premise to develop Eisenmenger's syndrome is the presence of a shunt. Aortic coarctation is the only option that does not contain a shunt, and therefore does not cause Eisenmenger's syndrome.

Question 8
What is the name of the congenital anomaly shown in Fig. 16.3, an apical 4-chamber view on transthoracic echocardiography?

A. Double inlet left ventricle
B. Cor triatriatum
C. Supravalvular mitral ring
D. Atrial septal defect
E. Subaortic membrane

Answer: B. Cor triatriatum. Figure 16.3 illustrates cor triatriatum, a congenital thin fibromuscular membrane that divides the left (cor triatriatum sinister, more common) or right atrium (cor triatriatum dextrum). Double inlet left ventricle refers to when both the left and right atrium is connected to the left ventricle, often with a hypoplastic or absent right ventricle. Supravalvular mitral ring is a result of abnormal connective tissue ridge that often leads to stenosis on the atrial side of the mitral valve. Atrial septal defect refers to a defect in the interatrial septum allowing blood flow between left and right atria. Subaortic membrane is a thin discrete membrane or fibromuscular ridge on the left ventricular side of the aortic valve, often causing outflow tract obstruction.

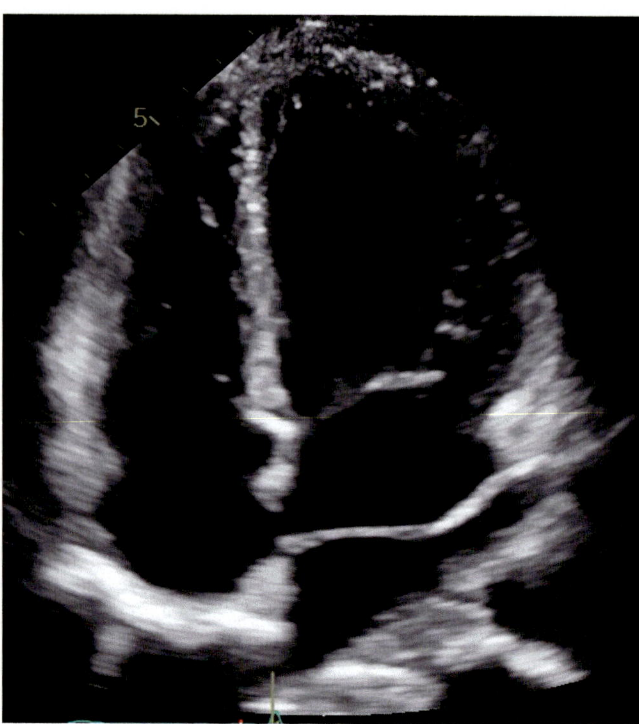

Fig. 16.3 Apical 4-chamber view

Question 9

What is the classical cause of delayed visualization of bubbles seen in the left atrium in a venous agitated saline test injection into the right heart from a peripheral intravenous line (occurring after 3–5 heart beats from when bubbles appear in the right atrium)?

A. Patent foramen ovale
B. Atrial septal defect
C. Ventricular septal defect
D. Patent ductus arteriosus
E. Intrapulmonary arteriovenous shunting

Answer: E. Intrapulmonary arteriovenous shunting. Agitated saline test is a method to evaluate for patent foramen ovale. A positive test with bubbles appearing in the left atrium from the right atrium suggests its presence. In patients with patent foramen ovales and atrial septal defects, the bubbles typically cross early within 1–3 heart beats from arriving in the right atrium to being in the left atrium. For ventricular septal defects, bubbles do not enter the left heart unless there is significant bidirectional flow, and then would need mitral regurgitation to get into the left atrium so is very unlikely. Patients with patent ductus arteriosus, which is a left-to-right shunt at the aorta to pulmonary artery level would not have bubbles appearing going backwards into the left atrium. In intrapulmonary arteriovenous shunting, the bubbles goes from right atrium, right ventricle, pulmonary artery then to pulmonary veins and into the left atrium, without going through the lungs so there is no dissipation of bubbles, hence the delayed positive test.

Question 10

Type B interruption of the aortic arch is defined by failure of formation of the aorta in which aortic segment?

A. Proximal to the brachiocephalic trunk
B. Between the brachiocephalic trunk and left common carotid artery
C. Between the left common carotid artery and left subclavian artery
D. Distal to the left subclavian artery
E. The different types are not defined by anatomical location.

Answer: C. Between the left common carotid artery and left subclavian artery. The different types of interruption of the aortic arch is defined by location. Type A is located distal to the left subclavian artery, type B between the left common carotid artery and left subclavian artery, and type C between the brachiocephalic trunk and the left common carotid artery. Amongst the subtypes, type B has the strongest association with DiGeorge Syndrome.

Question 11

What is the most likely type of defect illustrated in Fig. 16.4 (and Video 16.1), a subcostal view on transthoracic echocardiography?

A. Sinus venosus atrial septal defect
B. Ostium primum atrial septal defect
C. Ostium secundum atrial septal defect
D. Subpulmonary ventricular septal defect
E. Muscular ventricular septal defect

Answer: B. Ostium primum atrial septal defect. The location of Doppler color flow in Fig. 16.4 and Video 16.1 is seen crossing from the left to right atrium through the interatrial septum very close to the mitral and tricuspid valves, typical for ostium primum atrial septal defects (ASD). Secundum ASDs are located in the middle of the interatrial septum, and sinus venosus ASD at the junction between superior vena cava and right atrium, furthest away from the atrioventricular valves. Perimembranous and muscular ventricular septal defects are located in the in the membranous and muscular portions of the interventricular septum.

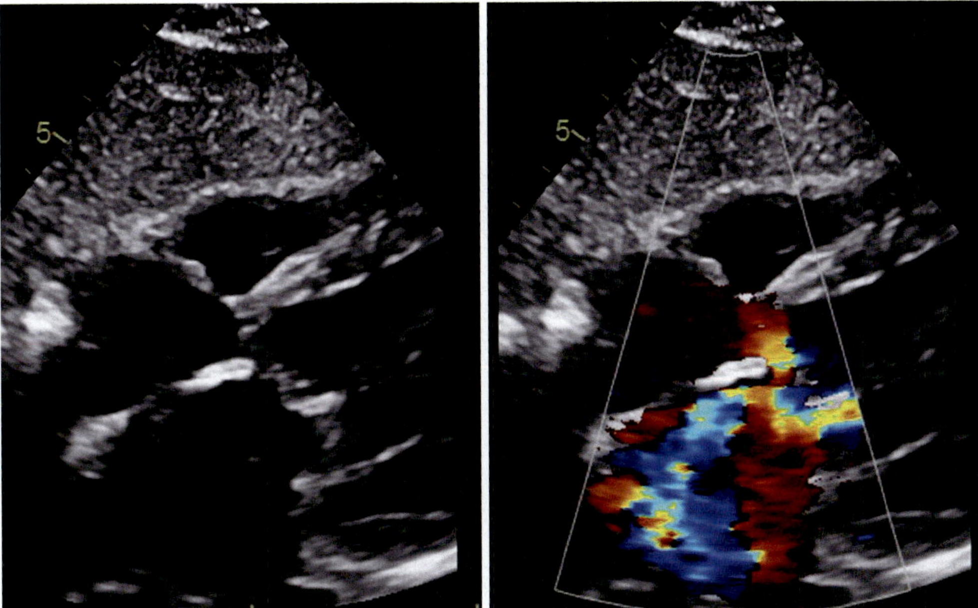

Fig. 16.4 Subcostal view without color Doppler (left panel) and with color Doppler (right panel)

Question 12
Which of the following is not associated with Ebstein's anomaly?

A. Tricuspid regurgitation
B. Lithium intake during pregnancy
C. Anomalous pulmonary venous drainage
D. Atrial septal defect
E. Wolf-Parkinson-White syndrome

Answer: C. Anomalous pulmonary venous drainage. Ebstein's anomaly affects the tricuspid valve leaflets with high rates of tricuspid regurgitation. In pregnant women who take lithium medications, their offspring have a higher risk of being born with Ebstein's anomaly. Ebstein's anomaly is also associated with both atrial septal defect and Wolf-Parkinson-White syndrome, but not with anomalous pulmonary venous drainage.

Question 13
What is the congenital abnormality seen on Fig. 16.5 (and Video 16.2), a parasternal short axis view on transthoracic echocardiography?

A. Cleft mitral valve
B. Parachute mitral valve
C. Bicuspid aortic valve
D. Ebstein's anomaly
E. Congenitally corrected transposition of the great arteries

Answer: A. Cleft mitral valve. Figure 16.5 and Video 16.2 illustrate a mitral valve cleft, a congenital mitral valve anomaly that involve partial splitting of the anterior or posterior mitral valve leaflet associated with mitral regurgitation. A parachute mitral valve is another rare congenital mitral valve anomaly where its shortened chordae tendinae all converge to one papillary muscle origin, causing stenosis from restricted opening. Figure 16.5 illustrates the mitral valve and not the aortic valve so is not a bicuspid aortic valve. The relative positions of the mitral and tricuspid valves cannot be determined on this image, and therefore Ebstein's anomaly and congenitally corrected transposition of the great arteries cannot be diagnosed.

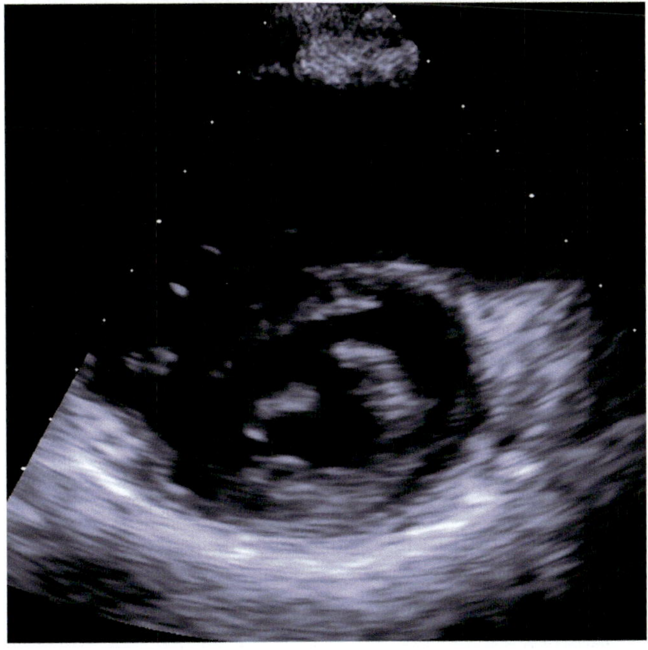

Fig. 16.5 Parasternal short axis

Question 14

Which of the following cardiovascular abnormalities is not associated with Turner's syndrome?

A. Ebstein's anomaly
B. Bicuspid aortic valve
C. Aortic coarctation
D. Aortic aneurysm
E. Anomalous pulmonary venous drainage

Answer: A. Ebstein's anomaly. Turner's syndrome is a genetic syndrome associated with a wide range of cardiovascular anomalies, including bicuspid aortic valve (with stenosis and/or regurgitation), aortopathies including aortic aneurysm and dissection, aortic coarctation, septal defects, mitral valve prolapse and anomalous pulmonary venous drainage. It is not associated with Ebstein's anomaly.

Question 15

Which of the following is not a complication of ventricular septal defect (VSD)?

A. Infective endocarditis
B. Arrhythmia
C. Aortic regurgitation
D. Systemic hypertension
E. Double-chambered right ventricle

Answer: D. Systemic hypertension. Many studies have shown increased risk of endocarditis in unoperated VSDs (where endocarditis is one of the indications for closure). Arrhythmias can develop in VSD patients, both atrial and ventricular. Aortic regurgitation also occurs more frequently in SVDs especially infundibular type because of deficiency in the septum supporting the right or left aortic valve cusp leading to prolapse and regurgitation during diastole. The left to right volume load from VSD accentuating pulmonary flow can cause pulmonary hypertension but not systemic hypertension. Gradual development of right ventricular muscle bundle hypertrophy on the margins of a membranous VSD can lead to a double-chambered right ventricle with higher proximal chamber pressure and lower distal chamber pressure.

Question 16

Which of the following is not associated with the condition observed in Fig. 16.6 and Video 16.3?

A. Aortic stenosis
B. Aortic valve endocarditis
C. Aortic dissection
D. Aortic coarctation
E. None of the above

Answer: E. None of the above. Figure 16.6 and Video 16.3 show a bicuspid aortic valve (BAV). BAV often become calcified and at earlier (middle-) age, which may manifest as aortic stenosis, regurgitation or both. It is the commonest cause of aortic stenosis in younger patients. It is associated with a higher risk of infective endocarditis in many observational studies. BAV's relationship with aortopathy is also well-established, with thoracic aortic aneurysms and dissection at a smaller dimensions on average than without BAV, and is also associated with aortic coarctation.

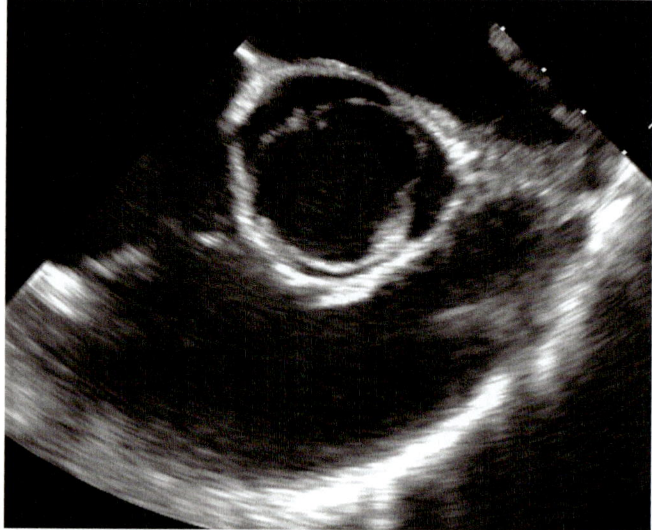

Fig. 16.6 Mid-esophageal view at 45 degrees on transesophageal echocardiography

Question 17

Agitated saline was injected into a left arm intravenous line of a patient, and bubbles were seen in the left atrium very soon after. The patient had chronically low oxygen saturations of around 88% despite the absence of chronic lung disease. What is the most likely congenital anomaly that would account for these findings?

A. Anomalous pulmonary veins to the right atrium
B. Patent ductus arteriosus
C. Left superior vena cava and unroofed coronary sinus
D. Ventricular septal defect
E. Congenitally corrected transposition of great arteries

Answer: C. Left superior vena cava and unroofed coronary sinus. Agitated saline does not get into the left atrium in anomalous pulmonary venous drainage, patent ductus arteriosus, ventricular septal defects (although all are examples of left-to-right shunting), or congenitally corrected transposition of great arteries. When there is a left superior vena cava that drains into the coronary sinus, there also would not be venous blood flow to the left atrium, unless there is an unroofed coronary sinus as in this case, which causes bubbles in the left atrium and right-to-left shunting leading to hypoxemia.

Question 18

What is the definition of an Ebstein's anomaly?

A. ≥5 mm/m² offset between the anterior tricuspid leaflet and the anterior mitral leaflet
B. ≥8 mm/m² offset between the septal tricuspid leaflet and the anterior mitral leaflet
C. ≥10 mm/m² offset between the posterior tricuspid leaflet and the anterior mitral leaflet
D. ≥12 mm/m² offset between the anterior tricuspid leaflet and the posterior mitral leaflet
E. ≥15 mm/m² offset between the septal tricuspid leaflet and the posterior mitral leaflet

Answer: B. ≥8 mm/m² offset between the septal tricuspid valve leaflet and the anterior mitral valve leaflet. This is the definition of Ebstein's anomaly, an offset of >8 mm/m² between the septal tricuspid leaflet and the anterior mitral leaflet indexed to body surface area.

Question 19

Which anatomical structure(s) need to be most thoroughly evaluated in presence of the type of atrial septal defect (ASD) seen in Fig. 16.7 and Video 16.4, each showing a bicaval view on transesophageal echocardiography?

A. Left atrial appendage
B. Pulmonary veins
C. Mitral valve
D. Aortic valve and aorta
E. Superior vena cava

Answer: B. Pulmonary veins. Figure 16.7 and Video 16.4 show a sinus venosus ASD, within the interatrial septum and adjacent to the superior vena cava. The most common congenital cardiovascular anomaly associated with sinus venosus ASDs are anomalous right pulmonary venous connections. For example, a superior defect is sometimes associated with the right superior pulmonary vein connecting to the superior vena cava, while an inferior defect is sometimes associated with the right inferior pulmonary vein draining into the inferior vena cava. It is therefore important to evaluate all the pulmonary veins whether they empty into the left atrium or elsewhere. Abnormalities in the other structures are not associated with sinus venosus atrial septal defects.

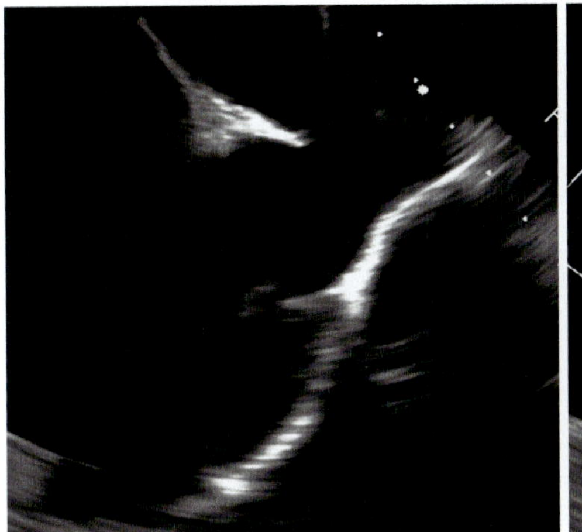

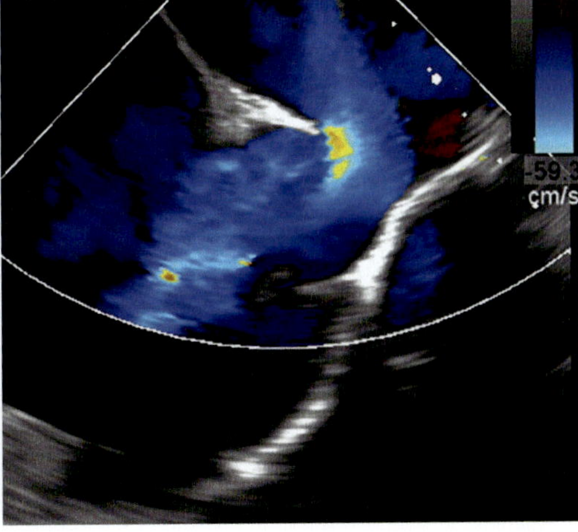

Fig. 16.7 Mid-esophageal bi-caval view at 90 degrees on transesophageal echocardiography without color Doppler (left panel) and with color Doppler (right panel)

Question 20

Which of the following echocardiographic features does not support closing a secundum atrial septal defect (ASD)?

A. Right-to-left shunting
B. Large defect
C. Right atrial dilation
D. Right ventricular enlargement
E. Pulmonary flow: systemic flow (Qp/Qs) of 1.6

Answer: A. Right-to-left shunting. The current American Heart Association/American College of Cardiology guidelines for adult congenital heart disease 2018 recommends that closure of secundum ASD be considered in patients with left-to-right shunt, right atrial and/or right ventricular enlargement, large defect, Qp/Qs $\geq$ 1.5 and functional impairment. If these factors are present, closure is more favorable in the presence of pulmonary arterial systolic pressure < 50% systemic blood pressure and pulmonary vascular resistance is <1/3 systemic vascular resistance. Right-to-left shunting (Eisenmenger syndrome) with confirmed pulmonary arterial hypertension on invasive hemodynamic assessment are contraindications to ASD closure.

Question 21

A patient presents with congenital pulmonary stenosis. Two-dimensional and echocardiographic measurements show right ventricular outflow tract diameter of 2.0 cm, peak velocity of 4 m/s and mean velocity of 3 m/s. What is the peak gradient across the pulmonary valve?

A. 16 mmHg
B. 27 mmHg
C. 36 mmHg
D. 48 mmHg
E. 64 mmHg

Answer E: 64 mmHg. Peak gradient (PG) across a valve can be estimated using the modified Bernouli eq. PG = 4 × (peak systolic velocity)^2. In this case, this would be $4 \times 4^2 = 64$ mmHg.

Question 22

What is the most likely diagnosis given Fig. 16.8 (continuous wave Doppler) and Video 16.5 (color Doppler) in a patient with and normal pulmonary arterial pressures on a subsequent right heart catheterization study?

A. Ebstein's anomaly
B. Right heart failure
C. Pulmonary valve stenosis
D. Atrial septal defect
E. Ventricular septal defect

Answer: E. Ventricular septal defect. In Video 16.5, the color Doppler jet appears very high above the tricuspid valve, separate to it, and with a visual appearance most consistent with mild or moderate severity (in contrast to a large proximal isovelocity surface area and severe TR). There was also some diastolic flow. Furthermore, in Fig. 16.8 there was a large pressure gradient of 93 mmHg without apparent RV remodeling and normal pulmonary arterial pressures on a subsequent right heart catheterization study. The jet most likely originates from a restrictive ventricular septal defect. It produces such high gradients because of the pressure difference between the left and right ventricle through a small defect. Apical displacement of the septal leaflet often with right heart overload is seen in Ebstein's anomaly (not seen here). The right ventricular size and function are normal here, which is inconsistent with right heart failure. Although pulmonary valve stenosis can cause high TR velocities with normal pulmonary arterial systolic pressures, we do not have pulmonary valve Doppler measurements here to make that diagnosis. The jet passes through the right ventricle, tricuspid valve then right atrium meaning it cannot be an atrial septal defect.

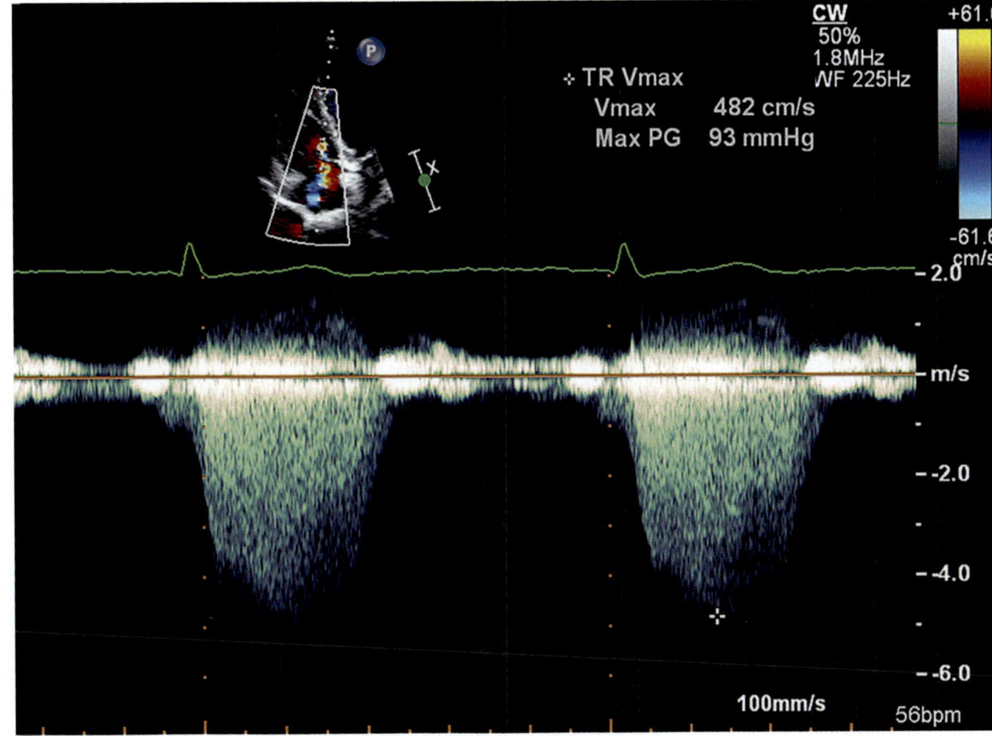

Fig. 16.8 Continuous wave Doppler

Question 23
Which of the following is not an indication or supporting factor for closure of a patent ductus arteriosus (PDA)

A. Left atrial enlargement
B. Right ventricular enlargement
C. Large left-to-rights shunt
D. Pulmonary arterial systolic pressure less than 50% of systemic arterial systolic pressure
E. Pulmonary vascular resistance less than 1/3 systemic vascular resistance

Answer: B. Right ventricular enlargement. The latest American Heart Association/American College of Cardiology guidelines for adult congenital heart disease 2018 recommends that PDA closure be considered in patients with left-to-right shunt, left atrial or left ventricular enlargement (from high left-sided cardiac output). Pulmonary arterial systolic pressure less than 50% of systemic arterial systolic pressure, and pulmonary vascular resistance less than 1/3 systemic vascular resistance are favorable supporting factors when indications are present for closure. The shunt from a PDA does not generally affect the right heart and therefore right ventricular enlargement does not occur and this is not an indication or supporting factor for closure of a PDA.

Question 24
Which of the following is not a complication of atrial septal defects (ASD)?

A. Left heart failure
B. Arrhythmia
C. Tricuspid regurgitation
D. Pulmonary hypertension
E. Paradoxical embolism

Answer: A. Left heart failure. Arrhythmias are common in ASD and this risk is not eliminated with closure. Chronic left to right shunting can lead to right ventricular volume overload and failure (rather than left heart failure), and functional tricuspid regurgitation. The elevated pulmonary flow from shunting can lead to pulmonary hypertension, and Eisenmenger Syndrome when end-stage. Venous thromboembolism may travel to the right heart and cross the ASD into the systemic circulation leading to strokes and other arterial system emboli, coined paradoxical emboli.

Question 25

What is the most likely diagnosis in Fig. 16.9, suprasternal view looking at the aortic arch and descending aorta, without color Doppler (left panel) and with color Doppler (right panel).

A. Right-sided aortic arch
B. Interrupted aortic arch
C. Thoracic aortic aneurysm
D. Aortic coarctation
E. Left subclavian artery stenosis

Answer: D. Aortic coarctation. Figure 16.9 shows narrowing in the proximal descending aorta and flow acceleration across the narrowing on color Doppler, indicating aortic coarctation. A right-sided aortic arch on this view would turn leftwards when going down. An interrupted aortic arch means that part of the aorta doesn't form completely and there is a missing gap. A thoracic aortic aneurysm would not cause accelerated flow. The left subclavian artery is a branch of the aortic arch and would head upwards and rightwards on this view, and not where the accelerated blood flow is seen.

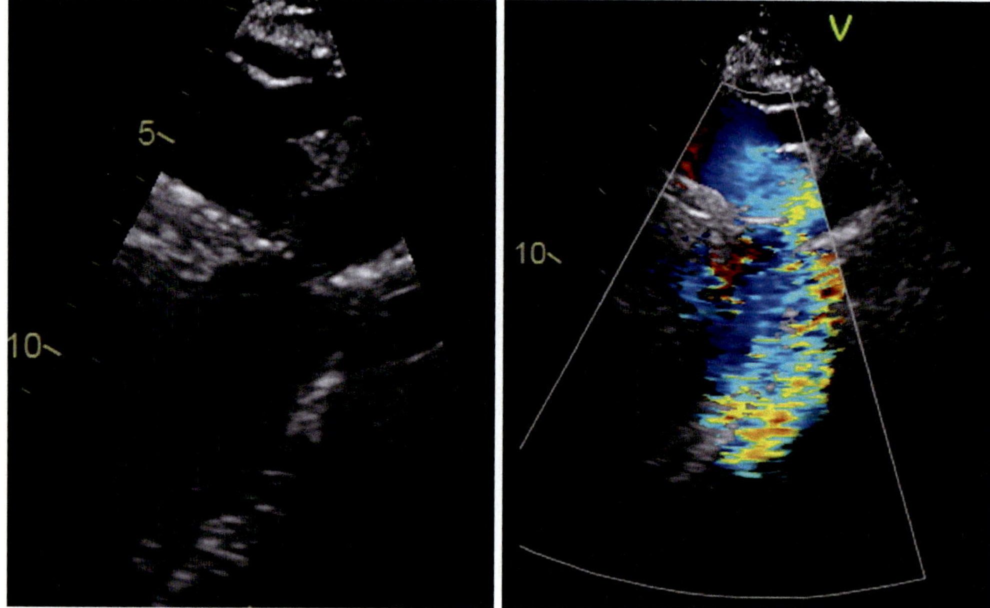

Fig. 16.9 Suprasternal view looking at the aortic arch and descending aorta, without color Doppler (left panel) and with color Doppler (right panel)

Question 26
Which of the following echocardiographic parameters support closing a ventricular septal defect (VSD)?

A. Right-to-left shunting
B. High peak gradient across the VSD
C. Progressive aortic regurgitation
D. Left atrial dilation
E. Pulmonary flow: systemic flow (Qp/Qs) of 1.3

Answer: C. Progressive aortic regurgitation The latest American Heart Association/American College of Cardiology guidelines for adult congenital heart disease 2018 recommends that VSD be considered in patients with left-to-right shunt, left ventricular enlargement, Qp/Qs ≥ 1.5, progressive aortic regurgitation because of perimembranous or supracristal VSD and history of infective endocarditis. If these factors are present, closure is more favourable in the presence of pulmonary arterial systolic pressure < 50% systemic blood pressure and pulmonary vascular resistance is <1/3 systemic vascular resistance. Right-to-left shunting (Eisenmenger syndrome) with confirmed pulmonary arterial hypertension on invasive hemodynamic assessment is a contraindication to closure. High peak gradient across the VSD suggests a smaller restrictive VSD without significant hemodynamic shunting and therefore not require closure. Left ventricular and right ventricular dilation, but not left atrial dilation, may be encountered as part of VSD pathophysiology with large shunts.

Question 27
Which of the following congenital malformation is not part of Shone's complex?

A. Supravalvular mitral membrane
B. Parachute mitral valve
C. Subaortic stenosis
D. Bicuspid aortic valve
E. Aortic coarctation

Answer: D. Bicuspid aortic valve. Shone's complex or syndrome is a rare association between four left-sided cardiovascular defects of obstructive nature, namely supravalvular mitral membrane, parachute mitral valve, subaortic stenosis and aortic coarctation. Although bicuspid aortic valve can also cause aortic stenosis (and regurgitation), it is not part of the typical spectrum of lesions in Shone's complex.

Question 28
What is the most likely diagnosis demonstrated by Fig. 16.10 and Video 16.6, an apical 4-chamber view on transthoracic echocardiography?

A. Atrioventricular septal defects
B. Gerbode defect
C. Ebstein's anomaly
D. Tetralogy of Fallot
E. Congenitally corrected transposition of the great arteries

Answer: E. Congenitally corrected transposition of the great arteries. An important finding on this apical 4-chamber view in Fig. 16.10 and Video 16.6 is that the "tricuspid" valve, which is anatomically more apically displaced than the mitral valve, appears on the right side of the image and associated with the systemic circulation ventricle (normally on the left side of the image). The commonest reason for this is congenitally corrected (or L-loop) transposition of the great arteries, where blood flows from the pulmonary veins and left atrium through the tricuspid valve to the systemic ventricle (morphologically right ventricle) then to the aorta, and returns via the systemic veins and right atrium through the mitral valve then the pulmonic ventricle (morphologically left ventricle). Atrioventricular septal defects are a type of septal defect involving both the interatrial and interventricular septum. A Gerbode defect is a rare septal defect causing blood flow from the left ventricle to the right atrium, made possible because the tricuspid valve is more apically displaced than the mitral valve. Ebstein's anomaly is a congenital anomaly with excessive septal displacement of the tricuspid valve. Tetralogy of Fallot encompasses the four features of overriding aorta, pulmonary stenosis, ventricular septal defect and right ventricular hypertrophy.

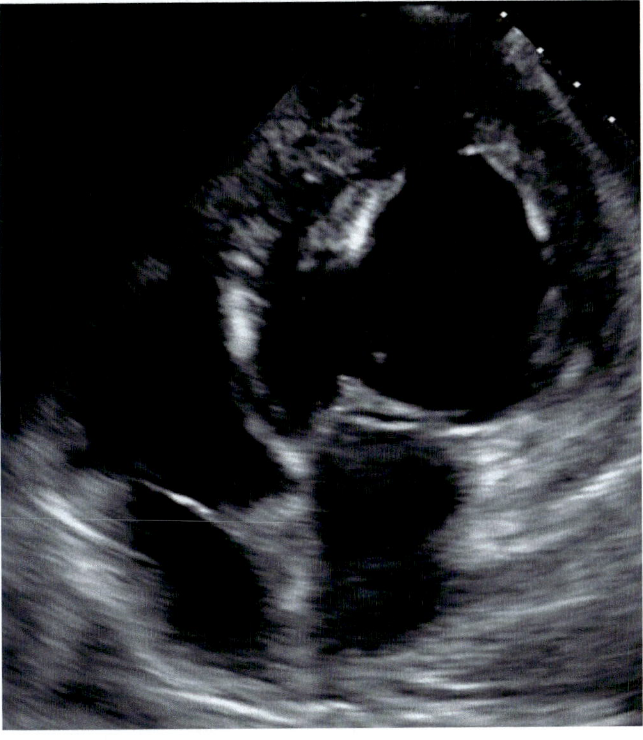

Fig. 16.10 Apical 4-chamber view

Question 29
Pulmonary valve replacement is often required in adulthood for patients with severe pulmonary regurgitation following surgical repair of Tetralogy of Fallot (TOF) in infancy. Which of the following is not an indication for pulmonary valve replacement in that setting?

A. Dyspnea
B. Severe right ventricular systolic dysfunction and dilation
C. Right ventricular systolic pressure < 2/3 systemic arterial systolic pressure
D. Other residual lesions requiring surgical interventions
E. Sustained arrhythmias

Answer: C. Right ventricular systolic pressure < 2/3 systemic arterial systolic pressure. The latest American Heart Association/American College of Cardiology guidelines for adult congenital heart disease 2018 recommends that patients with history of TOF repair with pulmonary regurgitation be considered for pulmonary valve replacement in the presence of symptoms. Also, any two of (1) mild/moderate left or right ventricular dysfunction, (2) severe right ventricular dilation, (3) right ventricular systolic pressure > 2/3 systemic arterial systolic pressure because of outflow tract obstruction, (4) progressive reduction in objective exercise tolerance. Surgery may also be considered if patients develop sustained tachyarrhythmias, or if there are other residual lesions requiring surgical interventions.

Question 30
Which of the following is least likely to occur after surgery for the congenital anomaly seen in Fig. 16.11 and Video 16.7 of the mid-transesophageal long axis views during systole on transesophageal echocardiography?

A. Pulmonary valve stenosis
B. Ventricular septal defect
C. Heart block
D. Recurrence after surgery
E. Infective endocarditis

Answer: A. Pulmonary valve stenosis. Figure 16.11 and Video 16.7 demonstrate a subaortic membrane with stenosis as can be seen from accelerated Doppler flow across it proximal to the aortic valve. Surgery for subaortic membranes are associated with an elevated risk of causing ventricular septal defects, aortic regurgitation and heart block peri-operatively, and particularly high risk of membrane recurrence requiring repeat procedures long-term as well as infective endocarditis. This operation relieves left ventricular outflow tract obstruction and is not associated with pulmonary valve stenosis.

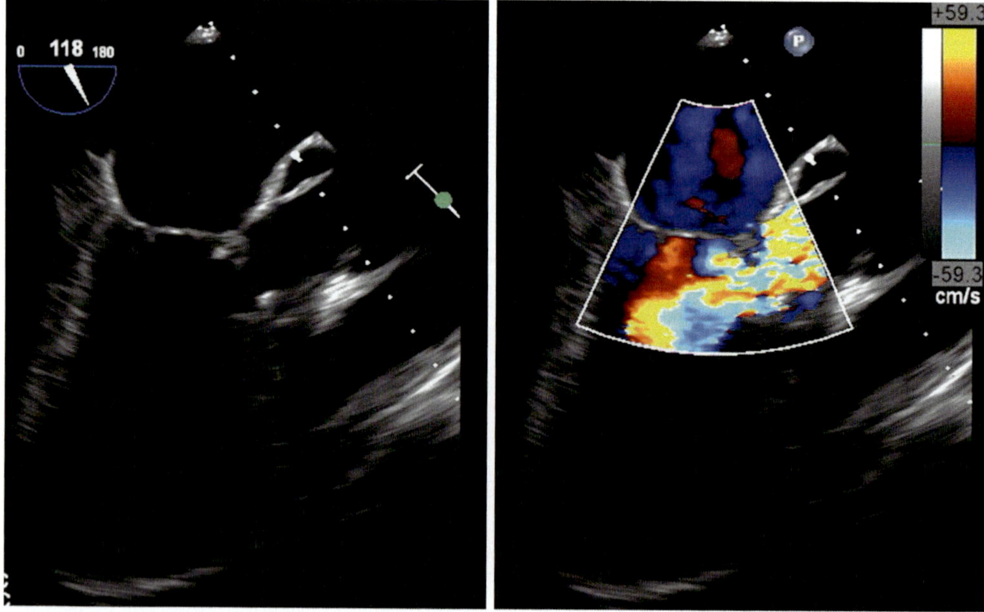

Fig. 16.11 Mid-esophageal view at 135 degrees (long axis) view during systole on transesophageal echocardiography without color Doppler (left panel) and with color Doppler (right panel)

Further Reading

Eidem BW, Johnson J, Lopez L, Cetta F. Echocardiography in pediatric and adult congenital heart disease. 3rd ed. Philadelphia, PA: Wolters Kluwer; 2021.

Li W, Henein M, Gatzoulis MA. Echocardiography in adult congenital heart disease. 1st ed. London, UK: Springer-Verlag; 2007.

Warnes CA, Williams RG, Bashore TM, et al. ACC/AHA 2008 guidelines for the management of adults with congenital heart disease: a report of the American College of Cardiology/American Heart Association Task Force on Practice Guidelines (Writing Committee to Develop Guidelines on the Management of Adults With Congenital Heart Disease). Developed in Collaboration With the American Society of Echocardiography, Heart Rhythm Society, International Society for Adult Congenital Heart Disease, Society for Cardiovascular Angiography and Interventions, and Society of Thoracic Surgeons. J Am Coll Cardiol. 2008;52(23):e143–263.

Wasserman MA, Shea E, Cassidy C, et al. Recommendations for the adult cardiac sonographer performing echocardiography to screen for critical congenital heart disease in the newborn: from the American Society of Echocardiography. J Am Soc Echocardiogr. 2021;34(3):207–22.

Abdominal Ultrasound

17

Madiha Syed, David R. Jury, and Nakul Kumar

Question 1

A resident in the ICU is examining a 35-year-old patient with urosepsis and acute kidney injury (AKI) to evaluate for obstructive causes of AKI. The resident reports he is only able to see the liver, spleen and diaphragm and is unable to see the kidney. He is holding the probe with the marker pointing to the head and probe at right anterior axillary line. Which of the following maneuvers could the student perform to improve image acquisition:

1. Move the probe to the right mid axillary line
2. Angle the transducer beam posteriorly
3. Move the patient into left lateral decubitus position (if imaging the right kidney)
4. Move the probe to fourth intercostal space at the anterior axillary line

Select the best answer:

A. 1 only
B. 1,3 and 4
C. 1,2 and 3
D. All of the above

Answer: C.

Key Point: The kidney is a retroperitoneal structure and requires the scanner to place the probe in the mid axillary line with the beam directed posteriorly.

Rationale: The kidney is a retroperitoneal organ and located posteriorly in the abdomen. A mistake often made by novice scanners is to start the scan too anteriorly. Ideally the probe should be placed in mid to posterior axillary line with the probe beam angulated posteriorly. The diaphragm is an important landmark and can help to orient the scanner. Most patients in the ICU are lying supine which causes the diaphragm to be pushed up; for retroperitoneal organs the transducer probe may need to be wedged between the patient and the bed. In some cases where it is difficult to obtain images patient can be turned into the lateral decubitus position to make scanning easier [1, 2].

Question 2

The following image was obtained from a patient in the right mid axillary plain with the probe angled posteriorly. Identify structures A and B (Fig. 17.1).

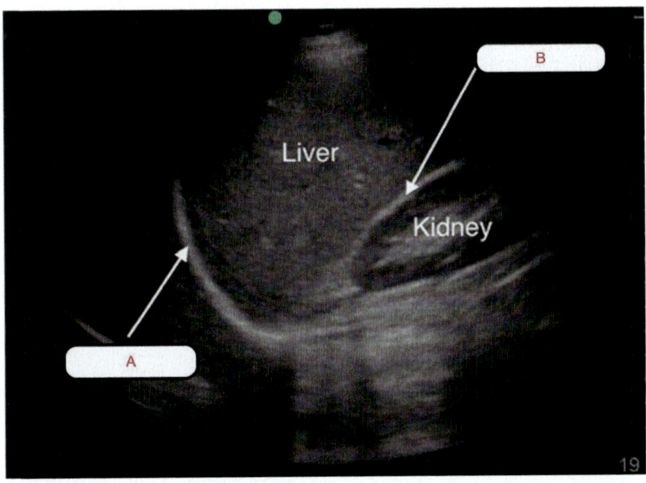

Fig. 17.1 Abdominal ultrasound (Reprinted from Minami T. Abdominal Ultrasound and Genitourinary Ultrasound in the Intensive Care Unit. In: Jankowich M, Gartman E (eds). Ultrasound in the Intensive Care Unit. Respiratory Medicine. New York, NY: Humana Press; 2015: 249–272. With permission from Springer Nature)

M. Syed (✉) · D. R. Jury · N. Kumar
Department of Intensive Care & Resuscitation, Cleveland Clinic Foundation, Cleveland, OH, USA
e-mail: syedm3@ccf.org; juryd@ccf.org; kumarn6@ccf.org

R. Sreedharan et al. (eds.), *Critical Care Echocardiography*, https://doi.org/10.1007/978-3-031-45731-9_17

A. Morrison's pouch and hepatorenal recess
B. Diaphragm and hepatorenal recess
C. Lesser omental sac and Morrison's pouch
D. Diaphragm and splenorenal recess

Answer: B.

Key Point: The space between the liver and kidney is known as the hepatorenal recess or Morrison's pouch. The liver is located inferior to the diaphragm which separates it from the pleural cavity.

Rationale: The space between the liver and kidney is known as the hepatorenal recess. It can be identified by placing the ultrasound in the mid to posterior axillary line and angling the beam posteriorly. This space is also called Morrison's pouch and is a potential space where fluid can accumulate in the abdomen [1].

Question 3

A 64-year-old male patient with colon cancer and sigmoid perforation is admitted to the ICU after post laparoscopic hemicolectomy. His postoperative course is complicated by abdominal sepsis, respiratory failure and acute kidney injury. On postoperative day 5 his urine output decreases despite his Cr improving to 0.9 mg/dL from 3.2 mg/dL. Urine output over the last 3 h has been 0 cc. The nurse obtains a bladder scan and asks you to review the image. The next best step in management will be: (Fig. 17.2)

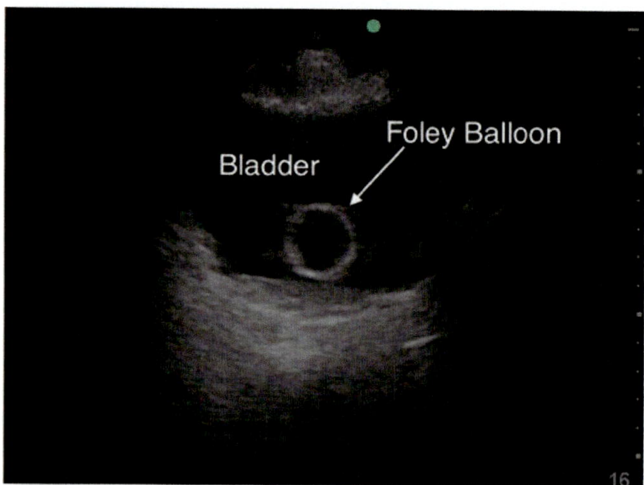

Fig. 17.2 Bladder ultrasound (Reprinted from Minami T. Abdominal Ultrasound and Genitourinary Ultrasound in the Intensive Care Unit. In: Jankowich M, Gartman E (eds). Ultrasound in the Intensive Care Unit. Respiratory Medicine. New York, NY: Humana Press; 2015: 249–272. With permission from Springer Nature)

A. Administer 500 cc fluid bolus
B. Obtain a formal renal and bladder ultrasound
C. Change the Foley catheter
D. Consult urology

Answer: C.

Key Point: In a normal bladder with a Foley catheter there is no anechoic space seen around the catheter as the bladder is drained and empty.

Rationale: Anuria and oliguria are common problems in ICU patients. Often the first step is to troubleshoot the indwelling catheter. Bladder ultrasound demonstrating a full bladder in a patient with oliguria and anuria points toward a distal obstruction (bladder outlet, urethra or Foley catheter). If the Foley catheter or bulb is visualized surrounded by anechoic space (fluid) then the likely cause is an obstructed Foley catheter; this should be flushed or replaced. If the bladder is visualized collapsed around the Foley catheter and patient is anuric; this would be indicative of a more proximal problem or absence of urine production (intrinsic renal or pre-renal etiology) [1, 3].

Please use the vignette below to answer Questions 4 and 5.

A 39-year-old female with polycystic kidney disease status post remote kidney transplant presented to emergency room with hematuria 5 days after biopsy of the transplanted kidney. Biopsy was done to assess for chronic rejection as her creatinine appeared to be slowly increasing over the last year (From 0.9 to 1.8 mg/dL). The patient states that she had been doing well but noticed hematuria and outpatient lab work showed an increase in creatinine from 1.9 mg/dL (baseline) to 3.5 mg/dL. Her vitals were as follows: HR 82 beats/min, BP 141/72 mmHg, RR 12 breaths/min, SpO^2 97%. Her lab work in the ED showed Hb 10.1 g/dL, wbc 7.3, platelet count 191,000. Electrolyte levels were normal, blood urea nitrogen level was 55 mg/dL. Renal Ultrasound with doppler was obtained (Fig. 17.3).

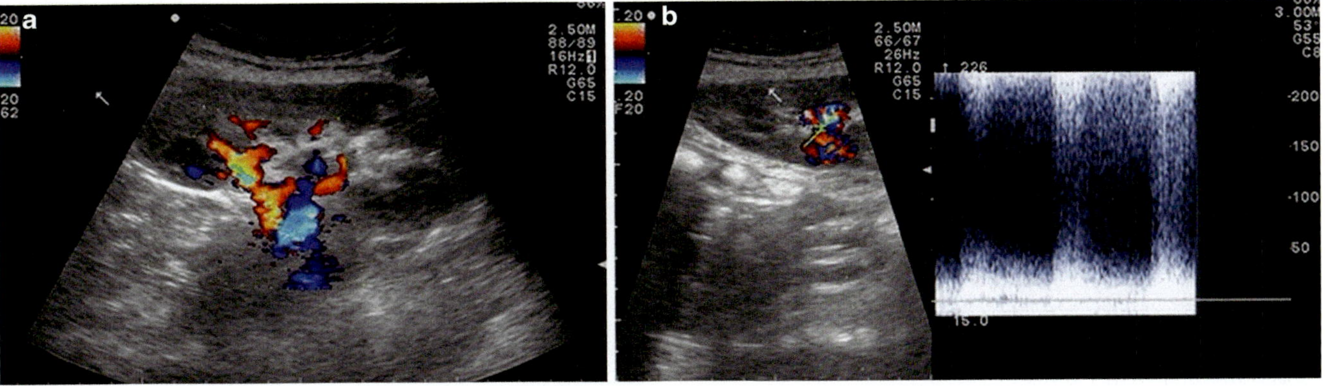

Fig. 17.3 2-D and Color Doppler Ultrasound of transplanted kidney (**a** and **b**) (Reprinted from Richenberg J. Kidney Trauma. In: Hamm B, Ros PR (eds). Abdominal Imaging. Heidelberg, Germany: Springer-Verlag; 2013: 1779–1794. With permission from Springer Nature)

Question 4
Based on the color flow doppler imaging what is the most likely diagnosis?

A. Renal artery stenosis
B. Acute on chronic rejection
C. Post -biopsy arteriovenous fistula
D. Renal artery laceration

Question 5
What would be the next best step in management?

A. Fluid bolus with 500 cc of normal saline
B. Emergent consult to interventional radiology
C. Increase immunosuppression dose
D. Admit for Observation

Answer: Question 4: C.; Question 5: D.

Key Point: Arteriovenous fistula can occur after percutaneous biopsy of the transplanted kidney. In most cases these resolve spontaneously and do not require surgical intervention.

Rationale: Arteriovenous fistulas can occur after kidney biopsy in native and transplanted kidneys. The incidence in native kidney biopsy is lower (0.3–6%) than transplanted ones (10–16%). Arteriovenous fistulas can be asymptomatic or present with hematuria, hypertension and renal insufficiency. The image in Fig. 17.3 shows an upper pole AV fistula after biopsy and color doppler shows chaotic flow. Diagnosis of renal artery stenosis requires flow characteristics proximal and distal to the stenosis to be assessed with doppler. It also requires abdominal and flank views. The patient does not have a renal artery laceration as hemoglobin level and vitals are within normal limits. This patient could have rejection, however, that is a pathological diagnosis. The gold standard for the diagnosis of arteriovenous fistulas is angiography, however, ultrasound is less invasive and does not require contrast exposure.

The management of arteriovenous fistula is mainly conservative in 80% of cases (most resolve spontaneously), in some cases where renal indices don't improve embolization by interventional radiology might be necessary [4–6].

Use the vignette below to answer Questions 6 and 7.

A 35-year-old female is brought to the ICU for monitoring after she sustained a blunt trauma in motor vehicle accident in which she was the passenger. She was initially hypotensive on arrival with improvement in vital signs with blood transfusion and intravenous fluids. Abdominal CT imaging showed a grade 1 liver laceration and bilateral pulmonary contusions. An image from the initial FAST exam is shown below (Fig. 17.4).

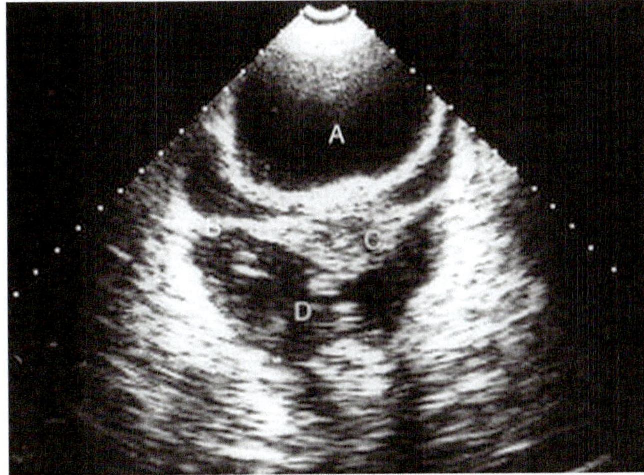

Fig. 17.4 Abdominal ultrasound (Reprinted from Lichtenstein DA. Urinary Tract. In: Lichtenstein DA (ed). Whole Body Ultrasonography in the Critically Ill. Heidelberg, Germany: Springer-Verlag; 2010: 69–76. With permission from Springer Nature)

Question 6

Figure 17.4 shows ______________ultrasound view in the abdomen. (Fill in the blank)

A. Left lower quadrant
B. Transvaginal
C. Subcostal
D. Bladder (Transverse)

Question 7

Match the labels in column 1 to the structures on column 2 based on the anatomical locations depicted on the image:

COLUMN 1

LABEL
A
B
C
D

COLUMN 2

STRUCTURE
Broad ligament
Uterus
Bladder
Hemorrhagic effusion

Answer: Question 6: D; Question 7: A-Bladder, B-Broad ligament, C-Uterus, D-Hemorrhagic Effusion.

Key Point: Fig. 17.4 **shows a transverse view of the bladder obtained in the suprapubic area This is a standard view in the FAST exam. The image shows hemoperitoneum (debris in the anechoic fluid) in a patient with blunt trauma.**

Rationale: The image shows a supra pubic transverse view of the bladder which is a standard view in the FAST exam. The bladder is examined in both longitudinal and transverse view in the FAST exam. The patient experienced blunt trauma and sustained a liver laceration, as a result she developed a hemoperitoneum. The hemo-peritoneum appears as coarse debris in the anechoic fluid surrounding the bladder, uterus and uterine ligaments. The uterus appears as a circular dense structure behind the bladder. Below is a normal suprapubic view in a female patient [7, 8] (Fig. 17.5).

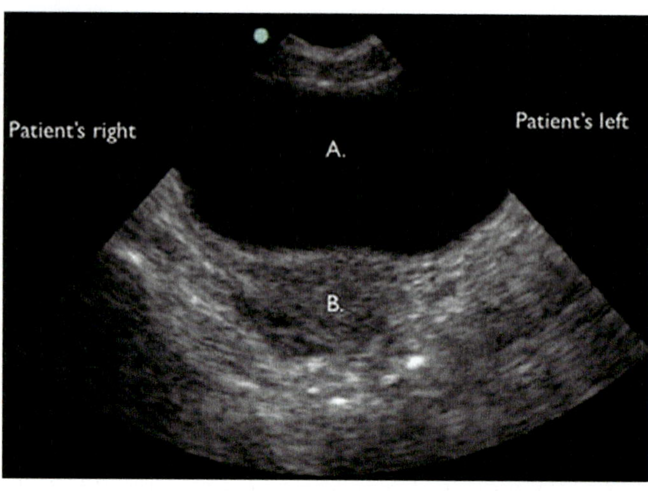

Fig. 17.5 Suprapubic view of the bladder (**A**) and uterus (**B**) in a female patient (Reprinted from Woods AN. Ultrasound in Trauma Critical Care. In: Jankowich M, Gartman E (eds). Ultrasound in the Intensive Care Unit. Respiratory Medicine. New York, NY: Humana Press; 2015: 295–321. With permission from Springer Nature)

Question 8

A 62-year-old male with diabetes and asthma is on the nursing floor with inability to urinate 7 hours after hernia repair surgery. The following images (Figs. 17.6 and 17.7) are obtained.

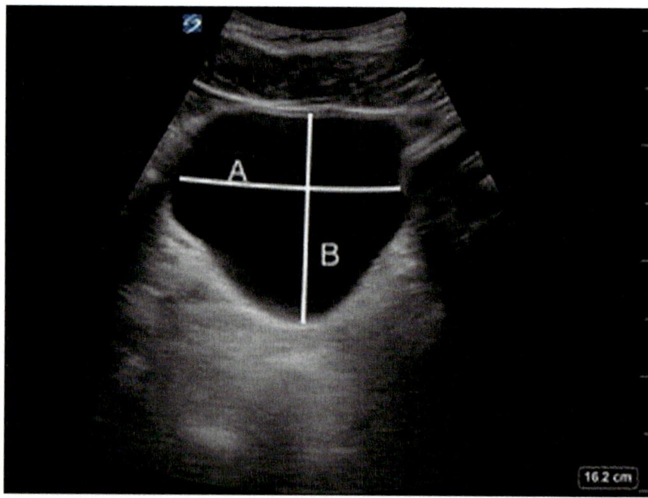

Fig. 17.6 Bladder ultrasound—Transverse view (Reprinted from Creditt A, Joyce M. Renal and Bladder Ultrasound. In: Creditt A, Tozer J, Vitto M, Joyce M, Taylor L (eds). Clinical Ultrasound: A Pocket Manual. Cham: Switzerland: Springer Nature; 2018:167–184. With permission from Springer Nature)

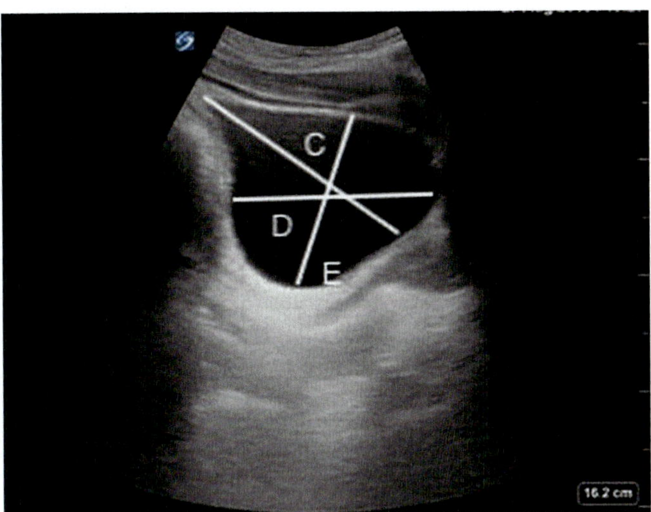

Fig. 17.7 Bladder ultrasound—Sagittal view (Reprinted from Creditt A, Joyce M. Renal and Bladder Ultrasound. In: Creditt A, Tozer J, Vitto M, Joyce M, Taylor L (eds). Clinical Ultrasound: A Pocket Manual. Cham: Switzerland: Springer Nature; 2018:167–184. With permission from Springer Nature)

How would you calculate the bladder volume?

A. Bladder volume = A × B × C × 0.52
B. Bladder volume = A × B × C × 0.75
C. Bladder volume = E × D × B × 0.52
D. Bladder volume = E × D × B × 0.75

Answer: B.

Key Point: The ellipsoid method for measuring bladder volume uses the formula

$$\text{Bladder volume} = A\left(\text{width}\right) \times B\left(\text{depth}\right) \times C\left(\text{length}\right) \times 0.75\left(\text{ml}\right)$$

Rationale: Acute urinary retention can be a common problem in patients that undergo general anesthesia or in the emergency room. Bladder ultrasound provides a quick and easy way to assess whether there is distal versus proximal disease. Bladder volume is calculated by measuring the depth and width in the suprapubic transverse/cross sectional view and the height is measured in the longitudinal/sagittal view. Most ultrasound machines have bladder volume calculators.

There are multiple methods of calculating bladder volume with varying degrees of accuracy, the prolate ellipsoid method (height × width × depth × 0.75) provides a reasonable estimate and it is easy to perform compared to other methods (e.g. double ellipsoid method, double area method etc.). Normal capacity of the bladder is 400–600 mls. A normal post void residual volume is less than 50 cm^3 [2, 3, 9–11].

Question 9

A 62-year-old male patient with gout, hypertension and diabetes is admitted to the ICU for septic shock. He is on norepinephrine at 10 mcg/min. His vitals show: HR 79 beats/min, BP 99/72 mmHg, RR 15 breaths/min, SpO^2 94%. He is confused on exam and urine output has been low. His labs show: white cell count 18,000 cells/L, Hemoglobin 12.1 g/dL, urine analysis is positive for leucocytes, bacteria, leucocyte esterase and nitrites. He is started on broad spectrum antibiotics and renal/bladder ultrasound is ordered. Which of the following are TRUE regarding imaging of acute pyelonephritis?

1. The kidneys get enlarged and swollen
2. Increased blood flow velocity is commonly seen in the renal artery
3. Cortical and medullary differentiation is lost
4. Hypoechoic renal parenchyma
   A. 1 and 3
   B. 1,3 and 4
   C. 1,2 and 4
   D. All of the above

Answer: B.

Key Point: Key features of acute pyelonephritis on ultrasound include enlargement of kidney and renal pyramids, loss of corticomedullary differentiation, hypoechoic renal parenchyma

Rationale: Acute pyelonephritis normally does not require imaging for routine cases and in 80% of the cases the kidney will appear normal. In the remaining 20% of cases the following abnormalities might be seen enlarged swollen kidneys, loss of corticomedullary differentiation, hypoechoic renal parenchyma, dilation of collecting system without obstruction and loss of renal sinus fat. Absence/decreased color flow instead of increased flow is seen in pyelonephritis. Increased echogenicity of the surrounding renal fat is indicative of the inflammatory response of the surrounding tissue. Small abscesses/focal pyelonephritis can be seen best with CT and not US [7, 11, 12].

Question 10

A 35 year old female presents to the ED with fever, chills and flank pain. Her vital signs on admission are HR 110 beat/min, BP 99/65 mmHg, RR 13 breaths/min, SpO2 98%. Her labs show leucocyte count 21,000 per liter, Hemoglobin 12.1 g/dL, platelets 231,000. Urine analysis showed moderate bacteria, positive nitrite and leucocyte esterase. The following image was seen on renal and bladder ultrasound evaluation (Fig. 17.8).

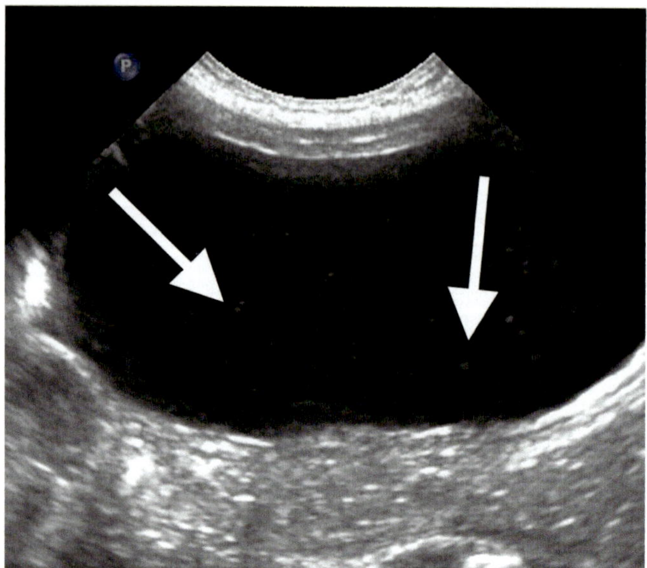

Fig. 17.8 Bladder ultrasound (Reprinted from Joseph W. McQuaid et al. Bladder debris on renal and bladder ultrasound: A significant predictor of positive urine culture, Journal of Pediatric Urology, Volume 13, Issue 4,2017, Pages 385.e1-385.e5. With permission from Elsevier)

What is indicated by the arrows in Fig. 17.8?

A. Artifacts
B. Bladder stones
C. Microbial gas
D. Blood clots

Answer: C.

Key Point: Microbial gas and pyuria can appear as multiple hyperechoic elements floating in the bladder.

Rationale: Pyuria is commonly associated with urinary tract infections and pyelonephritis. It can present as echogenic debris in the bladder. Blood clots and bladder stones are also echogenic but are larger in size and may have irregular boundaries. In the supine position pyuria and blood can collect in a gravity dependent manner and form an echogenic layer in the bladder [7] (Fig. 17.9).

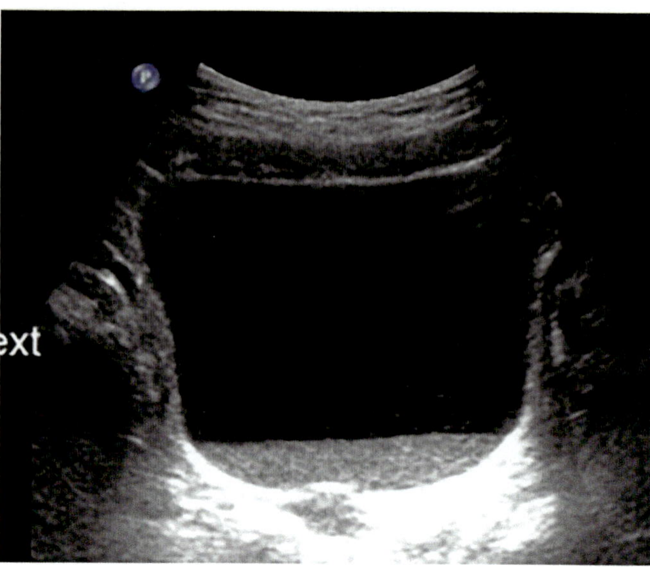

Fig. 17.9 Bladder ultrasound (Reprinted from Joseph W. McQuaid et al.Bladder debris on renal and bladder ultrasound: A significant predictor of positive urine culture, Journal of Pediatric Urology, Volume 13, Issue 4,2017, Pages 385.e1-385.e5. With permission from Elsevier)

Question 11

An 82-year-old male with hypertension, bladder cancer and diabetes is admitted to the ICU after a motor vehicle accident. He sustained a grade 2 liver laceration and fifth and sixth rib fractured. He has mild tachycardia but hemodynamics are normal. Initial labs showed mild anemia (Hemoglobin 11.1 g/dL) and urine analysis positive for microscopic hematuria. He is complaining of right sided chest pain and right flank pain. Renal ultrasound in performed and the following images are seen: (Figs. 17.10 and 17.11).

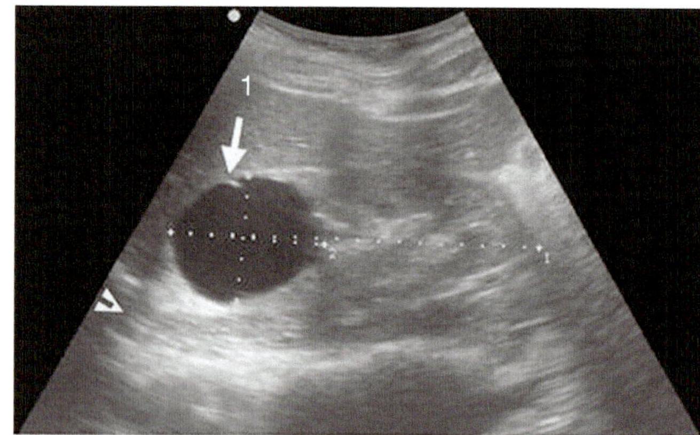

Fig. 17.10 Renal ultrasound—right kidney (Reprinted from Wang LJ. Renal Cystic Disease. In: Key Diagnostic Features in Uroradiology. Cham, Switzerland: Springer Nature; 2015: 97–139. With permission from Springer Nature)

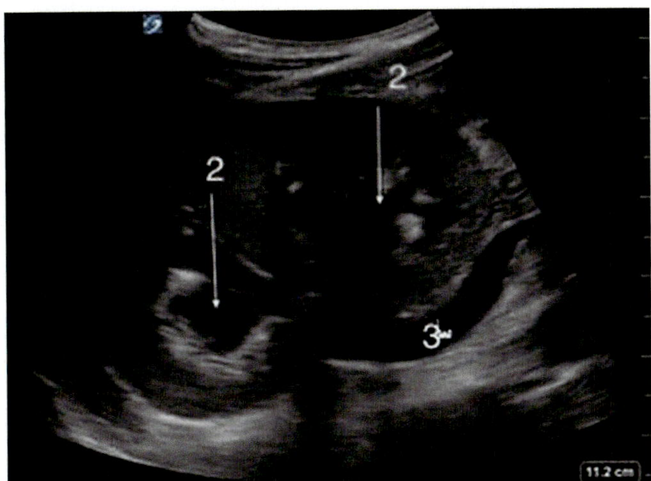

Fig. 17.11 Renal ultrasound—left kidney (Reprinted from Creditt A, Joyce M. Renal and Bladder Ultrasound. In: Creditt A, Tozer J, Vitto M, Joyce M, Taylor L (eds). Clinical Ultrasound: A Pocket Manual. Cham: Switzerland: Springer Nature; 2018:167–184. With permission from Springer Nature)

What findings are shown by structured marked 1, 2 and 3?

A. 1 = Renal cyst, 2 = mild hydronephrosis, 3 = hydroureter
B. 1 = Renal hematoma, 2 = mild hydronephrosis, 3 = hydroureter
C. 1 = Renal cyst, 2 = mild hydronephrosis, 3 = normal ureter
D. 1 = Adrenal cyst,2 = moderate hydronephrosis, 3 = hydroureter

Answer: A.

Key Point: Structure 1 is a renal cyst; it has a smooth thin wall with posterior enhancement. Structure 2 shows mild hydronephrosis which is characterized by blunting and enlargement of calyceal fornices, but renal papillae can still be seen. Structure 3 is a hydroureter; normally the ureter is not seen on ultrasound, when it is dilated it becomes more easily identifiable.

Rationale: Renal cysts are incidental findings that can be seen on ultrasound; their detection is increasing due to the widespread use of imaging in medicine. They are seen frequently in elderly patients. Simple cysts are structures found in the renal parenchyma that may distort the architecture. They are thin walled, round or oval in shape, lack internal echoes and may show posterior enhancement. They normal do not require further investigation or follow up. Complex cysts may be multiple in number, contain thick septations, calcification and solid components; they require further evaluation and follow up [3, 13–16].

Hydronephrosis severity is classified according to grades 0–4:

Grade: No dilation, calyceal walls are opposed to each other.
Grade 1: Dilation of renal pelvis without dilation of calyces, no parenchymal atrophy.
Grade 2: Mild dilation of renal pelvis and dilation of calyces, no parenchymal atrophy.
Grade 3: Moderate dilation of renal pelvis and calyces, blunting of fornices and flattening of papillae, mild cortical thinning may be seen.
Grade 4: Gross dilation of renal pelvis and calyces (appear ballooned), loss of border between pelvis and calyces and renal atrophy/cortical thinning.

Question 12
Which of the following is FALSE regarding ultrasound evaluation of the spleen?

A. In the supine patient; the probe should be held at the mid to posterior axillary line at the subxiphoid level to image the spleen.
B. Anterior angulation of the probe at the posterior axillary line will optimize visualization of the splenorenal recess.
C. The normal spleen is more hyperechoic than the kidneys and iso to hyperechoic compared to the liver.
D. Focal lesions detected on splenic ultrasound are usually subtle and non-specific.

Answer: B.

Key Point: Imaging of the spleen renal recess requires the probe to be placed in the mid to posterior axillary line at the subxiphoid level with the probe angulated posteriorly. This is because the kidney is a retroperitoneal organ and the spleen is an intraperitoneal organ.

Rationale: Answers A, C and D regarding splenic ultrasound are correct. The spleen is a homogenous appearing structure on ultrasound; its echogenicity is slightly more than the kidney and it is iso to hyperechoic compared to the liver. The spleen is oriented obliquely downward and anterior from the level of spinous process of the tenth or eleventh thoracic vertebra to the left mid-axillary line with its long axis paralleling the tenth rib. Imaging of the spleen requires the patient to be supine or in the right lateral decubitus position. The probe beam needs to be angled posteriorly if the splenorenal recess needs to be evaluated due to the retroperitoneal location of the kidney [17–19].

Please use the vignette below to answer Questions 13 and 14.

A 22-year-old cyclist collided with a car while making a right turn at an intersection. He is now in the ICU for management of polytrauma. The following image is from his left upper quadrant FAST exam in the emergency room (Fig. 17.12).

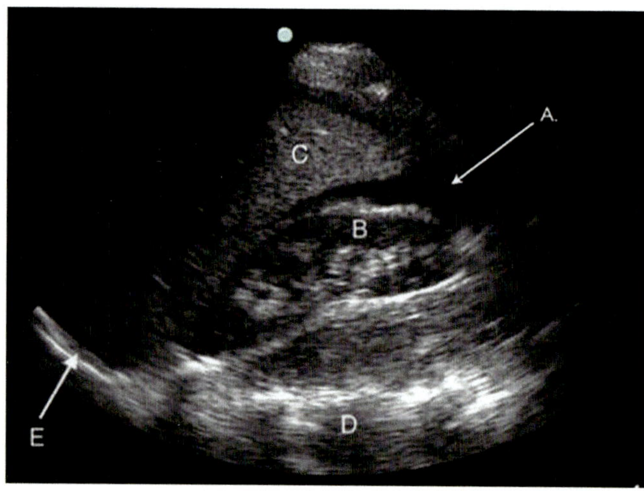

Fig. 17.12 Abdominal ultrasound (Reprinted from Woods AN. Ultrasound in Trauma Critical Care. In: Jankowich M, Gartman E (eds). Ultrasound in the Intensive Care Unit. Respiratory Medicine. New York, NY: Humana Press; 2015: 295–321. With permission from Springer Nature)

Question 13

Match the following labels with the structures:

A. ________.

B. ________.

C. ________.

D. ________.

E. ________.

Pleural effusion	Spine	Spleen
Diaphragm	Kidney	Liver
Renal medulla	Free fluid	

Question 14

Which of the following is/are TRUE regarding ultrasound imaging of splenic injury/trauma:

1. The sensitivity of ultrasound for detecting splenic trauma is approximately 70–80%; highest sensitivity with injuries grade III or higher.
2. Splenic laceration/hematoma may present with areas of both increased and decreased echogenicity.
3. In the LUQ free fluid flows preferentially into the subphrenic area than the splenorenal area
4. Small hematomas and lacerations can be missed on ultrasound and require Computed Tomography (CT) for accurate grading.

Answers

A. 1 only
B. 2 and 3
C. 1,2 and 4
D. All of the above

Answer: Question 13: A- free fluid, B-Kidney, C-Spleen, D- Spine, E- Diaphragm;

Question 14: D.

Key Point: The spleen is frequently injured in blunt trauma. The image (Fig. 17.12) **shows free fluid in the abdomen after splenic injury; free fluid preferentially collects in the subphrenic space. Computed tomography (CT) is required for accurate grading of splenic injury.**

Rationale: The spleen is frequently injured in blunt trauma. Ultrasonography of spleen lacerations and hematomas can present with both increased or decreased echogenicity. Hematomas are usually hyperechoic but develop decreased echogenicity with time and finally become anechoic due to degradation of blood products. Peri splenic fluid and subcapsular hematoma present as hypo to anechoic areas surrounding the spleen. The sensitivity of ultrasound to detect splenic injury is highest with grade 3 or higher injuries. Computed tomography has a sensitivity of 96–100% for splenic injury and grading of splenic injury is done on CT [8, 18, 20, 21].

Please use the vignette below to answer Questions 15 and 16.

68-year-old female with past medical history of hypertension, diabetes mellitus type 2, rheumatoid arthritis (on chronic steroids) is admitted to the ICU with septic shock. She is postoperative day 10 from an emergent bowel resection for sigmoid perforation associated with acute diverticulitis. She is currently on a norepinephrine infusion at 10 micrograms/min and broad spectrum antibiotics. The following image is seen on the left upper quadrant ultrasound exam (Fig. 17.13).

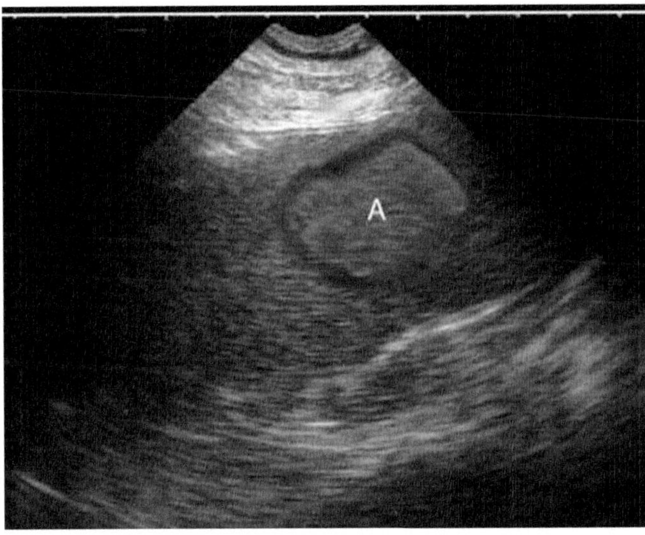

Fig. 17.13 Abdominal ultrasound-left upper quadrant (Reprinted from Lichtenstein DA. Various Targets in the Abdomen (Spleen, Adrenals, Pancreas, Lymph Nodes). In: Lichtenstein DA (ed). Whole Body Ultrasonography in the Critically Ill. Heidelberg, Germany: Springer-Verlag; 2010:77–81. With permission from Springer Nature)

Question 15

Identify structure A in Fig. 17.13:

A. Splenic infarct
B. Splenic hematoma
C. Splenic neoplasm
D. Splenic abscess

Question 16

What would be the next best step in management?

A. Continue antibiotics and monitoring in the ICU
B. Consult to surgery for splenectomy
C. Consult to interventional radiology for CT guided drainage
D. Computed tomography (CT) for grading and staging of the lesion

Answers: Question 15: D.; Question 16: C.

Key Point: Splenic abscess typically appears as a hypoechoic mass in the parenchyma, occasionally they can be isoechoic with a thin hypoechoic border of enhancement. Splenectomy is the gold standard, however, in order to preserve the spleen percutaneous drainage has been successful in patients with amenable anatomy (as shown in the image).

Rationale: Splenic abscess is an uncommon lesion with a high mortality due to delayed detection and treatment. Hematogenous spread from endocarditis or another source is usually the most common route of infection. Clinical symptoms are non-specific—fever and left upper quadrant pain. On ultrasound the lesions are hypoechoic but can be iso echoic with a rim of enhancement as seen in Fig. 17.13. Management includes broad spectrum antibiotic and drainage; treatment with antibiotics alone carries a mortality of 50%. Classically management would include splenectomy, however, with advances in radiology and in attempt to preserve the spleen percutaneous drainage can be performed. Percutaneous drainage is successful in uni or bilocular lesions with a thick wall and no septations. If there are multiple lesions, severe coagulopathy, septation, multiple abscesses, difficult anatomy (location near hilum/vessels)—surgery remains the gold standard [19, 22–24].

Question 17

Which of the following statements is TRUE regarding gastric ultrasound:

1. Right lateral decubitus position is the most accurate in quantifying gastric volumes.
2. A liner array, high frequency (5–12 MHz) probe can be used for gastric ultrasound in low body weight or pediatric patients.
3. The gastric fundus is the easiest to visualize with gastric ultrasound and should be used to measure gastric volume.
4. The same formula for gastric volume can be utilized in obese (BMI > 35) and non-obese patients.

Select your answer from the following regarding which statements are TRUE:

A. 2 and 3
B. 1,2 and 4
C. 1,2 and 3
D. All of the above

Answer: B.

Key Point: Statements 1, 2 and 4 are true (see details below). The gastric fundus is located in the left upper quadrant, inferior to the diaphragm, anterior to the left kidney and posterior to the spleen. It is a difficult area to image due to its deep location and limited acoustic window due to the overlying ribs.

Rationale: Gastric ultrasound can be performed in the supine, sitting or right lateral decubitus position. The right lateral decubitus position allows fluid to collect with gravity in the antrum and provides the most accurate volume measurements. The fundus is a difficult area to image due to its location, the antrum is the easiest. The same mathematical model can be used to measure gastric volumes in obese (BMI > 35) and non-obese patients. Curved array low frequency (2–5 MHz) probes are used for adults and linear/high frequency probes can be used for pediatric /low body weight patients [25, 26].

Question 18

A 75-year-old nursing home resident with history of dementia, hypertension, diabetes and chronic kidney disease is admitted to the ICU for agitation requiring dexmedetomidine infusion. He is diagnosed with acute cholecystitis and is febrile but hemodynamically stable. The following gastric ultrasound is performed to assess his NPO status prior to proceeding to OR for laparoscopic cholecystectomy. Based on the ultrasound, how long should the anesthesia and surgical team wait prior to proceeding with surgery? (Fig. 17.14)

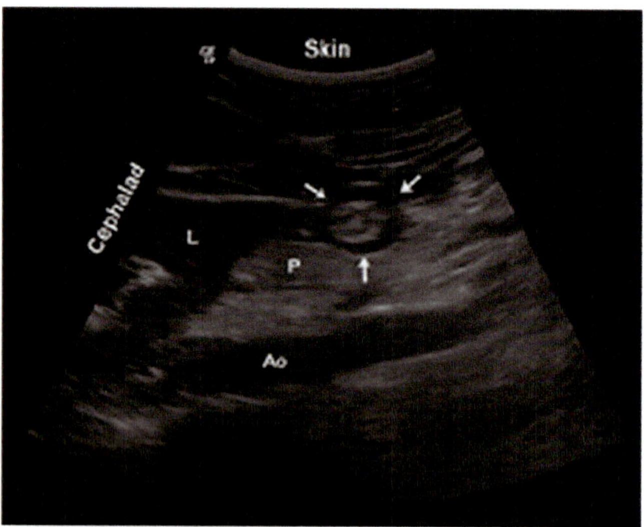

Fig. 17.14 Gastric ultrasound, L = liver, P = pancreas (Reprinted from Cubillos J, Tse C, Chan VWS, Perlas A. Bedside ultrasound assessment of gastric content: an observational study. *Can J Anesth/J Can Anesth* 2012;59(4):416–423. With permission from Springer Nature)

A. Proceed to surgery now
B. Wait 2 h
C. Wait 6 h
D. Wait 8 h

Answer: A.

Key Point: This image shows the gastric antrum in the sagittal plane (structure marked with arrows) with a "target" or "bull's eye" appearance, which is consistent with an empty stomach.

Rationale: Gastric Ultrasound can be used to assess gastric contents prior to procedures with moderate to deep sedation or general anesthesia to evaluate risk of aspiration. When the volume of gastric contents is greater than 1.5 mL/kg the risk of aspiration increased. It is useful in patients with cognitive deficiency, uncertain status or language barrier. Other features associated with the empty stomach on ultrasound is lack of peristalsis, thick prominent muscularis propria, and none to a very small volume of clear content [25–28].

Question 19

A 62-year-old male patient with multiple myeloma and chronic kidney disease is recovering from pneumonia and respiratory failure in the ICU. He sustains an accidental fall and has a pathologic fracture of his femur. The orthopedic surgeon wants to expedite his surgery and is asking whether he would be ready for anesthesia in an hour. The nurse mentions that the patient finished breakfast 1 hr ago. The following gastric ultrasound is obtained. Based on the image, when will it be safe for the patient to go to the OR? (Fig. 17.15a, b)

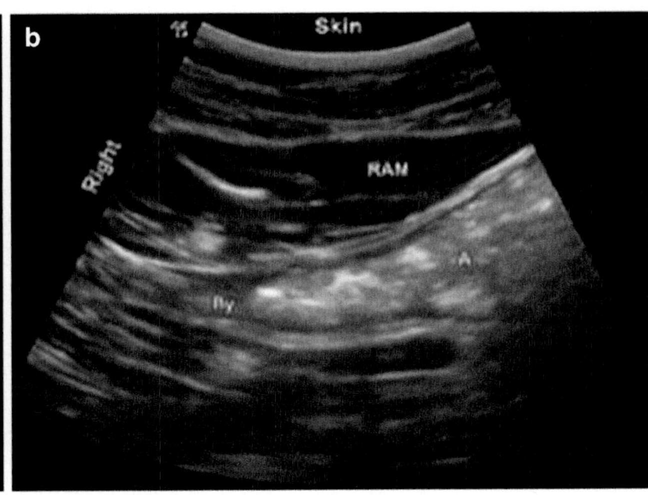

Fig. 17.15 (**a**) Gastric ultrasound—sagittal view. L = liver, P = pancreas = inferior vena cava (**b**) Gastric Ultrasound- Axial view. A = antrum, Py = pylorus, RAM = rectus abdominis muscle (Reprinted from Cubillos J, Tse C, Chan VWS, Perlas A. Bedside ultrasound assessment of gastric content: an observational study. *Can J Anesth/J Can Anesth* 2012;59(4):416–423. With permission from Springer Nature)

A. Patient can go now; the fracture repair is an urgent procedure.
B. Wait 1 h
C. Wait 5 h
D. Wait 7 h

Answer: D.

Key Point: The ultrasound images show hyperechoic and heterogenous content in the gastric antrum consistent with a meal. The wall of the antrum is thin, and it appears round and distended. Given that the patient just ate a meal and the procedure is urgent but not emergent; the patient will have to wait 7 h (for a total of 8 h of NPO time) prior to going to surgery.

Rationale: Clinical decisions regarding timing of surgery and anesthesia are often based on when the patient has consumed a drink or a meal. The time from a meal is used to decide when it would be safest to proceed with anesthesia with the lowest aspiration risk. Gastric ultrasound can reliably show contents of the stomach. Immediately after a meal the antrum can take on a "frosted glass" appearance due to the food bolus mixing with air and creating ring down artifacts. An hour or 2 later the antrum would appear round and circular with hyperechoic and heterogenous contents as seen in the images [25–27].

Question 20

A 22-year-old female with diabetes mellitus type 1 is admitted with septic shock to the emergency room. She was being treated outpatient for a urinary tract infection. She is on norepinephrine and was intubated for increased work of breathing. Her current vitals are: Blood pressure 92/64 mmHg, hear rate 108 beats/min, respiratory rate 21 breaths/min and SpO^2 98%. Her lab work showed leukocytosis 21,000 per mm^3, lactate 4.9 mg/dL, Creatinine 1.7 mg/dL, and Blood urea nitrogen 38 mmol/liter. She has received 30 mL/kg fluid bolus, blood and urine cultures are pending and CT abdomen and chest are ordered. She has received vancomycin and piperacillin-tazobactam for antibiotic coverage. The resident obtains the following abdominal ultrasound image A and then a close-up image B (Fig. 17.16).

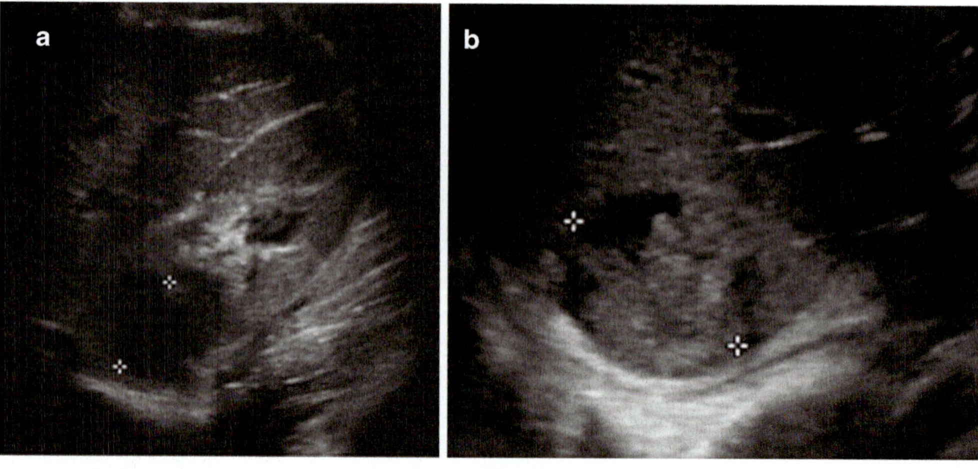

Fig. 17.16 Renal US (**a**) and (**b**) (Reprinted from Scionti A, Rossi P, Gulino P, et al. Acute Pyelonephritis. In: Miele V, Trinci M. (eds) Imaging Non-traumatic Abdominal Emergencies in Pediatric Patients. Cham, Switzerland: Springer Nature; 2016; 265. With permission from Springer Nature)

Based on the image what is the diagnosis?

A. Complex renal cyst
B. Fungal ball
C. Acute pyelonephritis
D. Renal abscess

Answer: D.

Key Point: Fig. 17.16 **shows a renal abscess; on ultrasound they appear as a hypoechoic/anechoic lesion with septae or debris inside the abscess cavity.**

Rationale: Renal abscesses are a common complication of pyelonephritis. They form due to concomitant vasospasm and inflammation resulting in necrosis of tissue and formation of an infected fluid collection. Renal ultrasound shows a hypoechoic/anechoic structure which may have septations. Occasionally air or debris can be seen in the abscess cavity. Pyelonephritis usually appears with focal loss of the regional corticomedullary differentiation on ultrasound. These are usually hypoechoic but can be hyperechoic as well. Complex renal cysts would not present with septic shock and fever. A fungal ball would be a rare presentation in the kidney, its usually diagnosed in immunocompromised individuals [29–33].

Question 21

A 39-year-old male with past medical history of Crohn's disease (on chronic steroids), diabetes type 1, hypertension is admitted with fever, hypotension and flank pain. He is on norepinephrine at 10 mcg/min and broad-spectrum antibiotics. His creatinine was 2.8 mg/dL, lactate 3.7 mg/dL and white blood cell count 24, ooo/ μL^3. His urine output has decreased to 30 mL over the last 4 hours. Renal ultrasound is obtained of the right and left kidney (Fig. 17.17).

What is shown in the ultrasound in Fig. 17.17?

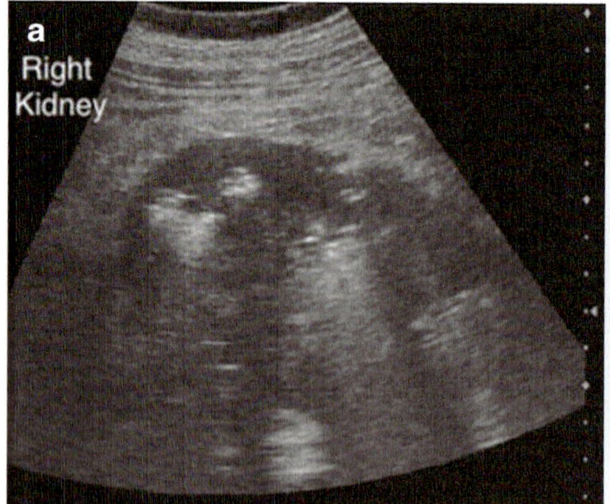

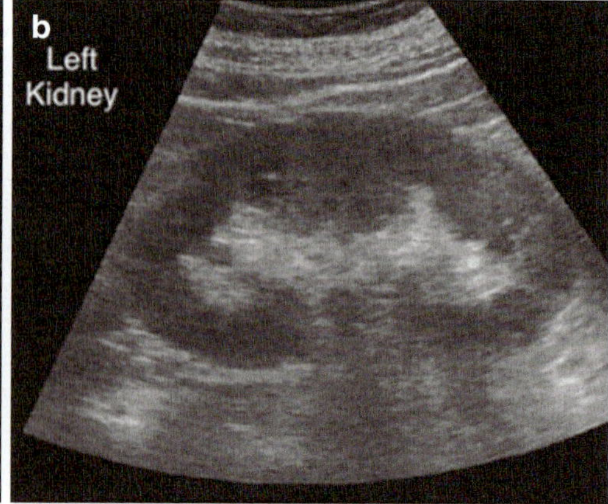

Fig. 17.17 Right Kidney (**a**) and Left kidney (**b**) ultrasound (Reprinted from Oyen R. Imaging of Pyelonephritis. In: Cova M, Stacul F (eds). Pain Imaging. Cham, Switzerland: Springer Nature. 2019: 303–322. With permission from Springer Nature)

A. Staghorn Calculus
B. Acute pyelonephritis
C. Emphysematous pyelonephritis
D. Moderate hydronephrosis

Answer: C.

Key Point: Emphysematous pyelonephritis and staghorn calculi can appear similar on ultrasound with hyperechoic appearance. However, staghorn calculi have distinctive, echo free "clean" shadow whereas shadowing with emphysematous pyelonephritis is associated with ring down artifacts due to air in the renal parenchyma.

Rationale: Emphysematous pyelonephritis is considered a urologic emergency and has a high mortality rate. It is a severe necrotizing, acute bacterial infection; most common causative organism is *E. coli*. It usually occurs in patients with diabetes and urinary tract obstruction associated with calculi. In Fig. 17.17 shows a normal left kidney but emphysematous pyelonephritis in the right kidney. There are multiple streaky hyperchoic streaks in the right kidney associated with ring down artifacts. See Fig. 17.18—white arrows indicate ring down artifact. The ring down shadows are somewhat hazy or "dirty". In staghorn calculi the shadows are "clean" and dark secondary to the content of the staghorn calculus (Figs. 17.17 and 17.18).

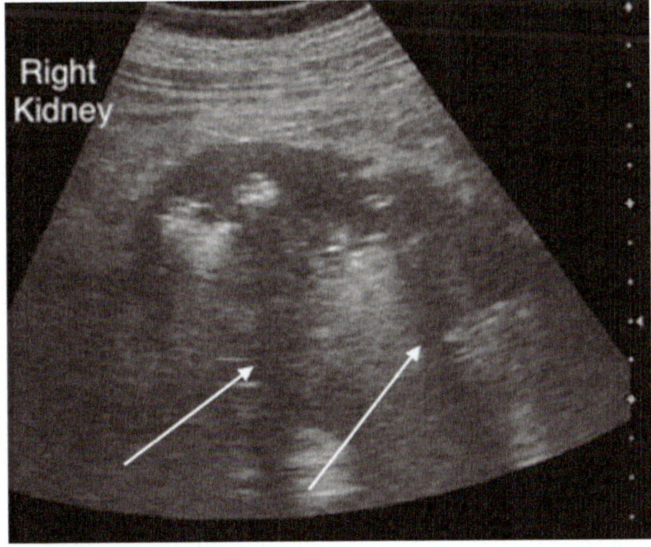

Fig. 17.18 Left kidney ultrasound (Reprinted from Oyen R. Imaging of Pyelonephritis. In: Cova M, Stacul F (eds). Pain Imaging. Cham, Switzerland: Springer Nature. 2019: 303–322. With permission from Springer Nature)

For Questions 22, 23, and 24 please refer to the vignette below.

54-year-old female with a past medical history of diabetes, hypertension, asthma and chronic pancreatitis presents to the emergency room with acute onset of abdominal pain, nausea and vomiting of 5 hours duration. On exam, she appears in obvious discomfort and is hypotensive and tachycardic with significant tenderness in the epigastric region. Point of care abdominal ultrasound is performed with the findings as pictured below (Fig. 17.19).

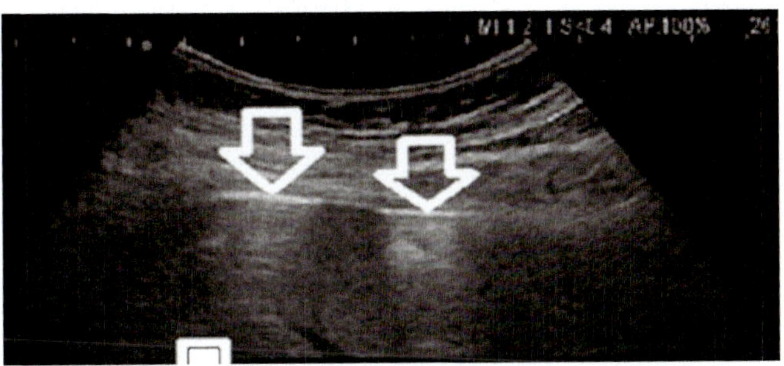

Fig. 17.19 Abdominal ultrasound (Reprinted from Cortellaro F, Perani C, Guarnieri L, et al. Point-of-Care Ultrasound in the Diagnosis of Acute Abdominal Pain. In: Aseni P, De Carlis L, Mazzola A, Grande A (eds). Operative Techniques and Recent Advances in Acute Care and Emergency Surgery. Cham, Switzerland: Springer Nature; 2019: 383–401. With permission from Springer Nature)

Question 22

What is the best point of care ultrasound technique to assess for abdominal free air?

A. Patient in supine position with thorax elevated 10–20°. Attention first to left upper quadrant with transducer placed longitudinally to left paramedian epigastric region overlying the spleen.
B. Patient in supine position with thorax elevated 10–20°. Attention first to right upper quadrant with transducer placed longitudinally to right paramedian epigastric region overlying the liver.
C. Patient in supine position with thorax elevated 20–30°. Attention first to umbilical region with transducer placed longitudinally moving cephalad to epigastric region overlying the liver.
D. Patient in supine position with thorax elevated 10–20°. Attention first to right upper quadrant with transducer placed longitudinally to far right hypochondriac region overlying the liver.

Answer: B.

Key point: Abdominal ultrasound in an acute abdomen can be quite painful and views obtained need to be done efficiently to offer clinical guidance while minimizing patient's discomfort.

Rationale: Slight elevation of the thorax in a supine patient allows free intraperitonel air (FIA) to collect at the anterior aspect of the liver adjacent to the abdominal wall; where FIA is most easily identified without confounding loops of bowel. By starting paramedian to the epigastric space the ultrasonographer is most likely to quickly visualize FIA if it is present [34–36].

Question 23

What do the arrows in Fig. 17.19 indicate?

A. Ring down artifact.
B. Free air with enhanced peritoneal stripe sign (EPSS).
C. Incorrect positioning of probe over thoracic cavity with A lines and rib shadowing.
D. Air bubbles in perihepatic fluid.

Answer: B.

Key point: Enhanced peritoneal stripe sign (EPSS) with reverberation artifact is suggestive of free intraperitoneal air (FIA).

Rationale: Ultrasound is superior to plain radiograph in detecting FIA from a perforation in the upper gastrointestinal tract. When using EPSS with reverberation artifact as a marker of FIA, the sensitivity and specificity of ultrasound and plain film was similar for lower gastrointestinal perforation [34, 35].

Question 24

Which of the following is TRUE regarding intraluminal bowel gas versus intraperitoneal free air?

A. Intraluminal bowel air moves with BOTH respiration and peristalsis.
B. Intraluminal bowel air moves with peristalsis ONLY.
C. Intraluminal bowel air moves with respiration ONLY.
D. Intraluminal bowel air can ONLY be differentiated with X-ray films.

Answer: A.

Key point: Intraluminal bowel air must be ruled out when diagnosing free intraperitoneal air (FIA).

Rational: Reflections of air that are intraluminal will move as the bowel contracts and relaxes with peristalsis. Hyperechoic intraluminal gas will also move with respiration. FIA under the abdominal wall will not move with either respiration or peristalsis [34, 37].

For Questions 25 and 26 please refer to the vignette below.

A 24-year-old male with past medical history significant for occasional cannabis use presents to the emergency department with nausea, malaise and right lower quadrant (RLQ) pain of 36-hours duration. Physical exam reveals tenderness and guarding in the RLQ. Abdominal point of care ultrasound (POCUS) is performed.

Question 25

What are the abdominal POCUS findings that suggest acute appendicitis? (Fig. 17.20)

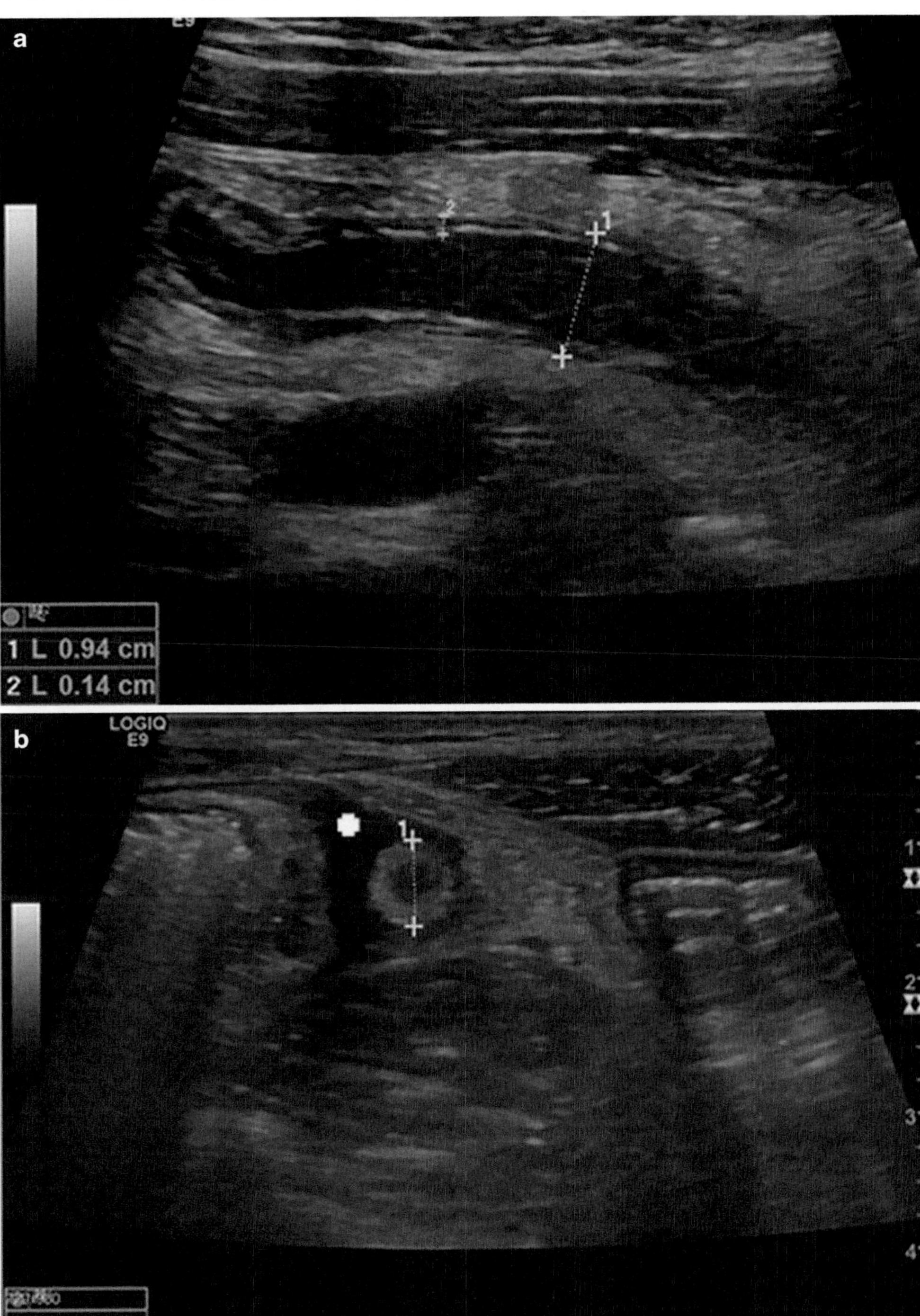

Fig. 17.20 Abdominal ultrasound (**a**) Longitudinal View (**b**) Transverse View (Reprinted from Mostbeck G, Adam EJ, Nielsen MB, et al. How to diagnose acute appendicitis: ultrasound first. Insights Imaging. 2016;7(2):255–263. With permission from Creative Commons License 4.0: http://creativecommons.org/licenses/by/4.0/)

A. A compressible tubular structure with a target sign, greater than 6 mm diameter, regular mucosa, no intraperitoneal fluid, normal omentum.
B. A non-compressible tubular structure with a target sign, greater than 6 mm diameter, irregular mucosa, intraperitoneal fluid, thickened omentum.
C. A non-compressible tubular structure with a target sign, greater than 3 mm diameter, irregular mucosa, intraperitoneal fluid, thickened omentum.
D. A non-compressible tubular structure with proximal acoustic shadowing, irregular mucosa, intraperitoneal fluid, normal omentum.

Answer: B.

Key point: Acute appendicitis usually presents with the following ultrasound findings: non compressible appendix (may be compressible if perforated), diameter > 6 mm, single wall thickness greater than or equal to

3 mm, target sign, appendicolith, hypervascularity in early stages and hypo to avascularity in abscess and necrosis.

Rational: When there is concern for acute appendicitis abdominal POCUS is recommend as the first imaging technique. When the appendix is visualized, abdominal POCUS is 100% sensitive and 85% specific for acute appendicitis. Difficulty in visualization can be encountered due to pain, obesity or bowel gas. Direct findings are mentioned above; indirect findings can be free fluid around the appendix, local abscess formation, increased echogenicity of local mesentery, enlarged mesenteric lymph nodes and signs of secondary bowel obstruction. Please see Table 17.1 for further details [38, 39].

Table 17.1 Acute appendicitis–ultrasound findings

Real-time US signs of acute appendicitis	
Direct signs	Indirect signs
Non-compressibility of the appendix	Free fluid surrounding appendix
Perforation: Appendix might be compressible	Local abscess formation
Diameter of the appendix >6 mm	Increased echogenicity of local mesenteric fat
Single wall thickness ≥ 3 mm	Enlarged local mesenteric lymph nodes
Target sign:	Thickening of the peritoneum
Hypoechoic fluid-filled lumen	Signs of secondary small bowel obstruction
Hyperechoic mucosa/submucosa	
Hypoechoic muscularis layer	
Appendicolith: Hyperechoic with posterior shadowing	
Colour doppler and contrast-enhanced US:	
Hypervascularity in early stage of AA	
Hypo-to avascularity in abscess and necrosis	

Adapted from Mostbeck G, Adam EJ, Nielsen MB, et al. How to diagnose acute appendicitis: ultrasound first. Insights Imaging. 2016;7(2):255–263. With permission from Creative Commons License 4.0: http://creativecommons.org/licenses/by/4.0/

Question 26

What is the graded compression technique for the evaluation of acute appendicitis? (Fig. 17.21)

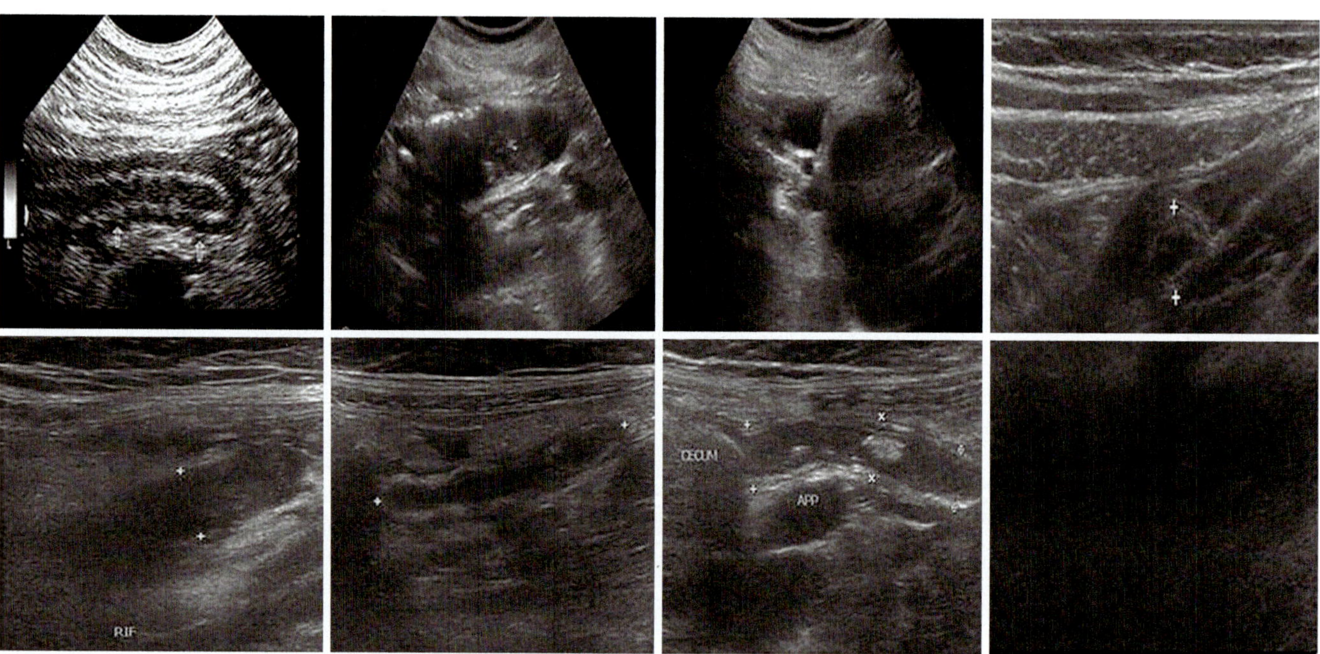

Fig. 17.21 Abdominal ultrasound (Reprinted from Shirah BH, Shirah HA, Alhaidari WA, et al. The role of preoperative graded compression ultrasound in detecting acute appendicitis and influencing the negative appendectomy rate. Abdom Radiol 2017; 42(1): 109–114. With permission from Springer Nature)

A. Apply steady pressure to the right iliac fossa slowly pushing normal loops of bowel away from the probe to reveal the appendix.
B. Applying then releasing slight pressure onto the right hypochondriac region with the probe oriented parasagittaly pushing normal loops of bowel away to reveal the appendix.
C. Steady pressure is applied to the right lumbar region transducer placed longitudinally to reveal the appendix.
D. Applying then releasing slight pressure to the hypogastric region slowly pushing normal loops of bowel away from the probe to reveal the appendix.

Answer: A.

Key point: The graded compression technique is performed by slowly and firmly compressing the anterior abdominal wall to displace the abdominal loops and locate the appendix.

Rational: The graded compression technique is performed with the patient in the supine position, scanning in the area of maximal pain indicated by the patient. Scanning is done in the right iliac fossa which corresponds to the anatomic location of the appendix. The graded compression technique increases sensitivity and specificity of abdominal POCUS for acute appendicitis diagnosis (sensitivity 89%, specificity 100%) and reduces the rate of negative appendectomy (no pathological findings upon physical inspection of the removed appendix) [38, 40].

Question 27

A twelve-year-old girl with no significant medical history presents to the emergency room with a one-day history of nausea and vomiting and worsening abdominal pain. Abdominal point of care ultrasound (POCUS) is performed. From the image below what is this most suggestive of? (Fig. 17.22)

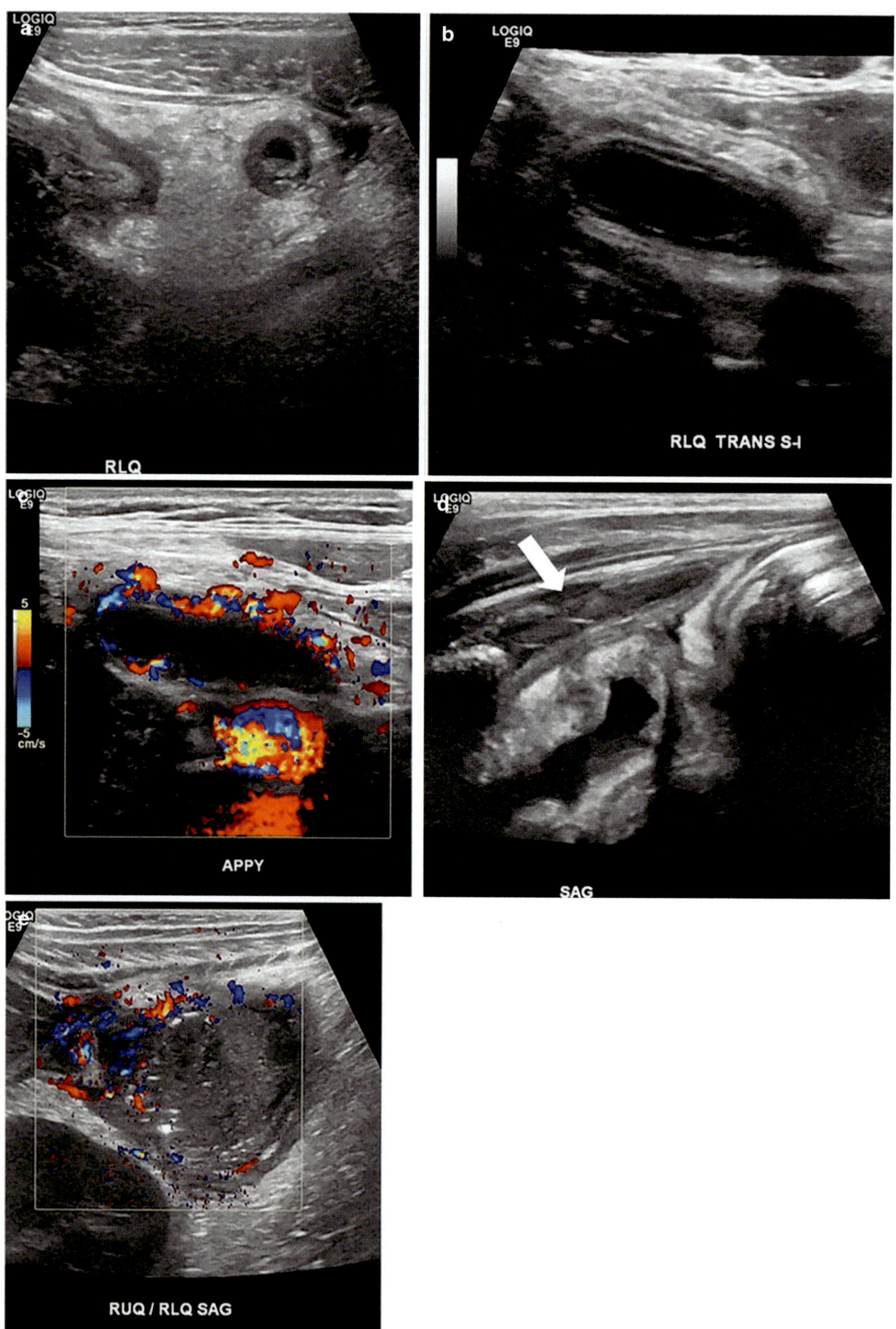

Fig. 17.22 Abdominal ultrasound (**a**–**e**). (Reprinted from Riedesel EL, Weber BC, Shore MW, et al. Diagnostic performance of standardized ultrasound protocol for detecting perforation in pediatric appendicitis. Pediatr Radiol 2019; 49(13): 1726–1734. With permission from Springer Nature)

A. Free air
B. Acute cholecystitis
C. Ovarian pedicle torsion
D. Perforated appendicitis

Answer: D.

Key point: Acute appendicitis is the most common surgical emergency in the pediatric population. Perforation is a surgical emergency.

Rational: The typical abdominal POCUS findings of an acute appendicitis do not have strong sensitivity for perforation. However, thinning and hyperemia of the appendix wall and a loculated fluid collection in the right lower quadrant are highly specific (>90%) for appendiceal perforation [38, 41].

Question 28

A 43-year-old woman with a past medical history of hypertension, diabetes mellitus and morbid obesity presents to the emergency department with malaise, vomiting and abdominal pain. She describes the abdominal pain as "severe cramps" for 12 hrs duration. Patient has an elevated white blood cell count of 22,000 cells/mm^3. Abdominal point of care ultrasound (POCUS) is performed demonstrating intraluminal bowel gas and otherwise equivocal results and lack of a Murphy's sign. What's the next appropriate step?

A. Admit to the regular nursing floor and observe.
B. STAT abdominal CT.
C. Admit to the regular nursing floor and perform serial abdominal POCUS.
D. Discharge home with prescription for analgesia.

Answer: B.

Key point: Acute abdominal pain with a moderate clinical suspicion and equivocal abdominal POCUS requires further imaging as abdominal POCUS in not the gold standard for diagnosing abdominal pathology.

Rational: Abdominal POCUS is not the gold standard for visualizing abdominal pathology. Age, obesity, abdominal pain and intraluminal air can make visualization of pathology challenging. Abdominal POCUS's merit lies in its timely ability to collect information and its lack of ionizing radiation. Equivocal abdominal POCUS exams with moderate index of suspicion must be further evaluated by abdominal computed tomography (CT) [34, 38].

For Questions 29 and 30 please refer to the vignette below.

A 52-year-old male with past medical history of hypertension and chronic obstructive pulmonary disease presents to the emergency department with a 48-hour history of abdominal pain and fevers. Physical exam is positive for tenderness to right upper quadrant and jaundiced appearance. Abdominal point of care ultrasound (POCUS) is performed to evaluate for acute cholecystitis (AC).

Question 29

The correct technique is:

A. With a curvilinear, low-frequency (2–5 MHz) probe; examination should begin by applying then releasing slight pressure onto the right hypochondriac region with the probe oriented para-sagittaly pushing normal loops of bowel away to reveal the gallbladder; asking the patient to assess for point of maximum tenderness.
B. With a curvilinear, low-frequency (2–5 MHz) probe; examination should begin at the with transducer placed longitudinally moving cephalad and laterally to the right subcostal margin to localize the gallbladder; asking the patient to assess for point of maximum tenderness.
C. With a curvilinear, low-frequency (2–5 MHz) probe; examination should begin at the xyphoid process and follow the right subcostal margin to localize the gallbladder; asking the patient to assess for point of maximum tenderness.
D. With a curvilinear, low-frequency (2–5 MHz) probe; examination should begin at right midaxillary line to the right iliac fossa to localize the gallbladder; asking the patient to assess for point of maximum tenderness.

Answer: C.

Key point: Abdominal ultrasound in an acute abdomen can be painful and views obtained need to be done efficiently to offer clinical guidance while minimizing patent's discomfort.

Rational: With proper technique abdominal POCUS is 88% sensitive, 87% specific for diagnosing gall stones. Gallstones in combination with pain when the sonographer presses directly over the gallbladder (sonographic Murphy's sign) has a 92% positive predictive value and 100% negative predictive value for acute cholecystitis [38, 42, 43].

Question 30

The major criteria of abdominal POCUS for acute cholecystitis are? (Fig. 17.23)

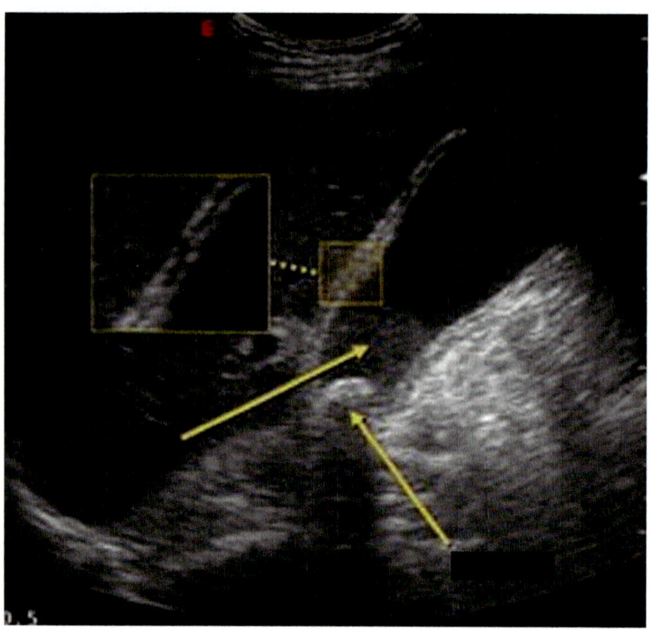

Fig. 17.23 Abdominal ultrasound (Reprinted from Zenobii MF, Accogli E, Domanico A, et al. Update on beside ultrasound (US) diagnosis of acute cholecysitits (AC). Intern Emerg Med 2016; 11(2):261–264. With permission from Springer Nature)

A. Pain when the sonographer presses directly over the gallbladder (sonographic Murphy's sign), gallstones, dilatation of the gallbladder (hydrops), air in the gallbladder wall.
B. Pain when the sonographer presses directly over the gallbladder (sonographic Murphy's sign), gallstones, biliary sludge or pus, air in the gallbladder wall.
C. Pain when the sonographer presses directly over the gallbladder (sonographic Murphy's sign), gallstone, hyperemic gall bladder wall (color doppler), air in the gallbladder wall.
D. Pain when the sonographer presses directly over the gallbladder (sonographic Murphy's sign), gallstones, gallbladder wall edema, air in the gallbladder wall.

Answer: D.

Key point: Pain when the sonographer presses directly over the gall bladder (sonographic Murphy's sign), gallstones, gallbladder wall edema or thickening > 3 mm, pericholecystic fluid, air in the gallbladder wall are the major criteria.

Rational: Dilatation of the gallbladder (hydrops) > 5 cm in transverse diameter, biliary sludge or pus are minor criteria. Hyperemic gall bladder wall is a supportive finding. Identification of two major with one minor criterion can increases sensitivity and specificity to 98% for acute cholecystitis [38, 43].

Question 31

Abdominal point of care ultrasound is performed. What view is this and what are the clinical findings? (Fig. 17.24)

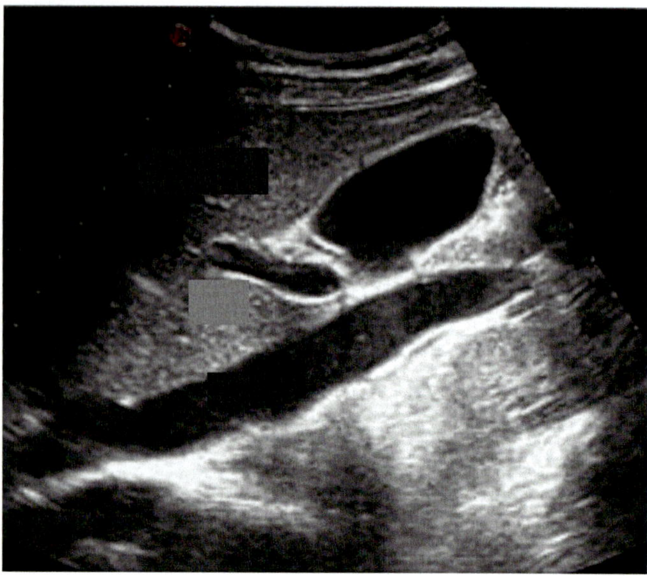

Fig. 17.24 Abdominal ultrasound (Reprinted from Zenobii MF, Accogli E, Domanico A, et al. Update on beside ultrasound (US) diagnosis of acute cholecysitits (AC). Intern Emerg Med 2016; 11(2):261–264. With permission from Springer Nature)

A. Right transverse subcostal scan of the gallbladder. Dilation of the gallbladder.
B. Right oblique intercostal scan of the gallbladder. Normal abdominal POCUS findings.
C. Right longitudinal subcostal scan of the gallbladder. Normal abdominal POCUS findings.
D. Right transverse subcostal scan of the gallbladder. Normal abdominal POCUS findings.

Answer: C.

Key point: Visualization of the gallbladder in three planes is necessary to identify the major and minor criteria of acute cholecystitis or objectively rule them out.

Rational: Small gallstones of less than 5 mm can be challenging to visualize and may not produce acoustic shadowing. Visualization of the gallbladder in three planes can increase sensitivity for gallstones [38, 43].

Question 32

A 37-year-old female with past medical history of gastroesophageal reflux disease presents to the emergency room with a 24-h history of abdominal pain and fevers. Physical exam is noted for tenderness in the right upper quadrant. Abdominal point of care ultrasound (POCUS) performed to evaluate for acute cholecystitis demonstrates a Murphy's sign. What clinical finding is noted from the image below and what is your next step in management? (Fig. 17.25)

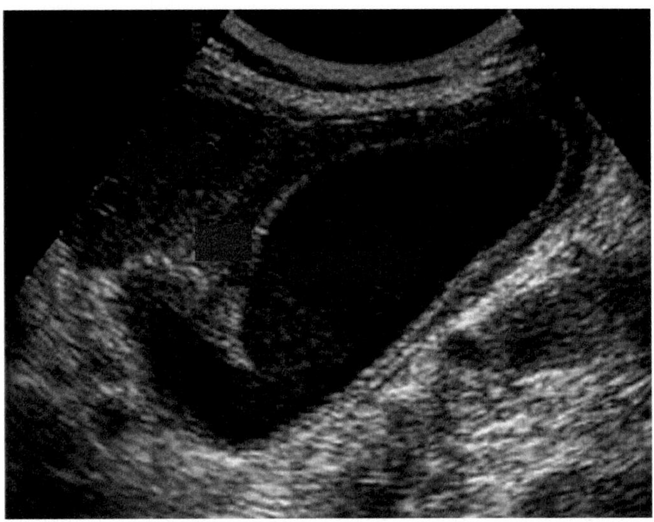

Fig. 17.25 Abdominal ultrasound (Reprinted from Zenobii MF, Accogli E, Domanico A, et al. Update on beside ultrasound (US) diagnosis of acute cholecysitits (AC). Intern Emerg Med 2016; 11(2):261–264. With permission from Springer Nature)

A. Acalculous acute cholecystitis and urgent surgical consult.
B. Acalculous acute cholecystitis and admit to regular nursing floor for observation.
C. Ambiguous POCUS exam and stat abdominal computed tomography.
D. Normal gallbladder without signs of acute cholecystitis; obtain a HIDA scan.

Answer: A.

Key point: Five percent of acute cholecystitis lacks gallstones on abdominal POCUS. When sludge is visualized within the gallbladder associated with tenderness on sonographic imaging (Murphy's sign)—this is suggestive of acalculous acute cholecystitis.

Rational: This image demonstrates sludge within the neck of the gallbladder. With a positive Murphy's sign this is suggestive of acalculous acute cholecystitis an urgent surgical consult is warranted. If abdominal POCUS is equivocal but the clinical presentation is suggestive of acalculous cholecystitis further imaging in the form of a hepatobiliary iminodiacetic acid scan (HIDA) is the next best test [38, 43, 44].

Question 33

A 69-year-old male presents to his primary care physician with malaise and weight loss. On exam he is jaundiced with tenderness at the right costal margin on abdominal exam. Abdominal point of care ultrasound was performed. What clinical finding is noted from the image below and what is your next step in management? (Fig. 17.26)

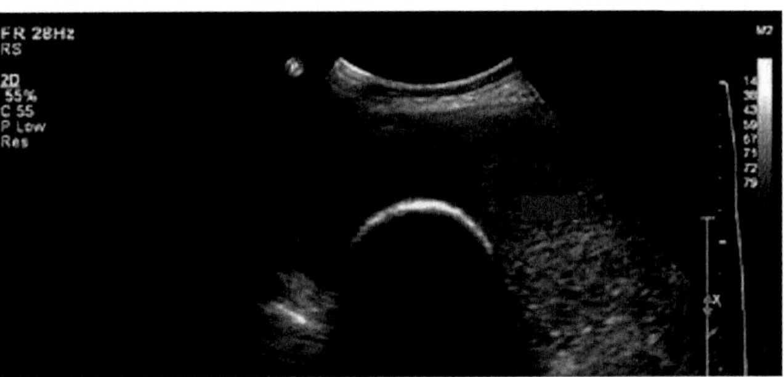

Fig. 17.26 Abdominal ultrasound (Reprinted from Cox M, Patel M, Joneja U, et al. Focal disruption in the wall of the porcelain gallbladder: a sign of gallbladder carcinoma. Intern Emerg Med 2017; 12:891–893. With permission from Springer Nature)

A. Poor abdominal POCUS technique. Place patient in supine position with thorax elevated 10–20°. Attention first to right upper quadrant with transducer placed longitudinally to right paramedian epigastric region overlying the liver.
B. Poor abdominal POCUS technique. Place patient in supine position, steady pressure applied to the right iliac fossa slowly pushing normal loops of bowel away from the probe to reveal the appendix; asking the patient to assess for point of maximum tenderness.
C. Calcified wall of gallbladder with posterior acoustic shadowing, obtain abdominal computed tomography scan.
D. Calcified wall of gallbladder with posterior acoustic shadowing, obtain stat consult for surgical emergency.

Answer: C.

Key point: Fig. 17.26 **shows calcified gallbladder wall. Calcified wall of gallbladder is associated with development of carcinoma.**

Rational: Often an incidental finding, calcified wall of gallbladder with posterior acoustic shadowing (porcelain gallbladder), is associated with development of carcinoma. Further imaging is warranted to look for focal disruption of gallbladder wall and associated calcifications [38, 45].

Question 34

A 68-year-old male with past medical history significant for coronary artery disease, chronic obstructive pulmonary disease and diabetes mellitus presented to the emergency department with a 3 days of right upper quadrant (RUQ) abdominal pain and nausea. On exam he appears jaundiced and is acutely tender to palpation of his RUQ. Abdominal point of care ultrasound (POCUS) is performed with the findings as pictured below. What does this signify and what is your next step? (Fig. 17.27)

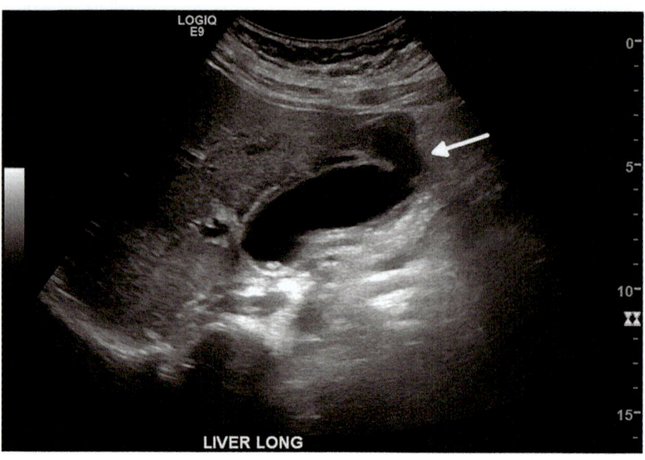

Fig. 17.27 Abdominal ultrasound (Reprinted from Dugdale P. Biliary Imaging for Gallstone Disease. In: Cox M, Eslick G, Padbury R (eds). The Management of Gallstone Disease. Cham, Switzerland: Springer Nature; 2018: 21–51. With permission from Springer Nature)

A. Acute cholecystitis; surgical consult.
B. Acute appendiceal perforation; stat surgical consult.
C. Acute cholecystitis with perforation; stat surgical consult.
D. Equivocal abdominal POCUS; HIDA scan.

Answer: C.

Key point: Gallbladder perforation is a rare complication that necessitates prompt surgical attention.

Rational: Gallbladder perforation is a life-threatening condition. It is associated with male gender, systemic disease and chronic steroid use. The most specific abdominal POCUS finding is a visualization of a gallbladder wall defect (the hole sign.) Less common is the visualization of gallstones outside of the gallbladder [46, 47].

Question 35

What is visualized in the abdominal point of care ultrasound (POCUS) below? (Fig. 17.28)

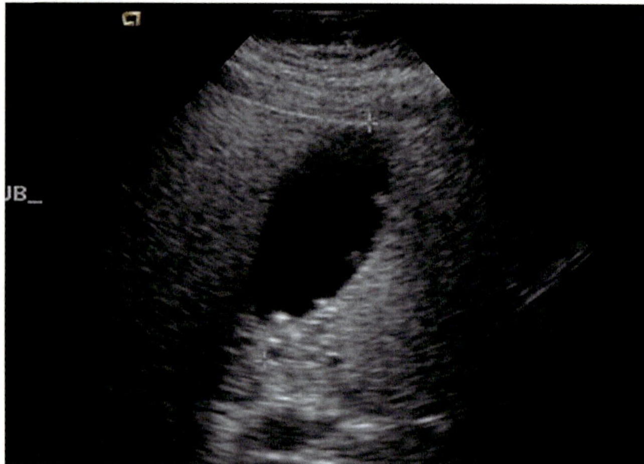

Fig. 17.28 Abdominal ultrasound (Reprinted from Elliott T. Gallbladder Polyps, Sludge and Adenomyomatosis. In: Cox M, Eslick G, Padbury R (eds). The Management of Gallstone Disease. Cham, Switzerland: Springer Nature; 2018: 137–146. With permission from Springer Nature)

A. Gallstones.
B. Gallbladder polyps.
C. Gallbladder pseudopolyps.
D. Sludge within the gallbladder.

Answer: B.

Key point: Gallbladder polyps are a common finding of abdominal POCUS. Risk stratification based on size, symptoms and demographics determine next steps.

Rational: Gallbladder polyps are a common abdominal POCUS finding, with a prevalence as high as 9.5%. Risk stratification and next steps are based upon size, acute cholecystitis symptoms, patients age, history of primary sclerosing cholangitis, Indian descent and sessile nature of the polyp. These factors determine if cholecystectomy vs serial abdominal POCUS exams should be performed [48, 49].

Question 36

58-year-old man with a history of primary sclerosing cholangitis (PSC), recurrent waxing and waning abdominal pain over several years presents to his primary care provider with mild abdominal pain. Abdominal point of care ultrasound (POCUS) is performed. What are the findings imaged below and what is the next best step in management? (Fig. 17.29).

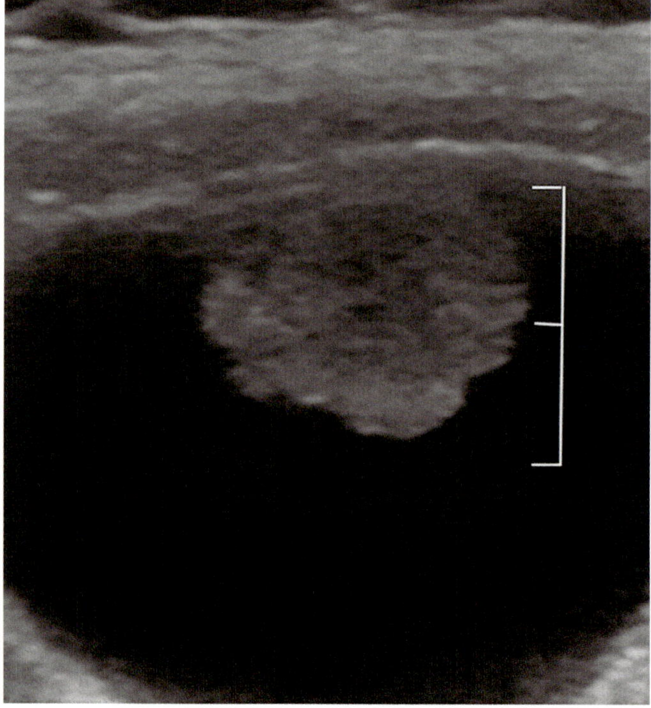

Fig. 17.29 Abdominal ultrasound (Reprinted from Choi TW, Kim JH, Park SJ, et al. Risk stratification of gallbladder polyps larger than 10 mm using high-resolution ultrasonography and texture analysis. Eur Radiol 2017;28(1): 196–205. With permission from Springer Nature)

A. Greater than 10 mm polyp, refer for cholecystectomy independent of other factors.
B. Greater than 10 mm polyp, with age and history of PSC refer for cholecystectomy.
C. Greater than 10 mm polyp, follow up abdominal POCUS at 6 months, and yearly thereafter.
D. Greater than 10 mm polyp, follow up abdominal POCUS at 1 year, and biannually thereafter.

Answer: A.

Key point: Large polyps (>10 mm), present an increased risk of malignancy. Cholecystectomy is indicated independent of other factors.

Rational: Joint guidelines from European Society of Gastrointestinal and Abdominal Radiology, European Association for Endoscopic Surgery and other Interventional Techniques, International Society of Digestive Surgery—European Federation and the European Society of Gastrointestinal Endoscopy have created the following guidelines regarding the management of gall bladder polyps [48–50] (Fig. 17.30).

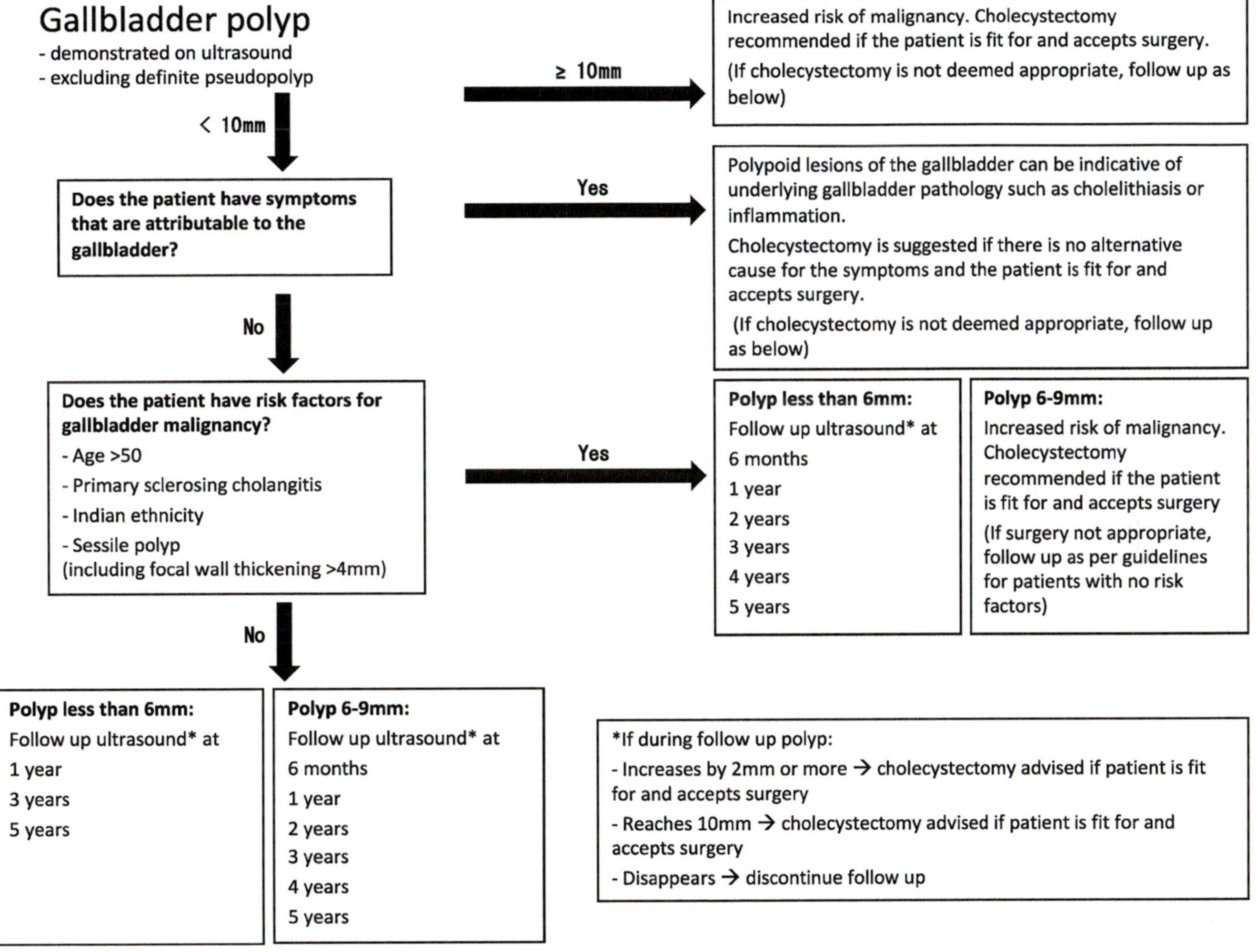

Fig. 17.30 Abdominal ultrasound (Reprinted from Wiles R, Thoeni RF, et al. Management and follow-up of gallbladder polyps. Euro Rad 2017; 27(9):3856–3866. With permission from Springer Nature)

Question 37

A 42-year-old man with no significant past medical history presents to his primary care provider with mild abdominal pain. Abdominal point of care ultrasound (POCUS) is performed. What are the findings and what is your next step? (Fig. 17.31).

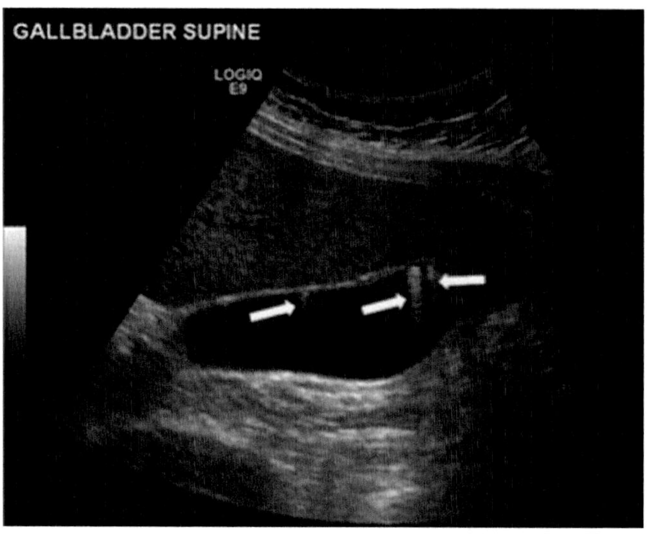

Fig. 17.31 Abdominal ultrasound (Reprinted from Wiles R, Thoeni RF, et al. Management and follow-up of gallbladder polyps. Euro Rad 2017; 27(9):3856–3866. With permission from Springer Nature)

A. Less than 6 mm polyp, refer for cholecystectomy.
B. Less than 6 mm pseudopolyp, no need for follow up.
C. Less than 6 mm polyp, follow up abdominal POCUS at 6 months, and yearly thereafter.
D. Less than 6 mm polyp, follow up abdominal POCUS at 1 year, and biannually thereafter.

Answer: B.

Key point: Pseudopolyps can demonstrate reverberation (comet tail) artifact posterior to the lesion. Pseudopolyps do not require follow up.

Rational: Pseudopolyps are usually less than 1 cm in size; they are non-cancerous, cholesterol filled growths. Pseudopolyps when demonstrating reverberation (comet tail) artifact posterior to the lesion do not present a risk of malignancy themselves and are not subject to the abdominal POCUS surveillance guidelines. However, not all pseudopolyps will have this feature making distinguishing them from true polyps challenging [48, 49].

Question 38

A 57-year-old woman presented to emergency department with a three-day history of right upper quadrant pain. On exam abdomen is tender to palpation and she appears jaundiced. Abdominal point of care ultrasound (POCUS) is performed with the following image produced. What is this suggestive of? (Fig. 17.32)

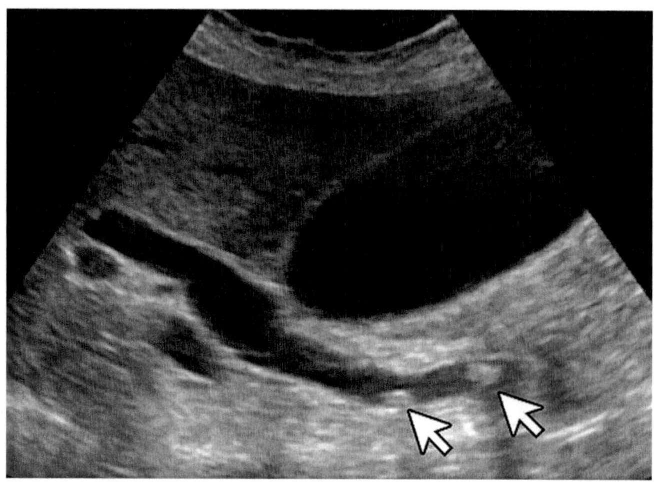

Fig. 17.32 Abdominal ultrasound (Reprinted from Burrowes DP, Choi HH, Rodgers SK, et al. Utility of ultrasound in acute pancreatitis. Abdom Radiol (NY) 2020; 45(5):1253–1264. With permission from Springer Nature)

A. Dilated distal common bile duct with echogenic intraluminal foci producing posterior acoustic shadowing consistent with choledocholithiasis.
B. Right portal vein branch demonstrating intrahepatic biliary dilatation.
C. Extraluminal gallbladder stones with posterior acoustic shadowing suggestive of gall bladder perforation with abscess formation.
D. Pneumobilia within a dilated distal common bile duct from gas forming organisms.

Answer: A.

Key point: Choledocholithiasis can be diagnosed on abdominal POCUS from echogenic intraluminal foci producing posterior acoustic shadowing causing a fluid-filled distended bile duct.

Rational: There are two types of choledocholithiasis:

1. Primary—stones developing within common bile duct, relatively rare, occurs in endemic areas (East Asia).
2. Secondary—migration of stones from gall bladder, which is more common.

Scanning requires skill in identifying common bile duct and following it to the ampulla of Vater. If stones are <5 mm they will be hard to visualize and may not cast acoustic shadows. Abdominal POCUS is only 50–80% sensitive for choledocholithiasis, it is 99% sensitive for common bile duct dilatation and 95% specific for choledocholithiasis. Abdominal POCUS is more sensitive than computed tomography for primary biliary disease [51, 52].

Question 39

A 57-year-old woman presented to emergency room with a three-day history of right upper quadrant pain. On exam she is tender to palpation and appears jaundiced. Amylase level 385 U/L and lipase 600 U/L. Abdominal point of care ultrasound (POCUS) is performed with the following image produced. What is this suggestive of and what is the next best step in management? (Fig. 17.33)

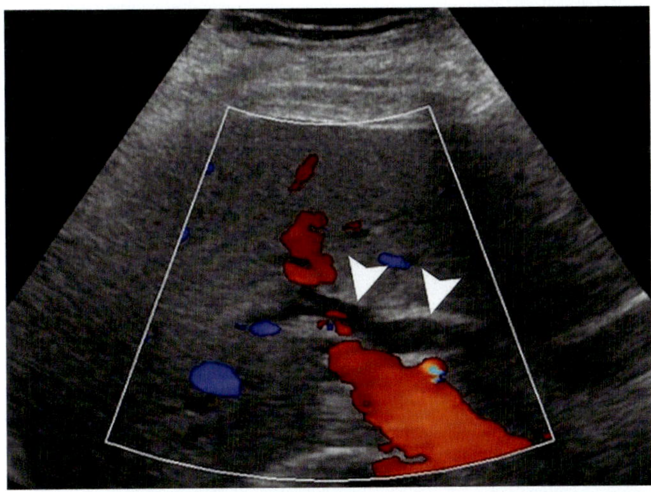

Fig. 17.33 Abdominal ultrasound (Reprinted from Burrowes DP, Choi HH, Rodgers SK, et al. Utility of ultrasound in acute pancreatitis. Abdom Radiol (NY) 2020; 45(5):1253–1264. With permission from Springer Nature)

A. Dilated distal common bile duct with echogenic intraluminal foci producing posterior acoustic shadowing consistent with choledocholithiasis. Proceed with therapeutic endoscopic retrograde cholangiopancreatography (ERCP).
B. Intrahepatic biliary dilatation. Proceed with diagnostic magnetic resonance cholangiopancreatography (MRCP).
C. Extraluminal gallbladder stones with posterior acoustic shadowing suggestive of gall bladder perforation with abscess formation, STAT surgery consult.
D. Pneumobilia within a dilated distal common bile duct from gas forming organisms, appropriate antibiotics and gastrointestinal consult.

Answer: B.

Key point: Abdominal POCUS is at best, 80% sensitive for choledocholithiasis. With moderate clinical suspicion MRCP is the next best step.

Rational: Abdominal POCUS is at best, 80% sensitive for choledocholithiasis. ERCP is an invasive procedure that carries risk of bleeding cholangitis, pancreatitis and perforation. With moderate clinical suspicion MRCP is the next best step. If choledocholithiasis is imaged with MRCP then clinical decision to proceed to ERCP can be made [51–53].

Question 40

An abdominal point of care ultrasound (POCUS) is performed. What is the structure identified? (Fig. 17.34a)

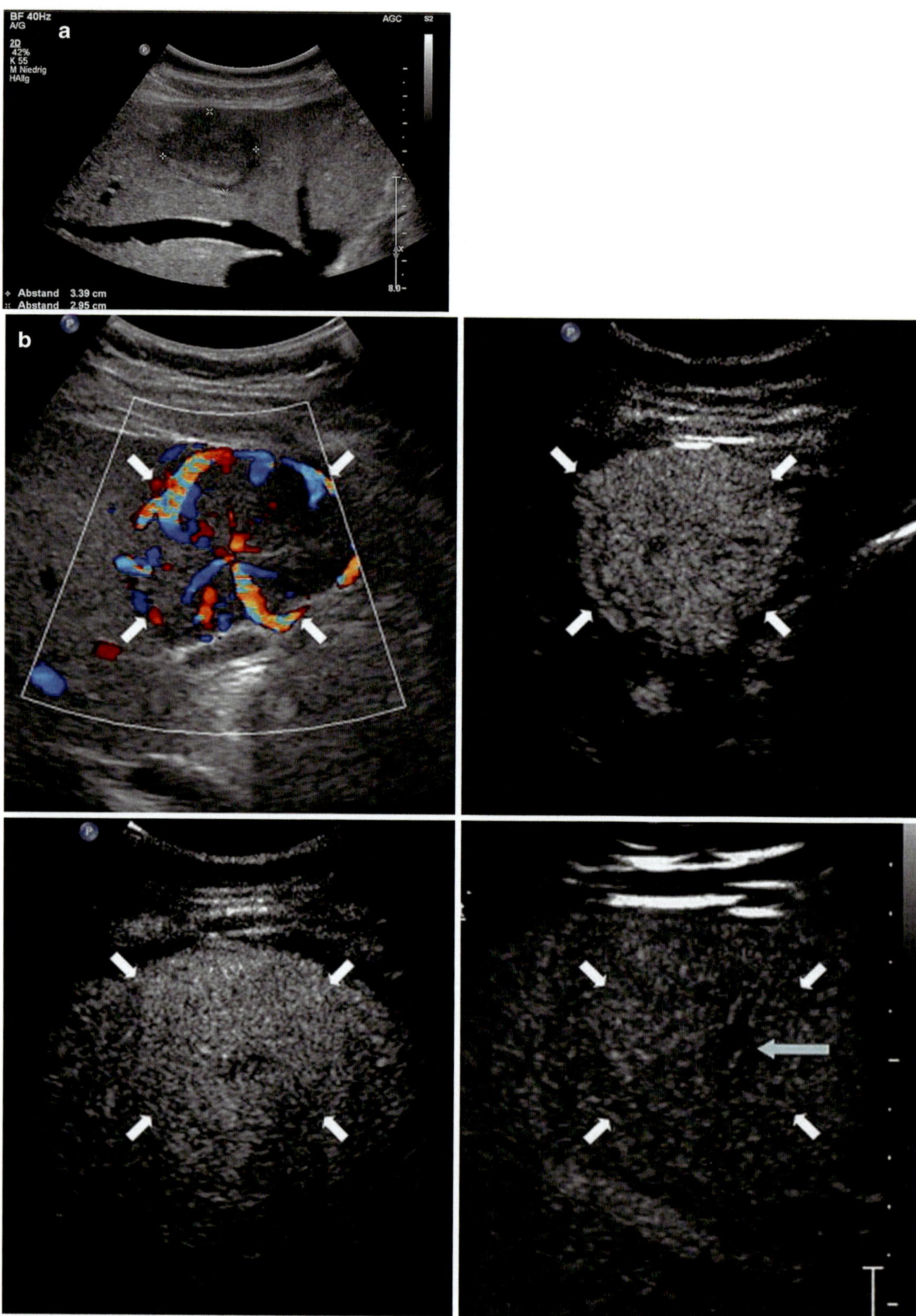

Fig. 17.34 (**a**) Abdominal ultrasound; (**b**)Abdominal ultrasound (**a**) (Reprinted from Kaltenbach TEM, Engler P, Kratzer W, et al. Prevalence of benign focal liver lesions: ultrasound investigation of 45,319 hospital patients. Abdominal Radiology 2016;41: 25–32. With permission from Creative Commons License 4.0: https://creativecommons.org/licenses/by/4.0/). (**b**) (Reprinted from Kong WT, Wang WP, Huang BJ, et al. Contrast-Enhanced Ultrasound in Combination with Color Doppler Ultrasound Can Improve the Diagnostic Performance of Focal Nodular Hyperplasia and Hepatocellular Adenoma. Ultrasound in Medicine & Biology 2015; 41(4): 944–951. With permission from Elsevier)

A. Hepatic cyst
B. Hepatic hemangioma
C. Focal nodular hyperplasia (FNH)
D. Hepatic adenoma

Answer: C.

Key point: Abdominal POCUS frequently observes incidental focal liver lesion. Differentiation of lesions as malignant or benign is important to determine next steps.

Rational: The image shows focal nodular hypoplasia. These lesions are benign and characterized by a red brown or tan mass composed of bening hepatocytes laced within fibrous septa (sometimes extending from a central stellate scar). On ultrasound these lesions have a non-homogenous appearance and may have a central feeding arterial vessel. On color and power doppler they have spoke-wheel distribution (see Fig. 17.34b). Table 17.2 shows characteristics of common hepatic "incidentalomas" in the liver and key features [54–56] (Fig. 17.34b).

Table 17.2 Criteria used to diagnose each lesion type

Liver lesion	Criteria
Focal fatty sparing	*Localization*
	Adjacent to the porta hepatis (segment IV)
	Gallbladder fossa
	Adjacent to the falciform ligament
	B-mode presentation
	Fatty liver
	Hypoechoic lesion
	Sharp edge
Hemangioma	Hyperechoic
	Sharp edge
	Round or oval form
	No blood flow in Doppler and Power Doppler-Mode
Cyst	Echo empty
	Posterior acoustic enhancement
	Border shadow sign
	Hyperechoic outlet echo
FNH	Spoke-wheel distribution in Doppler and Power-Doppler
	Central feeding arterial vessel
	Inhomogeneous
Adenoma	Hypoechoic/isoechoic
	Difficult to define

Reprinted from Kaltenbach TEM, Engler P, Kratzer W, et al. Prevalence of benign focal liver lesions: ultrasound investigation of 45,319 hospital patients. Abdominal Radiology 2016;41: 25–32. With permission from Creative Commons License 4.0: https://creativecommons.org/licenses/by/4.0/

Question 41

An abdominal point of care ultrasound is performed. What is the identified structure? (Fig. 17.35)

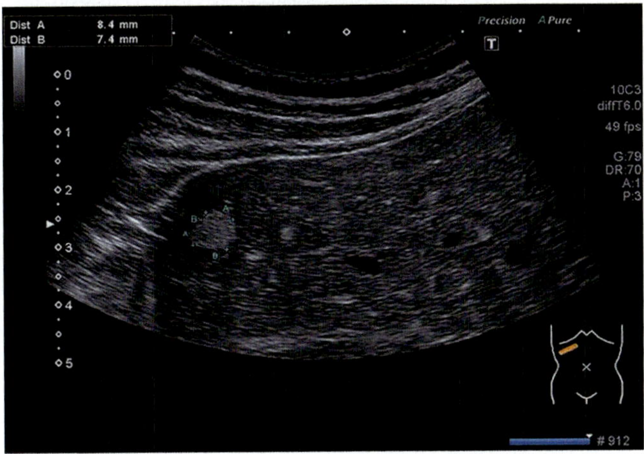

Fig. 17.35 Abdominal ultrasound (Reprinted from Kaltenbach TEM, Engler P, Kratzer W, et al. Prevalence of benign focal liver lesions: ultrasound investigation of 45,319 hospital patients. Abdominal Radiology 2016;41: 25–32. With permission from Creative Commons License 4.0: https://creativecommons.org/licenses/by/4.0/)

A. Hepatic cyst
B. Hepatic hemangioma
C. Focal nodular hyperplasia (FNH)
D. Hepatic adenoma

Answer: B.

Key point: Hepatic hemangiomas are hyperechoic round or oval structures. They have a sharp boundary and do not show any internal flow on doppler or power doppler.

Rational: Hemangiomas are composed of large blood-filled spaces line by flat endothelial cells and separate by fibrous septa. Due to the multiple interfaces between these surfaces they appear hyperechoic. Hemangiomas may also show posterior acoustic enhancement. Please see Table 17.2 in the answer to question 41 for differentiating features of other common benign hepatic lesions [54, 55, 57].

Question 42

A 27-year-old female with past medical history of reflux presents with epigastric pain. She has normal vital signs on examination. She is on multivitamins and oral contraceptives. An abdominal point of care ultrasound is performed. What is the finding shown on abdominal ultrasound? (Fig. 17.36)

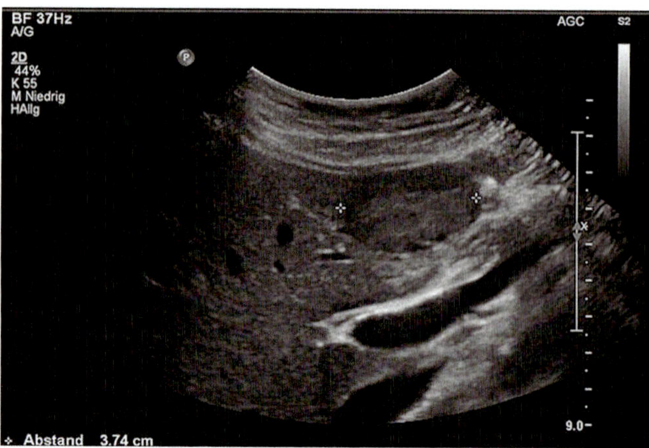

Fig. 17.36 Abdominal ultrasound (Reprinted from Kaltenbach TEM, Engler P, Kratzer W, et al. Prevalence of benign focal liver lesions: ultrasound investigation of 45,319 hospital patients. Abdominal Radiology 2016;41: 25–32. With permission from Creative Commons License 4.0: https://creativecommons.org/licenses/by/4.0/)

A. Hepatic cyst
B. Hepatic hemangioma
C. Focal nodular hyperplasia (FNH)
D. Hepatic adenoma

Answer: D.

Key point: Hepatic adenomas usually present as a solitary, well demarcated, heterogenous mass with variable echogenicity.

Rational: Hepatic adenomas are benign, hormone induced liver tumors. They are usually solitary (70–80%), often large at the time of diagnosis and are at risk for hemorrhage. Frequently seen in women on oral contraceptive pills. Also have association with obesity, anabolic steroid use, metabolic syndrome and glycogen storage diseases [54, 55].

Question 43

A 58-year-old male with a past medical history of obesity, smoking, chronic obstructive pulmonary disease and chronic pain presents to the emergency department with a 2-day history of abdominal pain that has been increasing in intensity. Abdominal point of care ultrasound (POCUS) is performed. What is the identified ultrasound finding as depicted in the image below? (Fig. 17.37)

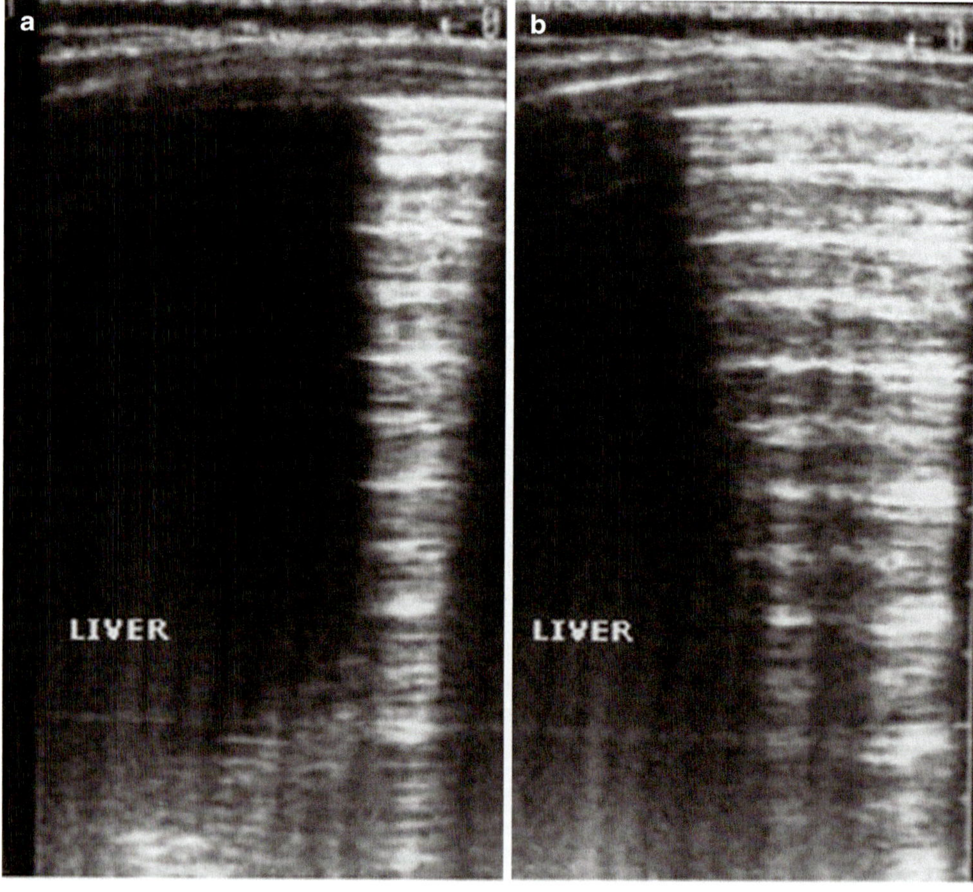

Fig. 17.37 Abdominal ultrasound (**a** and **b**) (Reprinted from Karahan O, Kurt A, Yikilmaz A, Kahriman G. New method for the detection of intraperitoneal free air by sonography: scissors maneuver. J Clin Ultrasound. 2004 Oct;32(8):381–5. With permission from John Wiley & Sons)

A. This is a normal abdominal ultrasound exam.
B. This is pseudopneumoperitoneum (Chilaiditi syndrome).
C. This is air within the lungs obscuring the costophrenic recess during inspiration (curtain sign).
D. This is pockets of free intraperitoneal air (FIA) migrating in response to abdominal wall deformation from the ultrasound probe (scissors maneuver).

Answer: D.

Key point: The scissors maneuver increases the sensitivity and specificity of identifying free intraperitoneal air (FIA).

Rational: The scissors maneuver is a relatively new sonographic technique used to detect intraperitoneal free air superficial to the liver; the maneuver consists of applying and then releasing pressure onto the abdominal wall with the caudal part of the linear-array probe (oriented para-sagittaly). The scissors maneuver is 90% sensitive and 100% specific for FIA [58–60].

For Questions 44, 45, 46 and 47, refer to the vignette below.

A 38 -year-old man presents to the emergency room after a motor vehicle collision where he was a restrained, front-seat driver travelling at approximately 50 miles/hr. On arrival, he complains of chest, back and abdominal pain. He is tachycardic with a heart rate of 135 beats/min and blood pressure of 110/63 mmHg. He has visible ecchymosis over his lower left chest and upper abdomen from impact with the steering wheel. An E-FAST exam was performed at the bedside with the image shown below (Fig. 17.38).

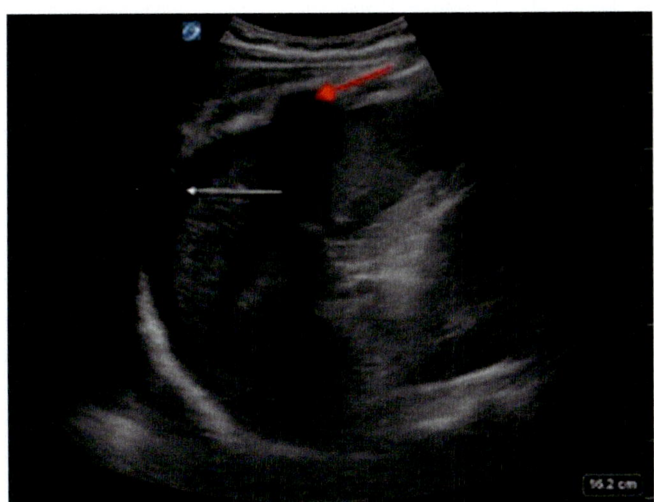

Fig. 17.38 Abdominal E – FAST (Reprinted from Creditt AB, Vitto M. Extended Focused Assessment with Sonography for Trauma. In: Creditt A, Tozer J, Vitto M, Joyce M, Taylor L (eds). Clinical Ultrasound: A Pocket Manual. Cham, Switzerland: Springer Nature. 2018: 19–45. With permission from Springer Nature)

Question 44

Which of the following is the most appropriate orientation for ultrasound probe placement on the abdomen to achieve this view?

A. Mid-axillary line on the left 8–10th intercostal space with the marker pointed towards the head.
B. Mid-axillary line on the right 8–10th intercostal space with the marker pointed towards the feet.
C. Mid clavicular line on the left 6–7th intercostal space with the marker pointed towards the feet.
D. Mid-axillary line on the right 8–10th intercostal space with the marker pointed towards the head.

Answer: A.

Key Points: Knowledge of landmarks and orientation for ultrasound probe placement is critical for appropriate high-quality image acquisition.

Rationale: An E-FAST exam has multiple views that are performed in succession. Improper probe placement will slow down diagnosis and patient management. Obtaining a view of the diaphragm and spleen simultaneously is necessary as blood will collect in this location first in the left upper quadrant [61, 62].

Question 45

The patient continues to deteriorate with worsening tachycardia and hypotension, and loss of consciousness. What would be the most likely diagnosis?

A. Intra-abdominal hemorrhage
B. Pericardial effusion
C. Large hemothorax
D. Diaphragmatic rupture

Answer: A.

Key Points: Rapid recognition of intra-abdominal bleeding and clinical deterioration is vital to improve chances for patient survival following a severe traumatic injury.

Rationale: Identification of free intraabdominal fluid and likely hemoperitoneum has a high sensitivity and specificity. In a patient with hemodynamic collapse, this sensitivity is increased, and management can be instituted promptly to improve chances for survival. It is critical to image the diaphragm above the spleen as fluid may not always collect in the splenorenal recess first [61, 63].

Question 46
Name the structure pointed by the red arrow and the type of artifact it is creating?

A. Free fluid; enhancement artifact.
B. Soft tissue calcification; reverberation artifact.
C. Bone; attenuation artifact.
D. Free Air; ring down artifact.
E. Foreign object, not an artifact.

Answer: C.

Key Points: Awareness of ultrasound artifacts can help with probe orientation and avoid false diagnosis.

Rationale: Attenuation occurs due to the gradual loss of signal intensity as ultrasound waves pass through a medium. Some structures, for instance, bone have a high attenuation coefficient and are difficult to penetrate leading to a hypoechoic area behind the structure. Rib shadowing and attenuation is a major factor in transthoracic and upper abdominal imaging. The LUQ is particularly susceptible to rib shadowing impacting image acquisition [64, 65].

Question 47
Which of the following is the most sensitive location for identification of hemoperitoneum from a splenic injury on an E-FAST exam of a supine adult male patient?

A. Splenorenal recess
B. Hepatorenal recess
C. Spleno-diaphragmatic recess
D. Recto-vesicular space

Answer: B.

Key Points: Morrison's Pouch (also known as the hepatorenal recess) is the most sensitive location for free fluid in the abdomen.

Rationale: A splenic injury and bleeding will first present itself as a collection in the hepatorenal recess (Morrison's pouch) due to its more dependent location prior to presenting in the left upper quadrant during an E-FAST exam. In children, the pelvis is the most sensitive location for fluid collection [61, 62].

Question 48
Which of the following is **TRUE** regarding differentiating a pericardial fat pad from a pericardial effusion while performing an E-FAST exam?

A. A pericardial effusion will have a speckled appearance, and only appear anterior to the right ventricle; A pericardial fat pad can be circumferential and anechoic.
B. An epicardial fat pad will be posterior to the left ventricle in the parasternal long axis view, but not present on the subcostal view.
C. Pericardial effusions have a speckled appearance and the appearance can differentiate between blood and fluid
D. Pericardial fat will be echogenic; pericardial effusions are anechoic and motionless.

Answer: D.

Key Points: Distinguishing normal anatomic findings from true pathology is critical, especially in decompensating patients and could save extra procedures and cost.

Rationale: An epicardial fat pad is typically seen anterior to the right ventricle in a parasternal long axis view, but can be seen circumferentially as well, becoming a confounder when assessing for a pericardial effusion. Combining multiple views looking for pericardial effusion posterior to the left ventricle can avoid this confusion and save valuable time in assessing a hemodynamically unstable patient [61, 66].

For Questions 49, 50, and 51, refer to the vignette below.

A 46-year-old obese female presents to the ED after falling off a horse. On arrival, she complains of pain over her left chest. She is tachycardic with a heart rate of 120 and a blood pressure of 150/80. Physical exam reveals bruising and tenderness to palpation over her right flank and lower abdomen. A chest x-ray shows a non-displaced fourth and fifth rib fracture with no visible pneumothorax.

Question 49
Which of the following echocardiographic signs is correctly paired with its associated lung pathology?

A. The barcode sign on B mode echocardiography, represents pulmonary edema.
B. The seashore sign on M mode echocardiography represents normal lung tissue.
C. The presence of B lines on B mode echocardiography indicates normal lung tissue.
D. The presence of comet tail artifacts on M-mode echocardiography represents a pneumothorax.

Answer: B.

Key Points: Echocardiographic signs of a pneumothorax are important to recognize. The seashore sign is seen on M-mode echocardiography and represents normal lung.

Rationale: Pneumothorax can be seen on ultrasound with a relatively high sensitivity and specificity. The barcode sign is seen on M-mode echocardiography and represents a pneumothorax. The loss of lung sliding, along with visualization of lung point all indicate the presence of a pneumothorax [61, 67, 68].

Question 50
After admission to the ICU, the patient becomes progressively more tachycardic associated with worsening lower

abdominal pain. An E-FAST exam is performed and the image in Fig. 17.39 is seen. Which of the following is **TRUE**?

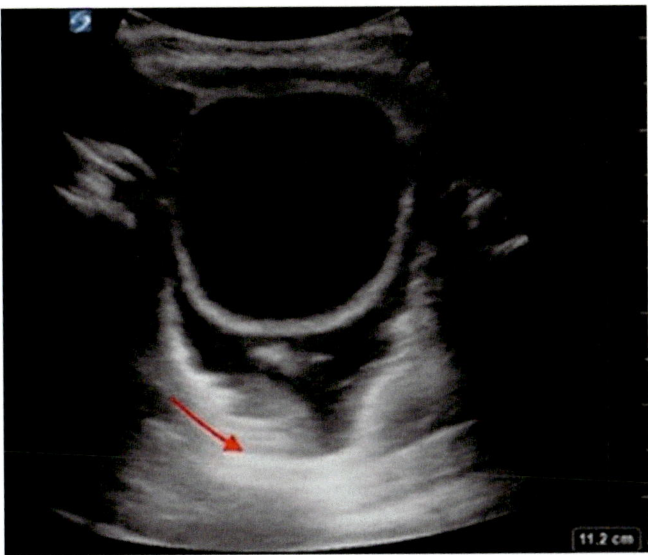

Fig. 17.39 Abdominal ultrasound (Reprinted from Creditt AB, Vitto M. Extended Focused Assessment with Sonography for Trauma. In: Creditt A, Tozer J, Vitto M, Joyce M, Taylor L (eds). Clinical Ultrasound: A Pocket Manual. Cham, Switzerland: Springer Nature. 2018: 19–45. With permission from Springer Nature)

A. The hypoechoic area posterior to the bladder represents attenuation artifact.
B. This image represents fluid in the retroperitoneal space.
C. There is a high probability of an anechoic fluid in the hepatorenal recess.
D. Pelvic imaging is not a routine component of an E-FAST exam.
E. Bleeding can be ruled out as the cause of this patient's decompensation.

Answer: C.

Key Point: A pelvic ultrasound in E-FAST will show fluid around the bladder, which remains intraperitoneal.

Rationale: Hepatorenal recess (Morrison's Pouch) is the most sensitive location for free fluid collection in the abdomen and is the most sensitive place for intra-abdominal bleeding to collect on an ultrasound exam. This is seen on a RUQ imaging during an E-FAST exam. If free fluid is seen around the bladder in the supine position, there is a high likelihood of free fluid in the hepatorenal recess as fluid collects there first due to gravity [61, 62, 69].

Question 51

What is the reason for the posterior hyperechoic area marked by the red arrow?

A. Attenuation
B. Reverberation
C. Enhancement
D. Sidelobe

Answer: C.

Key Points: Recognition of ultrasound artifacts is important to decrease the risk of false positive identification of pathology. Image quality can be improved by adjusting for expected artifacts.

Rationale: The ultrasound assumes an equal depth and density of soft tissue across all its scan lines. When sound energy travels through structures that produce less attenuation than their surrounding structures, the deeper tissue reflects stronger and is seen as a brighter, hyperechoic structure [64, 70].

Question 52

What is the difference between the original FAST and updated E-FAST exams?

A. The original FAST exam performed 3 abdominal windows; The E-FAST performs 3 abdominal windows and 1 subcostal window for the heart.
B. The original FAST exam was unable to see the pleural spaces bilaterally.
C. The E-FAST can rule out a pneumothorax with higher sensitivity/specificity than a chest x-ray.
D. The E-FAST exam includes a parasternal short axis view of the heart.

Answer: C.

Key Points: Knowing all the views for performing an efficient E-FAST is important in a critically ill patient with hemodynamic instability.

Rationale: The original FAST exam included three abdominal views in the right upper quadrant, left upper quadrant, pelvis and a subcostal view to assess for pericardial effusions. In 2004, the FAST was extended to E-FAST (addition of right and left anterior thoracic views) to allow for rapid recognition of pneumothoraces. Multiple studies have shown ultrasound as a better tool for assessment of a pneumothorax with high sensitivity and specificity compared to chest x-ray [62, 69].

For Questions 53, 54, and 55, refer to the vignette below.

A 44-year-old male with a history of hypertension presents to the hospital after a gunshot wound to the left anterior chest. In the emergency room a left sided chest tube is placed for a hemothorax and he is admitted to the trauma ICU. He is tachycardic with a heart rate of 137 beats/min and a blood pressure of 100/60 mmHg. An E-FAST exam is performed with the following images: (Figs. 17.40 and 17.41).

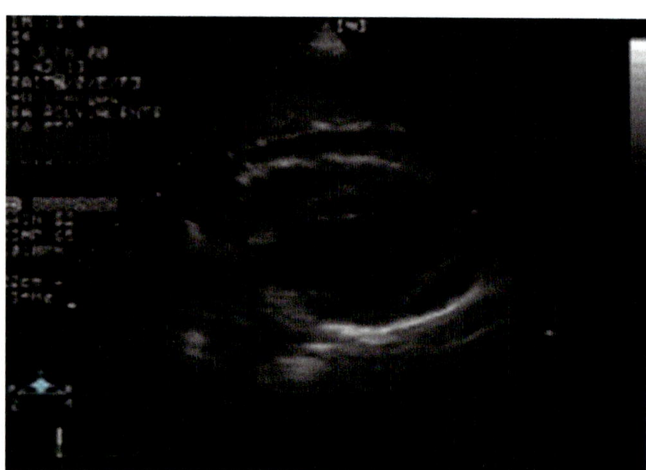

Fig. 17.40 E- FAST exam (Reprinted from Vilacosta I, Cañadas V, San Román JA, Vignon P. Acute Aortic Syndrome: Acute Aortic Diseases in Hemodynamically Unstable Patients. In: Backer D, Cholley BP, Slama M, Vieillard-Baron A, Vignon P (eds.) Hemodynamic Monitoring Using Echocardiography in the Critically Ill. Heidelberg, Germany: Springer-Verlag; 2011: 247–271. With permission from Springer Nature)

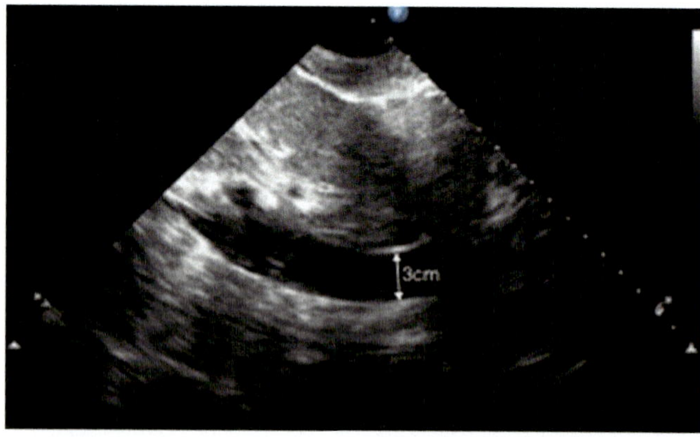

Fig. 17.41 E- FAST exam (Reprinted from Nair GB, Mathew JP. Critical Care Echocardiography: Pericardial Disease, Tamponade, and Other Topics. In: Jankovich M, Gartman E (eds). Ultrasound in the Intensive Care Unit. Respiratory Medicine. New York, NY: Humana Press; 2015: 147–173. With permission from Springer Nature)

Question 53

Which of the following is the most sensitive sign for the pathology seen during an echocardiographic exam of this patient?

A. Right atrial collapse during systole.
B. Right atrial collapse during diastole.
C. Right ventricular collapse during systole.
D. Right ventricular collapse during diastole.

Answer: A.

Key Point: Rapid recognition of cardiac tamponade is crucial for management of a rapidly deteriorating patient.

Rationale: It is important to differentiate a pericardial effusion from cardiac tamponade as the latter has significant hemodynamic consequences, while an effusion can become a confounder in the diagnosis of a decompensating patient. As the right atrium has the lowest intracardiac pressures, thus right atrial collapse becomes the most sensitive sign for the onset of cardiac tamponade. Collapse of the right atrium occurs before the right ventricle; the collapse of the right atrium occurs in systole in tamponade as the right atrial pressure is lowest with the x descent and the intracavitary pressure falls below the intrapericardial pressure [66, 71, 72].

Question 54

The patient becomes increasingly dyspneic, hypotensive and tachycardic. His heart sounds distant, with visible jugular venous distension. Which of the following is the most specific echocardiographic sign for the late stage pathology in this patient?

A. Right atrial collapse during systole
B. Right atrial collapse during diastole
C. Right ventricular collapse during systole
D. Right ventricular collapse during diastole

Answer: D.

Key Point: Identifying signs of cardiac tamponade can aid in diagnosis and guide management decisions.

Rationale: Right ventricular collapse during diastole is a late finding with significant hemodynamic consequences. Once present, an emergent bedside procedure such as a pericardiocentesis may be necessary to avoid complete hemodynamic collapse prior to definitive management [66, 71, 72].

Question 55

If an M-Mode scan line was passed through the vessel seen in Fig. 17.41, the tracing would show which of the following?

1. Diameter reduction of >50% during inspiration
2. Diameter reduction of >50% during expiration
3. Diameter reduction of <50% during inspiration
4. Diameter reduction of <50% during expiration
   A. 1 and 2
   B. 3 and 4
   C. 1 and 4
   D. 2 and 3

Answer: B.

Key Points: IVC imaging as an adjunct to subcostal views during trauma can aid in the differentiation of shock.

Rationale: IVC diameter is a key representation of right heart pressure and volume. Although it is not as helpful in isolation, combined with a clinical picture and other signs obtained through an E-FAST exam, it can help with rapid diagnosis for the cause of hemodynamic collapse in a patient. In cardiac tamponade, the IVC is dilated with minimal respiratory variation due to high intracardiac pressures impeding venous return [66, 73].

For Questions 56 and 57, refer to the vignette below.

A 57-year-old male with a history of uncontrolled hypertension, hyperlipidemia, cocaine abuse, and diabetes is admitted to the emergency room with a 3 day history of epigastric and back pain which started after a night out with friends. It is associated with nausea and vomiting that has been getting progressively worse in the past 24 hrs. He is tachycardic and hypotensive in the emergency room with decreased lower extremity pulses. An abdominal ultrasound is performed and the following image is seen (Fig. 17.42).

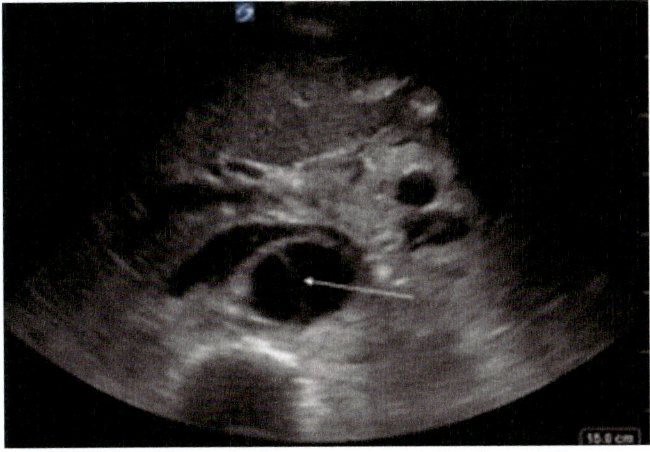

Fig. 17.42 Abdominal US (Reprinted from Creditt AB, Joyce M. Abdominal Aortic Aneurysm Ultrasound. In: Creditt A, Tozer J, Vitto M, Joyce M, Taylor L (eds). Clinical Ultrasound: A Pocket Manual. Cham, Switzerland: Springer Nature. 2018: 135–147. With permission from Springer Nature)

Question 56

Which of the following techniques is most likely to aid in identification of the true lumen in abdominal aortic dissection?

A. Two-dimensional imaging will show intimal flap movement into the true lumen during systole.
B. On M-mode imaging of the descending aorta, the larger lumen is usually the false lumen.
C. The larger false lumen will likely have higher velocity blood flow than the smaller true lumen.
D. The true lumen will show aliasing on color-flow doppler assessment

Answer: B.

Key Points: An aortic dissection with infrarenal involvement can be seen on abdominal ultrasonography and aid in the rapid diagnosis of an unstable patient.

Rationale: Acute aortic dissection is an emergency and should receive prompt treatment. The true lumen is most likely the narrower lumen. This is most likely in the setting of decreased mesenteric blood flow due to a static or dynamic obstruction from a large dissection flap, leading to the symptoms seen in this patient. The intimal flap moves in unison with the outer wall and usually moves towards the false lumen in systole [74, 75].

Question 57

The patient develops worsening shortness of breath and hypotension, with a widening pulse pressure. Which of the following findings would support the need for urgent surgical intervention?

A. Loss of holodiastolic flow on pulse wave doppler in the false lumen.
B. Steep systolic upstroke on pulse wave doppler with continuation of low velocity flow during diastole in the true lumen.
C. Aliasing systolic flow on pulse wave doppler in the true lumen.
D. Holodiastolic flow reversal on pulse wave doppler in the true lumen.

Answer: D.

Key Points: Identification of a Stanford Type A versus Type B dissection is critical as they require different management and different mortality risks.

Rationale: An acute aortic dissection associated with holodiastolic flow reversal in the descending aorta suggests severe aortic regurgitation. This would be classified as a Stanford Type A dissection requiring surgical intervention [74–76].

Question 58

A 66-year-old male with a history of hypertension, and former smoking presents to the hospital with complaints of gradually worsening epigastric and back pain for the past 2 months. A CT of the abdomen/pelvis shows an infra-renal abdominal aortic aneurysm. An abdominal ultrasound is performed with the image shown below. Which of the following best describes the management of this pathology? (Fig. 17.43)

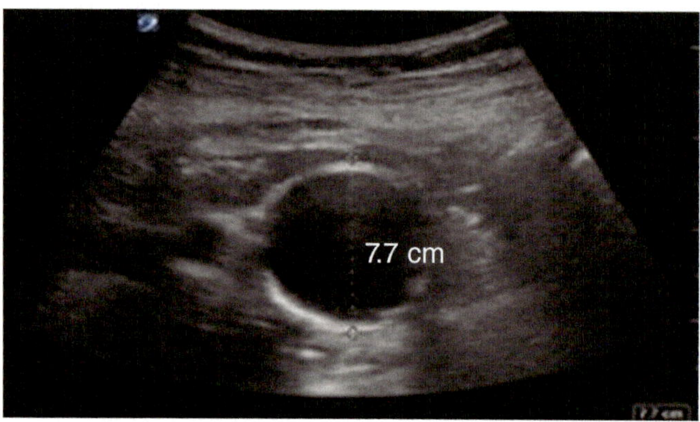

Fig. 17.43 Abdominal ultrasound (Reprinted from Creditt AB, Joyce M. Abdominal Aortic Aneurysm Ultrasound. In: Creditt A, Tozer J, Vitto M, Joyce M, Taylor L (eds). Clinical Ultrasound: A Pocket Manual. Cham, Switzerland: Springer Nature. 2018: 135–147. With permission from Springer Nature)

A. Surgical management is deferred until vessel size is larger than 8.0 cm.
B. A symptomatic patient is a surgical candidate regardless of vessel diameter.
C. Open surgical intervention is the only option for vessels of this size.
D. Endovascular repair was indicated when the vessel diameter reached 5 cm in this patient.

Answer: B.

Key Point: Surgical repair is recommended for aneurysm > 5.5 cm, rate of enlargement > 1 cm/year or symptomatic aneurysm of any size.

Rationale: The goal of elective abdominal aortic aneurysm repair is to reduce risk of rupture and prolong life. Identification of appropriate surgical candidates is important in patients with abdominal aortic aneurysms. An abdominal aortic vessel diameter > 5.5 cm in asymptomatic patients, or presence of symptoms with any size aortic aneurysm is an indication for surgical intervention. Risk of rupture increases as aneurysm size enlarges [75, 77, 78].

For Questions 59 and 60, refer to the following vignette:

A 35-year-old G3P2 female presents to the emergency room with lower abdominal pain, nausea, vomiting for the past 4 days. She is also experiencing intermittent vaginal bleeding for the past week. She is unsure of her last menstrual period but states it was at least 6 weeks ago. A urine B-HCG level is positive. She is tachycardic with a blood pressure of 118/65. The ultrasound examinations performed are shown below (Figs. 17.44 and 17.45).

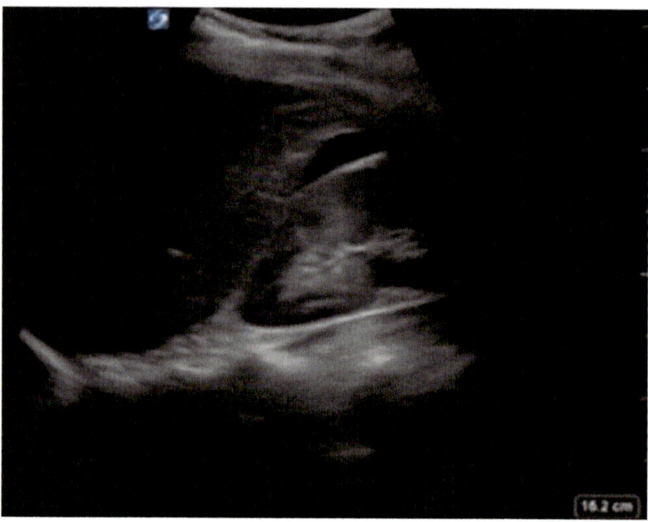

Fig. 17.44 Ultrasound (Reprinted from Creditt AB, Vitto M. Extended Focused Assessment with Sonography for Trauma. In: Creditt A, Tozer J, Vitto M, Joyce M, Taylor L (eds). Clinical Ultrasound: A Pocket Manual. Cham, Switzerland: Springer Nature. 2018: 19–45. With permission from Springer Nature)

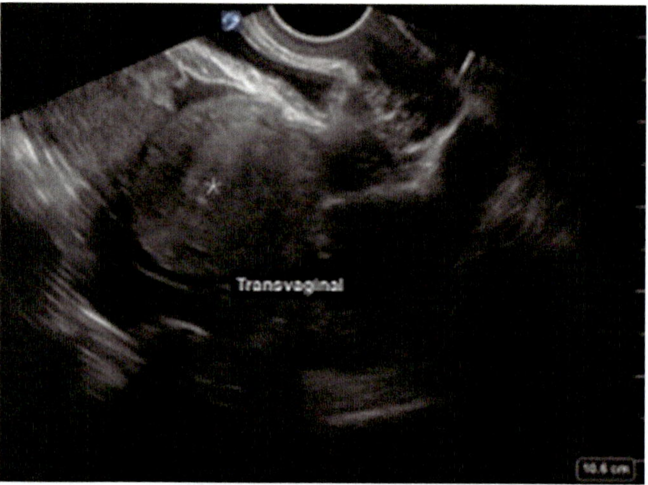

Fig. 17.45 Ultrasound (Reprinted from Tozer J, Creditt AB. Obstetric Ultrasound. In: Creditt A, Tozer J, Vitto M, Joyce M, Taylor L (eds). Clinical Ultrasound: A Pocket Manual. Cham, Switzerland: Springer Nature. 2018: 213–236. With permission from Springer Nature)

Question 59
Which of the following is true?

A. This patient has a low risk of hemodynamic instability and should be managed conservatively.
B. A transvaginal exam is not indicated in this circumstance.
C. The volume of free fluid present does not determine risk of ectopic pregnancy.
D. This patient will require an emergent surgical consultation.

Answer: D.

Key Point: Transvaginal ultrasound showing no gestational sac coupled with positive HCG is considered strongly predictive of ectopic pregnancy.

Rationale: Free fluid extending to Morrison's pouch coupled with large volume pelvic fluid and clinical history has a nearly 100% sensitivity for ectopic pregnancy. This patient will require an emergency surgical consultation for intra-abdominal bleeding. A transvaginal exam will help reveal the amount of free fluid present in the pelvis and the lack of a gestational sac to confirm the diagnosis. Most reliable diagnosis of ectopic pregnancy is to visualize the extrauterine gestation, however, this may not be present in 15–35% cases. Fig. 17.45 shows the yolk sac behind the empty uterus (marked by the asterisk) [79, 80].

Question 60
Which of the following is **TRUE** regarding the ultrasound image obtained in Fig. 17.44?

A. This was performed in the right lower quadrant along the mid axillary line with marker towards the head.
B. The liver is a heterogeneous structure and thus causes attenuation artifact for deeper structures.
C. Free fluid is seen as anechoic collection and should not be present in this location normally.
D. The diaphragm is not visible in this image and is necessary to make a diagnosis.

Answer: C.

Key Point: In the supine patient free fluid collects first in the hepatorenal recess due to gravity dependent drainage.

Rationale: The hepatorenal recess (Morrison's pouch) does not normally contain free fluid and is very sensitive for intra-abdominal fluid accumulation. The liver is a homogenous structure and allows for improved imaging to deeper structures due to lower ultrasound attenuation, sometimes leading to enhancement artifacts. The delineation of the diaphragm will help in establishing a diagnosis but is not required for free fluid identification if already present in the hepatorenal recess [79, 81].

Question 61
When performing a pelvic transabdominal ultrasound on a female patient, which of the following is most likely to be **TRUE**?

A. An empty bladder will provide better acoustic imaging.
B. A linear probe with a range of 5–12 MHz is the optimal imaging tool.
C. Free fluid in the rectouterine pouch is a normal finding.
D. A transvaginal ultrasound is only indicated if an intrauterine pregnancy is identified.

Answer: C.

Key Point: A small amount of free fluid in the rectouterine pouch (pouch of douglas) is normal in females of childbearing age.

Rationale: A transvaginal ultrasound has higher sensitivity and specificity for abnormal pelvic findings and is usually indicated if evidence of uterine or pregnancy related abnormalities are suspected. A curvilinear probe with a range of 3.5–5 Mhz is optimal and a full bladder will improve transabdominal imaging by decreasing attenuation for deeper structures [79, 80].

For Questions 62 and 63, refer to the vignette below:

A 27-year-old G2P1 30-week pregnant female with a history of prior cesarean section presents to the emergency room with intermittent spotting and vaginal bleeding that began a few hours ago. She denies abdominal pain, nausea, vomiting or fevers. She has a heart rate of 105 beats per minute with a blood pressure of 102/63 mmHg. Fetal heart tones are present at 145 beats per minute. A transabdominal ultrasound is performed with the following image (Fig. 17.46).

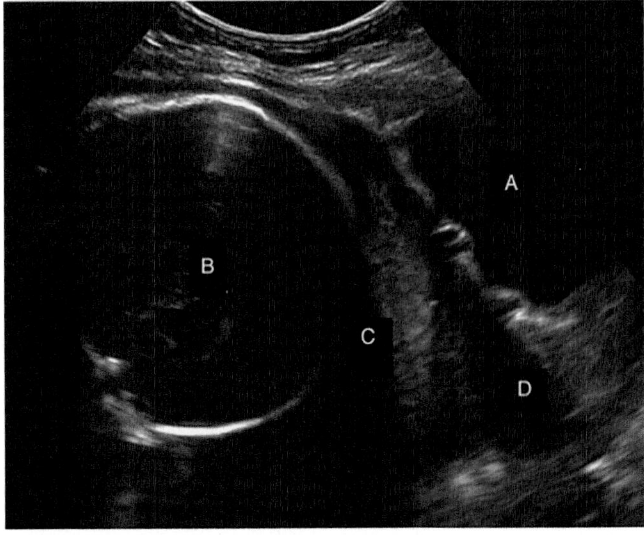

Fig. 17.46 Abdominal ultrasound (Reprinted from Oyelese Y, Canterino JC. Placenta Previa and Placenta Accreta. In: Sheiner E (ed.) Bleeding During Pregnancy: A Comprehensive Guide. New York, NY: Springer Nature; 2011: 135–150. With permission from Springer Nature)

Question 62
The structure labeled as A represents which of the following structures?

A. Physiologic free fluid in the pelvis
B. Bladder
C. Ovarian cyst
D. Intraabdominal bleeding

Answer: B.

Key Points: Bladder identification is key in helping probe positioning and imaging.

Rationale: Fluid is anechoic, and urine present in the bladder will appear as such. A full bladder can enhance imaging of posterior structures. Alternatively, it can become a hindrance during specific examination when full, such as in examination of improper placental implantation due to the pressure applied to the cervical os [79, 82].

Question 63
Which of the following is TURE when performing pelvic ultrasonography in this patient?

A. Place the patient in a sitting position for the duration of the exam.
B. Amniotic fluid present between the cervix and presenting part of the fetus excludes placenta previa.
C. Transvaginal imaging is an absolute contraindication for this patient.
D. A full bladder is necessary for appropriate identification of placenta previa.

Answer: B.

Key Point: Examination of the location and properties of the placenta is essential in diagnosing placenta previa. In a normal uterus there is no placental tissue between the fetus and cervix; the space is filled with anechoic fluid.

Rationale: Understanding the findings that rule out placenta previa is important in assessing pregnant patients with vaginal bleeding. A supine or even Trendelenburg position can help improve visualization by moving the fetus cephalad. Transvaginal imaging is not an absolute contraindication and can be performed safely according to ACOG guidelines. In the image, a complete posterior placenta previa (structure marked C) is seen between the fetal head (structure marked B) and the cervix (structure marked D). Amniotic fluid, which will be anechoic on ultrasound, should normally be present between the presenting part of the fetus and the cervix and would rule out placenta previa [82, 83].

Question 64
A 31-year-old G4P3 female presents to the emergency room with worsening abdominal pain over the past few hours. She has a history of hypertension, smoking and is 34 weeks pregnant. Her past two deliveries were by cesarean section. The patient has a heart rate of 125 beats per minute with a blood pressure of 140/74. There is scant vaginal bleeding on initial examination. Her abdomen is also tender to palpation. Fetal heart tones show a heart rate of 150 with variable decelerations. Abdominal ultrasonography is performed to aid with diagnosis with the image shown (Fig. 17.47).

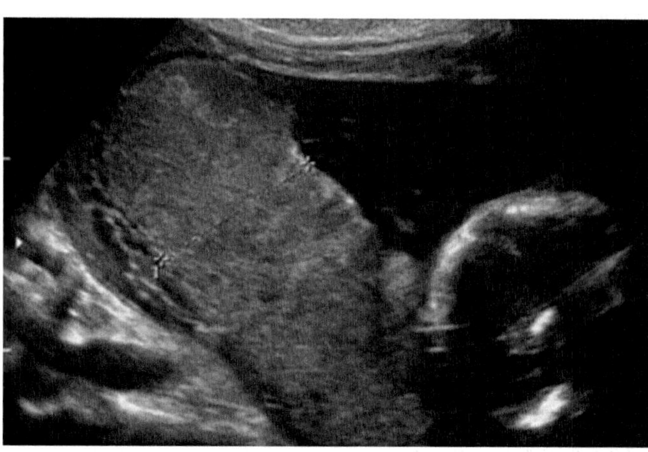

Fig. 17.47 Abdominal ultrasound (Reprinted from Wielgos M, Jarmuzek P, Pietrzak B. Abruptio Placenta. In: Malvasi A, Tinelli A, Di Renzo G. (ed.) Management and Therapy of Late Pregnancy Complications. Cham, Switzerland: Springer Nature; 2017: 37–52. With permission from Springer Nature)

Which of the following pathological findings associated with this patient are **TRUE**?

A. Lack of vaginal bleeding on presentation rules out emergent pathology.
B. Placenta previa is present in this patient leading to the clinical finding.
C. Retroplacental bleeding is likely and no further confirmatory testing is needed.
D. Free floating echogenic material in the amniotic fluid would be a reassuring sign.

Answer: D.

Key Point: The sonographic findings of placental abruption include: retroplacental hematoma, intra placental anechoic areas, thickening of the placental over 5.5 cm and separation and rounding of placental edges.

Rationale: Placental abruption is an emergency and should be identified quickly. Ultrasonography can expedite the diagnosis especially when frank vaginal bleeding and hypotension are not initially present. Although ultrasound sensitivity for visualization of a hematoma is <50%, it can help differentiate between placental abruption and placenta previa. Subchorionic, retroplacental, parenchymal, pre-placental bleeding can be visualized and aid in diagnosis [79, 84, 85].

Question 65

A 35-year-old G4P2 27-week pregnant female presents to the emergency room for abdominal pain, nausea, and vomiting that started 4 hrs ago. She states the pain feels like constant contractions and has noticed decreased fetal movement since the pain started. She has had a small amount of vaginal bleeding since the pain began. A transabdominal ultrasound is performed with the image shown below (Fig. 17.48).

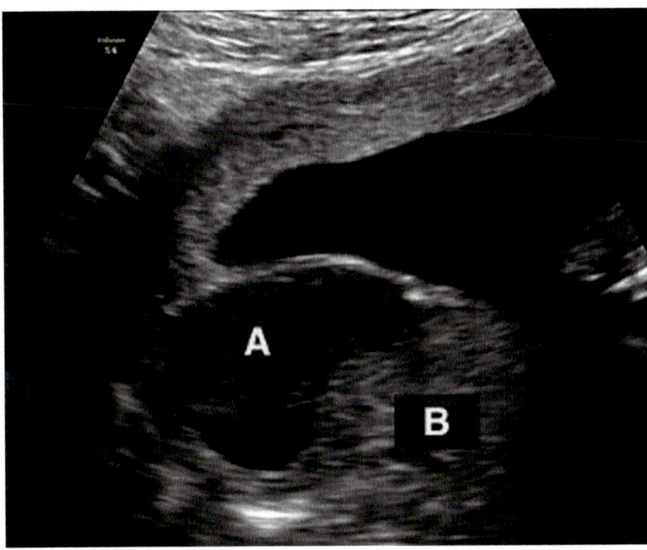

Fig. 17.48 Ultrasound (Reprinted from Wielgos M, Jarmuzek P, Pietrzak B. Abruptio Placenta. In: Malvasi A, Tinelli A, Di Renzo G. (ed.) Management and Therapy of Late Pregnancy Complications. Cham, Switzerland: Springer Nature; 2017: 37–52. With permission from Springer Nature)

Which of the following is true regarding the structures labeled in the image?

A. Structure 'A' is a normal finding
B. Structure 'B' represents new-onset bleeding and current hemodynamic instability
C. The size of structure A has no importance in the prognosis of this patient
D. Structure 'A' suggests the patient is at high risk for hemodynamic instability

Answer: D.

Key Points: A placental abruption is a clinical diagnosis and treatment should not be delayed, to avoid fetal and maternal morbidity.

Rationale: Ultrasound imaging can show hematoma formation in multiple locations around the placenta to help with diagnosis of placental abruption. This image shows a marginal hematoma, and the patient requires an urgent operation to save the fetus and avoid maternal morbidity as hemodynamic instability is inevitable. If the measured size of the hematoma exceeds 50 mL, there is a higher risk for poor prognosis for both mother and fetus. Structure 'B' shows the placenta detached from the uterine wall [79, 84, 85].

For Questions 66 and 67, refer to the vignette below:

A 68-year-old male presents to the emergency room with fever, abdominal pain, distension, nausea, vomiting that has progressively worsened for the past 3 days. He has a history of multiple prior abdominal surgeries. He is diffusely tender to palpation of the abdomen. He is tachycardic with a heart rate of 120 beats/min and a blood pressure of 93/47 mmHg. Laboratory workup shows a lactic acidosis of 4 mmol/L and white blood cell count of 23,000 cells/μL. An abdominal CT scan is ordered, and an ultrasound is performed in the interim with the image shown below (Fig. 17.49).

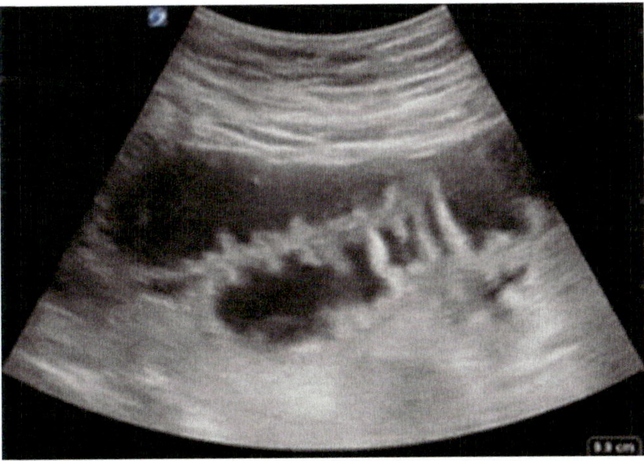

Fig. 17.49 Abdominal ultrasound (Reprinted from Creditt AB, Vitto M. Abdominal Ultrasound. In: Creditt A, Tozer J, Vitto M, Joyce M, Taylor L (eds). Clinical Ultrasound: A Pocket Manual. Cham, Switzerland: Springer Nature. 2018: 185–195. With permission from Springer Nature)

Question 66
Which of the following is TRUE regarding small bowel imaging on ultrasound?

A. A paralytic ileus will show decompressed bowel with wall thickening.
B. The presence of dilated small bowel loops is the most sensitive and specific finding on ultrasound for an SBO.
C. Prominent plicae circulares indicate normal bowel function is intact.
D. Jejunum is considered dilated when >1.5 cm and ileum is considered dilated when >1 cm.

Answer: B.

Key Points: Knowing the findings of small bowel obstruction on ultrasound will help expedite care for a patient and may help avoid an unnecessary CT scan.

Rationale: Clinical signs in addition to the ultrasound findings can help establish a diagnosis of small bowel obstruction much faster than formal CT with contrast imaging. Dilation of jejunal loops >2.5 cm and ileum >1.5 cm, with increased peristalsis, collapsed colonic lumen, and bowel wall edema are all signs of small bowel obstruction. Dilated proximal bowel with collapsed distal bowel can also help identify a transition point. In contrast, a paralytic ileus will have dilated small and large bowel with hypomotility and will generally lack bowel wall thickening [34, 86, 87].

Question 67
Which of the following is most likely TRUE about this patient's abdominal ultrasound?

A. Echogenic material within the bowel lumen moving in a whirling pattern.
B. Conniventes valvulae are most commonly seen in ileal obstructions and not jejunal obstructions.
C. A large bowel obstruction is 4–5 times more likely than a small bowel obstruction.
D. Abdominal X-ray will have a higher sensitivity and specificity in detecting this small bowel obstruction.
E. A CT scan of the abdomen is not needed.

Answer: A.

Key Points: Ultrasound findings suggesting small bowel obstruction include a to-and-fro pattern of fluid and echogenic material within the bowel lumen, which will move in a whirling pattern.

Rationale: Multiple findings will be present on ultrasound in this patient with an acute small bowel obstruction. Conniventes valvulae (plicae circulares) are present in the small bowel and are most prominently seen in jejunum during a small bowel obstruction. A small bowel obstruction is 4–5 times more likely than a large bowel obstruction and is definitely present in this patient. Despite a high sensitivity and specificity of ultrasound findings of small bowel obstruction, a CT scan of the abdomen and pelvis is still standard of care and will not only confirm the diagnosis of a small bowel obstruction, but also help with identifying the location of obstruction for surgical approach and prognostication of the disease process [34, 86, 87].

References

1. Minami T. Ultrasound in the intensive care unit. In: Jankowich M, Gartman E, editors. Abdominal ultrasound and genitourinary ultrasound in the intensive care unit. New York, NY: Humana Press; 2015. p. 249–72.
2. Hensley B, St-Cyr Bourque J, Noble VE. General diagnostic abdominal sonography. In: Brown SM, Blaivas M, Hirshberg EL, Kasal J, Pustavoitau A, editors. Comprehensive critical care ultrasound. 1st ed. Mount Prospect, IL: Society of Critical Care Medicine; 2015. p. 125.
3. Creditt A, Joyce M. Renal and bladder ultrasound. In: Creditt A, Tozer J, Vitto M, Joyce M, Taylor L, editors. Clinical ultrasound: a pocket manual. Cham: Switzerland: Springer Nature; 2018. p. 167–84.
4. Lubomirova M, Krasteva R, Bogov B, Paskalev E. Incidence of A-V fistulas after renal biopsy of native and transplanted kidney—two Centers experience. Open Access Maced J Med Sci. 2015;3(2):241–4.
5. Hamm B, Ros PR. Chapter 112—Kidney trauma. In: Abdominal imaging. Springer-Verlag Berlin Heidelberg. 2013: 1790–1791.
6. Harrison KL, Nghiem HV, Coldwell DM, Davis CL. Renal dysfunction due to an arteriovenous fistula in a transplant recipient. JASN. 1994;5(6):1300–6.
7. Lichtenstein DA. Urinary tract. In: Lichtenstein DA, editor. Whole body ultrasonography in the critically ill. Heidelberg, Germany: Springer; 2010. p. 69–76.
8. Woods AH. Ultrasound in trauma critical care. In: Jankowich M, Gartman E, editors. Ultrasound in the intensive care unit. Respiratory medicine. New York, NY: Humana Press; 2015. p. 295–321.
9. Dicuio M, Pomara G, Menchini Fabris F, Ales V, Dahlstrand C, Morelli G. Measurements of urinary bladder volume: comparison of five ultrasound calculation methods in volunteers. Arch Ital Urol Androl. 2005;77(1):60–2.
10. Hvarness H, Skjoldbye B, Jakobsen H. Urinary bladder volume measurements: comparison of three ultrasound calculation methods. Scand J Urol Nephrol. 2002;36(3):177–81.
11. Kao HW, Wu CJ. Ultrasound of renal infectious disease. J Med Ultrasound. 2008;16(2):113–22.
12. Schneider F, Pahernik S. Kidney and renal pelvis: inflammation. In: Hamm B, Ros PR, editors. Abdominal Imaging. Heidelberg, Germany: Springer; 2013. p. 1739–44.
13. Mazziotti S, Cicero G, D'Angelo T, et al. Imaging and management of incidental renal lesions. Biomed Res Int. 2017;2017:1854027.
14. Eknoyan GA. Clinical view of simple and complex renal cysts. JASN. 2009;20(9):1874–6.
15. Keays MA, Guerra LA, Mihill J, et al. Reliability assessment of Society for Fetal Urology ultrasound grading system for hydronephrosis. J Urol. 2008;180(4):1680–2.
16. Wang LJ. Renal cystic disease. In: Key diagnostic features in uroradiology. Cham, Switzerland: Springer Nature; 2015: 97–139.

17. Vancauwenberghe T, Snoeckx A, Vanbeckevoort D, Dymarkowski S, Vanhoenacker FM. Imaging of the spleen: what the clinician needs to know. Singap Med J. 2015;56(3):133–44.
18. Catalano OA, Soricelli A, Salvatore M. Spleen anatomy, function and development. In: Hamm B, Ros PR, editors. Abdominal Imaging. Heidelberg, Germany: Springer; 2013. p. 1479–94.
19. Lichtenstein DA. Various targets in the abdomen (spleen, adrenals, pancreas, lymph nodes). In: Lichtenstein DA, editor. Whole body ultrasonography in the critically ill. Heidelberg, Germany: Springer; 2010. p. 77–81.
20. Richards JR, McGahan JP, Jones CD, et al. Ultrasound detection of blunt splenic injury. Injury. 2001;32(2):95–103.
21. Ganguli S. Spleen: trauma, vascular, and interventional radiology. In: Hamm B, Ros PR, editors. Abdominal Imaging. Heidelberg, Germany: Springer; 2013. p. 1523–32.
22. Chun JY, Kim YH. Spleen infectious and inflammatory disorders. In: Hamm B, Ros PR, editors. Abdominal imaging. Heidelberg, Germany: Springer; 2013. p. 1511–22.
23. Thanos L, Dailiana T, Papaioannou G, et al. Percutaneous CT-guided drainage of splenic abscess. Am J Roentgenol. 2002;179(3):629–32.
24. Divyashree S, Gupta N. Splenic abscess in immunocompetent patients managed primarily without splenectomy: a series of 7 cases. Perm J. 2017;21:16–139.
25. Van de Putte P, Perlas A. Ultrasound assessment of gastric content and volume. BJA: Br J Anaesth. 2014;113(1):12–22.
26. El-Boghdadly K, Wojcikiewicz T, Perlas A. Perioperative point-of-care gastric ultrasound. BJA Educ. 2019;19(7):219–26.
27. Cubilos J, Tse C, Chan VW, Perlas A. Bedside ultrasound assessment of gastric content: an observational study. Can J Anaesth. 2012;59(4):416–23.
28. Kruisselbrink R, Gharapetian A, Chaparro LE, Ami N, Richler D, Chan VWS, Perlas A. Diagnostic accuracy of point-of-care gastric ultrasound. Anesth Analg. 2019;128(1):89–95.
29. Scionti A, Rossi P, Gulino P, Semeraro A, Defilippi C, Tonerini M. Acute pyelonephritis. In: Miele V, Trinci M, editors. Imaging non-traumatic abdominal emergencies in pediatric patients. Cham, Switzerland: Springer Nature; 2016. p. 255–68.
30. Praz V, Burruni R, Meid F, Wisard M, Jichlinski P, Tawadros T. Fungus ball in the urinary tract: a rare entity. Can Urol Assoc J. 2014;8(1–2):E118-20.
31. Ödev K, Turgut AT, MacLennan GT. Inflammatory conditions of the kidney. In: Dogra V, MacLennan G, editors. Genitourinary radiology: kidney, bladder and urethra. London, UK: Springer; 2013. p. 65–93.
32. Oyen R. Imaging of pyelonephritis. In: Cova M, Stacul F, editors. Pain imaging. Cham, Switzerland: Springer Nature; 2019. p. 303–22.
33. Ubee SS, McGlynn L, Fordham M. Emphysematous pyelonephritis. BJU Int. 2011;107(9):1474–8.
34. Abu-Zidan FM, Cevik AA. Diagnostic point-of-care ultrasound (POCUS) for gastrointestinal pathology: state of the art from basics to advanced. World J Emerg Surg. 2018;13:47.
35. Jiang L, Wu J, Feng X. The value of ultrasound in diagnosis of pneumoperitoneum in emergent or critical conditions: a meta-analysis. Hong Kong J Emerg Med. 2019;26(2):111–7.
36. Cortellaro F, Perani C, Guarnieri L, et al. Point-of-care ultrasound in the diagnosis of acute abdominal pain. In: Aseni P, De Carlis L, Mazzola A, Grande A, editors. Operative techniques and recent advances in acute care and emergency surgery. Cham, Switzerland: Springer Nature; 2019. p. 383–401.
37. Hefny AF, Abu-Zidan FM. Sonographic diagnosis of intraperitoneal free air. J Emerg Trauma Shock. 2011;4(4):511–3.
38. Khan MAB, Abu-Zidan FM. Point-of-care ultrasound for the acute abdomen in the primary health care. Turkish J Emerg Med. 2020;20(1):1–11.
39. Mostbeck G, Adam EJ, Nielsen MB, et al. How to diagnose acute appendicitis: ultrasound first. Insights Imaging. 2016;7(2):255–63.
40. Shirah BH, Shirah HA, Alhaidari WA, et al. The role of preoperative graded compression ultrasound in detecting acute appendicitis and influencing the negative appendectomy rate. Abdom Radiol. 2017;42(1):109–14.
41. Riedesel EL, Weber BC, Shore MW, et al. Diagnostic performance of standardized ultrasound protocol for detecting perforation in pediatric appendicitis. Pediatr Radiol. 2019;49(13):1726–34.
42. Villar J, Summers SM, Menchine MD, et al. The absence of gallstones on point-of care ultrasound rules out acute cholecystitis. J Emerg Med. 2015;49(4):487–0.
43. Zenobii MF, Accogli E, Domanico A, et al. Update on beside ultrasound (US) diagnosis of acute cholecysitits (AC). Intern Emerg Med. 2016;11(2):261–4.
44. Kaoutzanis C, Davies E, Leichtle SW, et al. Abdominal ultrasound versus hepato-imino diacetic acid scan in diagnosing aucte cholecystitis—what is the real benefit? J Surg Res. 2014;188(1):44–52.
45. Cox M, Patel M, Joneja U, et al. Focal disruption in the wall of the porcelain gallbladder: a sign of gallbladder carcinoma. Intern Emerg Med. 2017;12:891–3.
46. Dugdale P. Biliary imaging for gallstone disease. In: Cox M, Eslick G, Padbury R, editors. The management of gallstone disease. Cham, Switzerland: Springer Nature; 2018. p. 21–51.
47. Shapira-Rootman M, Mahamid A, Reindrop N, et al. Diagnosis of gallbladder perforation by ultrasound. Clin Imaging. 2015;39(5):827–9.
48. Elliott T. Gallbladder polyps, sludge and adenomyomatosis. In: Cox M, Eslick G, Padbury R, editors. The management of gallstone disease. Cham, Switzerland: Springer Nature; 2018. p. 137–46.
49. Wiles R, Thoeni RF, et al. Management and follow-up of gallbladder polyps. Eur Radiol. 2017;27(9):3856–66.
50. Choi TW, Kim JH, Park SJ, et al. Risk stratification of gallbladder polyps larger than 10 mm using high-resolution ultrasonography and texture analysis. Eur Radiol. 2017;28(1):196–205.
51. Burrowes DP, Choi HH, Rodgers SK, et al. Utility of ultrasound in acute pancreatitis. Abdom Radiol (NY). 2020;45(5):1253–64.
52. O'Connor OJ, Neill SO, Maher MM. Imaging of biliary tract disease. Am J Roentgenol. 2011;197(4):W551–8.
53. Talukdar R. Complications of ERCP. Best Pract Res Clin Gastroenterol. 2016;30(5):793–805.
54. Kaltenbach TEM, Engler P, Kratzer W, et al. Prevalence of benign focal liver lesions: ultrasound investigation of 45,319 hospital patients. Abdom Radiol (NY). 2016;41(1):25–32.
55. Virmani J, Kumar V, Kalra N, et al. Characterization of primary and secondary malignant liver lesions from B-mode ultrasound. J Digit Imaging. 2013;26(6):1058–70.
56. Kong WT, Wang WP, Huang BJ, et al. Contrast-enhanced ultrasound in combination with color doppler ultrasound can improve the diagnostic performance of focal nodular hyperplasia and hepatocellular adenoma. Ultrasound Med Biol. 2015;41(4):944–51.
57. Kim KW, Kim TK, Han JK, et al. Hepatic hemangiomas: spectrum of US appearances on gray-scale, power Doppler, and contrast-enhanced US. Korean J Radiol. 2000;1(4):191–7.
58. Hoffmann B, Nürnberg D, Westergaard MC. Focus on abnormal air: diagnostic ultrasonography for the acute abdomen. Eur J Emerg Med. 2012;19(5):284–91.
59. Karahan O, Kurt A, Yikilmaz A, Kahriman G. New method for the detection of intraperitoneal free air by sonography: scissors maneuver. J Clin Ultrasound. 2004;32(8):381–5.
60. Wichmann MW. Diverticular disease. In: Wichmann M, McCullough T, Roberts-Thomson I, Maddern G, editors. Gastroenterology for general surgeons. Cham, Switzerland: Springer Nature; 2019. p. 13–20.

61. Creditt AB, Vitto M. Extended focused assessment with sonography for trauma. In: Creditt A, Tozer J, Vitto M, Joyce M, Taylor L, editors. Clinical ultrasound: a pocket manual. Cham, Switzerland: Springer Nature; 2018. p. 19–45.
62. Giannasi G. Ultrasound exam approach in trauma patients. In: Sarti A, Lorini F, editors. Textbook of echocardiography for intensivists and emergency physicians. Cham, Switzerland: Springer Nature; 2019. p. 513–32.
63. Kameda T, Taniguchi N. Overview of point-of-care abdominal ultrasound in emergency and critical care. J Intensive Care. 2016;4:53.
64. Sethi J, Halvorson K. Principles of ultrasound for the intensivist. In: Jankowich M, Gartman E, editors. Ultrasound in the intensive care unit. respiratory medicine. New York, NY: Humana Press; 2015. p. 1–18.
65. Vitto M, Creditt AB. Introduction: basic ultrasound principles. In: Creditt A, Tozer J, Vitto M, Joyce M, Taylor L, editors. Clinical ultrasound: a pocket manual. Cham, Switzerland: Springer Nature; 2018. p. 1–18.
66. Lorini FL, Cerutti S, Di Dedda G. Pericardium and pericardial disease. In: Sarti A, Lorini FL, editors. Textbook of echocardiography for intensivists and emergency physicians. Cham, Switzerland: Springer Nature; 2019. p. 117–23.
67. Cipani S, Marini F. Acute dyspnea. In: Sarti A, Lorini FL, editors. Textbook of echocardiography for intensivists and emergency physicians. Cham, Switzerland: Springer Nature; 2019. p. 351–61.
68. Lichtenstein DA. Pneumothorax. In: Whole body ultrasonography in the critically ill. Heidelberg, Germany: Springer-Verlag; 2010: 163–178.
69. Lichtenstein DA. Peritoneum. In: Whole body ultrasonography in the critically ill. Heidelberg, Germany: Springer; 2010. p. 33–40.
70. Edelman S. Ultrasound physics. In: Edelman S, editor. Understanding ultrasound physics. Woodlands, TX: ESP; 2016. p. 1–38.
71. Tozer J, Creditt AB, Joyce M. Cardiac ultrasound. In: Creditt A, Tozer J, Vitto M, Joyce M, Taylor L, editors. Clinical ultrasound: a pocket manual. Cham, Switzerland: Springer Nature; 2018. p. 47–73.
72. Nair GB, Mathew JP. Critical care echocardiography: pericardial disease, tamponade, and other topics. In: Jankovich M, Gartman E, editors. Ultrasound in the intensive care unit. Respiratory medicine. New York, NY: Humana Press; 2015. p. 147–73.
73. Mayo PH. Pericardial effusion and cardiac tamponade. In: Backer D, Cholley BP, Slama M, Vieillard-Baron A, Vignon P, editors. Hemodynamic monitoring using echocardiography in the critically ill. Heidelberg, Germany: Springer; 2011. p. 151–62.
74. Vilacosta I, Cañadas V, San Román JA, Vignon P. Acute aortic syndrome: acute aortic diseases in hemodynamically unstable patients. In: Backer D, Cholley BP, Slama M, Vieillard-Baron A, Vignon P, editors. Hemodynamic monitoring using echocardiography in the critically ill. Heidelberg, Germany: Springer; 2011. p. 247–71.
75. Creditt AB, Joyce M. Abdominal aortic aneurysm ultrasound. In: Creditt A, Tozer J, Vitto M, Joyce M, Taylor L, editors. Clinical ultrasound: a pocket manual. Cham, Switzerland: Springer Nature; 2018. p. 135–47.
76. Zoghbi W, Adams D, Bonow RO, et al. Recommendations for noninvasive evaluation of native valvular regurgitation: a report from the American Society of Echocardiography developed in collaboration with the Society for Cardiovascular Magnetic Resonance. J Am Soc Echocardiogr. 2017;30(4):303–71.
77. Lichtenstein DA. Aorta. In: Whole body ultrasonography in the critically ill. Heidelberg, Germany: Springer-Verlag; 2010: 83–88.
78. Brewster DC, Cronenwett JL, Hallet JW Jr, et al. Guidelines for the treatment of abdominal aortic aneurysms. Report of a subcommittee of the Joint Council of the American Association for Vascular Surgery and Society for Vascular Surgery. J Vasc Surg. 2003;37(5):1106–17.
79. Tozer J, Creditt AB. Obstetric ultrasound. In: Creditt A, Tozer J, Vitto M, Joyce M, Taylor L, editors. Clinical ultrasound: a pocket manual. Cham, Switzerland: Springer Nature; 2018. p. 213–36.
80. Nickels LC. Ultrasound for ectopic pregnancy. In: Ganti L, editor. Atlas of emergency medicine procedures. New York, NY: Springer Nature; 2016. p. 643–7.
81. Harlev A, Wiznitzer A, Sheiner E. Ectopic pregnancy. In: Sheiner E, editor. Bleeding during pregnancy: a comprehensive guide. New York, NY: Springer Nature; 2011. p. 45–63.
82. Oyelese Y, Canterino JC. Placenta previa and placenta accreta. In: Sheiner E, editor. Bleeding during pregnancy: a comprehensive guide. New York, NY: Springer Nature; 2011. p. 135–50.
83. Nickels LC, De Portu G. Ultrasound for placenta previa. In: Ganti L, editor. Atlas of emergency medicine procedures. New York, NY: Springer Nature; 2016. p. 659–62.
84. Ananth CV, Kinzler WL. Placental abruption. In: Sheiner E, editor. Bleeding during pregnancy: a comprehensive guide. New York, NY: Springer Nature; 2011. p. 119–33.
85. Wielgos M, Jarmuzek P, Pietrzak B. Abruptio placenta. In: Malvasi A, Tinelli A, Di Renzo G, editors. Management and therapy of late pregnancy complications. Cham, Switzerland: Springer Nature; 2017. p. 37–52.
86. Iacobellis F, Laccetti E, Romano F, Altiero M, Scaglione M. Imaging of bowel obstruction and bowel perforation. In: Cova MA, Stacul F, editors. Pain Imaging. Cham, Switzerland: Springer Nature; 2019. p. 323–46.
87. Creditt AB, Vitto M. Abdominal ultrasound. In: Creditt A, Tozer J, Vitto M, Joyce M, Taylor L, editors. Clinical ultrasound: a pocket manual. Cham, Switzerland: Springer Nature; 2018. p. 185–95.

Vascular Ultrasound

18

Matthew Tabbut, Alexander Daves, Greg Adams, and Charles McCombs

Question 1
A 79-year-old female is admitted with bilateral lower extremity swelling and pain. As you perform the point-of-care ultrasound you note that this vessel is non-compressible. What is your next step in management? (Fig. 18.1).

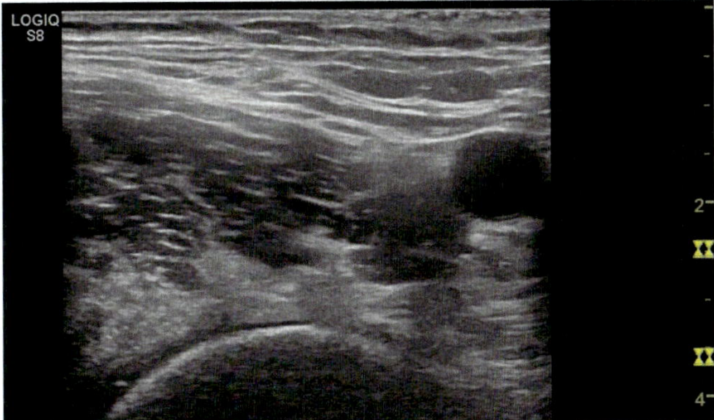

Fig. 18.1 Lower extremity vasculature at the level of the mid femoral vein

A. Comprehensive ultrasound
B. Move your transducer medially
C. Initiate anticoagulation
D. CT venogram of the iliac veins

Answer B: Move your transducer medially

The vessel imaged in this view is the common femoral artery which is immediately lateral to the common femoral vein. Veins are characterized by being thin-walled, anechoic and compressible. Arteries will have a thicker wall and typically appear with hyperechoic intima and adventitia layers with a hypoechoic media layer. Evaluation of the proper vessel should be performed before additional imaging is needed.

Question 2
Which vein is indicated by the arrow in Fig. 18.2?

A. Greater Saphenous Vein
B. Common Femoral Vein
C. Femoral Vein
D. Deep Femoral Vein

Answer D: Deep Femoral Vein.

M. Tabbut (✉)
Division of Emergency Ultrasound, Department of Emergency Medicine, MetroHealth Medical Center, Cleveland, OH, USA

Case Western Reserve University School of Medicine, Cleveland, OH, USA

Department of Emergency Medicine, The MetroHealth System, Cleveland, OH, USA
e-mail: mtabbut@metrohealth.org

A. Daves
Department of Emergency Medicine, Mountain View Hospital, Las Vegas, NV, USA

G. Adams
Department of Emergency Medicine, University of Colorado Health, Aurora, CO, USA

C. McCombs
Department of Pediatric Emergency Medicine, Nationwide Children's Hosptial, Columbus, OH, USA

R. Sreedharan et al. (eds.), *Critical Care Echocardiography*, https://doi.org/10.1007/978-3-031-45731-9_18

Fig. 18.2 Image of the lower extremity vasculature at the level of the proximal thigh

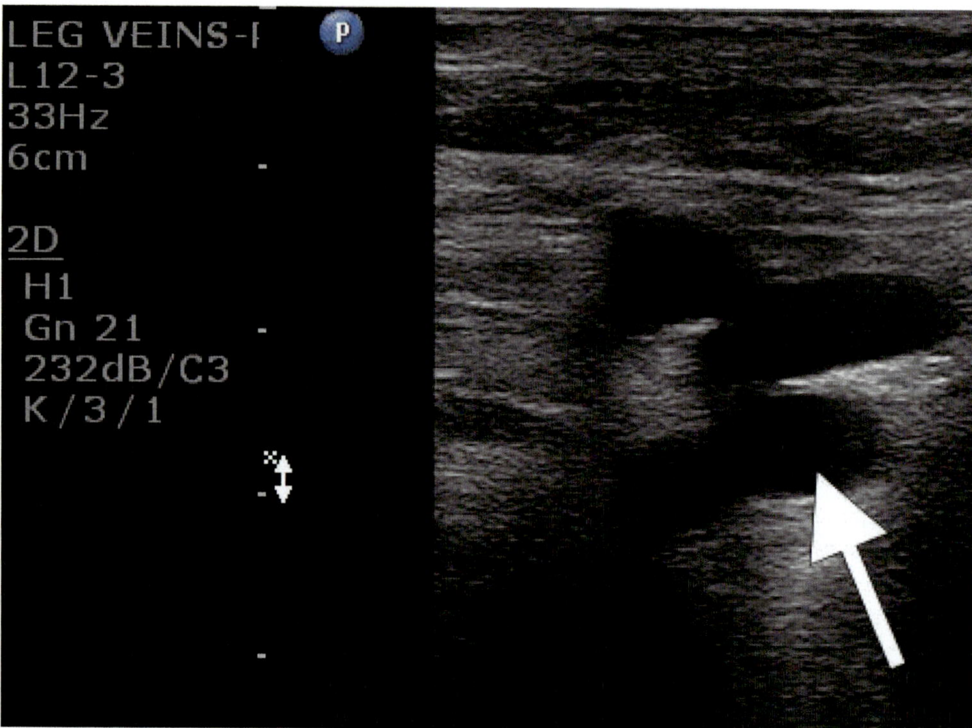

In this image the vein indicated is the deep femoral vein. The common femoral vein bifurcates in the proximal thigh into the femoral vein and the deep femoral vein. Drains blood from the medial thigh. Typically, this vessel is only visualized for a few cm beyond the bifurcation of the common femoral vein. Since it runs deep in the musculature of the thigh, the rate of isolated thrombosis in the deep femoral vein is low [1, 2].

Question 3
Which vessel is indicated by the arrow in Fig. 18.3?

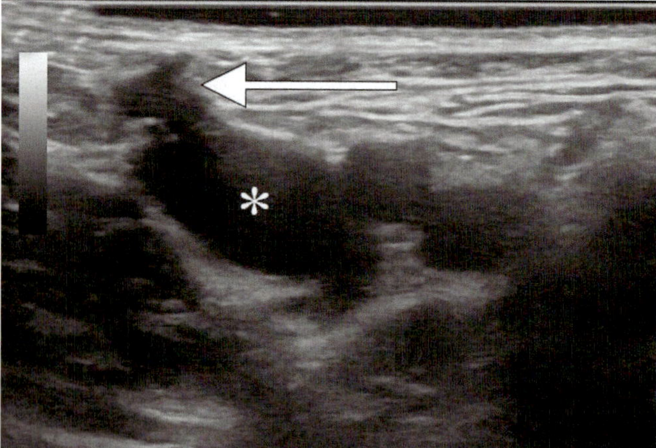

Fig. 18.3 Image of the lower extremity vasculature at the level of the proximal thigh

A. Greater Saphenous Vein
B. Common Femoral Vein
C. Femoral Vein
D. Deep Femoral Vein

Answer A: Greater Saphenous Vein.

This image shows the proximal portion of the deep venous system at the junction of the greater saphenous vein (arrow) and the common femoral vein (star). The GSV runs along the medial aspect of the leg and drains into the common femoral vein in the inguinal region. While it is technically a superficial vein, thrombi at or near the junction of the GSV and common femoral vein are often anticoagulation given the likelihood of propagation into the deep femoral system [1, 3].

Question 4
Which vessel is indicated by the star in Fig. 18.3?

A. Greater Saphenous Vein
B. Common Femoral Vein
C. Femoral Vein
D. Deep Femoral Vein

Answer B: Common Femoral Vein.

See answer to Question 3. The common femoral vein runs in parallel to the common femoral artery and is formed by the union of the femoral vein and the deep femoral vein in the thigh. It is joined medially by the greater saphenous vein and becomes the iliac vein as it passes through the inguinal canal. The common femoral vein runs medial to the common femoral artery [1].

Question 5

At what level is Fig. 18.4?

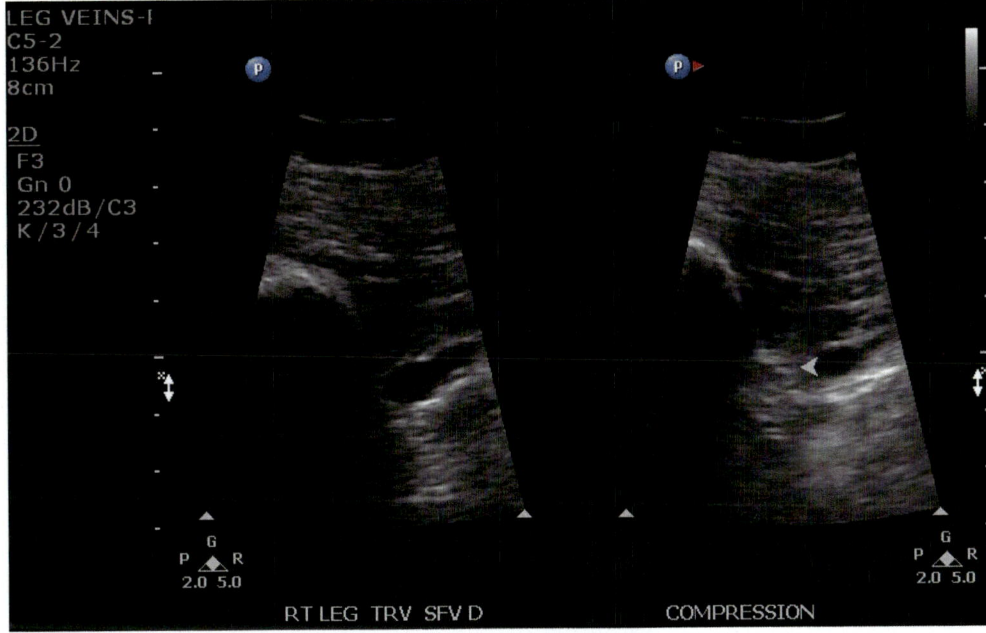

Fig. 18.4 Image of the lower extremity vasculature adjacent to the femur

A. Proximal thigh
B. Distal thigh
C. Popliteal fossa
D. Calf

Answer B: Distal Thigh.

This image is obtained of the femoral vein in the distal thigh. As the femoral vein descends the leg it travels medially and enters the popliteal fossa through the adductor canal. Sonographically, this the femoral vein will be in close proximity to the distal femur. Unless the patient is exceptionally thin, the femur is not well visualized in proximity to the vasculature in the proximal thigh or popliteal fossa.

Question 6

A critically ill 67-year-old male is in the intensive care unit for septic shock, respiratory failure and hypotension. As you begin to place an internal jugular central venous catheter you notice the following on your ultrasonographic survey prior to placement. Which of the following is the next best step? (Fig. 18.5)

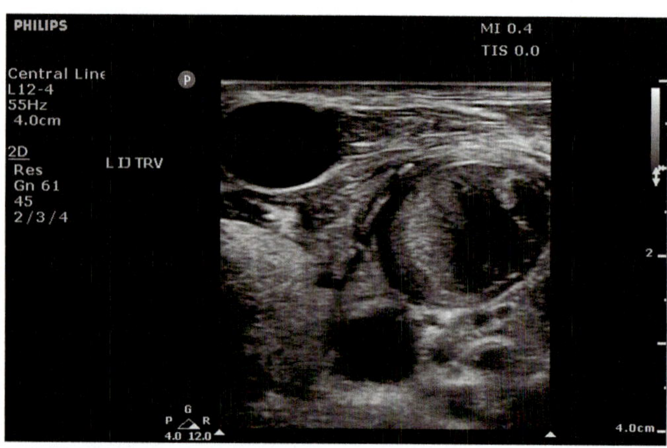

Fig. 18.5 Image of the left internal jugular vein

A. Attempt to pass the guidewire through the obstruction
B. Change to left subclavian access site
C. Change to contralateral internal jugular access site
D. Immediate thrombolysis

Answer C: Change to contralateral internal jugular access site.

This image shows an echogenic thrombus within the left internal jugular vein causing distension of the vein as well as dilation of the external jugular vein (seen in the superficial tissues on the left side of the screen. For reference, the thyroid is seen on the left of the image and the common carotid artery is between the thyroid and the internal jugular vein. Attempted cannulation at this site will likely not be successful requiring changing target vessel for catheterization. While moving to the left subclavian vein is a possibility, selecting the contralateral vessel may be a better solution.

Question 7

A 30-year-old male presents to your clinic for right hand swelling and pain on a follow up visit after a recent admission for cellulitis. He states that he had an IV placed in the hand which is the location of his pain. An upper extremity duplex ultrasound is performed showing the image below. What is the next step of management? (Fig. 18.6)

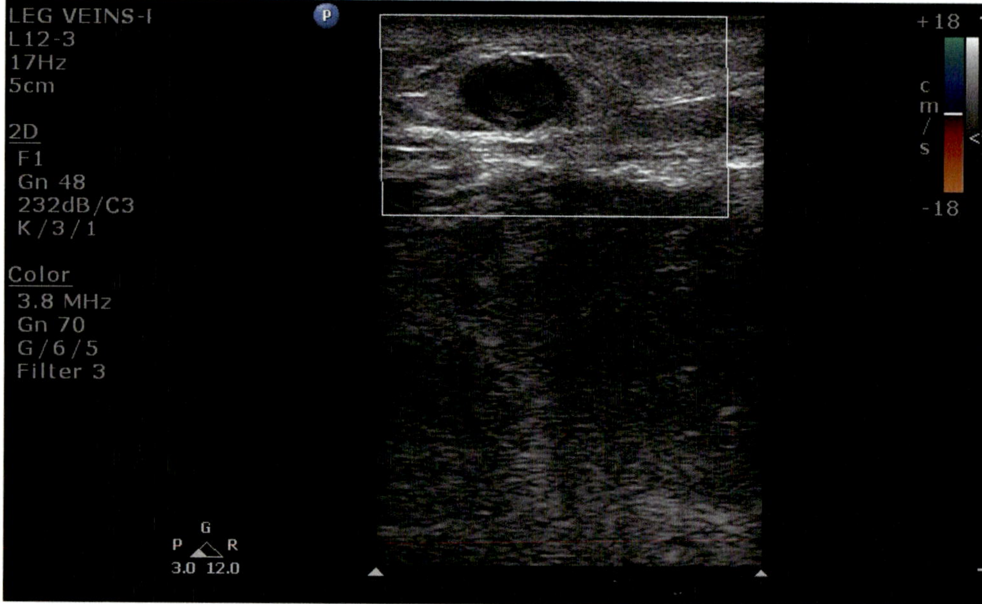

Fig. 18.6 Image of the right forearm over a palpable cord

A. Anticoagulation
B. NSAIDs and observation
C. Symptomatic pain control
D. Thrombectomy

Answer B: NSAIDs and observation.

This patient was found to have a superficial thrombus in the median cubital vein as a complication of his IV placement in the hospital. Superficial veins are typically treated with NSAIDs, warm compresses and observation. However, if there is extensive clot burden, these may need systemic anticoagulation. Thrombectomy in this context would not be indicated [4].

Question 8

A 65-year-old male is admitted to the ICU for respiratory failure secondary to severe multifocal pneumonia. He is in the intensive care unit for 8 days requiring HFNC and NIPPV. He is eventually transferred to the floor and then discharged 3 days later to a skilled nursing facility on IV antibiotics via PICC line. One week later, he complains of upper extremity swelling and paresthesias. An ultrasound is done showing a brachial vein thrombosis extending into the axillary vein. Which of the following would be considered this patient's primary risk factor for DVT development?

A. Immobilization
B. Presence of a foreign body
C. Smoking
D. Undiagnosed malignancy

Answer B: Presence of a foreign body.

This patient has multiple risk factors for deep venous thrombosis; however, for upper extremity deep venous thrombosis, the overriding risk factor is the presence of a foreign body: in this case, a PICC line. A recent study by Rokosh et al. found that 88% of UE DVTs were attributable to the presence of central venous access; whereas only 60% could be attributed to malignancy, 31% to smoking, 19% to immobilization – the latter of which is a much lesser concern in a non-intubated patient in the upper extremities [5].

Question 9

Which of the following upper extremity veins is considered a deep upper extremity vein?

A. Axillary Vein
B. Basilic Vein
C. Cephalic Vein
D. Median Cubital Vein

Answer A: Axillary Vein.

The axillary vein is the only vein listed that is considered a deep vein. The other options are considered superficial veins for the purposes of diagnosis deep venous thrombosis [6].

Question 10

A 55-year-old female is intubated in the intensive care unit for respiratory failure due to pneumonia. This is her eighth day intubated. Family complains that her left lower extremity appears swollen to them. Comprehensive ultrasound is currently unavailable, and you elect to perform a point-of-care evaluation of the left lower extremity. Which of the following methods is the most appropriate approach to take in evaluating for DVT in this patient?

A. Comprehensive whole leg ultrasonography including calf veins
B. 2-point exam
C. Sequential compression ultrasound
D. D-dimer laboratory testing with anticoagulation if positive

Answer C: Sequential compression ultrasound.

In this patient with concern for DVT, ultrasound evaluation of the lower extremity veins is indicated. Guideline for the evaluation of DVT include sequential compression of the deep venous system using grayscale ultrasound with color doppler. While comprehensive whole-leg ultrasound performed in a vascular lab or radiology suite would be appropriate, limited point-of-care ultrasound has been shown to be safe and effective in evaluating for DVT. At the beside this is usually abbreviated to grayscale compression ultrasound interrogating points sequentially down the deep venous system. Literature is conflicted about the safety of the 2 point technique. While D-dimer is usually elevated in the setting of DVT, it is not specific for the diagnosis and should prompt ultrasound imaging when positive where there is clinical concern for DVT [2, 7, 8].

Question 11

After performing the appropriate point-of-care exam, you discover a non-occlusive isolated mid-femoral vein thrombus. Which of the following methods would have been unable to identify the thrombus?

A. 2-point compression exam
B. Color Doppler
C. Spectral Doppler
D. Whole leg ultrasonography

Answer A: 2-point compression exam.

This patient had an isolated femoral vein thrombus. Two-point compression of the lower extremity is a focused examination that evaluates only the common femoral vein and the popliteal vein for venous thrombosis. A study by Adhikari, et al. found that 5.5% of thrombi in their population was isolated to the femoral vein. An additional study by Maki et al. reported up to 22% isolated femoral vein thrombi. The doppler methods each would have suggested the presence of a thrombus outside or inside the view of the transducer, and whole leg ultrasonography would have required interrogation of the mid femoral vein and would not have missed a DVT in this location [2, 9].

Question 12

What is the most reliable way of excluding venous thrombus?

A. 2D Compression
B. Color Doppler
C. Spectral Doppler
D. Augmentation

Answer A: 2D Compression.

The ultimate hallmark of intra-luminal thrombosis is a loss of compression. In the absence of thrombus, compression of the vein with the transducer shoulder result in collapse of the lumen and complete apposition of the walls of the vein. Generally complete compression is sufficient to evaluate the lower extremity vasculature for the presence a DVT. This is the best method of excluding thrombus. In cases that are unclear, color doppler can be added to evaluate for intraluminal filling defects. Spectral doppler and augmentation are supplemental techniques designed to evaluate for thrombus outside the region accessible by ultrasound.

Question 13

A 36-year-old female presents to the Emergency Department 1 week after being discharged from a prolonged hospitalization in the ICU and general medical floor for urosepsis. She complains of right leg swelling and pain. The right leg is scanned. Which technique can be used to confirm the findings? (Fig. 18.7)

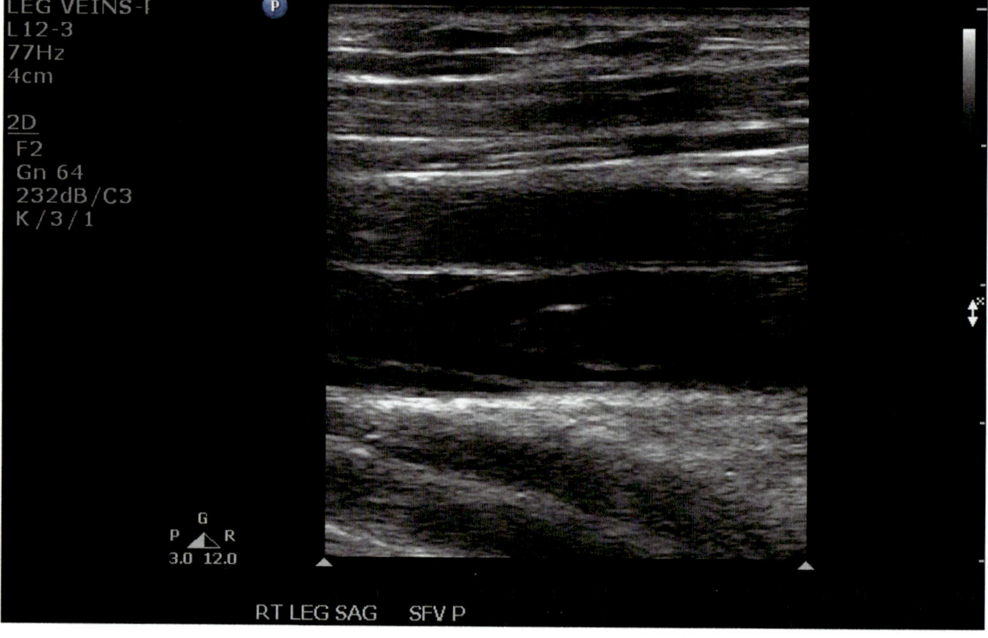

Fig. 18.7 Sagitally oriented image of the right leg at the level of the proximal femoral vein

A. Compression in long axis
B. Color doppler
C. Repeat scanning in 1 week
D. Spectral doppler

Answer B: Color Doppler.

This patient presents with an acute thrombus in the femoral vein. While the diagnosis can be made using 2D grayscale imaging and compression alone, the presence of DVT can be confirmed using color doppler. To evaluate for a filling defect in the vessel lumen. However, care must be taken to ensure proper doppler settings (i.e. PRF optimized for venous flow and color gain). Compression of the vessel in long axis is not considered standard protocol. It is difficult to obtain adequate compression in long axis. Repeating the scan in 1 week is unnecessary as an acute thrombus is clearly visible in the area of concern. Spectral doppler is unnecessary in this scan as the thrombus is clearly visible. There is no need to quantify the velocity of blood flow around the thrombus. Additionally, we are not evaluating for a thrombus outside the area of concern.

Question 14

A 54-year-old female is admitted to the ICU for acute respiratory failure due to COPD. As part of her initial workup in the ICU overnight she received a bedside vascular ultrasound. The overnight resident expressed difficulty confirming findings using doppler. What should be changed to improve image acquisition? (Fig. 18.8)

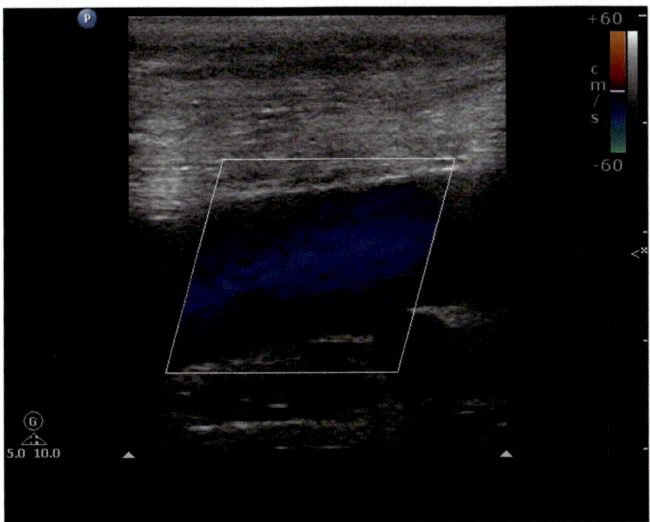

Fig. 18.8 Image of a lower extremity vein using color doppler

A. Lower scanning frequency
B. Increase grayscale gain
C. Adjust pulse repetition frequency
D. Change the angle of insonation

Answer C: Adjust pulse repetition frequency.

In this image the pulse repetition frequency is set to measure arterial velocities rather than venous velocities. The pulse-repetition frequency is the rapidity with which the probe sends pulsed signals. This can be adjusted for the expected velocity in the area of interest. In order to accurately display higher velocities, a higher PRF is needed. Conversely a lower PRF is needed to measure slower velocity as the slow velocity is lost in the background noise when the PRF is set too high. These signals are then removed by the linked wall filter. Ideally venous PRF should be set in the single digit range. Changing the scanning frequency and grayscale gain will have no effect on the doppler image displayed. Optimizing the angle of insonation is important for accurate doppler assessment but will not affect the PRF relative to the velocity of blood flow [10].

Question 15

A 32-year-old male is being scanned in the Emergency Department with concern for thrombus based on echogenic material in the vessel. Color doppler is applied to confirm findings. What adjustment should be made to improve Fig. 18.9?

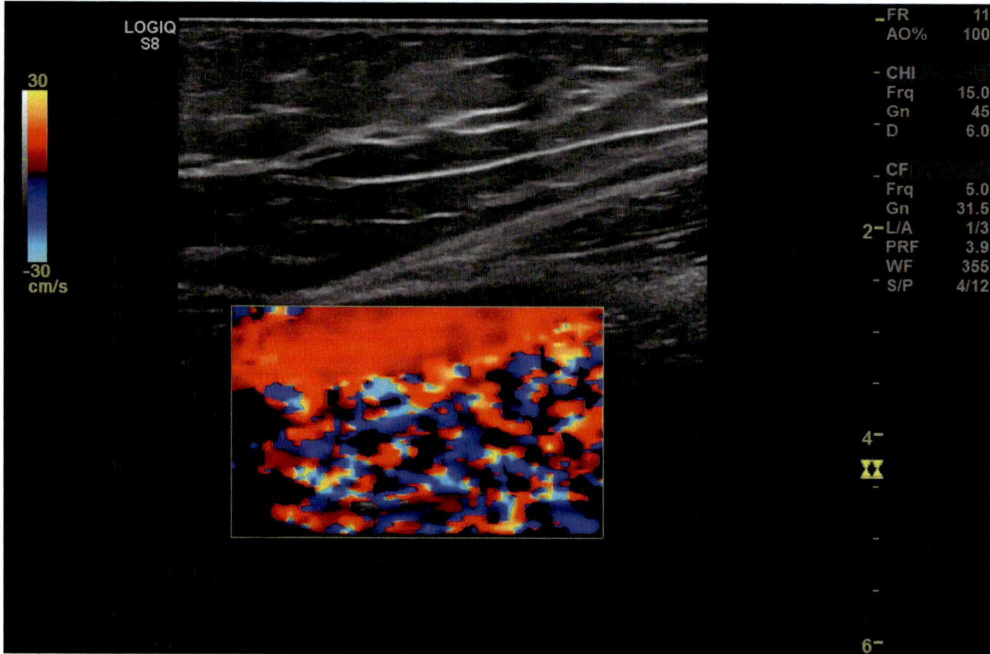

Fig. 18.9 Image of a lower extremity vein using color doppler

A. Adjust color gain
B. Adjust the pulse repetition frequency.
C. Adjust the beam angle
D. Increase the scanning frequency

Answer A: Adjust color gain.

This patient has echogenic material within the lumen of the vessel suspicious for thrombus. The best confirmation is lack of compressibility resulting from the echogenic material. Color doppler can be used to help confirm the presence or absence of a thrombus by looking for a filling defect. However, this technique can provide false information if the doppler settings are not adjusted appropriately. This image is over-gained resulting in bleed-over not only of the thrombus but also of the vessel walls. The pulse repetition frequency is appropriately set for venous flow. The angle of insonation either physically with the probe or electronically with beam steering can affect the accuracy of the doppler image resulting in an artificially diminished filling. It will not result in doppler bleed-over.

Question 16

A 33-year-old, pregnant female was transferred overnight to the ICU for sudden onset respiratory distress and hemodynamic instability. She was intubated for respiratory distress and placed on vasopressors for blood pressure management. A vascular ultrasound is being performed to evaluate for possible DVTs. What can be done to optimize the color doppler image? (Fig. 18.10)

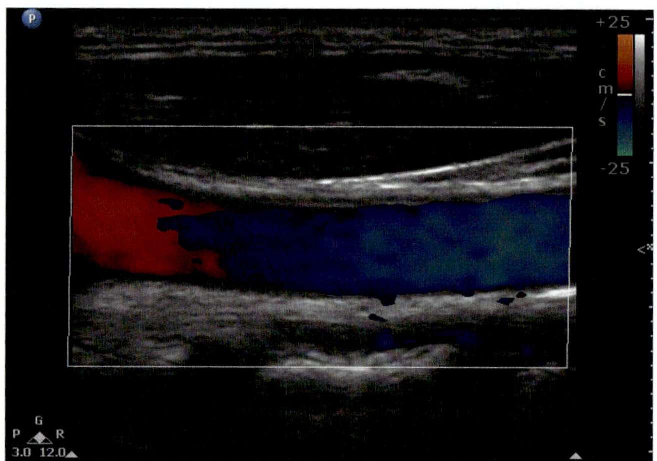

Fig. 18.10 Image of a vein using color doppler

A. Increase the color gain
B. Adjust the pulse repetition frequency
C. Change the angle of insonation
D. Change the focal zone

Answer C: Change the angle of insonation.

In this image there is no doppler signal at the area of interest because the doppler signal is being measured perpendicular to the direction of blood flow. Velocity is best measured when the ultrasound beam is parallel to the direction of flow. When angle of insonation and the direction of flow differ, this angle needs to be incorporated into the doppler equation (ΔF = (Fr-Ft) = (2 × Ft × V × cosθ)/c: *Fr = Frequency received, Ft = Frequency transmitted, V = flow velocity, c = speed of sound in medium, θ = angle created by direction of flow and ultrasound beam*). When the angle of insonation is perpendicular (θ = 90°) to the direction of flow, cosθ = 0 making the change in frequency unmeasurable. As angles approach 90°, the accuracy of doppler velocity measurement decreases. Angle of insonation relative to blood flow should be kept to less than 60°. This can be accomplished by adjusting the angle of the probe (heel-toe manipulation) or through electronic beam steering on the machine. Adjusting the color gain and PRF can have effects on the doppler image produced but will not overcome the effects of measuring velocities perpendicular to the direction of flow. Adjusting the focal zone will improve the grayscale image but does not significantly affect the doppler image produced.

Question 17

A 28-year-old female was admitted to the ICU after sudden hemodynamic instability. PE is among the concerns for her decompensation. A bedside ultrasound was performed which showed no visible thrombus and normal compression between the common femoral vein and popliteal vein. This image was obtained during valsalva. What should be done next? (Fig. 18.11)

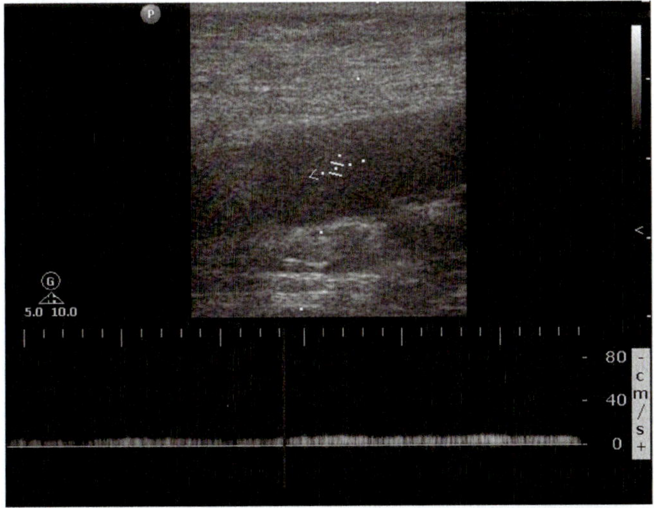

Fig. 18.11 Spectral doppler of the common femoral vein in long axis

A. Repeat ultrasound in 24 hrs
B. CT venography
C. Comprehensive duplex ultrasound
D. Impedance plesmithography

Answer B: CT venography.

This image shows lack of augmentation with Valsalva concerning for either intraluminal or extraluminal obstruction of the iliac veins. Normally, changes in venous flow with either deep respiration or Valsalva can be visualized using pulse-wave doppler of the common femoral vein. An obstruction of flow will cause a dampening or obliteration of this velocity flow change. Pelvic thrombi are not directly visible with ultrasound. Additional imaging studies such as CT venography, MR venography and contrast venography are needed to further evaluate for thrombus. While pulse-wave doppler can suggest obstruction, cross-sectional imaging is necessary to differentiate intraluminal vs extraluminal obstruction. Additionally, a partially occlusive thrombus will not necessarily change the pulse wave doppler tracing, so care must be taken when a pelvic thrombus is suspected despite normal or dampened tracing.

Question 18

A 32-year-old female is intubated in the ICU after complicated repair of her right mid-shaft femur fracture. You notice increased swelling in the right leg. On exam the wound is clean, dry and intact. Her leg compartments are soft and she has normal 2+ distal pulses. As part of your evaluation you perform a point-of-care ultrasound. What is your diagnosis? (Fig. 18.12)

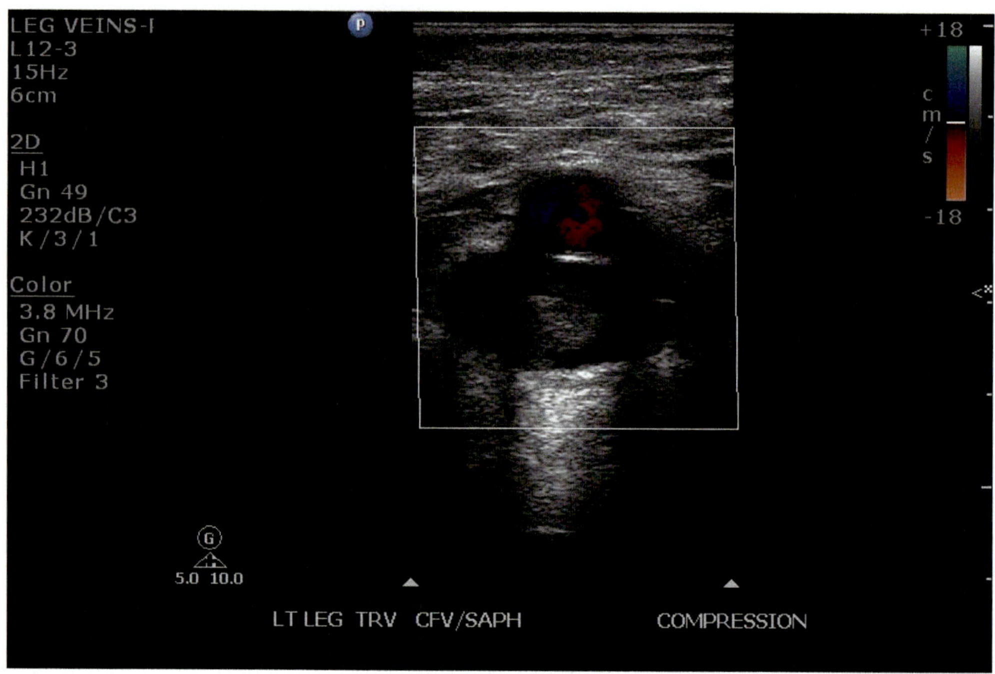

Fig. 18.12 Transverse image of the common femoral vein with color doppler

A. Compartment syndrome
B. Surgical hardware infection
C. Acute DVT
D. Post-surgical edema

Answer C: Acute DVT.

This patient has findings consistent with an acute DVT. Normally venous vasculature should be thin-walled, anechoic and compressible. When present, a DVT appears as echogenic material within the lumen of the vessel that precludes compression of the vein. Often veins with acute DVTs will be distended compared to the contralateral vessel. This patient is a high risk for DVT being immobilized and recently post-op from an orthopedic procedure. While complications of orthopedic injuries and surgery include infection, compartment syndrome and arterial compromise, this patient does not demonstrate any findings suggestive of these complications.

Question 19

A 54-year-old male is admitted to the hospital after sustaining a splenic laceration from a motor vehicle accident. On hospital day 2 he complains of pain in his left lower extremity. A bedside ultrasound is performed. What is the diagnosis? (Fig. 18.13)

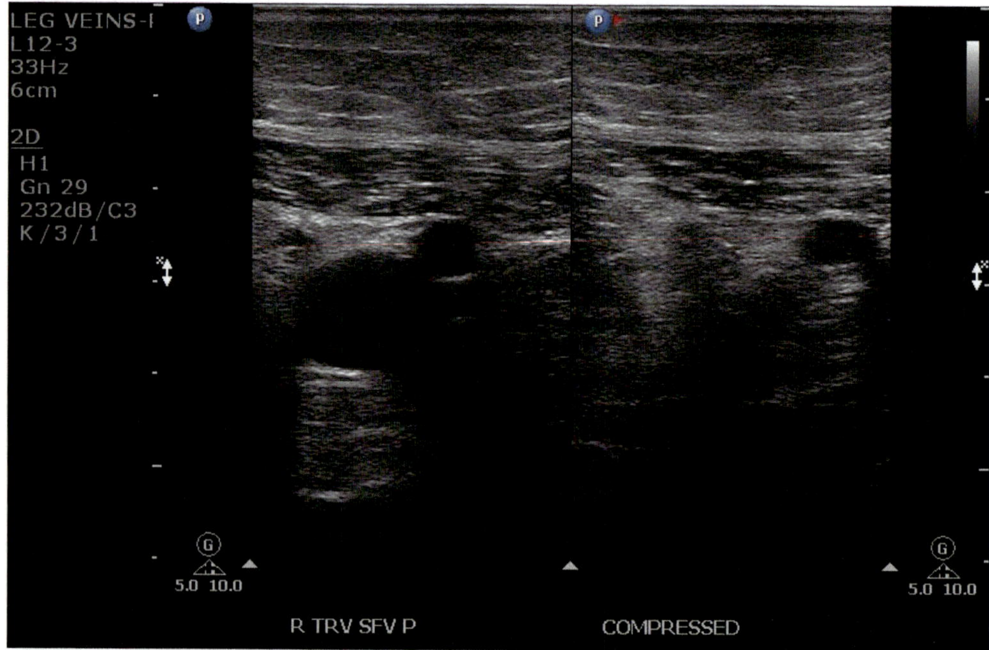

Fig. 18.13 Image of the right proximal femoral vein in transverse orientation with and without compression

A. Acute DVT
B. Chronic DVT
C. No DVT
D. Arterial dissection

Answer C: No DVT.

The image of this patient demonstrates and pre and post compression view of the femoral vein demonstrating complete collapsibility. Normal veins are thin walled, anechoic and collapsible as demonstrated by complete obliteration of the vessel and apposition of the vessel walls with compression. Presuming collapsibility throughout the deep venous system, an acute DVT can be confidently excluded. An acute thrombus will often appear as echogenic material within the vessel that prevents collapsibility. A chronic thrombus may take a variety of appearances but will likely appear adherent to the vessel wall. While the patent portion of the vessel lumen in an acute or chronic thrombus may collapse, there will be no apposition of the vessel walls [11].

Question 20

A 73-year-old patient presents to your clinic. He had a recent hospitalization for unilateral right-sided DVT complication by a pulmonary embolism. He was initially put on heparin and transitioned to warfarin before discharge. He is at your clinic today for a one-month follow up from his hospitalization. His right lower extremity still appears somewhat edematous compared with the left and you elect to evaluate the extremity in the office with point-of-care ultrasound. Which of the following best describes the images obtained? (Fig. 18.14)

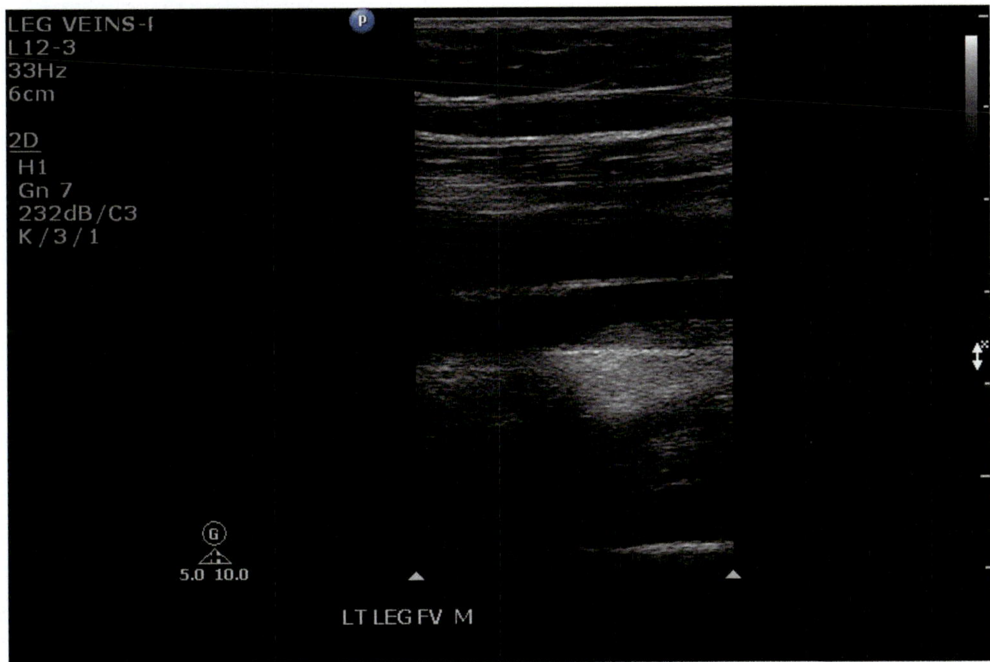

Fig. 18.14 Image of the left mid-femoral artery (top) and mid-femoral vein (bottom)

A. Inadequate image quality
B. Chronic thrombus
C. New acute thrombosis.
D. Resolution of prior DVT

Answer B: Chronic thrombus.

This ultrasound image demonstrates recanalization of a thrombus in the femoral vein. According to an article by Karande et al., in chronic thrombosis, the vein is incompressible, narrow, irregular and shows echogenic thrombus attached to the venous walls. This image is of adequate quality and does not demonstrate resolution of DVT, which would show a totally anechoic venous lumen that collapses with compression. An acute thrombosis may or may not be echogenic but is generally not adherent to the vessel wall [12].

Question 21

A 42-year-old female presents the Emergency department with groin pain. A bedside ultrasound is performed showing a thrombus in the greater saphenous vein at the junction with the common femoral vein. What is the next best step in management?

A. Discharge with repeat ultrasound in 1 week.
B. Initiate anticoagulation
C. Consult interventional radiology for catheter directed tPA
D. NSAIDs and warm compresses

Answer B: Initiate anticoagulation.

This patient has a thrombus in the greater saphenous vein. While the greater saphenous is generally considered a superficial vein, thrombi at or near the junction of the common femoral vein are anticoagulated as the likelihood of propagation in to the deep femoral system is high. Without limb threatening sequalae, intra-arterial thrombolysis is not indicated. Repeat imaging is appropriate for patients with superficial thrombi to ensure non-propagation. NSAIDs and warm compresses are indicated in patients with superficial thrombophlebitis without significant clot burden [13, 14].

Question 22

A 69-year-old male with a history of peripheral artery disease, hypertension and diabetes is admitted for acute hypoxic respiratory failure. On ICU day 2 he was noted to have worsening edema and cyanosis of his left lower extremity with decreased dorsalis pedis and posterior tibial pulses. What is the most likely diagnosis? (Fig. 18.15)

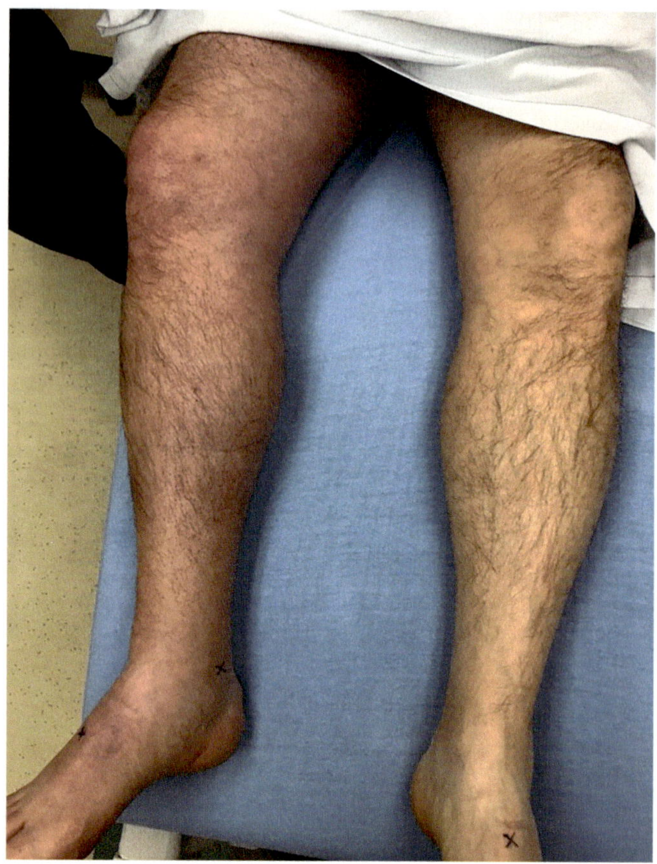

Fig. 18.15 Image showing edema and mottling of the right lower extremity. (Courtesy of Jon Schrock, MD)

A. Non-occlusive DVT
B. Lower extremity cellulitis
C. Phlegmasia cerulia dolens
D. Arterial embolism

Answer C: Phlegmasia cerulia dolens.

This patient presents with phlegmasia cerulia dolens (PCD). PCD is a condition where the deep veins and collaterals are completely occluded causing extremity swelling and ischemia. The diagnosis is made with CT or ultrasound showing thrombosis within the venous vasculature which would differentiate it from arterial thrombosis or embolism. Occlusion at this location prevents blood return from the affected extremity causing a more overt presentation and subsequently worse outcomes as this is a limb-threatening diagnosis [15].

Question 23

What definitive therapy for the above patient is most likely to be effective?

A. Thrombectomy
B. Catheter directed thrombolysis
C. Heparinization
D. Factor Xa Inhibitors

Answer B: Catheter directed thrombolysis.

Catheter directed thrombolysis offers a targeted approach to reduction in clot burden in patients with severe disease states such as pulmonary embolism with hemodynamic instability and large vessel DVT. It reduces the risk of bleeding as smaller volumes of thrombolytic medications are used, and there is a more rapid reduction in clot burden. There have not been a significant number of studies directly comparing thrombolysis and thrombectomy, but there are several organizations that have recommended this therapy in guideline statements [15–17].

Question 24

A 24-year-old female presents to the emergency department with proximal thigh pain and painful erythema of her calf. On exam swelling and tenderness are noted at the proximal thigh. The following images were obtained while scanning in the affected area (transverse and longitudinal images of a lymph node). What is the most appropriate treatment? (Fig. 18.16).

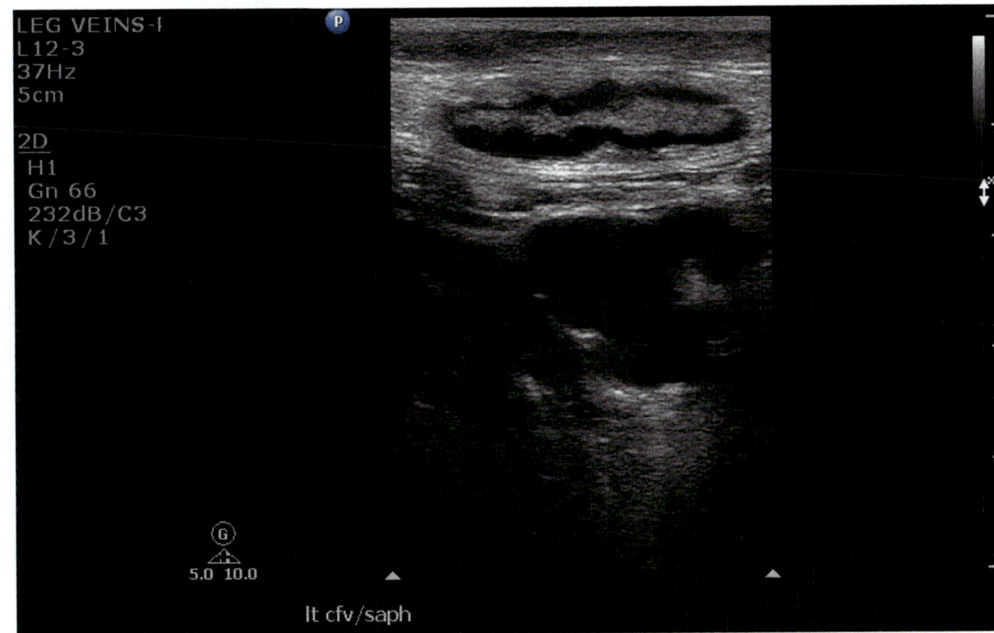

Fig. 18.16 Image of the proximal left thigh showing lymph node (superficial) and proximal vasculature (deep)

A. Initiate heparin
B. Consult vascular surgery for thrombectomy
C. Initiate antibiotics for lower extremity cellulitis
D. Consult interventional radiology for biopsy

Answer C: Initiate antibiotics for lower extremity cellulitis.

This image shows sonographic evidence of a lymph node. Most likely this patient is suffering from a lower extremity cellulitis rather than venous thrombus. The best decision at this time would be to treat the patient for a presumed infection with cellulitis. If the lymph node persists after treatment a biopsy could be done for further evaluation.

Question 25

A 48-year-old male presents to the emergency department with posterior knee pain for 1 week. This non-compressible structure was seen in the medial popliteal fossa. What is the most likely diagnosis? (Fig. 18.17)

A. Joint effusion
B. Baker cyst
C. Pseudoaneurysm
D. Popliteal vein distal to an occlusive DVT

Answer B: Baker cyst.

Bakers cysts are fluid filled structures near the knee that are most commonly caused by inflammation of the gastrocnemius-semimembranosus bursa. This bursa is found between the semimembranosus muscle and the popliteal vasculature and can communicate with the knee joint. These cysts are often asymptomatic but when ruptured can present similarly to deep vein thrombosis with patients often complaining of swelling, pain and stiffness [18].

Question 26

A 37-year-old morbidly obese female presents with pain and swelling in her left lower extremity. Her anatomy is difficult to define due to the presence of significant amounts of subcu-

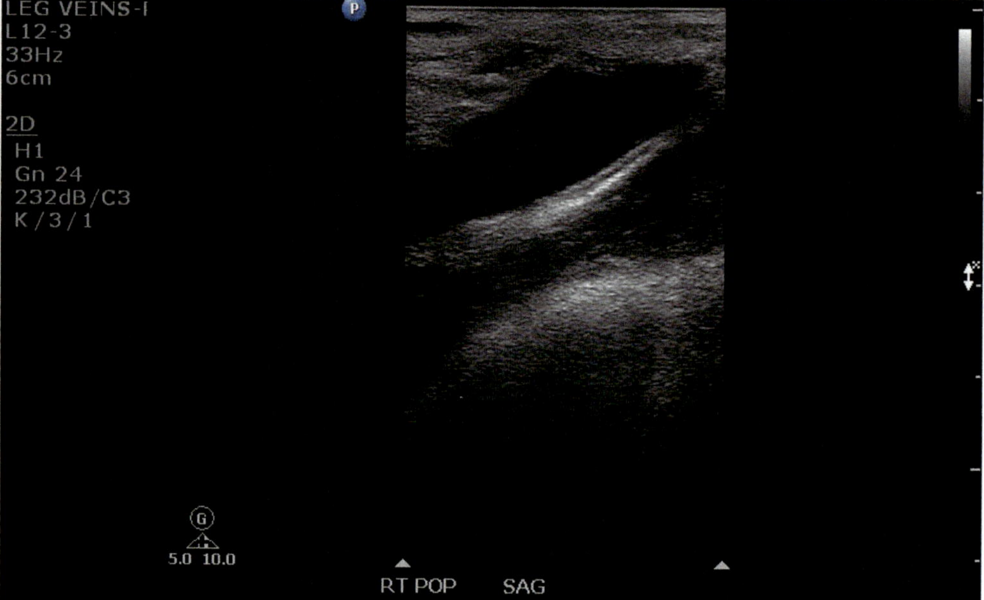

Fig. 18.17 Sagittal image of the popliteal fossa

taneous tissue. What can be done to increase tissue penetration?

A. Increase the transducer frequency
B. Change to the curvilinear transducer
C. Increase deep field gain
D. Add color doppler

Answer B: Change to the curvilinear transducer.

Scanning legs with thick subcutaneous tissue can pose a particular sonographic challenge as the linear transducer typically used for DVT ultrasound has a limited ability to penetrate owing to its higher frequency. Additionally, adipose tissue has a propensity to attenuate sound waves decreasing the amplitude of reflected waves. Thus, lowering the frequency or changing to a lower frequency transducer will allow for greater penetration. Changing the deep field gain will increase the machine sensitivity to returning waves in the deep field but will not necessarily increase penetration. Adding color doppler may help in identifying vasculature in the deep field but will not increase tissue penetration.

Question 27

A 48-year-old female is being scanned for lower extremity pain and swelling in the thigh as indicated in Fig. 18.18. What anatomical variant is shown here?

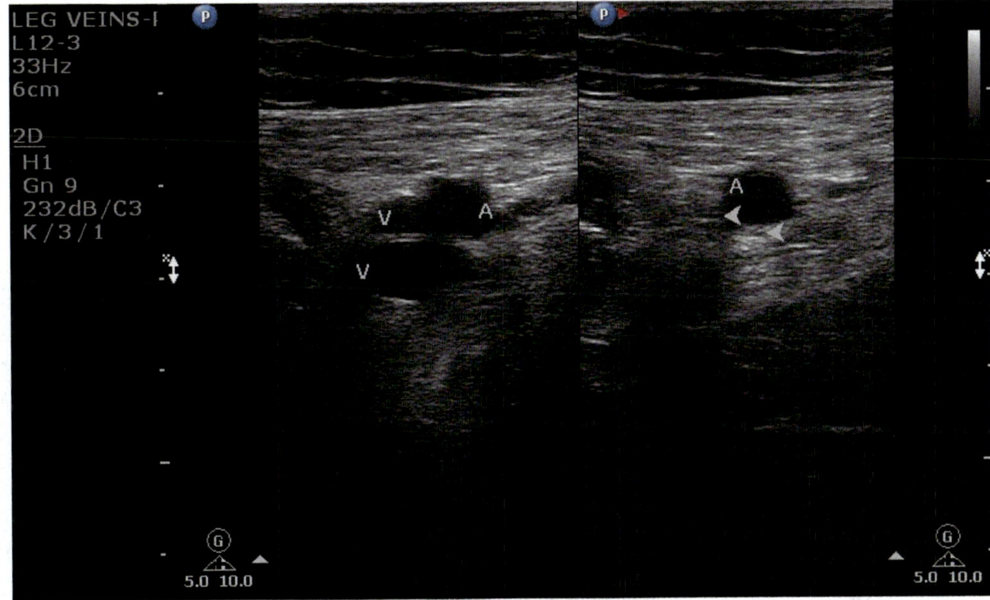

Fig. 18.18 Image of the mid femoral vein in transverse orientation

A. Mirror artifact
B. Duplication of the femoral vein
C. Collateralization of deep venous system
D. Distalization of the deep femoral vein

Answer B: Duplication of the femoral vein.

The image supplied shows a duplication of the femoral vein. This is a common anatomical variant seen in the lower extremity and one study demonstrated duplication of the femoral vein occurs in 10% of studied patients. Both limbs of a duplicated system can develop thrombus and need to be individually interrogated [19, 20].

Question 28

A 53-year-old female presents to the ED with right groin pain 1 week after having a left heart catheterization. You note a pulsatile area to the right inguinal area. The rest of the limb appears warm and well perfused with 2+ distal pulses. You perform a point-of-care ultrasound evaluation of the region and see the following. Which of the following does this represent? (Fig. 18.19)

A. Arterio-venous fistula
B. Phlegmasia alba dolens
C. Pseudoaneurysm
D. Reactive lymph node

Answer C: Pseudoaneurysm.

Pseudoaneurysms of the femoral artery often arise from repeated punctures. Arterial puncture is a known iatrogenic cause of pseudoaneurysm. The characteristic finding is a color doppler image with a bidirectional appearance of flow, often referred to as "ying-yang." Pulsed doppler will demonstrate to-and-fro movement of fluid in the neck of the pseudoaneurysm [21].

Question 29

You are on overnight call to the intensive care unit when you admit a 42-year-old female in diabetic ketoacidosis. On your initial evaluation, the patient complains of left lower extremity swelling. Comprehensive ultrasound is unavailable and you elect to perform a point-of-care evaluation of the affected extremity. While attempting to apply compression to the mid-

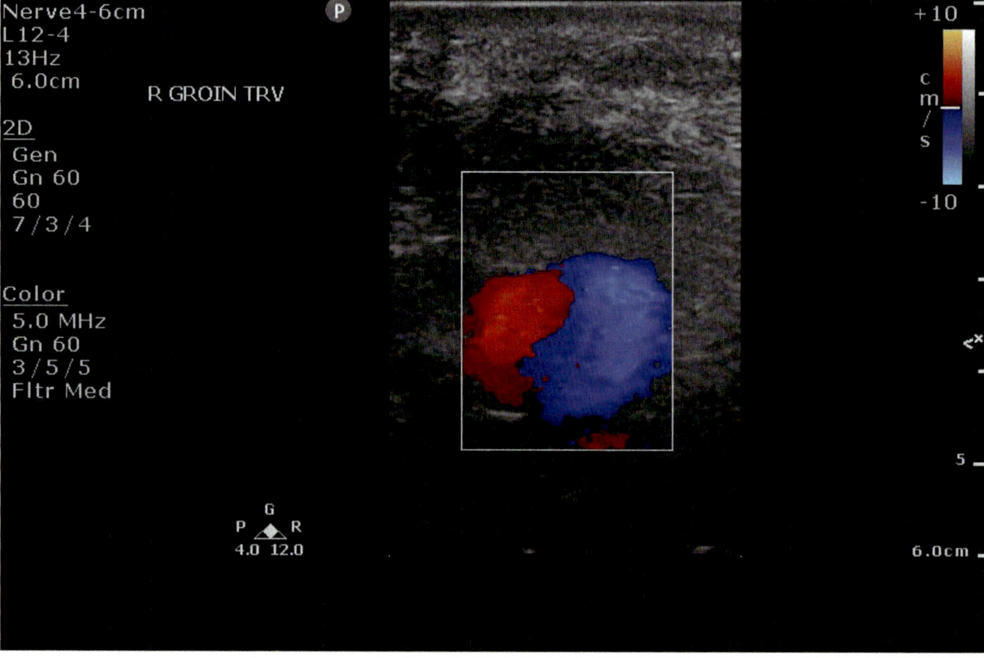

Fig. 18.19 Image of the right groin in transverse orientation with color doppler

distal femoral vein, you are unable to fully compress the vein. You attempt switching to a lower frequency on the curvilinear probe but are still unable to fully compress the vein. You suspect this is due to the patient's body habitus. What other adjunctive techniques might be useful in evaluating for DVT?

A. Move rotationally around the leg to look for less attenuation through other structures
B. Increase compressive force on the vessel in question
C. Switch to a higher frequency transducer
D. Wrap the non-scanning hand around the patient's leg and compress from both sides

Answer D: Wrap the non-scanning hand around the patient's leg and compress from both sides.

Patients that are morbidly obese are often more technically challenging to image. Often, depth has to be increased beyond the ability of a linear probe's resolution and may require changing to a lower frequency transducer. Even with the use of a lower frequency transducer, the operator may not be able to apply enough pressure anteriorly to compress the vein, assuming good visualization of the vein with the transducer. In this case, placing the non-scanning hand posteriorly and compressing in both directions will often allow enough force to be directed at the vein to compress it. The other methods listed may help improve visualization of the vein but will not help with compression of the vein.

Question 30

As you utilize the appropriate technique to compress in the patient, you find a focal area in the region distal to the midpoint of the thigh that does not compress. The areas immediately proximal and distal do compress well and there is good color flow throughout the vessel. Which areas were you find non-compressible?

A. Adductor canal
B. Inguinal ligament
C. Lesser saphenous vein
D. Saphenous fascia

Answer A: Adductor canal.

According to a 1990 article written by Wright et al. in the Journal of Vascular Surgery, segmental incompressibility of the superficial femoral vein often occurs within the adductor canal. The deep veins should be compressible at all other sites listed [22].

References

1. Moore KL, Dalley AF. Clinically oriented anatomy. 5th ed. Hoboken, NJ: Wiley; 2006. p. 581–3.
2. Adhikari S, et al. Isolated deep vein thrombosis: implications for 2-point compression ultrasonography of the lower extremity: a randomized controlled trial. Ann Emerg Med. 2015;66(3):262–6.
3. Kim S, Patel N, Thapar K, Pandurangadu AV, Bahl A. Isolated proximal greater saphenous vein thrombosis and the risk of propegation to deep vein thrombosis and pulmonary embolism. Vasc Health Risk Manag. 2018;14:129–35.
4. Kearon C, et al. Antithrombotic therapy for vte disease: chest guideline and expert panel report. Chest. 2016;149:315–52.
5. Rokosh R, et al. High prevalence and mortality associated with upper extremity deep venous thrombosis in hospitalized patients at a tertiary care center. Ann Vasc Surg. 2019;65:55–65.
6. Heil J, et al. Deep vein thrombosis of the upper extremity. Dtsch Arztebl Int. 2017;114:244–9.
7. Bernardi E, et al. Serial 2-point ultrasonography plus d-dimer vs. whole leg color coded doppler ultrasonography for diagnosing suspected symptomatic deep vein thrombosis: a randomized controlled trial. JAMA. 2008;6:36–43.
8. Zuker-Herman R, Ayalon Dangur I, Berant R, Sitt EC, Baskin L, Shaya Y, Shiber S. Comparison between two-point and three-point compression ultrasound for the diagnosis of deep vein thrombosis. J Thromb Thrombolysis. 2018;45(1):99–105.
9. Maki D, et al. Distribution of thrombi in acute lower extremity deep venous thrombosis: implications for sonography and CT with MR venography. Am J Roentgenol. 2000;175:1299–301.
10. Terslev L, et. Al. Settings and artifacts relevant for doppler ultrasound in large vessel vasculitis. Arthritis Res Ther. 2017;19:167.
11. Crisp J. Compression ultrasonography of the lower extremity with portable vascular ultrasonography can accurately detect deep venous thrombosis in the emergency department. Ann Emerg Med. 2010;56:601–10.
12. Karande GY, Hedgire SS, Sanchez Y, et al. Advanced imaging in acute and chronic deep vein thrombosis. Cardiovasc Diagn Ther. 2016;6(6):493–507.
13. Blaivas M. Point-of-care ultrasonographic deep venous thrombosis evaluation after just ten minutes' training: is this offer too good to be true? Ann Emerg Med. 2010;56(6):611–3.
14. Blumberg RM, Barton E, Gelfand ML, Skudder P, Brennan J. Occult deep venous thrombosis complicating superficial thrombophlebitis. J Vasc Surg. 1998;27(2):338–43.
15. Jaff MR. Management of massive and submassive pulmonary embolism, iliofemoral deep vein thrombosis, and chronic thromboembolic pulmonary hypertension: a scientific statement from the American Heart Association. Circulation. 2011;123(16):1788–830.
16. Kearon C, Akl EA, Comerota AJ, et al. Antithrombotic therapy for VTE disease: antithrombotic therapy and prevention of thrombosis, 9th ed: American College of Chest Physicians Evidence-Based Clinical Practice Guidelines [published correction appears in Chest. 2012 Dec;142(6):1698-1704]. Chest. 2012;141(2 Suppl):e419S–96S. https://doi.org/10.1378/chest.11-2301.
17. Elsharawy M, Elzayat E. Early results of thrombolysis vs anticoagulation in iliofemoral venous thrombosis. A randomised clinical trial. Eur J Vasc Endovasc Surg. 2002;24(3):209–14.
18. Handy JR. Popliteal cysts in adults: a review. Semin Arthritis Rheum. 2001;31(2):108–18.
19. Simpson WL, Krakowsi DM. Prevalence of lower extremity venous duplication. Indian J Radiol Imaging. 2010;20(3):230–4.
20. Dona E, Fletcher JP, Hughes TM, Saker K, Batiste P, Ramanathan I. Duplicated popliteal and superficial femoral veins: incidence and potential significance. Aust N Z J Surg. 2000;70(6):438–40.
21. Sayit A, et al. Delayed superficial femoral artery Pseudoaneurysm following penetrating trauma in a young patient with sonographic findings. West Afr J Radiology. 2016;23:132–5.
22. Wright D, et al. Pitfalls in lower extremity venous duplex scanning. J Vasc Surg. 1990;11:675–9.

19 Devices, Foreign Bodies, and Intra Cardiac Masses

Katarzyna Gil, Rob Montgomery, and Patrick Collier

Question 1

In patients with left ventricular assist devices (LVADs),

A. The aortic valve should remain closed
B. The aortic valve should at least open intermittently
C. The LVAD speed should be set low enough to allow aortic valve opening with every heartbeat
D. Aortic valve opening should not occur at any LVAD speed in patients with extremely poor native left ventricular function
E. Aortic regurgitation does not occur in systole

Answer: B. The aortic valve should at least open intermittently. It is important to evaluate the degree of aortic valve opening while assessing LVADs [1]. The valve should be characterized as either closed, opening with every cardiac cycle or opening intermittently. LVAD speed should be set low enough to allow at least intermittent aortic valve opening, although in patients with poor LV function such opening may not occur at any LVAD speed. The frequency and duration of aortic valve opening are most accurately assessed by recording several (~6) cardiac cycles using M-mode at a slow sweep speed (25–50 mm/s). Continuously closed aortic cusps have been associated with the development of aortic root thrombosis and LVAD-associated aortic regurgitation. Timing of LVAD-associated aortic regurgitation is often continuous (systolic and diastolic, rather than only diastolic) and thus may result in larger regurgitant volumes than what might be expected based upon the jet appearance alone.

Question 2

A 32-year-old patient with nonischemic cardiomyopathy status post HeartMate II LVAD implantation three months ago is admitted to the hospital due to shortness of breath. Which of the following findings are present on her transthoracic echocardiography (Fig. 19.1)?

A. Aortic valve opening and non-continuous aortic regurgitation
B. Aortic valve opening and continuous aortic regurgitation
C. Little or no aortic valve opening and non-continuous aortic regurgitation
D. Little or no aortic valve opening and continuous aortic regurgitation
E. None of these

Answer: D. Little or no aortic valve opening and continuous aortic regurgitation. Continuous aortic regurgitation is shown here in Fig. 19.1 (top and bottom left panels show diastolic phase aortic regurgitation while the top right panel shows systolic phase aortic regurgitation as indicated by the red line on the associated electrocardiogram). The bottom right panel demonstrates little or no aortic valve opening over several (~6) cardiac cycles using M-mode at a slow sweep speed (25–50 mm/s). New-onset aortic regurgitation in patients with LVAD has an adverse effect on LVAD performance, morbidity and mortality [1]. Another example of no aortic valve opening and continuous aortic regurgitation is highlighted in Videos 19.1 and 19.2.

Supplementary Information The online version contains supplementary material available at https://doi.org/10.1007/978-3-031-45731-9_19.

K. Gil
Ohio State University Wexner Medical Center, Columbus, OH, USA
e-mail: Katarzyna.Gil@osumc.edu

R. Montgomery · P. Collier (✉)
Robert and Suzanne Tomsich Department of Cardiovascular Medicine, Sydell and Arnold Miller Family Heart and Vascular Institute, The Cleveland Clinic Foundation, Cleveland, OH, USA
e-mail: MONTGOR4@ccf.org; colliep@ccf.org

R. Sreedharan et al. (eds.), *Critical Care Echocardiography*, https://doi.org/10.1007/978-3-031-45731-9_19

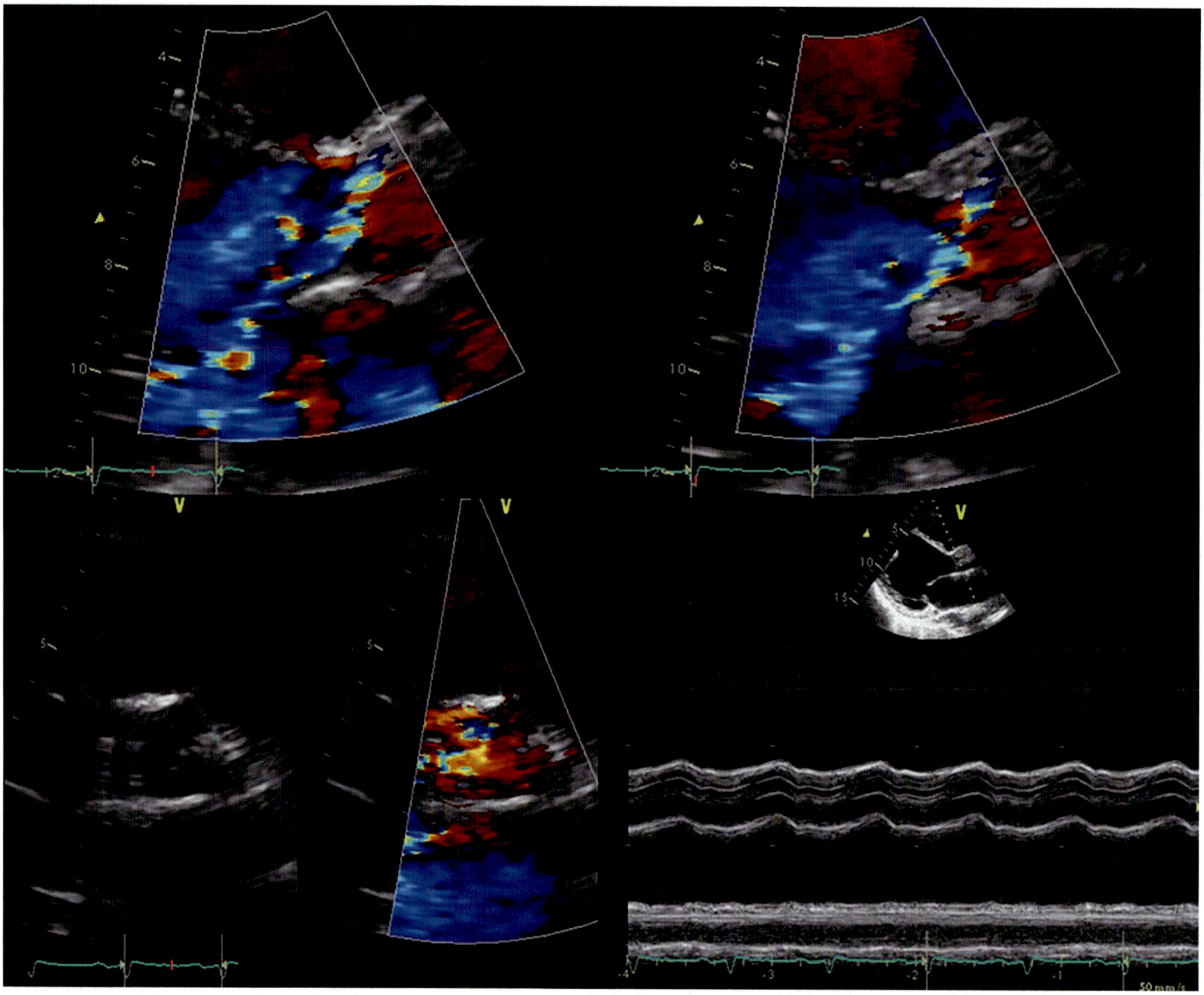

Fig. 19.1 Transthoracic echocardiographic views in a patient post HeartMate II LVAD implantation

Question 3

A 44-year-old patient with recently diagnosed ischemic cardiomyopathy was admitted to the hospital due to cardiogenic shock. A temporary CentriMag biventricular device was inserted and the patient was placed on the heart transplant list. There was no evidence of bacteremia. Transthoracic echocardiography (Fig. 19.2) demonstrated:

A. Thrombus on the aortic cannula
B. Thrombus on the left ventricular cannula
C. Vegetation on the aortic cannula
D. Vegetation on the left ventricular cannula
E. Left ventricular apical tendon

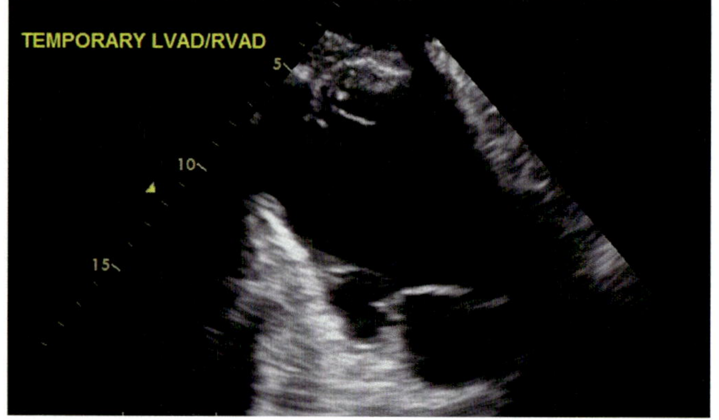

Fig. 19.2 Apical view

Answer: B. Thrombus on the left ventricular cannula. Transthoracic echocardiography (Fig. 19.2) demonstrates a filamentous echodensity attached to the left ventricular cannula. The differential diagnosis of such a finding includes thrombus, vegetation, degenerative changes, surgical material and tumors. Clinical correlation is advised in all such cases to help interpret the findings clinically. In this case, thrombus appears to be the most probable diagnosis due to the relatively recent implantation of the assist device together with the lack of bacteremia. The CentriMag biventricular assist device can be used for peri-operative or post-cardiotomy circulatory support in patients with heart failure [2]. Cannulae are inserted either through a midline sternotomy or through a right mini-thoracotomy.

Question 4

A 45-year-old patient with nonischemic cardiomyopathy status post LVAD implantation is admitted to the hospital due to fever. Doppler interrogation of the outflow LVAD cannula should reveal:

A. Uni-directional flow with peak systolic flow velocities around 1 m/s
B. Uni-directional flow with peak systolic flow velocities around 2 m/s
C. Bi-directional flow with peak systolic flow velocities around 1 m/s
D. Bi-directional flow with peak systolic flow velocities around 2 m/s
E. None of these

Answer: A. Uni-directional flow with peak systolic flow velocities around 1m/s. Doppler interrogation of the outflow LVAD cannula should reveal low-velocity, unidirectional flow. Velocities above 2 m/s are considered abnormal and warrant further consideration for possible obstruction.

Question 5

A 45-year-old patient with nonischemic cardiomyopathy status post LVAD implantation is admitted to the hospital due to fever. Transesophageal echocardiography (Fig. 19.3) demonstrates:

A. Normal inflow LVAD cannula peak velocity
B. Normal outflow LVAD cannula peak velocity
C. Elevated inflow LVAD cannula peak velocity
D. Elevated outflow LVAD cannula peak velocity
E. None of these

Answer: D. Elevated outflow LVAD cannula peak velocity. The terminal portion of the outflow graft and its anastomosis to the ascending aorta can be visualized using trans-thoracic echocardiography (high left parasternal long-axis view) or transesophageal echocardiography (modified long-axis view) (Fig. 19.3). Spectral and color Doppler interrogation of the outflow LVAD cannula should reveal low-velocity (~1 m/s), unidirectional flow [1]. Outflow-graft-velocity benchmarks are not available but in general, are dependent on the caliber of the cannula. For example, normal flow velocities through Heart-Mate II outflow grafts are lower than through smaller-caliber HeartWare (now off the market) outflow grafts (16 mm vs 10 mm diameters respectively). Typically, velocities above 2 m/s are considered abnormal and warrant further consideration for possible obstruction.

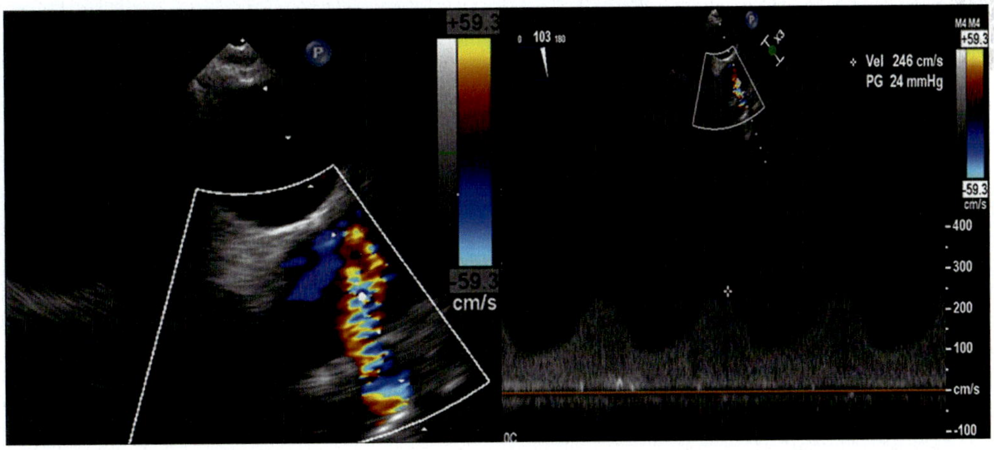

Fig. 19.3 Transesophageal echocardiographic views with color Doppler (left panel) and with Continuous Wave Doppler (right panel)

Question 6

A 45-year-old patient with nonischemic cardiomyopathy status post HeartMate II implantation is admitted to the hospital due to dizziness. Transthoracic echocardiography demonstrates:

A. Normal inflow LVAD cannula peak velocity
B. Elevated outflow LVAD cannula peak velocity
C. Elevated inflow LVAD cannula peak velocity
D. Elevated outflow LVAD cannula peak velocity
E. None of these

Answer: C. Elevated inflow LVAD cannula peak velocity. Fig. 19.4 demonstrates turbulent color Doppler at the inflow LVAD cannula in an apical long-axis view (left panel) with elevated continuous wave Doppler velocities (right panel) around 2.5ms consistent with elevated inflow LVAD cannula peak velocity. Apically inserted inflow cannula can be visualized on parasternal and apical views [1]. Spectral and color Doppler interrogation of the HM-II inflow cannula should reveal laminar, unidirectional flow from the LV to the inflow cannula, with no evidence of turbulence or regurgitation [1]. Pulsed and CW spectral Doppler interrogation may require off-axis modification of a standard parasternal, apical, or short-axis view and should reveal low peak velocity [1].

Question 7

Which of the following statements regarding spectral and color Doppler interrogation of LVAD inflow cannula is true?

A. HM II - laminar, unidirectional flow with peak systolic flow velocities below 1.5 m/s; HVAD - laminar, unidirectional flow with peak systolic flow velocities below 1.7 m/s
B. HM II - laminar, unidirectional flow with peak systolic flow velocities below 1.7 m/s; HVAD - laminar, unidirectional flow with peak systolic flow velocities below 1.5 m/s
C. HM II - laminar, unidirectional flow with peak systolic flow velocities below 1.5 m/s; HVAD - velocities cannot be measured due to Doppler artifacts
D. HM II - velocities cannot be measured due to Doppler artifacts; HVAD - laminar, unidirectional flow with peak systolic flow velocities below 1.5 m/s
E. None of these

Answer: C. HM II - laminar, unidirectional flow with peak systolic flow velocities below 1.5 m/s; HVAD - velocities cannot be measured due to Doppler artifacts. HM-II inflow-cannula peak systolic flow velocities are typically below 1.5 m/s and higher velocities suggest obstruction. HVAD inflow-cannula velocities cannot be measured due to Doppler artifacts [1].

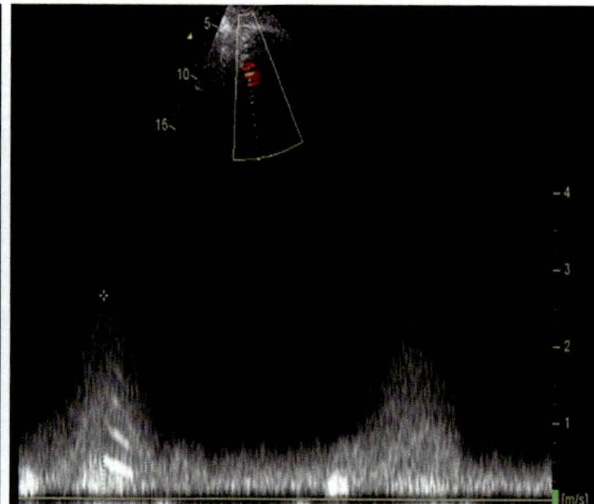

Fig. 19.4 Transthoracic echocardiographic views in a patient post HeartMate II LVAD implantation

Question 8

72-year-old patient with nonischemic cardiomyopathy underwent HM II implantation as destination therapy. Fig. 19.5 shows transthoracic echocardiographic findings most consistent with which of the following?

A. Normal outflow LVAD cannula peak velocity
B. High-velocity spectral Doppler with aliased color-flow at the inflow orifice due to malposition, suction event/other inflow obstruction
C. Decreased outflow cannula peak velocity
D. Decreased inflow cannula peak velocity (markedly reduced peak systolic and nadir diastolic velocities) suggestive of internal inflow-cannula thrombosis or more distal obstruction within the system
E. None of these

Answer: D. Decreased inflow cannula peak velocity (markedly reduced peak systolic and nadir diastolic velocities) suggestive of internal inflow-cannula thrombosis or more distal obstruction within the system. Inflow LVAD cannula peak velocity is low (bottom right panel in Fig. 19.5) despite what appears to be good Doppler alignment raising the possibility of internal inflow-cannula thrombosis or more distal obstruction within the system. Doppler flow velocity profile may appear relatively continuous (decreased phasic /pulsatile pattern).

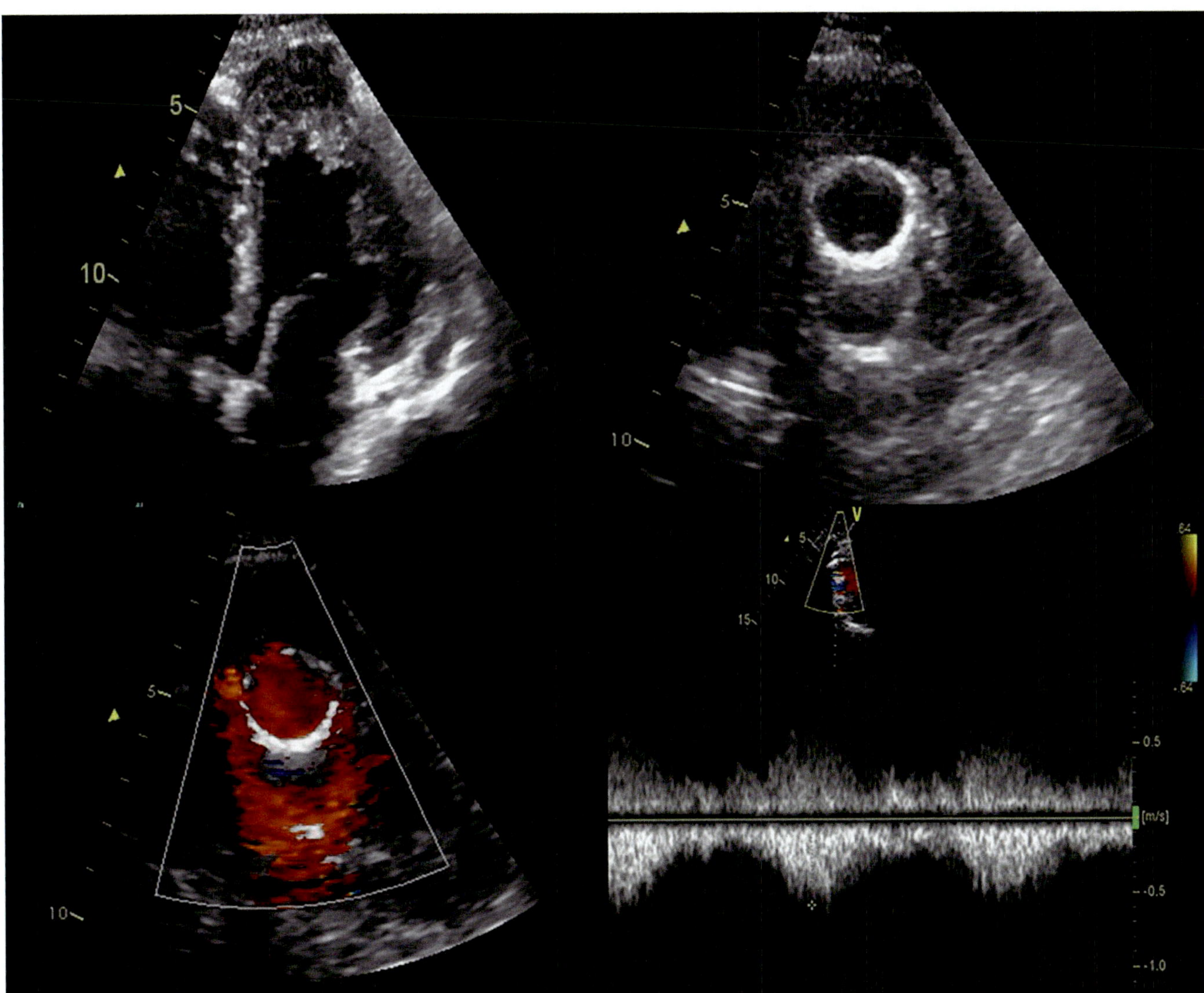

Fig. 19.5 Transthoracic echocardiographic views in a patient post HeartMate II LVAD implantation

Question 9
Echocardiography in a patient with a LVAD allows direct visualization of the following?

A. Distal inflow cannula, proximal outflow graft, mechanical impeller
B. Proximal inflow cannula, distal outflow graft
C. Proximal inflow cannula, distal outflow graft, mechanical impeller
D. Proximal inflow cannula, proximal outflow graft
E. None of these

Answer: B. Proximal inflow cannula, distal outflow graft Echocardiography allows direct visualization of the proximal inflow cannula at the left ventricular apex, and the distal outflow graft at the ascending aorta. Echocardiography does not allow direct visualization of the proximal outflow graft nor the mechanical impeller [1].

Question 10
Turbulent color Doppler flow through HM II inflow cannula or significant peak systolic velocity variability suggests:

A. Mechanical obstruction by the interventricular septum
B. Mechanical obstruction by LV trabeculations
C. Mechanical obstruction by the sub-mitral apparatus
D. None of these
E. All of these

Answer: E. All of these Any turbulence of flow on spectral and color Doppler analysis of inflow HM II cannula or significant peak systolic velocity variability suggests mechanical obstruction [1]. It can be caused by the interventricular septum, LV muscular trabeculations or the sub-mitral apparatus [1].

Question 11
A "suction event" is:

A. A sudden decrease in arterial oxygen saturation after LVAD implantation in patients with PFO or other right-to-left shunt
B. A condition in which a segment of LV myocardium occludes the inflow cannula and reduces pump inflow
C. Is usually related to over-pumping of the right ventricle
D. Cannot be corrected without surgical revision
E. All of these

Answer: B. A condition in which a segment of LV myocardium occludes the inflow cannula and reduces pump inflow. Signs of a suction event include a decrease in LV size (typically <3 cm), leftward interventricular septum shifting, inlet cannula flow impedance, worsening tricuspid regurgitation due to septal shifting and/or right ventricular enlargement. Such a "suction event" can be corrected by reducing the pump speed and identifying and treating the underlying cause of the event [1].

Question 12
A "suction event" can result from:

A. Hypovolemia
B. Cardiac tamponade
C. Right ventricular failure
D. None of these
E. All of these

Answer: E. All of these. A "suction event" (whereby a segment of LV myocardium occludes the inflow cannula and reduces pump inflow) is usually related to excessive LVAD speeds (where the interventricular septum shifts leftward to impede flow into the inflow cannula), or clinical scenarios such as hypovolemia, cardiac tamponade, right ventricular failure (Videos 19.3 and 19.4) [1]. As stated, it can be corrected by reducing the pump speed and identifying and treating the underlying cause of the event [1].

Question 13
Angulation of the LVAD inflow cannula towards the interventricular septum:

A. Has to be avoided
B. Some angulation might be acceptable
C. Is acceptable in patients with a small left ventricle
D. Is acceptable in patients with a small right ventricle
E. Is always acceptable

Answer: B. Some angulation might be acceptable An inflow cannula should be positioned within the LV apex and directed towards the mitral valve [1]. Some angulation towards the interventricular septum might be acceptable [1]. An excessive angulation might require surgical revision after decrease in LV size [1]. Direct contact of the interventricular septum and cannula might cause ventricular arrhythmia and inflow cannula-flow obstruction [1]. Echocardiographic findings suggesting inflow cannula-flow obstruction include high-velocity color or spectral Doppler at inflow orifice with aliased color-flow Doppler and continuous wave Doppler velocity > 1.5 m/s [1].

Question 14
In patients with LVAD and suspected inflow-cannula obstruction:

A. Inflow-cannula and outflow-cannula spectral Doppler velocities may be elevated
B. Inflow-cannula spectral Doppler velocities may be decreased, and outflow-cannula Doppler velocities may be elevated

C. Inflow-cannula spectral Doppler velocities may be elevated, and outflow-cannula velocities may be decreased
D. Inflow-cannula and outflow-cannula spectral Doppler velocities may be decreased
E. None of these.

Answer: C. Inflow-cannula spectral Doppler velocities may be elevated, and outflow-cannula velocities may be decreased. In patients with inflow-cannula obstruction, inflow-cannula spectral Doppler velocities may be elevated since blood accelerates proximal to the obstruction [1]. Outflow-cannula velocities may be decreased or peak velocities may vary [1]. Transesophageal echocardiography might visualize vegetations or thrombi obstructing cannulas [1].

Question 15
Tamponade in patients with LVAD:

A. May mimic right ventricular failure
B. Should be suspected in the presence of pericardial effusion/hematoma, small left/right ventricle size, and high-flow alarms
C. Should be suspected if right ventricular outflow tract cardiac output is high and fails to vary with pump speed changes
D. None of these
E. All of these

Answer: A. May mimic right ventricular failure. Cardiac tamponade in patients with LVAD may mimic right ventricular failure [1]. Cardiac tamponade should be suspected in presence of pericardial effusion/hematoma, small left/right ventricle size, and low-flow alarms [1]. Typically, right ventricular outflow tract cardiac output is low and fails to vary with pump speed changes [1].

Question 16
In patients with LVAD and mechanical obstruction of the outflow graft, which of the following statements is true?

A. Inflow-cannula spectral Doppler velocities may be normal or decreased, and outflow-cannula spectral Doppler velocities must be normal or increased
B. Inflow-cannula spectral Doppler velocities may be normal or decreased, and outflow-cannula spectral Doppler velocities may be normal, decreased or increased
C. Inflow-cannula spectral Doppler velocities may be normal or decreased, and outflow-cannula spectral Doppler velocities must be normal or decreased
D. A ramp study is not helpful
E. None of these

Answer: B. Inflow-cannula spectral Doppler velocities may be normal or decreased, and outflow-cannula spectral Doppler velocities may be normal, decreased or increased. Mechanical obstruction of the outflow graft might result from its malposition, kinking, external compression or thrombosis [1]. Depending on the degree of obstruction, inflow-cannula spectral Doppler velocities may be normal or decreased [1]. The outflow-cannula velocities may be normal or decreased if sampled significantly proximal or distal to the obstruction or increased if sampled in the area of obstruction [1]. A ramp study might be extremely helpful by revealing attenuation of change in LV size, the degree of AV opening and flow changes with changes in pump speeds which could indicate mechanical obstruction of the outflow graft [1].

Question 17
High-flow alarms in patients with LVADs can be caused by:

A. Right ventricular failure, significant aortic regurgitation, systemic arterial vasodilation
B. Significant aortic regurgitation, systemic arterial vasodilation, pump thrombosis
C. Right ventricular failure, inflow/outflow-cannula obstruction, significant aortic regurgitation
D. Significant aortic regurgitation, cardiac tamponade, pump thrombosis
E. None of these

Answer: B. Significant aortic regurgitation, systemic arterial vasodilation, pump thrombosis. High-flow alarms are caused by significant aortic regurgitation, systemic arterial vasodilation, pump thrombosis and recovery of native LV function [1]. Low-flow alarms can be caused by suction events, right ventricular failure, hypovolemia, cardiac tamponade, inflow/outflow-cannula obstruction, hypertension and arrhythmias [1].

Question 18
Echocardiographic signs of primary LVAD pump dysfunction secondary to thrombosis include:

A. Decreased LV end-diastolic diameter, a septal shift towards the right ventricle, increased AV opening, decreased diastolic spectral Doppler velocities through inflow and outflow cannulas
B. Increased LV end-diastolic diameter, a septal shift towards the right ventricle, increased AV opening, decreased systolic spectral Doppler velocities through inflow and outflow cannulas
C. Increased LV end-diastolic diameter, a septal shift towards the right ventricle, increased AV opening, decreased diastolic spectral Doppler velocities through inflow and outflow cannulas
D. Cannot be recognized without a ramp study
E. None of these

Answer: C. Increased LV end-diastolic diameter, a septal shift towards the right ventricle, increased AV opening, decreased diastolic spectral Doppler velocities through inflow and outflow cannulas. Echocardiographic signs of primary LVAD pump dysfunction secondary to thrombosis include failure to unload the left ventricle (manifesting as increased LV end-diastolic diameter, a septal shift towards the right ventricle and increased AV opening). Depending on the degree of obstruction, inflow-cannula spectral Doppler velocities may be normal or decreased [1]. The outflow-cannula velocities may be normal or decreased if sampled significantly proximal or distal to the obstruction or increased if sampled in the area of obstruction [1]. Echo findings such as the above can suggest LVAD pump dysfunction secondary to thrombosis. Sometimes, thrombus can be directly visualised (see Video 19.5) which highlights a case of outflow-cannula thrombosis). A ramp study might be extremely helpful by revealing attenuation of change in LV size, the degree of AV opening and flow changes with changes in pump speeds which could provide additional information to indicate mechanical obstruction of the outflow graft [1].

Question 19

In patients with continuous flow-LVAD:

A. Left ventricular end-systolic diameter is the most accurate measure of left ventricular unloading
B. Left ventricular end-diastolic diameter is the most accurate measure of left ventricular size
C. Left ventricular end-diastolic volume is the most accurate measure of left ventricular size
D. Left ventricular end-systolic volume is the most accurate measure of left ventricular unloading
E. None of these

Answer: C. Left ventricular end-diastolic volume is the most accurate measure of left ventricular size. Left ventricular end-diastolic diameter is the most reproducible measure of left ventricular unloading in patients with continuous flow-LVAD [1]. The LV end-diastolic volume is the most accurate measure of LV size in those patients [1]

Question 20

Persistence of significant mitral regurgitation after LVAD implantation:

A. May indicate outflow cannula malposition
B. May indicate inadequate LV unloading
C. Is expected
D. Can be corrected by reducing the pump speed
E. None of these

Answer: B. May indicate inadequate LV unloading. Persistence of significant mitral regurgitation after LVAD implantation may indicate inadequate (too low) LVAD speed, inflow cannula malposition and interference with subvalvular apparatus, inadequate LV unloading or LVAD malfunction [1].

Question 21

Speed-change testing involving low pump speeds in patients with a LVAD:

A. Should not be performed in patients on oral anticoagulation
B. Is associated with risk of embolic events
C. Can be continued if a "suction event" event occurs
D. Can safely be performed if anticoagulation therapy is inadequate
E. Can safely be performed in the presence of a possible intra-cardiac or aortic root thrombus

Answer: B. Is associated with risk of embolic events. One of the settings in which a speed-change test occurs is a problem-focused (ramp) exam and ideally requires an experienced and knowledgeable member of the mechanical circulatory support team to be immediately available to solve potential problems and recognize key safety endpoints. Speed-change testing involving low pump speeds can only be performed if a patient is on anticoagulation [1]. In general, strong consideration should be given to deferring speed-change exams if baseline imaging shows a possible intra-cardiac or aortic root thrombus. The procedure is associated with risk of embolic events with sudden AV opening given presence of aortic root thrombus or pump thrombi [1]. The test has to be stopped if there is appearance of a suction event, new symptoms, hypertension or cannula flow reversal [1].

Question 22

27-year-old patient with peripartum cardiomyopathy was admitted to the hospital with cardiogenic shock. An Impella CP was placed. Reduced flows were noted and the initial transthoracic echocardiography image is shown in Fig. 19.6 (left panel). The Impella device was repositioned and the subsequent transthoracic echocardiography image is shown in Fig. 19.6 (right panel). No further Impella flow alarms were noted and exit Impella flow was noted above the aortic valve.

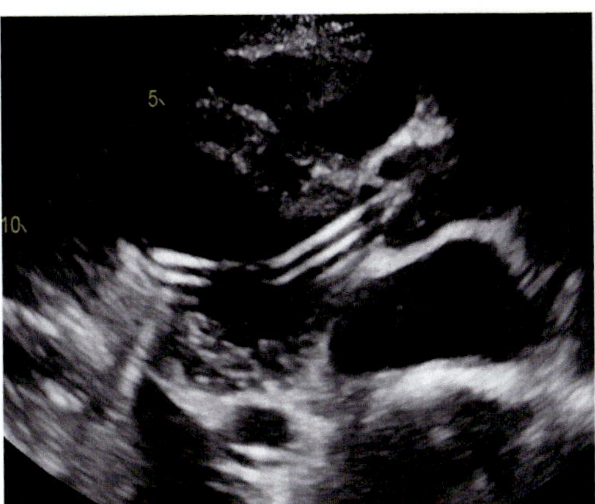

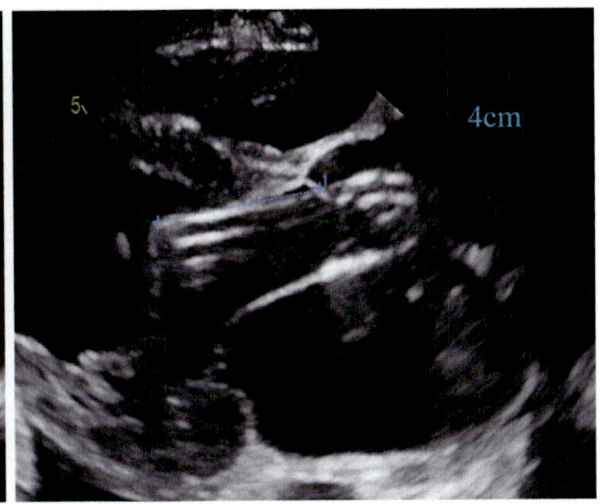

Fig. 19.6 Modified parasternal long axis view of the left ventricle in a patient post Impella CP implantation

Transthoracic echocardiography images in Fig. 19.6 (left panel; right panel) demonstrate an Impella catheter position that is:

A. An optimal Impella position in the left panel
B. A suboptimal Impella position in the right panel
C. The Impella catheter inlet area should be placed 3.5–4.0 cm below the aortic annulus
D. Impella position cannot be adequately assessed by echocardiography
E. These echo images are non-diagnostic

Answer: C. The Impella catheter inlet area should be placed 3.5–4.0 cm below the aortic annulus. The Impella catheter should be angled towards the left ventricular apex away from the heart wall, and it should not be obstruct the mitral valve. The Impella catheter inlet area should be placed 3.5–4.0 cm below the aortic annulus [1]. Absence of Impella flow alarms and exit Impella flow noted above the aortic valve is further support for adequate Impella catheter position. Another example of a case involving Impella catheter-related malposition due to impingement on the mitral valve and severe mitral regurgitation is shown in Videos 19.6, 19.7 and 19.8.

Question 23
In patients receiving Impella catheter support:

A. The aortic valve always opens
B. The aortic valve is always closed
C. Net forward flow can be obtained by calculating right ventricular outflow tract stroke volume and cardiac volume with Doppler methods
D. Pump's color flow artifact should lie proximal to the annulus
E. The Impella catheter inlet area should be placed 5 cm below the aortic annulus.

Answer: C. Net forward flow can be obtained by calculating right ventricular outflow tract stroke volume and cardiac volume with Doppler methods. In patients receiving Impella catheter support, the aortic valve may be partially open or closed as with other LVADs [1]. Net forward flow can be obtained by calculating right ventricular outflow tract stroke volume and cardiac volume with Doppler methods [1]. Pump's color flow artifact should lie distal to the annulus [1]. The Impella catheter inlet area should be placed 3.5–4.0 cm below the aortic annulus [1].

Question 24
A 62-year-old patient with non-ischemic cardiomyopathy status post ICD implantation presents acutely with a saddle pulmonary embolism on CT which also reported suspicion for intra-cardiac masses. Trans-thoracic imaging was technically difficult and images were non-diagnostic. Transesophageal echocardiography was performed. A saddle pulmonary embolism was also evident by transesophageal echocardiography (Video 19.9). In Fig. 19.7, additonal large serpiginous echodensities were identified and these were located:

A. On the device lead, tricuspid valve and in the inferior vena cava extending into the right atrium
B. On the device lead, tricuspid valve and in the superior vena cava extending into the right atrium
C. On the mitral valve and in the inferior vena cava extending into the right atrium
D. On the aortic valve and in the superior vena cava extending into the right atrium
E. On the interatrial septum and in the right atrium

Answer: B. On the device lead, tricuspid valve and in the superior vena cava extending into the right atrium. Fig. 19.7 shows transesophageal echocardiographic images of bi-caval views where the superior vena cava is towards the right and the inferior vena cava is towards the left. The left

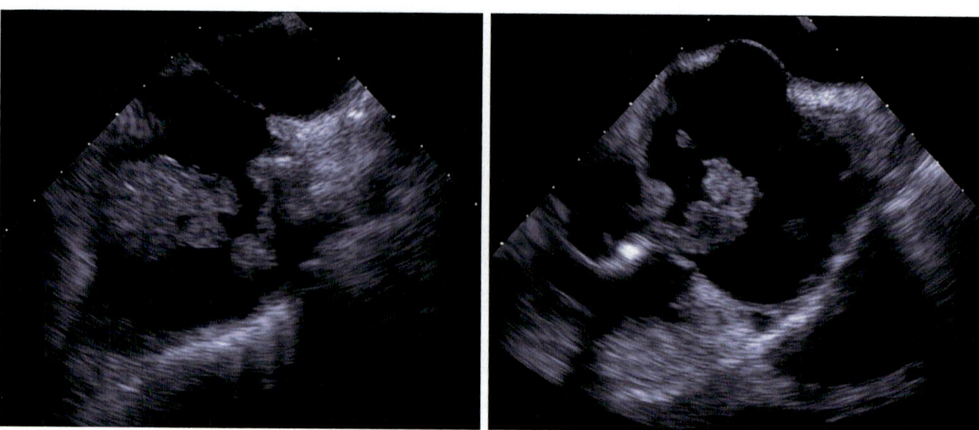

Fig. 19.7 Transesophageal echocardiographic bi-caval views (90 degrees)

panel shows large serpiginous echodensities within in the right atrium as well as in the superior vena cava extending into the right atrium. The right panel shows large serpiginous echodensities on the device lead and on the tricuspid valve. The mitral and aortic valves are not seen in these bi-caval views. The interatrial septum appears free of echodensities. In the presence of a persistent foramen ovale, right atrial echodensities may extend across the interatrial septum (eg. clot in transit) and may cause paradoxical embolism.

Question 25

Masses on leads of cardiovascular implantable electronic devices:

A. Are found in 70% of echocardiographic studies imaging intra-cardiac leads
B. Differential diagnosis includes vegetation, thrombus and fibrinous strands
C. Clinical correlation is generally not important to make a definitive diagnosis
D. Are most often related to side-lobe artifact
E. Are most often related to mirror artifact

Answer: B. Differential diagnosis includes vegetation, thrombus and fibrinous strands. Masses on device leads are reported in 14% of echocardiographic studies imaging leads [3]. The incidence of thrombi on device leads has been reported to be as a high as 48% on autopsies [3]. The differential diagnosis includes vegetation, thrombus and fibrinous strands [3]. Clinical correlation is necessary in every case to make a definitive diagnosis. Reverberations from right ventricular intra-cardiac device leads occasionally may mimic masses in other cardiac chambers.

Question 26

Figure 19.8 shows an echodensity marked with an asterisk (*) represents:

A. Right ventricular lead of a permanent pacemaker
B. Temporary pacing lead
C. Leadless pacemaker
D. Pulmonary valve calcification
E. Prominent tricuspid valve sub-valvular apparatus

Answer: C. Leadless pacemaker. Leadless pacemakers are implanted directly into the right ventricle (Video 19.10). The

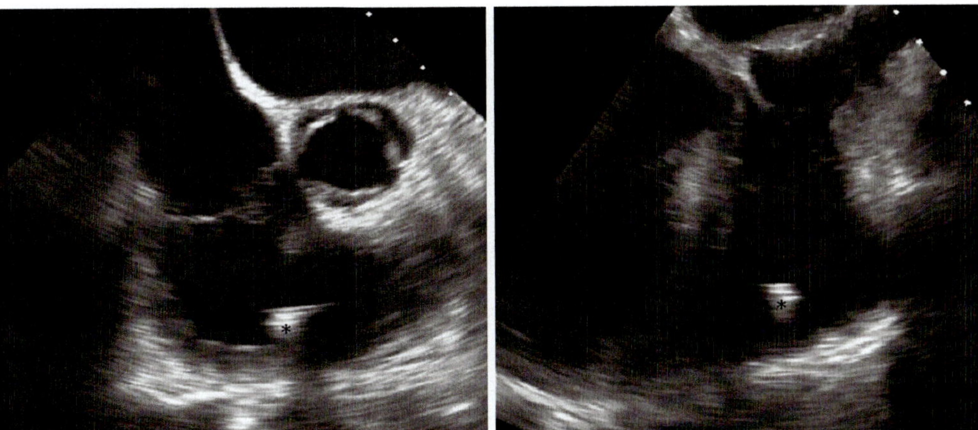

Fig. 19.8 Transesophageal echocardiographic views

absence of leads avoids risks such as venous obstruction and makes infective endocarditis, tricuspid regurgitation less likely. Pocket complications such as infection or hematoma are also avoided.

Question 27

A 45-year-old patient with a dual chamber pacemaker underwent routine echocardiography that revealed a normally functioning tricuspid valve. No signs of bacteremia were noted. Fig. 19.9 shows an echodensity marked with an asterisk (*) that most likely represents:

A. Right atrial lead prolapsing into the right ventricle during diastole
B. Chiari network
C. Right ventricular lead prolapsing into the right atrium during systole
D. Prominent Eustachian Valve
E. Vegetation

Answer: A. Right atrial lead prolapsing into the right ventricle during diastole. Fig. 19.9 shows similar images in the top panels with and without color, and similar images in the bottom panels with and without color. Red forward flow across the tricuspid valve in the top panel implies that the top panel color compare images are diastolic images. Blue reverse flow across the tricuspid valve in the bottom panel implies that the bottom panel color compare images are systolic images. The echodensity marked with an asterisk (*) is seen to be in the right atrium in the bottom images in systole, and in the right ventricle in the top images (diastole), therefore most likely represents a right atrial lead prolapsing into the right ventricle during diastole. A Chiari network and the Eustachian Valve represent right atrial structures while vegetation is also a less likely differential given the images and clinical scenario.

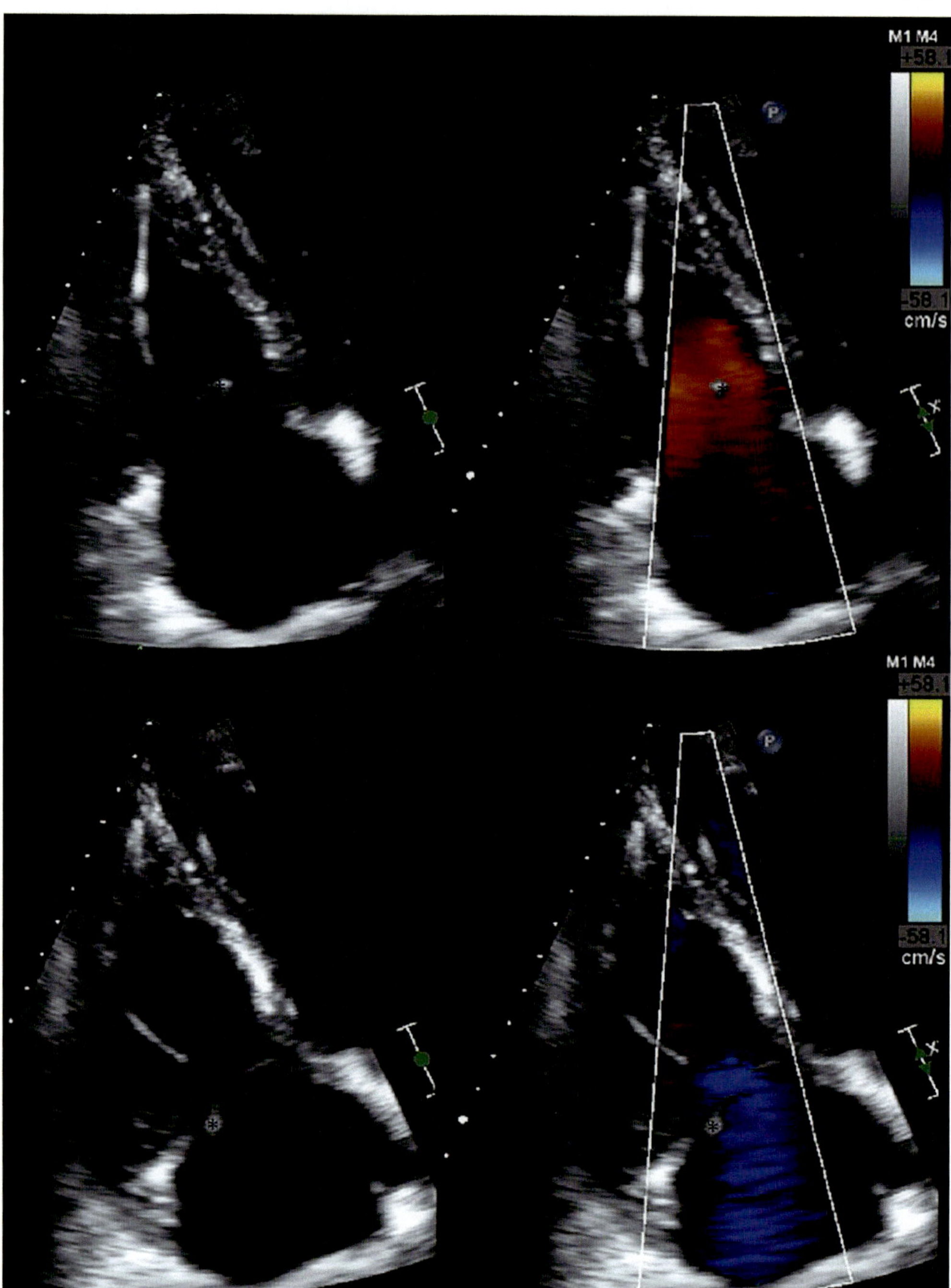

Fig. 19.9 Transthoracic echocardiographic views

Question 28
What are the characteristics of myxoma on transthoracic echocardiography?

A. It is a lobulated and well-defined mass often attached to the interatrial septum via a stalk
B. It is often associated with hemopericardium
C. It is a homogenous mass without foci of calcification
D. It is a broad attached mass with limited mobility
E. It never causes functional mitral stenosis

Answer: A. It is a lobulated and well-defined mass often attached to the interatrial septum via a stalk. Myxomas are the most common benign tumor of the heart and are usually well circumscribed, lobulated, round or oval, mobile masses with smooth margins attached to the endocardial surface by a stalk (see Video 19.11) [4]. They are often heterogeneous with foci of calcification. Myxomas are often confused with thrombi [4]. Large and even giant left atrial myxomas have been described and have been associated with functional mitral stenosis.

Question 29

Myxomas are most often located in (in order of decreasing frequency):

A. Left atrium, right atrium, left ventricle, right ventricle
B. Right atrium, left atrium, right ventricle, left ventricle
C. Left ventricle, left atrium, right atrium, right ventricle
D. Left atrium, left ventricle, right atrium, right ventricle
E. Left atrium, right ventricle, right atrium, left ventricle

Answer: A. Left atrium, right atrium, left ventricle, right ventricle. Myxomas are most often located in the left (almost 90%) and right (15%) atrium [4]. A smaller number are equally split between the left and right ventricles (5% each) [4].

Question 30

A papillary fibroelastoma visualized on an echocardiographic study is usually:

A. Located on the upstream size of the valve only
B. Immobile
C. Calcified
D. Small size and highly mobile
E. A lobulated and well-defined mass often attached to the interatrial septum via a stalk

Answer: D. Small size and highly mobile. Papillary fibroelastomas are rare, benign, small, well circumscribed and pedunculated tumors of the endocardium that most often originate from left-sided heart valves [5]. A lobulated and well-defined mass often attached to the interatrial septum via a stalk would most likely be a myxoma. Fibroelastomas are the most common valve-associated tumors (85–90%), are may be confused with vegetations and Lambl's excrescences [4]. Unlike vegetations, fibroelastomas are usually attached to the downstream side of the valve [4]. They rarely cause valvular dysfunction, but thrombus formed on their surface may cause cerebral, retinal, coronary and pulmonary embolic events [5].

Question 31

A 54-year-old patient with hypertension underwent a routine echocardiographic study. There is no fever, bacteremia or weight loss. Transthoracic echocardiography (Fig. 19.10) demonstrates a mobile well circumscribed echodensity:

A. On the tricuspid valve
B. On the pulmonary valve
C. Associated with severe pulmonary stenosis
D. Associated with severe tricuspid regurgitation
E. With an appearance most consistent with papillary fibroelastoma, less likely myxoma

Answer: E. With an appearance most consistent with papillary fibroelastoma, less likely myxoma. These transthoracic echocardiographic images show the pulmonary valve; top left, parasternal short axis view; top right, zoomed parasternal short axis view; bottom left, showing the pulmonary artery and pulmonary artery bifurcation; bottom right, continuous wave Doppler showing a degree of pulmonary valve regurgitation and mildly increased systolic forward flow velocities suggesting mild pulmonary valve stenosis.

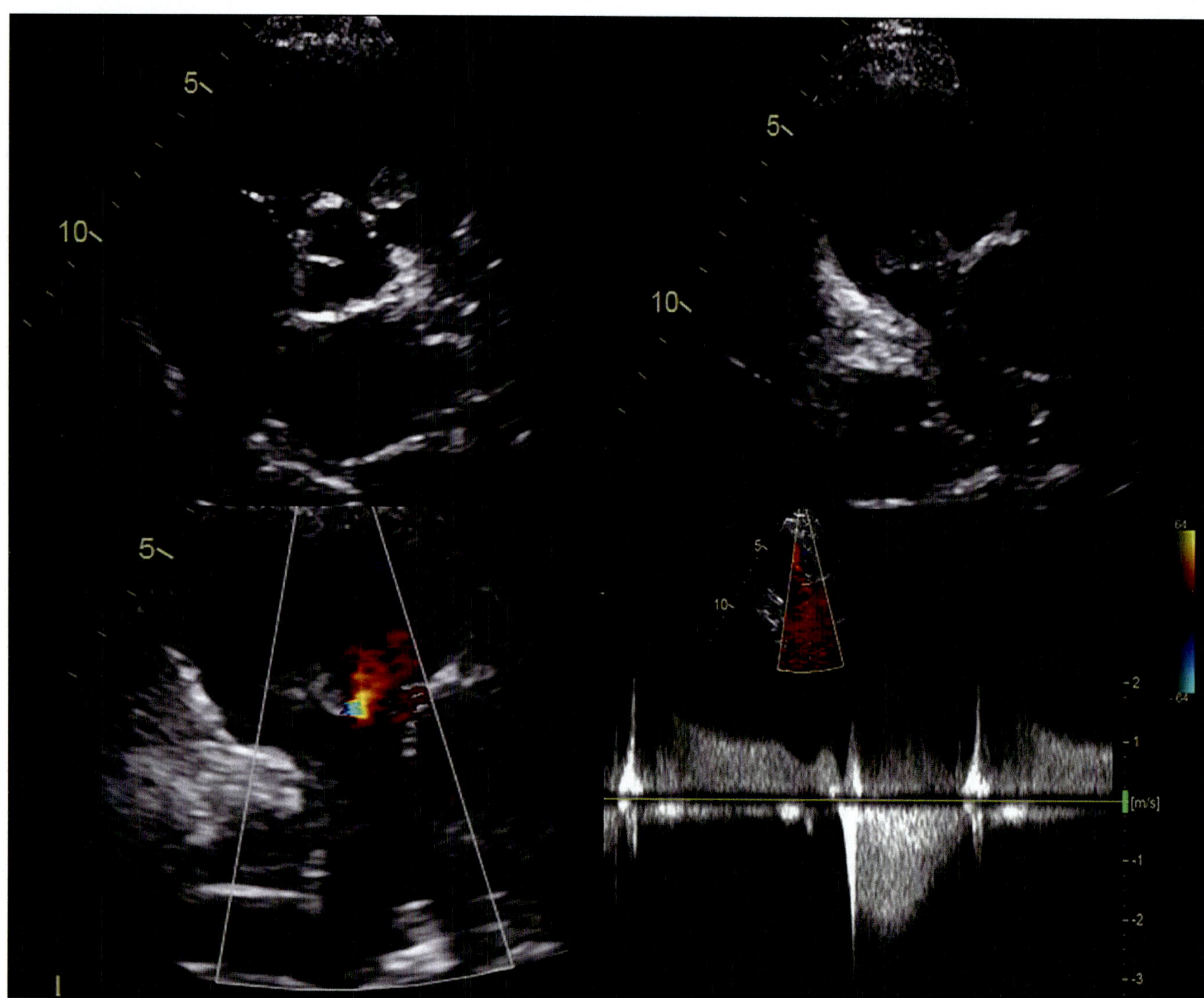

Fig. 19.10 Transthoracic echocardiographic views

Question 32

The transthoracic images in Fig. 19.11 demonstrate:

A. Pulmonary vein thrombus
B. Eustachian valve
C. Right ventricular pacemaker lead
D. Cor triatriatum sinister
E. Cor triatriatum dexter

Answer: B. Eustachian valve. The transthoracic images in Fig. 19.11 demonstrate a right atrial echodensity consistent with an Eustachian valve, which is a leaf-like linear structure at the junction of inferior vena cava and right atrium, that is directed towards the foramen ovale (See Videos 19.12 and 19.13). Cor triatriatum dexter is a very rare congential anomaly sinistrum resulting from persistence of the right venous valve and results in partitioning the right atrium into two separate chambers. Cor triatriatum sinistrum is a left atrial structure.

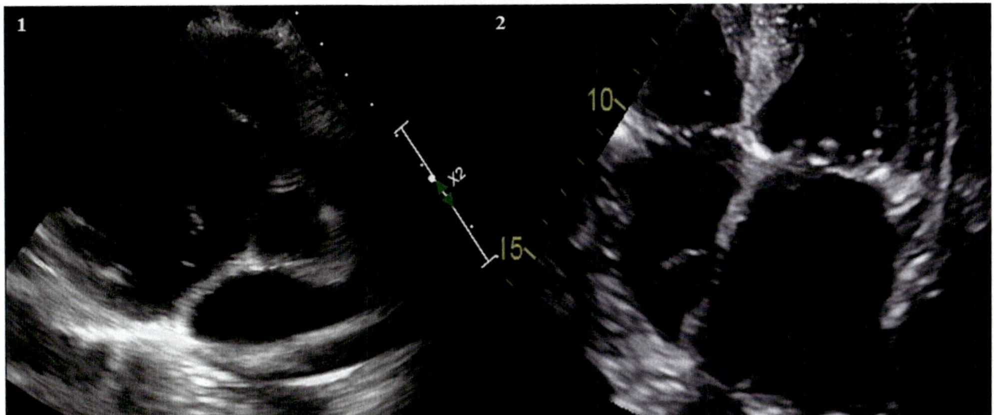

Fig. 19.11 Transthoracic echocardiographic views

Question 33
The Eustachian valve is a remnant of the embryonic:

A. superior vena caval valve
B. inferior vena caval valve
C. tricuspid valve
D. coronary sinus valve
E. cor triatriatum dexter

Answer: B. inferior vena caval valve. The Eustachian valve is a leaf-like linear structure at the junction of inferior vena cava and right atrium, and a remnant of the embryonic inferior vena caval valve that is directed towards the foramen ovale. The equivalent valve for the coronary sinus is the Thebesian valve.

Question 34
The Chiari network:

A. Can cause problems during percutaneous procedures
B. Can be confused for a flail tricuspid valve leaflet
C. Is thought to be a variant of the Eustachian valve
D. All of these
E. None of these

Answer: D. All of these. The Chiari network is a freely mobile membranous structure in the right atrium attached along the ridge connecting vena cavae and interatrial septum [6]. It is believed to be a variant of Eustachian valve but more mobile and thinner [6]. The Chiari network might be confused for a tricuspid vegetation, a flail tricuspid valve leaflet, thrombus and pedunculated tumors [6]. Entrapment of right-heart catheters in Chiari network has been reported [6].

Question 35
A 43-year-old man presents with drenching night sweats, fatigue and a subjective fever for 2 weeks. Chest x-ray findings were consistent with a recent upper respiratory infection but also showed an enlarged cardiac silhouette. On further questioning, he reports exertional dyspnea and dizziness with standing that has worsened over the prior 2 months. An echocardiogram was performed and showed a large right atrial mass (Fig. 19.12). An F-FDG PET [7] scan showed intense uptake in the right atrium with no other sites identified. A cardiac CT showed an intra-cardiac mass invading the right atrial wall with vascular supply from the right coronary artery. Biopsy of this mass is most likely to show:

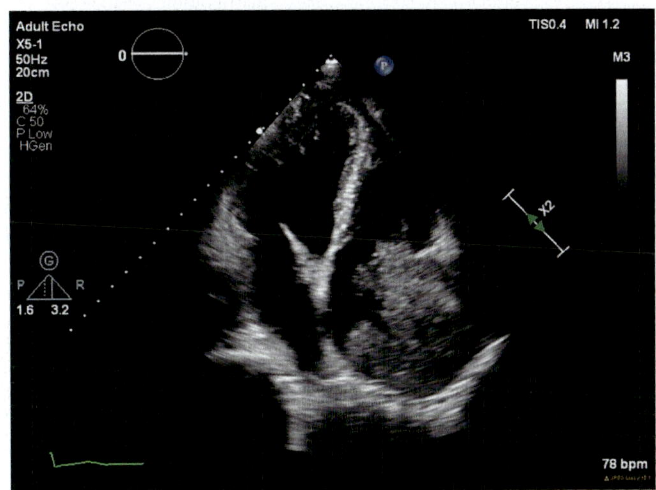

Fig. 19.12 Modified apical 4 chamber view

A. Angiosarcoma
B. Rhabdomyosarcoma
C. Atrial Myxoma
D. Primary cardiac lymphoma
E. Liposarcoma

Answer: A. Angiosarcoma. Secondary cardiac tumors are considered the most frequent cardiac neoplasms. Amongst primary cardiac tumours, the vast majority are benign, with myxomas being the most common. Myxomas may be associated with obstructive symptoms, but are not associated with invasion of other tissues. Overall, primary malignant neoplasms of the heart are rare but the most common are sarcomas (accounting for up to 90% of primary cardiac malignancies). Roughly one quarter of these sarcomas are angiosarcomas. Angiosarcomas are infiltrative hypervascular tumors that tend to occur in the right atrium and may lead to obstructive symptoms. Surgical resection is commonly recommended though prognosis is poor [8]. Less common sarcomas are leiomyosarcomas, rhabdomyosarcomas, liposarcomas, and osteosarcomas. After sarcomas, primary cardiac lymphomas are the next most common primary malignant neoplasm of the heart.

Question 36

A 50-year-old woman undergoes routine transthoracic echocardiography (Fig. 19.13) for the evaluation of paroxysmal atrial fibrillation. This subxiphoid view shows:

A. Lipomatous hypertrophy of the interatrial septum
B. Lipoma
C. Liposarcoma
D. Rhabdomyoma
E. Fibroma

Answer: A. Lipomatous hypertrophy of the interatrial septum. Figure 19.13 demonstrates lipomatous hypertrophy of the interatrial septum, characterized by excessive fat accumulation in the limbus of the fossa ovalis of the septum. The fossa ovalis is spared in lipomatous hypertrophy of the interatrial septum giving the dumbbell appearance. Lipomatous hypertrophy of the interatrial septum is differentiated from lipomas in that it is not encapsulated [9]. Very rarely, if very exuberant, lipomatous hypertrophy of the interatrial septum can cause obstructive physiology (most commonly to the vena cavae), in which case surgical options can be considered. Liposarcoma is a rare primary malignant tumor of the heart which is associated with tissue plane infiltration and invasion. Rhabdomyoma are intramural tumors often multiple and involving the interventricular septum that more commonly affect children, are highly associated with tuberous sclerosis, and frequently regress during early childhood. Fibromas are intramural usually solitary tumors often involving the interventricular septum that typically do not regress and may contain calcifications.

Question 37

The most common primary cardiac tumor in children is:

A. Teratoma
B. Myxoma
C. Hemangioma
D. Rhabdomyoma
E. Liposarcoma

Answer: D. Rhabdomyoma. In contrast to adults where the most common primary cardiac tumors are myxomas, the most common primary cardiac tumor in children is a rhabdomyoma, accounting for 45% of tumors [10]. Ninety percent of cardiac tumors in children are benign. Other common primary cardiac tumors in children are fibromas, teratomas and myxomas.

Question 38

A 35-year-old woman with a history of resistant hypertension, irregular menses, progressive weight gain and right sided back pain undergoes an echocardiogram which shows a right atrial mass extending from the inferior vena cava. Cross sectional imaging is most likely to show:

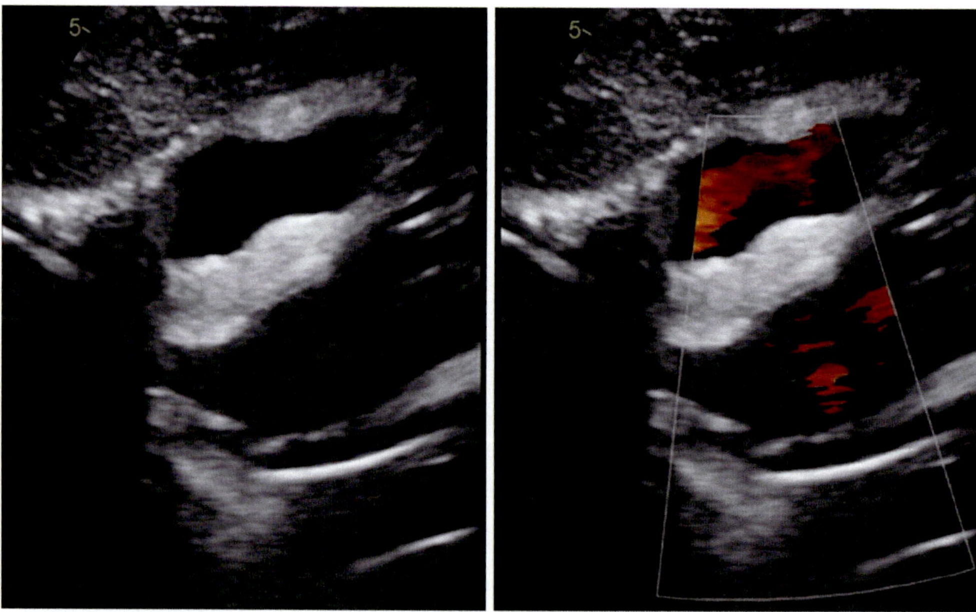

Fig. 19.13 Subcostal views without color Doppler (left panel) and with color Doppler (right panel)

A. Adrenocortical carcinoma
B. Renal cell carcinoma
C. Wilm's Tumor
D. Hepatocellular carcinoma
E. Liposarcoma

Answer: D. Adrenocortical carcinoma While all these entities have metastatic potential to the heart via intravascular tumor extension into the inferior vena cava, the patient's clinical syndrome is most consistent with a functional adrenal tumor [11].

Question 39
Which of these statements is false?

A. Metastatic spread to the heart via the lymphatic system, while documented, is exceedingly rare compared to hematogenous spread and direct tumor invasion.
B. The pericardium tends to be spared as a site of tumor metastases.
C. Secondary cardiac tumors are around 40 times more common than primary cardiac tumors.
D. Melanoma are amongst the malignancies with the highest proclivity to cardiac metastasis.
E. Lung cancers are amongst the malignancies with the highest proclivity to cardiac metastasis.

Answer: B. The pericardium tends to be spared as a site of tumor metastases. In principle, all malignancies have metastatic potential to spread to the heart (though cancers of the central nervous symptoms are not known to spread to the heart). The manner of spread can be hematogenous or direct/intravascular invasion, rarely lymphatic. The most common cancers to metastasize are carcinomas of the lung, the breast and the esophagus, malignant lymphoma, leukemia, and malignant melanoma. Of these lung, breast and esophagus carcinomas are thought to spread via the lymphatic system and as such affect the pericardium commonly [12].

Question 40
Which of the following statements about the finding on this echocardiogram in Fig. 19.14 is false?

A. Two key echocardiographic features indicating high risk for embolization are protrusion into the left ventricular cavity and free mobility.
B. Anticoagulation is associated with significant reduction with risk of systemic embolization
C. This condition is an absolute contraindication to cardioversion.
D. Use of contrast, doubles the rate of detection of these masses

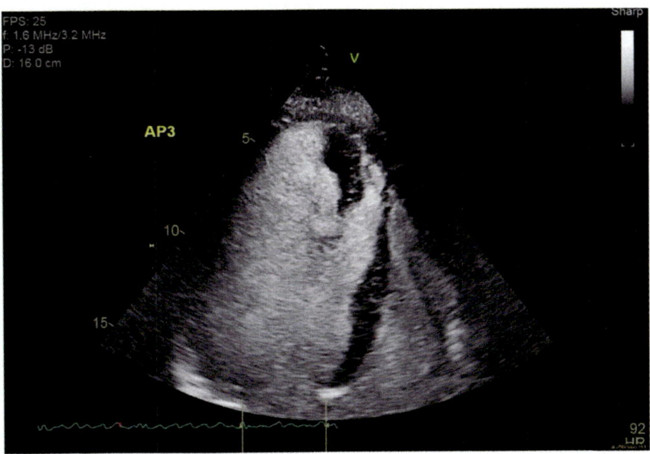

Fig. 19.14 Modified apical 3 chamber view

E. The most sensitive cardiac imaging modality of detection is cardiac magnetic resonance imaging, but specificity for this finding is high with echo and cardiac magnetic resonance imaging.

Answer: C. This condition is an absolute contraindication to cardioversion. While hesitance regarding cardioversion in the presence of apical left ventricular thrombus is understandable, there is little data to support such concerns. Case series suggest that risk of systemic embolization with cardioversion is low in the proper setting [7].

Question 41
A 25-year-old woman undergoing CT abdomen-pelvis is incidentally found to have a well-defined, spherical mass next to the pericardial space of the right atrium consistent with a pericardial cyst. An echocardiogram is performed (Fig. 19.15). Which is true regarding diagnosis and management?

A. The rim of the cyst is echodense and well circumscribed and the interior has an echodensity similar to soft tissue on echocardiography
B. Pericardial cysts tend to be found along the right costophrenic angle but can occur anywhere along the heart border.
C. Pericardial cysts require serial surveillance with yearly MRI or CT to evaluate for malignant transformation, though resection is often offered regardless of symptoms.
D. Pericardial cysts are known to continually and slowly expand, usually at rate of 2–5 mm/year in diameter.
E. Pericardial cysts are associated with a high likelihood of cardiac tamponade and constrictive physiology

Answer: A. Pericardial cysts tend to be found along the right costophrenic angle but can occur anywhere along

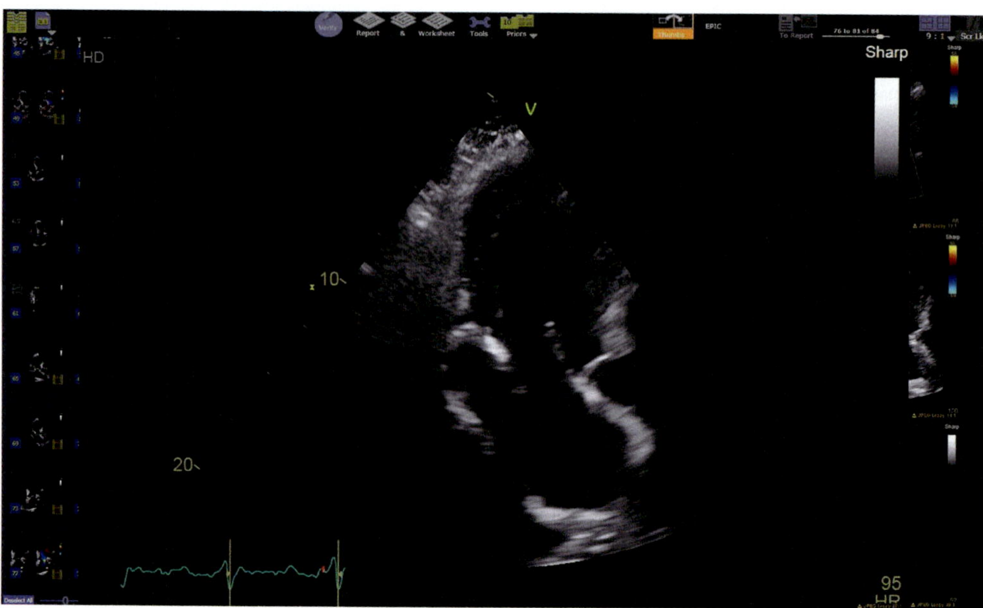

Fig. 19.15 Transthoracic echocardiographic view

the heart border.. The majority of pericardial cysts are asymptomatic. Case series of pericardial cysts suggest that they tend to remain asymptomatic and largely stable in size of time and that life-long serial imaging is not needed [13].

Question 42
A 45-year-old woman with a history of Cushing's syndrome and prior atrial myxoma resection is found to have a recurrent atrial myxoma on routine echocardiography. Exam is notable for multiple intensely pigmented dark blue nevi. She reports that her two children have similar medical issues. What genetic disorder is this patient's presentation most consistent with?

A. Carney complex
B. Uhl's syndrome
C. Peutz-Jeghers syndrome
D. McCune-Albright syndrome
E. Gorlin syndrome

Answer: A. Carney Complex. This complex is a rare autosomal dominant syndrome that involves inactivating mutations of the PRKAR1A gene which is associated with abnormalities in skin pigmentation, endocrine tumors (commonly Sertoli tumors, primary pigmented nodular adrenal cortical disease, thyroid adenoma) and cardiac myxomas. Case series have shown increased recurrence rate of myxomas in Carney complex [14].

Question 43
A 57-year-old coal miner presents to the emergency department with several weeks of fevers, chills, shortness of breath and weight loss. In the course of her workup an echocardiogram is obtained which shows a small left atrial mass not consistent with thrombus or vegetation. This mass most likely represents:

A. Myxoma
B. Fibroma
C. Lipoma
D. Sarcoma
E. Metastasis

Answer: E. Metastasis. The majority of cardiac tumors are those that have metastasized from outside of the heart. While there are certain classic findings on echocardiography that may suggest a primary cardiac tumor, in the absence of such finding metastasis must strongly be considered. Of note, some atrial myxomas are known to secrete IL-6, which can lead to constitutional symptoms.

Question 44
An otherwise healthy 63-year-old asymptomatic woman undergoes an echocardiogram for evaluation of a murmur. The echocardiogram shows a 1.5 cm, mobile, pedunculated and stippled mass attached to the aortic side of the aortic valve. Which statement is false about this patient's condition?

A. Surgical excision is not recommended unless symptoms or evidence of valve dysfunction are noted.
B. Lambl's excrescences have the same histologic appearance of this mass but are differentiated by being linear in appearance rather than pedunculated.
C. For such masses that are over 1 cm, there may be an increased risk for embolic phenomenon that may be lessened by resection.

D. One third of such masses are seen only on transesophageal echocardiography.
E. This mass more likely represents a papillary fibroelastoma than a myxoma

Answer: A. Surgical excision is not recommended unless symptoms or evidence of valve dysfunction are noted. The described mass has characteristics most consistent with a papillary fibroelastoma (See Videos 19.14, 19.15 and 19.16). Because of the risk of thromboembolism, such patients with low surgical risk are commonly recommended to undergo excision of left sided papillary fibroelastomas at experienced surgical centers. There is weak observational single center data regarding surgical excision versus medical management of papillary fibroelastomas showing reduction in future stroke risk with excision. Of the papillary fibroelastomas observed in this study, around one-third were only seen on transesophageal echocardiography.

Question 45
A 67 year old patient in cardiogenic shock following acute coronary syndrome was placed on venoarterial extracorporeal membrane oxygenation (VA ECMO). Low flow alarms prompted an echocardiographic assessment as in Fig. 19.16 which demonstrate

A. The inflow cannula is directed towards and may be abutting the septum
B. There is chamber collapse associated with cardiac tamponade physiology
C. There is outflow cannula thrombus
D. There is kinking of the outflow cannula
E. None of the above

Answer: A. The inflow cannula is directed towards and may be abutting the septum. Echocardiographic assessment in the setting of VA ECMO low flow alarms may be helpful to work throught differential diagnoses such as cannula obstruction, cardiac tamponade and others. In this case the tip of the VA ECMO cannula was abutting the inter-atrial septum (Video 19.17) and causing low flow alarms. Under trans-esophageal echocardiographic guidance, the tip of the VA ECMO cannula was withdrawn to a position free within the right atrium (Videos 19.18 and 19.19) correcting flow with no further alarms.

Question 46
Extracorporeal membrane oxygenation (ECMO) cannulation:

A. Should be guided by transthoracic echocardiography as a method of choice
B. Should be guided by transesophageal echocardiography as a method of choice
C. Should be guided by intra-cardiac echocardiography as a method of choice
D. Should be guided by fluoroscopy as a method of choice
E. None of these

Answer: E. None of these. Spatial resolution of transthoracic echocardiography is not high enough for guiding ECMO cannulation [15]. Fluoroscopy and transesophageal echocardiography are used in guiding ECMO cannulation, but none of these methods is recommended as superior [16].

Question 47
An Avalon veno-venous extracorporeal membrane oxygenation (VV-ECMO) catheter is:

A. A single-lumen catheter with superior vena caval inflow and inferior vena caval (IVC) outflow
B. A single-lumen catheter with inferior vena caval inflow and superior vena caval (IVC) outflow
C. A dual-lumen catheter with bi-caval inflow drainage ports and a right atrial outflow port
D. A dual-lumen catheter with superior vena caval inflow and inferior vena caval (IVC) outflow

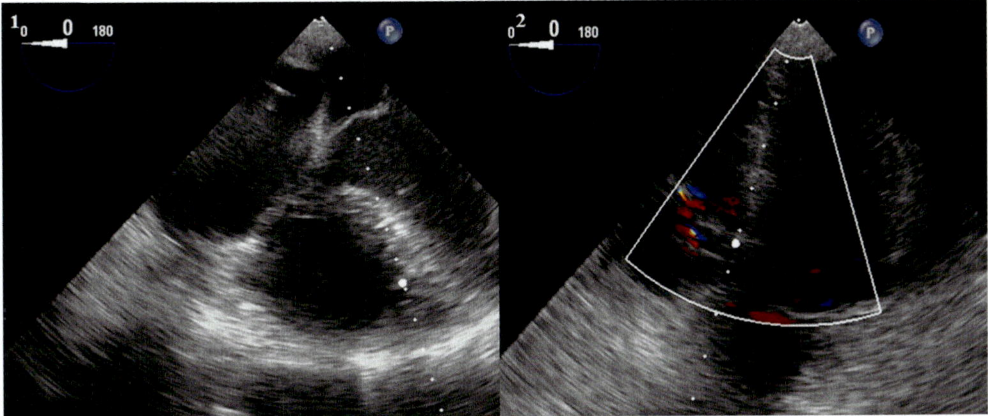

Fig. 19.16 Transesophageal echocardiographic views without color Doppler (left panel) and with color Doppler (right panel)

E. A triple-lumen catheter with inferior vena caval inflow and superior vena caval (IVC) outflow

Answer: C. A dual-lumen catheter with bi-caval inflow drainage ports and a right atrial outflow port. An Avalon catheter is **single** VV-ECMO **catheter** which can simultaneously drain venous blood from the central circulation (superior and inferior vena cavas) to deliver oxygenated blood directly into the heart [17]. It is inserted peripherally via the right internal jugular vein and has a dual-lumen construction (one for venous inflow, one for venous outflow) which requires careful positioning utilizing fluoroscopy or echocardiography. The proximal inflow drainage port is positioned in the SVC, and the distal inflow drainage port is positioned in the IVC below the hepatic veins [17]. The outflow port should be positioned in the right atrium and oriented in front of the tricuspid valve [16]. Blood is removed from both SVC and IVC, passed through an oxygenator and returned into the right atrium [16].

Question 48

An Avalon catheter insertion under guidance of transesophageal echocardiography may be challenging since:

A. Looping of the guidewire in the right atrium and the right ventricle may occur
B. Presence of the guidewire in both caval veins does not preclude its looping in the right atrium and the right ventricle
C. Transesophageal echocardiography does not allow continuous surveillance of the course and position of the guidewire
D. Following catheter insertion, rotation or displacement of the catheter needs to be avoided as this may result in re-circulation and ineffective support
E. All of these

Answer: E. All of these. Avalon catheter insertion under guidance of transesophageal echocardiography may be challenging since transesophageal echocardiography does not allow for continuous surveillance of the entire course and position of the guidewire in one image which thus may become looped at a point outside of the image [18]. Following catheter insertion, rotation or displacement of the catheter needs to be avoided as this may result in re-circulation and ineffective support.

Question 49

Predictors of successful VA-ECMO weaning include:

A. Aortic VTI > 5 cm
B. LVEF > 15%
C. Lateral mitral annulus peak systolic velocity > 6 cm/s
D. Global longitudinal strain less negative than −5%
E. All of the above

Answer: C. Lateral mitral annulus peak systolic velocity > 6 cm/s. Predictors of successful VA-ECMO weaning include aortic VTI ≥ 10 cm, LVEF > 20–25%, and lateral mitral annulus peak systolic velocity > 6 cm/s [19].

Question 50

Physicians monitoring patients on VA-ECMO with echocardiography should look closely for:

A. Increase in LV size
B. Migration of cannulae through the interatrial septum
C. Presence of intra-cardiac and intravascular thrombi
D. All of these
E. None of these

Answer: D. All of these. Patients on VA-ECMO require constant echocardiographic monitoring [20]. Echocardiography enables rapid assessment of cannula positioning, cardiac filling and cardiac function. ECMO cannulae can migrate through the interatrial septum [20]. Outside the heart, cannulae can obstruct venous drainage causing liver congestion and SVC syndrome [20]. An increase in LV size can suggest the need for inotropic support, or an additional mechanical device, to promote forward flow [20]. Since risk of intra-vascular and intra-cardiac thrombosis is increased on VA-ECMO, ascending aorta, left ventricle and pulmonary veins should be closely inspected for presence of thrombi (Video 19.20) [20].

References

1. Stainback RF, Estep JD, Agler DA, et al. Echocardiography in the management of patients with left ventricular assist devices: recommendations from the American Society of Echocardiography. J Am Soc Echocardiogr. 2015;28(8):853–909.
2. Gregoric ID, Cohn WE, Akay MH, La Francesca S, Myers T, Frazier OH. CentriMag left ventricular assist system: cannulation through a right minithoracotomy. Tex Hear Inst J. 2008;35(2):184–5.
3. Chang D, Gabriels J, Laighold S, Williamson AK, Ismail H, Epstein LM. A novel diagnostic approach to a mass on a device lead. Hear Case Rep. 2019;5(6):306–9.
4. Pepi M, Evangelista A, Nihoyannopoulos P, et al. Recommendations for echocardiography use in the diagnosis and management of cardiac sources of embolism. Eur J Echocardiogr. 2010;11(6):461–76.
5. Generali T, Tessitore G, Mushtaq S, Alamanni F. Pulmonary valve papillary fibroelastoma: management of an unusual, tricky pathology. Interact Cardiovasc Thorac Surg. 2013;16(1):88–90.
6. Kim MJ, Jung HO. Anatomic variants mimicking pathology on echocardiography: differential diagnosis. J Cardiovasc Ultrasound. 2013;21(3):103–12.

7. Bangalore S, Petre L, Herweg B, et al. Cardioversion in patients with left ventricular thrombus is not associated with increased thromboembolic risk. J Am Soc Echocardiogr. 2006;19(4):438–40.
8. Reardon MJ, Walkes JCM, DeFelice CA, Wojciechowski Z. Cardiac autotransplantation for surgical resection of a primary malignant left ventricular tumor. Tex Hear Inst J. 2006;33(4):495–7.
9. Simons M, Cabin H, Jaffe C. Lipomatous hypertrophy of the atrial septum: Diagnosis by combined two-dimensional echocardiography and computerized tomography. Am J Cardiol. 1984;54(3):465–6.
10. Bruce CJ. Cardiac tumours: diagnosis and management. Heart. 2011;97(2):151–60.
11. Quencer KB, Friedman T, Sheth R, Oklu R. Tumor thrombus: Incidence, imaging, prognosis and treatment. Cardiovasc Diagn Ther. 2017;7(Suppl 3):S165–77.
12. Reynen K, Köckeritz U, Strasser RH. Metastases to the heart. Ann Oncol. 2004;15(3):375–81.
13. Alkharabsheh S, Gentry JL, Khayata M, et al. Clinical features, natural history, and management of pericardial cysts. Am J Cardiol. 2019;123(1):159–63.
14. Stratakis CA, Kirschner LS, Carney JA. Clinical and molecular features of the carney complex: diagnostic criteria and recommendations for patient evaluation. J Clin Endocrinol Metab. 2001;86(9):4041–6.
15. Kapoor P. Echocardiography in extracorporeal membrane oxygenation. Ann Card Anaesth. 2017;20(5):S1–3.
16. Banfi C, Pozzi M, Siegenthaler N, et al. Veno-venous extracorporeal membrane oxygenation: cannulation techniques. J Thorac Dis. 2016;8(12):3762–73.
17. Betancor J, Xu B, Rehman KA, et al. Transesophageal echocardiographic guidance of venovenous extracorporeal membrane oxygenation cannula (avalon cannula) repositioning. Case. 2017;1(4):150–4.
18. Ngai CW, Ng PY, Sin WC. Bicaval dual lumen cannula in adult veno-venous extracorporeal membrane oxygenation—clinical pearls for safe cannulation. J Thorac Dis. 2018;10(Suppl 5):S624–8.
19. Zhang Z. Echocardiography for patients undergoing extracorporeal cardiopulmonary resuscitation: a primer for intensive care physicians. J Intensive Care. 2017;5(1):1–9.
20. Victor K, Barrett NA, Gillon S, Gowland A, Meadows CIS, Ioannou N. Critical care echo rounds extracorporeal membrane oxygenation. Echo Res Pract. 2015;2(2):D1–D11.

Echocardiography for Cardiac Arrest

20

Courtney M. Smalley, Matthew R. Dettmer, Matthew C. Kostura, and Samuel J. Tate

Clinical Pearls

1. Point-of-care ultrasound can be a useful adjunct in cardiopulmonary arrest.
2. Two types of image acquisition can be used: transthoracic echocardiography and transesophageal echocardiography.
3. Bedside ultrasound can help assess for cardiac contractility in ventricular tachycardia, ventricular fibrillation, asystole, and pulseless electrical activity.
4. Reversible causes of cardiac arrest that can be identified with bedside ultrasound are the following: tamponade, pulmonary embolism, hypovolemia and tension pneumothorax.
5. The SHoC protocol (Sonography in Hypotension and Cardiac Arrest) can be used to help guide imaging during cardiac arrest.
6. The four "F's" associated with the SHoC protocol are fluid, form, function, and filling.
7. Asystole on the rhythm strip in association with no cardiac movement on bedside ultrasound has the lowest chance of survival.
8. The four views for transthoracic echocardiography are subxiphoid, parasternal long axis, parasternal short axis, and apical four chamber views.
9. The five views recommended views for transesophageal echocardiography in cardiac arrest are midesophageal four chamber, midesophageal long axis, transgastric short axis, and bicaval views.
10. Transesophageal echocardiography in cardiac arrest has the following advantages over transthoracic echocardiography: the ability to continue compressions while assessing the ultrasound image, the quality of the compressions can be assessed in real time, emphysema and body habitus are not a barrier to obtaining windows, and the patient can be cardioverted while probe is in place.

Question 1
The primary purpose of utilizing point-of-care ultrasound in the setting of cardiac arrest for non-shockable rhythms such as pulseless electrical activity (PEA) and asystole are to find all of the following reversible causes except:

A. Tamponade
B. Pulmonary embolism
C. Volume overload
D. Hypovolemia

Answer: C.

Key Point: Point-of-care ultrasound should be used during cardiac arrest to identify reversible causes.

Rationale: The four main reversible causes in cardiac arrest are tamponade, pulmonary embolism, hypovolemia and tension pneumothorax. By utilizing point-of-care ultrasound during an arrest, life threatening causes can be identified and acted upon by performing pericardiocentesis in the setting of tamponade, thrombolytics in the setting of pulmonary embolism, fluids in the setting of hypovolemic shock, and chest tube placement in the setting of pneumothorax [1].

Supplementary Information The online version contains supplementary material available at https://doi.org/10.1007/978-3-031-45731-9_20.

C. M. Smalley (✉) · M. C. Kostura
Emergency Services Institute, Cleveland Clinic Health System, Cleveland, OH, USA
e-mail: smallec@ccf.org; kosturm@ccf.org

M. R. Dettmer
Emergency Services Institute, Respiratory Institute, Cleveland Clinic Health System, Cleveland, OH, USA
e-mail: dettmem2@ccf.org

S. J. Tate
Department of Emergency Medicine, University of California Davis Health, Davis, CA, USA
e-mail: sjtate@ucdavis.edu

R. Sreedharan et al. (eds.), *Critical Care Echocardiography*, https://doi.org/10.1007/978-3-031-45731-9_20

Question 2

Which of the following point-of-care ultrasound views paired with its goal for identification is considered a core view when utilizing the SHoC protocol for Cardiac Arrest?

A. Lung view—identify absence of lung sliding consistent with pneumothorax and/or pleural fluid
B. IVC view—identify filling status
C. Subxiphoid cardiac view—identify pericardial fluid
D. Aorta view—identify dissection flap

Answer C.

Key Point: The core views as defined in the SHoC protocol (Sonography in Hypotension and Cardiac Arrest) are the subxiphoid and parasternal cardiac views to assess for pericardial fluid, ventricular form, and ventricular function.

Rationale: The core views were defined as point-of-care ultrasound views that should be performed routinely for all patients. Supplementary views, defined as views which are only performed on a case by case basis, were defined as lung views to assess for pneumothorax or pleural fluid and IVC views to assess for filling. Additional ultrasound views, defined as exams performed which additional investigation is required, include endotracheal tube confirmation, proximal leg ultrasound for DVT, and sources of blood loss in the abdomen (AAA, peritoneal, pelvic free fluid) [2] (Fig. 20.1).

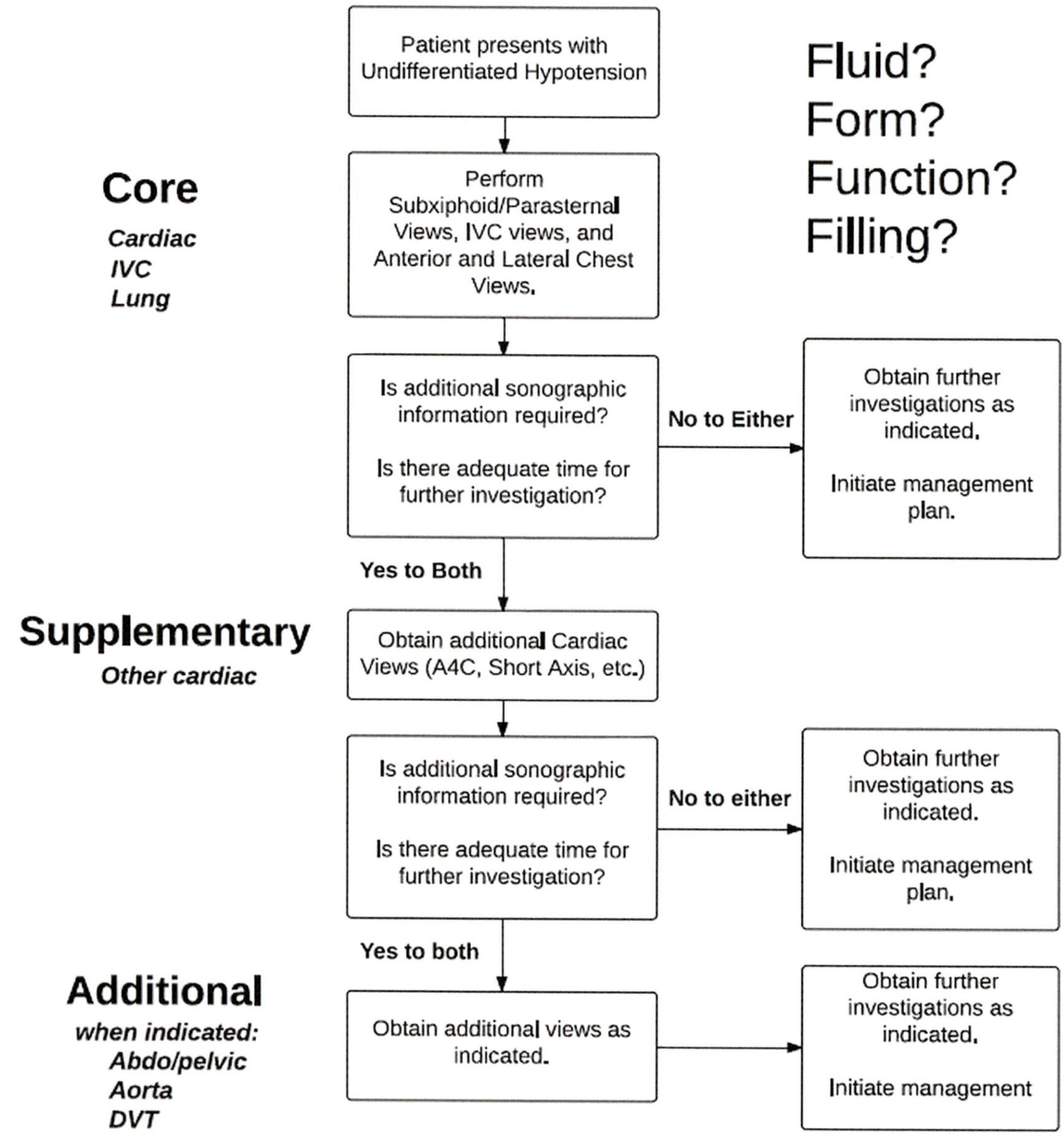

Fig. 20.1 SHoC Ultrasound Protocol

Question 3
When interpreting point-of-care ultrasound views during cardiac arrest, it is important to investigate the "4Fs"as described in the SHoC protocol for Cardiac Arrest. Which of the following is not one of the "4Fs"?

A. Flow
B. Form
C. Function
D. Filling

Answer: A.
Key Point: The SHoC protocol for Cardiac Arrest (Sonography in Hypotension and Cardiac Arrest) states that it is important to investigate the "4Fs": fluid, form, function, and filling.

Rationale: The core views of the SHoC protocol (Sonography in Hypotension and Cardiac Arrest) are the subxiphoid and parasternal cardiac views which assess for 3 of the 4Fs. 1) **Fluid** = pericardial fluid; **Form** = ventricular form/right heart abnormalities; **Function** = is there cardiac contractility. The 4th "F", **Filling**, can be assessed by performing a supplementary views of the IVC views to assess for filling [2].

Question 4
A 70-year-old male with a past medical history of chronic obstructive pulmonary disease, acute coronary syndrome, and hypertension is brought in by EMS in cardiac arrest. Per report, patient was at home watching television when he got up and his wife witnessed him collapse in front of her. He was pulseless and wife immediately started CPR. Paramedics were called and upon arrival, AED was placed that showed no shockable rhythm. ACLS was continued and the patient was brought to your emergency department intubated with CPR in progress for 9 minutes. During a pulse check, you place a probe on the patient to investigate the heart. Which of the following is the poorest prognostic indicator on point-of-care ultrasound for return to spontaneous circulation (ROSC)?

A. Subxiphoid cardiac view demonstrating pericardial effusion
B. Parasternal long access view demonstrating fine ventricular fibrillation
C. Apical four chamber cardiac view demonstrating organized cardiac rhythm during pulse check without a femoral pulse
D. Subxiphoid cardiac view demonstrating no spontaneous cardiac movement

Answer: D.
Key Point: Asystole has the lowest OHCA survival rate.

Rationale: Less than 8% of patients survive an OHCA compared to 40% of patients with a shockable rhythm. Patient with PEA have even lower survival rate (6%), [3, 4].

Question 5
Clinical indications for utilizing point-of-care ultrasound during cardiac arrest include all of the following except:

A. Identification of reversible etiologies of cardiac arrest
B. Utilization of transesophageal echocardiography to get real-time feedback on the quality of chest compressions
C. Determine if there is spontaneous cardiac movement during pulse checks
D. As a marker to help guide when a patient should be intubated

Answer: D.
Key Point: Point-of-care ultrasound during cardiac arrest assist in identifying cardiac movement, reversible causes of cardiac arrest, and effectiveness of interventions.

Rationale: Integrating point-of-care ultrasound when performed during the rhythm assessment in the appropriate time frame can assist in identifying cardiac movement or rhythm in patients presenting with cardiac arrest. Transthoracic echo and transesophageal echo can assist in identification of reversible causes of arrest. When utilizing transesophageal echo, the clinician can obtain real-time feedback on the quality of compressions. While reversible causes of cardiac arrest, such as tension pneumothorax, can be identified with bedside ultrasound, current guidelines do not utilize point-of-care ultrasound as a marker for when a patient should have a definitive airway [1, 5].

Questions 6–8

An 82 y/o female with a past medical history of CLL, congestive heart failure, and atrial fibrillation arrives to your emergency department with shortness of breath. Patient states he has been noticing increasing leg swelling for the last week. Shortly after arriving, a nurse notifies you that patient is becoming somnolent. You arrive to the room and find the patient pulseless and apneic. Pulseless electrical activity is noted on monitor and ACLS is initiated. During the pulse check, you place an ultrasound probe on the patient to assess the heart and see the image below (Fig. 20.2).

Question 6
Which view has been obtained in the image above?

A. Transthoracic Subxiphoid View
B. Transesophageal Midesophageal Long Axis View
C. Transesophageal Transgastric Short AxisView
D. Transthoracic Apical Four Chamber View

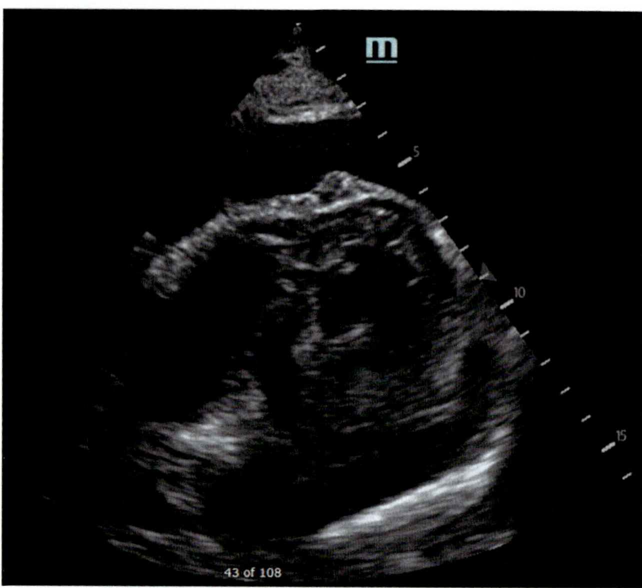

Fig. 20.2 TTE Pericardial Effusion

Answer: A.

Key Point: Transthoracic subxiphoid view is the preferred view in cardiac arrest.

Rationale: Transthoracic subxiphoid view is the quickest view available to determine the etiology of cardiac arrest and the least likely of all the transthoracic cardiac views to interfere with chest compressions. A Transthoracic Apical Four chamber view can be difficult to obtain while CPR is in progress due to lack of access to the fifth and sixth intercostal space on the chest. While transesophageal views can be advantageous in the setting of cardiac arrest, they may take longer to acquire given insertion time of the probe.

Question 7

What is the likely etiology behind this patient's cardiac arrest?

A. Ruptured Abdominal Aortic Aneurysm
B. Pulmonary Embolism
C. Pericardial Tamponade
D. Hypovolemic Shock

Answer: C.

Key Point: The image demonstrates a large pericardial effusion surrounding the heart in the transthoracic subxiphoid view.

Rationale: In pulseless electrical activity, it is important to consider pericardial tamponade as the etiology behind cardiac arrest. While ruptured abdominal aortic aneurysm can be an etiology behind cardiac arrest, it does not usually present on point-of-care ultrasound as pericardial effusion, but rather as enlarged abdominal aorta or free fluid in the peritoneal cavity. Point-of-care ultrasound can be utilized to determine risk of pulmonary embolism as primary etiology behind cardiac arrest, although this presents as significant right ventricular dilation and bowing into the left ventricle. Profound hypovolemic shock can present in cardiac arrest, however, these patients have a flattened IVC and not pericardial fluid around the heart.

Question 8

The most successful location to perform emergency pericardiocentesis when utilizing bedside ultrasound is the following:

A. Using ultrasound, place needle in the subxiphoid area 1 cm inferior to the xiphocostal angle and aim toward the right shoulder at a 45-degree angle
B. Using ultrasound, find the area with the largest fluid collection in the parasternal view and place needle 1 cm lateral to sternal border at the left fifth or sixth intercostal space
C. Using ultrasound, place needle at the apex of the heart and introduce the needle 1 cm lateral to and below the apical heartbeat, aim at the left shoulder
D. Using ultrasound, place needle 1 cm lateral to the right of the sternal border at the fifth or sixth intercostal space and aim toward subxiphoid area

Answer: B.

Key Point: The most successful view when performing pericardiocentesis using point-of-care ultrasound will be utilizing the view that has the largest fluid collection.

Rationale: There are 3 views for which pericardiocentesis can be performed using bedside ultrasound. In the subxiphoid view, the needle should be placed in the subxiphoid area 1 cm inferior to the xiphocostal angle and aim toward the **left** shoulder at a 45-degree angle. Using the apical ultrasound view, the needle should be placed at the apex of the heart and the needle should be introduced 1 cm lateral to and below the apical heartbeat while aim at the **right** shoulder. Lastly, using the parasternal view, find the area with the largest fluid collection under ultrasound should be identified and the needle should be inserted until fluid returns. This is usually 1 cm lateral to sternal border at the left fifth or sixth intercostal space. Performing pericardiocentesis by placing the needle to the right of the sternal border and aiming toward the subxiphoid area is not considered a standard method of performing pericardiocentesis [6, 7].

Questions 9–10

81 y/o male with an unknown past medical history arrives to the hospital in cardiac arrest. Per EMS, paramedics were called to house for respiratory distress. When they arrived at the house, patient had agonal respirations and was pulseless. CPR was initiated, IO access obtained, and ACLS was initiated with 2 rounds of epinephrine prior to arrival to the emergency department. Care was transferred to the emergency department team and 2 min of compressions were performed prior to pulse check. During pulse check, no femoral pulse was palpated and the following video clip was obtained using bedside ultrasound (Video 20.1).

Question 9
What rhythm is this patient currently in?

A. Pulseless Electrical Activity
B. Asystole
C. Ventricular tachycardia
D. Ventricular fibrillation

Answer: A.

Key Point: When reviewing this video clip, the patient has one unorganized beat consistent with pulseless electrical activity.

Rationale: Pulseless electrical activity is defined as an electrocardiogram demonstrating a heart rhythm but with no palpable pulse. In a study performed by the SHoC- ED investigators, POCUS was compared to ECG tracings for mechanical activity and found ultrasound was better at determining presence of mechanical activity when compared to ECG [8].

Question 10
The maximum amount of time recommended for obtaining bedside ultrasound images during a pulse check is the following:

A. 3 s
B. 5 s
C. 10 s
D. 20 s

Answer: A.

Key Point: Current guidelines recommend a pulsecheck of no more than 10 s.

Rationale: One recent study in 2019 found that the use of point-of-care ultrasound during cardiac arrest was significant in increasing the duration of pulse checks to greater than 10 s. It is important that physicians recognize that when available, ultrasound can assist with the diagnosis and treatment of reversible causes of cardiac arrest but current guidelines recommend that a well-trained operator should be able to obtain these views in under 10 s to minimize time without CPR [9–11].

Questions 11–12

A 64-year-old female arrives to the ED via EMS with chief complaint of sudden onset chest pain and shortness of breath. EMS is unable to establish an IV and the patient arrives to the ED in respiratory distress. Per EMS she was hypoxic with oxygen saturations near 80% on room air but this improved to 95% on a non-rebreather. Vitals on arrival to the ED are otherwise notable for a heart rate of 112, blood pressure of 74/52 mmHg, temperature of 97 °F (36.1 °C), respiratory rate of 24, oxygen saturation of 96% on a non-rebreather mask. Past medical history includes obesity, hypertension, hyperlipidemia, and throat cancer in remission status post radiation 3 years ago. She has had no prior surgeries. The patient denies smoking or illicit drugs, and occasionally drinks alcohol.

Pertinent exam findings include a cardiac exam with tachycardic rate, regular rhythm, no murmurs, and thready radial pulses. On pulmonary exam she is tachypneic and in respiratory distress with rapid shallow breathing but clear breath sounds throughout both lung fields. She has no significant edema or calf tenderness on musculoskeletal exam.

ECG and a limited bedside transthoracic echocardiogram images are obtained and shown below. On the dynamic images you note the left ventricular ejection fraction initially looks adequate. As you step out of the room to place orders, the nurse calls you back in because the patient's blood pressure has dropped and he cannot find a pulse. You initiate CPR (Figs. 20.3 and 20.4).

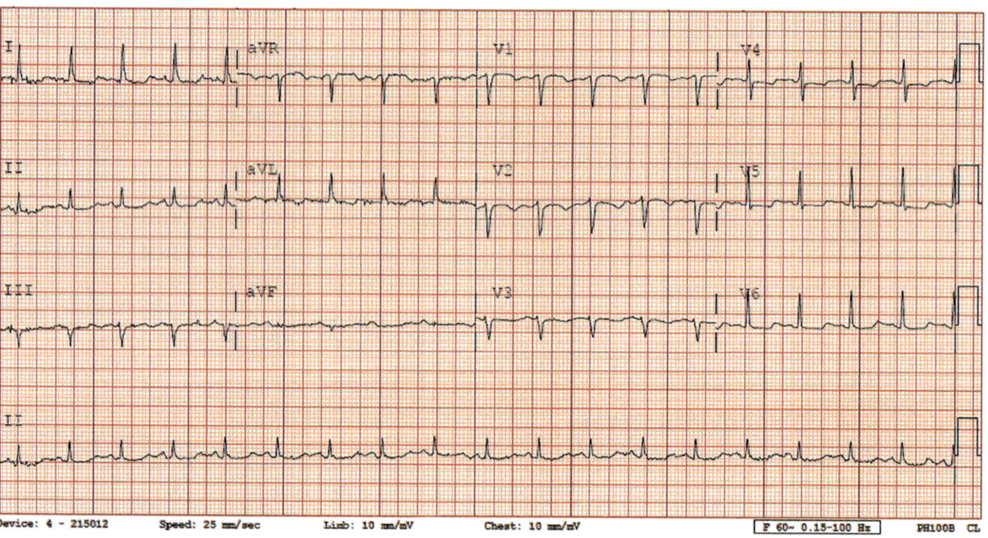

Fig. 20.3 EKG Sinus Tachycardia

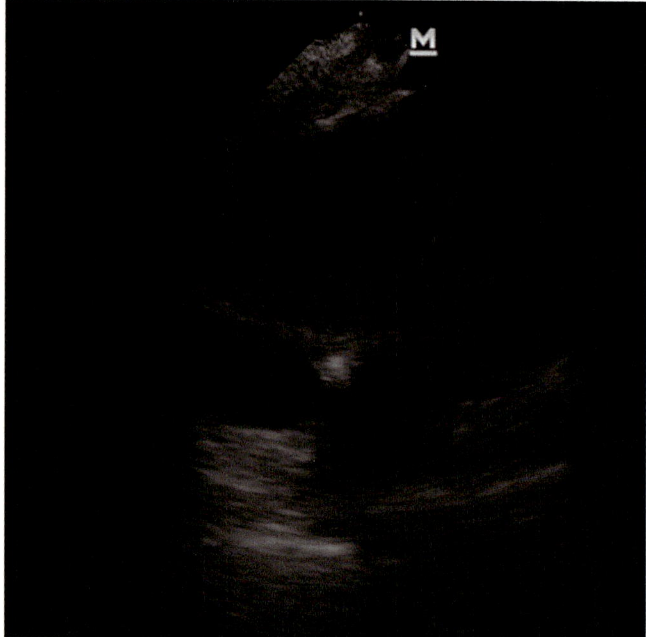

Fig. 20.4 TTE RV Strain Apical4

Question 11

Prior to the loss of pulses, what type of shock is most likely responsible for the patient's hypotension?

A. Neurogenic Shock
B. Cardiogenic Shock
C. Obstructive Shock
D. Distributive Shock

Answer: C.

Key Point: Acute right ventricular enlargement on ultrasound in the setting of acute cardiac arrest, indicates a massive pulmonary embolism which is a type of obstructive shock.

Rationale: The picture above is of an apical 4 chamber view for a transthoracic echocardiogram. Relative to the left ventricle, the right ventricle is enlarged. In the acute setting of a patient who has not had a prolonged down time, right ventricular dilatation indicates a massive pulmonary embolism as the likely cause. Pulmonary embolism is a type of obstructive shock, because a massive clot in the lungs is preventing blood from reaching the left ventricle. In neurogenic shock, the patient should be bradycardic and hypotensive, commonly as a result of a traumatic spine injury. In cardiogenic shock, one would expect global cardiac dysfunction or a significantly decreased left systolic ejection fraction on echocardiogram. In distributive shock, such as sepsis, hypotension is due to extravasation of fluids from the inflammatory response. A patient with distributive shock would also be hypotensive and tachycardic, but one would not expect them to have an enlarged right ventricle [5, 12].

Question 12
A peripheral IV is established in the right antecubital fossa and resuscitation according to ACLS protocol is underway. Based on the patient's presentation and the most likely diagnosis, what additional therapies should be given?

A. Stat Cardiac Catheterization if ROSC is obtained
B. 1 amp of Calcium Chloride
C. IV Lidocaine
D. Alteplase 100 mg IV if the patient has no contraindications to thrombolytics

Answer: D.
Key Point: Treatment of a massive pulmonary embolism is thrombolytics.
Rationale: Of the answer choices above, thrombolytics is the best choice. While the patient is still undifferentiated, based on the echocardiogram showing right ventricle dilatation with no known underlying pulmonary history, massive pulmonary embolism is a likely cause of her cardiac arrest. While there is some conflicting evidence as to benefit of thrombolytics for undifferentiated cardiac arrest, if a massive pulmonary embolism is suspected, thrombolytics could treat the underlying cause. The ECG above shows non-specific ischemic findings, but no definitive STEMI. There are no signs of hyperkalemia on ECG, so without labs, calcium chloride is not the best choice. IV Lidocaine could be considered if the patient's rhythm shows ventricular tachycardia, but there is no evidence of this at this point in the cardiac arrest and it is not recommended as first line by ACLS guidelines. In prospective trials and randomized control trials, lidocaine was less effective than amiodarone in improving hospital admission rates after out-of-hospital cardiac arrest due to shock-refractory ventricular fibrillation or polymorphic ventricular tachycardia [12–14].

Question 13
Which of the following echocardiogram findings is least likely to be associated with an underlying acute massive pulmonary embolism?

A. Aortic Stenosis
B. McConnell's Sign
C. Flattening of the intra-ventricular septum
D. Enlarged right ventricle

Answer: A.
Key Point: McConnell's Sign, flattened intra-ventricular septum, and an enlarged right ventricle are all associated with right heart strain caused by a massive pulmonary embolism.
Rationale: While cardiac ultrasound is not sensitive to rule out pulmonary embolism, secondary findings of right heart strain from an acute massive pulmonary embolism can be seen on echocardiogram and may prompt further work up. Other causes of right heart strain on ultrasound include pulmonary hypertension, and chronic lung pathology. Findings of right heart strain on echocardiogram include an enlarged right ventricle, flattening of the intra-ventricular septum due to elevated right ventricular pressures, or hypokinesis of the right ventricular free wall with preservation of the apex which is also known as McConnell's sign. Early studies of McConnell's sign report a sensitivity of 77% and a specificity of 94% for pulmonary embolism, but further studies showed a lower sensitivity [15, 16] (Fig. 20.5).

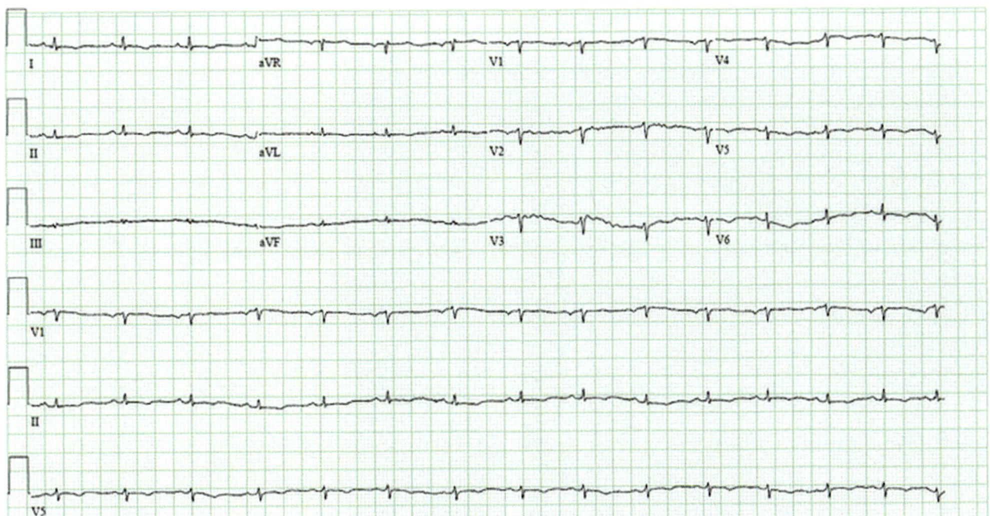

Fig. 20.5 EKG Sinus Tachycardia

Questions 14–15

A 55-year-old female with a past medical history of metastatic breast cancer s/p mastectomy on oral immunotherapy presents via EMS with shortness of breath. On arrival to the ED the patient is in respiratory distress and BiPAP was placed by EMS. Oxygen saturations are 94% on the BiPAP and she is too short of breath to speak. She is afebrile and blood pressure on arrival to the ED is 100/55 mmHg. An ECG is obtained as shown below. The patient's work of breathing is not improving while on non-invasive positive pressure ventilation and she is subsequently intubated. Shortly after intubation, you cannot find a pulse and CPR is started according to ACLS protocol.

Question 14
Based on the patient's history and ECG what finding is most likely to be found on be bedside echocardiogram?

A. Enlarged right ventricle
B. Wall motion abnormalities
C. Mitral regurgitation
D. Pericardial effusion

Answer: D.

Key Point: Diffuse low voltage on ECG is a sign of a pericardial effusion.

Rationale: The ECG above shows diffuse low voltage. While this is sometimes caused by a large body habitus, another common cause of a low voltage ECG is a pericardial effusion. There are no ECG findings to indicate right heart strain so based on ECG one would not expect to find an enlarged right ventricle. There are also no specific ECG findings to indicate ischemia isolated to a specific coronary artery, so focal wall motion abnormalities would also not be an expected finding based on this ECG. Electrical alternans can also been seen with a pericardial effusion and cardiac tamponade [12, 17].

Questions 14–15 Continued

At the first pulse check after 2 min of CPR, no pulse is palpated, and the monitor shows the following cardiac rhythm. The last dose of epinephrine was given 1 min ago. A limited transthoracic echocardiogram is attempted and the following parasternal long axis view is obtained (Figs. 20.6 and 20.7).

Question 15
What is the most appropriate next step?

A. Bedside pericardiocentesis
B. Resume chest compressions
C. Defibrillation at 200 J biphasic energy
D. Epinephrine 1 mg IV

Answer: B.

Key Point: Minimizing interruptions in CPR is a key metric in high quality basic life support (BLS).

Rationale: In the above scenario, the patient has no pulse, and the rhythm presented is not ventricular tachycardia nor ventricular fibrillation. Therefore this is a "Pulseless Electrical Activity (PEA)" scenario and according to ACLS guidelines one should resume compressions and give epinephrine every 3–5 min. No shock would be advised per ACLS guidelines. Based on the ultrasound findings, cardiac tamponade is a likely cause of the cardiac arrest and one

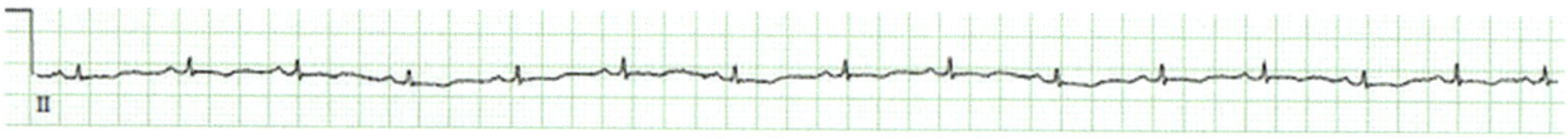

Fig. 20.6 EKG Sinus Tachycardia

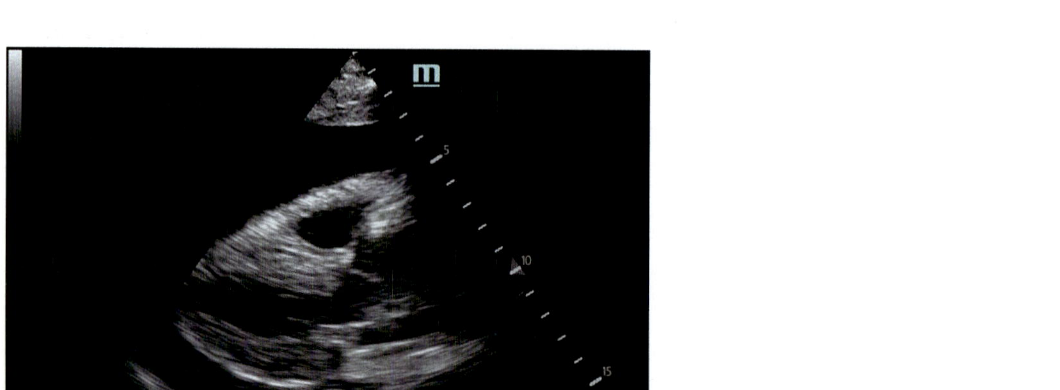

Fig. 20.7 TTE Pericardial Effusion

should prepare for a bedside pericardiocentesis to treat the underlying cause of the cardiac arrest. However the next best step is to resume chest compressions and perform good basic life support care until equipment is ready to perform the pericardiocentesis [13].

Question 16
In which of the following scenarios would an emergent pericardiocentesis be most indicated as the next step?

A. Bedside cardiac ultrasound shows a 2 cm circumferential pericardial effusion and there is a high suspicion for an underlying type A acute aortic dissection
B. Cardiomegaly is noted on chest X ray of a patient presenting with atraumatic shortness of breath, and a less than 1 cm pericardial effusion is seen on ultrasound
C. Patient presents with orthopnea, but no rales on exam, and bedside echocardiogram shows a 2.5 cm circumferential pericardial effusion with right ventricular collapse in diastole
D. Patient has electrical alternans on ECG, and a swinging heart with pericardial effusion that causes right atrial collapse in 1/3 of the cardiac cycle on bedside cardiac ultrasound

Answer: C.

Key Point: Right ventricular collapse in diastole with a pericardial effusion is an ominous sign for cardiac tamponade.

Rationale: Of the four choices, choices A and C are most concerning for cardiac tamponade. However if a patient has an underlying type A aortic dissection, then emergent surgical management is the treatment of choice and a pericardiocentesis could potentially delay surgical care. If surgical management is not promptly available, pericardiocentesis of small temporizing amounts can be considered, but should never delay definitive surgical management. The European Society of Cardiology developed a scoring system for triage and management of pericardial effusions based on underlying etiology, clinical presentation, and imaging findings. Choice C would total to the highest score, indicating an emergent pericardiocentesis would be indicated. Progressive worsening signs of cardiac tamponade on ultrasound are right atrial collapse in 1/3 or greater of the cardiac cycle, followed by right ventricular collapse in diastole, followed by left atrial collapse which is most specific for cardiac tamponade [12, 17].

Question 17
Which of the following techniques is recommended when performing an emergent pericardiocentesis?

A. Use dynamic ultrasound guidance and direct the needle to the area of the largest fluid collection closest to the skin surface
B. Using agitated saline to verify that you are in the correct space is contraindicated, because injection of saline will worsen tamponade.
C. The optimal approach is inserting the needle between 3 to 5 cm lateral to the sternum.
D. Ideally if time allows, a patient with cardiac tamponade should be intubated and sedated prior to performing the pericardiocentesis.

Answer: A.

Key Point: Dynamic ultrasound guidance to direct the needle to the largest fluid pocket can minimize complications of an emergent pericardiocentesis.

Rationale: Of the above choices, A is the recommended safest technique for performing a pericardiocentesis. Choice B is incorrect, as using agitated saline can be used to confirm you are in the correct space if you are unsure. If you withdrawal fluid first, then reinject with a smaller amount of agitated saline (usually 5 mL), then the risk of inducing tamponade is low. In choice C, inserting the needle between 3 to 5 cm lateral to the sternum risks lacerating the internal mammary artery or causing a pneumothorax and should be avoided if possible. Choice D is incorrect, because placing the patient on positive pressure ventilation will cause an increase in intrathoracic pressure. High intrathoracic pressures may decrease preload and RV return and may result in full cardiac tamponade physiology and cardiac arrest. Ideally the patient would not be intubated and on positive pressure ventilation as one wants to maintain adequate preload, to help prevent cardiac tamponade and hemodynamic collapse [6, 12].

Questions 18–20

A 78-year-old female arrives to the ED in cardiac arrest. She has a history of coronary artery disease, COPD, diabetes, and hypertension and suffered a witnessed cardiac arrest by a family member who states the patient had sudden onset of chest pain, and subsequently passed out while cooking in the kitchen. CPR was started by the family member on scene, and continued by EMS. She has been given 2 rounds of epinephrine and received on electrical defibrillation for ventricular fibrillation by EMS prior to arrival to the ED. A supraglottic airway device was placed by EMS and chest rise is present with bag ventilations. As the patient is transferred to the ED gurney, a backboard is placed, CPR is continued, and Epinephrine 1 mg is given via an intraosseous line that EMS placed

Question 18

As you direct the continuation of CPR on this patient according to ACLS protocol, you consider performing a transesophageal echocardiogram. Transesophageal echocardiogram (TEE) during resuscitation of a patient in cardiac arrest can be used to do all of the following EXCEPT:

A. Access for cardiac activity during pauses in CPR
B. Identify the presence of ventricular thrombus during cardiac arrest which may indicate the patient could benefit from thrombolytics
C. Identify right ventricular dilation which is 98% specific for an acute pulmonary embolism during cardiac arrest
D. Access the quality of CPR during chest compressions

Answer: C.

Key Point: All of the above choices are benefits of using cardiac ultrasound to guide resuscitation, but there are many other causes of right ventricular dilation besides a pulmonary embolism.

Rationale: While TEE may be used to identify right ventricular dilation, this finding is not sensitive nor specific for an acute pulmonary embolism. Many patients who suffer cardiac arrest may develop signs of RV strain simply due to a prolonged hypoxic period. In the study by Teran et al., right ventricular dilatation was seen in 30% of the cohort, but the authors felt it was unlikely that this high percentage of patients had an acute pulmonary embolism. All of the other responses describe some of the advantages of performing a TEE during CPR. In particular the mid-esophageal long axis view can assess for valve opening and proper left ventricular compression during CPR to dynamically guide chest compressions. TEE can identify the presence or absence of cardiac squeeze during pauses in CPR as well as potential underlying causes of cardiac arrest such as a left ventricular thrombus or a pericardial effusion [5, 10].

Question 19

What step must be done in this patient prior to performing the transesophageal echocardiogram?

A. Removal of the pre-hospital airway device and placement of a definitive airway
B. Establish IV access
C. Establish central venous access in the left femoral vein
D. Electrical Defibrillation

Answer: A.

Key Point: In order to place a transesophageal ultrasound probe, one needs a clear path down the esophagus.

Rationale: While electrical defibrillation and attempts to establish better venous access on the patient may be part of the resuscitation effort, these steps are not required before doing a transesophageal echocardiogram. However, most pre-hospital airway devices have a balloon or a portion of the device that blocks the esophagus and thus would hinder placement of the ultrasound probe. Therefore the pre-hospital device should be removed and a more definitive airway established before placing the ultrasound probe down the esophagus [17].

Question 20

After the third round of CPR you obtain the following view with your transesophageal ultrasound probe. No pulse is palpated and the cardiac rhythm on your external monitoring device shows asystole. However, you note fine ventricular fibrillation on your ultrasound. What view is obtained and based on your ultrasound findings, what therapy might the patient benefit from? (Fig. 20.8)

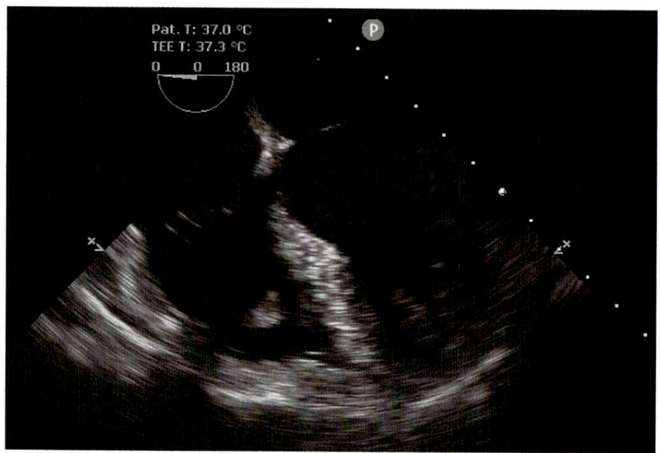

Fig. 20.8 TEE Mid-Esophageal 4 Chamber

A. Mid-esophageal 4 chamber view, electrical defibrillation
B. Mid-esophageal 4 chamber view, thrombolytics
C. Mid-esophageal long axis view, electrical defibrillation
D. Mid-esophageal long axis view, thrombolytics

Answer: A.

Key Point: One must understand the ideal views to obtain when performing TEE as they may show reversible causes of cardiac arrest.

Rationale: The view above shows all 4 chambers of the heart. In a mid-esophageal long axis view only 3 chambers of the heart are generally seen (right ventricle, left ventricle, and left atrium) and the aortic root should be seen as well. One of the proposed uses of transesophageal echocardiogram in cardiac arrest is for the detection of fine ventricular fibrillation. If this is noted on the echocardiogram, then electrical defibrillation would be the most reasonable next step.

Questions 21–24

A 43-year-old woman is brought in by EMS after being found unresponsive and apneic in bed by a family member. CPR was initiated on scene by the family member. On arrival by EMS, her initial rhythm was asystole, and blood glucose was 10 mg/dL. She was given one amp of D50, epinephrine, and bicarbonate in route to the ED. On arrival to the ED she does not have a palpable pulse and the initial rhythm is pulseless electrical activity (PEA).

Question 21
ACLS continues for PEA Arrest. You are unable to see the heart on transthroacic echocardiography (TTE) due to significant air obstructing the view and are considering trans-esophageal echo (TEE). Which of the following is a contraindication to TEE probe placement?

A. History of esophageal stricture
B. History of esophageal obstruction
C. Poor airway control
D. All of the above

Answer: D.

Key Point: TEE must not be placed in patients with absolute contraindications including esophageal obstruction, esophageal stricture, or poor airway control.

Rationale: Before the decision to place the TEE probe, careful consideration of the patient's risk versus benefit should be weighed. Absolute contraindications including esophageal obstruction and esophageal stricture can cause esophageal injury or perforation leading to significant complications. Additional contraindications to TEE include poor airway control or lack of a definitive airway [18].

Question 22
TEE can be potentially placed in all of the following except?

A. Patient with a Cervical spine injury
B. Patient with an Esophageal Ring
C. Patient with severe coagulopathy
D. Patient with Esophageal varices

Answer: B.

Key Point: Esophageal obstructions are an absolute contraindications and an esophageal ring is a potential causes of obstruction. The risks and benefits of placement should be considered if there are relative contraindications.

Rationale: Relative contraindications do not necessarily preclude placement of the TEE probe, but placement should be weighed against the increased risk of the procedure. Relative contraindications include: severe coagulopathy, upper GI bleeding, history of esophageal surgery or varices, and cervical spine injury. If cervical spinal injury is suspected, particular care should be given during TEE probe intubation and it may be helpful to have a second provider provide jaw thrust or laryngoscopy while immobilization is maintained [18].

Question 23
After consideration of the risks and benefits as well as absolute and relative contraindications of placement, the TEE probe was placed during arrest. You are able to view the heart during CPR and are offering guidance to CPR givers to optimize their efforts. Which of the following anatomic parameters during CPR that has shown promise in successful resuscitation after cardiac arrest: (Video 20.2)

A. LVOT opening during the compression phase of CPR
B. Movement of RV free wall toward septum
C. Ejection fraction during CPR
D. Aortic root diameter difference between compressive and relaxed phases of CPR

Answer: A.

Key Point: Emerging evidence suggests left ventricular outflow tract opening during CPR is associated with improved outcomes.

Rationale: Although there is limited data in TEE specific guidance of CPR, according to a retrospective cohort study, patients with an LVOT that opened during the compressive phase of CPR had a significantly higher survival to hospital admission [19, 20].

Question 24
Evaluation of the cause of the patient's PEA arrest is undertaken during active CPR and pulse checks. The three main cardiac views in resuscitative TEE are:

A. Mid-esophageal 4 chamber, mid-esophageal long axis, and the transgastric short axis
B. Mid-esophageal 4 chamber, transgastric long axis, and the transgastric short axis
C. Mid-esophageal 5 chamber, mid-esophageal long axis, and the transgastric short axis
D. Transgastric long axis, mid-esophageal ascending aortal short axis, and mid-esophageal bicaval view

Answer: A.

Key Point: Resuscitative TEE obtains limited views that are similar to standard views obtained in TTE.

Rationale: The workhorse views to help identify or exclude cardiac pathology leading to arrest include mid-esophageal 4 chamber, mid-esophageal long axis and the transgastric short axis. These views are similar to the TTE views of the apical four chamber, the parasternal long axis, and the parasternal short axis respectively. These views were proposed as they were able to "efficiently capture the scope of ED cardiac ultrasound" including evaluation of pericardial effusion, LV/RV size and function, assessment of fluid status, and guidance of procedures [21, 22].

Questions 25–27

A 65-year-old male with history of ischemic cardiomyopathy (EF 15%) status post ICD placement, CAD, obesity, DM, ESRD newly on hemodialysis, COPD, DVT/PE (status post IVC filter) presents to the ED after a witnessed cardiac arrest. Initial rhythm was PEA for EMS. ACLS is continued and ROSC is obtained just as TEE is being placed. The patient is hypotensive after ROSC and an evaluation of the possible causes of cardiac arrest is initiated (Video 20.3).

Question 25
The likely etiology of this patient's hypotension based this image is:

A. Obstructive Shock
B. Hypovolemic Shock
C. Cardiogenic Shock
D. Cardiac Tamponade

Answer: C.

Key Point: TEE has been shown to identify potential causes of hypotension and lead to immediate management changes to improve hypotension.

Rational: This image shows a heart with significantly diminished ejection fraction. There is also a non-anatomic, bright hyperechoic line running through the right side of the heart consistent with his know ICD wire. This can sometimes be confused as the edge of the free wall and thus the blood in the RV can be mistakenly interpreted as a pericardial effusion. This mid esophageal 4 chamber view does not show an effusion. Although the right ventricle is large, there is no bowing of the septum toward the LV and thus this patient's hypotension is unlikely from obstructive shock. TEE has been shown to identify the cause of hypotension as well as leading to changes in management in about 30–50% of patients [23, 24].

Question 26
You would like to move from the mid-esophageal 4 chamber view (ME4C) to the mid-esophageal long axis view (MELAX) for further interrogation of the heart. To move from the ME4C to the MELAX one must: (Video 20.4)

A. Increase the omniplane from 0 to 110-160 degrees
B. Decrease the omniplane from 110-160 to 0 degrees
C. Rotate the probe to the patient's right
D. Advance the probe and increase the omniplane to 110–160 degrees**Answer: A.**

Key Point: From the mid-esophageal probe position, only rotation of the omniplane is necessary from 0 to 110–160 degrees.

Rational: Of the four TEE windows proposed for resuscitative TEE by Arntfield et al., three of the four are obtained at the mid esophageal depth. From the ME4C view the omniplane can be advanced to 110–160 degrees to obtain the MELAX view [22, 25].

Question 27
After ROSC, the patient was noted to be hypotensive and had a significantly depressed ejection fraction on TEE. In a patient with cardiogenic shock, the best choice for an initial pressor is:

A. Dopamine
B. Norepinephrine
C. Dobutamine
D. Either B or C

Answer: D.

Key Point: Although limited strong evidence of initial pressor choice in cardiac shock exists, dopamine has been associated with more arrhythmias than alternative pressors.

Rational: Dopamine has more associated arrhythmias and is therefore a poor choice for initial management. Either dobutamine or norepinephrine would be good choices to initiate in this patient with cardiogenic shock. Dobutamine has strong B1 adrenergic properties and is therefore a strong inotropic agent, but has the side effect of causing a decrease in systemic vascular resistance. Norepinephrine was studied extensively in septic shock patients and has proven superiority over alternative agents for this indication. Norepinephrine has strong alpha 1 and moderate B1 adrenergic activity with fewer arrhythmias than alternative agents [26].

Questions 28–30

A 70-year-old male with unknown medical history presents with a witnessed arrest at work. Initial rhythm for EMS was ventricular fibrillation, and he received multiple defibrillations in route. A King Airway was placed by EMS which was exchanged with an ET tube in the resuscitation room. Initial rhythm was ventricular fibrillation on the monitor. TEE was placed (Video 20.5).

Question 28
To maximize utility of compressions, direction should be given to the person giving compressions to move the area of maximal compression to:

A. Ventricular side of the aortic valve
B. Over the aortic valve itself
C. Over the ascending aorta
D. Over the right atria

Answer: A.

Key Point: Moving the area of maximal compression of CPR to over the ventricles can potentially increase utility of CPR and was associated with successful resuscitation.

Rational: Although limited evidence exists on the real time guidance of CPR, there is evidence to suggest that obtaining CPR that maximizes LVOT opening is associated with ROSC. Practically, moving the CPR maximal force, or the area of maximal compression, inferior to the Aortic valve and therefore overlying the ventricles can help maximize LVOT opening. Compressive forces over the aortic valve, ascending aorta, or the right atria are all areas that may obstruct the opening of the LVOT and therefore be less successful resuscitations [19].

Question 29
After continuing ACLS for approximately 25 min, you obtain these videos on pulse check. Your recommendation based on this is: (Video 20.6)

A. Low likelihood of survival, step resuscitation efforts
B. Defibrillate
C. Perform pericardiocentesis
D. Give code dose epinephrine

Answer: A.

Key Point: With no kinetic cardiac activity on ultrasound, the likelihood of survival is very low.

Rational: These views at pulse check show no kinetic cardiac activity. Previous studies have shown no ROSC with the absence of kinetic cardiac activity on ultrasound. A new larger study suggests that there may be some people who will obtain ROSC who presented with no kinetic cardiac activity, but a very low survival to hospital discharge (0.6%). This brings into question the previous data giving credence to stopping all efforts if no kinetic cardiac activity is seen as there were no survivors identified in previous papers. With this patient, the likelihood of survival after full resuscitation efforts and no continued cardiac activity are consistent with a reasonable endpoint to resuscitation efforts [27, 28].

Question 30
Consider instead if after continuing ACLS for approximately 25 min, you obtain this view on pulse check. Your recommendation based on this is: (Video 20.7)

A. Low likelihood of survival, step resuscitation efforts
B. Defibrillate
C. Perform pericardiocentesis
D. Give code dose epinephrine**Answer: B.**

Key Point: This patient has organized cardiac activity consistent with pulseless ventricular tachycardia which would necessitate defibrillation according to ACLS.

Rational: Although studies are limited, interpreting cardiac rhythm on transesophageal echocardiography has been described and may have a role in conjunction with cardiac monitor to assess pulse. In this patient there is organized, regular cardiac activity, although limited mechanical movement. This is consistent with ventricular tachycardia. According to ACLS, defibrillation with 120–200 J Biphasic defibrillation is recommended for pulseless ventricular tachycardia [10, 20].

Questions 31–32

A 35-year-old male presents to the emergency department by ambulance as a trauma activation. He is lethargic and unable to provide history. Per emergency medical services personnel, he was in a witnessed altercation and sustained a stab wound to the chest. On arrival, his vital signs are HR: 135, BP: 85/40, RR 35, T 36.0, SpO_2 92% on room air. His airway reflexes are intact and he has bilateral breath sounds. He has intact, thread distal pulses. IV access is obtained and fluid resuscitation initiated. On exam, he has a single wound to the anterior chest. There are no other signs of trauma. An extended focused assessment with sonography in trauma (FAST) scan is performed (Fig. 20.2).

Question 31
Which view is present on the transthoracic echo image above?

A. Parasternal Short Axis.
B. Parasternal Long Axis.
C. Apical 4-chamber.
D. Subxiphoid.

Answer: D.

Key Point: Subxiphoid long axis shows pericardial effusion.

Rational: During a FAST exam, routinely a transthoracic subxiphoid view is obtained to assess for the presence of pericardial effusion [29].

Question 32

A complete extended-FAST scan is obtained, which shows an absence of free peritoneal fluid and no pleural effusion. Despite IV fluid resuscitation, patient's blood pressure begins to decline and he becomes pulseless. High quality CPR is initiated immediately and the patient is emergently intubated. During the first pulse check, the patient's heart is visualized with bedside ultrasound. Based on the image provided above, prompt management of which emergent conditions should be considered a priority?

A. intra-abdominal hemorrhage.
B. hemothorax.
C. cardiac tamponade.
D. pulmonary contusion.

Answer: C.

Key Point: Collapse of the right ventricle in the setting of pericardial effusion is consistent with cardiac tamponade.

Rational: In the absence of other findings, a pericardial effusion in an unstable patient who has sustained penetrating injury to the chest should raise concern for cardiac tamponade. The second image shows collapse of the right ventricle, consistent with cardiac tamponade. Tamponade management should be considered a priority in this patient with an otherwise negative FAST scan [29, 30].

Questions 33–34

A 65-year-old female with history of metastatic breast cancer is admitted to the medical intensive care unit (MICU) from the oncology floor with hypotension. On arrival to the MICU, her vital signs are: HR 135, BP 85/40, RR 40, T 36.5, SpO_2 85% on non-rebreather mask at 15 L/m. On exam, she is in significant respiratory distress, has clear lungs on auscultation, no abdominal pain, 3+ pitting edema in bilateral lower extremities. IV access is obtained. 12-lead EKG shows new right bundle branch block. Portable CXR shows no significant infiltrate, edema, pneumothorax, or pleural effusion.

Diagnostic evaluation of bilateral lower extremities reveal echogenic, non-compressible right femoral vein.

Question 33

What is the reported sensitivity of bedside ultrasound in the evaluation of lower extremity deep vein thrombosis?

A. <30%.
B. 30–50%.
C. 50–70%.
D. >70%.

Answer: D.

Key Point: Bedside ultrasound can be used in the evaluaton of deep venous thrombosis in critical ill patients.

Rational: In a recent meta-analysis of the accuracy of bedside ultrasound performed by emergency physicians for the diagnosis of DVT, mean weighted sensitivity was reported as 96.1%, with no study reporting a sensitivity lower than 70% [31].

Question 34

The patient becomes increasingly somnolent and develops PEA arrest. ACLS protocol with high quality CPR is initiated. At the first pulse check, a bedside echocardiogram is performed. Which view is demonstrated in the image below? (Fig. 20.9).

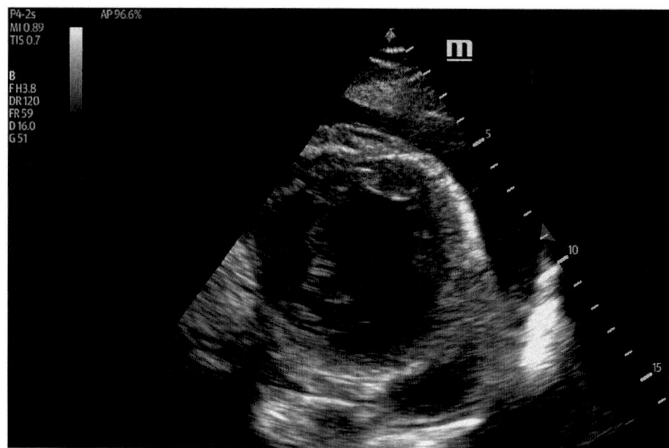

Fig. 20.9 TTE Right Ventricular Strain

A. Transthoracic parasternal short axis view.
B. Tranesophageal mid-esophaegeal long axis view.
C. Tranesophageal bicaval view.
D. Transthoracic subxiphoid view.

Answer: A.

Key Point: The view demonstrated in the image above is a transthoracic parasternal short axis view.

Rational: The presented cardiac view is a transthoracic parasternal short axis window, which is the preferred window in which to compare right ventricular and left ventricular diameters. In this image, the right ventricle is showing evidence of a "D sign", indicating bowing of the septum into the left ventricle.

Question 35
A right ventricular to left ventricular diameter of what value is suggestive of right ventricular dilation?

A. < 0.35.
B. 0.35–0.5.
C. 0.5–0.65.
D. >0.65.

Answer: D.

Key Point: > 0.65 right to left ventricular diameter is suggestive of right ventricular dilation.

Rational: In this image, the right ventricle is showing evidence of a "D sign", indicating bowing of the septum into the left ventricle. Additionally, the right ventricle to left ventricular diameter is >0.65 [30, 32].

Question 36
In the absence of contraindications, administration of which therapy should be a priority?

A. systemic heparin.
B. broad spectrum antibiotics.
C. systemic thrombolytics.
D. chest tube placement.

Answer: C.

The presented cardiac view is a parasternal short axis window, which is the preferred window in which to compare right ventricular and left ventricular diameters. In a prospective observational study of 103 patients presenting to the emergency department with suspected pulmonary embolus, mean RV:LV diameter was 0.71 in patients with pulmonary embolus and 0.48 in patients without pulmonary embolus ($p < 0.0001$). In this patient with a clinical history suggestive of pulmonary embolus, findings of DVT and RV dilation, pulmonary embolus as cause of cardiac arrest should be considered. Current guidelines recommend the administration of systemic thrombolytics for unstable patients with pulmonary embolus [30–33].

Question 37
An 80-year-old with history of prior ischemic stroke, diabetes mellitus type II, hypertension, and recurrent aspiration events is found unresponsive and pulseless at his nursing facility. CPR is initiated in the field, his airway is secured, and the patient is brought to the emergency department. On the first pulse check, the patient is noted to be in PEA. A bedside ultrasound is obtained (Video 20.8).

Which of the following is present in the view provided?

A. pericardial effusion.
B. hyperdynamic left ventricle.
C. cardiac standstill.
D. dilated right ventricle.**Answer: C.**

Key Point: Bedside ultrasound can be used to identify cardiac standstill.

Rational: The presented image demonstrates a parasternal long view of the heart. There is no motion noted in the cardiac wall, as such this video represents cardiac standstill. Presence of cardiac standstill in cardiac arrest is strongly associated with failure to achieve return of spontaneous circulation (ROSC). Systematic review identified presence of cardiac activity on bedside ultrasound as being associated with ROSC (RR 4.35 (95% CI 2.2-8.63) [30, 34, 35].

Questions 38–41

A 65-year-old male is brought to the emergency department in cardiac arrest. Adult cardiac life support is ongoing. On arrival, high quality CPR is continued. On the first pulse check, no carotid pulse is palpated. Cardiac monitor does not reveal any organized cardiac activity. Simultaneously, bedside echocardiogram is performed which shows diffuse quivering of the entire myocardium (Video 20.9).

Question 38
In addition to restarting high quality CPR, which of the following is the next appropriate action.

A. Endotracheal intubation
B. Initiate therapeutic hypothermia
C. Prepare for and administer defibrillation at 200 J
D. Consult for emergent cardiac catheterization

Answer: C.

Key Point: The transthoracic subxiphoid view shows diffuse quivering of the entire myocardium consistent with ventricular fibrillation.

Rational: For patients in cardiac arrest, categorization of rhythm is critical as prompt defibrillation for patients with ventricular fibrillation (VF) or pulseless ventricular tachycardia (VT) is associated with improved outcomes. During cardiopulmonary resuscitation (CPR), clinical distinction between asystole and fine VF maybe challenging. Identification of disorganized cardiac activity, as shown in the provided clip may help the provider identify VF. If VF is identified in the arresting patient, immediate defibrillation is indicated [36, 37].

Question 39

An action is taken. On the next pulse check, cardiac monitor reveals organized, narrow complex rhythm. No carotid pulse is palpated. In addition to continuing high quality CPR, which of the following are indicated?

A. Prepare for and administer defibrillation at 200 J
B. Consider reversible causes of cardiac arrest
C. Initiate therapeutic hypothermia
D. Obtain non-contrast computed tomography (CT) scan of patient's brain

Answer: B.

Key Point: Point-of-care echocardiography can be used to identify reversible causes of cardiac arrest.

Rational: Following defibrillation, the patient has an organized, narrow complex rhythm but no palpable pulse, indicating that the patient is demonstrating pulseless electrical activity. In addition to continuing high quality CPR, it is appropriate to consider and treat any reversible causes of the patient's arrest [1].

Question 40

Additional ultrasound images are obtained. The patient remains pulseless with organized rhythm on the cardiac monitor. Based on the image below, which of the following is the next appropriate action? (Fig. 20.10)

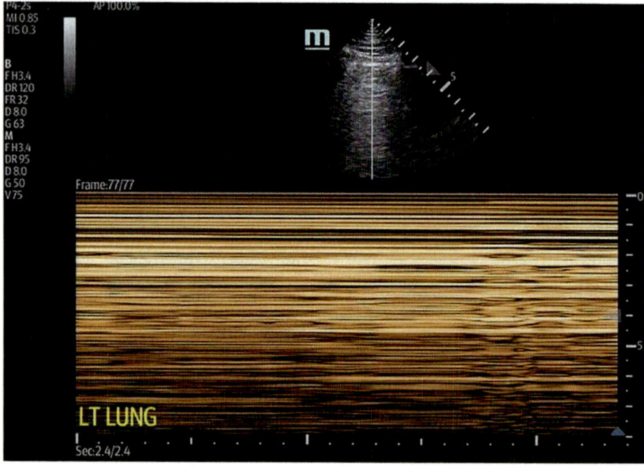

Fig. 20.10 Left Lung Pneumothorax

A. Ultrasound-guided pericardiocentesis
B. Systemic thrombolysis
C. Cardiac catheterization
D. Emergent thoracostomy on affected side

Answer: D.

Key Point: Tension pneumothorax can be a reversible cause of cardiac arrest.

Rational: In this case, lung ultrasound is performed to evaluate for pneumothorax—the view presented shows pleura with absent lung sliding, suggestive of pneumothorax. As the patient remains in cardiac arrest, management of this pneumothorax via thoracostomy is indicated [38–40].

Question 41

The advantages of using tranesophageal echocardiography over transthoracic echocardiography in cardiac arrest are all of the following except:

A. The quality of chest compressions can be assessed in real time
B. Cardioversion can take place while the probe is in place
C. There are no risk of complications
D. Body habitus is not a barrier in obtaining windows

Answer: C.

Key Point: Transesophageal echocardiography has a small risk of esophageal perforation with probe insertion.

Rational: The advantages of using transesophageal echocardiography in cardiac arrest are the following: Compression can continue without any interruption, the quality of the compressions can be assessed in real time, emphysema and body habitus are not a barrier to obtaining windows, and cardioversion can occur while the probe is in place [20].

References

1. Blanco P, Martínez BC. Point-of-care ultrasound in cardiopulmonary resuscitation: a concise review. J Ultrasound. 2017;20(3):193–8.
2. Atkinson P, Bowra J, Milne J, Lewis D, Lambert M, Jarman B, et al. International Federation for Emergency Medicine Consensus Statement: Sonography in hypotension and cardiac arrest (SHoC): an international consensus on the use of point of care ultrasound for undifferentiated hypotension and during cardiac arrest – CORRIGENDUM. CJEM. 2017;19(04):327.
3. Chan P, McNally B, Tang F, Kellermann A. Recent trends in survival from out-of-hospital cardiac arrest in the United States. Circulation. 2014;130(21):1876–82.
4. Parish DC, Dinesh Chandra KM, Dane FC. Success changes the problem: why ventricular fibrillation is declining, why pulseless electrical activity is emerging, and what to do about it. Resuscitation. 2003;58(1):31–5.
5. Teran F, Dean A, Centeno C, Panebianco N, Zeidan A, Chan W, et al. Evaluation of out-of-hospital cardiac arrest using transesophageal echocardiography in the emergency department. Resuscitation. 2019;137:140–7.
6. Tsang T, Freeman W, Sinak L, Seward J. Echocardiographically guided pericardiocentesis: evolution and state-of-the-art technique. Mayo Clin Proc. 1998;73(7):647–52.
7. Roberts J, Thomsen T, Custalow C, Roberts HJ, Hedges. Clinical procedures in emergency medicine: expert consult—online and print. s: Elsevier; 2014.
8. Atkinson P, Keyes A, O'Donnell K, Beckett N, Banerjee A, Fraser J, et al. Do electrocardiogram rhythm findings predict cardiac activity during a cardiac arrest? A study from sonography in cardiac arrest

and hypotension in the emergency department (SHoC-ED). Cureus. 2018;10:e3624.

9. Huis Int Veld M, Allison M, Bostick D, Fisher K, Goloubeva O, Witting M, et al. Ultrasound use during cardiopulmonary resuscitation is associated with delays in chest compressions. Resuscitation. 2017;119:95–8.
10. Link M, Berkow L, Kudenchuk P, Halperin H, Hess E, Moitra V, et al. Part 7: adult advanced cardiovascular life support. Circulation. 2015;132(18 suppl 2):S444–64.
11. Soar J, Nolan J, Böttiger B, Perkins G, Lott C, Carli P, et al. European Resuscitation Council Guidelines for Resuscitation 2015. Resuscitation. 2015;95:100–47.
12. Walls R, et al. "Shock." rosen's emergency medicine: concepts and clinical practice. 9th ed. Philadelphia, PA: Elsevier; 2018. p. 68–76.
13. Al-Khatib S, Stevenson W, Ackerman M, Bryant W, Callans D, Curtis A, et al. 2017 AHA/ACC/HRS guideline for management of patients with ventricular arrhythmias and the prevention of sudden cardiac death: executive summary. Circulation. 2018;138(13):e272.
14. Chatterjee S, Chakraborty A, Weinberg I. Thrombolysis for pulmonary embolism and risk of all-cause mortality, major bleeding, and intracranial hemorrhage: a meta-analysis. J Vasc Surg. 2014;60(4):1094.
15. Mediratta A, Addetia K, Medvedofsky D, Gomberg-Maitland M, Mor-Avi V, Lang RM. Echocardiographic diagnosis of acute pulmonary embolism in patients with Mcconnell's sign. Echocardiography. 2016;33(5):696–702.
16. McConnell MV, Solomon SD, Rayan ME, Come PC, Goldhaber SZ, Lee RT. Regional right ventricular dysfunction detected by echocardiography in acute pulmonary embolism. Am J Cardiol. 1996;78(4):469–73.
17. Long B, Alerhand S, Maliel K, Koyfman A. Echocardiography in cardiac arrest: an emergency medicine review. Am J Emerg Med. 2018;36(3):488–93.
18. Lumb P. Journal of critical care: 2014. J Crit Care. 2014;29(1):160–1.
19. Catena E, Ottolina D, Fossali T, Rech R, Borghi B, Perotti A, et al. Association between left ventricular outflow tract opening and successful resuscitation after cardiac arrest. Resuscitation. 2019;138:8–14.
20. Blaivas M. Transesophageal echocardiography during cardiopulmonary arrest in the emergency department. Resuscitation. 2008;78(2):135–40.
21. Fair J, Mallin M, Mallemat H, Zimmerman J, Arntfield R, Kessler R, et al. Transesophageal echocardiography: guidelines for point-of-care applications in cardiac arrest resuscitation. Ann Emerg Med. 2018;71(2):201–7.
22. Arntfield R, Pace J, McLeod S, Granton J, Hegazy A, Lingard L. Focused transesophageal echocardiography for emergency physicians—description and results from simulation training of a structured four-view examination. Crit Ultrasound J. 2015;7(1):27.
23. Heidenreich P, Stainback R, Redberg R, Schiller N, Cohen N, Foster E. Transesophageal echocardiography predicts mortality in critically Ill patients with unexplained hypotension. J Am Coll Cardiol. 1995;26(1):152–8.
24. van der Wouw P, Koster R, Delemarre B, de Vos R, Lampe-Schoenmaeckers A, Lie K. Diagnostic accuracy of transesophageal echocardiography during cardiopulmonary resuscitation. J Am Coll Cardiol. 1997;30(3):780–3.
25. Denault A, Vegas A, Lamarche Y, Tardif J, Couture P. Basic transesophageal and critical care ultrasound. Boca Raton, FL: CRC Press; 2017. p. 32–4.
26. van Diepen S, Katz J, Albert N, Henry T, Jacobs A, Kapur N, et al. Contemporary management of cardiogenic shock: a scientific statement from the American Heart Association. Circulation. 2017;136(16):e232.
27. Salen P, Melniker L, Chooljian C, Rose J, Alteveer J, Reed J, et al. Does the presence or absence of sonographically identified cardiac activity predict resuscitation outcomes of cardiac arrest patients? Am J Emerg Med. 2005;23(4):459–62.
28. Gaspari R, Weekes A, Adhikari S, Noble V, Nomura J, Theodoro D, et al. Emergency department point-of-care ultrasound in out-of-hospital and in-ED cardiac arrest. Resuscitation. 2016;109:33–9.
29. Melniker L, Leibner E, McKenney M, Lopez P, Briggs W, Mancuso C. Randomized controlled clinical trial of point-of-care, limited ultrasonography for trauma in the emergency department: the first sonography outcomes assessment program trial. Ann Emerg Med. 2006;48(3):227–35.
30. Walley PE, Walley KR, Goodgame B, Punjabi V, Sirounis D. A practical approach to goal-directed echocardiography in the critical care setting. Crit Care. 2014;18(6):681.
31. Pomero F, Borretta V, Bonzini M, Melchio R, Douketis J, Fenoglio L, et al. Accuracy of emergency physician–performed ultrasonography in the diagnosis of deep-vein thrombosis. Thromb Haemost. 2013;109(01):137–45.
32. Quezada C, Bikdeli B, Barrios D, Barbero E, Chiluiza D, Muriel A, et al. Meta-analysis of prevalence and short-term prognosis of hemodynamically unstable patients with symptomatic acute pulmonary embolism. Am J Cardiol. 2019;123(4):684–9.
33. Mansencal N, Vieillard-Baron A, Beauchet A, Farcot J, El Hajjam M, Dufaitre G, et al. Triage patients with suspected pulmonary embolism in the emergency department using a portable ultrasound device. Echocardiography. 2008;25(5):451–6.
34. Blaivas M, Fox JC. Outcome in cardiac arrest patients found to have cardiac standstill on the bedside emergency department echocardiogram. Acad Emerg Med. 2001;8(6):616–21.
35. Wu C, Zheng Z, Jiang L, Gao Y, Xu J, Jin X, et al. The predictive value of bedside ultrasound to restore spontaneous circulation in patients with pulseless electrical activity: a systematic review and meta-analysis. PLoS One. 2018;13(1):e0191636.
36. Amaya SC, Langsam A. Ultrasound detection of ventricular fibrillation disguised as asystole. Ann Emerg Med. 1999;33(3):344–6.
37. Querellou E, Meyran D, Petitjean F, Le Dreff P, Maurin O. Ventricular fibrillation diagnosed with trans-thoracic echocardiography. Resuscitation. 2009;80(10):1211–3.
38. Lichtenstein D, Meziere G, Biderman P, Gepner A. The "lung point": an ultrasound sign specific to pneumothorax. Intensive Care Med. 2000;26(10):1434–40.
39. Gilbert TB, McGrath BJ, Soberman M. Chest tubes: indications, placement, management, and complications. J Intensive Care Med. 1993;8(2):73–86.
40. Yarmus L, Feller-Kopman D. Pneumothorax in the critically ill patient. Chest. 2012;141(4):1098–105.

21 Ultrasonography for Procedural Guidance

Ronny Munoz-Acuna, Akiva Leibowitz, and Somnath Bose

Question 1

Clinical stem: A 62 y/o male with a PMH of HTN and CAD undergoes a resection of a distal pancreatic mass, 3 days later initiates with abdominal pain, and develops hypotension and acidosis refractory to fluid resuscitation, patient is started on pressors and antibiotics and transferred to the ICU. Given that the patient now is on norepinephrine and vasopressin with a weak pulse, decision was made to place a CVL and an arterial line. Select all that apply to the appropriate technique for CVL insertion:

A. US probes best suited for CVC placement are small linear probes with high-frequency transducers (5–15 MHz)
B. Landmark techniques can account for anatomic variations at the CVC insertion site
C. Short axis technique is superior to long axis technique
D. The use of US for CVC placement in the IJV does not reduce the total rate of complications compared with conventional landmark techniques

Answer: A.

Key point: US-guided technique decreases complications during IJL CVL placement.

Rationale: The use of US for CVC placement in the IJV reduces the total rate of complications compared with conventional landmark techniques (US (4.0%) vs landmark (13.5%); risk ratio (95% confidence interval (CI)) 0.29 (0.17–0.52)). For SV the use of US resulted in a reduced rate of accidental arterial puncture (US (0.8%) vs landmark (5.9%); risk ratio (95% CI) 0.21 (0.06–0.82)) and hematoma formation (US (1.2%) vs landmark (6.6%); risk ratio (95% CI) 0.26 (0.09–0.76)). For FV US compared with the landmark technique increased the overall success rate (US (89.0%) vs landmark (78.9%); risk ratio (95% CI) 1.11 (1.00–1.23)) and the success rate with the first attempt (US (85.0%) vs landmark (48.7%); risk ratio (95% CI) 1.73 (1.34–2.22)) [1–3].

R. Munoz-Acuna
Department of Anesthesia, Critical Care and Pain Medicine, Beth Israel Deaconess Medical Center, Harvard Medical School, Boston, Massachusetts, USA

Department of Anesthesia, Critical Care and Pain, Yale New Haven Hospital, Yale School of Medicine, New Haven, USA
e-mail: ronny.munoz-acuna@yale.edu

A. Leibowitz · S. Bose (✉)
Department of Anesthesia, Critical Care and Pain Medicine, Beth Israel Deaconess Medical Center, Harvard Medical School, Boston, Massachusetts, USA
e-mail: aleibow1@bidmc.harvard.edu; sbose2@bidmc.harvard.edu

R. Sreedharan et al. (eds.), *Critical Care Echocardiography*, https://doi.org/10.1007/978-3-031-45731-9_21

Question 2

The structure marked in Fig. 21.1 corresponds to:

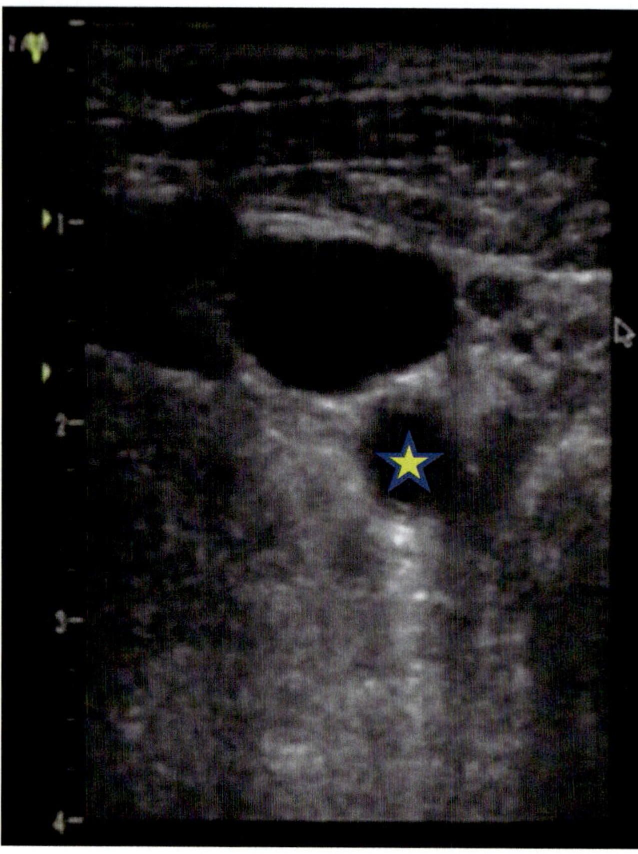

Fig. 21.1 US image obtained by placing a linear probe on the anterior cervical triangle. Personal Archive

A. EJV
B. IJV
C. Common carotid artery
D. Sternocleidomastoid muscle

Answer: C.

Key point: The IJV is anterolateral to the CA in 92%, >1 cm lateral to the carotid in 1%, medial to the carotid in 2%, and outside of the path predicted by landmarks in 5.5% of patients.

Rationale: The IJ is classically described as exiting the external jugular foramen at the base of the skull posterior to the internal carotid and coursing toward an anterolateral position (in relation to the carotid) as it travels caudally [4, 5] (Fig. 21.2).

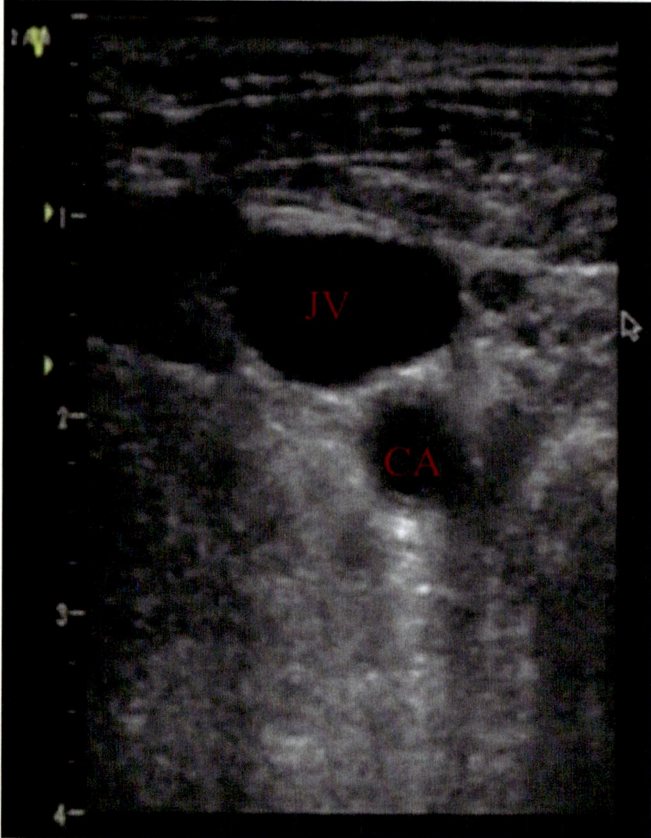

Fig. 21.2 US image obtained by placing a linear probe on the anterior cervical triangle depicting the following structures: CA: carotid artery, JV: Jugular vein. Note how the JV is anterolateral to the CA. Personal Archive

Question 3

Before placement one of the vessels is assessed using pulse wave doppler obtaining the following trace, this is indicative of which vessel (Fig. 21.3):

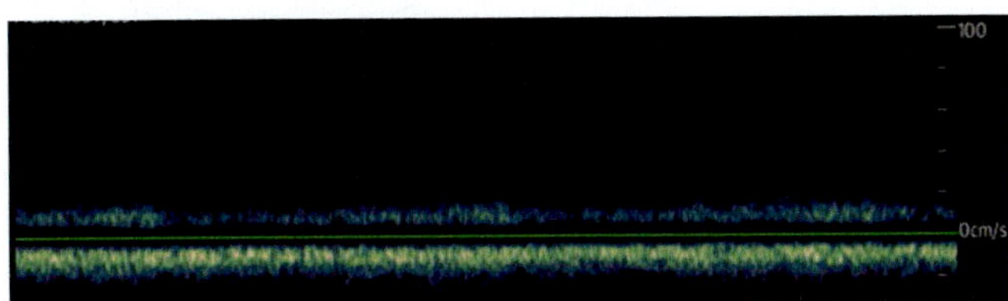

Fig. 21.3 Pulsed- wave Doppler sonography. Personal Archive

A. Internal Carotid Artery
B. External Carotid Artery
C. Internal Jugular Vein
D. AV malformation

Answer: C

Key point: Doppler US can be used to help differentiate between arterial and venous structures.

Rationale: The IJ vein has an elliptical shape and is larger and more collapsible with modest external surface pressure than the carotid artery (CA), which has rounder shape, thicker wall, and smaller diameter. Color flow Doppler demonstrates pulsatile blood flow in an artery in either SAX or LAX orientation. A small pulsed-wave Doppler sample volume within the vessel lumen displays a characteristic systolic flow within an artery, while at the same velocity range displays bi-phasic systolic and diastolic flow and a reduced velocity in a vein [5].

Question 4

According to Fig. 21.4, the reason for not placing a CVL in this position is:

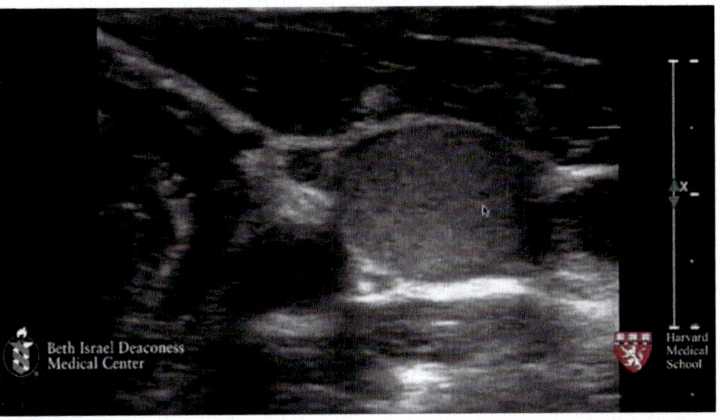

Fig. 21.4 Ultrasound image obtained with linear probe in the anterior cervical triangle, while holding continuous but gentle pressure. Personal Archive

A. Venous Thrombosis
B. Hematoma
C. Dissection
D. Arterial Thrombosis

Answer: A

Key point: US examination can help assess the patency of the vessels, and to define an appropriate target for CVL placement [6, 7].

Rationale: Several US findings are associated with vein thrombus in which the vein cannulation should be avoided:

- Thrombus visualized in the lumen of the vein.
- Vein cannot be completely compressed.
- Absence of spontaneous flow in the vein.
- Absence of flow did phases with respiration.
- Presence of increased collaterals, with a high suspicion of thrombus.

Question 5

For a patient with limited access a decision is made to place a line in the common femoral vein, which is located within the "femoral triangle" in the inguinal-femoral region. The borders of this area are the following:

A. Inguinal ligament laterally, the adductor longus medially, and the sartorius muscle superiorly.
B. Inguinal ligament medially, the adductor longus superiorly, and the sartorius muscle laterally.
C. Inguinal ligament superiorly, the adductor longus laterally, and the sartorius muscle medially.
D. Inguinal ligament superiorly, the adductor longus medially, and the sartorius muscle laterally.

Answer: D

Key point: The femoral triangle is formed by the inguinal ligament superiorly, the adductor longus medially, and the sartorius muscle laterally.

Rationale: The common femoral vein lies within the "femoral triangle" in the inguinal-femoral region. When obtaining the central venous access in the femoral vein, the key anatomical landmarks to identify in the inguinal-femoral region are the inguinal ligament and the femoral artery pulsation. This region is bordered by the inguinal ligament superiorly, the adductor longus medially, and the sartorius muscle laterally. It is important to understand the relationship of structures within the inguinal-femoral region which can be remembered by using the mnemonic "NAVEL." Moving laterally to medially, (N) femoral nerve, (A) femoral artery, (V) femoral vein, (E) empty space, (L) lymphatics [8].

Question 6

During a subclavian vein canulation using ultrasound guidance the following image is obtained, the structure marked with an asterisk corresponds to (Fig. 21.5):

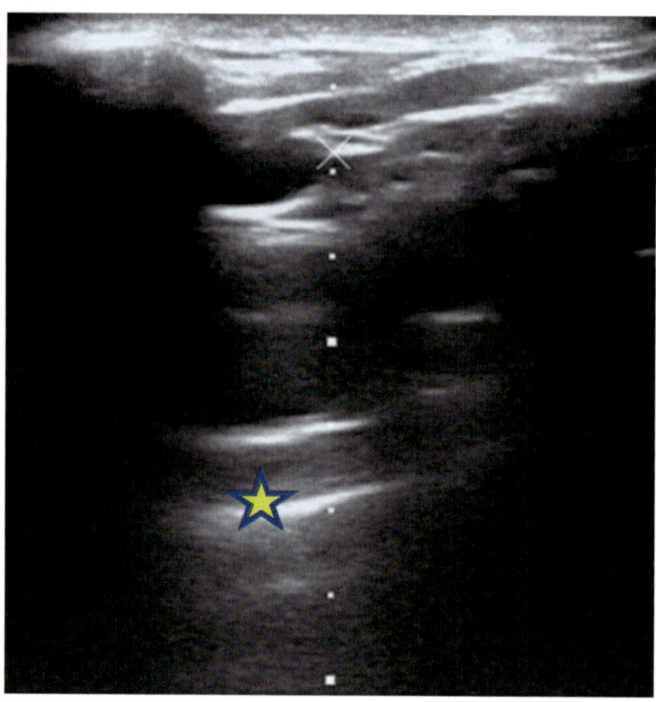

Fig. 21.5 Image depicting sonography of the subclavian long-axis approach for central venous canulation. Personal Archive

A. Subclavian vein
B. Subclavian artery
C. Axillary Nerve
D. Pleura

Answer: D.

Key point: The lung and pleural cavity lie deep and inferior to the subclavian vein and are particularly vulnerable to accidental puncture on the left chest (as compared to the right) where the apex of the lung can extend above the first rib.

Rationale: The subclavian vein is the continuation of the axillary vein as it courses beneath the clavicle. It travels superiorly starting at the lateral border of the first rib, then under the clavicle medially until it joins the internal jugular vein. The subclavian artery runs superior and posterior to the subclavian vein. It can be accessed from a supraclavicular or an infraclavicular approach. Ultrasound-guided subclavian vein access is a safe, effective and efficient option for central venous cannulation. Using ultrasound can decrease the time to cannulation in addition to many of the feared complications. However, more data and practice with the technique may be required for providers to feel comfortable with this underutilized access option [9–11].

Question 7

In a hypotensive patient, a decision is made to place an arterial line for close hemodynamic monitoring and blood draws. Which of the following is true regarding arterial lines?

A. Risk of major complications is less than 1% after placement of an arterial line, independent of the vessel used.
B. Femoral arterial lines have an increased risk of sepsis secondary to being closer to the perianal area.
C. Axillary arterial lines have a higher incidence of causing embolism to the brain.
D. Incidence of pseudoaneurysm is greater after placement of an arterial line in the brachial artery.

Answer: A.

Key point: Incidence rates for major complications such as permanent ischemic damage, sepsis and pseudoaneurysm formation are low and similar for the radial, femoral and axillary arteries. They occur in fewer than 1% of cases.

Rationale: The most frequently used site is the radial artery because of its well documented low complication rates and easy access Although temporary occlusion is reported quite frequently, serious ischemic damage was reported in only two studies, with a mean complication rate of 0.09%. Other major complications such as pseudoaneurysm and sepsis were reported to occur in a mean of 0.09% and 0.13% of cases, respectively. The second most frequently cannulated artery is the femoral artery where serious ischemic complications were reported in only one study, and the mean complication rate was 0.18%. The incidence rates for other major complications such as pseudoaneurysm and sepsis (0.3% and 0.44%, respectively), The third most cannulated artery in the present review of the literature was the axillary artery, and no difference in complications when compared to radial or femoral arteries [12].

Question 8

Regarding the proper technique for a radial arterial line insertion. The following statement is true:

A. A curvilinear ultrasound is recommended for correct visualization of the vessels.
B. A biphasic doppler waveform that changes with breathing is characteristic of an arterial signal.
C. Arteries can be differentiated from a vein applying smooth yet constant pressure in the transducer.
D. The longitudinal approach is superior to the transverse approach for placing an arterial line.

Answer: C.

Key point: Arterial cannulation using an US is effective and safe, although adequate training of the clinician is required.

Rationale: Ultrasound guidance has emerged as a valuable adjunct for radial artery catheter placement. The advantages of ultrasound guidance include real-time visualization of landmarks, improved pre-procedure planning, reduction in complications, less time spent at the bedside, and improved first-attempt success rates. Disadvantages of ultrasound guidance include equipment cost, equipment availability, limited availability of experts to train providers, and the cost of training providers. There are three methods when cannulating an artery: transverse, longitudinal and static technique (does not use real time assistance). The best method to use is still unclear, and the best strategy may be to utilize whichever technique the operator is most comfortable and experienced utilizing [13].

Question 9

The following statement is false regarding benefits of using US for arterial lines placement:

A. Real-time visualization of landmarks.
B. Improved pre-procedure planning.
C. Reduction in complications.
D. Less time spent at the bedside.
E. Improved first-attempt success rates.
F. Less incidence of catheter related infections.

Answer: F.

Key point: although US guided a-line placement has several benefits, reducing the incidence of infections is not one of them.

Rationale: The advantages of ultrasound guidance include real-time visualization of landmarks, improved pre-procedure planning, reduction in complications, less time spent at the bedside, and improved first-attempt success rates. Disadvantages of ultrasound guidance include equipment cost, equipment availability, limited availability of experts to train providers, and the cost of training providers [13].

Question 10

Ultrasound guidance should be considered for the following group of patients

A. Patients without a palpable radial pulse
B. Patients who have undergone prior attempts
C. Patients with coagulopathy or abnormal clotting factors
D. Patients with severe hypotension
E. Patients with radial artery as the only available site
F. All of the above

Answer: F.

Key point: Although there is no absolute indication for using ultrasound when placing arterial lines, certain populations may benefit from this approach.

Rationale: In patients who present difficult vascular access, ultrasound guidance is effective for establishing both venous and arterial access. Proper training is essential for successful utilization of ultrasound guidance. The radial artery can be difficult to cannulate, especially for those not experienced in the procedure. We support the use of ultrasound guidance to reduce insertion-related complications. Ultrasound guidance has become the standard of care for placement of internal jugular vein central venous catheters and peripherally inserted central catheters; current evidence suggests that ultrasound guidance should be the standard of care for radial artery cannulation as well. The technique can easily be used for arterial puncture and may reduce morbidity associated with arterial puncture and assist in success for patients who are considered "tough sticks." [12, 13].

Question 11

During an axillary line placement under ultrasound guidance the following image is obtained. The structure marked with (*) (Fig. 21.6):

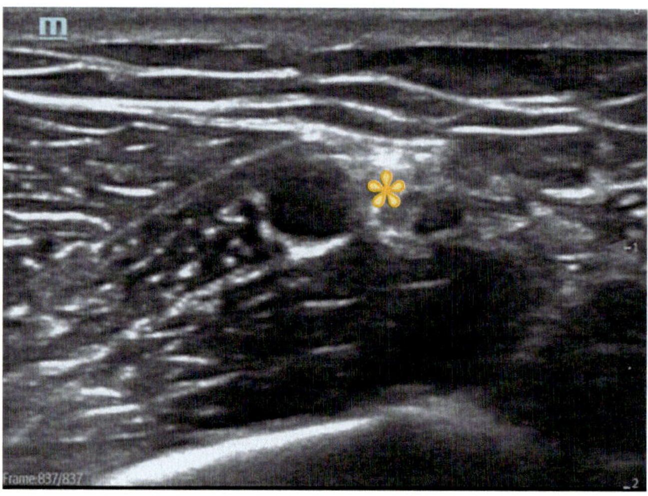

Fig. 21.6 Ultrasound image using a linear probe of the axillary fossa. Personal Archive

A. Innervates the palm and the volar aspects of the lateral 3.5 digits.
B. Innervates the dorsal 1.5 digits and palmar aspects of the proximal hand.
C. Innervates the posterior and lateral arm, the posterior forearm and the dorsal aspect of the lateral 3.5 fingers.
D. Is responsible for sensation along the lateral forearm.

Answer: A.

Key point: The median nerve medial to the biceps and brachialis and lateral to the brachial artery, is located in close relation to the axillary artery and may be punctured inadvertently when placing arterial axillary lines.

Rationale: The median nerve emerges from the lateral and medial cords and carries fibers from C5-T1. It runs medial to the biceps and brachialis and lateral to the brachial artery. It enters the forearm under the biceps aponeurosis and through the two heads of pronator teres. It gives rise to the anterior interosseous nerve in the forearm and then continues distally through the carpal tunnel. The median nerve is responsible for cutaneous innervation of the palm (via the palmar cutaneous nerve branching before the carpal tunnel), and the volar aspects of the lateral 3.5 digits (via superficial digital branches) [14, 15].

Question 12

A 78-year-old female with DM2 and COPD, complains of 7 days of fever and SOB. She deteriorates rapidly in the ED and is intubated and admitted to the ICU. Vitals are as follows: HR 105/min, Sinus Tachycardia, NIBP 90/45, Sat O2: 92% with FiO2 of 80% and 16 cmH20 of PEEP. Chest X-Ray shows a "veiling opacity" of the right lung field. Lung US is performed at bedside: Which of the following statements is correct?

A. Effusions as small as 50 cc can be visible in supine CXR.
B. Physical examination is 70% accurate diagnosing pleural effusion.
C. Position of the probe has no effect in measuring the pleural effusion volume.
D. Lung ultrasound is more accurate than supine radiography and is as accurate as a CT for the diagnosis of pleural effusion.

Answer: D.

Key point: Thoracic US is more reliable than physical exam and CXR at diagnosing pleural effusion and is as accurate as CT according to international guidelines.

Rationale: Pleural effusions as small as 50 mL can be visible in upright lateral CXR images, but conventional posteroanterior images require a volume of at least 200 mL A diagnostic accuracy of 91% for thoracic ultrasound, compared with 56% for the physical examination, and 33% for X-ray examination has been reported regarding diagnosing of pleural effusion. Consequently, the International Consensus Conference on Lung Ultrasound stated, "for the detection of effusion, lung ultrasound is more accurate than supine radiography and is as accurate as CT" [16, 17].

Question 13

Which findings of the thoracic ultrasound may point towards this effusion being a transudate?

A. Anechoic, non-septated, normal pleural thickness
B. Hyperechoic, septated, increased pleural thickness
C. Anechoic, non septated, air bronchograms, irregular pleural thickness
D. Hyperechoic, air bronchograms, increased pleural thickness

Answer: A.

Table 21.1 Ultrasonographic characteristics of exudates vs transudates. Adapted from Yang PC, Luh KT, Chang DB, Wu HD, Yu CJ, Kuo SH. Value of sonography in determining the nature of pleural effusion: analysis of 320 cases. AJR Am J Roentgenol. 1992 Jul;159(1):29–33

	Exudate	Transudate
Internal echogenicity	Anechoic, non-septated or septated. Hemothorax can be hyperechogenic. Septated or non-septated.	Usually non septated and homogenous
Pleural thickness	Thickened	Normal
Other	Pneumothorax, consolidation, air bronchogram	Generally bilateral

Key Point: TUS may help elucidate the etiology of the pleural effusion, given that exudates and transudates have different ultrasonographic findings.

Rationale: Effusions can be divided into anechoic, complex non-septated, and complex septated. Anechoic effusions are echo-free, complex non-septated have echogenic material inside the effusion and complex septated have floating fibrin strands or septa inside the effusion. Transudates are usually anechoic, Exudates have septations or internal echogenicity and are associated with pleural thickness (>3 mm) and lung changes. Furthermore, homogenously echogenic effusions are typical of hemothorax or empyema [17, 18] (Table 21.1).

Question 14

After transthoracic ultrasound evaluation, the pleural fluid is deemed to be an exudate and a thoracentesis is planned. Regarding this procedure the following statement is true:

A. Real time US guidance has less complications than post marking technique.
B. Aspiration of pleural fluid is not an aseptic technique.
C. The thoracentesis needle is inserted into the intercostal space at the superior margin of the inferior rib so as not to damage the neurovascular bundle.
D. In order to prevent re-expansion pulmonary edema (RPE), no more than 2.5 L should be aspirated.

Answer: C.

Key point: Real time US is not superior to postmarking technique for thoracocentesis.

Rationale: When possible, patients getting thoracentesis should be placed in an upright sitting position with arms elevated or in a supine position with an arm behind the head. In this position, effusion gravitates down to the lower part of the chest, leading to an increased safety margin (depth of pleural effusion). The correct placement of the needle is visualized in real-time and is continuously monitored. Direct needle guidance is technically more challenging and did not seem to be a safer procedure than the site marking technique. Pleural aspiration should be a full aseptic technique using a small-bore needle, a syringe, and a tubing system. A needle is inserted into the intercostal space at the inferior rib's superior margin, not to damage the neurovascular bundle. Aspiration should be terminated should the patient develop a cough or complain of chest discomfort. To prevent re-expansion pulmonary edema (RPE), no more than 1.5 L should be aspirated [17, 19].

Question 15

Which of the following is true, regarding the proper technique for thoracocentesis:

A. The needle is inserted along the superior edge of the rib to avoid vascular or neural damage.
B. The needle is inserted along the inferior edge of the rib to avoid vascular or neural damage.
C. Color doppler cannot be used to visualize the presence of vessels in the intercostal space.
D. Local infection surrounding the insertion site of the thoracentesis needle (e.g. cellulitis, herpes zoster) is not a contraindication for thoracocentesis.

Answer: A.

Key point: US use help to avoid vascular or neural puncture of the intercostal veins, arteries and nerves.

Rationale: The best puncture site is where the operator can visualize each anatomical structure (i.e., diaphragm, pleural, organs) and can measure the maximum distance between visceral and parietal pleural (increasing the safety margin). To minimize the risk of neurovascular bundle injury the needle must aim to the upper rib margin perpendicular to pleura, with the transducer to follow the needle trajectory under direct needle guidance. The needle must be advanced slowly under direct visualization. Aspiration of fluid with a syringe confirms the correct position using the site marking technique. For direct needle guidance, the correct position of the needle tip is visualized in real-time and constantly monitored [20].

Question 16

According to the following US image (Fig. 21.7), the best place for a thoracocentesis should be:

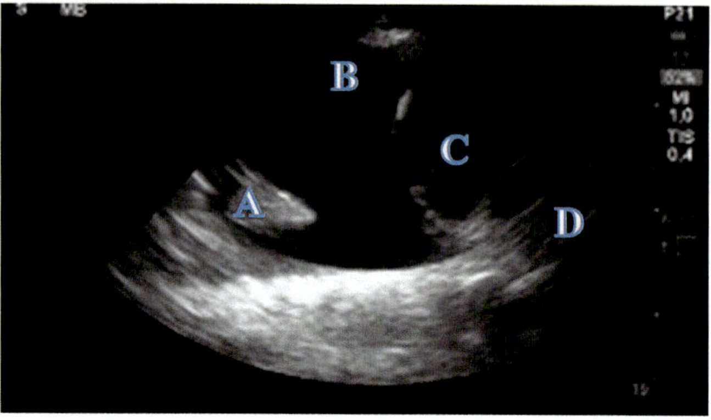

Fig. 21.7 Thoracic ultrasound using a curvilinear probe. Personal Archive

A. A
B. B
C. C
D. D

Answer: B.

Key point: The best puncture site is where the operator can visualize each anatomical structure and can measure the maximum distance between visceral and parietal pleural.

Rationale: Thoracocentesis be carried out in the safety triangle, almost always at the posterior axillary line if aiming for effusion [and performed under image guidance. The safety triangle is bordered by the lateral edge of the pectoralis major, the lateral edge of the latissimus dorsi and a line along the fifth intercostal space at the level of the nipple. The best puncture site is, in fact, the place where the operator can visualize each anatomical structure (i.e., diaphragm, pleural, and organs) and where the operator can measure the maximum distance between visceral and parietal pleural (increasing the safety margin). One of the most commonly used US methods for estimation of pleural effusion volume (V) V (mL) = 20 × Sep (mm) [17].

Question 17

A 45-year-old male, with a PMH of EtOH cirrhosis, presents with low grade fever, tachycardia, altered mental status, found to have increased INR, and AKI stage II. Patients is admitted to the ICU where he is intubated overnight. During morning rounds, he is found to have a distended abdomen, with caput medusa. A curvilinear probe is placed, showing a moderate amount of ascites. Which of the following is true regarding the use of US in paracentesis:

A. US guided paracentesis should only be attempted in the LLQ.
B. Mild coagulopathy or thrombocytopenia are contraindications for paracentesis.
C. Emptying the bladder, either by having the patient void or placing a Foley catheter, is indicated prior to paracentesis.
D. Patients with known or new onset ascites and clinical signs of SBP can get treated with antibiotics avoiding getting a paracentesis.

Answer: C.

Key point: Bedside US aids in the diagnosis and management of patients with both worsening ascites and SBP. Bedside US facilitates the rapid diagnosis and subsequent safe drainage of ascites, even when fluid pockets are small.

Rationale: The most common location for ascites is the suprapubic region, both in males and females. Following this, the site of the largest pockets of ascites can be individually identified in each patient. There is a correlation between the smallest fluid depth measurement ("SFD"—the distance from the most superficial bowel loop to the abdominal wall and the volume of drained paracentesis fluid (1 L for each 1 cm increase in the SFD). With the knowledge gained by bedside US, the procedure can then be more safely performed. The only absolute contraindications to paracentesis are: clinically evident fibrinolysis or disseminated intravascular coagulation. US-guided paracentesis does not generally need to be preceded by laboratory evaluation for coagulopathy or thrombocytopenia [21, 22].

Question 18

Which of the following statements regarding the US-guided technique for paracentesis is true?

A. A 10 MHz curvilinear or phased array probe is recommended for this initial assessment.
B. Ascites will typically appear dark (anechoic) on US examination.
C. The best location for placement of the paracentesis needle is generally where the abdominal wall is the thickest.
D. The Word Gastroenterology Organization states that at least 100 mL of fluid is necessary for diagnostic paracentesis.

Answer: B.

Key point: Prior to the paracentesis procedure, the US should be used to identify ascites and search for the largest fluid pockets. A 3 MHz curvilinear or phased array probe is recommended for this initial assessment. A determination is then made regarding the amount of ascites present and the likelihood that the fluid can be safely aspirated. The World Gastroenterology Organization states that at least 20 mL of fluid is necessary for diagnostic paracentesis. The best location for placement of the paracentesis needle is generally where the abdominal wall is thinnest. The paracolic gutter areas may be the sites with the least wall thickness, especially in patients with a high BMI [22, 23].

Question 19

Regarding the risks and benefits of the different techniques for US-guided paracentesis the following is true:

A. There is no difference in the incidence of complications between blind and US-guided paracentesis.
B. Most common complications of either technique include failed acquisition of ascites fluid, laceration of a vascular structure with hemorrhage into the peritoneal cavity and needle puncture of bowel or bladder.
C. Static technique allows for real time visualization of needle entrance in the peritoneal space.
D. The ascites "safety zone", is the ascites filled space that lies below the bowel.

Answer: B.

Key point: US guided paracentesis in real time is the preferred technique for paracentesis, it has been shown to be more effective especially in patients with a small amount of ascites.

Rationale: There are two general techniques for incorporating the US in the paracentesis procedure: h static and dynamic. The dynamic approach utilizes a sterile probe cover so that US may be used to guide and monitor needle insertion into the peritoneal space in real-time. Available evidence supports US use before the paracentesis procedure for site planning and the avoidance of procedural complications. These are most commonly defined as the failed acquisition of ascites fluid, laceration of a vascular structure with bleeding into the peritoneal cavity, and needle puncture of bowel or bladder. The risk of complications becomes even more critical in patients with smaller volumes of ascites. One can then determine the "ascites safety zone," or the fluid-filled region below the abdominal wall and above the bowel and mesentery, into which a needle can be safely placed [22, 24].

Question 20

There are several complications associated with paracentesis, such as vascular injury. Which of the following is true regarding the use of US for this procedure?

A. Vascular structures can first be identified using B-mode US, or grey scale imaging, by looking for the typical rounded appearance of artery and vein then color doppler US can be used to confirm the presence of vascular structures.
B. The curvilinear probe should be used to identify critical vascular structures within the abdominal wall.
C. Anatomical location of the inferior epigastric artery and vein is consistent between patients.
D. The hemorrhagic complication rate related to paracentesis in most available studies lies between 10% and 20%.

Answer: A.

Key point: A linear probe can be used to asses vasculature and avoid vascular puncture during the procedure to avoid hemorrhagic complications.

Rationale: The hemorrhagic complication rate related to paracentesis in most available studies lies between 1% and 2%. The high-frequency linear probe should be used to identify critical vascular structures within the abdominal wall. Therefore, accurate identification of abdominal wall vascular structures is essential to avoiding a hemorrhagic procedural complication. Vascular structures can first be identified using B-mode US, or greyscale imaging, by looking for the typical rounded appearance of artery and vein. Color Doppler US can then be used to confirm the presence of vascular structures [25, 26].

Question 21

Which of the following is true regarding US use for the assessment of ascites?

A. Simple ascites is identified by hyperechoic fluid on the US and is immobile to patient changes in position.
B. Hyperechoic fluid or multiple septum are usually encountered in complex ascites.
C. Tuberculosis, pseudomyxoma, or hemorrhage can be visualized as simple ascites.
D. Most cases of complex ascites have <250/uL PMN.

Answer: B.

Key point: Visual characteristic of the peritoneal fluid on the US can help differentiate between simple and a complex ascites.

Rationale: Simple ascites is characterized by anechoic fluid, filling the space between organs and bowel without mass effect. Fluid is mobile with patient's position change and compresses with transducer pressure. Complex ascites is recognized by internal echoes and multiple septa, with loculated pockets of fluid [27, 28] (Table 21.2).

Table 21.2 Causes of ascites. Adapted from Huang L, Xia H, Zhu S. Ascitic Fluid Analysis in the Differential Diagnosis of Ascites: Focus on Cirrhotic Ascites. Journal of clinical and translational hepatology. 2014

	Cirrhosis	CHF	Malignancy	SBP
Appearance	Clear straw	Clear, pale yellow	Milky or bloody	Cloudy or turbid
TP	<25 g/L	<25 g/L	>25 g/L	>25 g/L
SAAG	>1.1 g/dL	>1.1 g/dL	<1.1 g/dL	<1.1 g/dL
LDH	nl	nl	↑	↑
Glucose	nl	nl	↓	↓
Cell counts	nl	nl	Varies	>250/uL or nL

Question 22

The following condition is not an absolute contraindication for paracentesis:

A. Refusal by a competent and informed patient.
B. Active infection over the site of needle insertion.
C. Acute abdomen requiring surgical intervention.
D. Coagulation disorders.

Answer: D.

Key point: Coagulation disorders are relative contraindications for paracentesis.

Rationale: Although many patients undergoing paracentesis have baseline coagulopathy or thrombocytopenia, the use of fresh-frozen plasma or platelet concentrates is not recommended before paracentesis. The costs and risks associated with such transfusion probably exceed any benefit. Bleeding complications secondary to paracentesis are rare and, when present, are usually mild and self-limited. In one case series, the rate of severe bleeding was 0.19%, with a death rate of 0.016%. Of note, bleeding complications were not associated with coagulopathy or thrombocytopenia [29].

Question 23

A 45-year-old male with a history of asthma and type 1 DM, is admitted to the ICU in the setting of COVID-19 pneumonia. He tolerated HFNC for a couple hours, but since he is deteriorating quicky the decision to intubate him is made. Using a linear probe to perform a neck ultrasound the following image is obtained (Fig. 21.8). Which are the correctly labeled structures.

A. A – Right IJV, B – Airway
B. B – Esophagus, D – Carotid
C. A – Carotid, C – Esophagus
D. C – Esophagus, B – Airway

Answer: B.

Key point: US can be helpful identifying the different structures in the neck, vessels, muscles, cartilages, esophagus and airway.

Rationale: Usage of upper airway ultrasound is useful in dealing with critically ill patients especially in airway management because of its portability, non-invasiveness, cost effectiveness, and reproducibility [30]. Use of US for airway include:

- Assessment of airway anatomy for difficult intubation,
- ETT and LMA placement and depth, a
- Assessment of airway size,
- Ultrasound-guided invasive procedures such as percutaneous needle cricothyroidotomy and tracheostomy,
- Prediction of post extubation stridor
- Left double-lumen bronchial tube size, and detecting upper airway pathologies

Question 24

After intubation the following US image is obtained (Fig. 21.9), you would expect the following:

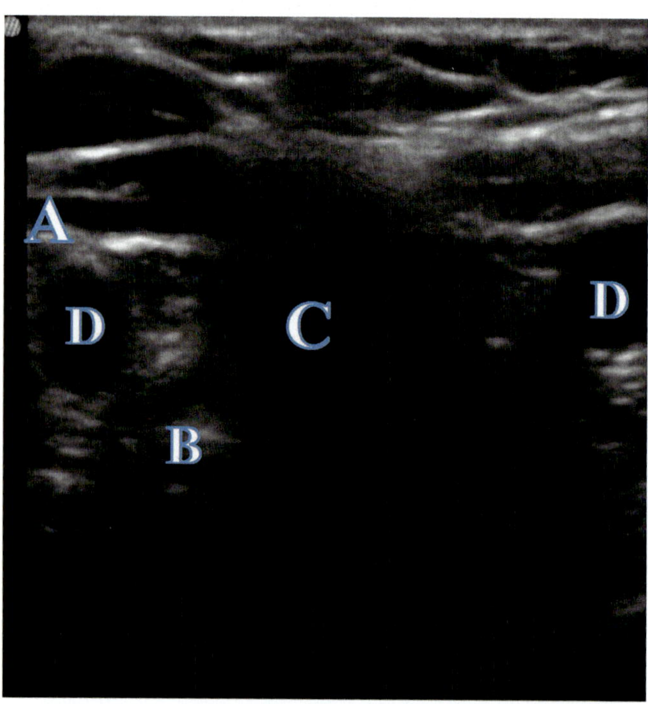

Fig. 21.8 Sonographic evaluation of the neck using a linear probe. Image courtesy of Yannis Amador MD

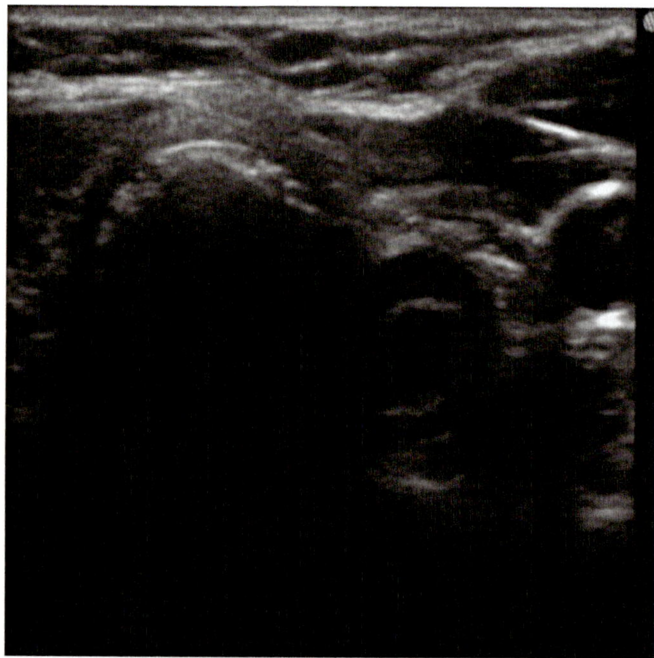

Fig. 21.9 Sonographic evaluation of intubation with real-time ultrasonography. Image courtesy of Yannis Amador MD

A. Absent capnography with no lung sounds
B. ETCO >30 mmHg with normal capnography waveform
C. High pressures with increased airway resistance
D. ETCO <30 mmHg with a normal capnography waveform

Answer: A.

Key Point: US can be used to identify endotracheal and esophageal intubation.

Rationale: Ultrasound is a reliable tool for assessment of the subglottic airway. Upper airway ultrasonography can also be advantageous in situations involving cardiovascular arrest, bronchoconstriction or circumstances in which capnography or end-tidal carbon dioxide measurement (ETCO2) may be faulty. ETT position in trachea is seen as two hyperechoic lines which is described as "double tract" or "double lumen" sign [31].

Question 25

After the tube is advanced into the trachea, the stylet is removed, and the balloon is inflated. After a couple minutes patient oxygen saturation drops to the low 90 s, with high peak pressures noted on the ventilator screen. The following images are obtained (Fig. 21.10), which would be the most probable diagnosis.

A. Massive Hemothorax
B. Pleural Effusion
C. Esophageal intubation
D. Right mainstem bronchial intubation.

Answer: D.

Key point: Absence of lung sliding can be seen in several conditions, following intubation, with concomitantly high peak pressures make a right mainstem intubation the most likely diagnosis.

Rationale: Most cases occur in the right mainstem bronchus, but about 5% may occur in the left mainstem bronchus. If chest radiography is delayed or unavailable, suboptimal ventilation and oxygenation in these patients may occur if the endotracheal tube (ETT) position is not promptly determined. The two most common approaches are to scan the anterior neck to determine the position of the tube and the balloon in the trachea. The second approach is observing "lung sliding" which is the result of the movement of the pleural lining against each other when lung expansion occurs. Bilateral lung sliding confirms tracheal intubation, whereas lack of sliding on either side may indicate contralateral endobronchial intubation. This can also be accomplished by documenting diaphragmatic excursion on sonography [31, 32].

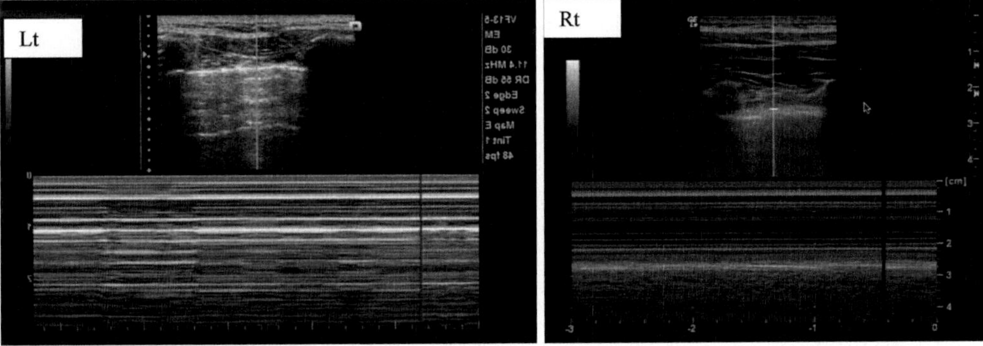

Fig. 21.10 M-mode of left and right hemithoraces. Image courtesy of Yannis Amador MD

Question 26

During neck US the following image is obtained (Fig. 21.11), the correct place for a cricothyroidotomy is:

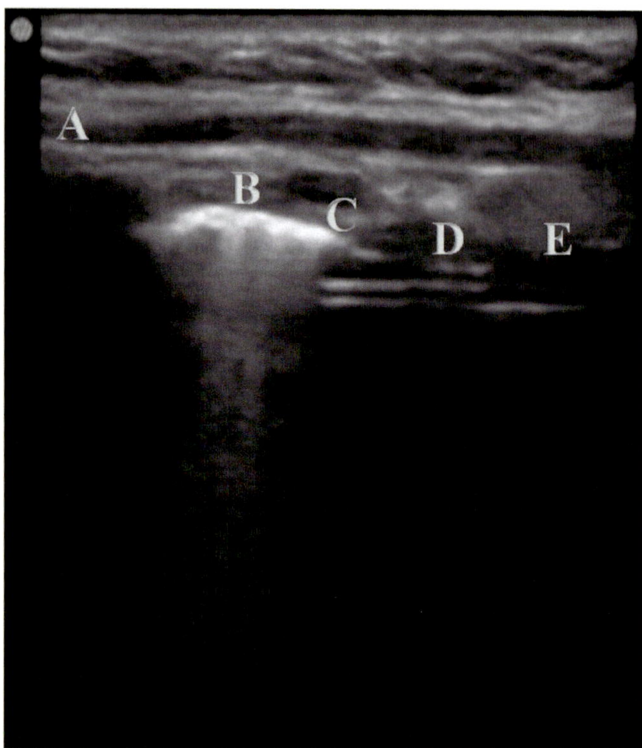

Fig. 21.11 Longitudinal view of a ultrasonographic evaluation of the neck using a linear probe. Image courtesy of Yannis Amador MD

A. A
B. B
C. C
D. D
E. E

Answer: B.

Key point: the cricothyroid membrane appears as a white line with echo lines deep to it which corresponds to reverberation artefacts.

Rationale: The inability to identify the cricothyroid membrane by inspection and palpation contributes substantially to cricothyrotomy's high failure rate. Before initiating airway management, the potential ease or difficulty of performing cricothyrotomy and tracheostomy should be evaluated, and an attempt should be made to identify the cricothyroid membrane. The cricothyroid membrane can be identified as a whiite line with white echo reverberation s below, located between the thyroid and cricoid cartilage. Also seen in the image below are the tracheal rings and the ETT tube in the trachea [31] (Fig. 21.12).

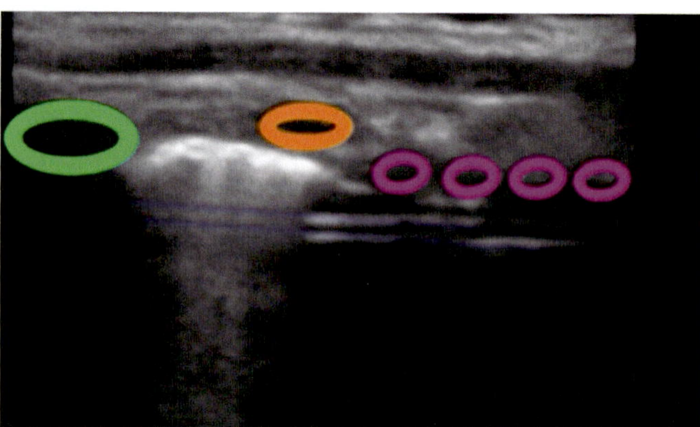

Fig. 21.12 Longitudinal view of a ultrasonographic evaluation of the neck using a linear probe Acoustic window is visualized under the cricothyroid membrane, between the thyroid and cricoid cartilages. Image courtesy of Yannis Amador MD

Question 27

After an intubation attempt utilizing a high definition linear probe the following image is obtained (Fig. 21.13). Given the findings shown in this image the following is expected:

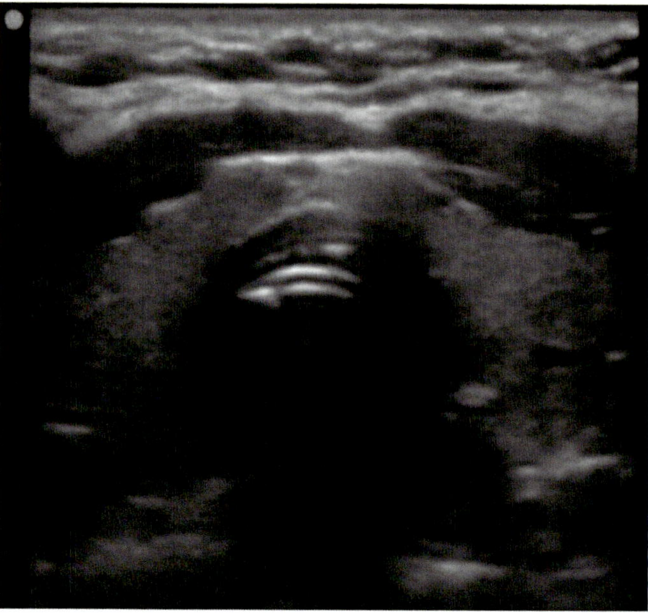

Fig. 21.13 Real time imaging of intubation using a linear probe positioned in the anterior neck. Short-axis view. Image courtesy of Yannis Amador MD

A. No breath sounds on physical exam
B. Absence of ETCO2
C. Substantial air leak as measured by the ventilator
D. Normal capnography waveform

Answer: D.

Key point: ETT tube in the trachea can be recognized by the double contour sign.

Rationale: The likely reason that airway US has gained attention is the ease at which images can be obtained. Airway US for ETT confirmation is best used when the end-tidal CO2 monitor is not accurate, radiology is unavailable, the patient arrives intubated and requires airway confirmation, or the patient does not respond as expected after intubation [31].

Question 28

A 35 y/o patient with a history of Multiple Sclerosis and Migraine, is admitted with severe ARDS to the ICU, he remains severely hypoxic after protective lung mechanical ventilation is stablished, and a trial of prone positioning and inhaled prostaglandin was attempted. A follow up echo also shows severe myocarditis with profound LV dysfunction. The decision is made to place this patient on VA-ECMO. A TTE is attempted obtaining the following image. Regarding the following US image (Fig. 21.14), the following is true:

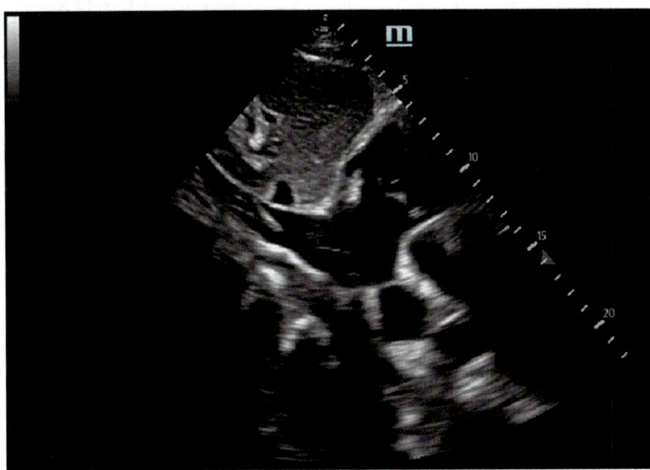

Fig. 21.14 Subcostal view using a phase array probe. Personal Archive

A. Structure corresponds to SVC and return cannula and should be pulled back.
B. Structure corresponds to IVC and venous drain cannula and is well positioned.
C. Structure corresponds to IVC and venous drain cannula and should be advanced 5 cm.
D. Structure corresponds to IVC and venous drain cannula and should be pulled back 5 cm.

Answer: B.

Key point: Transthoracic echocardiography may allow appropriate visualization of ECMO cannula.

Rationale: For venovenous ECMO, the femoral drainage cannula should be in the right atrium just beyond the cavoatrial junction. Owing to its shorter length, the jugular return cannula tip is positioned within the superior vena cava, near its right atrial junction. Sufficient distance between cannula usually prevents occurrence of recirculation, which worsens patient's oxygenation, as reinjected blood is immediately suctioned by the drainage cannula. Turbulent flow entering the drainage cannula suggests recirculation, in which case cannula repositioning may improve oxygenation [33, 34].

Question 29

In this same patient, given the severe LV dysfunction a decision is made to place an IMPELLA 5.0 in the operating room. Back in the ICU, the patient's vasopressor requirements start escalating, a bedside TTE is performed obtaining the following image (Fig. 21.15). According to the image the following decision needs to be made:

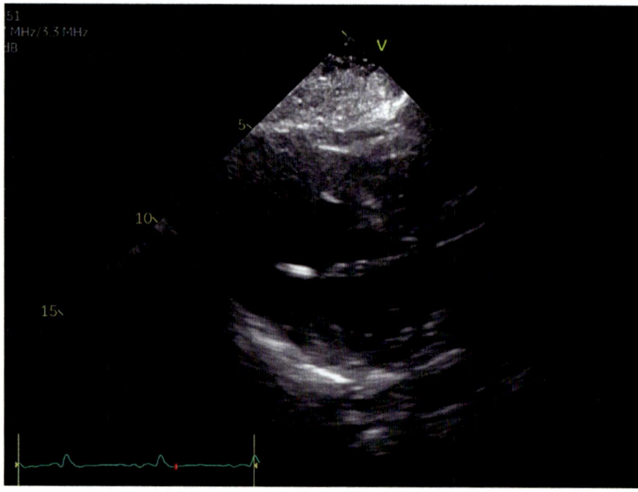

Fig. 21.15 Focused TTE. Parasternal long-axis view. Personal Archive

A. Replace Impella cannula
B. Evacuate LV thrombus
C. Pull back 5 cm the Impella cannula
D. Cannula is well placed, look for other causes

Answer: D.

Key point: Ideally US should be performed before MCS start to verify there are no contraindications, every time the catheter is repositioned, and periodically to assess for myocardial recovery.

Rationale: There are several indications for echocardiography for Impella LVAD support [35, 36] (Table 21.3).

Question 30

All of the following US findings may provide evidence that the patient is ready to be weaned from VA ECMO except:

A. LVOT VTI >12.5
B. Tissue velocity imaging (**TVI**) E/e' < 12
C. RV dilation
D. No interventricular dependence.
E. LVEF ≥ 20–25%

Answer: C.

Key point: US can be used for management of patients on VA ECMO undergoing weaning.

Rationale: For a successful VA ECMO weaning strategy, the etiology of cardiac failure must be compatible with myocardial recovery. Patient should be hemodynamically stable: Any significant metabolic disturbances must be resolved and a pulsatile arterial waveform existent for at least 24 hours. Ideally, MAP >60 mmHg in the absence of, or with low doses of catecholamines. Pulmonary function should not be severely impaired. If PaO2/FiO2 < 100 mmHg with ECMO oxygenator set at 21%, bridging the patient from VA- to VV-ECMO may be considered. The patient must tolerate a full weaning trial where the ECMO flow is gradually decreased to 66% and 33% of its baseline value and then to a minimum of 1–1.5 L/min. Doppler-echocardiographic assessment should ideally demonstrate a LVEF of ≥20–25%, an aortic VTI of ≥12 cm, and a TDSa ≥6 cm/s [37].

Table 21.3 Indications for the echocardiographic evaluation in patients receiving circulatory mechanical support. Adapted from Catena E, Milazzo F, Merli M, Paino R, Garatti A, Colombo T, et al. Echocardiographic evaluation of patients receiving a new left ventricular assist device: the Impella ® recover 100. Eur J Echocardiogr. 2004 Dec 1;5(6):430–7

Before implantation	During implantation	After implantation
• Exclude anatomic contraindications • Large atheroma in the ascending aorta • Aneurysm in the ascending aorta • Stenosis or regurgitation of aortic valve • Fibromuscular narrowing of left ventricular outflow tract • Myxomatous mitral valve • PFO or interatrial defect • Evaluate right and left ventricular function • Determinate the degree of mitral and tricuspid regurgitation • Optimize left ventricular filling	• Verify the appropriate direction of the cannula • Verify the appropriate position of the inlet of the cannula • Verify the appropriate position of the outlet of the pump • Exclude right to left atrial shunting • Optimize right and left ventricular filling	• Assess the patency of the cannula • Verify the appropriate position of the cannula • Monitorize loading and function of right and left ventricles • Monitorize mitral regurgitation

References

1. Brass P, Hellmich M, Kolodziej L, Schick G, Smith AF. Ultrasound guidance versus anatomical landmarks for internal jugular vein catheterization. Cochrane Database Syst Rev. 2015;1:CD006962.
2. Saugel B, Scheeren TWL, Teboul J-L. Ultrasound-guided central venous catheter placement: a structured review and recommendations for clinical practice. Crit Care. 2017;21(1):225.
3. Leibowitz A, Oren-Grinberg A, Matyal R. Ultrasound guidance for central venous access: current evidence and clinical recommendations. J Intensive Care Med. 2020;35(3):303–21. https://doi.org/10.1177/0885066619868164. Epub 2019 Aug 6
4. McGee DC, Gould MK. Preventing complications of central venous catheterization. N Engl J Med. 2003;348(12):1123–33.
5. Troianos CA, Hartman GS, Glas KE, Skubas NJ, Eberhardt RT, Walker JD, et al. Guidelines for performing ultrasound guided vascular cannulation: recommendations of the American Society of Echocardiography and the Society of Cardiovascular Anesthesiologists. J Am Soc Echocardiogr. 2011;24(12):1291–318.
6. Yardim H, Erkoc R, Soyoral YU, Begenik H, Avcu S. Assessment of internal jugular vein thrombosis due to central venous catheter in Hemodialysis patients: a retrospective and prospective serial evaluation with ultrasonography. Clin Appl Thromb Hemost [Internet]. 2012;18(6):662–5.
7. Kornbau C, Lee KC, Hughes GD, Firstenberg MS. Central line complications. Int J Crit Illn Inj Sci. 2015;5(3):170–8.
8. Castro D, Martin Lee LM, Bhutta BS. Femoral vein central venous access. In: StatPearls [Internet]. Treasure Island (FL): StatPearls Publishing; 2020 [cited 2020 Nov 3]. Available from: http://www.ncbi.nlm.nih.gov/books/NBK459255/
9. Brass P, Hellmich M, Kolodziej L, Schick G, Smith AF. How do ultrasound guidance and anatomical landmarks compare for subclavian or femoral vein catheterization? Cochrane Database Syst Rev. 2015;1:CD011447.
10. Fragou M, Gravvanis A, Dimitriou V, et al. Real-time ultrasound-guided subclavian vein cannulation versus the landmark method in critical care patients: a prospective randomized study. Crit Care Med. 2011;39(7):1607–12.
11. Lanspa MJ, Fair J, Hirshberg EL, Grissom CK, Brown SM. Ultrasound-guided subclavian vein cannulation using a micro-convex ultrasound probe. Ann Am Thorac Soc. 2014;11(4):583–6. https://doi.org/10.1513/AnnalsATS.201311-414BC. PMID: 24611628; PMCID: PMC4225800
12. Scheer BV, Perel A, Pfeiffer UJ. Clinical review: complications and risk factors of peripheral arterial catheters used for hemodynamic monitoring in anesthesia and intensive care medicine. Crit Care. 2002;6(3):199–204.
13. Miller AG, Bardin AJ. Review of ultrasound-guided radial artery catheter placement. Respir Care. 2016;61(3):383–8.
14. Htet N, Vaughn J, Adigopula S, Hennessey E, Mihm F. Needle-guided ultrasound technique for axillary artery catheter placement in critically ill patients: a case series and technique description. J Crit Care. 2017;41:194–7.
15. Patel M, Varacallo M. Anatomy, shoulder and upper limb, arm nerves. In: StatPearls [Internet]. Treasure Island (FL): StatPearls Publishing; 2020 [cited 2020 Nov 3]. Available from: http://www.ncbi.nlm.nih.gov/books/NBK547735/
16. Volpicelli G, Elbarbary M, Blaivas M, Lichtenstein DA, Mathis G, Kirkpatrick AW, et al. International evidence-based recommendations for point-of-care lung ultrasound. Intensive Care Med. 2012;38(4):577–91.
17. Brogi E, Gargani L, Bignami E, Barbariol F, Marra A, Forfori F, et al. Thoracic ultrasound for pleural effusion in the intensive care unit: a narrative review from diagnosis to treatment. Crit Care. 2017;21(1):325.
18. Yang PC, Luh KT, Chang DB, Wu HD, Yu CJ, Kuo SH. Value of sonography in determining the nature of pleural effusion: analysis of 320 cases. AJR Am J Roentgenol. 1992;159(1):29–33.
19. Mayo PH, Goltz HR, Tafreshi M, Doelken P. Safety of ultrasound-guided thoracentesis in patients receiving mechanical ventilation. Chest. 2004;125(3):1059–62.
20. Vetrugno L, Guadagnin GM, Orso D, Boero E, Bignami E, Bove T. An easier and safe affair, pleural drainage with ultrasound in critical patient: a technical note. Crit Ultrasound J. 2018;10(1):18.
21. McVay PA, Toy PT. Lack of increased bleeding after paracentesis and thoracentesis in patients with mild coagulation abnormalities. Transfusion. 1991;31(2):164–71.
22. Ennis J, Schultz G, Perera P, Williams S, Gharahbaghian L, Mandavia D. Ultrasound for detection of ascites and for guidance of the paracentesis procedure: technique and review of the literature. IJCM. 2014;05(20):1277–93.
23. Tirado A, Wu T, Noble VE, Huang C, Lewiss RE, Martin JA, et al. Ultrasound-guided procedures in the emergency department-diagnostic and therapeutic asset. Emerg Med Clin North Am. 2013;31(1):117–49.
24. Nazeer SR, Dewbre H, Miller AH. Ultrasound-assisted paracentesis performed by emergency physicians vs the traditional technique: a prospective, randomized study. Am J Emerg Med. 2005;23(3):363–7.
25. Sharzehi K, Jain V, Naveed A, Schreibman I. Hemorrhagic complications of paracentesis: a systematic review of the literature. Gastroenterol Res Pract [Internet]. 2014 [cited 2020 Oct 22];2014. Available from: https://www.ncbi.nlm.nih.gov/pmc/articles/PMC4280650/
26. Gharahbaghian L, Williams S, Perera P, Ennis J, Schultz G, Mandavia D. Ultrasound for detection of ascites and for guidance of the paracentesis procedure: technique and review of the literature. Int J Clin Med. 2014;5(20):720–6.
27. Sahani DV, Samir AE. Abdominal imaging E-book: expert radiology series. Philadelphia, PA: Elsevier Health Sciences; 2010.
28. Huang L, Xia H, Zhu S. Ascitic fluid analysis in the differential diagnosis of ascites: focus on cirrhotic ascites. J Clin Transl Hepatol. 2014;2(1):58–64.
29. Barr L. Basic ultrasound-guided procedures. Crit Care Clin. 2014;30(2):275–304.
30. Osman A, Sum KM. Role of upper airway ultrasound in airway management. J Intensive Care. 2016;4(1):52.
31. You-Ten KE, Siddiqui N, Teoh WH, Kristensen MS. Point-of-care ultrasound (POCUS) of the upper airway. Can J Anesth/J Can Anesth. 2018;65(4):473–84.
32. Blaivas M, Tsung JW. Point-of-care sonographic detection of left endobronchial main stem intubation and obstruction versus endotracheal intubation. J Ultrasound Med. 2008;27(5):785–9.
33. Douflé G, Roscoe A, Billia F, Fan E. Echocardiography for adult patients supported with extracorporeal membrane oxygenation. Crit Care. 2015;19(1):326.
34. Viau-Lapointe J, Douflé G. Transthoracic view of extracorporeal membrane oxygenation cannulae. Am J Respir Crit Care Med. 2018;199(10):e39–40.
35. Anderson BB, Collard CD. Images in anesthesiology: proper positioning of an Impella 2.5 and CP heart pump. Anesthesiology. 2017;127(6):1014.
36. Catena E, Milazzo F, Merli M, Paino R, Garatti A, Colombo T, et al. Echocardiographic evaluation of patients receiving a new left ventricular assist device: the Impella ® recover 100. Eur J Echocardiogr. 2004;5(6):430–7.
37. Bailleul C, Aissaoui N. Role of echocardiography in the management of veno-arterial extra-corporeal membrane oxygenation patients. J Emerg Crit Care Med. 2019;3:25.

States of Shock

22

Orlando Garner, Ali Omranian, Purvesh R. Patel, and Pralay K. Sarkar

Abbreviations

AP4C	Apical 4 chamber
IVC	Inferior Vena Cave
PLAPS	Posterolateral alveolar and/or pleural syndrome
PLAX	Parasternal long access
POCUS	Point of care ultrasound
PSAX	Parasternal short access
PW	Pulse wave doppler
SC4C	Subcostal 4 chambers
TAPSE	Tricuspid annular plane systolic excursion
TTC	Takotsubo cardiomyopathy
TV	Tidal volume
VTI	Velocity time interval

Question 1

A 35-year-old woman, 32-weeks pregnant, presented to the emergency department complaining of shortness of breath that began 1 week ago. She felt lightheaded on the day of presentation and decided to come to the emergency room. Her antenatal period had been uneventful. Vital signs disclosed pulse of 120 bpm, blood pressure of 75/48 mmHg, respiratory rate of 35 per minute, temperature of 98 F and an oxygen saturation of 87% on room air. She appeared to be in moderate respiratory distress and fatigued. Chest auscultation revealed a flow murmur in left upper sternal border and clear breath sounds bilaterally. Gravid uterus was palpated without any tenderness. A chest x-ray was normal. Point-of-care ultrasound was performed, and the following images are obtained.

Videos 22.1, 22.2 and 22.3.

What is the best next step in her management?

A. Bolus crystalloids at 30 ml/kg of actual body weight
B. Initiate norepinephrine for a target mean arterial pressure greater than 65 mmHg
C. Infuse tissue plasminogen activator (t-PA)
D. To obtain CT Pulmonary angiogram

Answer: C. Infuse tissue plasminogen activator (t-PA)

Rationale: Hyperdynamic LV function associated with a "D" septum on parasternal short-axis (PSAX, Video 22.2), dilated RV in apical 4-chamber (A4C, Video 22.3) and PSAX accompanied by a thin RV wall, usually <5 mm thick, suggests acute right ventricular pressure overload. In acute massive PE, McConnell's sign can be seen; it is characterized by apical RV contraction with midchamber wall akinesia, consistent with acute RV pressure overload. Left common femoral vein showed an occlusive thrombus (Video 22.1). Clear CXR and normally aerated lung on point-of-care ultrasound support diagnosis of PE. Systemic thrombolysis is recommended in patients with acute massive pulmonary embolism with Shock without bleeding risk, including pregnant patients. CT PA confirmation is not needed for thrombolysis.

In a critically ill patient without an alternative diagnosis, demonstration of RV strain and presence of DVT provide sufficient clinical ground for thrombolysis without additional delay for CT confirmation (Choice C). Attempt for CT confirmation leads to delay along with risk of transporting a hypotensive patient (choice D is wrong).

Supplementary Information The online version contains supplementary material available at https://doi.org/10.1007/978-3-031-45731-9_22.

O. Garner · A. Omranian · P. R. Patel
Division of Pulmonary and Critical Care Medicine, Baylor College of Medicine, Houston, TX, USA
e-mail: ali.omranian@bcm.edu; purvesh.patel@bcm.edu

P. K. Sarkar (✉)
Division of Pulmonary and Critical Care Medicine, Baylor College of Medicine, Houston, TX, USA

Division of Pulmonary, Critical Care and Sleep Medicine, Department of Medicine, Baylor College of Medicine,, Houston, TX, USA
e-mail: pralay.sarkar@bcm.edu

R. Sreedharan et al. (eds.), *Critical Care Echocardiography*, https://doi.org/10.1007/978-3-031-45731-9_22

In acute right ventricular failure, inappropriate volume resuscitation can cause further rapid deterioration (Choice A). While norepinephrine can be started as a temporizing measure to obtain a target central blood pressure while thrombolysis is being initiated or in progress (choice B), thrombolysis is the best next management step.

Question 2 and 3

A 89-year-old female with dementia, hypertension and CKD presented from nursing home to the emergency room with acute onset dyspnea and wheezing over 2 h. At triage patient's temperature was 99.2 °F, blood pressure was 110/80, pulse rate was 124/min, respiration rate was 26/min, saturation was 97% on 4 L/min nasal cannula, GCS was 15. On examination, patient was in mild respiratory distress with few bilateral expiratory wheezing. Transthoracic echocardiogram from 6 month back showed normal LV function with ejection fraction of 55%, normal RV size and function, bioprosthetic AVR with normal function, mild to moderate TR with RVSP of 25 mmHg. Abnormal laboratory findings shows WBC count of 12.9, mildly elevated troponin at 0.68 and positive urinalysis with WBC count of 147/HPF with moderate leucocyte esterase and negative nitrates.

Lung ultrasound showed bilateral A-line pattern.

Bedside echocardiogram was performed and representative images Videos 22.4 and 22.5

Question 2: What is the next best step in the management of this patient?

A. IV fluid resuscitation with goal of 30 cc/kg of crystalloids.
B. Broad-spectrum IV antibiotics for suspected sepsis.
C. Bedside DVT study.
D. IV furosemide 80 mg.

Answer: C. Bedside DVT study.

Rationale: Video 22.4 is a parasternal short axis view that shows normal left ventricular function. Right ventricle is dilated and there is 2D echo evidence of RV volume overload. Additionally, apical four chamber view (Video 22.5) shows reduced contractility of right ventricular free wall with preserved contraction of right ventricular apical part (McConnel's Sign).

Therefore, there is high concern for acute pulmonary embolism as the cause of cor-pulmonale. Searching for DVT will be the most reasonable action at bedside (choice C). Volume resuscitation will be inappropriate in presence of RV strain (Choice A is wrong).

While a diagnosis of UTI can be suspected based on the urinalysis, it does not explain the hypoxemia in presence of normal lung ultrasound. Septic shock is less likely in this patient and immediate broad spectrum antibiotics (choice B) is not the most relevant next step.

Question 3: What is the best treatment option for this patient?

A. To administer 100 mg IV tissue plasminogen activator.
B. To administer reduced dose (50 mg) IV tissue plasminogen activator.
C. To perform ultrasound assisted catheter directed thrombolysis (EKOS).
D. To start intravenous unfractionated heparin therapy.

Answer: D. To start intravenous unfractionated heparin therapy

Rationale: The clinical and echocardiographic picture is consistent with a diagnosis of submassive pulmonary embolism. She is hemodynamically stable and maintaining acceptable oxygenation. Therefore, an immediate thrombolysis is not indicated. Similarly, catherter directed thromolysis is not standard of care in submassive pulmonary embolism and should be decided only on case by case basis. Systemic anticoagulation will be the most appropriate next treatment step.

Question 4

A 76-year-old-male was admitted to Medical ICU with a clinical picture of aspiration pneumonia, respiratory failure requiring mechanical ventilation, and septic shock. His significant other medical history included hypertension, diabetes mellitus and a prior stroke with residual right hemiparesis. He was slowly improving until day 10 of MICU stay, when he became hemodynamically unstable: developed atrial fibrillation with rapid ventricular response. Though the heart rate was controlled with Amiodarone infusion, he continued to have hypotension requiring escalating vasopressor support to maintain an acceptable mean arterial blood pressure. A day prior to these clinical developments, he underwent debridement of a right foot wound and gastrostomy tube placement. While the procedure was uneventful, he has bleeding from the gastrostomy site with a drop in hemoglobin.

On physical examination, vital signs disclosed heart rate of 90 bpm, blood pressure of 80/45 mm Hg, temperature 98 F. Chest auscultation disclosed normal S1 and S2; a superimposed S3 was appreciated. Diffuse crackles were heard bilaterally on lung auscultation. Site of gastrostomy tube looked clean. There was no tenderness to abdominal palpation. Laboratory parameters were notable for Hemoglobin of 6.7 gm/dL (8.1 gm/dL prior to surgery);

serum lactic acid of 4 mmoL/L (normal 0.5–2.2 mmoL/L); serum Troponin I of 0.28 ng/mL (normal <0.04 ng/mL).

Ultrasound examination was performed for evaluation of shock:

Videos 22.6 and 22.7.

Question 4: What is the most likely cause of shock in this patient?

A. Septic shock
B. Hypovolemic shock
C. Cardiogenic shock
D. Obstructive shock

Answer: C. Cardiogenic shock

Rationale: This elderly patient developed shock after several days in ICU. Given the clinical context, there were several potential causes of shock in this patient. He was being treated for sepsis and showed improvement; therefore, worsening sepsis and septic shock was considered less likely (Choice A). Given the bleeding from gastrostomy site and ~ 2 gm/dL drop in hemoglobin, significant internal bleeding and hypovolemic shock could be considered; however, a IVC diameter of >2 cm argued against hypovolemia as the cause of shock (choice B). Echocardiography also showed hypokinesis involving inferior and lateral walls of left ventricle. Elevated troponin level and new regional wall motion abnormality established diagnosis of acute myocardial infarction in this patient with multiple risk factors for coronary artery disease. Presence of spontaneous echo contrast in IVC suggested a low flow status in the current clinical context, also consistent with a diagnosis of cardiogenic shock (choice C).

Question 5 and 6

Clinical stem:

A 26-year-old previously healthy male has been unwell for 3 days with fever, body ache and runny nose. He presented to emergency room with 1-day history of dyspnea. On initial evaluation, his room air saturation was found to be 86% and CXR showed bilateral diffuse alveolar infiltrates. Rapid test for Influenza A was positive. He was intubated and placed on mechanical ventilation. Following intubation, he developed hypotension and received 2 L fluid bolus. Following transfer to medical ICU, he continued to be hypotensive and vasopressors were added. He continued to be mechanically ventilated, deeply sedated with propofol infusion and paralyzed with cisatracturium infusion. He developed refractory hypoxemia with oxygen saturation of 85% despite being on 100% FiO2 on the ventilator, with PEEP of 14 cm H2O. At the time of this evaluation, vital signs were heart rate of 130/min, blood pressure 90/45 mmHg and SaO2 of 89%. Ventilator settings were as follow: tidal volume set at 5 ml/kg of ideal body weight, respiratory rate of 24/min, PEEP 14 and FiO2 of 100%, with a plateau pressure of 32 cm of H20. Physical examination revealed an acutely ill young male with bilateral diffuse crackles and decreased heart sounds on auscultation; abdomen was soft with positive bowel sounds. POCUS was performed for comprehensive assessment of refractory hypoxemia and shock.

Video 22.8.

Image 22.1.

Question 5: What is the most likely cause of shock in this patient?

A. Septic shock
B. Obstructive shock
C. Hypovolemic shock
D. Cardiogenic shock

Answer: B. Obstructive shock

Rationale: Acute Cor pulmonale or acute right heart failure can result from increased resistance in the pulmonary circulation or direct injury to myocardium. Increased acute

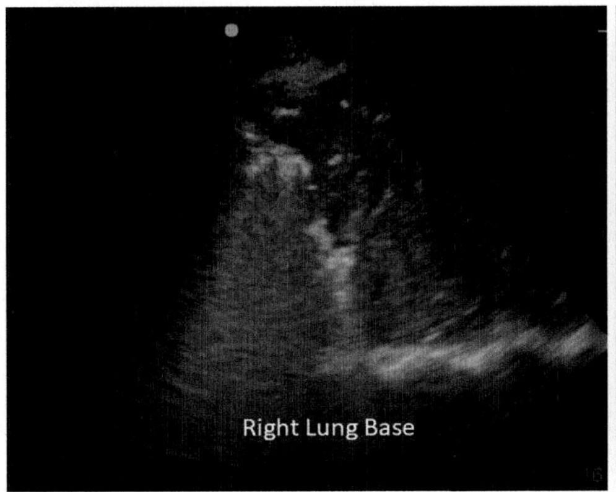

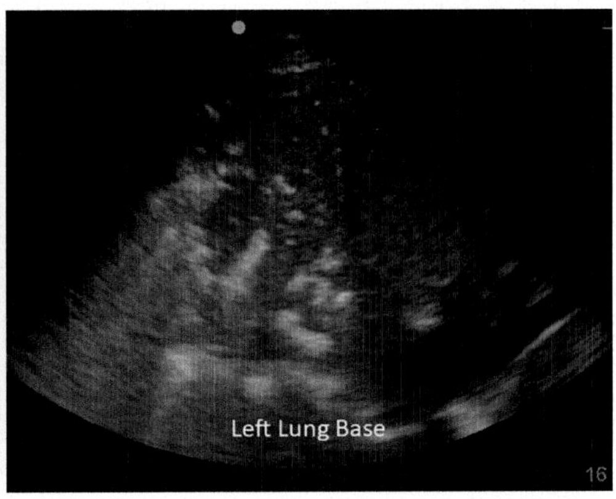

Image 22.1 Lung ultrasound right basal region

pulmonary circulation resistance can be caused by ARDS, profound hypoxia or high pressures on mechanical ventilation which can result in subsequent hemodynamic instability. Parasternal short axis view shows dilated right ventricle with septal flattening, suggesting RV pressure overload. In the given clinical circumstances, these findings will suggest acute cor pulmonale. Therefore, the shock is likely to be obstructive in nature (Choice B).

Question 6: What is the next best step in the management of hypotension in this patient?

A. To increase vasopressor dose
B. To increase PEEP
C. To administer additional volume
D. To place the patient in prone position

Answer: D. To place the patient in prone position

Rationale: This patient has acute cor pulmonale. Therefore, additional volume resuscitation, vasopressors are unlikely to improve right ventricular function and improve shock. The patient also has refractory hypoxemia and lung ultrasound shows dense basal areas of consolidation, contributing to shunt physiology and hypoxemia. Given the hemodynamic instability, further increase in PEEP or recruitment maneuvers cannot be performed. Prone positioning can help both oxygenation and improve right ventricular size and function (Choice D).

Question 7 and 8
Clinical stem:

A 56 year old woman was admitted with right pyelonephritis, sepsis and septic shock. She had lactic acidosis and acute kidney injury at the time of presentation. She was admitted to ICU. Initial evaluation at the time of the ICU admission with shock showed normal cardiac function, IVC diameter of 1.2 cm. She received volume resuscitation and was started on vasopressor support. Her hemodynamic parameters and urine output improved after initial management.

On Day 3 of illness, she continued to require vasopressor support: Norepinephrine 15 mcg/min and Vasopressin 0.04 IU/min. Her heart rate was 100/min; mean arterial pressure (MAP) or 70 mm Hg; CVP of 10 mm Hg. On examination, her extremities felt cold and she had mild confusion. Urine output has been 120 mL over last 8 hours. Serum lactic acid was 3 mg/dL.

Bedside ultrasound and Echocardiography is performed for hemodynamic assessment. IVC diameter was 2.3 cm (not shown). Lung ultrasound showed Representative clips images are shown below:

See Videos 22.9 and 22.10.

See Images 22.2 and 22.3.

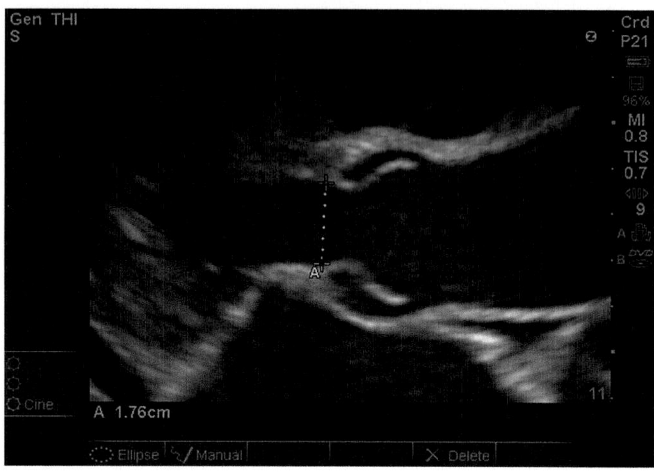

Image 22.2 LVOT diameter

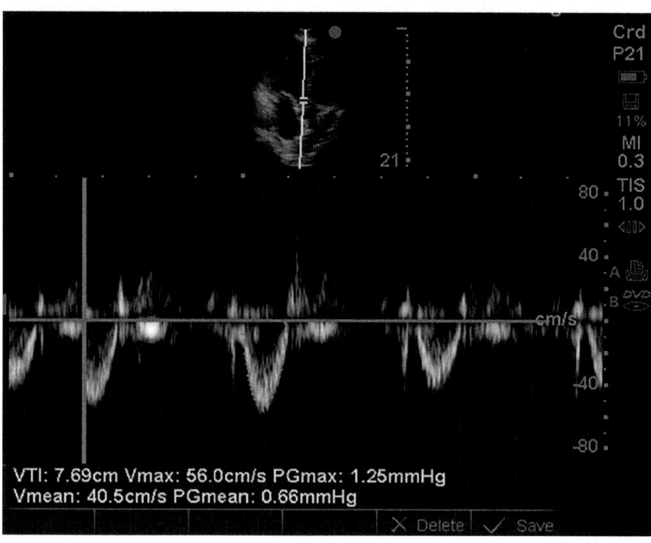

Image 22.3 LVOT VTI

Question 7:
Calculate the systemic vascular resistance.

A. 800 dyn·s·cm^{-5}.
B. 1200 dyn·s·cm^{-5}.
C. 2580 dyn·s·cm^{-5}.
D. 1800 dyn·s·cm^{-5}.

Correct answer: C. 2580 dyn ·s·cm^{-5}.

Question 8: What is the next best step in the hemodynamic management of this patient?

A. To increase dose of Norepinephrine
B. To start Phenylephrine
C. Volume resuscitation
D. Dobutamine infusion

Correct answer: D. Dobutamine infusion

Rationale: From the description of the clinical picture, it is evident that on day 3 of illness, the patient continues to have features of shock. Therefore, a fresh assessment of cause of shock was needed. Based on the data provided, left ventricular stroke volume and cardiac output can be measured:

$$SV(mL) = LVOT\ cross-sectional\ area(cm^2) \times VTI(cm).$$

$$Cardiac\ output(CO, L/min) = SV \times HR/min.$$

Once CO is known, systemic vascular resistance (SVR) can be calculated from the hemodynamic data available:

SVR ($dyn \cdot s \cdot cm^{-5}$) = [MAP (mm Hg) – CVP (mm Hg) ÷ CO] × 80.

In this case, the calculated SVR is 2580 $dyn \cdot s \cdot cm^{-5}$ (Normal 700–1600 $dyn \cdot s \cdot cm^{-5}$).

As the SVR is already high and clinical examination suggests vasoconstriction e.g., cold extremities, further increase in vasopressor dose or addition of another vasopressor will be inappropriate management; therefore, choices A and B in Question 2 are wrong. IVC diameter is 2.2 cm and does not clearly suggest hypovolemia. Both the parasternal long axis (PSL) view (Video 22.9) and apical four chamber (A4C) view (Video 22.10) suggest reduced LV function. Therefore, low SV and CO are mostly from reduced LV function. An inotrope will be the most appropriate next step in management (choice D).

Question 9

A 58 year old man with a new diagnosis of AIDS presents with subacute history of cough and dyspnea. He was found to have multiple pulmonary opacities and mediastinal lymphadenopathy.

He developed respiratory failure and was intubated. Subsequent bronchoscopy and biopsy confirmed a diagnosis of small cell lung cancer. In the second week of ICU stay, patient developed a new fever, with leukocytosis and hypotension. A diagnosis of sepsis from acute calculous cholecystitis was made. He was started on appropriate antibiotics. After volume resuscitation, he was started on vasopressor support for management of septic shock. An emergent image guided cholecystostomy was performed for source control. On day 3 after diagnosis of septic shock, the patient continued to require multiple vasopressors: Norepinephrine 1 mcg/kg/min, Vasopressin 0.04 IU/min. His blood pressure is 100/70 mm Hg, heart rate is 110/min. He had oliguria. Serum lactate was noted to be increasing after initial normalization. Serum AST and ALT were noted to be increasing.

The following table summarizes important laboratory parameters:

Lab parametery	Day 1	Day 3
Lactate (mmoL/L)	2.5	5.9
AST (IU/L)	91	899
ALT (IU/L)	67	222

An echocardiographic evaluation was undertaken and relevant clips are shown.

See Videos 22.11 and 22.12.

See Image 22.4.

Question 9: What is the next best step in management of this patient?

A. To increase Norepinephrine dose
B. To change Norepinephrine to Phenylephrine
C. To start Epinephrine infusion
D. To decrease Norepinephrine dose
E. To start Dobutamine infusion

Answer: D. To decrease Norepinephrine dose

Rationale: The echocardiographic assessment shows normal left ventricular systolic function. Right ventricle is dilated though has normal function. Therefore, Dobutamine infusion has no role. Dilated right ventricle and IVC diameter of >2.5 cm will suggest that the patient might have become volume overloaded from resuscitation with potential adverse consequences, including congestive hepatopathy.

Rising lactate, persistent oliguria and a biochemical picture consistent with ischemic injury to liver should also prompt review of the vasopressor dose as excessive doses of vasopressor can cause organ ischemia.

In this case, reducing the dose of norepinephrine dose will be the most prudent next step.

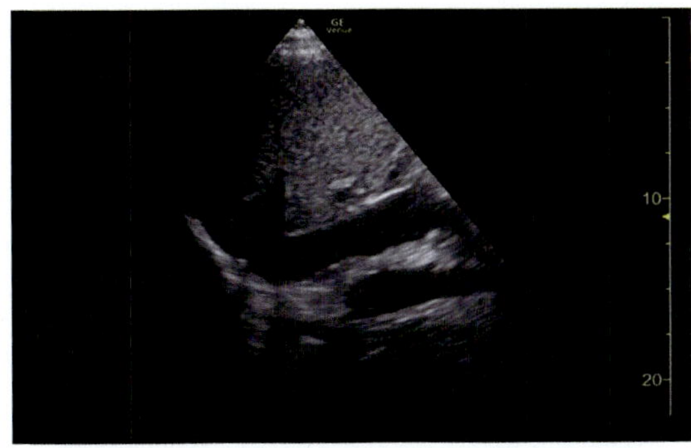

Image 22.4 IVC

Question 10

A 42-year-old woman had a diagnosis of multiple myeloma for which she had received multiple lines of chemotherapy without any sustained remission. She presented with fever, acute GI symptoms (cramps, nausea, vomiting, diarrhea) and clinical picture of septic shock. At admission, she also had AKI. A urinary tract infection was subsequently found as the cause of sepsis.

After admission to ICU, she received volume resuscitation and vasopressor support with initial improvement in blood pressure and urinary output. Approximately 48 hrs from her initial presentation, she continued to require high doses of vasopressor support to maintain MAP >65 mm Hg. Serum lactic acid was noted to be 4.80 mg/dL. Serum AST was 3249 IU/mL (92 IU/mL at admission), serum ALT was 1562 IU/mL (81 IU/mL). INR increased to 3.8 from 1.4 at the time of admission. The vasopressor doses at the time of assessment were: Norepinephrine 30 mcg/min; Vasopressin 0.04 U/hour; Phenylephrine 60 mcg/min.

An ultrasound assessment was undertaken to evaluate the persistent shock state of the patient and worsening organ function. Representative clips are shown.

See Video 22.13

See Image 22.5.

Question 10: What is the next best step in the management of this patient?

A. To change Norepinephrine infusion to Epinephrine infusion
B. To add Dobutamine infusion
C. To reduce vasopressor dose
D. Diuresis
E. A and C
F. C and D
G. B and D

Answer: F.

Key Point: If there is delay in resolution of shock with or without worsening organ function, repeated echocardiographic assessments are necessary to accurately identify the most likely cause.

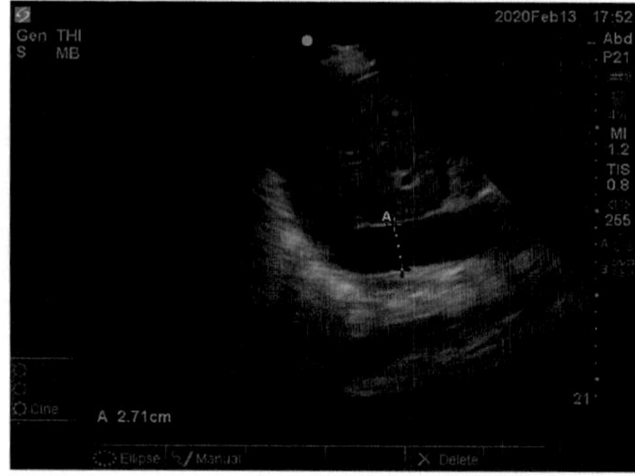

Image 22.5 IVC

Rationale: The parasternal short axis view shows diastolic flattening of interventricular septum, suggesting right ventricular volume overload. IVC is 2.5 cm. These findings together with rapidly worsening liver function would suggest that patient has developed right ventricular dysfunction from volume resuscitation, leading to congestive hepatopathy. Use of multiple vasopressor at this stage will only worsen the organ dysfunction. Reducing the dose of vasopressor and diuresis are the appropriate actions to take. Choice F is therefore right. The LV systolic function is preserved and therefore inotropic support is not necessary. In this patient with reduction in dose of vasopressor and diuresis, there was rapid improvement in lactic acidosis, liver function and coagulopathy.

Question 11–13

Clinical stem: A 60-year-old woman, an executive in a multinational corporation, had significant history of alcohol abuse. She was otherwise in good health. She was investigated for chest pain ~1 months prior to this admission. An echocardiogram performed at that time of the health check-up had shown normal left ventricular function. Coronary angiogram did not show any significant coronary artery disease at the same time.

This occasion, she was admitted with complaints of fatigue, chronic cough (? duration), new acute diarrhea and tremor. Initial laboratory parameters were notable for an abnormal liver function panel: AST > ALT, hyperbilirubinemia, elevated ALP and GGT, mildly elevated INR and WBC count. Biliary ultrasound did not show any obstructive pathology except for stable dilatation of common bile duct (compared to an ultrasound 2 years ago). A subsequent CT abdomen showed hypodense areas in liver of unclear etiology, some ascites and colonic thickening. CT chest showed bilateral upper and mid-zone ground glass opacities with small bilateral pleural effusion.

She was treated during first few days of hospital stay with broad spectrum antibiotics with presumed pulmonary source of infection. A diagnosis of alcoholic hepatitis was also considered to explain the liver function abnormalities.

On day 5 of hospitalization, rapid response team was called when patient had tachypnea and acute desaturation. A new encephalopathy was also noted. She was transferred to MICU. Rising leucocytosis was noted as well. Over next 24 hrs, overall clinical status deteriorated. Patient developed rapidly worsening renal and hepatic function, developed coagulopathy and became hemodynamically unstable with systolic blood pressure decreasing from 130 mm Hg to 105 mm Hg with MAP of 68 mm Hg. Heart rate was 94/min. Her encephalopathy had worsened. EKG showed sinus tachycardia and low voltage. Serum Troponin was borderline elevated.

A bedside echocardiogram was performed to assess her shock.

See Video 22.14.

See Image 22.6.

A continuous wave Doppler interrogation through the left ventricular outflow tract showed a velocity of 3 m/s.

Question 11: What is pathophysiology of the cardiac dysfunction in this patient?

A. Acute platelet aggregation and occlusion of epicardial coronary arteries
B. Rupture of atherosclerotic plug in epicardial coronary arteries with superimposed acute thrombosis
C. Myocardial hibernation from sepsis
D. Systemic cytokine storm from acute liver failure
E. Catecholamine surge

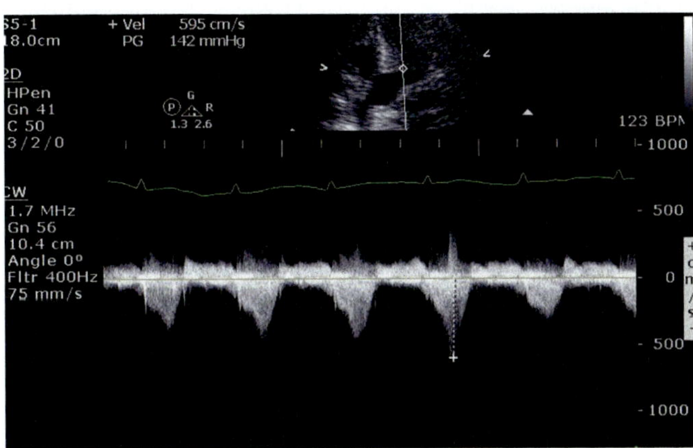

Image 22.6 CW doppler across LVOT

Answer: E.

Question 12: Which of the following medications can worsen hemodynamic status in this patient?

A. Furosemide
B. Phenylephrine infusion
C. Esmolol infusion
D. Dobutamine infusion

Answer: D.

Question 13: What will be the next best step in management of this patient?

A. Cardiac catheterization to rule out acute coronary syndrome
B. Esmolol infusion
C. Norepinephrine infusion
D. Intra-aortic balloon pump
E. Left ventricular assist device

Key Point:

Unexplained liver function abnormality should have searched for a broad based cause including ischemic hepatitis. Presence of bilateral pleural effusion 5 days before clinical deterioration should have been a clue to evaluate cardiac function.

Rationale: The echocardiographic clips show reduced LV function with preserved basal contractility and apical hypokinesis. This pattern of findings, along with recent normal echo and cardiac catheterization results, would point to a diagnosis of Takotsubo or stress cardiomyopathy. Most accepted hypothesis of stress cardiomyopathy is that a catecholamine surge leads, through multiple mechanisms, e.g., direct catecholamine toxicity, adrenoceptor-mediated damage, epicardial and microvascular coronary vasoconstriction and/or spasm, and increased cardiac workload, to myocardial damage. Therefore, E is the correct answer in Question 11.

Continuous wave Doppler of LVOT shows dynamic LVOT obstruction, revealed by increased LVOT flow velocity. Use of an inotropic agent will worsen the obstruction. Therefore, Dobutamine infusion will be detrimental and should be avoided. D is the correct answer in Question 12.

In view of LVOT obstruction, Esmolol infusion can be tried to improve hemodynamic status of this patient. By reducing contractility, short acting beta blockers can improve LVOT obstruction, cardiac output and blood pressure. Therefore, B is the correct answer in question 13.

Question 14
Clinical stem:

A 45-year-old female with past medical history of morbid obesity, sleep apnea, type 2 diabetes mellitus and hypertension presents to the emergency department because of lethargy. According to her family she was last seen in her usual state of health last night when she went to sleep, and they became concerned when she did not wake up in the morning. Vital signs disclose pulse of 85 bpm, respiratory rate of 12 breaths per minute, temperature 98.5F, blood pressure of 115/86 mmHg and $Sp0_2$ of 95% on room air. Physical examination finds a lethargic, obese woman with clear breath sounds bilaterally, S1 and S2 within normal limits, soft abdomen and Glasgow coma scale of 6/15. An arterial blood gas finds a pH of 7.24, P_aCO_2 of 96 mmHg, HCO_3–45 mEq/L and a P_aO_2 75 mmHg and rapid sequence intubation is performed to ventilate patient. Initial ventilator settings are tidal volume of 7 ml/kg of ideal body weight, respiratory rate of 25, FiO_2 of 0.5 and PEEP of 5. Shortly after intubation patient becomes hemodynamically unstable and mean arterial pressure drops to 50 mmHg. POCUS is performed to evaluate her hemodynamic status. Relevant images are shown below and the following is found.

See Video 22.15.

See Image 22.7.

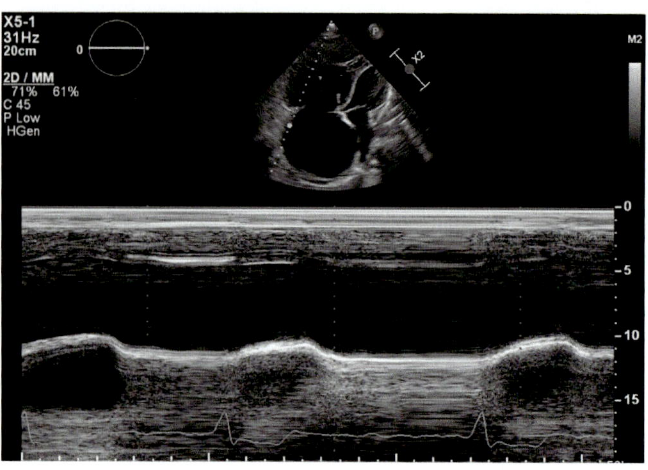

Image 22.7 TAPSE

Q14: Which hemodynamic parameter would help determine the cause of this patient's shock?

(a) Pulmonary artery ejection time
(b) TAPSE
(c) Stroke volume variation at RVOT
(d) Pulse pressure variation from an arterial line

Answer: (b) TAPSE.

Key point: The patient has RV failure as evidenced by a TAPSE of <10 mm possibly from long-standing pulmonary hypertension from untreated sleep apnea which caused hemodynamic instability after being placed on mechanical ventilation.

Rationale: The cause of hemodynamic instability is probably caused by RV failure as evidenced by a dilated RV, and septal flattening which are echocardiographic signs of RV dysfunction. This was most likely caused by long standing sleep apnea and obesity hypoventilation, causing pulmonary hypertension. RV dysfunction was further exacerbated by invasive positive pressure ventilation. The patient has a decreased RV systolic function, as estimated by TAPSE which is easily measured at bedside with POCUS. TAPSE is measured in M-mode from an apical 4-chamber view by having the cursor line intersect the lateral tricuspid annulus which results in a sawtooth pattern, with the value being represented by the height of each wave. Normal values range from 22–24 mm, with decreased RV function being defined by a TAPSE less than 17 mm.

Question 15
Clinical stem:

A middle aged man was brought to the emergency room (ER) by emergency medical services (EMS). The patient was in a shopping mall when he collapsed. As per eyewitness account, he was seen to clutch his chest, appeared to be in pain and then fell down and lost his consciousness. Cardiopulmonary resuscitation was started by a bystander before EMS arrived to continue resuscitation. ROSC was achieved after 5 min of resuscitation. The initial cardiac rhythm was noted to be sinus tachycardia.

After ROSC was achieved, he was intubated in the field. He was sedated and paralyzed as he started waking up and was transported to the emergency room.

On initial assessment in ER, his blood pressure was 80/50 mm Hg and heart rate was 110/min. His oxygen saturation was 87% on FIO2 of 100%. Extremities appeared cold. He appeared dehydrated. Though his medical history was unknown, a medication bottle of Amlodipine was found in his pocket.

An immediate ultrasound assessment of his shock state and respiratory failure was undertaken. Representative clips are shown in Video 22.16.

See Video 22.16.

Question 15:

What is the most likely category of shock in this patient?

A. Hypovolemic shock
B. Cardiogenic shock
C. Obstructive shock
D. Distributive shock
E. Neurogenic shock

Answer: C. Obstructive shock.

Key Point:

In a patient with shock, a whole body ultrasound approach will help to identify causes of shock accurately.

Rationale: This patient presented with a clear picture of shock. Echo showed normal right and left ventricular function, making cardiogenic shock unlikely. Based on the history, there is no suggestion of hypovolemia. Lack of IVC size variation will also be an evidence against hypovolemia. Similarly, no cause of distributive or neurogenic shock is found in the clinical presentation of the patient. The lung ultrasound shows lung point, a confirmatory finding for diagnosis of pneumothorax. This case highlights the importance of a systematic and whole body approach with critical care ultrasonography and interpretation of ultrasound findings in light of the clinical presentation.

Question 16
Clinical stem:

A 65-year-old male was found down in his apartment and brought to the emergency department by relatives. He was last seen normal 3 days ago and was only complaining of a headache at the time. Relatives at bedside stated that he had coronary artery disease with stent placement 8 years ago. He also had hypertension. His medications included low dose Aspirin and Metoprolol. He had history of heavy alcohol consumption for many years. Initial vital signs disclosed a heart rate of 80 bpm, respiratory rate of 17, temperature of 98.5 F and blood pressure of 118/66 mmHg. Initial evaluation finds him to be well-nourished male, drowsy with no focal neurological deficit, Chest auscultation was unremarkable. Abdomen was soft with quiet bowel sounds. He was intubated for airway protection. Initial work-up showed hemoglobin of 7.1 gm/dL, elevated lactic acid level and elevated serum troponin. EKG showed T-wave inversion in V3-V6. Patient was being admitted to coronary care unit with suspicion of non-STEMI when his blood pressure dropped to 65/40 mmHg and pulse increased to 110 bpm range.

POCUS is performed at bedside to assess the source of shock further and the following images are obtained.

See Videos 22.17 and 22.18.

Q16: What is the next best step to manage this patient's shock?

(a) To administer Aspirin and Clopidogrel for acute coronary syndrome
(b) Immediate coronary angiography and revascularization
(c) Volume resuscitation
(d) To start Norepinephrine infusion

Key point: The patient has hypovolemic shock as evident from complete effacement of LV cavity at the end of systole.

Rationale: Though this patient has known history of coronary artery disease and EKG changes and elevated troponin can point towards fresh cardiac ischemia, echocardiography shows normal global LV systolic function. Therefore, cardiogenic shock is ruled out.

Left upper quadrant ultrasound showed large fluid filled stomach. In presence of anemia and ultrasound evidence of volume depletion, hemorrhagic shock from upper GI bleeding should be the most likely diagnosis.

Question 17
Clinical stem:

A 68-year-old female presents to the emergency department complaining of worsening shortness of breath for the past two weeks that is exacerbated by moderate physical activity and a dry cough. She denies fever, chills, diaphoresis, chest pain, hemoptysis, sick contacts. She has a past medical history of morbid obesity, type 2 diabetes mellitus and right knee osteoarthritis for which she requires a cane to ambulate. Current medications are acetaminophen as needed, topical naproxen gel and maximum dose metformin.

Physical examination discloses a heart rate of 55 bpm, blood pressure of 85/50, temperature of 97.5 F and a respiratory rate of 28 bpm. She is in moderate respiratory distress with accessory muscle use, an S3 is appreciated on auscultation with crackles throughout both lung fields. The rest of the examination is normal. Point of care cardiac ultrasound is performed, and the parasternal long axis images reveal the following findings.

See Video 22.19.

See Image 22.8.

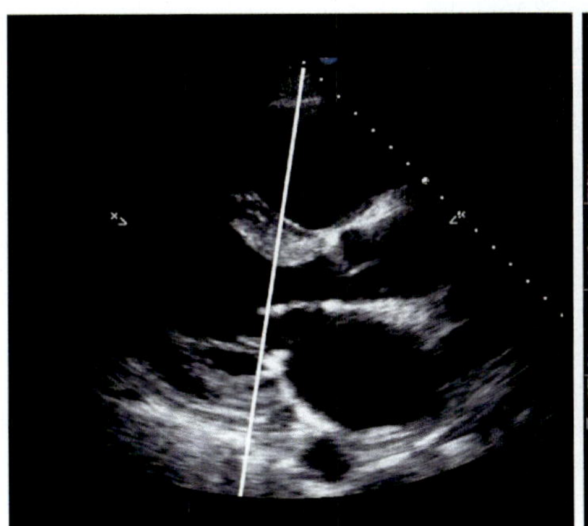

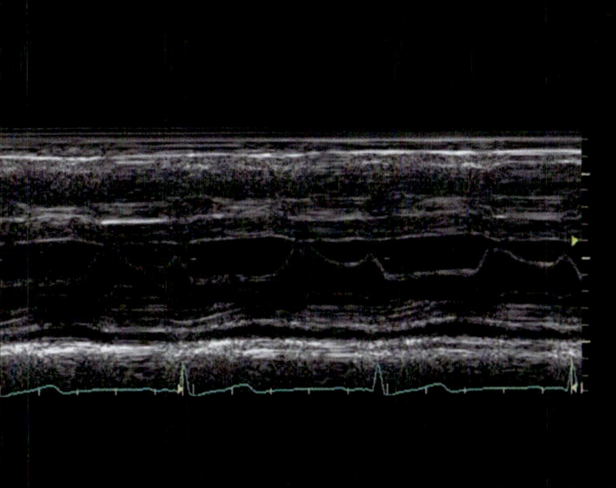

Image 22.8 PLAX M mode at mitral leaflet

Question 17: What is the patient's estimated ejection fraction?

A. LVEF >60%
B. LVEF >40%
C. LVEF <40%
D. LVEF <25%

Answer C.

Key Point: When the anterior mitral valve leaflet is within 1 cm of the septum it corresponds with an LVEF greater than >40%.

Rationale: A visually estimated left ventricular ejection fraction (LVEF) is comparable to a quantitative, calculate LVEF.

When assessing left ventricular systolic function three characteristics are paramount: (1) Endocardial excursion, which is if the endocardium moves symmetrically towards the center of the chamber. (2) Increase in myocardial thickness by 40% in all left ventricular segments during systole. (3) Septal motion of the anterior mitral valve leaflet tip within 1 cm from the septum.

Question 18
Clinical stem:

A 40-year-old female arrives to the hospital after a neighbor called an ambulance after finding her collapsed in her front yard. First responders found her to be hypotensive and obtunded, she was intubated in the field for airway protection. Her vital signs upon presentation to the emergency department disclose a pulse of 120 bpm, 20 breaths per minute, blood pressure of 83/45 mmHg and temperature 103.2, SaO2 92%. Ventilator settings were assist control mode tidal volume at 8 mL/kg of ideal body weight, PEEP 15, FiO2 0.5, respiratory rate 20. Peak airway pressure was 22 cm H2O Physical examination showed a sedated, obese, female patient, with clear breath sounds bilaterally though reduced in right basal region, normal heart sounds, patient was grimacing when abdomen is palpated and has a RASS -2. Blood pressure did not improve after 2 L of lactated Ringer's bolus. POCUS was performed while waiting for laboratory results. IVC was 2.1 cm in diameter.

See Image 22.9.

See Video 22.20.

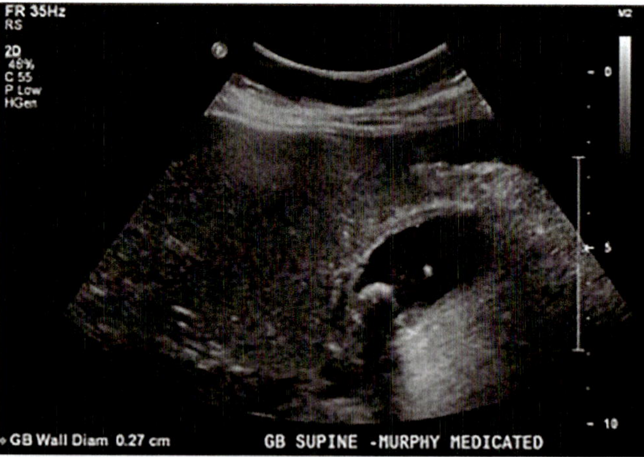

Image 22.9 Gallbladder

Question 19: What type of shock does the patient have?

A. Cardiogenic shock
B. Obstructive shock
C. Septic shock
D. Hypovolemic shock

Answer D.

Key point: Patient likely has septic shock from acute cholecystitis as evidenced by gallbladder wall thickening.

Rationale: The source of septic shock is likely from acute cholecystitis. Acute cholecystitis is evidenced in ultrasound by the presence of gallstones, sonographic Murphy's sign, gallbladder wall thickening >3 mm and pericholecystic fluid. Gallstones and sonographic Murphy's sign has a positive predictive value >90% and a negative predictive value >95%. Gallbladder wall thickness > 3 mm is most likely due from cholecystitis, although there can be false positives from ascites, congestive heart failure, hepatitis and nonfasted states.

Questions 19 & 20
Clinical Stem:

A 42-year-old female with past medical history of HTN, DM, SLE and associated mild pulmonary hypertension was admitted to the hospital with report of worsening dyspnea for past 4 weeks. Patient's lupus was complicated by lupus nephritis and chronic renal failure (CKD stage V). Her follow-up has been irregular with last follow-up being more than a year ago. Patient's prior echocardiography was suggestive of ePASP of 43 to 48 mmHg, LV ejection fraction of 65%. On examination, the patient was in mild respiratory distress. Temperature was 98.1 °F, pulse rate was 69/min, respiration rate was 22/min, blood pressure was 110/75 and saturation was 91% on BiPAP with FIO2 of 80%. ABG showed PaO2 of 59 mm Hg on the same setting. Serum lactate was 3 mg/dL.

A portable chest x-ray showed clear lung fields. Bedside ultrasound and echocardiography were performed for hemodynamic assessment. Representative clips are shown below:

See Video 22.21

Question 19: What is the cause of hypoxemia in this patient?

A. Intracardiac shunt.
B. Increased dead space.
C. Intrapulmonary shunt.
D. V-Q mismatch.

Answer A. Intracardiac shunt.

Key point: In a patient with pulmonary hypertension, significant hypoxemia should lead to a search from right to left shunt.

Rationale: Based on clinical history, prior echo findings and current echo imaging, a diagnosis of pulmonary hypertension is clear. The clinical scenario also suggests RV failure (relative hypotension, elevated lactate).

From the AP4C view, the right atrium is dilated with bowing out of septum towards left. There is also a thinned out portion of the septum. SC4C view with color Doppler shows flow across the interatrial septum. In agitated saline contrast study, there is appearance of saline contrast in left sided chambers within 3 heart beats, confirming the diagnosis of right to left intracardiac shunt.

Question 20: What is the next best step in the management of this patient?

A. Start continuous intravenous furosemide.
B. Start inhaled nitric oxide.
C. Start intravenous dobutamine.
D. Call interventional cardiology consult immediately.

Answer: A.

Rationale: This patient has severe pulmonary hypertension with suggestion of right heart failure and right to left shunt.

Early management should include diuresis as the mainstay of decompensated right heart failure. Role of inhaled nitric oxide is not established in management of decompensated right heart failure. Although an inotropic agent can be used along with diuretics, diuresis is a prime measure for controlling right heart failure.

In the presence of decompensated right heart failure, closure of PFO will lead to acute worsening of heart failure and is therefore not advised.

Question 21
Clinical stem:

A 67-year-old male with a medical history of diabetes mellitus and end-stage renal disease on hemodialysis presents to the hospital for acute confusion. According to his family members, he has been progressively getting more confused and difficult to arouse for the past 2 days. He has not missed his regular hemodialysis sessions. Vital signs disclose a pulse of 92 bpm, respiratory rate of 24 per minute, temperature of 100.8 F, blood pressure of 82/55 mmHg and a saturation of oxygen of 90% on room air. Examination finds a lethargic, chronically ill appearing male with chest auscultation finding tachycardic albeit with normal heart sounds and crackles in posterior right lower lung field, abdomen is soft, nontender and there is an AV fistula on the right arm without any obvious signs of inflammation. Lab work is remarkable for white blood cells of 12,000/mL, hemoglobin of 8 mg/dL lactate of 6 mmoL/L and an anion gap of 15, chest X ray is pending. In the interim, POCUS is performed, and relevant images are in the following video (Video 22.22).

See Video 22.22.

Question 21: What is the next step in management?

A. Start Dobutamine infusion
B. Transfuse packed red blood cells
C. Bolus crystalloids at 30 ml/kg of actual body weight and start broad-spectrum antibiotics
D. Start norepinephrine infusion

Answer C.

Key point: According to the Surviving Sepsis Campaign guidelines, patients with septic shock should receive 30 mL/kg of crystalloids and broad-spectrum antibiotics should be initiated promptly.

Rationale: Patient has septic shock, as evidenced by lung ultrasonography of right hemithorax with a large area of consolidation and adjacent pleural effusion with few internal strands. He also appears to be hypovolemic, with subcostal view revealing a small and collapsible inferior vena cava and end-systolic cavity obliteration of LV.

Question 22
Clinical stem:

A 54-year-old male with past medical history of nonischemic cardiomyopathy (NICMP) with a continuous flow left ventricular assist device (CF-LVAD) presents to the emergency department after there was an alarm in his device. He admits to feeling short of breath, without any chest pain and feeling. Initial vital signs find a heart rate of 65 on telemetry, mean arterial pressure of 45 mmHg, respiratory rate 25, temperature of 98.5 and saturation of oxygen of 90% on room air. LVAD speed is 2300 rpm, flow is 1.7 L/m and power is 2.3 watts. Physical examination discloses finds a positive hum on chest auscultation, diffuse bilateral crackles, no tenderness to abdominal palpation, site of driveline insertion without signs of infection and there is +1 lower extremity edema. Serum lactate is elevated and serum creatinine is elevated from baseline. POCUS findings are shown below (Video 22.23):

See Video 22.23

Question 22: What is the best next step?

A. Increase pump speed
B. Start inotropic support
C. Bolus tPA
D. Give 1 L bolus of lactated ringer

Answer: A.

Key point: Patient is having low flows with POCUS signs of dilated cardiac chambers and plethoric IVC suggesting that the LVAD speeds might be too low.

Rationale: The patient has features of shock. The increase in size of both ventricles and plethoric IVC with low flows and MAPs are suggestive of possible low speeds and increasing the speed, then reassessing with POCUS after this change is made can be an appropriate maneuver but should be done under the guidance of the team that placed the LVAD.

Question 23
Clinical stem:

A 65-year-old-male with known medical history of uncontrolled hypertension, heavy smoking and stage III CKD, presented to the emergency department complaining of sharp, chest and upper abdominal pain starting on the day of admission without any alleviating or exacerbating factors. His pulse rate was 120 bpm, respiration was 30 per minute, temperature was 97.8 F and blood pressure is 89/43 mmHg. He was in severe distress from pain, diaphoretic with generalized pallor. Chest auscultation revealed faint heart sounds. There was tenderness to abdominal palpation with rebound and quiet bowel sounds. A point of care ultrasound is performed and reveals the following images.

See Videos 22.24 and 22.25.

Question 23: What would be the next best step?

A. Start norepinephrine infusion
B. CT Pulmonary angiogram
C. Emergent TEE
D. Consult vascular surgery

Answer: D.

Key point: In a highly suggestive clinical scenario, unequivocal evidence of hypovolemia should initiate plan in line of management of ruptured aortic aneurysm.

Rationale: The clinical history, along with clear evidence of hypovolemia point to a diagnosis of ruptured aortic aneurysm. Surgical management should be planned without delay. Therefore, D is the right choice. POCUS also is an excellent tool in identification of abdominal aortic aneurysms. Very small IVC and normal RV on echo would be strong evidence against a diagnosis of acute massive pulmonary embolism; so CTPA I unnecessary and will consume critical time with additional risk of transportation of a very ill and unstable patient. TEE may give complementary information by showing thoracic aorta, but not necessary in this particular case where patient has already developed hemorrhagic shock. There is no suggestion of distributive shock. Norepinephrine will be harmful in a hypovolemic patient.

Questions 24 & 25
Clinical stem:

A 74 y.o. male with known medical history of type 2 diabetes mellitus, coronary artery disease with prior history of percutaneous coronary intervention, heart failure with reduced ejection fraction (LVEF 45–49%, 2 months prior to current admission), presented with complaints of complaining of 2 days of substernal chest pain and DOE. He also complained of mild epigastric pain associated with nausea, vomiting, and poor oral intake. His home medication included Furosemide, Spironolactone, Lisinopril and Metoprolol. Blood pressure was 125/82 mm Hg; pulse was 92/min, regular; RR 18/min, oxygen saturation 96% on room air. On examination, he was alert and oriented, speech clear and appropriate with no neurological deficits. Airway was patent, respirations symmetric and unlabored with no use of accessory muscles; there were scattered rhonchi on auscultation. Heart examination revealed S1, S2, with no murmurs, rubs or gallops.

Initial lab studies showed Na 116, K 5.4; Cl 77, BUN 25, creatinine 1.8 (baseline 0.8). AST 918 IU/L, ALT 749 IU/L. INR 1.3; Lactic acid was 3.4 mmol/L.

Initial bedside ultrasound assessment showed IVC of 1.3 cm, severely reduced global LV systolic function and bilateral A-line pattern on lung ultrasound.

Question 24: What is the next best step in management of this patient?

A. IV fluid bolus
B. To start Norepinephrine infusion
C. To start Dobutamine infusion
D. To check B-natriuretic peptide and before administering IV fluid

Correct answer: A.

After initial volume resuscitation with 2 L of crystalloids, ~ 8 hrs later, lactic acid was noted to be 7.3 mmol/L, AST 1817 IU/L, ALT 1209 IU/L, INR 2.3. He continued to be hemodynamically stable without any tachycardia. Urine output was <100 mL in previous 6 hrs.

A repeat echocardiogram assessment was performed.

See Video 22.26.

Question 25: What is the most likely cause of his worsening liver function?

A. Low cardiac output from decreased preload
B. Low cardiac output from decreased LV contractility
C. Congestive changes from right ventricular failure
D. Volume overload from earlier volume resuscitation

Correct answer: D.

Key Point: Even in patients with heart failure, hypovolemia can be a prominent reason in etiology of shock and should be recognized. Management of shock needs multiple reassessments over initial hours to decide the treatment option. In this patient.

Rationale: The patient was on treatment with diuretics. There was also history of poor oral intake for several days. IVC size was <1.5 cm. Hyponatremia and hypochloremia would also point to excessive use of diuretics. Overall, clinical, echocardiographic and laboratory parameters at admission gave a clear indication of hypovolemia. Therefore, in spite of severe reduction in global LV systolic function, volume resuscitation should be the first course of action. There was no suggestion on pulmonary edema on clinical evaluation and lung ultrasound; this gave more room for volume administration in spite of poor LV function. Therefore, answer A is correct in question 1.

In the repeat assessment, the IVC is ~2 cm, suggesting improvement in volume status. Worsening lactic acid level, oliguria and rising liver enzymes would suggest that the shock has not resolved. Reduced VTI suggests that stroke volume and cardiac output were low. Reduced VTI after adequate volume resuscitation and severely reduced LV contractility would suggest that low cardiac output is driven to a significant extent by reduced LV contractility. Beta blocker therapy likely masked compensatory tachycardia that could normally be expected in a person with low cardiac output and shock. Therefore, B is the correct choice in question 2.

At this stage, a trial of an inotropic agent is warranted.

Question 26
Clinical stem:

A 23-year-old female is evaluated after a rapid response is called for hypotension after being admitted to the hospital that same night for pyelonephritis. She has received 4 L boluses of normal saline but her blood pressure modestly responded to these interventions and she has already received a dose of ceftriaxone. Upon your examination patient complains of left flank pain and subjective fever, her vital signs disclose pulsations of 115 bpm, temperature of 104 F, respiratory rate of 26 per minute and a blood pressure of 85/63 mmHg. Physical examination finds a toxic appearing patient, chest auscultation within normal limits and she had left costovertebral angle tenderness. Laboratory work shows a white blood cell count of 12,300, lactate of 5, creatinine of 2 (baseline 0.9 2 months ago) and uranalysis positive for wbc of 20 m/L, 5–6 RBC + nitrites and leukocyte esterase. A POCUS is performed at bedside with the following findings.

See Video 22.27.

Question 26: What is the next best step in the care of this patient?

A. To give an additional liter of NS
B. To broaden coverage to piperacillin-tazobactam
C. To start norepinephrine infusion
D. To transfer patient to the intensive care unit

Answer C.

Key point: The patient has septic shock from a complicated UTI caused by obstructing nephrolithiasis resulting in hydronephrosis and is no longer fluid responsive.

Rationale: Renal ultrasonography can detect and grade obstructive uropathy and hydronephrosis. Large renal calculi can also be identified. When clinical suspicion is high, unilateral hydronephrosis can be considered obstructive from a possible calculus. The patient in this case has already received a considerable amount of IV crystalloids and her IVC indicates that she is volume replete, therefore administering more IV fluids may be detrimental. Starting a vasopressor infusion will be the next best step for management of shock.

Question 27
Clinical stem.

A 45-year-old male with known history of end-stage renal disease on chronic hemodialysis, presented to the emergency department for worsening shortness of breath that began 5 days ago. He states that he had missed his regular hemodialysis sessions due to lack of transportation. Initial hemodynamic parameters showed a HR of 90/min and blood pressure of 160/90 mm Hg. CXR showed mild perihilar congestion. As his fistula was not function, a right femoral temporary hemodialysis catheter was placed and the patient was taken to the hemodialysis unit. A rapid response was called 1 hour later for an acute change in mental status and hypotension. Vital signs disclose HR of 110ts per minute, respiratory rate of 25 per minute, temperature 98 F, Sa02 of 92% on 3 L/min oxygen and blood pressure 90/67 mm Hg. Physical examination finds a chronically ill male in moderate respiratory distress, with jugular venous distension, crackles bilaterally and distant heart sounds but an LVS4 could be appreciated, abdomen was soft and there was bilateral pedal edema. Labs disclose hemoglobin of 7.5 mg/dL, white blood cells of 7 × 10^9/L, troponins of 0.04 ng/mL, BNP of 800 ng/L and EKG find nonspecific ST segment abnormalities in lateral leads. A POCUS is performed.

See Video 22.28.

Question 27: What is the most likely cause of hypotension in this patient?

A. Pericardial effusion and cardiac tamponade
B. Acute myocardial infarction
C. Excessive volume removal through hemodialysis
D. Deep issue bleeding**Answer: D.**

Key point: Even in a patient with pericardial effusion and some echocardiographic sign of tamponade physiology, a complete assessment is necessary to reveal additional causes.

Rationale: This patient has a small pericardial effusion with RA collapse which might suggest tamponade physiology. However, IVC is very small, arguing against tamponade and suggesting hypovolemia. At presentation, the patient had peripheral edema and pulmonary congestion, suggesting volume overload. It is unlikely that volume removal in <1 h on hemodialysis ill cause hypovolemia and shock. Given that the patient had a new placement of femoral dialysis catheter, local deep tissue bleeding or retroperitoneal bleeding is the most likely cause of hypotension in this patient.

Patients who have tamponade physiology have collapse of RA during ventricular systole, RV during ventricular diastole and a plethoric IVC. Tamponade can be ruled out if the IVC has a collapse of 50% or more with inspiration.

Questions 28 & 29
Clinical Stem:

64-year-old female with past medical history of hypertension, dyslipidemia, CAD (status post PCI in 4 years back), NASH presented to the emergency room with 1 week of nausea, vomiting and generalized weakness. Patient was admitted to medical ICU for hypotension (shock) and AKI. On admission, patient's vital signs were temperature 98.7 °F, pulse rate 120/min, respiration rate 24/min, blood pressure 60 s over 40 s. Patient was found to have acute kidney injury with BUN of 64 mg/dL and serum creatinine of 10.6 mg/dL (serum creatinine 0.91 mg/dL 1-month back). Patient's other pertinent laboratory findings were troponin elevation at 0.13 ng/mL, ALT 332 IU/L, AST 433 IU/L, total bilirubin 3.5 mg/dL with direct 1, lactic acid 5.2, WBC count 8.5×10^3/mL. On examination, patient was in mild discomfort secondary to nausea, sclera was icteric and lungs were clear.

Goal directed echocardiography performed for evaluation of the shock and pertinent images are shown below: Videos 22.29, 22.30 and 22.31.

See Videos 22.29, 22.30 and 22.31

Question 28: What is the type of shock?

A. Cardiogenic shock
B. Distributive shock
C. Obstructive shock
D. Hypovolemic shock

Answer: D.

Question 29: What is the pathophysiology of this shock?

1. Bacterial factors, inflammatory cytokines, complement anticoagulation cascade activation associated decreased peripheral vascular resistance.
2. Hypovolemia
3. Gastrointestinal bleeding
4. Retro-peritoneal bleeding

Answer: c.

Key: The LV cavity is small with hyperdynamic LV systolic function. This along with <1cm IVC is highly suggestive of hypovolemia

Rationale: The LV cavity is small with hyperdynamic LV systolic function. This along with <1cm IVC is highly suggestive of hypovolemia. Gastric ultrasound shows echogenic material inside gastric cavity, which in a cirrhotic patient is highly suggestive of gastrointestinal bleeding

Question 30
Clinical stem: A 35-year-old female is being evaluated for acute onset shortness of breath that began three days ago. She states that previously she was able to jog 2 miles daily without any difficulty. She has a history of asthma for which she takes an albuterol inhaler as needed but has not been working during this particular episode. Current vital signs show a pulse rate of 105 bpm, respiratory rate 23 breaths per minute, blood pressure of 80/50 mmHg and a temperature of 100.8 F. She is obese, neck examination for JVD is difficult due to her body habitus, chest auscultation reveals tachycardia with regular rhythm, with S1 and S2 heard appropriately but difficult to assess due to prominent adipose tissue, lungs sound clear bilaterally, her abdomen is soft and non-tender and she has trace pedal edema. Point-of-care-ultrasound is performed at bedside and the following images are obtained:

See Video 22.32.

Other ultrasound findings included bilateral A-line pattern on lung ultrasound and IVC diameter of 2.4 cm.

Question 30: Which is the best next step in management of her dyspnea?

A. Emergent needle decompression
B. Bolus of crystalloids at 30 ml/kg
C. Urgent pericardiocentesis
D. Start methylprednisolone and continuous albuterol nebulization

Answer C.

Key point: Patient has pericardial tamponade and requires emergent pericardiocentesis.

Rationale: A normal pericardium contains approximately 10 mL of serous fluid, effusions of this sac are mostly seen as an anechoic strip that encircle the heart. Tamponade occurs when the pressure in the pericardium supersedes the pressure of one or more cardiac chambers. Ultrasound findings of tamponade include collapse of the right atrium during systole and right ventricle during diastole and an engorged inferior vena cava (IVC) due to elevated right heart pressures. A dilated IVC is 97% sensitive for tamponade and its absence argues greatly against tamponade.

Question 31
Clinical stem:

A 55-year-old female patient with past medical history of type 2 diabetes mellitus and cryptogenic cirrhosis is evaluated for a distended, moderately tender abdomen accompanied by generalized weakness that began 2 days prior to admission. She usually undergoes outpatient paracentesis every week with her last one being 6 days prior to admission, in which around 3 L ascetic fluid was removed without complications; no studies were sent. Vital signs disclose pulsations of 125 beats per minute, respiratory rate of 16 per minute, temperature of 98.6 F and blood pressure of 85/63 mmHg. Physical examination finds a pale and jaundiced female with clear breath sounds bilaterally, tachycardia with normal s1 and s2, abdomen is tensely distended, tender to palpation, no organomegaly appreciated, various spider angiomata noticed with a hematoma on the site of previous paracentesis and quiet bowel sounds. Lab work show a hemoglobin of 5.5 g/dL (previously 9 g/dL), platelets of 35 × 10^3/mL, white blood cell count 9 × 10^9/L (stable), INR of 3, lactate of 5 mg/dL. POCUS is performed at bedside. LV and RV function is found to be normal. **Other relevant images are shown in Video 22.33.**

See Video 22.33.

Question 31: Besides giving blood products, what is the next best step?

A. Repeat paracentesis
B. Insert central venous catheter
C. Consult interventional radiology
D. Start broad spectrum antibiotics

Answer: C.

Key point: Patient is undergoing hemorrhagic shock from hemoperitoneum likely a complication from previous paracentesis.

Rationale: All types of peritoneal free fluid appear to be anechoic on POCUS but if there is clotted blood or other debris it may appear more echogenic due to the increased proteinaceous material. Additionally, strands or loculations are often seen. Patient also has signs of hypovolemia as evidenced by a very small IVC (virtual IVC); this coupled with the acute anemia point towards a hemorrhagic shock as the etiology of the hemodynamic instability. Consulting interventional radiology for embolization of a bleeding vessel is the most appropriate next step.

See Video 22.34.

Question 32
Clinical stem:

A 74y.o. woman with 80 pack-year smoking history presented with 1-month history of progressive shortness of breath, dry cough and episodes of streaky hemoptysis. CXR and CT chest showed a large right upper lobe mass and large right pleural effusion. The pleural effusion was drained with improvement in dyspnea. Next day morning, she underwent bronchoscopy which showed infiltrative mass in right upper lobe bronchus with near total occlusion; biopsy was obtained from the right upper lobe mass. Six hour after bronchoscopy and biopsy, she developed acute shortness of breath, and sustained a cardiac arrest from which she was successfully revived after 4 min of resuscitation. Copious blood tinged secretions were noted in the endotracheal tube after she was intubated during the code. Post-resuscitation, heart rate was noted to be 64/min, blood pressure 106/70 mm Hg, oxygen saturation 96% on FIO2 40% and her airway pressure was 21 cm H20 on AC/VC mode with TV of 400 mL and peak flow rate of 60 L/min. On examination, breath sound was diminished on right side. Post resuscitation she underwent an echocardiogram, the images from which are shown in Video 22.34.

Question 32: What is the most likely cause of acute decompensation and cardiac arrest in this patient?

A. Obstructive shock from acute massive pulmonary embolism
B. Obstructive shock from tension pneumothorax after biopsy
C. Hemorrhagic shock from bleeding into the airways
D. Distributive shock from post-obstructive pneumonia
E. Obstructive shock from acute valvular obstruction

Answer E.

Key Point: Some rare valvular pathology can cause sudden hemodynamic collapse.

Rationale: The patient's deterioration was sudden and there are many potential explanations in this case. The echo shows a large heterogeneous mass attached to the atrial side of the anterior leaflet of the mitral valve. Some parts of the mass are independently mobile. In a patient with known cancer, tumor thrombus should be considered. Sudden occlusion of mitral valve with the mass likely caused the cardiac arrest in this patient (choice E). While acute massive pulmonary embolism is possible, restoration of hemodynamic parameters to normal after resuscitation will be unusual. The PSS view also shows normal RV size with no septal flattening, thereby ruling out massive pulmonary embolism (choice A). Tension pneumothorax similarly should not improve on its own. Also, endobronchial biopsy from an endoscopically visible tumor usually does not cause pneumothorax (choice B is wrong). Significant airway bleeding is usually manifested by hemoptysis and hypoxemia. The symptoms before and after resuscitation and ability to ventilate and oxygenate the patient after resuscitation will point against this diagnosis (choice C). The time line of events does not fit a diagnosis of sepsis and septic (distributive) shock (choice D).

Question 33 & 34
Clinical Stem

A 66-year-old male with past medical history of type 2 diabetes mellitus, chronic kidney disease stage II and hypertension presents to the emergency department complaining of shortness of breath for the past week, that has increased in severity over the past two days. Shortly after his arrival the patient decompensates and requires to be intubated immediately. He is placed on assist control mechanical ventilation (VC-CMV) with a tidal volume of 6 ml/kg of ideal body weight, respiratory rate of 15, PEEP of 5 and FiO2% of 100%. His vital signs are as follows, heart rate of 125 bpm, Sp02 92% on 100% FiO2, a mean arterial pressure (MAP) of 45 mmHg and a temperature of 99 F. Physical examination disclose a mechanically ventilated patient sedated on dexmetomidine at a RASS of −2, heart sounds are distant but with a discernible S1 and S2, with a regular rhythm, decreased breath sounds in the left hemithorax, with mild crackles, abdomen is soft and non-tender, lower extremities disclose pedal edema of 1 + .Basic lab work has been sent and a chest x-ray is pending. He is given 2 L of lactated ringers with a transient, short lived improvement to the MAP, prompting a norepinephrine infusion to support his blood pressure. You are called to the bedside to evaluate the nature of his shock and you obtain the following images. IVC is measured 1.4 cm.

See Image 22.10.

See Video 22.35.

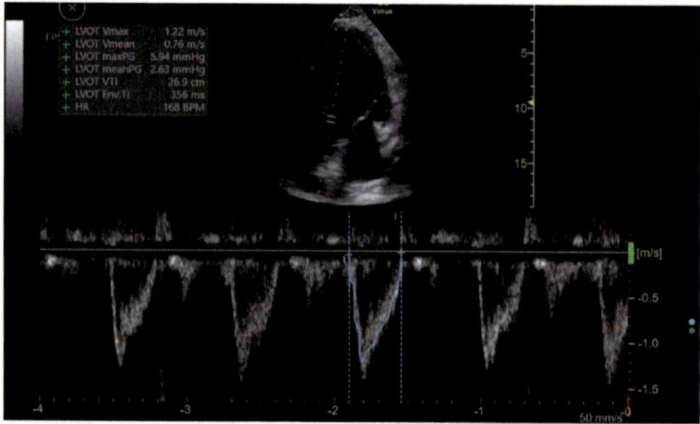

Image 22.10 Increase LVOT VTI

Question 33: What is the nature of this patient's shock?

A. Obstructive shock from massive pulmonary embolus.
B. Septic shock from possible community acquired pneumonia (CAP).
C. Cardiogenic shock from decompensated heart failure with reduced ejection fraction (HFrEF).
D. Hemorrhagic shock from upper gastro-intestinal bleed (UGIB).

Answer B.

Key Points: Sepsis is a high output low resistance hemodynamic state. Heart and lung ultrasound complement each other in diagnosis of shock.

Rationale: The patient has an infiltrate and atelectasis in the left lower lobe with adjacent pleural effusion. PLAPS is a typical ultrasound finding in pneumonia. When coupled with a hyperdynamic left ventricle with a collapsible inferior vena cava it suggests septic shock.

Obstructive shock causes increase in IVC size. LVOTI VTI is supposedly lower than 18 cm/s in cardiogenic shock. Hemorrhagic or hypovolemic shock leads to underfilled cardiac chambers, thin IVC (<1.2 cm) and low VTI. Increased VTI is seen in septic shock.

Question 34:

The patient becomes persistently hypoxic on the ventilator and currently has a P/F ratio of 70 mmHg and you deeply sedate and paralyze him resolving the hypoxia. The nurse calls you for increasing norepinephrine requirements after deep sedation is obtained and is asking if you want to start another vasopressor. The following images is obtained prior to passive leg raise test (PLR).

See Image 22.11.

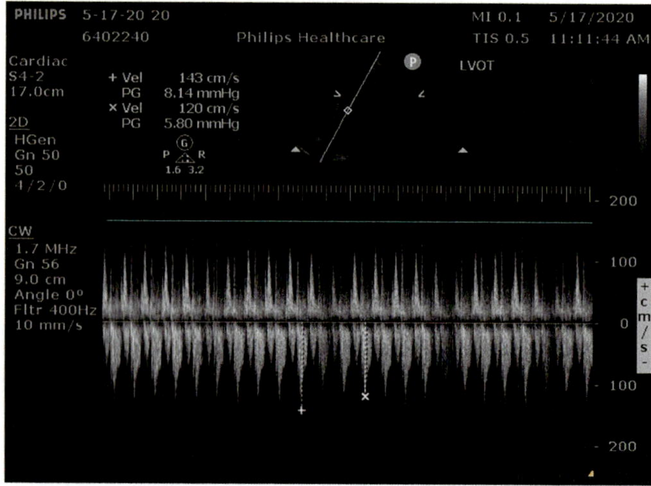

Image 22.11 Aortic peak velocity measurement

Question 34: What is the best next step?

A. Start vasopressin.
B. Decrease PEEP.
C. Give more crystalloids.
D. Lighten sedation.

Answer C.

Key point: Aortic peak velocity and VTI variation >12–14% correlates with volume responsiveness.

Rationale: Passive leg raise (PLR) is a none invasive maneuver that can be done at bedside to assess responsiveness to IV fluid bolus. LVOT VTI is expected to increase with PLR.

The other echocardiographic finding which correlates with volume responsiveness is aortic peak velocity variation. Once sweep speed is decreased more doppler waves are captured in one screen over a few respiration cycles. Aortic peak velocity of pulse wave (PW) doppler with respiration variation of >12–14% in a passive state like our patient who's paralyzed with neuromuscular blockade correlates with volume responsiveness.

On another note, volume responsiveness does not always mean necessity of IV fluid administration. Other clinical findings should be considered once initial volume expansion is achieved.

Question 35

Clinical Stem:

A 42 years old female with past medical history of diabetes mellitus type 2 and obesity who's been admitted to telemetry floor for 7 days with diagnosis of hypoxemic respiratory failure secondary to COVID 19 pneumonia is transferred to medical ICU after increasing in oxygen requirement. Heated humidified high flow therapy with FiO2 100% is started. She's being treated with empiric antibiotics, dexamethaosone as well as diuretics. In physical exam she's awake and follows command but appears distressed and have labored breathing. Lung auscultation reveals diminished air entry in upper lungs and bibasilar crackles. Cardiac exam is unremarkable except for sinus tachycardia.

Vital signs are as follows, blood pressure 110/68 mmHg, heart rate 145/min, respiratory rate 34/min, temperature 100.1, SpO2 90%.

Chest X-ray shows alveolar opacities in both lungs, more prominent in lower lungs.

Respiratory support for an hour fails to improve her clinical condition. ABG is obtained revealing pH 7.28 pCo2 52, PaO2 62 mmHg, SpO2 91. Pertinent labs are lactic acid 3.2 mmol/L (normal <2 mmol/L) and serum glucose 380 mg/dL. Patient is subsequently intubated with use of videoscopic laryngoscope. Fentanyl 25mcg, Etomidate 30 mg and Rocuronium 100 mg is used for RSI. However shortly after intubation ventilator is alarming with high peak pressure. 10 min later blood pressure which is monitored through a transduced arterial line drops to 80/44 mmHg and continues to decline. Patient is bradycardic and heart rate is slowly going down. Epinephrine infusion is immediately started. An ultrasound exam of heart and lungs are done. There's no pericardial effusion, in AP4C view LV appears to have sluggish contractility, RV appears to have the same size as LV and IVC is 1.8 cm with minimal respiration variation. Right lung ultrasound is unremarkable. Left lung ultrasound is shown in Video 22.36.

See Image 22.12.

See Video 22.36.

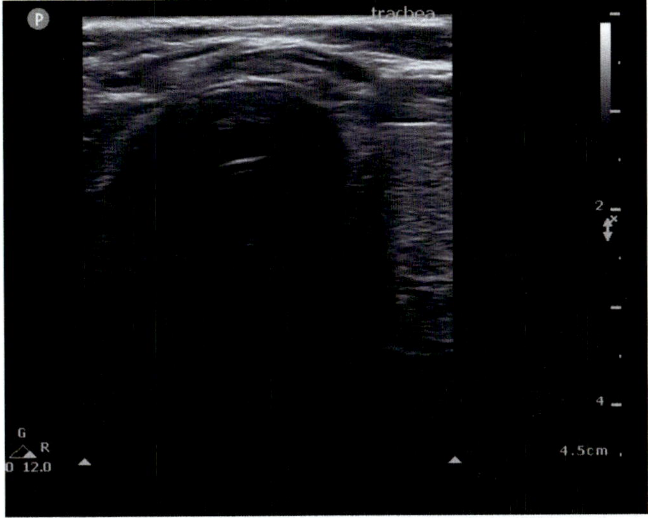

Image 22.12 Trachea

Question 35: Which of the following explains the critical decompensation?

A. obstructive shock due to tension pneumothorax.
B. septic shock due to hospital acquired pneumonia, with septic cardiomyopathy.
C. RV dysfunction secondary to COVID19 pneumonia.
D. Dead space ventilation.

Answer D.

Keypoint: Acidosis and respiratory gas exchange issues could lead to acute shock.

Rationale: This patient is developing ARDS and hypoxemia secondary to COVID19 infection. The hemodynamic changes appearing after intubation are either related to intubation complications, sedatives side effect or respiratory acidosis and hypoxemia due to dead space ventilation.

Absence of A-lines rules out pneumothorax. ARDS and severe hypoxemia can explain increase in RV size and pressure. RV dysfunction is reported in COVID19 pneumonia and is a possibility however it doesn't explain the acutely diminished LV contractility and bradycardia. Lung ultrasound shows ET tube placement in trachea. Normal right lung findings but absence of left pleural motion which altogether suggest right main stem intubation.

Right main stem intubation leads to delivery of the entire tidal volume to one lung. In a normal lung this complication may not cause an acute problem. Considering the low lung compliance in ARDS, right lung ventilation will lead to remarkable increase in peak pressure which subsequently will cause alarming ventilator and early cycling of the breath before the set tidal volume is delivered. Basically, patient will receive lower TV leading to hypocapnia and hypoxemia which will progress to suppression of myocardial activity and cardiac arrest if not corrected quickly. Lung ultrasound is very useful in diagnosing this scenario.

Question 36
Clinical Stem.

A 22-year-old female, who' s29 weeks pregnant, G1P0, with no known medical problem, presented to the referring hospital with respiratory failure. She was intubated and diagnosed with SARS-COVID19 pneumonia. And emergently delivered via cesarean section due to her critical condition and was transferred to a quaternary referral hospital on Post OP day 1, for ECMO evaluation. She has severe hypoxemia with PF ratio of 70. Her chest x ray revealed bilateral patchy opacities, midline trachea and optimal position of ET tube. Ventilator is set at VC-CMV mode, tidal volume 350 (6 mL/kg), PEEP 12, FiO2 100%, RR 20. Her plateau pressure in 24cmH2O. She is deeply sedated to RASS –5 with propofol infusion 40 mcg/kg/min, midazolam infusion 8 mg/h and fentanyl infusion 200mcg/hr. Rocuronium infusion is started as well as inhaled epoprostenol arginine (VELETRI) 200mcg/hr. Prone positioning is planned. She's hypotensive requiring norepinephrine. Bedside ultrasound exam is done, and the images are shown.

See Images 22.13, 22.14 and 22.15.

See Video 22.37.

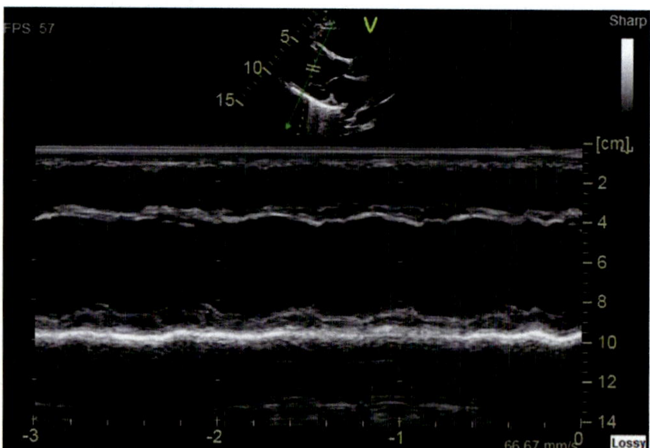

Image 22.13 PSLX

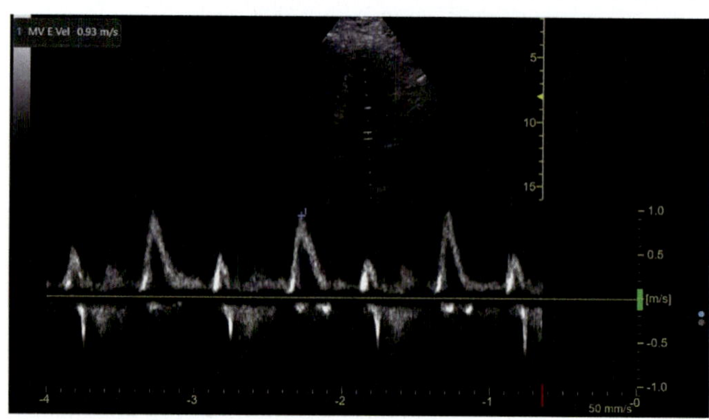

Image 22.14 Mitral Doppler peak velocity (E)

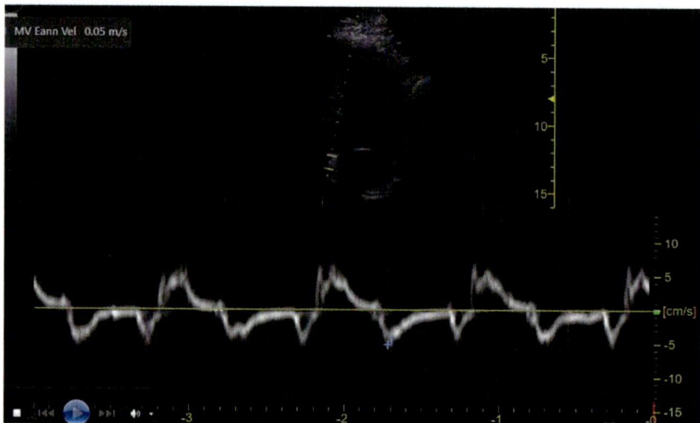

Image 22.15 Mitral TDI (e')

Question 36: What is most likely cause of her shock?

A. Post op hemorrhage shock.
B. Cardiogenic shock.
C. Vasodilatory shock secondary to sepsis or high dose sedation.
D. Obstructive secondary to Corpulmonale acute right heart failure.

Answer B.

Keypoint: The patient has sonographic evidence of possible Takotsubo cardiomyopathy (TTC) as demonstrated by the hypodynamic left ventricle (LV) and increased chamber size.

Rationale: It has been reported that COVID-19 can have cardiac manifestations, including RV failure and TTC and clinicians should have a high level of suspicion in these cases. Ultrasonographic manifestations of TTC include wall motion abnormalities in apical and midventricular segments, depressed ejection fraction and diastolic dysfunction evidenced by E'/e ratio. Right ventricle (RV) strain can also be observed, with the RV mirroring the LV in what is called a reverse McConnell's sign.

With possibly no coronary artery disease at age of 22, acute decompensation in LV systolic function with wall motion abnormalities could suggest Takatsubo. In this exam, M-mode in PSLX clearly shows minimal changes from systole to diastole. Same pattern is seen in AP4C view with midventricular hypokinesis. E is around 120 and e' is around 10. E/e' = 12 which is more suggestive of elevated filling pressures of L heart (normal E/e' < 8).

Suggested Reading

Guyatt GH, Akl EA, Crowther M, et al. Executive summary: antithrombotic therapy and prevention of thrombosis, 9th ed: American College of Chest Physicians evidence-based clinical practice guidelines. Chest. 2012;141(2 Suppl):7S–47S.

Lodato JA, Ward RP, Lang RM. Echocardiographic predictors of pulmonary embolism in patients referred for helical CT. Echocardiography. 2008;25(6):584–90.

McConnel MV, Solomon SD, Rayan ME, et al. Regional right ventricular dysfunction detected by echocardiography in acute pulmonary embolism. Am J Cardiol. 1996;78(4):469–73.

Thygesen K, Alpert JS, Jaffe AS, et al. Third universal definition of myocardial infarction. Nat Rev Cardiol. 2012;9(11):620–33.

Schmitt J, Duray G, Gersh BJ, Hohnloser SH. Atrial fibrillation in acute myocardial infarction: a systematic review of the incidence, clinical features and prognostic implications. Eur Heart J. 2009;30(9):1038–45.

Vieillard-Baron A, Charron C, Caille V, Belliard G, Page B, Jardin F. Prone positioning unloads the right ventricle in severe ARDS. Chest. 2007;132(5):1440–6.

Jardin F, Vieillard-Baron A. Right ventricular function and positive pressure ventilation in clinical practice: from hemodynamics subsets to respirator settings. Intensive Care Med. 2003;29:1426–34.

Lewis JF, Kuo LC, Nelson JG, Limacher MC, Quinones MA. Pulsed Doppler echocardiographic determination of stroke volume and cardiac output: clinical validation of two new methods using the apical window. Circulation. 1984;70(3):425–31.

Grossman W, Baim D. Grossman's cardiac catheterization, angiography, and intervention, 6th Edition. Page 172, Tabe 8.1

Pelliccia F, Kaski JC, Crea F, Camici PG. Pathophysiology of Takotsubo syndrome. Circulation. 2017;135(24):2426–41.

Medina de Chazal H, Del Buono MG, Keyser-Marcus L, et al. Stress cardiomyopathy diagnosis and treatment: JACC state-of-the-art review. J Am Coll Cardiol. 2018;72(16):1955–71.

Bossone E, D'andrea A, D'alto M, et al. Echocardiography in pulmonary arterial hypertension: from diagnosis to prognosis. J Am Soc Echocardiogr. 2013;26(1):1–14.

Lang RM, Badano LP, Mor-Avi V, et al. Recommendations for cardiac chamber quantification by echocardiography in adults: an updated from the American society of echocardiography and the European association of cardiovascular imaging. J Am Soc Echocardiogr. 2015;28:1–39.e14

Lichtenstein D, Meziere G, Biderman P, Gepner A. The "lung point": an ultrasound sign specific to pneumothorax. Intensive Care Med. 2000;26(10):1434–40.

Kameda T, Nobuyuki T. Overview of point-of-care abdominal ultrasound in emergency and critical care. J Intensive Care. 2016;4:53.

Johnson BK, Tierney DM, Rosborough TK, et al. Internal medicine point-of-care ultrasound assessment of left ventricular function correlates with formal echocardiography. J Clin Ultrasound. 2016;44(2):92–9. 2

Unluer EE, Karagoz A, Akoglu H, Bayata S. Visual estimation of bedside echocardiographic ejection fraction by emergency physicians. West J Emerg Med. 2014;15(2):221–6.

Ralls PW, Colletti PM, Lapin SA, et al. Real-time sonography in suspected acute cholecystitis: prospective evaluation of primary and secondary signs. Radiology. 1985;155767:–771.

Villar J, Summers S, Menchine M, et al. The absence of gallstones on point-of-care ultrasound rules out acute cholecystitis. J Emerg Med. 2015;49(4):475–80.

Rhodes A, Evans LE, Alhazzani W, et al. Surviving sepsis campaign: international guidelines for management of sepsis and septic shock:2016. Intensive Care Med. 2017;43(3):304–77. https://doi.org/10.1007/s00134-017-4683-6. Epub 2017 Jan 18

Allen SJ, Sidebotham D. Postoperative care and complications after ventricular assist device implantation. Best Pract Res Clin Anaesthesiol. 2012;26:231–46.

Pratt AK, Shah NS, Boyce SW. Left ventricular assist device management in the ICU. Crit Care Med. 2014;42:158–68.

Scolleta S, Biagioli B, Franchi F, Muzzi L. Echocardiography and hemodynamic monitoring tools for clinical assessment of patients on mechanical circulatory support. In: Komamura K, editor. Recent advances in the field of ventricular assist devices. Croatia: InTech; 2013.

Rubano E, Mehta N, Caputo W, Paladino L, Sinert R. Systematic review: emergency department bedside ultrasonography for diagnosing suspected abdominal aortic aneurysm. Acad Emerg Med. 2013;20(2):128–38.

Smith-Bindman R, Aubin C, Bailitz J, et al. Ultrasonography versus computed tomography for suspected nephrolithiasis. N Engl J Med. 2014;371(12):1100–10.

Dalziel PJ, Noble VE. Bedside ultrasound and the assessment of renal colic: a review.

Otto CM. Pericardial disease. In: Otto CM, editor. Textbook of clinical echocardiography. 4th ed. Philadelphia: PA. Saunders; 2009. p. 242–58.

Spodick DH. Acute cardiac tamponade. N Engl J Med. 2003;349:684–90.

Salen P, Melanson SW, Heller MB. The focused abdominal sonography for trauma (FAST) examination: considerations and recommendations for training physicians in the use of a new clinical tool. Acad Emerg Med. 2007;7:162–8.

Seif D, Perera P, Mailhot T, Riley D, Mandavia D. Bedside ultrasound in resuscitation and the rapid ultrasound in shock protocol. Crit Care Res Pract. 2012;2012:503254.

Bussani R, De-Giorgio F, Abbate A, Silvestri F. Cardiac metastases. J Clin Pathol. 2007;60(1):27–34.

Miller A, Mandeville J. Predicting and measuring fluid responsiveness with echocardiography. Echo Res Pract. 2016;3(2):G1–G12. https://doi.org/10.1530/ERP-16-0008.

Douglas IS, Alapat PM, Corl KA, et al. Fluid response evaluation in sepsis hypotension and shock: a randomized clinical trial [published online ahead of print, 2020 Apr 27]. Chest. 2020;20:30768–6. https://doi.org/10.1016/j.chest.2020.04.025. S0012-3692

Senussi M, Kantamneni P, Latifi M, Omranian A, Krveshi L, Barakat A, Masri A, Schmidhofer M. Protocolized tracheal and thoracic ultrasound for confirmation of endotracheal intubation and positioning. Crit Care Explor. 2020;2(9):e0225. https://doi.org/10.1097/CCE.0000000000000225.

Minhas AS, Scheel P, Garibaldi B, et al. Takotsubo Syndrome in the setting of COVID-19 infection [published online ahead of print, 2020 May 1]. JACC Case Rep. 2020; https://doi.org/10.1016/j.jaccas.2020.04.023.

Citro R, Lyon AR, Meimoun P, et al. Standard and advanced echocardiography in takotsubo (stress) cardiomyopathy: clinical and prognostic implications. J Am Soc Echocardiogr. 2015;28(1):57–74. https://doi.org/10.1016/j.echo.2014.08.020.

Index

R. Sreedharan et al. (eds.), *Critical Care Echocardiography*, https://doi.org/10.1007/978-3-031-45731-9

M

N

O

U

V

Printed by Printforce, the Netherlands